Comm

Haemo	0
	0
Mean	8
Platel	8
White	6
neu	6
lym	16
eos	16

Blood gases

	kPa	mmHg	
pH 7.35–7.45			p173, p658
P_aO_2	>10.6	75–100	p173, p658
P_aCO_2	4.7–6	35–45	p173, p658
Base excess ±2mmol/L			p173, p658

U&E etc (urea and electrolytes) *If outside this range, consult:*

sodium	135–145mmol/	p666
potassium	3.5–5mmol/L	p668
creatinine	70–150µmol/L	p292 & p294
urea	2.5–6.7mmol/L	p292 & p294, p661 (eGFR)
calcium	2.12–2.65mmol/L	p670
albumin	35–50g/L	p678
proteins	60–80g/L	p678

LFTs (liver function tests)

bilirubin	3–17µmol/L	p242
alanine aminotransferase, ALT	3–35iu/L	
aspartate transaminase, AST	3–35iu/L	p242
alkaline phosphatase	30–35iu/L (*adults*)	p242

'Cardiac enzymes' For troponins, see p81 & p104.

creatine kinase	25–195iu/L	p104 (p538)
lactate dehydrogenase, LDH	70–250iu/L	p104

Lipids and other biochemical values

cholesterol	<6mmol/L *desired*	p682
triglycerides	0.5–1.9mmol/L " "	p682
amylase	0–180*somorgyi* u/dL	p584
C-reactive protein, CRP	<10mg/L	p679
glucose, fasting	3.5–5.5mmol/L	p190
prostate specific antigen, PSA	0–4ng/mL	p681
T4 (total thyroxine)	70–140mmol/L	p200
TSH	0.5–~5mu/L	p200

For all other reference intervals, see p741

Contents

From the preface to the first edition

This book, written by junior doctors, is intended principally for medical student and house officers. The student becomes, imperceptibly, the house officer. For hir we wrote this book not because we know so much, but because we know w remember so little. For the student the problem is not simply the quantity c information, but the diversity of places from which it is dispensed. Trailing eager behind the surgeon, the student is admonished never to forget alcohol withdrawa as a cause of post-operative confusion. The scrap of paper on which this is writte spends a month in the white coat pocket before being lost for ever in the laundry At different times, and in inconvenient places, a number of other causes may b presented to the student. Not only are these causes and aphorisms never brough together, but when, as a surgical house officer, the former student faces a cor fused patient, none is to hand.

We aim to encourage the doctor to enjoy his patients: in doing so we believe h will prosper in the practice of medicine. For a long time now, house officers hav been encouraged to adopt monstrous proportions in order to straddle simultane ously the diverse pinnacles of clinical science and clinical experience. We hope tha this book will make this endeavour a little easier by moving a cumulative memor burden from the mind into the pocket, and by removing some of the fears that ar naturally felt when starting a career in medicine, thereby freely allowing the doc tor's clinical acumen to grow by the slow accretion of many, many days and night

R.A.H. & J.M.L. 198

Preface to the seventh edition

Who needs handbooks? With so many wonderful guidelines emanating from nat ional institutions and Royal Colleges, and so much evidence-based medicine on th web, the idea of a handbook might appear redundant. But just how wonderful ar all these guidelines? Let us look at the evidence: in one study of a quiet day on ca 18 patients were seen by one doctor, who made 44 diagnoses. The guideline advising on these conditions ran to 3679 pages. All these guidelines no doub needed to be read carefully and in full. Carefully! In full!! Just what planet are w on if we expect this to happen? Pluto, it turns out. Each day on Pluto lasts 153.3 hours. Allowing 2 minutes a page and a few seconds for reflection, this is jus long enough to digest the necessary guidelines. From this we conclude that ever junior doctor should be provided with breathing apparatus to survive in the rare fied atmosphere which gives rise to guidelines, as well as a team of readers to giv advice as he or she works at the bedside. Pie in the sky? Not quite. Here on Eart the answer lies in your own hands as you read this, and OUP put it there in the hop and certain knowledge that this bird in your hand is worth *at least* two on Plut

We welcome Tom Turmezei and Chee Kay Cheung, who breathe new life int this edition—which goes to press 21 years after our first edition. We are awa that by being 21 we may be regarded as being almost established: we would f rather continue to enjoy the fate of our first edition, which was banned from tw medical schools—so far as we could tell for making learning medicine too eas Or perhaps it was for saying that we should work for our patients, not our consul ants. To revive this sense of the subversive we have run comments orthogonal the text (sometimes literally and sometimes metaphorically)—to act as a count to our more Panglossian sentiments, which might otherwise fatuously indicate th everything is for the best in the best of all possible wards. Voltaire, the creator Panglos, like all true saprophytes (*Candida* included), fed for ever off decayi matter (the effete French Court)—whereas we take our nourishment from t living wells of knowledge embodied in Medline, the BMJ, and the *New Englar Journal of Medicine*.

This edition embodies countless changes—the most obvious being the additic of a Radiology chapter—and the introduction of colour images throughout the te But the main thing we bring to our readers is a friend in the pocket—weari bright new underclothes, and freshly recommitted to the task of being yo champion, your mentor, and your fond support—come what may.

Conflicts of interest

This volume has been critically appraised by two doctors (JML & JABC) who have no contact with commercial interests such as pharmaceutical companies. In order to reassure readers, and in the light of recent studies which have shown that writers of guidelines often have overt and covert connections with drug companies, we wish to place on record that there has been no covert pressure to exclude or include certain drugs in this text, they have adhered to a policy of not seeing representatives from any such commercial company, and neither are they in receipt of any gifts, grants, or hospitality from such companies.

Drugs (and how to keep abreast of changes)

While every effort has been made to check this text, it is still possible that errors have been missed. Also, dosage schedules are continually being revised and new side-effects recognized. Oxford University Press makes no representation, expressed or implied, that drug dosages in this book are correct. For these reasons, the reader is strongly urged to consult the most recently published *British National Formulary*, and the pharmaceutical company's *data sheet* (summaries of product characteristics/SPC; www.Medicines.org.uk) before administering any of the drugs recommended in this book. Unless stated otherwise, drug doses and recommendations are for the *non-pregnant adult* who is *not breast-feeding*.

Corrections are posted on the web at www.oup.com/OHCM. See also the *What's new* section of www.bnf.org.

Readers are also reminded of the need to keep up to date, and that this need can only ever be partly addressed by printed texts such as this.

Acknowledgements

We would like to record our heartfelt thanks to our advisers on specific sections—each is acknowledged on chapter's first page.

For checking the text we thank, and admire the fortitude of, Judith Collier, David Knight, Ahmad Mafi and Thomas Jaconelli. We particularly thank our drug reader, Dr Steve Emmett, for his painstaking work checking drug dosages.

IBW would like to acknowledge his clinical mentors Jim Holt and John Cockcroft. We also thank Dr P Scally and Dr J Harper for providing x-ray plates, as well as for many thoughtful comments on the whole text. For further help we thank Dr J Burke, Dr Omid Zarghom, and Professor J McCormack.

The British Lending Library and staff at the Cairns Library, Oxford, and at Worthing Postgraduate Library have been most helpful in tracing references.

We would like to thank the staff of OUP for their help and support. It is a particular pleasure to document here the enormous contribution made to this and many other Oxford Handbooks by Alison Langton, whose steadfast support since OHCM's conception in 1981 has been a model of fair and creative publishing.

Readers' comments These have formed a vital part of our endeavour to provide an accurate, comprehensive, and up-to-date text. We sincerely thank the many students, doctors and other health professionals who have found the time and the generosity to write to us on our Reader's Comments Cards (enclosed) or via the web. These have now become so numerous that they cannot all be listed here.

3rd-party web addresses We disclaim any responsibility for 3rd-party content.

Symbols and abbreviations

► ►►	this fact or idea is important. ►►don't dawdle!—prompt action saves lives
💣	incendiary (controversial) topic
[ ]	non-*BNF* drug dose
💾	reference available on our website www.oup.com/OHCM
♂:♀	male-to-female ratio. ♂:♀=2:1 means twice as common in males
@1234567	search Medline (pubmed.gov) with '1234567' to get an abstract (omit the '@')
∵ ~	on account of (∴ means *therefore*; ~ means *approximately*)
-ve +ve	negative and positive, respectively
↑ ↓ ↔	increased, decreased, and normal, respectively (eg serum level)
Δ; ΔΔ	diagnosis; ΔΔ means differential diagnosis (list of possibilities)
A_2	aortic component of the second heart sound
A2A	angiotensin-2 receptor antagonist (p283; = AT-2, A2R, and AIIR)
Ab	antibody
ABC	airway, breathing, and circulation: basic life support (see inside back cover)
ABG	arterial blood gas (P_aO_2, P_aCO_2, pH, HCO_3^-)
ABPA	allergic bronchopulmonary aspergillosis
Ac	*ante cibum* (before food)
ACE(i)	angiotensin-converting enzyme (inhibitors)
ACTH	adrenocorticotrophic hormone
ADH	antidiuretic hormone
ad lib	*ad libitum*; as much/as often as wanted (Latin for *at pleasure*)
AF	atrial fibrillation
AFB	acid-fast bacillus
AFP or α-FP	alpha-fetoprotein
Ag	antigen
AIDS	acquired immunodeficiency syndrome
Alk phos	alkaline phosphatase (also ALP)
ALL	acute lymphoblastic leukaemia
AMA	antimitochondrial antibody
AMP	adenosine monophosphate
ANA	antinuclear antibody
ANCA	antineutrophil cytoplasmic antibody
APTT	activated partial thromboplastin time
AR	aortic regurgitation
ARA	angiotensin receptor antagonist (p301; also AT-2, A2R, and AIIR)
ARDS	acute respiratory distress syndrome
ARF	acute renal failure
AS	aortic stenosis
ASD	atrial septal defect
ASO(T)	antistreptolysin O (titre)
AST	aspartate transaminase
AT-2	angiotensin-2 receptor blocker (p283; also AT-2, A2R, and AIIR)
ATN	acute tubular necrosis
ATP	adenosine triphosphate
AV	atrioventricular
AVM	arteriovenous malformation(s)
AXR	abdominal x-ray (plain)
Ba	barium
BAL	bronchoalveolar lavage
Bd	*bis die* (twice a day)
BKA	below-knee amputation
BMJ/BMA	*British Medical Journal/British Medical Association*
BNF	*British National Formulary*
BP	blood pressure
bpm	beats per minute (eg pulse)
Ca	cancer
CABG	coronary artery bypass graft
cAMP	cyclic adenosine monophosphate (AMP)
CAPD	continuous ambulatory peritoneal dialysis
CBD	common bile duct
CC	creatinine clearance (also CrCl)
CCF	congestive cardiac failure (ie left and right heart failure)
CCU	coronary care unit
CHB	complete heart block
CHD	coronary heart disease (related to ischaemia and atheroma)
CI	contraindications
CK	creatine (phospho)kinase (also CPK)
CLL/CML	chronic lymphocytic leukaemia/chronic myeloid leukaemia
CMV	cytomegalovirus
CNS	central nervous system
COC	combined oral contraceptive, ie (o)estrogen + progesterone
COPD	chronic obstructive pulmonary disease
CPAP	continuous positive airways pressure
CPR	cardiopulmonary resuscitation
CRF	chronic renal failure
CRP	c-reactive protein
CSF	cerebrospinal fluid
CT	computer tomography
CVP	central venous pressure

CVS	cardiovascular system
CXR	chest x-ray
d	day(s) (also expressed as /7)
DC	direct current
DIC	disseminated intravascular coagulation
DIP	distal interphalangeal
dl	decilitre
DoH (or DH)	department of health (UK)
DM	diabetes mellitus
DU	duodenal ulcer
D&V	diarrhoea and vomiting
DVT	deep venous thrombosis
DXT	deep radiotherapy
E-BM	evidence-based medicine and its journal published by the BMA
EBV	Epstein–Barr virus
ECG	electrocardiogram
Echo	echocardiogram
EDTA	ethylene diamine tetraacetic acid (eg in FBC bottle)
EEG	electroencephalogram
ELISA	enzyme linked immunosorbant assay
EM	electron microscope
EMG	electromyogram
ENT	ear, nose, and throat
ERCP	endoscopic retrograde cholangiopancreatography; see also MRCP
ESR	erythrocyte sedimentation rate
ESRF	end-stage renal failure
EUA	examination under anaesthesia
FB	foreign body
FBC	full blood count
FDP	fibrin degradation products
FEV_1; F_iO_2	forced expiratory volume in 1st sec; F_iO_2: partial pressure of O_2 in inspired air
FFP	fresh frozen plasma
FroM	full range of movements
FSH	follicle-stimulating hormone
FVC	forced vital capacity
g	gram
GA	general anaesthetic
GAT (Sanford)	Sanford *guide to antimicrobial therapy* www.sanfordguide.com
GB	gall bladder
GC	gonococcus
GCS	Glasgow coma scale
GFR	glomerular filtration rate eGFR, p661
GGT	gamma glutamyl transpeptidase
GH	growth hormone
GI	gastrointestinal
GP	general practitioner
G6PD	glucose-6-phosphate dehydrogenase
GTN	glyceryl trinitrate
GTT	glucose tolerance test (also OGTT: oral GTT)
GU(M)	genitourinary (medicine)
h	hour
HAV	hepatitis A virus
Hb	haemoglobin
HBsAg/HBV	hepatitis B surface antigen/hepatitis B virus
HCC	hepatocellular cancer
Hct	haematocrit
HCV (HDV)	hepatitis C virus (HDV is hepatitis D virus)
HDL	high-density lipoprotein, p683
HHT	hereditary haemorrhagic telangiectasia
HIDA	hepatic immunodiacetic acid
HIV	human immunodeficiency virus
HOCM	hypertrophic obstructive cardiomyopathy
HONK	hyperosmolar nonketotic (diabetic coma)
HRT	hormone replacement therapy
HSV	herpes simplex virus
IBD	inflammatory bowel disease
IBW	ideal body weight, p434
ICP	intracranial pressure
IDA	iron-deficiency anaemia
IDDM	insulin-dependent diabetes mellitus
IFN-α	alpha interferon
IE	infective endocarditis
Ig	immunoglobulin
IHD	ischaemic heart disease
IM	intramuscular
INR	international normalized ratio (prothrombin ratio)
IP	interphalangeal
IPPV	intermittent positive pressure ventilation
ITP	idiopathic thrombocytopenic purpura
ITU	intensive therapy unit
iu	international unit

IVC	inferior vena cava
IV(I)	intravenous (infusion)
IVU	intravenous urography
JAMA	*Journal of the American Medical Association*
JVP	jugular venous pressure
K	potassium
KCCT	kaolin cephalin clotting time
Kg	kilogram
Kpa	kiloPascal
L	litre
LAD	left axis deviation on the ECG; also left anterior descending coronary artery
LBBB	left bundle branch block
LDH	lactate dehydrogenase
LDL	low-density lipoprotein, p683
LBW	lean body weight, p434
LFT	liver function test
LH	luteinizing hormone
LIF	left iliac fossa
LKKS	liver, kidney (R), kidney (L), spleen
LMN	lower motor neurone
LP	lumbar puncture
LUQ	left upper quadrant
LV	left ventricle of the heart
LVF; LVH	left ventricular failure; left ventricular hypertrophy
μg	microgram
MAI	*Mycobacterium avium intracellulare*
MAOI	monoamine oxidase inhibitors
mane	morning (from Latin; the 'e' may be written 'é', but purists frown on this)
MC & S	microscopy, culture and sensitivity
MCP	metacarpo-pharangeal
MCV	mean cell volume
MDMA	3,4-methylenedioxymethamphetamine
ME	myalgic encephalomyelitis
MET	meta-analysis
mg	milligram
MI	myocardial infarction
min(s)	minute(s)
mL	millilitre
mmHg	millimetres of mercury
MND	motor neurone disease
MRCP	magnetic imaging cholangiopancreatography (also Member of Royal College of Physicians)
MRI	magnetic resonance imaging
MRSA	methicillin-resistant *Staphylococcus aureus* (p408)
MS	multiple sclerosis (do not confuse with mitral stenosis)
MSU	midstream urine
NAD	nothing abnormal detected
NBM	nil by mouth
ND	notifiable disease
NEJM	*New England Journal of Medicine*
ng	nanogram
NG(T)	nasogastric (tube)
NHS	National Health Service (UK)
NICE	National Institute for Health and Clinical Excellence www.nice.org.uk
NIDDM	non-insulin-dependent diabetes mellitus
NMDA	*N*-methyl-*D*-aspartate
NNT	number needed to treat, for 1 extra satisfactory result (p650)
Nocte	at night
NR	normal range—the same as reference interval
NSAIDs	non-steroidal anti-inflammatory drugs
N&V	nausea and/or vomiting
od	*omni die* (once daily)
OD	overdose
OGD	oesophagogastroduodenoscopy
OGS	oxogenic steroids
OGTT	oral glucose tolerance test
OHCS	*Oxford Handbook of Clinical Specialties*, 7[e] OUP, Collier & Longmore
om; on	*omni mane* (in the morning); *omni nocte* (at night)
OPD	out-patients department
ORh−	blood group O, Rh negative
OT	occupational therapist
OTM/S	*Oxford Textbook of Medicine* (OUP 4[e], 2003)/*Surgery* (2000)
P_2	pulmonary component of second heart sound
P_aCO_2	partial pressure of carbon dioxide in arterial blood
PAN	polyarteritis nodosa
P_aO_2	partial pressure of oxygen in arterial blood
PBC	primary biliary cirrhosis
PCP	*Pneumocystis carinii* (*jiroveci*) pneumonia
PCR	polymerase chain reaction (DNA diagnosis)
PCV	packed cell volume
PE	pulmonary embolism
PEEP	positive end-expiratory pressure

PERLA	pupils equal and reactive to light and accommodation
PEF(R)	peak expiratory flow (rate)
PID	pelvic inflammatory disease
PIP	proximal interphalangeal (joint)
PMH	past medical history
PND	paroxysmal nocturnal dyspnoea
PO	*per os* (by mouth)
PPF	purified plasma fraction (albumin)
PPI	proton pump inhibitor, eg omeprazole, lansoprazole, etc.
PR	*per rectum* (by the rectum)
PRL	prolactin
PRN	*pro re nata* (as required)
PRV	polycythaemia rubra vera
PSA	prostate specific antigen
PTH	parathyroid hormone
PTT	prothrombin time
PUO	pyrexia of unknown origin
PV	*per vaginam* (by the vagina; the route for pessaries)
PVD	peripheral vascular disease
qds; qqh	*quater die sumendus* (to be taken 4×daily); qqh *quarta quaque hora:* every 4h
R	right
RA	rheumatoid arthritis
RAD	right axis deviation on the ECG
RBBB	right bundle branch block
RBC	red blood cell
RCT	randomized control trial
RFT	respiratory function tests
Rh	Rh; not an abbreviation, but derived from the rhesus monkey
RIF	right iliac fossa
RUQ	right upper quadrant
RV	right ventricle of heart
RVF	right ventricular failure
RVH	right ventricular hypertrophy
℞	*recipe* (treat with)
S or sec	second(s)
S1, S2	first and second heart sounds
SBE	subacute bacterial endocarditis (IE is *infective endocarditis*)
SC	subcutaneous
sd	standard deviation
SE	side-effect(s)
SL	Sublingual
SLE	systemic lupus erythematosus
SOB	short of breath (SOB(O)E: short of breath on exercise)
SPC	summary of product characteristics (SPC; www.medicines.org.uk)
SpO_2	peripheral oxygen saturation (%)
SR	slow-release (also called MR, modified-release)
Stat	*statim* (immediately; as initial dose)
STD/STI	sexually-transmitted disease or sexually-transmitted infection
SVC	superior vena cava
Sy(n)	syndrome
T°	temperature
$T_{½}$	biological half-life
T3; T4	triiodothyronine; T4 is thyroxine
TB	tuberculosis
tds	*ter die sumendus* (to be taken 3 times a day)
TFTs	thyroid function tests (eg TSH)
TIA	transient ischaemic attack
TIBC	total iron binding capacity
tid	*ter in die* (3 times a day)
TPR	temperature, pulse, and respirations count
TRH; TSH	thyroid-releasing hormone; TSH means thyroid-stimulating hormone
U	units
UC	ulcerative colitis
U&E	urea and electrolytes and creatinine—in plasma, unless stated otherwise
UMN	upper motor neurone
URT(I)	upper respiratory tract (infection)
US(S)	ultrasound (scan)
UTI	urinary tract infection
VDRL	venereal diseases research laboratory (syphilis serology)
VE	ventricular extrasystole
VF	ventricular fibrillation
VMA	vanillyl mandelic acid (HMMA)
$\dot{V}/\dot{Q}$	ventilation/perfusion ratio
VSD	ventriculo-septal defect
VT	ventricular tachycardia
WBC; WCC	white blood cell; white blood cell count
wk(s)	week(s)
WR	Wassermann reaction
yr(s)	year(s)
ZN	Ziehl–Neelsen (stain for acid-fast bacilli, eg mycobacteria)

Other abbreviations are given on pages where they occur: also, consult the *index*.

Prologue to clinical medicine: Dag Hammarskjöld on teamwork

Good doctors are good team players, because health care is complex, and nobody knows everything; and nobody knows how to relate to every patient and his or her unique needs. Because we are all fallible, we all see many examples of poor teams, where bad communication, power struggles, and personality clashes lead to poor outcomes. Stress, overwork, and resource restrictions contribute to this, but not inevitably. So it is worthwhile, at the outset of this journey through clinical medicine, to commit oneself to being a good team member. 3 rules help: (1) All members are valuable; none is irreplaceable, and members are valued for who they are, not just for the resources they bring. (2) 'Innocence is no excuse'—ie you may not be 'to blame' for a group's malfunction but in the end each member is responsible for everything. (3) Every member needs encouragement. Just how important this is, is shown by this comment from a well-known statesman:[1]

'He was impossible. It wasn't that he didn't attend to his work. But his manner brought him into conflict with everybody ... When the crisis came, and the whole truth had to come out, he laid the blame on us: in his conduct there was nothing, absolutely nothing to reproach. His self-esteem was so strongly bound up, apparently, with the idea of his innocence, that one felt a brute as one demonstrated, step by step, the contradictions in his defence, and, bit by bit, stripped him naked before his own eyes. But justice to others demanded it.

When the last rag of a lie had been taken from him, and we thought there was nothing more to be said, out it came with stifled sobs.

"But why did you never help me? You knew that I always felt you were against me. And fear and insecurity drove me further and further along the course for which you now condemn me. It's been so hard—everything. One day, I remember, I was so happy: one of you said that something I had produced was quite good—"

So, in the end, we were, in fact, to blame. We had not voiced our criticisms, but we had allowed them to stop us from giving him a single word of acknowledgement, and in this way had barred every road to improvement. It is always the stronger one who is to blame.'

1 *Markings*, p47. *Dag Hammarskjöld.* Translated by WH Auden, Faber.

Dedication

This work is dedicated to doctors everywhere, especially to those who are just starting out, or who are in the thick of it, or who are at the sharp end of a difficult decision.

The Old Hippocratic oath ~425BC

I swear by Apollo the physician, and Aesculapius and Health and All-heal, and all the gods and goddesses, that, according to my ability and judgment, I will keep this oath and stipulation—to reckon him who taught me this Art equally dear to me as my parents, to share my substance with him, and relieve his necessities if required; to look upon his offspring in the same footing as my own brothers, and to teach them this Art, if they shall wish to learn it, without fee or stipulation, and that by percept, lecture, and every other mode of instruction, I will impart a knowledge of the Art to my own sons, and those of my teachers, and to disciples bound by a stipulation and oath according to the law of medicine, but to none other.

I will follow that system of regimen, which, according to my ability and judgment, I consider for the benefit of my patients, and abstain from whatever is deleterious and mischievous.

I will give no deadly medicine to anyone if asked, nor suggest any such counsel; and in like manner I will not give to a woman a pessary to produce abortion. With purity and with holiness I will pass my life and practice my Art.

I will not cut persons labouring under the stone, but will leave this work to be done by men who are practitioners of this work.

Into whatever houses I enter, I will go into them for the benefit of the sick, and will abstain from every voluntary act of mischief and corruption; and, further, from the seduction of females, or males, of freemen or slaves.

Whatever, in connection with my professional practice, I see or hear, in the life of men, which ought not to be spoken of abroad, I will not divulge, as reckoning that all such should be kept secret.

While I continue to keep this oath unviolated, may it be granted to me to enjoy life and practice this Art, respected by all men, in all times. Should I violate this Oath, may the reverse be my lot.

A New Hippocratic oath ~2004AD

I promise that my medical knowledge will be used to benefit people's health; patients are my first concern. I will listen to them, and provide the best care I can. I will be honest, respectful, and compassionate towards all.

I will do my best to help anyone in medical need, in emergencies. I will make every effort to ensure the rights of all patients are respected, including vulnerable groups who lack means of making their needs known.

I will exercise my professional judgment as independently as possible, uninfluenced by political pressure or the social standing of my patient. I will not put personal profit or advancement above my duty to my patient.

I recognize the special value of human life, but I also know that prolonging life is not the only aim of health care. If I agree to perform abortion,[1] I agree it should take place only within an ethical and legal context.

I will not provide treatments that are pointless or harmful, or which an informed and competent patient refuses. I will help[2] patients find the information and support they want to make decisions on their care.

I will answer as truthfully as I can, and respect patients' decisions, unless that puts others at risk of substantial[3] harm. If I cannot agree with their requests, I will explain why.

If my patients have limited mental awareness, I will still encourage them to participate in decisions as much as they feel able. I will do my best to maintain confidentiality about all patients.

If there are overriding reasons preventing my keeping a patient's confidentiality I will explain them. I will recognize the limits of my knowledge and seek advice from colleagues as needed. I will acknowledge my mistakes.

I will do my best to keep myself and my colleagues informed of new developments, and ensure that poor standards or bad practices are exposed to those who can improve them.

I will show respect for all those with whom I work and be ready to share my knowledge by teaching others what I know. I will use my training and professional standing to improve the community in which I work.

I will treat patients equitably and support a fair and humane distribution of health resources. I will try to influence positively authorities whose policies harm public health.

I will oppose policies which breach internationally accepted standards of human rights. I will strive to change laws that are contrary to patients' interests or to my professional ethics.

While I continue to keep this Oath unviolated, may it be granted to me to enjoy life and the practice of the Art, respected by all, in all times.

After the BMA's *Revised Hippocratic Oath*, with changes:
1 The BMA draft did not cater for those believing that abortion is unethical.
2 The BMA wording was stronger here, requiring us to *ensure* that patients actually *receive* this information (often an impossibility).
3 The word *substantial* has been added to prevent a serious breach of confidentiality in the name of a slight benefit to another party. Contrary to the BMA's version, the last paragraph about enjoying life has been inserted from the old Oath. Other changes are minor.

Ideals

Decision and *intervention* are the essence of action: *reflection* and *conjecture* are the essence of thought: the essence of medicine is combining these realms in the service of others. We offer these ideals to stimulate both thought and action: like the stars, ideals are hard to reach, but they serve for navigation during the night. We choose Orion (fig 1) as our emblem for this navigation as he had miraculous sight (a gift from his immortal lover, Eos, to help him in his task of hunting down all dangerous things)—and, as his constellation is visible in the Northern *and* the Southern hemispheres (being at the celestial equator), he links our readers everywhere.

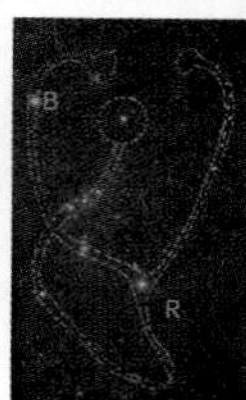

Fig 1. The constellation of Orion has 3 superb stars: *Bellatrix* (the bell of the stethoscope), *Betelgeuse* (B) and *Rigel* (R). The 3 stars near the crossover (Orion's belt) are Alnitak, Alnilam, and Mintaka.[1]

- Do not blame the sick for being sick.
- If the patient's wishes are known, comply with them.
- Work for your patients, not your consultant.
- Ward staff are usually right; respect their opinions.
- Treat the whole patient, not the disease, or the nurses.
- Admit people—not 'strokes', 'infarcts', or 'crumble'.
- Spend time with the bereaved; help them to shed tears.
- Give the patient (and yourself) time: time for questions, to reflect, to allow healing, and time to gain autonomy.
- Give patients the benefit of the doubt. Be optimistic. Optimistic patients who feel in charge, live longer.[2]
- Use ward rounds to boost patients' morale, not your own.
- Be kind to yourself: you are not an inexhaustible resource.
- Question your conscience—however strongly it tells you to act.

Ideal and less than ideal methods of care

A story illustrates the options: a man cut his hand and went round to his neighbou for help. This neighbour happened to be a doctor, but it was not the doctor but hi 3-year-old daughter who opened the door. Seeing that he was hurt and bleedinc she took him in, pressed her handkerchief over his wound, and reclined him, feet up in the nearest chair. She stroked his head and patted his hand, and told him abou her marigolds, and then about her frogs, and, after some time, was starting to te him about her father—when her father eventually appeared. He quickly turned th neighbour into a patient, and then into a bleeding biohazard, and then dispatche him to Casualty 'for suturing'. (The neighbour had no idea what this was.) H waited 3 hours in Casualty, had 2 desultory stitches, and 1 interview, with medical student who suggested a tetanus vaccination (to which he unfortunatel developed an allergic reaction). He returned to his doctor next door a few day later, praising his young carer, but not the doctor (who had turned him into patient), nor the hospital (who had turned him into an item on a conveyor belt), no the student who turned him into a question mark (does a 50-year-old man with full series of tetanus vaccinations need a booster at the time of injury?).

It was the 3-year-old who was his true nurse-cum-physician and universa health worker, who took him in on his own terms, cared for him, and gave him time and dignity. Question her instinct for care as you will: point out that it could have led to harm, and is, in any case, inadequate for scientific medicine, and that the hospita was just a victim of its own success. But remember that the story shows that *ther is*, as TS Eliot said, *at best, only a limited value in the knowledge derived fron experience*, eg the knowledge encompassed in this book. The child had the innate understanding and the natural compassion that we all too easily lose amid the science, the knowledge, and our stainless-steel universe of organized health care

The bedside manner and communication skills

Our bedside manner matters as it shows patients if they can *trust* us. Where there is no trust there is little healing. A good bedside manner is not static. It develops in the light of patients' needs. And it is grounded in the timeless virtues of honesty, humour, and humility in the presence of human weakness and human suffering.

The following are examples from an endless variety of phenomena which arise whenever doctors meet patients. One of the great skills (and pleasures) in medicine is to learn how our actions and attitudes influence patients, and how to take this knowledge into account when assessing the validity and significance of the signs and symptoms we elicit. What we receive from our patients is not 'hard evidence', but a much more plastic commodity, moulded as much by the doctor's attitude and the hospital or consulting room environment as by the patient's own hopes and fears. It is our job to adjust our attitudes and environment so that these hidden hopes and fears become manifest and the channels of communication are always open.

Anxiety reduction or intensification Simple explanation of what you are going to do often defuses what can be a highly charged affair. With children, try more subtle techniques, such as examining the abdomen using the child's own hands, or examining his teddy bear first (see p601).

Pain reduction or intensification Compare: 'I'm going to press your stomach. If it hurts, cry out' with 'I'm going to touch your stomach. Let me know what you feel' and 'Now I'll lay a hand on your stomach. Sing out if you feel anything.' The examination can be made to sound frightening, neutral, or joyful, and the patient will relax or tense up accordingly.

The tactful or clumsy invasion of personal space During ophthalmoscopy, eg we must get much nearer to the patient than is acceptable in normal social intercourse. Both doctor and patient may end up holding their breath, which helps neither the patient keep his eyes perfectly still, nor the doctor to carry out a full examination. Simply explain 'I need to get very close to your eyes for this.' (Not 'We need to get very close for this'—one of the authors was kissed repeatedly while conducting ophthalmoscopy by a patient with frontal lobe signs.)

Inducing trance-like states Watch a skilful practitioner at work palpating the abdomen: the right hand rests idly on the abdomen, far away from the part which hurts. He meets the patient's gaze: 'Have you ever been to the seaside?' His hand caresses rather than penetrates. 'Imagine you are back on the beach now, perfectly at ease, gazing at the blue, blue sky.' He presses as hard as he needs. 'Tell me now, where were you born and bred?' If he stops talking and frowns only during palpation of the epigastrium, something possibly quite useful has been discovered.

Communication All ideas are useless unless we communicate them. Be simple and direct. Avoid jargon; even words such as 'remission' and 'jaundice' are often misunderstood. In one study, 10% of patients said jaundice meant yellow vomit; see www.psychooncology.org. Give the most important details first. Check on retention and understanding. Be specific. 'Drink 6 cups of water daily' is better than 'Drink more fluids'. Give videos or written material with easy readability. Flesch's formula quantifies this: $F=206.835-(1.015 \times \text{ASL})-(84.6 \times \text{ASW})$ where ASL=average sentence length (number of words ÷ number of sentences) and ASW=average number of syllables/word. 100 is very easy; aim for >70. ***F*** for the first paragraph of this page is 71 but our second paragraph is much more complex: ***F***=39, as calculated by Microsoft Word's® automated Flesch score. It is sobering to display readability statistics for patient information leaflets imported into Word®, and then fun to see if you can re-edit to get a score of >70. ►Don't assume all patients can read: naming the pictures but not the words on our test chart (p51) reveals this tactfully.

Ensure harmonization between your view of what should be done and your patient's. We often talk of ***compliance*** with our regimens, when what we should talk of is ***concordance***, for concordance recognizes the central role of patient participation in all good plans of care.

Asking questions

No class of questions is 'correct'. Sometimes you need to ask one type of question, sometimes another. Get good at shifting from one kind to another, and you will soon learn to judge the most effective questions for the patient in front of you. The aim of asking questions is to *describe*, not from the point of view of intellectual imperialism ('If you can describe the world, you can have it'), but from the point of view of practical help: what cannot be described cannot be cured, and what is described but still cannot be cured can, at least, be shared, mitigated, and so partially overcome. Different kinds of questions either throw light on this issue, or obscure it, as in the 2 examples below.

Leading questions On seeing a bloodstained handkerchief you ask: 'How long have you been coughing up blood?' '6 weeks, doctor', so you assume haemoptysis for 6 weeks. In fact, the stain could be due to an infected finger, or to epistaxis (nose bleed). On finding this out later (and perhaps after expensive and unpleasant investigations), you will be annoyed with your patient for misleading you—whereas he was trying to be polite by giving the sort of answer you were obviously expecting. With such leading questions as these, the patient is not given an opportunity to deny your assumptions.

Questions suggesting the answer 'Was the vomit red, yellow, or black—like coffee grounds?'—the classic description of vomited blood. 'Yes, like coffee grounds, doctor.' The doctor's expectations and hurry to get the evidence into a pre-decided format have so tarnished the story as to make it useless.

Open questions The most open question is 'How are you?' This suggests no particular answer, so the direction a patient chooses offers valuable information. Other examples are gentle imperatives such as 'Tell me about the vomit' 'It was dark' 'How dark?' 'Dark bits in it' 'Like...?' 'Like bits of soil in it.' This information is gold, although it is not cast in the form of 'coffee grounds'.

Patient-centred questions 'What do you think is wrong?' 'Are there any other aspects of this we might explore?' 'Are there any questions you want to ask?' (a closed question). Better still, try 'What are the other things on your mind? How does having this affect you? What is the worst thing? It makes you feel...' (The doctor is silent.) ►Unless you become patient-centred your patient may never be fully satisfied with you, or fully cooperative.

Casting your questions over the whole family This is most useful in revealing if symptoms are caused or perpetuated by psychological mechanisms. They probe the network of causes and enabling conditions which allow nebulous symptoms to flourish in family life. 'Who else is important in your life? ... Are they worried about you? Who really understands you?' Until this sort of question is asked, illness may be refractory to treatment. Eg 'Who is present when your headache starts? Who notices it first—you or your wife? Who worries about it most (or least)? What does your wife do when (or before) you get it?' Think to yourself: *Who* is his headache? We note with fascination research showing that in clusters of hard-to-diagnose symptoms, it is the spouse's view of them that is the best predictor of outcome: if the spouse is determined that symptoms must be physical, the outcome is worse than if the spouse allows that some symptoms may be psychological.

Echoes Try repeating the last words said as a route to new intimacies, otherwise inaccessible, as you fade into the distance, and the patient soliloquizes '...I've always been suspicious of my wife.' 'Wife ...' 'My wife ... and her father together.' 'Together...' 'I've never trusted them together.' 'Trusted them together...' 'No, well, I've always felt I've known who my son's real father was... I can never trust those two together.' Without any questions you may unearth the unexpected, important clue which throws a new light on the history.

►*If you only ask questions, you will only receive answers in reply.* If you interrogate a robin, he will fly away: treelike silence may bring him to your hand.

What is the mechanism? Finding narrative answers

Like toddlers, we should always be asking '*Why?*'—not just to find ultimate causes, but to enable us to choose the simplest level for intervention. Some simple change early on in a chain of events may be sufficient to bring about a cure, whereas later on in the chain such opportunities may not arise.

For example, it is not enough for you to diagnose heart failure in your breathless patient. Ask: '*Why is there heart failure*?' If you do not, you will be satisfied with giving the patient an anti-failure drug—and any side-effects from this, such as uraemia or incontinence induced by diuretic-associated polyuria, will be attributed to an unavoidable consequence of necessary therapy.

If only you had asked '*What is the mechanism of the heart failure*?' you might have found a cause, eg anaemia coupled with ischaemic heart disease. You cannot cure the latter, but treating the anaemia may be all that is required to cure the patient's breathlessness. But do not stop there. Ask: '*What is the mechanism of the anaemia*?' You find a low MCV and a correspondingly low serum ferritin (p312)—and you might be tempted to say to yourself, I have the prime cause.

Wrong! Put aside the idea of prime causes, and go on asking '*What is the mechanism*?' Retaking the history (often the best 'investigation') shows a very poor diet. '*Why is the patient eating a poor diet*?' Is he ignorant or too poor to eat properly? You may find the patient's wife died a year ago, he is sinking into a depression, and cannot be bothered to eat. He would not care if he died tomorrow.

You come to realize that simply treating the patient's anaemia may not be of much help—so go on asking '*Why?*': 'Why did you bother to go to the doctor if you aren't interested in getting better?' It turns out he only went to see you to please his daughter. He is unlikely to take your drugs unless you really get to the bottom of what he cares about. His daughter is what matters and, unless you include her, all your initiatives may fail. Talk to her, offer help for the depression, teach her about iron-rich foods and, with luck, your patient's breathlessness may gradually begin to disappear. Even if it does *not* start to disappear, you are learning to stand in your patient's shoes and you may discover what will enable him to accept help. And this dialogue may help you to be a kinder doctor, particularly if you are worn out by endless lists of technical tasks which you must somehow fit into impossibly overcrowded days and nights. You never really know a man until you stand in his shoes and walk around in them. Harper Lee; *To Kill a Mockingbird*

Constructing imaginative narratives yielding new meanings Doctors are often thought of as being reductionist or mechanistic—but the above shows that asking '*Why?*' can enlarge the scope of our enquires into holistic realms. Another way to do this is to ask '***What does this symptom mean?***'—for this person, his family, and our world. A limp might mean a neuropathy, or falling behind with the mortgage, if you are a dancer; or it may represent a medically unexplained symptom which subtly alters family hierarchies both literally (on family walks) and metaphorically. Science is about clarity, objectivity, and theory in modelling reality. But there is another way of modelling the external world which involves subjectivity, emotion, ambiguity, and arcane relationships between apparently unrelated phenomena. The medical humanities (p19) explore this—and have burgeoned recently[4]—leading to the existence of two camps: humanities and science. If, while reading this you are getting impatient to get to the real nuts and bolts of technological medicine, you are in the latter camp. We are not suggesting that you leave it, only that you learn to operate out of both. If you do not, your professional life will be full of failures which you may deny or remain in ignorance of. If you *do* straddle both camps, there will also be failures, but you will realize what these failures *mean*, and you will know how to *transform* them. This transformation happens through dialogue and reflection. We would achieve more if we did less: every hospital should have a department of reflection and it should be visited as often as the radiology department. In fact every hospital has many such departments, carved out of our own minds—it's just that their entrances are blocked by piles of events, tasks and happenings.

Death: diagnosis and management

Death is Nature's master stroke, albeit a cruel one, because it allows genotypes space and opportunity to try on new phenotypes. The time comes in the life of any organ or person when it is better to start again from scratch rather than carry on with the weight and muddle of endless accretions. Our bodies and minds are these perishable phenotypes—the froth, which always turns to scum, on the wave of our genes. These genes are not really *our* genes. It is we who belong to them for a few decades. It is one of Nature's great insults that she should prefer to put *all* her eggs in the basket of a defenceless, incompetent neonate rather than in the tried and tested custody of our own superb minds. But as our neurofibrils begin to tangle, and that neonate walks to a wisdom that eludes us, we are forced to give Nature credit for her daring idea. Of course, Nature, in her careless way, can get it wrong: people often die in the wrong order (one of our chief roles is to prevent this mis-ordering of deaths, not the phenomenon of death itself).

So we must admit that, on reflection, dying *is* a brilliant idea, and one that it is most unlikely we could ever have thought of ourselves.

Causes of death Homicide, suicide, misadventure, or natural causes.

Diagnosing death Apnoea with no pulse[1] and no heart sounds, and fixed pupils.[2] If on a ventilator, brain death may be diagnosed even if the heart is still beating, via the ***UK brain death criteria*** which state that brain death is death of the brainstem, recognized by establishing:

- Deep coma with absent respirations (hence on a ventilator).
- The absence of drug intoxication and hypothermia (<35°C).
- The absence of hypoglycaemia, acidosis, and U&E imbalance.

Tests: All brainstem reflexes should be absent.

- Unreactive pupils. Absent corneal response (no blink to a cotton-wool touch).
- No vestibulo-ocular reflexes, ie no eye movement occurs after or during slow injection of 20mL of ice-cold water into each external auditory meatus in turn. Visualize the ear-drum first to eliminate false negative tests, eg due to wax.
- No motor response within the cranial nerve distribution should be elicited by adequate stimulation.
- No gag reflex or response to bronchial stimulation, and no respiratory effort on stopping the ventilator and allowing P_aCO_2 to rise to 6.7kPa.

Other considerations: Repeat tests after a suitable interval, eg 24h. Spinal reflexes are not relevant to diagnosing brain death; EEG is not required, nor is a neurologist. The doctor diagnosing brain death must be a consultant (or his deputy registered for >5yrs). The opinion of one other doctor (any) should also be sought.

US criteria for brain death are different: an EEG must confirm absence of cerebral activity if brain death is to be diagnosed within 6h of apparent cessation of brain activity. Diagnosis is allowed in cases of intoxication if isotope angiography shows absent cerebral circulation, or if the intoxicant has been metabolized.

Organ donation: The point of diagnosing brain death is partly that this allows organs (kidney, liver, cornea, heart, or lungs) to be donated and removed with as little hypoxic damage as possible. Don't avoid the topic with relatives. Many are glad to consent and to know that good can come after the death of a relative, that some part of the relative will go on living, giving a new life to another person.

After death Inform GP and the consultant. See the relatives. Sign death certificates promptly. If the cause is violence, injury, neglect, surgery, anaesthesia, alcohol, suicide, or poisoning, or is unknown, inform the Coroner/Procurator Fiscal.

1 Length of absence of circulation (important for non-heart-beating organ donation) before brain death occurs is controversial: 2 or 10min? *Lancet* 2000 **356** 528. * In USA, death of the *whole* brain is needed.
2 One of us (JML) keeps a red torch (with dark spots) in the shape of a ladybird in his pocket to conduct this ancient ceremony. It has now received so many dying eyebeams that it is invested with a fond glow that only the dead can impart to us, the living, who remain watching over them, quietly awaiting our own turn, spots before our eyes and wings at our feet, for the few seconds it takes to note *fixed dilated pupils*.

Facing death

People imagine that they are not afraid of death when they think of it while they are in good health (Marcel Proust). So, to get into the mood, as a thought experiment, place a finger in your left supraclavicular fossa, and feel there the craggy node of Virchow, telling of some distant gastric malignancy, as if it were a death warrant. Perhaps you have just 4 months left. Live with this 'knowledge' for a day or two, and see how it changes your attitude to family and friends on the one hand, and the million irrelevances which clutter our minds on the other.

As the week unfolds, you may experience thoughts and feelings that are new to you, but all too familiar to your patients. And as the months and years roll by, and you find yourself sitting opposite certain patients, put that finger once more on that metaphorical node and turn it over in your mind, and it will turn you, so you are sitting not opposite your patient but beside him. But there is only so much comfort you can bring in this way, as, in the end, you cannot tame death.

Whenever you find yourself thinking *it is better for him not to know,* suspect that you mean: *it is easier for me not to tell.* We find it hard to tell for many reasons: it distresses patients; it may hold up a ward round; we do not like acknowledging our impotence; telling reminds us of our own mortality and may unlock our previous griefs. We use many tricks to minimize the pain: *rationalization* ('He would not want to know'); *intellectualization* ('Research shows that 37% of people at stage 3 survive 2 years...'); *brusque honesty* ('You are unlikely to survive 1 month' and, so saying, the doctor rushes off to more vital things); *inappropriate delegation* ('Sister will explain it all to you when you are calmer'). Telling may help because:

- He already half knows but everyone shies away so he cannot discuss his fears (of pain, or that his family will not cope).
- There may be many affairs for the patient to put in order.
- To enable him to judge if unpleasant therapy is worthwhile.

►*Most patients are told less than they would like to know.*

What are his worries likely to be? Put yourself in the patient's place.

- Give some information, and then the opportunity to ask for more.
- Be sensitive to hints that he may be ready to learn more. 'I'm worried about my son.' 'What is worrying you most?' 'Well, it will be a difficult time for him, (pause) starting school next year.' Silence, broken by the doctor, 'I get the impression there are other things worrying you.' The patient now has the opportunity to proceed further, or to stop.
- Ensure that the GP and the nurses know what you have and have not said. Also make sure that this is written in the notes.

Stages of acceptance Accepting death takes time, and may involve passing through 'stages' on a path. It helps to know where your patient is on this path (but progress is rarely orderly and need not always be forwards: the same ground often needs to be recovered). At first there may be *shock* and *numbness*, then *denial* (which reduces anxiety), then *anger* (which may lead you to dislike your patient, but anger can have positive attributes, eg in energizing people—and it can trump fear and pain; it is different from mere hostility), then *grief*, and then, perhaps, *acceptance.* Finally there may be intense longing for death as the patient moves beyond the reach of worldly cares.[1]

Living wills and advance directives If a patient's views are known, comply with them. But these views change, are ambiguous, or hard to interpret, even if a *living will* exists. In one study of a will stating '*... with the development of any life threatening medical situation I should not be given active treatment such as antibiotics or ventilation ...*', 6 out of 12 health professionals said they would give antibiotics for pneumonia, as the will was not clear enough (eg had quality of life deteriorated enough to trigger the will?). Assume that living wills *do* have legal status; get help from colleagues or a judge if in doubt.

1 JS Bach 1727 *Ich habe genug*, Cantata No. 82, composed for the Feast of the Purification.

►Consult the *BNF* or *BNF for children* or your local equivalent before giving any drug with which you are not thoroughly familiar; check interactions meticulously.

Before prescribing, ask if the patient is allergic to anything. The answer is often 'Yes'—but do not stop here. Characterize the reaction, or else you risk denying a possibly life-saving, and very safe, drug such as penicillin because of a mild reaction, eg nausea. Is the reaction a ***true allergy*** (anaphylaxis, p780, or a rash?), a ***toxic effect*** (eg ataxia is inevitable if given large doses of phenytoin), or a ***predictable adverse reaction*** (eg GI bleeding from aspirin), or an ***idiosyncratic reaction***?

Remember *primum non nocere*: first do no harm (p746). The more minor the complaint, the more weight this dictum carries. The more serious the complaint, the more its antithesis comes into play: *nothing ventured, nothing gained.*

Prescribing in renal failure See p295. In **liver failure**, see p251.

Ten commandments ►These should be written on every tablet.

1 Explore alternatives to drugs—which often lead to doctor-dependency, paternalism, and medicalization of life. Drugs are also expensive: >£11 billion/yr[UK]; prices increase much faster than general inflation. There are 3 places to look:
The larder: lemon and honey for sore throats, rather than penicillin.
The blackboard: eg education about the self-inflicted causes of oesophagitis. Rather than giving expensive drugs, advise raising the head of the bed, and avoiding tight garments, too many big meals, smoking, and alcohol excess.
Lastly, look to yourself: giving a piece of yourself, some real sympathy, is worth more than all the drugs in your pharmacopoeia to patients who are frightened, bereaved, or weary of life. One of us (JML) for many years looked after a lady who was paranoid: monthly visits comprised an injection and a hug, no doubt always chaperoned, until one day mental health nurses took over her care. She was seen by a different nurse each month. They didn't know about hugging, so after a while she stopped cooperating, and soon it fell to me to certify her death.

2 Are you prescribing for a minor illness because you want to solve all problems? Patients may be happy just to know the illness *is* minor. Knowing this may make it acceptable. Some people do not believe in drugs, and you must find this out.

3 Decide if the patient is responsible. If he now swallows *all* the quinine pills you have so attentively prescribed for his cramps, death will be swift.

4 Know of other ways your prescription may be misused. Perhaps the patient whose 'insomnia' you so kindly treated is even now selling it on the black market or grinding up your prescription prior to injecting himself, desperate for a fix. Will you be suspicious when he returns to say he has lost his drugs?

5 Address these questions when prescribing off the ward:
- How many daily doses are there? 1–2 is *much* better than 4. Good doctors spend much time harmonizing complex regimens: the more you know about practical therapeutics the better for your patient. One reason for 'failure' of HIV drugs, for example, is that regimens are too complex. Drug companies know this, so keep abreast of new modified release (MR) preparations.
- The bottle/box: can the patient read the instructions—and can he open it?
- How will you know if the patient forgets to return (follow-up)?
- If the patient agrees, enlist the spouse's help in ensuring that he remembers to take the pills. Check, eg by counting the remaining pills at the next visit.

6 List the risks (side-effects, contraindications, interactions, risk of allergy). Of any new problem, always ask yourself: *Is this a side-effect?*

7 Agree with the patient on the risk : benefit ratio's favourability. Try to ensure there is true concordance (p3) between you and your patient.

8 Record how you will review the patient's need for each drug.

9 Quantify progress towards specified, agreed goals, eg pulse rate to mark degree of β-blockade; or peak flow to guide steroid use in asthma.

10 List benefits of *this* drug to *this* patient for *all* drugs taken. Specify what each drug is for—and co-operate with national computer schemes (eg the 'NHS spine') which aggregate drugs prescribed for your patient from *all* sources.

Prevention

Two mottoes: *The only good medicine is preventive medicine* and *If preventable... why not prevented?* During life on the wards you will have many opportunities for preventive medicine, and unconsciously you will pass most of them over, in favour of more glamorous tasks such as diagnosis, and clever interventions, involving probes, scalpels, and imaging. But if we imagine a ward where scalpels remain sheathed and the only thing being probed is our commitment to health, then preventive medicine comes to the fore, and it is our contention that such a ward might produce more health than some entire hospitals. The first step is to motivate your patient to take steps to benefit their own health by asking Socratic questions. 'Do you want to smoke?' 'What does your family think about smoking' 'Do you want your children to smoke?' 'Would there be any advantages in giving up?' 'Why is your health important to you?' 'Is there anything more important we can help with?' 'How would you spend the money you might save?' These types of questions along with specific strategies in prevention (p79) are more likely to produce change than withering looks and lectures on lung cancer or legs dropping off. In summary: in any preventive activity, get the patient on your side: make him *want* to change. Once you have done this, address the topics in the BOX (among others). Sometimes referral to other agencies is needed—eg for genetic counselling, contraception, and preconception advice (*OHCS* p2).

Examples of prevention
Primary prevention: (preventing occurrence)
Vaccination
Quit smoking advice
Binge drinking advice
Healthy eating advice
Safe(r) sex advice (HIV)
Screening for hypertension
Preconception folic acid to prevent spina bifida
Fluoride in water (caries)
Secondary prevention: (screening for 1st stages)
Cervical cytology
Mammography
Proteinuria in pre-eclampsia
Microalbuminuria in DM
Colonoscopy for polyps
Densitometry (osteoporosis)
Diet advice in impaired fasting glycaemia
Tertiary prevention: (preventing complications)
Aspirin after a stroke
Statins in angina
Retinal photography in DM
Hip protectors after falls
'Don't go barefoot' in those with diabetic neuropathy
Vitamin D in osteoporosis

The law of unintended consequences (Sod's law, p646) decrees that those whom you have to persuade the hardest to accept prevention by screening will be those to whom a complication befalls—such as colon perforation during colonoscopy to prevent cancers in those with UC or polyps. Or endoscopy will find an area of possible cancer in someone with Barrett's oesophagus (p686)—and a fit person dies of a post-op complication (oesophagectomy is dangerous). With this in mind, concentrate on those preventive activities which are simple, cheap, and have a complication rate approaching zero.

Individualized risk communication Risk communication which is done thoughtlessly and only dwelling on positive aspects can lead to bitterness, anger, and litigation. If communication is based on a person's individual risk factors for a condition (eg age, family history, smoking status, cholesterol level, eg using formulae such as that on p642), is risk communicated in ways that change behaviour? A 2003 Cochrane meta-analysis suggests 'not necessarily' (although uptake of screening tests *is* improved). At least this technique promotes dialogue, and dialogue opens doors, minds, and possibilities for choice. ***Informed participation*** is the aim, not passive acceptance of advice. It does not make much difference whether information is given as an absolute risk, or as a risk score, or categorized as high, medium, or low risk. See also 'Consent' p554.

Is this new drug any good? Analysis & meta-analysis

Research is a booming enterprise as seen from the inside (publications, impact factors, citations, grant income, large teams etc)[1]—but $billions go in and not much comes out. Very occasionally we recommend a new drug: on what grounds?

1 Does the research paper give a clear, clinically significant answer as well as a statistically significant answer in patients similar to those I treat?

2 Is the journal peer reviewed? Experts vet the paper before release (an imperfect process, as they have unknown axes to grind ± competing interests).

3 Are the statistical analyses valid? Much must be taken on trust as many analyses depend on sophisticated computing. Few papers, unfortunately, present 'raw' data. Look out for obvious faults by asking questions such as:

- Is the sample large enough to detect a clinically important difference, say a 20% drop in deaths from disease X? If the sample is small, the chance of missing such a difference is high. In order to reduce this chance to less than 5%, and if disease X has a mortality of 10%, >10,000 patients would need to be randomized. If a small trial which lacks power (the ability to detect true differences) *does* give 'positive' results, the size of the difference between the groups is likely to be exaggerated. (This is type I error; a type II error applies to results which indicate that there is no effect, when in fact there is.) ►So beware even quite big trials which purport to show that a new drug is as effective as an established treatment.
- Were the compared groups chosen randomly? Did randomization produce groups that were well matched? Were the treatments being compared carried out by practitioners equally skilled in each treatment?
- Was the study 'double blind' (both patient and doctor are unaware of which treatment the patient is having)? Could either have told which was given, eg by the metabolic effects of the drug?
- Was the study placebo- controlled? Good research can go on outside the realm of double-blind, randomized trials, but you need to be more careful in drawing conclusions—eg for intermittent symptoms, a bad time (prompting a consultation) is followed by a good time, making any treatment given in the bad phase appear effective. ***Regression towards the mean*** occurs in many areas, eg repeated BP measurement: because of transitory or random effects, most people having a high value today will have a less high value tomorrow—and most of those having a low value today will have a less extreme value tomorrow. This concept works at the bedside: if someone who is drowsy after a head injury has a high BP, and the next measurements are *higher still*, ie no regression to the mean, then this suggests a 'real' effect, such as ICP↑.
- Has time been allowed for criticism of the research to appear in the correspondence columns of the journal in question?

4 If I were the patient, would I want the new treatment?

5 What has the *National Institute for Clinical Excellence*[UK] (NICE) said? Note that NICE quite often changes its mind—a problem with all intelligent organizations.

Meta-analyses Systematic merging of similar trials *may* explain data inconsistencies. It is quicker and cheaper than doing new studies, and can establish generalizability of research.[10] *Be cautious!* In one study looking at recommendations of meta-analyses where there was a later 'definitive' big trial, it turned out that meta-analyses got it wrong 30% of the time, and 20% of good meta-analyses fail to avoid bias.[11] Don't assume that all meta-analyses, even those from the best stables, such as Cochrane, are free of bias owing to pharmaceutical funding.[12]

►A big well-planned trial may be worth centuries of uncritical medical practice; but a week's experience on the wards may be more valuable than years reading journals. This is the paradox in medical education: how can we trust our own experiences knowing they are all anecdotal; how can we be open to novel ideas but avoid being merely fashionable? A stance of wary open-mindedness may serve us best.

1 Charlton 2006 *Med Hypotheses* 66 1 *Is medical research a good way of spending money?* Possibly not.

Surviving house jobs

If some fool or visionary were to say that our aim should be to produce the greatest health and happiness for the greatest number of our patients, we would not expect to hear cheering from the tattered ranks of midnight house officers: rather, our ears are detecting a decimated groan—because these men and women know that there is something at stake in house-officership far more elemental than health or happiness: namely survival. Here we are talking about our own survival, not that of our patients. It is hard to think of a greater peacetime challenge than these first months on the wards. Within the first weeks, however brightly your armour shone, it will now be smeared and splattered if not with blood, then with the fallout from very many decisions which were taken without sufficient care and attention. Not that you were lazy, but *force majeure* on the part of Nature and the exigencies of ward life have, we are suddenly stunned to realize, taught us to be second-rate: for to insist on being first-rate in all areas is to sign a kind of death warrant for many of our patients, and, more pertinently for this page, for ourselves. Perfectionism cannot survive in our clinical world. To cope with this fact, or, to put it less depressingly, to flourish in this new world, don't keep re-polishing your armour (what are the 10 causes of atrial fibrillation—or are there 11?), rather furnish your mind—and nourish your body (regular food and drink make those midnight groans of yours less intrusive). Do not voluntarily deny yourself the restorative power of sleep. A good nap is the order of the day—and for the nights, sleep for as long as possible. Remember that sleep is our natural state in which we were first created, and we only wake to feed our dreams.

We cannot prepare you for finding out that you do not much like the person you are becoming, and neither would we dream of imposing on our readers a recommended regimen of exercise, diet, and mental fitness. Finding out what can lead you through adversity is the art of living. What will you choose: physical fitness, martial arts, poetry, karate, the sermon on the mount, juggling, meditation, yoga, a love affair—or will you make an art form out of the ironic observation of your contemporaries?

Many nourish their inner person through a religious belief, and attend mosque, church, synagogue, or temple. A multicultural society provides diversity and room for all branches of expression. Bear in mind not to compare yourself with your contemporaries. Those who make the most noise are often *not waving but drowning*. Plan recreation in advance. Start thinking about senior house officer jobs, and speak to the Regional Postgraduate Advisor in the specialty you select. Such enquiries supply energy to get you through the darker hours of house jobs, and may motivate you if the going gets tough. Not that this is any guarantee that the plans will work, but if your yoga, your sermons, and your fitness regimens turn to ashes in your mouth, then at least you will know the direction in which to spit. House jobs are not just a phase to get through and to enjoy where possible (there are often *many* such possibilities); they are also the anvil on which we are beaten into a new and perhaps rather uncomfortable shape. Luckily not all of us are made of iron and steel so there is a fair chance that, in due course, we will spring back into something resembling our normal shape, and, in so doing, we may come to realize that it was our weaknesses, not our strengths, which served us best.

House jobs can encompass tremendous up-and-down swings in energy, motivation, and mood, which can be precipitated by small incidents. If you are depressed for more than a day, speak to a sympathetic friend, partner, or counsellor to help you put it in perspective. ►When in doubt, communicate.

Quality, QALYs, and the interpretation of dreams

Resource allocation: who gets what Resource allocation is about cutting the health cake—whose size is *given*. What slice should go to transplants, new joints, and services for dementia? Cynics would say that this depends on how vociferous each group of patients (or doctors) is. Others try to find a rational way to allocate resources. Health economists (econocrats) have invented the QALY for this purpose. NB: Focusing on how to cut the cake diverts attention from how large the cake should be (is it better to spend money on space exploration or incontinence pads?)

How much is a life worth? Some countries will spend $2–10 million to find a man on a life-raft; others will spend nothing ('he's just one more mouth to feed').[13][14] Totalitarian capitalist states (eg China) will take a different view to liberal democracies. In France, one life is worth a hundred cherry trees, if the blossom is fine.[15]

What is a QALY? The essence of a QALY (Quality Adjusted Life Year) is that it takes a year of healthy life expectancy to be worth 1, but regards a year of unhealthy life expectancy to be worth <1. Its exact value is lower the worse the quality of life of the unhealthy person.[16] If a patient is likely to live for 8yrs in perfect health on an old drug, he gains 8 QALYs; if a new drug would give him 16yrs but at a quality of life rated by him at only 25% of the maximum, he would gain only 4 QALYs. The dream of a health economist is to buy most QALYs for his budget. As a rule of thumb, some heath assessment organizations (NICE[UK], controversially) *sometimes* keep an arbitrary figure in their head (such as £30,000/QALY).[17] If an intervention costs more than this, the reasons for recommending it have to be all the more explicit.

Cost per QALY♦ In various studies, with undeclared assumptions, this was (£):			
GP advice to stop smoking	220	Kidney transplant	4710
Preventing stroke by BP treatment	940	Breast cancer screening	5780
Pacemaker implantation	1100	Infliximab in Crohn's [18]	6700
Valve replaced		Heart transplant	7840
(eg for aortic stenosis)	1140	Home dialysis	17,260
Hip replacement (♀ aged 60–69)[19]	1470	Brain tumour surgery	107,780
CABG for LAD stenosis (p135)	2090	Interferon in MS (p488)♦	834,000

QALYs *do* help in rationing, but problems include pricing and invidiousness in choosing between the health of different people; a *huge* snag is that if we accept that the quality of our life is the quality of our relationships (Anthony Robbins), and that the value of relationships is unquantifiable (1 wife is good, but 2 wives are not *exactly* twice as good),[1] then we can see why bodies such as NICE get excoriated over issues such as dementia drugs, when apparently small objective improvements can cause disproportionate joy, as when a demented man becomes able to recall his son's name.[20][21]

The inverse care law and distributive justice

'Availability of good medical care tends to vary inversely with the need for it in the population served. This operates more completely where medical care is most exposed to market forces ... The market distribution of medical care exaggerates maldistribution of medical resources.'

There is much evidence in support of this famous thesis formulated by Tudor Hart,[22] and there is no doubt that if one wants to make a positive contribution to health, it is no good just discovering pathways, blocking receptors, and inventing drugs. The more this is done, the more urgent the need for distributive justice—that unyielding and perpetually problematic benchmark against which we are all judged.

If those who shout loudest get heard first, we need to know when to train our ears to be deaf—eg when deciding who to put on urgent and non-urgent operating lists. Unconsciously, we calibrate our lives to reduce stress. If we can learn the art of selective deafness, this need for the stressless life becomes less pressing, and, in the silence, we may come to know our professional values a little better.

1 This is an example of a **non-parametric quantity**, ie a quantity where simple ordering *may* be valid, but not operations such as addition or multiplication. Most medical statistics are assumed to be parametric; this is often false, invalidating much research. statsoft.com/textbook/stnonpar.html

Psychiatry on medical and surgical wards

►Psychopathology is common in colleagues, patients, and relatives. ►Seek help for your own problems. Find a sympathetic GP and register with her. You are not the best person to plan your assessment, treatment, and referral.

Current mental state ►OHCS p324. 'Move gently through her thoughts, as one might explore a new garden.[1] What is in bloom now? Where do those paths lead? What is under that stone? ***Focus on:*** Appearance; behaviour (anxious? suspicious?); speech (rate; content); mood; beliefs; hallucinations; orientation; memory (current affairs recall, monarch's name); concentration. Note the patient's insight and degree of rapport. Non-verbal behaviour often gives more valid clues than words alone.

Depression This is common, and often ignored, at great cost to wellbeing. Thinking 'I would be depressed in her situation' may sap our will to help, and as biological features (early waking, ↓appetite, ↓weight, loss of interest in sex and hobbies) are common on all wards, we may not realize just how bad things have got. ***The 2 'best questions' are:*** *'Have you been bothered by feeling down, depressed, or hopeless in the last month?'* If so, ask *'Have you been bothered by lack of interest or pleasure in doing things?'* If 'yes', depression is likely. There may also be guilt and feelings of worthlessness. ►*Don't think it's not your job to recognize and treat depression.* It is as important as pain. Try to arrange activities to boost the patient's morale and confidence, and keep him in touch with his fellows. Communicate your thoughts to other team members: nurses, physio- and occupational therapists, as well as relatives, if the patient wishes. Among these, your patient may find a kindred spirit who can give insight and support. ►If in doubt, try an antidepressant, and see if it helps, eg dosulepin 25–75mg at night, or lofepramine[2] 70mg/8–12h PO, if no hepatic or severe renal impairment. For *selective serotonin reuptake inhibitors* (eg fluoxetine, 20mg/24h), see OHCS p340. Remember that cognitive interventions are just as important as drugs (OHCS p370), so liaise with the patient's GP before discharge.

Alcohol This is a common cause of problems on the ward (both the results of abuse and the effects of withdrawal). See p274.

The violent patient Recognize early warning signs: tachypnoea, clenched fists, shouting, chanting, restlessness, repetitive movements, pacing, gesticulations. Your own intuition may be helpful here. At the first hint of violence, get help. If alone, make sure you are nearer the door than the patient.

- Do not be alone with the patient; summon the police or porters if needed.
- Try calming and talking with the patient. Do not touch him. Use your body language to reassure (sitting back, open palms, attentive).
- Get his consent; if unforthcoming, emergency treatment can still be given to save life, or serious deterioration. Enlist the help of nurses who know the patient.
- Use minimum force to achieve his welfare (but this may entail 6 strong men).

Causes: *anger, alcohol intoxication, drugs* (recreational; prescribed), *hypoglycaemia, delirium* (p476), *psychosis*. Do blood glucose, or give IV dextrose stat (p816). Before further tests, haloperidol may be needed: ~2mg IM (up to 10 or, rarely, 18mg stat; monitor pulse, T°, and BP every 15min–4h); maximum daily dose: 18mg.

If a rational adult refuses vital treatment, it may be as well to respect this decision, provided he is 'competent', ie he understands the consequences of his actions, and what you are telling him, is able to retain this information, and form the belief that it is true. Competence is rarely all or nothing, so don't hesitate to get the opinion of others. Enlist the persuasive powers of someone the patient respects.

Mental Health Acts Familiarize yourself with local procedures and laws pertaining to your country before your period of duty starts (OHCS p402). In England, Common Law allows restraining a patient who is being violent on the ward.

1 Ian McEwan 2001 *Atonement*, Vintage, 150.

2 Caution if: past heart disease, epilepsy, blood dyscrasias, prostatism, glaucoma, hyperthyroidism, or porphyria. CI: recent MI, heart block. SE: drowsiness, confusion, BP↓, pulse↑, vomiting, rash, LFT↑, marrow↓ ± anticholinergic SEs (dry mouth, constipation, vision↓, urine retention, sweating, tremor). Interactions: alcohol, anaesthetics (arrhythmias). Lofepramine is well tolerated. Wait 3wks for benefits to start.

The elderly patient in hospital

►Only in the past 3 centuries has life-expectancy risen much above 40 years. *Ar ageing population is a sign of successful social, health, and economic policies.*

Healthy ageing is not a contradiction as health is not just 'complete mental anc physical wellbeing (WHO) but also a process of adaptation, to changing environ ments, to growing up and ageing, to healing when damaged, to suffering, anc death. Health embraces the future so includes anguish and the inner resources tc live with it' (Illich, *OHCS* p470). ►Ageing is a continuum and is malleable representing cumulative effects of stressors (eg free radicals) and acquirec mechanisms for dealing with them (as important as genetic effects).

Beware ageism! Old age is associated with disease but doesn't cause it *per se.* Any deterioration is from treatable disease *until proved otherwise.*

1 Contrary to stereotype, most old people are fit. 80% of those over 85yrs olc do not live in institutions (95% if aged ~65yrs); 70% manage stairs and car bathe without help. Number of years in education and the number of co morbidities correlate inversely with difficulties in the activities of daily living.

2 With any problem, find the cause; don't always be thinking: *this is simply ageing.* Look (within reason) for treatable disease, ↓fitness, and social factors

3 Do not restrict treatment simply because of age. Old people vary. Age alone is a poor predictor of outcome and should not be used as a substitute for carefu assessment of each patient's potential for benefit and risk.

Characteristics of disease in old age There are differences of emphasis in the approach to old people compared with young people.

1 ***Multiple pathology:*** Several disease processes may coincide: find out whicl impinge on each complaint (eg senile cataract + arthritis = falls).

2 ***Multiple causes:*** One problem may have several causes. Treating each alone may do little good; treating all may be of much benefit.

3 ***Non-specific presentations:*** Some presentations are common in old people—eg the 'geriatric giants': incontinence (p604); immobility; instability (falls); anc dementia/confusion (p476 & p478). Any disease may present with these. Also typical signs and symptoms may be absent (myocardial infarction without ches pain; pneumonia, but no cough, fever, or sputum).

4 ***Rapid worsening if treatment is delayed:*** Complications are common.

5 ***More time is required for recovery:*** Points 4–6 reflect impairment ir homeostatic mechanisms and loss of 'physiological reserve'.

6 ***Impaired metabolism and excretion of drugs:*** Doses may need lowering, no least because there is often less tolerance to side-effects.

7 ***Social factors:*** These are central in aiding recovery and return to home.

Special points Assess all disabilities; get home details, eg stairs; access to toilet

- Drug concordance (p3): how many different tablets can he cope with? Probably not many more than 2. So which are the most important drugs? You may have to ignore other desirable remedies, or enlist the help of a friend, a spouse, or a pharmacist (who can batch morning, noon, and night doses in compartmentalized containers so complex regimens may be reduced to 'take the morning compartment when you get up, the noon compartment before lunch, etc').
- Social network (regular visitors; family and friends).
- Care details: what services are in operation?—meals delivered; community psychiatric or district nurse—who else is involved in the care?
- Speak to others (relatives; neighbours; carers; GP).
- Make a *careplan.* Include nutrition. If food is dumped beside a blind man, and no one helps cut it up, he may starve. A passing doctor may arrange a CT 'for cachexia' when what he needs is food and cataract surgery.

On examination: Do BP lying and standing (postural drop >20/10mmHg ≈ falls). Rectal exam: impaction ≈ overflow incontinence. Detailed CNS exam may be needed if presentation is non-specific. This tires patients, so consider doing in batches.

1 Cross-national studies are difficult—but see Ostir G 2006 *Arch Gerontol Geriatr* **42** 21.

Beyond the hospital: planning successful discharges (How to live and be frail in the community)

►*Start planning discharge from day 1.* A very common question on ward-rounds is: 'Will this patient get on OK at home?—we've got him as good as we can, but is discharge safe?' In answering this take into account:

- Does the patient live alone? Does any carer have support? Is he/she already exhausted by other duties (eg a handicapped toddler)?
- Is your patient in fact a carer for someone else even more frail?
- Most patients want to go home promptly. If not, find out why.
- Is the accommodation suitable? Stairs? Toilet on same floor?
- If toilet access is difficult, can he transfer from chair to commode?
- Can he open a tin, use the phone, plug in a kettle, cook soup?
- Is the family supportive—in theory or in practice?
- Are the neighbours friendly? 'But I would not trouble them'. Explore the validity of this sentiment by asking if they would want to know if they were reasonably fit, and a neighbour were in need.
- Are social services and community geriatric services well integrated? Or will the person who provides the lunch ignore the patient if she cannot gain access? Proper *case management programmes* with defined responsibilities, entailing integration of social and geriatric services really can help *and* save money (~20%). Such integration is rare but is possible in the UK thanks partly to the advent of Primary Care Trusts with overarching responsibilities for *both* medical *and* social care.

UK NHS national service framework (NSF) for older people

NSF'S ATTEMPT TO IMPROVE SERVICES BY CENTRAL COMMAND AND CONTROL: THE LEAST SUBTLE AND EFFECTIVE METHOD

There are 8 standards of care

http://bmj.com/cgi/content/full/326/7402/1300

1. ***Rooting out age discrimination:*** NHS services are to be provided regardless of age, on the basis of need alone. Social services will not use age in eligibility criteria or policies, to restrict access to available services.
2. ***Person-centred care:*** NHS services treat older people as individuals and enable them to make choices about their own care
3. ***Intermediate care:*** Older people will have access to intermediate care services at home or in designated care settings, to promote their independence by providing enhanced services from the NHS and councils to prevent unnecessary hospital admission. Rehabilitation services will enable early discharge from hospital and prevent premature or unnecessary admission to long-term residential care.
4. ***General hospital care:*** Older people's care in hospital is delivered through appropriate specialist care and by hospital staff who have the right set of skills to meet their needs.
5. ***Stroke:*** People who are thought to have had a stroke must have access to diagnostic services, and be treated appropriately by a specialist stroke service, and subsequently, with their carers, participate in a multi-disciplinary programme of secondary prevention and rehabilitation.
6. ***Falls:*** The NHS, working in partnership with councils, is required to take action to prevent falls and reduce fractures in older people and provide advice on fall prevention, through a specialist falls service.
7. ***Mental health in older people*** is to be promoted by access to integrated mental health services (from the NHS or councils) to ensure effective diagnosis, treatment, and support, for them and their carers.
8. ***The promotion of health and active life in older age:*** The health and well-being of older people are promoted through a coordinated programme of action led by the NHS with support from councils.

On being busy: Corrigan's secret door

Unstoppable demands, increasing expectations as to what medical care should bring, the rising number of elderly patients, coupled with the introduction of new and complex treatments all conspire, it might be thought, to make doctors ever busier. In fact, doctors have always been busy people. Sir James Paget, for example, would regularly see more than 60 patients each day, sometimes travelling many miles to their bedside. Sir Dominic Corrigan was so busy 160 years ago that he had to have a secret door made in his consulting room so that he could escape from the ever-growing queue of eager patients.

We are all familiar with the phenomenon of being hopelessly over-stretched, and of wanting Corrigan's secret door. Competing, urgent, and simultaneous demands make carrying out any task all but impossible: the house officer is trying to put up an intravenous infusion on a shocked patient when his 'bleep' sounds. On his way to the phone a patient is falling out of bed, being held in, apparently, only by his visibly lengthening catheter (which had taken the house officer an hour to insert). He knows he should stop to help but, instead, as he picks up the phone, he starts to tell Sister about 'this man dangling from his catheter' (knowing in his heart that the worst will have already happened). But he is interrupted by a thud coming from the bed of the lady who has just had her varicose veins attended to: however, it is not her, but her visiting husband who has collapsed and is now having a seizure. At this moment his cardiac arrest 'bleep' goes off, summoning him to some other patient. In despair, he turns to Sister and groans: 'There must be some way out of here!' At times like this we all need Corrigan to take us by the shadow of our hand, and walk with us through a metaphorical secret door, into a calm inner world. To enable this to happen, make things as easy as possible for yourself.

First, however lonely you feel, you are not usually alone. Do not pride yourself on not asking for help. If a decision is a hard one, share it with a colleague. Second, take any chance you get to sit down and rest. Have a cup of coffee with other members of staff, or with a friendly patient (patients are sources of renewal, not just devourers of your energies). Third, do not miss meals. If there is no time to go to the canteen, ensure that food is put aside for you to eat when you can: hard work and sleeplessness are twice as bad when you are hungry. Fourth, avoid making work for yourself. It is too easy for junior doctors, trapped in their image of excessive work and blackmailed by misplaced guilt, to remain on the wards reclerking patients, rewriting notes, or rechecking results at an hour when the priority should be caring for themselves. Fifth, when a bad part of the rota is looming, plan a good time for when you are off duty, to look forward to during the long nights.

However busy the 'on take', your period of duty will end. For you, as for Macbeth:

Come what come may,
Time and the hour runs through the roughest day.

Riding the wave

In *Macbeth*, toil and trouble go hand in hand, but sometimes we work best when we are busy. This is recognized in the aphorism that *if you want a job done quickly, give it to a busy (wo)man.* Observe your colleagues and yourself during a busy day. Sometimes our energy achieves nothing but our own inundation. At other times, by jettisoning everything non-essential, we get airborne, and accomplish marvellous feats. But note that what keeps us riding the wave of a busy day is not what we jettison but what we retain: humour, courtesy, and an ability to twinkle. A smile causes no delays, and reaches far beyond our lips.

Health and medical ethics

In our public medical personas, we often act as though morality consisted only in following society's conventions: we do this not so much out of laziness but because we recognize that it is better that the public think of doctors as old-fashioned or stupid, than that they should think us evil. But in the silences of our consultations, when it is we ourselves who are under the microscope, then, wriggle as we may, we cannot escape our destiny, which is to lead as often as to follow, in the sphere of ethics. To do this, we need to return to first principles, and not go with the flow of society's expectations. To give us courage in this enterprise, we can recall the aviator's and the seagull's law: it is only by *facing* the prevailing wind that we can become airborne, and achieve a new vantage point from which to survey our world.

Our analysis starts with our aim: to do good by making people healthy. ***Good***[1] is the most general term of commendation, and entails four cardinal duties:

1 Not doing harm. We owe this duty to all people, not just our patients.
2 Doing good by positive actions. We particularly owe this to our patients.
3 Promoting justice—ie distributing scarce resources fairly (p12) and respecting rights: legal rights, rights to confidentiality, rights to be informed, to be offered all the options, and to be told the truth.
4 Promoting autonomy. This is not universally recognized; in some cultures facing starvation, for example, it may be irrelevant, or even be considered subversive.

Health entails being sound in body and mind, and having powers of growth, development, healing, and regeneration. *How many people have you made healthy (or at least healthier) today?* And in achieving this, *how many cardinal duties have you ignored?* Herein lies a central feature of medicine. We cannot spend long on the wards or in our surgeries trying to 'make people healthy' before we have breached every cardinal duty—particularly (3) and (4). Does it matter? What is the point of having principles if they are regularly ignored? The point of having them is to provide a context for our negotiations with patients. If we want to be better doctors, there are many worse places to start than by trying to put these principles into action. Inevitably, when we try to, there are times when they conflict with each other. What should guide us when these principles conflict? It is not just a case of deciding off the top of one's head on the basis of the above analysis. It may be worthwhile aspiring to a synthesis—if you have the time (time will so often be what you do *not* have; but so often, in retrospect, when things have gone wrong, you realize that they would not have done so if you had *made* time).

Synthesis When we must act in the face of two conflicting duties, one of the duties is *not* a duty. How do we tell which one? Trying to find out involves getting to know our patients, and asking some questions:

- Are the patient's wishes being complied with?
- What do your colleagues think? What do the relatives think? Ask the patient's permission first. Have they his or her best interests at heart?
- Is it desirable that the reason for an action be universalizable? (That is, if I say this person is too old for such-and-such an operation, am I happy to make this a general rule for everyone?—Kant's 'law'.)[2]
- If an investigative journalist were to sit on a sulcus of mine, having full knowledge of my thoughts and actions, would she be bored or would she be composing vitriol for tomorrow's newspapers? If so, can I answer her, point for point? Am I happy with my answers? Or are they merely tactical devices?
- What would a patient's representative think—eg the elected chairman of a patient's participation group (OHCS p496)? These opinions are valuable as they are readily available (if a local group exists) and they can stop decision-making from becoming dangerously medicalized.

1 Don't think of good and evil as forever opposite; good can come out of evil, and vice versa: this fundamental mix-up explains why we learn more from our dissolute patients than we do from saints.
2 There are problems with universalizability: only intuition can suggest how to resolve conflicts between competing universalizable principles. Also, there is a sense in which all ethical dilemmas are unique, so no moral rules are possible or required—so they *cannot* be universal (Sartre, Nietzsche).

Difficult patients

'Unless both the doctor and the patient become a problem to each other, no solution is found.'[1] Jung's aphorism is untrue for half our waking lives: for an anaesthetist eg there is no need for the patient to become a problem in order for the anaesthetic to work. But, as with all the best aphorisms, being untrue is the least of the problems they cause us. Great aphorisms signify because they unsettle. Our settled and smug satisfaction at finishing a period of duty without any problems is so often a sign of failure. We have kept the chaos at bay, whereas, if we were greater men or women, we would have embraced it. Half our waking professional lives we spend as if asleep, on automatic, following protocols or guidelines to some trite destination—or else we are dreaming of what we could do if we had more time, proper resources, and perhaps a different set of colleagues. But if we had Jung in our pockets he would be shaking us awake, derailing our guidelines, and saluting our attempts to risk genuine interactions with our patients, however much of a mess we make of it, and however much pain we cause and receive. (Pain, after all, is the inevitable companion to lives led authentically.[2]) To the unreflective doctor, and to all average minds, this interaction is anathema, to be avoided at all costs, because it leads us away from anaesthesia, to the unpredictable, and to destinations which are unknown.

So, every so often, try being pleased to have difficult patients: those who question us, those who do not respond to our treatments, or who complain when these treatments *do* work. Very often, it will seem that whatever you say it is wrong: misunderstood, misquoted, and mangled by the mind you are confronting—perhaps because of fear, loneliness, or past experiences which you can only guess at. If this is happening, *shut up*—but don't *give up*. Stick with your patient. Listen to what he or she is saying and not saying. And when you have understood your patient a bit more, negotiate, cajole, and even argue—but don't bully or blackmail ('If you do not let your daughter have the operation she needs, I'll tell her just what sort of a mother you are . . .'). When you find yourself turning to walk away from your patient, turn back and say 'This is not going very well, is it? Can we start again?' And don't hesitate to call in your colleagues' help: not to win by force of numbers, but to see if a different approach might bear fruit. By this process, you and your patient may grow in stature. You may even end up with a truly satisfied patient. And a satisfied patient is worth a thousand protocols.

1 Carl Jung, *Memories, Dreams, Reflections*, 166 www.jelder.com/quotations/woundedhealer.html.

2 'Some say that the world is a vale of tears. I say it is a place of soul making'—John Keats, the first medical student to formulate these ideas about pain. They did not do him much good, because he died shortly after expressing them. But his ideas can do us good—perhaps if each day we try at least once for authentic interactions with a patient, unencumbered by professionalism, research interests, defensive medicine, a wish to show off to our peers, or a wish to get though the day with the minimum of fuss.

Medicine, art, and the humanities

Let us start with an elementary observation: *there are no justly famous living doctors*; indeed *there are no famous dead doctors*. The most famous doctors are either villains or those immortalized in literature—eg Dr Watson, Dr Frankenstein, and Dr Faustus.[1] Hereby we demonstrate the power of the written word. And it *is* an extraordinary power. When we curl up in an armchair and read for pleasure, we open the portals of our minds because we are alone. While we are reading, there is no point in dissembling. We confront our subject matter with a steady eye because we believe, that, while reading to ourselves, we cannot be judged. Then, suddenly, when we are at our most open and defenceless, literature takes us by the throat—and that eye which was so steady and confident a few minutes ago is now perhaps misting over, or our heart is missing a beat, or our skin is covered in a goose-flesh more papular than ever a Siberian winter produced. Once we have been on earth for a few decades, not much in our mundane world sends shivers down our spines, but the power of worlds of literature and art to do this ever grows.

There are, of course, doctors who are quite well known: Arthur Conan Doyle, William Carlos Williams, Somerset Maugham, and Anton Chekhov, and they are all artists. What about Sigmund Freud? Here is the exception which proves the rule—proves in the sense of testing, for he is not really an exception. We can accept him among the great only in so far as we view his oeuvre as an artistic oeuvre, rather than as a scientific one. Science has progressed for years without Freud, but, as art, his work and insights (such as the subconscious, which he 'invented') will survive: and survival, as Bernard Shaw pointed out, is the only test of greatness.

The reason for the ascendancy of art over science is simple. We scientists, in our humble way, are only interested in explaining reality. Artists are good at explaining reality too: but they also *create* it. Our most powerful impressions are produced in our minds not by simple sensations but by the association of ideas. It is a pre-eminent feature of the human mind that it revels in seeing something as, or through, something else: life refracted through experience, light refracted through jewels, or a walk through the woods transmuted into a Pastoral Symphony. Ours is a world of metaphor, fantasy, and deceit.

What has all this to do with the day-to-day practice of medicine? The answer lies in the word 'defenceless' above. When we read alone and for pleasure, our defences are down—and we hide nothing from the great characters of fiction. In our consulting rooms, and on the ward, we so often do our best to hide everything, beneath the white coat, or the avuncular bedside manner. So often, a professional detachment is all that is left after all those years inured to the foibles, fallacies, and frictions of our patients' tragic lives. It is at the point where art and medicine collide, that doctors can re-attach themselves to the human race and re-feel those emotions which motivate or terrify our patients. We all have an Achilles heel: that part of our inner self which was not rendered forever invulnerable to mortal cares when we were dipped in the waters of the river Styx as it flowed down the wards of our first disillusion. Art and literature, among other things, may enable this Achilles heel to be the means of our survival as thinking, sentient beings, capable of maintaining a sympathetic sensibility to our patients.

The American approach is to create Professors of Literature-in-Medicine and to conjure with concepts such as *the patient as text*, and most American medical schools do courses in literature in an attempt to inculcate ethical reasoning and speculation. Here, we simply intend to demonstrate, albeit imperfectly, in our writings and in our practice of medicine, that *every* contact with patients has an ethical and artistic dimension, as well as a technical one.

1 Of course Dr Faust, that famous charlatan, necromancer, and quack from medieval Germany, did have a real existence. In fact, there may have been two of them, who together gave rise to myths of devil-dealing, debauchery, and the undisciplined pursuit of science, without moral constraints.

2 Clinical skills

Contents

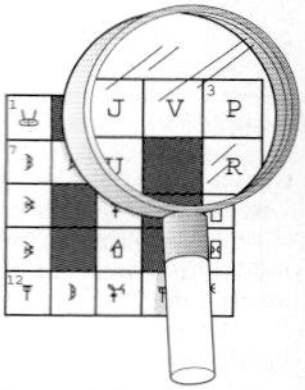

Fig 1. Skills acquired over years of training help us to unravel the clues that we pick up during history-taking and clinical examination. However, the clues are rarely straight: most are cryptic (eg clubbing, p56, caused by several underlying processes). Just as with crosswords, the satisfaction of completing the whole puzzle comes only after having put together the network of solved clues successfully. With practice we get quicker, slicker and better, just like the veteran solver. No wonder our elders seem to make such easy work of it all—see BOX opposite, *The patient now waiting for you ...*

Other relevant pages: Symptoms and signs (p52–p77); pre-op care (p552); acute abdomen (p580); lumps (p616–p624); hernias (p630–p633); varicose veins (p634); urine (p278); peripheral nerves (p444); dermatomes (p446).

In *OHCS*: Vaginal and other gynaecological examinations (*OHCS* p242); abdominal examination in pregnancy (*OHCS* p40); the history and examination in children and neonates (*OHCS* p100–p102); examination of the eye (*OHCS* p412); visual acuity (*OHCS* p414); eye movements (*OHCS* p422); ear, nose, and throat examination (*OHCS* p536); skin examination (*OHCS* p584); examination of joints—see the contents page to **Orthopaedics and trauma** (*OHCS* p656).

Principle sources: *Clinical Examination*, 4e, NJ Talley and S O'Connor, Blackwell Science, ISBN 0729537420; *Aids to Undergraduate Medicine*, 6e, JL Burton *et al*, Churchill, ISBN 0443056927.

We thank Dr TA Roper, who is our Specialist Reader for this chapter.

Advice and experience

►The way to learn physical signs is at the bedside, with guidance from an experienced colleague. This chapter is not intended as a substitute for this process: it is simply an *aide-mémoire*.

►We ask questions to get information to help with differential diagnosis. But we also ask questions to find out about the inner life and past exploits of our patients, so that they do not bore us, and so that we can respect them as individuals. The patient is likely to notice and reciprocate this respect, and this reciprocation is the foundation of most of our therapeutic endeavours. Our challenge is to identify with as broad a range of humanity as possible, without getting exhausted by the scale of this enterprise.

►'Truth lies not only in what is said, but also in who says it, to whom, why, how, and under what circumstances.' Vaclav Havel *Letters To Olga* (138)

The patient now waiting for you in cubicle 9 . . .

The first news of your next patient will often be via a phone call: 'There's an MI on the way in'—or 'There's someone dementing in cubicle 9'—or 'Can you take the overdose in resus?' On hearing such sanitized, dehumanized descriptions, our minds will start painting pictures, and the tone of these messages tends to colour these pictures. So when we arrive at the bedside, our mind is far from a *tabula rasa* or blank canvas on which the patient can paint his woes.

The mind is always painting pictures, filling in gaps, and falling into traps. Perception is an active process, for, as Marcel Proust, that life-long all-knowing patient, observed:[1]

> *We never see the people who are dear to us save in the animated system, the perpetual motion of our incessant love for them, which before allowing the images that their faces present to reach us catches them in its vortex, flings them back upon the idea that we have always had of them, makes them adhere to it, coincide with it.*

So if you want to know your patient, take snapshots of him from various angles, and briefly contemplate him in the round before Proust's vortex whisks you off track. Divest yourself of those prejudices and expectations which all good diagnosticians somehow ignore, and you will be all set for a Gestalt recognition (p188) of incipient myxoedema (the cause of the dementia in cubicle 9—see p189), jaundice, anaemia, or, perhaps more important, the recognition that the person in front of you is frightened, failing, or dying.

Embracing the oral tradition

The written word has been with us only for a few thousand years. Even during this phase in history, epics, stories, methods, and teaching have still been passed on by word of mouth through the practice of oral tradition. It may be surprising, therefore, that we rely so much on the written word, given that so many important nuances can be missed.

In a working culture that has shifted from continuing care by multi-talented individuals towards an ever-changing team in a string of handovers, we might do well to uphold this oral tradition. So to keep the chain strong and the care continuous, we should in the first instance strive to communicate face to face, at least when practical. In the least, to remain politic, we should continue to talk to each other—see MINIBOX.

Encourage 'The good...'
• Face to face handover • Clear histories • Civility
Avoid '...the bad...'
• Written handover • Hurrying • Abruptness
Prevent '...the ugly'
• Mismanagement • Missed investigations, results and procedures • Upset patients, carers and relatives

1 *The Guermantes Way* i p187 trans. CK Scott Moncrieff.

Taking a history

Taking (or receiving) histories is what most of us spend most of our profession life doing, and it is worth doing well. A good history is the biggest step towards th correct diagnosis. History-taking, examination, and treatment of a patient beg the moment one reaches the bedside. (The divisions imposed by our page titles a somewhat misleading). Try to put the patient at ease: a good rapport may reliev distress on its own. It often helps to shake hands. Always introduce yourself ar check whether the patient is comfortable. Be conversational rather tha interrogative in tone. General questions (age, occupation, marital status) help brea the ice and assess mental functions—sometimes important to establish early o

Presenting complaint (PC) 'What has been the trouble recently?' Record th patient's own words rather than eg 'dyspnoea'.

History of presenting complaint (HPC) When did it start? What was the firs thing noticed? Progress since then. Ever had it before? '<u>SOCRATES</u>' questions: sit onset (gradual, sudden); character; radiation; associations (eg nausea, sweating timing of pain/duration; exacerbating and alleviating factors; severity (eg scale (1–10, compared with childbirth, or with worst ever previous pain).

Direct questioning (DQ) Specific questions about the diagnosis you have in min (+ its risk factors, eg travel—p378) and a review of the relevant system.

Past medical history (PMH) Ever in hospital? Illnesses? Operations? As specifically about diabetes, asthma, bronchitis, TB, jaundice, rheumatic fever, hig BP, heart disease, stroke, epilepsy, peptic ulcer disease, anaesthetic problems.

Drug history (DH) Any tablets, injections? Any 'off-the-shelf' or 'over-the-counte drugs? Herbal remedies, the Pill? Ask the features of allergies: it may not have bee one, but on the other hand it may have been a minor reaction of sensitization any warning is given at all) before full-blown anaphylaxis.

Social history (SH) Probe without prying. 'Who else is there at home?' Job. Marit status. Spouse's job and health. Housing—any stairs at home? Who visits relatives, neighbours, GP, nurse? Are there any dependents at home? Mobility—ar walking aids needed? Who does the cooking and shopping? What can the patie not do because of the illness? The social history is all too often seen as dispensable adjunct, eg while the patient is being rushed to theatre, but vital clu may be missed about the quality of life and it is too late to ask when the surgeor hand is deep in the belly and she is wondering how radical a procedure to perforr It is worth cultivating the skill of asking a few searching questions of the admittir family doctor while you are conversing on the phone. If you are both busy, do no waste time on things you will shortly verify yourself but tap his knowledge of th patient and his 'significant others'. Remember: the GP is likely to be a specialist his patients, whom he may have known for decades. He may even hold a 'living wi or advance directive to reveal your patient's wishes if he cannot speak for himse

Alcohol, tobacco, recreational drugs How much? How long? When stopped? Th CAGE questionnaire is useful as a screening test for alcoholism (p274). Quanti smoking in terms of **pack-years**: 20 cigarettes/day for 1 year equals 1 pack-yea Smoking is forbidden among Sikhs, so be tactful. We all like to present ourselv well, so be inclined to double any stated quantities (**Holt's 'law'**).

Family history (FH) Areas of the family history may need detailed questioning, e to determine if there is a significant family history of heart disease you need to as about the health of the patient's grandfathers and male siblings, smoking, tenden to hypertension, hyperlipidaemia, and claudication before they were 60 years old, a well as ascertaining the cause of death. Ask about TB, diabetes, and other releva diseases. See BOX. ►**Be tactful when asking about a family history of malignanc**

Functional enquiry (p24) helps uncover undeclared symptoms. Some of this ma already have been incorporated into the history.

►Don't hesitate to retake the history after a few days: recollections change.

Drawing family trees to reveal dominantly inherited disease[1]

Advances in genetics are touching all branches of medicine. It is increasingly important for doctors to identify patients at high risk of genetic disease, and to make appropriate referrals. The key skill is drawing a family tree to help you structure a family history as follows:

1 Start with your patient. Draw a square for a male and a circle for a female. Add a small arrow (↗, see below) to show that this person is the *propositus* (the person through whom the family tree is ascertained).

2 Add your patient's parents, brothers, and sisters. Record basic information only, eg age, and if alive and well (a&w). If dead, note age and cause of death, and pass an oblique stroke through that person's symbol.

3 Ask the key question 'Has anybody else in your family had a similar problem as yourself?', eg heart attack/angina/stroke/cancer. Ask only about the family of diseases that relate to your patient's main problem. Do not record a potted medical history for each family member: time is too short.

4 Extend the family tree upwards to include grandparents. If you haven't revealed a problem by now, go no further—you are unlikely to miss important familial disease. If your patient is elderly it may be impossible to obtain good information about grandparents. If so, fill out the family tree with your patient's uncles and aunts on both the mother's and father's sides.

5 Shade those in the family tree affected by the disease. ● = an affected female; ■ = an affected male. This helps to show any genetic problem and, if there is one, will help demonstrate the pattern of inheritance.

6 If you have identified a familial susceptibility, or your patient has a recognized genetic disease, extend the family tree down to include children, to identify others who may be at risk, and who may benefit from screening. ►You must find out who is pregnant in the family, or may soon be, and arrange appropriate genetic counselling (*OHCS* p154).

The family tree below shows these ideas at work and indicates that there is evidence for genetic risk of colon cancer, meriting referral to a geneticist.

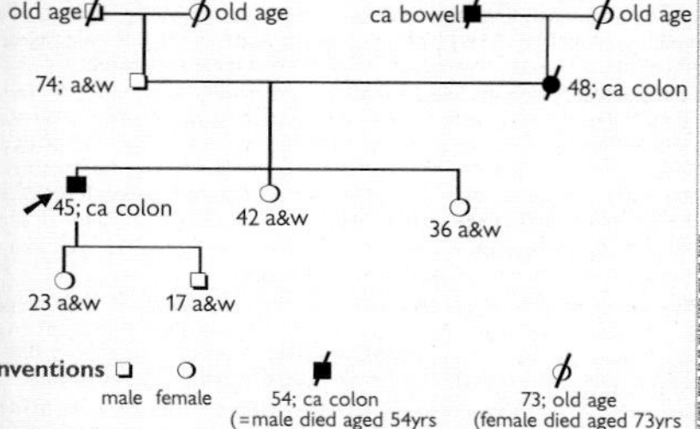

THIS PAGE OWES MUCH TO DR HELEN FIRTH, WHO WE THANK.

1 Use a different approach in paediatrics, and for autosomal or sex-linked disease. Ask if p... ...lated (consanguinity ↑risk of recessive diseases).

Functional enquiry

Just as skilled acrobats are happy to work without safety nets, so also olde clinicians may operate without the functional enquiry. But to do this you must be experienced enough to understand all the nuances of the presenting complaint.

General questions may be the most significant, eg in TB, endocrine problems, or cancer: •Weight loss •Night sweats •Any lumps •Fatigue/malaise/lethargy •Sleeping pattern[1] •Appetite •Fevers •Itch or rash •Recent trauma[2]

Cardio-respiratory symptoms Chest pain (p80). Exertional dyspnoea (=breathlessness): quantify exercise tolerance **and how it has changed**, eg stairs climbed, or distance walked, before onset of breathlessness. Paroxysmal nocturna dyspnoea (PND). Orthopnoea, ie breathlessness on lying flat (a symptom of left ventricular failure): quantify in terms of number of pillows the patient must sleep on to prevent dyspnoea. Oedema. Palpitations (awareness of heartbeats). Cough Sputum. Haemoptysis (coughing up blood). Wheeze.

Gut symptoms Abdominal pain (constant or colicky, sharp or dull; site; radiation duration; onset; severity; relationship to eating and bowel action; alleviating or exacerbating, or associated features). Other questions—think of symptoms throughout the GI tract, from mouth to anus:

- Swallowing (p232)
- Indigestion (p234)
- Nausea/vomiting (p232)
- Bowel habit (p238 & p240)
- Stool:
  - colour, consistency, blood, slime
  - difficulty flushing away (p272)
  - tenesmus or urgency

Tenesmus is the feeling of incomplete evacuation of the bowels (eg due to a tumou or irritable bowel syndrome). **Haematemesis** is vomiting blood. **Melaena** is alterec (black) blood passed PR (p244), with a characteristic smell.

Genitourinary symptoms Incontinence (stress or urge, p604). Dysuria (painfu micturition). Haematuria (bloody micturition). Nocturia (needing to micturate at night). Frequency (frequent micturition) or polyuria (the frequent passing of large volumes of urine). Hesitancy (difficulty starting micturition). Terminal dribbling.

Vaginal discharge (p406). Menses: frequency, regularity, heavy or light duration, painful. First day of last menstrual period (LMP). Number of pregnancies and births. Menarche. Menopause. Any chance of pregnancy now?

Neurological symptoms ***Special senses:*** Sight, hearing, smell, and taste. Seizures faints, 'funny turns'. Headache. 'Pins and needles' (paraesthesiae) or numbness Limb weakness ('Are your arms and legs weaker than normal?'), poor balance Speech problems (p46). Sphincter disturbance. Higher mental function and psychiatric symptoms (p46–p49). The important thing is to assess function: wha the patient can and cannot do at home, work, etc.

Musculoskeletal symptoms Pain, stiffness, swelling of joints. Diurnal variation i symptoms (ie with time of day). Functional deficit.

Thyroid symptoms ***Hyperthyroidism:*** Prefers cold weather, bad temperec sweaty, diarrhoea, oligomenorrhoea, weight↓ (though often ↑appetite), tremor palpitations, visual problems. ***Hypothyroidism:*** Depressed, slow, tired, thin hair croaky voice, heavy periods, constipation, dry skin, prefers warm weather.

►History-taking may seem deceptively easy, as if the patient knew the hard fact and the only problem was extracting them; but what a patient says is a mixture o hearsay ('she said I looked very pale'), innuendo ('you know, doctor, down below') legend ('I suppose I bit my tongue; it was a real fit, you know'), exaggeratio ('I didn't sleep a wink'), and improbabilities ('The Pope put a transmitter in m brain'). The great skill (and pleasure) in taking a history lies not in ignoring thes garbled messages, but in making sense of them.

1 Too sleepy? Think of myxoedema or narcolepsy. Early waking? Think of depression. Being woken by pai is always a serious sign. ►For the significance of the other questions here listed, see Chapter 3.

2 Trauma is not just important because something may be broken, but because even if it seems trivial, ·y provide the all-illuminating flash of insight which explains odd CNS features (eg post-traumat ·ural haemorrhage) or the vague prodromes of illnesses such as tetanus.

Presenting your findings—and the role of jargon

We are forever presenting patients to our colleagues, almost never questioning the mechanisms and motivations which permeate these oral exchanges—and sometimes send them awry. By some ancient right we assume authority to retell the patient's story at the bedside—not in our own words but in highly stylized medical code: 'Mr Hunt is a 19-year-old **Caucasian male**, a **known case of** Down's syndrome with little intelligible speech and an IQ of 60, **who complains of** paraesthesiae and weakness in his right **upper limb**... He **admits to drinking 21 units per week** and **other problems** are...'

Do not comfort yourself by supposing this ritualistic reinterpretation arises out of the need for brevity. If this were the reason, and we are speaking in front of the patient, all that is in bold above could be omitted, or drastically curtailed. The next easy conclusion to confront is that we purposely use this jargon to confuse or deceive the patient. This is only sometimes the case, and we must look for deeper reasons for why we are wedded to these medicalisms.

We get nearer to the truth when we realize that these medicalisms are used to sanitize and tame the raw data of our face-to-face encounters with patients—to make them bearable to us—so that we can **think** about the patient rather than having to **feel** for him or her. This is quite right and proper—but only sometimes. Usually what our patients need is sympathy, and this does not spring from cerebration. These medicalisms insulate us from the unpredictability of experiential phenomena. We need the illusion that we are treading on well-marked-out territory when we are describing someone's pain—a problematic enterprise, not least because if the description is objective it is invalid (pain is, *par excellence*, subjective), and if it is subjective, it is partly incommunicable.

These medicalisms enroll us into a half-proud, half-guilty brotherhood, cemented by what some call patronage and others call fear. This fear can manifest itself as intense loyalty so that, err as we may, we cling to our medical loyalties unto death (that of the patient, not our own). Language is the tool unwittingly used to defend this autocracy of fear. The modulations of our voice, the stylized vocabulary, and the casual neglect of logic and narrative order ensure, in the above example, that we take on board so little of our patient that we remain upright and afloat, above the whirlpools of our patients' lives. In this case, not a case at all, but a child, a family, a mother worried sick about what will happen to her son when she dies: a son who has never **complained** of anything, has never **admitted** to anything, expresses no **problems**—it is our problem that his hand is weak, and his mother's that he can no longer attend riding for the disabled, because she can no longer be away from home and do her part-time job. So when you next hear yourself declaim in one breath that 'Mr Smith is a 50-year-old Caucasian male with crushing central chest pain radiating down his left arm', take heed—what you may be communicating is that you have stopped thinking about this person—and pause for a moment. Look into your patient's eyes: confront the whirlpool.

Footnotes in History: Osler

One of the keys to enjoying medicine is an enthusiasm for involvement, which can be rewarded with the pleasure of sharing in the success of a treatment with a patient and colleagues alike. One outstanding man of medicine and shaper of medical history with such an enthusiasm was William Osler. He held the attitude that promoting equanimity and courtesy among patients and colleagues was an essential part of practice—he himself was a constant inspiration to his students and fellow teachers and also to his patients at a time when prognoses were generally poor. So if you are ever short of inspiration consider what may have been his, because aside from his many scientific contributions, Osler also wrote on the modern philosophies of medical education and patient care. For further insights, see www.whonamedit.com.

Physical examination

With a few exceptions (eg BP), physical examination is not a good screening test for detecting disease. Plan your examination to emphasize the areas that the history suggests may be abnormal. A few well-directed, problem-oriented minutes can save hours of fruitless physical examination. You will still be expected to examine all 4 major systems (cardiovascular, respiratory, abdominal, and neurological), but with time you will be adept at excluding any major pathology. Establish your own comprehensive routine—practice is the key.

Look at your patient as a whole to decide how sick he seems to be. Is he well or *in extremis*? Try to decide **why** you think so. Is he in pain? Does it make him lie still (eg peritonitis) or writhe about (eg colic)? What is the pattern of breathing: laboured; rapid; shallow; irregular; distressed? Is he obese or cachectic? Is his behaviour appropriate? Can you detect any unusual ***smell*** eg hepatic fetor (p250), cigarettes, alcohol? Also take a moment to look around the bed for other clues, eg inhalers, insulin administration kit, walking aids etc.

Specific diagnoses can often be made from ***the face and body habitus*** and these may be missed unless you stop and consider them: eg acromegaly, thyrotoxicosis, myxoedema, Cushing's syndrome, or hypopituitarism, see p188. Is there an abnormal distribution of body hair (eg bearded ♀, or hairless ♂) suggestive of endocrine disease? Is there anything about him to trigger thoughts about Paget's disease, Marfan's, myotonia, and Parkinson's syndrome? Look for rashes, eg the malar flush of mitral disease and the butterfly rash of SLE.

Assess the degree of ***hydration*** by examining the skin turgor (see BOX), the axillae, and mucous membranes. Sunken orbits may also occur in dehydration. Check peripheral perfusion: eg press the nose/finger and time capillary return (CR)—it should be <2s in a well-hydrated individual. Record the temperature, and BP (lying and standing may be compared to postural hypotension, a sign of shock).

Check for ***cyanosis*** (central and peripheral, p56). Is the patient ***jaundiced***? Yellow skin is unreliable and may be produced by the lemon tinge of uraemia, pernicious anaemia, carotenaemia (in all these cases the sclerae are not yellow), or caecal carcinoma. The sign of jaundice is yellow sclerae seen in good daylight. ***Pallor*** is a nonspecific sign and may be racial, familial, or cosmetic. ***Anaemia*** is assessed from the palmar skin creases (when spread) and conjunctivae (fig 1, p311)—usually pale if Hb <8–9g/dL: you cannot conclude anything from **normal** conjunctival colour; but if they are pale, the patient is probably anaemic. Koilonychia and stomatitis (sore, dry, inflamed skin around the mouth, particularly at its lateral edge) suggest iron deficiency. Anaemia with jaundice suggests malignancy or haemolysis. Pathological ***hyperpigmentation*** is seen in Addison's, haemochromatosis (slate-grey) and ***amiodarone***, ***gold***, ***silver***, and ***minocycline*** therapy.

Palpate for ***lymph nodes*** in the neck (from behind), axillae, groins, and epitrochlear region (rarely palpable, but significant if present)—see p64 for causes. Any ***subcutaneous nodules*** (p64, p617)?

Don't forget to look at the results of ***urinalysis*** and ***urine output charts*** where indicated. Look at the ***temperature chart***. Average temperature values are 36.8°C (mouth), 36.4°C (axilla), 37.3°C (rectum).[1] **Hypothermia** is defined as a core temperature <35°C; special thermometers may be needed to measure temperatures below this level. A morning temperature ≥37.3°C (mouth) or >37.7°C (rectum) constitutes a **fever**.[2] Note the periodicity of any fever (p376). Do not always believe the temperature chart—if you suspect that the patient has a fever (eg by back-of-the-hand on the forehead), take the temperature yourself.

Don't feel downheartened if you miss a clinical sign—inter-observer variation is a fact of life! Embrace the opportunity to ingrain what you have missed into your own subconscious routine, building up your skills with time and practice.

1 The accuracy of different non-invasive methods for measuring temperature is continually being assessed.
2 The nadir is at 6 AM, with a zenith at 6 PM; the mean amplitude of variability is 0.5°C.

The hands

A wealth of information can be gained from shaking hands and rapidly examining the hands of the patient. Is there a palsy or deformity—eg the patient may offer the other hand? Are they warm and well-perfused? Warm, sweaty hands signal hyperthyroidism while cold, moist hands may be due to anxiety. Are the rings tight with oedema? Lightly pinch the dorsum of the hand—persisting ridging of the skin means loss of tissue turgor (dehydration, or lack of connective tissue support from ageing). Are there any tar stains from tobacco use? Does the patient have difficulty releasing your hand after shaking it (dystrophia myotonica, p502)? Reluctance to let go is also a sign of loneliness.

Nails ***Koilonychia*** (spoon-shaped nails) suggests iron deficiency, fungal nail infection or Raynaud's. ***Onycholysis*** (nail destruction) is seen with hyperthyroidism, fungal infection, and psoriasis. ***Beau's lines*** (fig 1) are transverse furrows from temporary arrest of nail growth at times of ↑biological stress: malaria, typhus, rheumatic fever, Kawasaki disease, myocardial infarct, chemotherapy, Guillain–Barré & Raynaud's syndrome, trauma, high-altitude climbing, and deep sea diving.[3] As nails grow at ~0.1mm/d, the furrow's distance from the cuticle allows dating of the stress. ***Mees' lines*** are single white, transverse bands seen in arsenic poisoning or renal failure. ***Muehrcke's lines*** are paired white, parallel transverse bands (*without* furrowing)[4] seen eg in hypoalbuminaemia. ***Terry's nails:*** Proximal portion of nail is white/pink, nail tip is red/brown (causes: cirrhosis, chronic renal failure). ***Pitting*** is seen in psoriasis and alopecia areata.

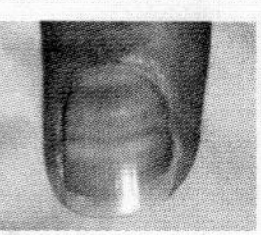

Fig 1. Beau's lines

Splinter haemorrhages are fine longitudinal haemorrhagic streaks (under nails), which in the febrile patient may suggest infective endocarditis. They may be normal—being caused, eg by gardening. ***Nail-fold infarcts*** are characteristically seen in vasculitic disorders.

Clubbing of the nails occurs with many disorders (p56). There is an exaggerated longitudinal curvature and loss of the angle between nail and nail-fold (ie no dip). Also the nail feels 'boggy'. The cause is unknown but may be due to ↑blood flow through multiple arteriovenous shunts in the distal phalanges.

Chronic paronychia is a chronic infection of the nail-fold and presents as a painful swollen nail with intermittent discharge. Treatment: keep nails dry; antibiotics, eg ***erythromycin*** 250mg/6h PO and ***nystatin*** ointment.

The hands Changes occur in many diseases. ***Palmar erythema*** is associated with cirrhosis, pregnancy, and polycythaemia. ***Pallor*** of the palmar creases suggests anaemia; ***pigmentation*** of the palmar creases (fig 2) is normal in Asians and blacks but is also seen in Addison's disease and Nelson's syndrome (↑ACTH after removal of the adrenal glands in Cushing's disease).[5] An odd rash on the knuckles (Gottren's papules) with dilated end-capillary loops at the nail-fold suggests dermatomyositis (p538). ***Dupuytren's contracture*** (fibrosis and contracture of palmar fascia, p690) is seen in liver disease, trauma, epilepsy, and ageing.[6] Swollen proximal interphalangeal (PIP) joints with distal (DIP) joints spared suggests rheumatoid arthritis; swollen DIP joints suggests osteoarthritis, gout, or psoriasis. Look for ***Heberden's*** (DIP, fig 3) and ***Bouchard's*** (PIP) 'nodes'—osteophytes (bone over-growth at a joint) seen with osteoarthritis.

Fig 2. Hyperpigmented palmar creases.

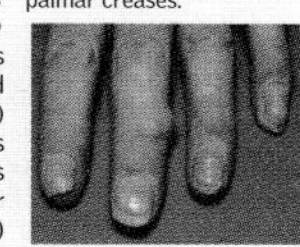

Fig 3. Heberden's node

History Ask about age, occupation, hobbies, sport, exercise and ethnic origin.

Presenting symptoms
- Chest pain (p80 & p772)
- Palpitations; dizziness; blackouts
- Ankle swelling
- Dyspnoea (p58)—exertional? orthopnoea? PND?

Past history
- Angina or MI
- Rheumatic fever
- Intermittent claudication

Ischaemic heart disease (IHD) risk factors
- Smoking
- Hypertension
- Diabetes mellitus
- Hyperlipidaemia
- Family history (1st degree relative <60yrs old with IHD.)

Drug history
- Previous and current regimens

Past tests and procedures:
- ECG
- Echocardiography
- Angiograms
- Cardiac scintigraphy
- Angioplasty/stents
- CABG (bypass grafts)

Appearance Ill or well? In pain? Dyspnoeic? Are they pale, cold, and clammy? Is there corneal arcus or xanthelasma (hyperlipidaemia (p682))? Is there a malar flush (mitral stenosis, low cardiac output)? Are there signs of Graves' disease (bulging eyes, goitre—p202)? Is the face dysmorphic, eg Down's syndrome, Marfan's syndrome (p698)—or Turner's, Noonan's, or William's syndromes (p139)? Can you hear the click of a prosthetic valve?

Hands Finger clubbing occurs in congenital cyanotic heart disease and endocarditis. Splinter haemorrhages, Osler's nodes (tender nodules in finger pulps) and Janeway lesions (red macules on palms) are signs of infective endocarditis. If found, examine the fundi for Roth's spots (retinal infarcts p376, fig 1). Are there nail-fold infarcts (vasculitis, p542) or nailbed capillary pulsation (Quincke's sign in aortic regurgitation)? Is there arachnodactyly (Marfan's) or polydactyly (ASD)? Are there tendon xanthomata (hyperlipdaemia)? **Pulse** See p30.

Blood pressure (see BOX) **Systolic BP** is the pressure at which the pulse is first heard as on cuff deflation; the **diastolic** is when the heart sounds disappear (Korotkov sound, K5) or become muffled (K4—use eg in the young, who often have no K5; state which you use). The ***pulse pressure*** is the difference between systolic and diastolic pressures. It is narrow in aortic stenosis and wide in aortic regurgitation. It also narrows in hypovolaemia and widens in septic shock. Defining hypertension is problematic: see p124. Examine the fundi for hypertensive changes (p125). **Shock** may occur if systolic <100mmHg (p778). ***Postural hypotension*** is defined as a drop in systolic >20mmHg or diastolic >10mmHg on standing (p68).

Jugular venous pressure See p30.

Praecordium Inspect for ***scars***: median sternotomy (CABG; valve replacement, congenital heart disease). Inspect for any pacemakers. Palpate the ***apex beat***. Normal position: 5th intercostal space in the mid-clavicular line. Is it displaced laterally? Is it abnormal in nature: **heaving** (caused by outflow obstruction, eg aortic stenosis or systemic hypertension), **thrusting** (caused by volume overload, eg mitral or aortic incompetence), **tapping** (mitral stenosis, essentially a palpable 1st heart sound), **diffuse** (LV failure, dilated cardiomyopathy) or **double impulse** (HOCM)? Is there dextrocardia? Feel for ***left parasternal heave*** (RV enlargement eg in pulmonary stenosis, cor pulmonale, ASD) or ***thrills*** (transmitted murmurs).

Auscultating the heart See BOX.

Lungs Examine the bases for creps & pleural effusions, indicative of cardiac failure.

Oedema Examine the ankles, legs, sacrum, torso for pitting oedema.

Abdomen Hepatomegaly and ascites in right-sided heart failure; pulsatile hepatomegaly with tricuspid regurgitation; splenomegaly with infective endocarditis.

Peripheral pulses Palpate radial, brachial, carotid, femoral, popliteal, dorsalis pedis and posterior tibial pulses. Feel for ***radio-femoral delay*** (coarctation of the aorta) and ***radio-radial delay*** (eg from aortic arch aneurysm). Auscultate for ***bruits*** over the carotids and elsewhere, particularly if there is inequality between pulses or absence of a pulse. Causes: atherosclerosis (elderly), vasculitis (young, p542).

Auscultating the heart

►If you spend time listening to the history, and feeling pulses, auscultation will hold few surprises: you will often already know the diagnosis. Feel for the pulse at the same time as you listen, either at the apex or in the carotid artery.

- Listen with bell and diaphragm at the apex (mitral area). Identify ***1st*** and ***2nd heart sounds***: are they normal? Listen for ***added sounds*** (p32) and ***murmurs*** (p34). Repeat at lower left sternal edge and in aortic and pulmonary areas (right and left of manubrium in the 2nd intercostal space)—and in both the left axilla (radiation of mitral incompetence) and over the carotids (radiation of aortic stenosis).
- Reposition the patient in the left lateral position: again feel the apex beat (is it tapping, as in mitral stenosis?) and listen specifically for a diastolic rumble of mitral stenosis. Sit the patient up and listen at the lower left sternal edge for the blowing diastolic sound of aortic regurgitation—accentuated at the end of expiration.

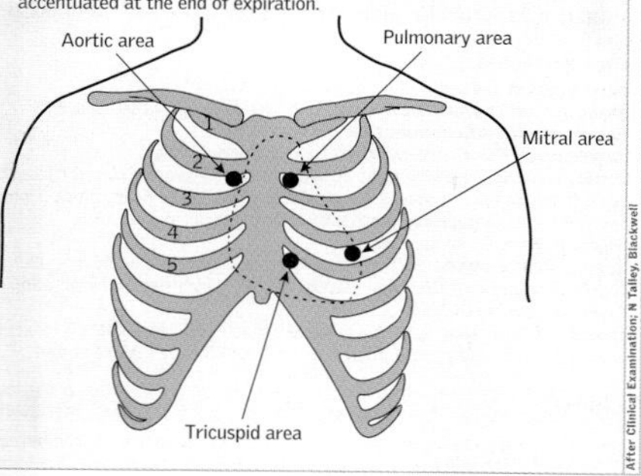

After Clinical Examination; N Talley, Blackwell

An unusual BP measurement

It is always important not to interpret a BP measurement in isolation (p124). We cannot be certain to diagnose hypertension (or hypotension) in isolation, as there may be many confounding factors such as pain, the 'white coat' effect, and the equipment used. Getting the cuff size right is very important, as too small will give an elevated reading and too large will give a low reading—the optimal cuff width is 40% of the arm circumference. If you suspect a BP reading to be anomalous check the equipment and review the observation chart for previous readings and other vital signs. Consider taking a manual reading with a different set yourself! Mercury sphygmomanometers are the type least likely to go wrong. See *regression towards the mean*, p10. Often a quiet chat with the patient will bring the BP down (both yours and your patient's)—and if you keep your ears open, the patient may reveal some new tangential but vital fact which the official history glossed over.

The jugular venous pressure

The internal jugular vein acts as a capricious manometer of right atrial pressure. Observe 2 features: the **height** (jugular venous pressure, JVP) and the **waveform** of the pulse. JVP observations are often difficult. Do not be downhearted if the skill seems to elude you. Keep on watching necks, and the patterns you see may slowly start to make sense—see BOX for the local venous anatomy. Relating the waveform to the arterial pulse (by concomitant palpation) will help to decipher patterns.

The height Observe the patient at 45°, with his head turned slightly to the left—good lighting and correct positioning makes the examination a lot easier. Look for the right internal jugular vein, which passes just medial to the clavicular head of sternocleidomastoid up behind the angle of the jaw to the ear lobes. The JVP is the vertical height of the pulse above the sternal angle. It is raised if >4cm. Pressing on the abdomen normally produces a transient rise in the JVP. If the rise persists throughout a 15s compression, it is a **positive abdominojugular reflux sign**.[1] This is a sign of right ventricular failure, reflecting inability to eject the increased venous return.

The waveform See BOX.

Abnormalities of the JVP

- ***Raised JVP with normal waveform:*** Fluid overload, right heart failure.
- ***Raised JVP with absent pulsation:*** SVC obstruction.
- ***Large a wave:*** Pulmonary hypertension, pulmonary stenosis.
- ***Cannon a wave:*** When the right atrium contracts against a closed tricuspid valve, large 'cannon' a waves result. ***Causes:*** complete heart block, single chamber ventricular pacing, ventricular arrhythmias/ectopics.
- ***Absent a wave:*** Atrial fibrillation.
- ***Large systolic v waves:*** Tricuspid regurgitation—look for earlobe movement.
- ***Constrictive pericarditis:*** High plateau of JVP (which rises on inspiration—Kussmaul's sign) with deep x and y descents.
- ***Absent JVP:*** When lying flat, the jugular vein should be filled. If there is reduced circulatory volume (eg dehydration, haemorrhage) the JVP may be absent.

Pulses

►Assess the radial pulse to determine rate and rhythm. **Character** and **volume** are best assessed at the brachial or carotid arteries. A **collapsing pulse** may also be felt at the radial artery when the patient's arm is elevated above his head.

Rate Is the pulse fast (≥100bpm, p112) or slow (≤60bpm, p110)?

Rhythm An irregularly irregular pulse occurs in AF or multiple ectopics. A regularly irregular pulse occurs in 2° heart block and ventricular bigeminus.

Character and volume

- ***Bounding pulses*** are caused by CO_2 retention, liver failure, and sepsis.
- ***Small volume pulses*** occur in aortic stenosis, shock, and pericardial effusion.
- ***Collapsing ('waterhammer') pulses*** are caused by aortic incompetence, AV malformations, and a patent ductus arteriosus.
- ***Anacrotic (slow-rising) pulses*** occur in aortic stenosis.
- ***Bisferiens pulses*** occur in combined aortic stenosis and regurgitation
- ***Pulsus alternans*** (alternating strong and weak beats) suggests LVF, cardiomyopathy, or aortic stenosis.
- ***Jerky pulses*** occur in HOCM.
- ***Pulsus paradoxus*** (systolic pressure weakens in inspiration by >10mmHg) occurs in severe asthma, pericardial constriction, or cardiac tamponade.

Peripheral pulses (See p28.) See p759 for ABG sampling.

1 This sign was first described by W Pasteur in 1885, in the context of tricuspid incompetence. The term 'hepatojugular reflux' later arose, but was replaced by 'abdominojugular reflux' (not *reflex*!), as pressure over the middle of the abdomen, as well as over the liver, can be used to elicit the sign.

The jugular venous pressure wave

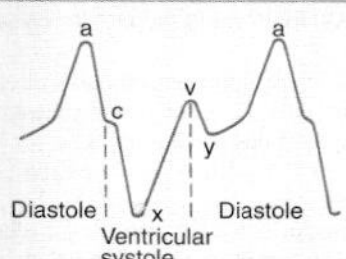

- a wave: atrial systole
- c wave: closure of tricuspid valve, not normally visible
- x descent: fall in atrial pressure during ventricular systole
- v wave: atrial filling against a closed tricuspid valve
- y descent: opening of tricuspid valve

The JVP drops as the x descent during ventricular systole because the right atrium is no longer contracting and the tricuspid valve is closed. This means that the pressure in the right atrium is dropping and this is reflected by the JVP.

The jugular venous systems

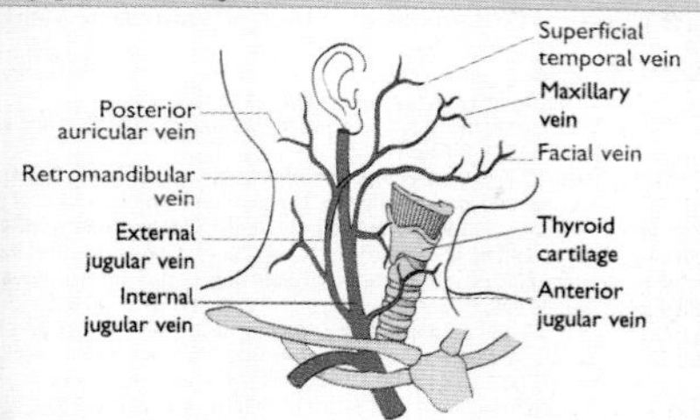

Is a pulse arterial or venous?

A venous pulse:

- Is not usually palpable.
- Is obliterated by finger pressure on the vessel.
- Rises transiently with pressure on abdomen (**abdominojugular reflux**) or on liver (**hepatojugular reflux**).
- Alters with posture and respiration.
- Usually has a double pulse for every arterial pulse.

Arterial pulse waveforms

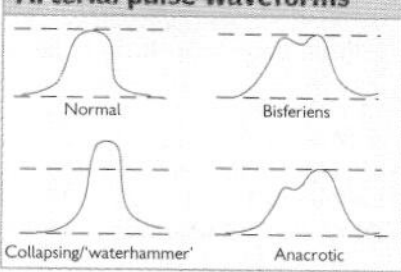

Inside the waterhammer Before the age of video games, the waterhammer was a popular toy that consisted of a vacuum tube half-filled with water. On inversion, the whoosh of water produced an intriguing hammer-blow as it rushed from end to end. This is the alternative name for Corrigan's (collapsing) pulse—ie one in which the upstroke is abrupt and steep, whose peak is reached early and with abnormal force—before a rapid downstroke (as blood whooshes back into the left ventricle through an incompetent aortic valve). Sometimes events conspire to put *us* in the waterhammer—rushing about in a vacuum tilted for the malicious pleasure of an unseen child. To let some air in, take a deep breath, and read all about Corrigan (p16).

The heart sounds

►Listen systematically: sounds then murmurs. While listening, palpate the carotic artery: S_1 is synchronous with the upstroke.

Heart sounds The 1st and 2nd sounds are usually clear. Confident pronouncements about other sounds and soft murmurs may be difficult. Even senior colleagues disagree with one another about the more difficult sounds and murmurs.

The 1st heart sound (S_1) represents closure of mitral (M_1) and tricuspid (T_1) valves. Splitting in inspiration may be heard and is normal.

In mitral stenosis, because the narrowed valve orifice limits ventricular filling there is no gradual decrease in flow towards the end of diastole. The valves are therefore at their maximum excursion at the end of diastole, and so shut rapidly leading to a loud S_1 (the 'tapping' apex). S_1 is also loud if diastolic filling time is shortened eg if the P-R interval is short, and in tachycardia.

S_1 is soft if the diastolic filling time is prolonged eg if the P-R interval is long, or if the mitral valve leaflets fail to close properly (ie mitral incompetence).

The intensity of S_1 is variable in AV block, AF, and nodal or ventricular tachycardia.

The 2nd heart sound (S_2) represents aortic (A_2) and pulmonary valve (P_2) closure. The most important abnormality of A_2 is softening in aortic stenosis.

A_2 is said to be loud in tachycardia, hypertension, and transposition, but a loud A_2 is probably not a useful clinical entity.

P_2 is loud in pulmonary hypertension and soft in pulmonary stenosis. **Splitting in inspiration** is normal and is mainly due to the variation with respiration of right heart venous return, causing the pulmonary component to be delayed. **Wide splitting** occurs in right bundle branch block, pulmonary stenosis, deep inspiration, mitral regurgitation, and VSD. **Wide fixed splitting** occurs in ASD. **Reversed splitting** (ie A_2 following P_2, with splitting increasing on expiration) occurs in left bundle branch block, aortic stenosis, PDA (patent ductus arteriosus), and right ventricular pacing. A single S_2 occurs in Fallot's tetralogy, severe aortic or pulmonary stenosis, pulmonary atresia, Eisenmenger's syndrome (p143), large VSD hypertension. NB: splitting and P_2 are heard best in the pulmonary area.

A 3rd heart sound (S_3) may occur just after S_2. It is low pitched and best heard with the bell of the stethoscope. S_3 is pathological over the age of 30yrs. A loud S_3 occurs in a dilated left ventricle with rapid ventricular filling (mitral regurgitation, VSD) or poor LV function (post MI, dilated cardiomyopathy). In constrictive pericarditis or restrictive cardiomyopathy it occurs early and is more high pitched ('pericardial knock').

A 4th heart sound (S_4) occurs just before S_1. Always abnormal, it represents atrial contraction against a ventricle made stiff by any cause, eg aortic stenosis, or hypertensive heart disease.

Triple and gallop rhythms A 3rd or 4th heart sound occurring with a sinus tachycardia may give the impression of galloping hooves. An S_3 gallop has the same rhythm as '**Ken**-tucky', whereas an S_4 gallop has the same rhythm as 'Tenne**ssee**'. When S_3 and S_4 occur in a tachycardia, eg with pulmonary embolism, they may summate and appear as a single sound, a summation gallop.

An ejection systolic click is heard early in systole with bicuspid aortic valves, and if BP↑. The right heart equivalent lesions may also cause clicks.

Mid-systolic clicks occur in mitral valve prolapse (p130).

An opening snap precedes the mid-diastolic murmur of mitral stenosis. It indicates a pliable (noncalcified) valve.

Prosthetic sounds are caused by nonbiological valves, on opening and closing: **rumbling sounds** ≈ ball and cage valves (eg Starr-Edwards); **single clicks** ≈ tilting disc valve (eg single disc: Bjork Shiley; bileaflet: St Jude—often quieter). Prosthetic mitral valve clicks occur in time with S_1, aortic valve clicks in time with S_2.

Clinical skills

The cardiac cycle

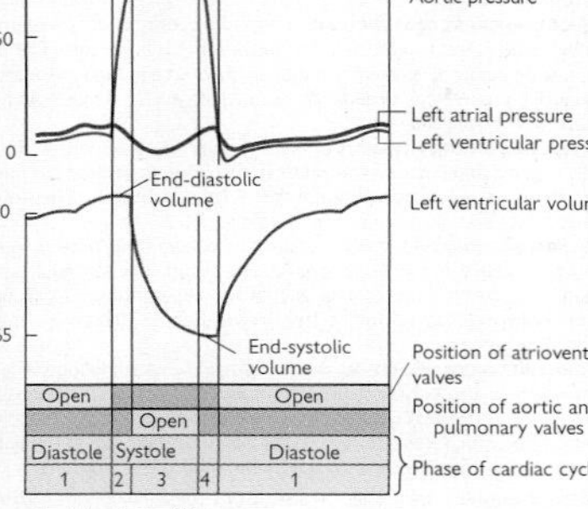

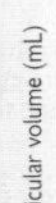

Cardiac murmurs[1]

- ► Always consider other symptoms and signs before auscultation and think: what d I expect to hear? But don't let your expectations determine what you hear.
- ► Use the stethoscope correctly: remember that the bell is good for low-pitche sounds (eg mitral stenosis) and should be applied **gently**. The diaphragm filter out low pitches, making higher pitched murmurs easier to detect (eg aorti regurgitation). NB: a bell applied tightly to the skin becomes a diaphragm.
- ► Consider any murmur in terms of **character**, **timing**, **loudness**, **area wher loudest**, **radiation**, and **accentuating manoeuvres**.
- ► When in doubt, rely on echocardiography rather than disputed sounds. (But sti enjoy trying to figure out the clinical conundrum!)

Character and timing

- ***An ejection-systolic murmur*** (ESM, crescendo–decrescendo) usually originate from the outflow tract and waxes and wanes with the intraventricular pressure ESMs may be innocent and are common in children and high output states (e tachycardia, pregnancy). Organic causes include aortic stenosis and sclerosis pulmonary stenosis, and HOCM.
- ***A pansystolic murmur (PSM)*** is of uniform intensity and merges with S_2. It i usually organic and occurs in mitral or tricuspid regurgitation (S_1 may also b soft in these), or a ventricular septal defect (p142). Mitral valve prolapse ma produce a late systolic murmur ± midsystolic click.
- ***Early diastolic murmurs (EDM)*** are high pitched and easily missed: listen for th 'absence of silence' in early diastole. An EDM occurs in aortic and, though rar pulmonary regurgitation. If the pulmonary regurgitation is secondary t pulmonary hypertension resulting from mitral stenosis, then the EDM is called Graham Steell murmur.
- ***Mid-diastolic murmurs (MDM)*** are low pitched and rumbling. They occur i mitral stenosis (accentuated presystolically if heart still in sinus rhythm rheumatic fever (Carey Coombs' murmur: due to thickening of the mitral valv leaflets), and aortic regurgitation (Austin Flint murmur: due to the fluttering c the anterior mitral valve cusp caused by the regurgitant stream).

Intensity All murmurs are graded on a scale of 1–6 (see TABLE), though in practic diastolic murmurs, being less loud, are only graded 1–4. Intensity is a poor guide t the severity of a lesion—an ESM may be inaudible in severe aortic stenosis.

Area where loudest Though an unreliable sign, mitral murmurs tend to be loudes over the apex, in contrast to the area of greatest intensity from lesions of th aortic (right 2nd intercostal space), pulmonary (left 2nd intercostal space) an tricuspid (lower left sternal edge) valves.

Radiation The ESM of aortic stenosis classically radiates to the carotids, in contras to the PSM of mitral regurgitation, which radiates to the axilla.

Accentuating manoeuvres

- ***Movements*** that bring the relevant part of the heart closer to the stethoscop accentuate murmurs (eg leaning forward for aortic regurgitation, left later position for mitral stenosis).
- ***Expiration*** increases blood flow to the left side of the heart and therefor accentuates left sided murmurs. ***Inspiration*** has the opposite effect.
- ***Valsalva manoeuvre*** (forced expiration against a closed glottis) decrease systemic venous return, accentuating mitral valve prolapse and HOCM, bu softening mitral regurgitation and aortic stenosis. ***Squatting*** has exactly th opposite effects. ***Exercise*** accentuates the murmur of mitral stenosis.

Non-valvular murmurs ***A pericardial friction rub*** may be heard in pericarditis. I is a superficial scratching sound, not confined to systole or diastole. ***Continuou murmurs*** are present throughout the cardiac cycle and may occur with a pater ductus arteriosus, arteriovenous fistula, or ruptured sinus of Valsalva.

1 **Heart murmurs in children** (See *OHCS* p137.)

Typical waveforms of common heart murmurs

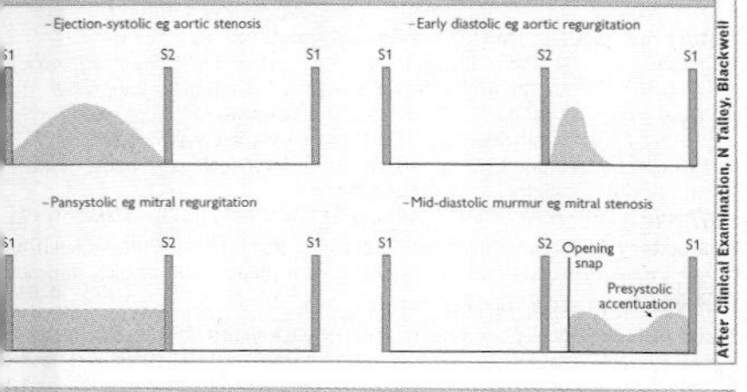

After Clinical Examination, N Talley, Blackwell

Grading intensity of heart murmurs

►The following grading is commonly used for murmurs—systolic murmurs from 1 to 6 and diastolic murmurs from 1 to 4, never being clinically >4/6.

Grade	Description
1/6	Very soft, only heard after listening for a while
2/6	Soft, but detectable immediately
3/6	Clearly audible, but no thrill palpable
4/6	Clearly audible, palpable thrill
5/6	Audible with stethoscope only partially touching chest
6/6	Can be heard without placing stethoscope on chest

Prosthetic valve murmurs

Prosthetic aortic valves: All types produce a degree of outflow obstruction and thus have an ESM. Tilting single disc (eg Bjork Shiley) and bileaflet (eg St Jude) valves do not completely close and allow a regurgitant stream during diastole, hence they have a low-intensity diastolic murmur. The intensity of this murmur increases as the valve fails. Ball and cage valves (eg Starr–Edwards) and tissue valves **do** close completely in diastole and so any diastolic murmur implies valve failure.

Prosthetic mitral valves: Ball and cage valves project into the left ventricle and can cause a low-intensity ESM as they interfere with the ejected stream. Tissue valves and bileaflet valves can have a low-intensity diastolic murmur. Consider any systolic murmur of loud intensity to be a sign of regurgitation and ∴ failure.

History Age, race, occupation. **Presenting symptoms**—as follows:

- ***Cough:*** (see BOX) Duration? Character (eg brassy/barking/hollow)? Nocturnal (≈asthma)? Exacerbating factors? Sputum/haemoptysis?
- ***Dyspnoea:*** (p58 & p770) Duration? Steps climbed/distance walked before onset? NYHA classification (p121)? Diurnal variation (≈asthma)?
- ***Hoarseness:*** (*OHCS* p568) eg due to laryngitis, recurrent laryngeal nerve palsy, Singer's nodules, or laryngeal tumour.
- ***Wheeze*** (p38) • ***Fever/night sweats*** (p60) • ***Chest pain*** (p80) • ***Stridor*** (p72)

Past history Ask about: Pneumonia/bronchitis; TB; atopy[1] (asthma/eczema/hay fever); previous CXR abnormalities; lung surgery; myopathy; neurological disorders

Family history Atopy?[1] Emphysema? TB?

Social history Quantify smoking in terms of **pack-years** (20 cigarettes/day for 1 year = 1 pack-year). Occupational exposure (farming, mining, asbestos exposure has possible serious compensatory implications? Animals at home (eg birds) Recent travel/TB contacts?

Drug history Respiratory drugs (eg steroids, bronchodilators)? Any other drugs, especially with respiratory SEs (eg ACE inhibitors, cytotoxics, β-blockers, amiodarone)

Examination Undress to the waist, and sit him on the edge of the bed.

Inspection Assess **general health**: is he unwell? Cachectic? Using accessory muscles of respiration, eg sternocleidomastoids, platysma, and strap muscles of the neck (infrahyoid)? Are there signs of respiratory distress (see below)? Is there stridor (p72)? Count the **respiratory rate** and note **breathing pattern**. Is there Kussmaul's (rapid, deep respiration, p62) or Cheyne–Stokes (apnoea alternating with hyperpnoea, p54) breathing? Look for **chest wall deformities** (p54). Inspect the chest for scars of past surgery, chest drains, or radiotherapy (skin thickening and tattoos demarcating the field of irradiation). Note **chest wall movement**: is it symmetrical? If not, pathology is on the restricted side. Is there paradoxical respiration (abdomen sucked in with inspiration; seen in diaphragmatic paralysis)

Examine the hands for clubbing (p56), peripheral cyanosis (p56), tar staining, and wasting/weakness of the intrinsic muscles—seen in T1 lesions (eg Pancoast tumour, p700). Palpate the wrist for tenderness (hypertrophic pulmonary osteoarthropathy, HPOA, from lung cancer). Check for asterixis (CO_2 retention flap). Palpate the pulse for a paradoxical character (weakens in inspiration; quantify in mmHg by measuring BP in inspiration and expiration, p30).

Regard the face Check for ptosis and a constricted pupil (Horner's syndrome, eg Pancoast's tumour, p700). Are the tongue and lips bluish (central cyanosis, p56)

Feel the trachea in the sternal notch (it should pass just to the right). If deviated concentrate on the upper lobes for pathology. Note the presence of **tracheal tug** (descent of trachea with inspiration, meaning severe airflow limitation). Palpate for **cervical lymphadenopathy** from behind, with the patient sitting forward.

Examining the chest (See p38.) If an abnormality is detected, try to localize it to the likely **segment** (see BOX). If this is not possible, state the **zone** of the finding.

Further examination Look at the JVP (p30) and examine the heart for signs of **cor pulmonale** (p186). Look at **temperature charts**. Inspect the **sputum** (See BOX Test peripheral O_2 **saturation** and PEFR at the bedside (p148).

Respiratory distress occurs if high negative intrapleural pressures are needed to generate air entry. Signs: tachypnoea, nasal flaring, tracheal tug (pulling of thyroid cartilage towards sternal notch in inspiration), the use of accessory muscles of respiration, intercostal, subcostal, and sternal recession, and pulsus paradoxus (p30

1 Atopy implies predisposition to, or concurrence of, asthma, hay fever and eczema with production of specific IgE on exposure to common allergens (eg house dust mite, grass, cats).

Clinical skills

Characteristic coughs

Coughing is a relatively nonspecific symptom, resulting from irritation anywhere from the pharynx to the lungs. The character of a patient's cough may, however, give some clues as to the underlying cause:

- ***Loud, brassy coughing*** suggests pressure on the trachea eg by a tumour.
- ***Hollow, 'bovine' coughing*** is associated with recurrent laryngeal nerve palsy.
- ***Barking coughs*** occur in acute epiglottitis.
- ***Chronic cough:*** Think of pertussis, TB, foreign body, asthma (eg nocturnal).
- ***Dry, chronic coughing*** may occur following acid irritation of the lungs in oesophageal reflux, and as a side-effect of ACE inhibitors.

►Do not ignore a change in character of a chronic cough; it may signify a new problem eg infection, malignancy.

Sputum examination

Always inspect any sputum produced, however unpleasant this task may be. Send suspicious sputum for microscopy (Gram stain and auramine/ZN stain, if indicated), culture, and cytology.

- ***Black carbon specks*** in the sputum suggests smoking, the most common cause of increased sputum production.
- ***Yellow/green sputum*** suggests infection eg bronchiectasis, pneumonia.
- ***Pink frothy sputum*** suggests pulmonary oedema.
- ***Bloody sputum (haemoptysis)*** may be due to malignancy, TB, infection, or trauma, and requires investigation for these causes. See p62.
- ***Clear sputum*** is probably saliva.

Surface pleural, lung and fissure markings

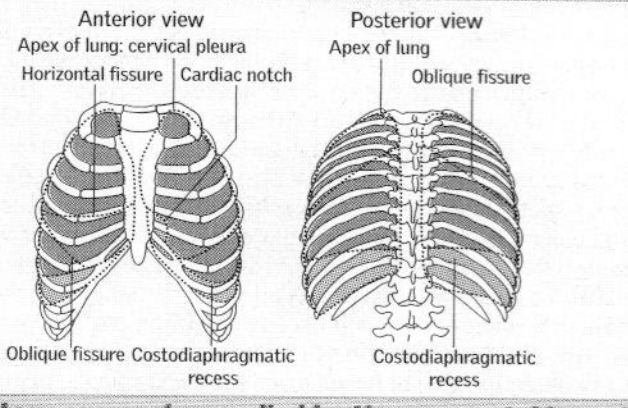

The respiratory segments supplied by the segmental bronchi

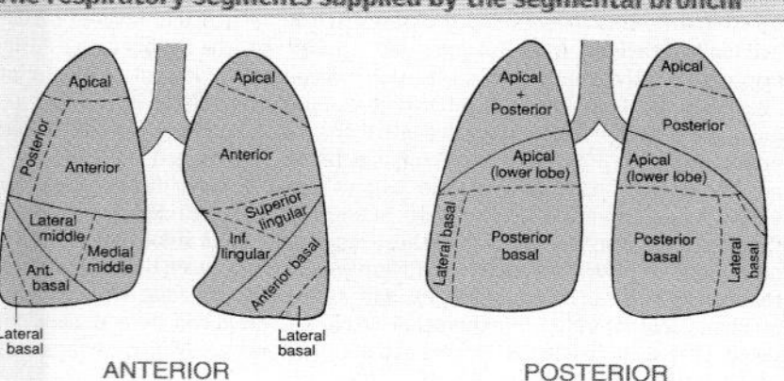

Examining the chest

Inspection General—see p36. Look for deformities of the spine (kyphoscoliosis) or chest wall (*pectus excavatum* or *carinatum*, p54), or scars from surgery.

Palpation ***Lymphadenopathy:*** Check for cervical lymphadenopathy from behind, with the patient sitting forward. ***Tracheal position:*** Is it central or displaced to one side (towards an area of collapse, away from a large pleural effusion or tension pneumothorax; slight deviation to the right is normal). ***Expansion:*** Use both hands to compare chest expansion on both sides; expansion <5cm on deep inspiration is abnormal. Reduced expansion implies pathology on that side. Test ***tactile vocal fremitus*** by asking the patient to repeat '99' while palpating the chest wall with the ulnar border of your hands over different respiratory segments, comparing similar positions over each lung in turn. Increased vocal fremitus implies consolidation, but is less sensitive than vocal resonance (see p76).

Percussion Percuss symmetrical areas of the anterior, posterior, and axillary regions of the chest wall. When percussing posteriorly, move the scapulae out of the way by asking the patient to move his elbows forward across his chest. Do not forget to percuss the supraclavicular fossae (lung apices). ***Causes of a dull percussion note:*** collapse, consolidation, fibrosis, pleural thickening, or pleural effusion (classically stony dull). The **cardiac dullness** is usually detectable over the left side of the chest. The **liver dullness** usually extends up to the fifth rib, right mid-clavicular line; if the chest is resonant below this level, it is a sign of lung hyperexpansion (eg asthma, emphysema). ***Causes of a hyperresonant percussion note:*** pneumothorax or hyperinflation (COPD).

Auscultation Listen with the diaphragm over symmetrical areas of the anterior, posterior, and axillary regions of the chest wall, and use the bell to auscultate over the supraclavicular fossae. ►Consider breath sounds in terms of **quality**, **intensity**, and the **presence of additional sounds**.

- ***Quality and intensity*** Normal breath sounds have a rustling quality and are described as vesicular. **Bronchial breathing** has a hollow quality; there is a gap between inspiration and expiration. Bronchial breath sounds occur where normal lung tissue has become firm or solid, eg consolidation, localized fibrosis, above a pleural effusion, or next to a large pericardial effusion (Ewart's sign, p140). It may be associated with increased tactile vocal fremitus, vocal resonance, and whispering pectoriloquy (p76). **Diminished breath sounds** occur with pleural effusions, pleural thickening, pneumothorax (fig 1, p735), bronchial obstruction, asthma, or COPD. The **silent chest** occurs in life-threatening asthma and is due to severe bronchospasm which prevents adequate air entry into the chest.
- ***Added sounds*** **Wheezes (rhonchi)** are caused by air passing through narrowed airways. They may be monophonic (a single note, signifying a partial obstruction of one airway, eg tumour) or polyphonic ('My chest sounds like a load of cats'—multiple notes, signifying widespread narrowing of airways of differing calibre, eg asthma, COPD). Wheezes may also be heard in left ventricular failure ('cardiac asthma'). **Crackles (crepitations)** are caused by the re-opening, during inspiration, of the small airways which have become occluded during expiration. They may be fine and high pitched if coming from distal air spaces (eg pulmonary oedema, fibrosing alveolitis) or coarse and low pitched if they originate more proximally (eg bronchiectasis). The timing of crackles is important; early inspiratory crackles suggest small airways disease (eg COPD), whereas late/pan-inspiratory crackles suggest disease confined to the alveoli. Crackles that disappear on coughing are insignificant. **Pleural rubs** are caused by movement of the visceral pleura over the parietal pleura, when both surfaces are roughened, eg by an inflammatory exudate. Causes include adjacent pneumonia or pulmonary infarction. **Pneumothorax click** is produced by a shallow left pneumothorax between the 2 layers of parietal pleura over-lying the heart and is heard during cardiac systole.

►Clinical examination has only a 50% sensitivity for picking up pneumonia (specificity 60–75%).

Some physical signs

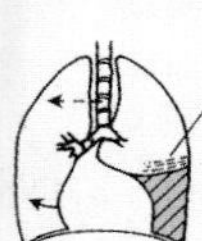

(There may be bronchial breathing at the top of an effusion)

Expansion: ↓
Percussion: Stony dull ↓
Air entry: ↓
Vocal resonance: ↓

PLEURAL EFFUSION

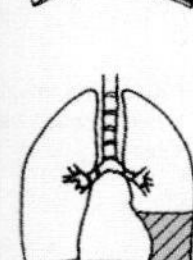

Trachea + mediastium central
Expansion ↓
Percussion note ↓
Vocal resonance ↑
Bronchial breathing ± coarse crackles (with whispering pectoriloquy)

CONSOLIDATION

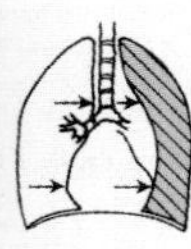

Expansion ↓
Percussion note ↓
Breath sounds ↓

EXTENSIVE COLLAPSE PNEUMONECTOMY/ LOBECTOMY

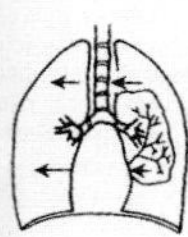

Expansion ↓
Percussion note ↑
Breath sounds ↓

PNEUMOTHORAX

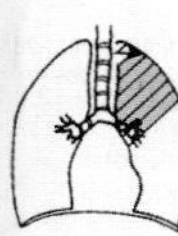

Expansion ↓
Percussion note ↓
Breath sounds bronchial ± crackles

FIBROSIS

Gastrointestinal history

Presenting symptoms
Abdominal pain (p52), distension
Nausea, vomiting, haematemesis
Dysphagia (p232)
Indigestion (dyspepsia, p58)
Recent change in bowel habit
Diarrhoea or constipation (p240)
Rectal bleeding (p70) or melaena (p244)
Appetite, weight change
Mouth ulcers (p230); Jaundice (p242)
Pruritus; Dark urine, pale stools

Social history
Smoking, alcohol, recreational drug use
Overseas travel, tropical illnesses
Contact with jaundiced persons
Occupational exposures
Sexual orientation

Past history
Peptic ulcer disease
Carcinoma
Jaundice, hepatitis
Blood transfusions, tattoos
Previous operations
Last menstrual period (LMP)

Past treatment
Steroids, the Pill
NSAIDs; antibiotics
Dietary changes

Family history
Irritable bowel syndrome (IBS)
Inflammatory bowel disease (IBD)
Peptic ulcer disease
Polyps, cancer
Jaundice

Examining the gastrointestinal system

Inspect (and smell) for signs of chronic liver disease:
- Hepatic fetor on breath (p250)
- Purpura (purple stained skin, p330)
- Spider naevi (fig 1, p253)
- Gynaecomastia
- Scratch marks
- Palmar erythema
- Clubbing (rare)
- Muscle wasting
- Jaundice
- Liver flap (asterixis, a coarse irregular tremor seen in hepatic failure)
- Leuconychia (hypoalbuminaemia)

Inspect for signs of malignancy, anaemia, jaundice, hard Virchow's node in left supraclavicular fossa (p614). Look at the abdomen. Note:
- Visible pulsation (aneurysm, p586)
- Striae (stretch marks, eg pregnancy)
- Peristalsis
- Distension
- Scars
- Genitalia
- Masses
- Herniae

If abdominal wall veins look dilated, assess **direction of flow**. In inferior vena cava (IVC) obstruction, flow below the umbilicus is up; in portal hypertension (*caput medusae*), flow radiates out from the umbilicus. ***The cough test:*** While looking at the face, ask the patient to cough. If this causes abdominal pain, flinching, or a protective movement of hands towards the abdomen, suspect peritonitis. (See BOX)

Genitourinary history

Presenting symptoms
Fever, loin/scrotal pain, dysuria, haematuria
Urethral/vaginal discharge (p406)
Sex—any problems? Painful intercourse (dyspareunia, *OHCS* p310)?
Menses: menarche, menopause, length of periods, amount, pain? Intermenstrual loss?
1st day of last menstrual period (LMP)?

Past history
Urinary tract infection
Renal colic
DM, BP↑, gout, analgesic use
Previous operations

Social history
Smoking
Sexual orientation

Detecting outflow obstruction (eg from prostatic hypertrophy). Ask:
- On wanting to pass water, is there delay before you start? **(Hesitancy)**
- Does the flow stop and start? Do you go on dribbling when you think you've stopped, even after giving it a good shake? **(Terminal dribbling)**
- Is your stream getting weaker? Can you hit the wall OK? **(Poor stream)**
- Do you ever pass water when you do not want to? **(Incontinence**—p604)
- Do you feel the bladder is not empty after passing water?[i]
- On feeling an urge to pass water, do you have to go at once? **(Urgency)**[i]
- Do you urinate often at night? **(Nocturia)**[i] In the day? How often? **(Frequency**

i = irritative (or 'filling') symptoms: they can be caused by eg UTI as well as obstruction; see p68.

Palpating and percussing the abdomen

►See also p52

Adjust the patient so that he is lying flat, with his head resting on only 1 pillow, and his arms at his side. Expose from 'nipples to knees', but remember to consider modesty. Make sure that the patient and your hands are warm.

Inspection See OPPOSITE. Is the abdomen moving with respiration? Count the respiratory rate (may be a marker of intra-abdominal disease); eg ↑ with 1 splinting of the diaphragm from distension; 2 fast, shallow breaths to avoid painful deeper inspiration; 3 respiratory compensation of metabolic acidosis; 4 shock.

Palpation While palpating, be looking at his face to assess any pain. First palpate gently through each quadrant, starting away from the site of the pain—otherwise everywhere may be uncomfortable! Note tenderness, guarding (involuntary tensing of abdominal muscles because of pain or fear of it), and rebound tenderness (greater pain on removing hand than on gently depressing abdomen: it is a sign of peritoneal inflammation); Rovsing's sign (appendicitis, p582); Murphy's sign (cholecystitis, p590).

Palpating the liver: Begin in the right iliac fossa with the patient breathing deeply. Use the radial border of the index finger to feel the liver edge, moving up 2cm at a time at each breath in. Assess its size (causes of hepatomegaly—p63), regularity, smoothness, and tenderness. Is it pulsatile (tricuspid regurgitation)? Confirm the lower border and define the upper border by percussion (normal upper limit is in 5th intercostal space): it may be pushed down by emphysema. Listen for an overlying bruit. ***The scratch test*** is an another way to find the lower liver edge: start with the diaphragm of the stethoscope over the right costal margin. Gently scratch the abdominal wall, starting in the right lower quadrant and working up towards the liver edge. A sharp increase in transmission of the scratch is heard when the lower border of the liver is reached.

Palpating the spleen: Start in the RIF, moving towards the left upper quadrant with each breath. **Features of the spleen differentiating it from kidney:** cannot get above it (ribs overlie its top); overlying percussion note is dull; it moves more with inspiration—towards the RIF; it may have a palpable notch on its medial side. If you suspect splenomegaly but cannot detect it, assess the patient in the right lateral position with your left hand pulling forwards from behind the rib cage. Is the percussion note dull in the mid-axillary line in the 10th intercostal space?

Palpating the kidneys: Try bimanually with the left hand under the patient to push it up in the renal angle. Attempt to ballot the kidney (ie bounce it gently but decisively between a hand applied to the loin and the other applied opposite, anteriorly). It moves only slightly with respiration.

Percussion If this induces pain, there may be peritoneal inflammation below (eg an inflamed appendix). Some experts use percussion first, before palpation, because even anxious patients do not expect this to hurt—so, if it does hurt, this is a very valuable sign. Percuss for the shifting dullness of ascites (p624): the level of right-sided flank dullness increases by lying on the right, and vice versa for lying on the left. Ultrasound is a more reliable way of detecting ascites.

Auscultation Bowel sounds: absence implies ileus; they are enhanced and tinking in bowel obstruction. Listen for bruits in the aorta, renal and femoral arteries.

Examine Mouth, tongue, rectum (p627), genitalia, and urine as appropriate.

Ordering the examination during clinical exams: It can be useful to auscultate before palpation/percussion, as bowel sounds induced by palpation may mask vascular bruits (you should not palpate deeply in the vicinity of bruits lest you damage an aneurysm)—and this is the preferred order in many places. In the UK you may be expected to auscultate last, especially during finals examinations. If you don't, you might need to explain, 'I am auscultating now to detect bruits which might be dangerous to palpate.'

The neurological system

History This should be taken from the patient and if possible, from a close frier or relative as well for corroboration/discrepancies. The patient's memor perception, or speech may be affected by the disorder making the history difficu to obtain. Note the progression of the symptoms and signs: gradual deterioratic (eg tumour) *vs* intermittent exacerbations (eg multiple sclerosis) vs rapid onset (e stroke). Ask about age, occupation and ethnic origin. Right- or left-hand dominan

Presenting symptoms

- ***Headache:*** (p448 & p768) Different to usual headaches? Acute/chronic? Spee of onset? Single/recurrent? Unilateral/bilateral? Associated aura (migrair p450)? Any meningism (p806)? Worse on waking (↑ICP)? Decreased conscio level? ►Take a 'worst-ever' headache very seriously. (See p735)
- ***Weakness:*** (p458) Speed of onset? Muscle groups affected? Sensory loss? A sphincter disturbance? Loss of balance? Associated spinal/root pain?
- ***Visual disturbance:*** (*OHCS* p410) eg blurring, double vision (diplopi photophobia, visual loss. Speed of onset? Any preceding symptoms? Pain in ey
- ***Special senses:*** Hearing (p456), smell, taste.
- ***Dizziness:*** (p454) Illusion of surroundings moving (vertigo)? Heari loss/tinnitus? Any loss of consciousness? Positional?
- ***Speech disturbance:*** (p46) Difficulty in expression, articulation, comprehension (can be difficult to determine)? Sudden onset or gradual?
- ***Dysphagia:*** (p232) Solids and/or liquids? Intermittent or constant? Difficulty coordination? Painful (odynophagia)?
- ***Fits/faints/'funny turns'/involuntary movements:*** (p452) Frequency? Dur ion? Mode of onset? Preceding aura? Loss of consciousness? Tongue bitin Incontinence? Any residual weakness/confusion? Family history?
- ***Skin sensation disturbance:*** Eg numbness, 'pins & needles' (paraesthesiae), pa odd sensations. Distribution? Speed of onset? Associated weakness?
- ***Tremor:*** (p72) Rapid or slow tremor? Present at rest? Worse on delibera movement? Taking β-agonists? Any thyroid problems? Any family history?

Cognitive state If there is any doubt about the patient's cognition, an object measure is a cognitive test—guessing has been shown to be inaccurate! T following 10 questions comprise the abbreviated mental test score (AMTS) commonly used screening questionnaire for cognitive impairment:

1. Tell patient an address to recall at the end (eg 42 West Street, Gateshead)
2. Age
3. Time (to nearest hour)
4. What year is it?
5. Recognize 2 people (eg doctor & nurse)
6. Date of birth
7. Dates of the Second World War
8. Name of present monarch
9. Name of hospital/institution
10. Count backwards from 20 to 1

A score of ≤6 suggests poor cogniti acute (delirium), or chronic (dement AMTS correlates well with the m detailed mini-mental state examinat (MMSE™). **NB:** deaf, dysphasic, depress and un-cooperative patients, as wel those who do not understand Engl will also get low scores. See TABLE, p for a longer dementia score test.

Past medical history Ask about meningitis/encephalitis, head/spine trau seizures, previous operations, risk factors for vascular disease (p462, hypertension, hyperlipidaemia, diabetes mellitus, smoking), and recent travel there any chance that the patient is pregnant (eclampsia, *OHCS* p48)?

Drug history Any anticonvulsant/antipsychotic/antidepressant medication? A psychotropic drugs (eg ecstasy)? Any medication with neurological side-effects ***isoniazid*** which can cause a peripheral neuropathy)?

Social and family history What can the patient do and not do, ie activities of d living (ADLs)? What is the Barthel Index score? Any neurological or psychia disease in the family? Any consanguinity?

Examining the neurological system

►The neurological system is usually the most daunting examination to learn, but the most satisfying once perfected. Learn at the bedside from a senior colleague, preferably a neurologist, and there is no substitute for practice. Be aware that books present ideal situations: often one or more signs are equivocal or even contrary to expectation; don't be put off, consider the whole picture, including the history; try re-examining the patient.

Higher mental function Conscious level (Glasgow coma scale, p776), orientation in time, place, and person, memory (short and long term). See opposite for the AMTS and p47 for the full mental test score (MTS).

Speech Is there alteration in voice sound (**dysphonia** eg in laryngitis, recurrent laryngeal nerve palsy, or vocal cord tumour)? **Dysphasia** & **dysarthria**: see p46?

Skull and spine Malformation. Signs of injury. Palpate scalp. If there is any question of spinal injury, **do not move the spine**: in-line immobilisation is required. Is there meningism (p806)? Auscultate for carotid/cranial bruits. Screening by listening for carotid bruits has a high specificity (91%) but a low sensitivity (56%), so if stenosis is suspected arrange a carotid ultrasound scan.

Motor system (upper or lower limb) ►It is essential to discriminate whether weakness is upper (UMN) or lower (LMN) motor neurone (p439).

Inspect for posture abnormality (eg 'pyramidal' posture of UMN lesions, p439), or involuntary movement, wasting, or fasciculation (muscle twitching, not moving the limb)?

Drift: Patient sitting, arms outstretched, eyes closed. Do arms drift downwards? Unequal drift is a valuable sign of subtle focal motor deficits, occurring in UMN weakness, cerebellar disease, and loss of proprioception (=**pseudoathetosis**).

Tone: Look for **hypotonia** (floppy) or **spasticity** (pressure fails to move joint until it gives way, like a clasp-knife), rigidity (lead pipe), rigidity + tremor (cogwheeling. Is there **clonus** (rhythmic muscle 'beats' on sudden stretching, eg gastrocnemius on ankle dorsiflexion) at wrist, patella, or ankle?

Power: (See p438) Oppose each movement. Ascertain the distribution of any weakness—which movements/nerve roots are affected (myotomes, p444)? Quantify strength of each movement eg using UK MRC scale (p439).

Reflexes: Brisk in UMN lesions, reduced/absent in LMN lesions. Biceps reflex: (C5–6), triceps (C7–8), supinator (C5–6), knee (L3–4 ± L2), ankle (S1–2), abdominals (lost in UMN lesions), plantars (up-going in UMN lesions). **Hoffman's reflex:** flexion of thumb and index finger on flicking the middle finger's pulp (p439).

Coordination: Finger–nose (touch nose with a finger), rub heel up and down shin, rapid alternating movements (eg rapidly pronate and supinate hand on dorsum of other hand; clumsiness in this (=**dysdiadochokinesis**) occurs in cerebellar lesions). Is there dyspraxia (p46)?

Gait: (See p459) Ask the patient to walk: normally; heel-to-toe; on heels; then on toes. Observe standing feet together ± squatting. If balance is worse on shutting the eyes, **Romberg's test** is +ve, implying abnormal joint position sense. If he cannot perform this even with eyes open, this may be cerebellar ataxia, but not Romberg's +ve.

Sensation ***Dorsal column:*** Light touch (cotton wool), vibration (128Hz tuning fork), joint position sense (=**proprioception**). ***Spinothalamic:*** pain (pin-prick) and temperature. Testing temperature sensation is not usually required, but can be performed with test tubes filled with hot and cold water. Determine if any sensory loss is below a spinal cord level (eg cord compression), or in a glove and stocking distribution (eg peripheral neuropathy)? See dermatomes on p446.

Cranial nerves See p44.

Cranial nerve examination

Approach to examining the cranial nerves Where is the lesion? Thi systematically. Is it in the brainstem (eg MS), or outside, pressing on the brainster Is it the neuromuscular junction (myasthenia) or the muscles (eg a dystrophy Cranial nerves may be affected singly or in groups. ►Face the patient (helps sp asymmetry). For causes of lesions, see BOX. For names of the nerves, see BOX, p4

I *Smell:* Test ability of each nostril to distinguish familiar smells, eg peppermi

II *Acuity* in each eye separately, and its correctability with glasses or pin-ho use chart on p51. ***Visual fields:*** Compare during confrontation with your ov fields or formally. Any losses/inattention? Sites of lesions: *OHCS* p428. ***Pupi*** (p68) Size, shape, symmetry, reaction to light (direct and consensual), a accommodation if reaction to light is poor. ***Ophthalmoscopy:*** (*OHCS*, p41 Darken the room. Instil ***tropicamide*** 0.5%, 1 drop, if needed (►check f history of glaucoma beforehand). Select the focusing lens for the best view the optic disc (pale? swollen?). This is found when the ophthalmoscope's dot light is reflected from the cornea at 9 o'clock (right disc) or 3 o'clock (le disc). Follow vessels outwards to view each quadrant; rack back through t lenses to inspect lens and cornea. If the view is obscured, examine the r reflex, with your focus on the margin of the pupil, to look for a cataract. Y will get a view of the fovea if you ask the patient to look at t ophthalmoscope's finest beam (after drops)—this is the sacred place: the or place with 6/6 vision. ►Pathology here merits prompt ophthalmic referra

III[P], IV & VI Eye movements. ***III palsy:*** Ptosis, large pupil, eye down and out. ***palsy:*** diplopia on looking down and in (often noticed on descending stairs head tilting compensates for this (ocular torticollis). ***VI nerve palsy:*** Horizon diplopia on looking out. ***Nystagmus*** is involuntary, often jerky, eye oscillatio Horizontal nystagmus is often due to a vestibular lesion (acute: nystagn away from lesion; chronic: towards lesion), or cerebellar lesion (unilate lesions cause nystagmus towards the affected side). If it is more in whiche eye is abducting, MS may be the cause (internuclear ophthalmoplegia, p64) also deafness/tinnitus, suspect a peripheral cause (eg VIII lesion, barotraur Ménière's, p454). If it varies with head position, suspect benign positio vertigo (p454). If it is up-and-down, ask a neurologist to explain what is goi on—upbeat nystagmus classically occurs with lesions in the midbrain or at base of the 4th ventricle, downbeat nystagmus in foramen magnum lesic Nystagmus lasting ≤2 beats is normal, as is nystagmus at the extremes of ga

V ***Motor palsy:*** 'Open your mouth': jaw deviates to side of lesion.
Sensory: Corneal reflex lost first; check all 3 divisions.

VII[P] ***Facial nerve lesions*** cause droop and weakness. As the forehead has bilate representation in the brain, only the lower two-thirds is affected in U lesions, but all of one side of the face in LMN lesions. Ask to 'raise yo eyebrows'; 'show me your teeth'; 'puff out your cheeks'. Taste can be tes (though rarely done) with salt/sweet solutions.

VIII ***Hearing:*** p456. Ask to repeat a number whispered in an ear while you blo the other. Perform Weber's and Rinne's tests (p456). ***Balance/vertigo:*** p4

IX[P] & X[P] ***Gag reflex:*** Touch the back of the palate with a spatula to elicit a reflex c traction. The afferent arm of the reflex involves IX; the efferent arm involve X lesions also cause the palate to be pulled to the normal side on saying '

XI ***Trapezii:*** 'Shrug your shoulders' against resistance.
Sternocleidomastoid: 'Turn your head to the left/right' against resistan

XII ***Tongue movement:*** The tongue deviates to the side of the lesion.

:auses of cranial nerve lesions

Any cranial nerve may be affected by diabetes mellitus; stroke; MS; tumours; sarcoidosis; vasculitis, p542, eg PAN (p543), SLE (p540); syphilis. Chronic meningitis (malignant, TB, or fungal) tends to pick off the lower cranial nerves one by one.

I Trauma; respiratory tract infection; frontal lobe tumour; meningitis.

II Field defects may start as small areas of visual loss (scotomas, eg in glaucoma). ***Monocular blindness:*** Lesions of one eye or optic nerve, eg MS, giant cell arteritis. ***Bilateral blindness:*** Methanol, tobacco amblyopia; neurosyphilis. **Field defects—*Bitemporal hemianopia:*** Optic chiasm compression, eg pituitary adenoma, craniopharyngioma, internal carotid artery aneurysm (fig 1, p440). ***Homonymous hemianopia:*** Affects half the visual field contralateral to the lesion in each eye. Lesions lie beyond the chiasm in the tracts, radiation, or occipital cortex, eg stroke, abscess, tumour.

Optic neuritis (pain on moving eye, loss of central vision, afferent pupillary defect, disc swelling from papillitis). **Causes:** Demyelination (eg MS); rarely sinusitis, syphilis, collagen vascular disorders.

Ischaemic papillopathy: Swelling of optic disc due to ischaemia of the posterior ciliary artery (eg in giant cell arteritis).

Papilloedema (swollen discs): 1 ↑ICP (tumour, abscess, encephalitis, hydrocephalus, benign intracranial hypertension); 2 retro-orbital lesion (eg cavernous sinus thrombosis, p472).

Optic atrophy (pale optic discs and reduced acuity): MS; frontal tumours; Friedreich's ataxia; retinitis pigmentosa; syphilis; glaucoma; Leber's optic atrophy; optic nerve compression.[18]

III[c] alone Diabetes; giant cell arteritis; syphilis; posterior communicating artery aneurysm (+ surgery);[19] idiopathic; ↑ICP (if uncal herniation through the tentorium compresses the nerve). 3rd nerve palsies without a dilated pupil are typically 'medical' (eg diabetes; BP↑). Early dilatation of a pupil implies a compressive lesion, from a 'surgical' cause (tumour; aneurysm) because the parasympathetic fibres run on the outer aspect of the nerve.

IV[c] alone Rare and usually due to trauma to the orbit.[20]

VI[c] alone MS, Wernicke's encephalopathy, false localizing sign in ↑ICP, pontine stroke (presents with fixed small pupils ± quadriparesis).[21]

V[c] ***Sensory:*** Trigeminal neuralgia (pain but no sensory loss, p449), herpes zoster, nasopharyngeal cancer, acoustic neuroma (p454). ***Motor:*** Rare.

VII ***LMN:*** Bell's palsy (p492), polio, otitis media, skull fracture, cerebello-pontine angle tumours eg acoustic neuroma, malignant parotid tumours, herpes zoster (Ramsay Hunt syndrome *OHCS* p652). ***UMN:*** (spares the forehead, because of its bilateral cortical representation) Stroke, tumour.

VIII (p454 & p456) Noise, Paget's disease, Ménière's disease, herpes zoster, acoustic neuroma, brainstem CVA, drugs (eg aminoglycosides).

IX, X, XII Trauma, brainstem lesions, neck tumours.[22]

XI Rare. Polio, syringomyelia, tumour, stroke, bulbar palsy, trauma, TB.

Groups of cranial nerves VIII, then V ± VI: Cerebellopontine angle tumours, eg acoustic neuroma (p454; facial weakness is, surprisingly, not a prominent sign). **V & VI** (Gradenigo's syndrome): Lesion (eg a complication of otitis media) at the apex of the petrous temporal bone ('petroapicitis' on MRI).[23] **III, IV & VI:** Stroke, tumours, Wernicke's encephalopathy, aneurysms, MS.[24] **III, IV, V_a & VI:** Cavernous sinus thrombosis, superior orbital fissure lesions (Tolosa–Hunt syndrome, *OHCS* p654). **IX, X & XI:** Jugular foramen lesion. ***ΔΔ:*** Myasthenia gravis, muscular dystrophy, myotonic dystrophy, mononeuritis multiplex (p494).

Remember that these cranial nerves carry parasympathetic fibres. Sympathetic fibres originate from the thoracic chain and run with the arterial supply to distribute about the body.

Structures passing through the cavernous sinus; see BOX, p49. NB: V_a is the only division of V to do so.

Speech and higher mental function

►Have mercy on those with dysphasia: they are suffocating because language the oxygen of the mind.[1]

Dysphasia (Impairment of language caused by brain damage) ***Assessment:***

1 If speech is fluent, grammatical and meaningful, dysphasia is unlikely.
2 **Comprehension:** Can the patient follow one, two, and several step command (touch your ear, stand up then close the door).
3 **Repetition:** Can the patient repeat a sentence?
4 **Naming:** Can he name common and uncommon things (eg parts of a watch)
5 **Reading and writing:** Normal? They are usually affected like speech dysphasia. If normal, the patient is unlikely to be aphasic—is he mute?

Classification: • ***Broca's (expressive) anterior dysphasia:*** Non-fluent spee produced with effort and frustration with malformed words, eg 'spoot' for 'spoo (or 'that thing'). Reading and writing are impaired but comprehension is relative intact. Patients understand questions and attempt to convey meaningful answe **Site of lesion:** infero-lateral dominant frontal lobe (see fig 1).

- ***Wernicke's (receptive) posterior dysphasia:*** Empty, fluent speech, like talki ragtime with phonemic (*flush* for *brush*) and semantic (*comb* for *brus* paraphasias/neologisms (may be mistaken for psychotic speech). He is oblivious errors. Reading, writing, **and** comprehension are impaired (replies a inappropriate). **Site of lesion:** posterior superior dominant temporal lobe.
- ***Conduction aphasia:*** (Traffic between Broca's and Wernicke's area interrupted.) Repetition is impaired; comprehension and fluency less so.
- ***Nominal dysphasia:*** Naming is affected in all dysphasias, but in nomir dysphasia, objects cannot be named but other aspects of speech are normal. Th occurs with posterior dominant temporoparietal lesions.

►Mixed dysphasias are common. Discriminating features take time to emerge aft an acute brain injury (fig 1). Consider speech therapy (of variable use).

Dysarthria Difficulty with articulation due to incoordination or weakness of t musculature of speech. Language is normal (see above). ***Assessment:*** Ask repeat 'British constitution' or 'baby hippopotamus'.

- ***Cerebellar disease:*** Ataxia speech muscles cause slurring (as if drunk) a speech irregular in volume and scanning or staccato in quality.
- ***Extrapyramidal disease:*** Soft, indistinct, and monotonous speech.
- ***Pseudobulbar palsy:*** (p498) Spastic dysarthria (**upper motor neurone**). Spee is slow, indistinct, and effortful ('Donald Duck' or 'hot potato' voice from bilate hemispheric lesions, MND (p498), or severe MS).
- ***Bulbar palsy:*** **Lower motor neurone** (eg facial nerve palsy, Guillain–Barré, M p498)—any associated palatal paralysis gives speech a nasal character.

Dysphonia Difficulty with speech volume due to weakness of respiratory muscl or vocal cords (Myasthenia, p504; Guillain–Barré syndrome, p694). It may precipitated in myasthenia by asking the patient to count to 100. Parkinson's giv a mixed picture of dysarthria and dysphonia.

Dyspraxia (Poor performance of complex movements despite ability to do ea individual component). Test by asking the patient to copy unfamiliar hand positio or mime an object's use, eg a comb. The term 'dyspraxia' is used in 3 other wa

- ***Dressing dyspraxia:*** The patient is unsure of the orientation of clothes on body. Test by pulling one sleeve of a sweater inside out before asking the patie to put it back on (mostly nondominant hemisphere lesions).
- ***Constructional dyspraxia:*** Difficulty in assembling objects or drawing- 5-pointed star (nondominant hemisphere lesions, hepatic encephalopathy).
- ***Gait dyspraxia:*** More common in the elderly; seen with bilateral frontal lesio lesions in the posterior temporal region, and hydrocephalus.

1 *You cannot say, or guess, for you know only a heap of broken images… connecting nothing with noth* TS Eliot, *The Wasteland*, 1922, Faber & Faber; ISBN 0571202

Problems with classifying dysphasias

The classical model of language comprehension occurring in Wernicke's area and language expression in Broca's area is too simple. Functional MRI studies show that the old idea that the processing of abstract words is confined to the left hemisphere, whereas concrete words are processed on the right is too simplistic.[1] It may be better to think of a mosaic of language centres in the brain with more or less specialized functions. There is evidence that tool-naming is handled differently and in a different area to fruit-naming. There are also individual differences in the anatomy of these mosaics. This is depressing for those who want a rigid classification of aphasia, but a source of hope to those who have had a stroke: recovery may be better than neuroimaging leads us to believe. So, where possible, be optimistic.

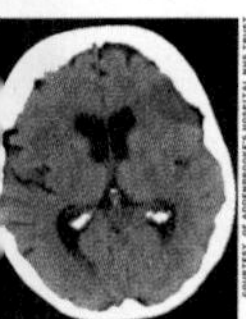

COURTESY OF ADDENBROOKE'S HOSPITAL NHS TRUST

Fig 1. CT of the brain without IV contrast medium, showing a low attenuation area in the frontal lobe, corresponding to an area of acute infarction. This patient was seen in the emergency department with a fractured right neck of femur: she had fallen on to her right side. After a few questions, it became clear that she was only saying the word 'yes' in conversation. Further assessment of her speech revealed that she was able to form a few phrases, but with difficulty and frustration at her errors. She intermittently understood 3-stage commands and repetition was reasonable, but she often misunderstood simple questions. On balance, she probably had an expressive dysphasia, but in the acute setting it was hard to tell.

The Blessed *Dementia Information–Memory–Concentration* test[2]

This is a quantifiable, standardized way of measuring someone's cognitive function. It is most useful for serial measurements, but like all such scores it is not perfect. Sensitivity and specificity for detecting dementia are both ~90%, though scores will varying according to underlying diagnosis (eg poorer sensitivity for detecting Alzheimer's disease), tester variability (meaning that a 2–3 point improvement eg on starting some new treatment may go undetected) and subject population. Making more than 10 errors signifies cognitive impairment:

Question	Score	Question	Score
Know his name	0 or 1	Type of place eg hospital	0 or 1
Know his age	0 or 1	Name of hospital	0 or 1
Time (to nearest hour is OK)	0 or 1	Name of ward	0 or 1
Time of day	0 or 1	Name of town	0 or 1
Day of the week	0 or 1	School	0 or 1
Date of month	0 or 1	(Former) occupation	0 or 1
Season	0 or 1	(Former) employer	0 or 1
Current year	0 or 1	Former town of work or home	0 or 1
Teach name and address and test recall after 5min:		Prime minister or head of government name	0 or 1
Mr. John Brown		Years of World War I	0 or 1
42 West Street	0 to 5	Years of World War II	0 or 1
Gateshead		Monarch/head of state's name	0 or 1
Recognises 2 people	0, 1 or 2	Months of year backwards	0, 1 or 2
Birthday	0 or 1	Count from 1 to 20	0, 1 or 2
Town of birth	0 or 1	Count from 20 to 1	0, 1 or 2
Name of spouse or sibling	0 or 1	**Maximum score**	**36**

NB: Including an 'informant report questionnaire' improves the efficiency of the mental test score as a screening tool for dementia. Another score that can be used to assess cognitive function is the mini-mental state examination (MMSE™), though recent copyright means that its use has become more restricted. See also the AMTS, p42.

1 While abstract words activate a sub-region of the left inferior frontal gyrus more strongly than concrete words, specific activity for concrete words can also be observed in the left basal temporal cortex.

2 Kafka's law: *In youth we take examinations to get into institutions. In old age to keep out of them.*

Psychiatric assessment

Introduce yourself, ask a few factual questions (precise name, age, marital statu job, and who is at home). These will help your patient to relax.

Presenting problem Then ask for the main problems which have led to th consultation. Sit back and listen. Don't worry whether the information is in convenient form or not—this is an opportunity for the patient to come out with h worries unsullied by your expectations. After 3–5min you should have a list of a the problems (each sketched only briefly). Read them back to the patient and ask there are any more. Then ask about:

History of presenting problem For each problem obtain details, both curre state and history of onset, precipitating factors, and effects on life.

Check of major psychiatric symptoms Check those which have not yet bee covered: **depression**—low mood, anhedonia (inability to feel pleasure), thoughts worthlessness/hopelessness, sleep disturbance with early morning waking, loss weight and appetite. Ask specifically about **suicidal thoughts and plans:** 'Have yc ever been so low that you thought of harming yourself?', 'What thoughts have yc had?' **Hallucinations** ('Have you ever heard voices when there hasn't been anyor there, or seen visions?'), and **delusions** ('Have you ever had any thoughts or belie which have struck you afterwards as bizarre?'); **anxiety** and **avoidance behavio** (eg avoiding shopping because of anxiety or phobias); **obsessional thoughts** ar **compulsive behaviour, eating disorders, alcohol** (see p274 for alcohol screenir tests) and **other drugs.**

Present circumstances Housing, finance, work, marriage, friends.

Family history Ask about health, personality, and occupation of parents ar siblings, and the **family's medical and psychiatric history.**

Background history Try to understand the presenting problem.

- ***Biography*** (relationships with family and peers as a child; school and wo record; sexual relationships and current relationships; and family). Previous wa of dealing with stress and whether there have been problems and sympton similar to the presenting ones.
- ***Premorbid personality*** (mood, character, hobbies, attitudes, and beliefs).

Past medical and psychiatric history

Mental state examination This is the state **now**, at the time of interview.

- ***Appearance:*** Clothing, glasses, headwear? Unkempt/meticulous?
- ***Observable behaviour:*** Eg excessive slowness, signs of anxiety.
- ***Mode of speech:*** Include the rate of speech, eg retarded or gabbling (pressure speech). Note its content. Flight of ideas? Knight's move? (See BOX)
- ***Mood:*** Note thoughts about harming self or others. Gauge your own respons to the patient. The laughter and grand ideas of manic patients are contagious, a to a lesser extent is the expression of thoughts from a depressed person.
- ***Beliefs:*** Eg about himself, his own body, about other people, and the future. No abnormal beliefs (delusions), eg that thoughts are overheard, and abnormal ide (eg persecutory, grandiose).
- ***Unusual experiences or hallucinations:*** Note modality, eg visual, auditory.
- ***Orientation:*** In time, place, and person. What is the date? What time of day it? Where are you? What is your name?
- ***Short-term memory:*** Give a name and address and test recall after 5min. Ma sure that he has got the address clear in his head before waiting the 5min.
- ***Long-term memory:*** Current affairs recall. Name of current political leade (p47). This tests many other CNS functions, not just memory.
- ***Concentration:*** Months of the year backwards.
- Note the degree of your ***rapport*** and the patient's ***insight*** into his current stat

Nonverbal behaviour Gesture, gaze and mutual gaze, expressions, tears, laught pauses (while listening to voices?), attitude (eg withdrawn).

Psychiatric symptoms

There are many different ways to think about psychiatric symptoms. One simple approach can be to consider negative and positive symptoms. ***Negative symptoms*** involve the absence of a behaviour, thought, feeling or sensation (eg lack of appetite, apathy, and blunted emotions in depression), whereas ***positive symptoms*** involve their presence when not normally expected (eg thought insertion, ie 'someone is putting thoughts into my head'). Understanding the difference between psychosis and neurosis is vital. ***Psychosis*** entails a thought disorder (eg thought insertion, thought broadcasting) ± delusions (abnormal beliefs which are held to despite all reasoning, and which run counter to the patient's culture) and abnormal perceptions (eg hallucinations), ***neurosis*** entails insight—if there are intrusive ideas or odd experiential phenomena the person knows that they are false or illusory (and may be triggered by stress etc).

Interesting abnormalities of speech include ***flight of ideas***, in which the speech races through themes, switching whimsically or through associations eg 'clang' association: 'Yesterday I went down to the local shop. I didn't hop (*clang*), but I walked. Kangaroos hop, don't they. My friend Joey wasn't there, though ...'. ***Knight's move*** is an unexpected change in the direction of speech or conversation (akin to the lateral component of the move of the knight's piece in chess) and ***neologism*** is the formation of new words. They may be normal or indicate an organic brain condition or a psychosis.

Many psychiatric symptoms in isolation, to a lesser degree of severity, or even in a different culture, may well be considered part of 'normal' behaviour. For example, where would we be without language embracing brave new words? [34] As with so many aspects of medicine, in psychiatry there is a vast spectrum of behaviour, thought and perception, at least one extreme of which is considered to be 'abnormal'. It is in part our challenge to attempt to interpret these symptoms with relevance, insight and impartiality so that we may best benefit our patients and not form opinions that are set in stone. On acute medical wards psychiatric symptoms are usually due to stress, drug or alcohol withdrawal, U&E imbalance, or medication. When in doubt, ask a psychiatrist to help. NB: it is normal for the bereaved to hear the voice of the person who has died.

►Beware of simplistic formulations, eg *If you talk to God, you are praying. If God talks to you, you have schizophrenia* (Dr Thomas Szasz). It is not the auditory phenomenon which makes the diagnosis of psychosis: what matters is what the patient believes about the phenomenon, and whether they are associated with a thought disorder or a delusion.

The contents of the cavernous sinus and the cranial nerve names

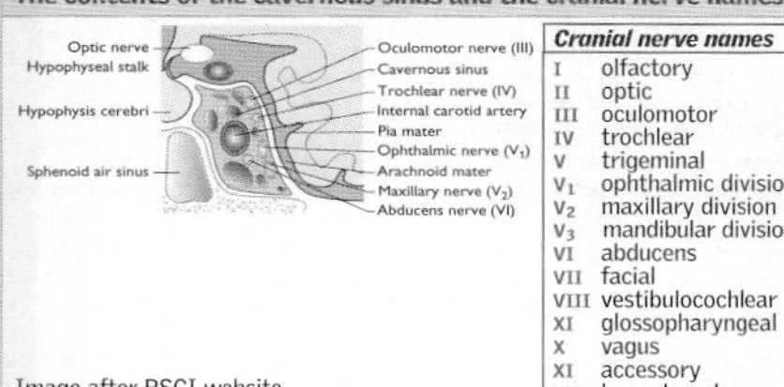

Image after RSCI website

Cranial nerve names	
I	olfactory
II	optic
III	oculomotor
IV	trochlear
V	trigeminal
V_1	ophthalmic division
V_2	maxillary division
V_3	mandibular division
VI	abducens
VII	facial
VIII	vestibulocochlear
XI	glossopharyngeal
X	vagus
XI	accessory
XII	hypoglossal

Method and order for routine examination

We all have our own system, sometimes based on these lines, but sometimes containing elements unique to each doctor, arising from his or her own interaction with countless past patients and their eccentricities. This fact is one reason why it is often so helpful to ask for second opinions: the same field may be ploughed again but yield quite a different harvest.

1 Look at the patient. Healthy, unwell, or *in extremis*? This vital skill improves with practice. ►Beware those who are sicker than they look, eg cardiogenic shock; cord compression; nonaccidental injury.
2 Pulse, BP; T°; infrared tympanic[IRT] & liquid crystal[LC] devices avoid mercury.[1]
3 Examine nails, hands, conjunctivae (anaemia), and sclerae (jaundice). Consider: Paget's, acromegaly, endocrine disease (thyroid, pituitary, or adrenal hypo/hyperfunction), body hair, abnormal pigmentation, skin.
4 Examine mouth and tongue (cyanosed; smooth; furred; beefy, eg rhomboid area denuded of papillae by *Candida*, after prolonged steroid inhaler use).
5 Examine the neck from behind: nodes, goitre.
6 Make sure the patient is at 45° to begin CVS examination in the neck: JVP; feel for character and volume of carotid pulse.
7 The praecordium. Look for abnormal pulsations. Feel the apex beat (character; position). Any parasternal heave or thrill? Auscultate (bell & diaphragm) apex in the left lateral position, then the other 3 areas (p29) and carotids. Sit the patient forward: listen during expiration.
8 Whilst sitting forward, look for sacral oedema.
9 Begin the respiratory examination with the patient at 90°. Observe (and count) respirations; note posterior chest wall movement. Assess expansion, then percuss and auscultate the chest with the bell.
10 Sit the patient back. Feel the trachea. Inspect again. Assess expansion of the anterior chest. Percuss and auscultate again.
11 Examine the breasts* (if indicated) and axillary nodes (p610).
12 Lie the patient flat with only one pillow. Inspect, palpate, percuss, and auscultate the abdomen.
13 Look at the legs: any swellings, perfusion, pulses, or oedema?
14 CNS exam: ***Cranial nerves:*** pupil responses; fundi; visual fields; visual acuity. Do corneal reflexes. 'Open your mouth; stick your tongue out; screw up your eyes; show me your teeth; raise your eyebrows.' ***Peripheral nerves:*** Look for wasting and fasciculation. Test tone in all limbs. 'Hold your hands out with your palms towards the ceiling and fingers wide. Now shut your eyes.' Watch for pronator drift. 'Keep your eyes shut and touch your nose with each index finger.' 'Lift your leg straight in the air. Keep it there. Put your heel on the opposite knee (eyes shut) and run it up your own shin.' You have now tested power, coordination, and joint position sense. Tuning fork on toes and index fingers to assess vibration sense.
15 Examine the gait and the speech.
16 Any abnormalities of higher mental function to pursue?
17 Consider rectal and vaginal examination.*
18 Examine the urine with dipstick and microscope if appropriate.

►***Remember the need for a chaperone for all intimate examinations.**

►**In general, go into detail where you find (or suspect) something to be wrong.**

1 IRT is better than forehead LC strips; LC is specific (100%) but not sensitive (39%).

He moved

all the brightest gems

faster and faster towards the

ever-growing bucket of lost hopes; had there been just one more year

of peace the battalion would have made a floating system of perpetual drainage.

A silent fall of immense snow came near oily remains of the recently eaten supper on the table.

We drove on in our old sunless walnut. Presently classical eggs ticked in the new afternoon shadows.

We were instructed by my cousin Jasper not to exercise by country house visiting unless accompanied by thirteen geese or gangsters.

The modern American did not prevail over the pair of redundant bronze puppies. The worn-out principle is a bad omen which I am never glad to ransom in August.

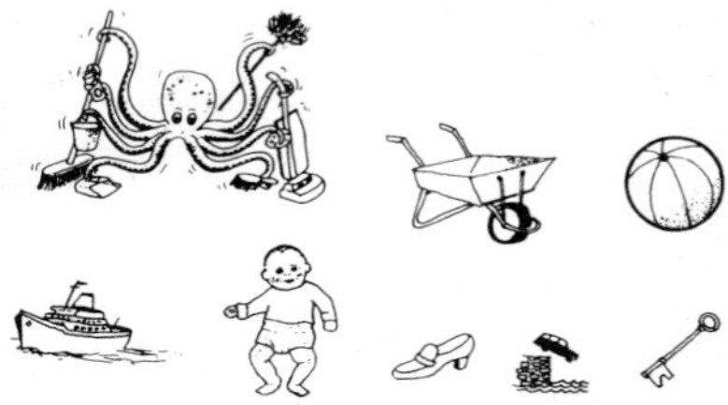

Snellen chart. For indication only, and not for diagnostic use at this scale. Snellen charts (at correct scale) are used by recording the smallest type accurately read or object named, at 30 cm.

3 Signs and symptoms

Symptoms are features which patients report. ***Physical signs*** are elicited at the bedside. Together, they constitute the features of the condition in that patient. Their evolution over time, and interaction with the physical, psychological, and social spheres comprise the natural history of any disease. Here, we discuss symptoms in isolation. This is unnatural—but a good first step in learning how to diagnose. All doctors have to know about symptoms and their relief: this is what doctors are for. This chapter is disappointing in trying to explain *combinations* of symptoms, as illnesses often do not fit into the 80-or-so features given below. It was this disappointment which was our stimulus to produce our electronic system, where over 20,000 signs, symptoms, and test results can be sifted in devious and diverse ways to help with difficult problems in differential diagnosis. See www.webmentorlibrary.com. So do not expect too much from this chapter: just a few common causes of common symptoms and signs.

Abdominal distension ***Causes:*** The famous five **Fs** (see BOX). Specific groups: ***Air*** is resonant on percussion. ***Ascites*** is free fluid in the peritoneal cavity. Signs: shifting dullness and fluid thrill (p41). The characteristic feature of ***pelvic masses*** is that you cannot get below them (ie their lower border is undefined). Causes of ***right iliac fossa masses:*** Appendix mass/abscess (p582), kidney mass, caecal cancer, a Crohn's or TB mass, intussusception, amoebic abscess or any pelvic mass.

Also see causes of ***ascites with portal hypertension*** (p624), ***hepatomegaly*** (p62), ***splenomegaly***, and ***other abdominal masses*** (p624).

Abdominal pain varies depending on the underlying cause. Examples: irritation of the mucosa (acute gastritis), smooth muscle spasm (acute enterocolitis), capsular stretching (liver congestion in CCF), peritoneal inflammation (acute appendicitis) and direct splanchnic nerve stimulation (retroperitoneal extension of tumour). The ***character*** (constant or colicky, sharp or dull), ***duration***, and ***frequency*** depend on the mechanism of production. The ***location*** and ***distribution*** of referred pain depend on the anatomical site. ***Time of occurrence*** and ***aggravating*** or ***relieving factors*** such as meals, defecation, and sleep also have special significance related to the underlying disease process. ►Evaluation of the acute abdomen is considered on p580. The site of the pain may provide a clue as to the cause:

- **Epigastric pain** Pancreatitis, gastritis or duodenitis, peptic ulcer, gall bladder disease, aortic aneurysm.
- **Left upper quadrant pain** Peptic ulcer, gastric or colonic (splenic flexure) ca, splenic rupture, subphrenic or perinephric abscess, renal (colic, pyelonephritis).
- **Right upper quadrant pain** Cholecystitis, biliary colic, hepatitis, peptic ulcer, colonic cancer (hepatic flexure), renal (colic, pyelonephritis), subphrenic or perinephric abscess.
- **Loin pain** Renal colic, pyelonephritis, renal tumour, perinephric abscess, pain referred from vertebral column.
- **Left iliac fossa pain** Diverticulitis, volvulus, colon cancer, pelvic abscess, inflammatory bowel disease, hip pathology, renal colic, urinary tract infection (UTI), cancer in undescended testis. *Gynae:* Torsion of ovarian cyst, salpingitis, ectopic pregnancy. **Right iliac fossa pain** All causes of left iliac fossa pain plus appendicitis and Crohn's ileitis, but usually excluding diverticulitis.
- **Pelvic pain** *Urological:* Urinary tract infection (UTI), urinary retention, bladder stones. *Gynae:* Menstruation, pregnancy, endometriosis (*OHCS* p288), salpingitis, endometritis (*OHCS* p274), torsion of ovarian cyst.
- **Generalised:** Gastroenteritis, irritable bowel syndrome, peritonitis, constipation.
- **Central:** Mesenteric ischaemia, abdominal aneurysm, pancreatitis.
- ***Remember referred pain:*** Myocardial infarct → epigastrium; pleural pathology.

Amaurosis fugax See p468.

Abdominal distension: the *Famous Five* Fs: Fat, flatus, fluid, faeces, and fetus

Air	Ascites	Solid masses	Pelvic masses
Intestinal obstruction (incl. faecal)	Malignancy[1]	Malignancy[1]	Bladder: full or Ca
	Cirrhosis	Lymph nodes	Fibroids; fetus
	Right heart failure	Aortic aneurysm	Ovarian cyst
Aerophagy (air swallowing)	Hypoproteinaemia (eg nephrotic)	Cysts: renal, pancreatic	Ovarian cancer
			Uterine cancer

Enid Blyton's *Famous Five* characters can generally solve any crime or diagnostic problem using 1950s methodologies steeped in endless school holidays, copious midnight feasts (always confection laden), and lashings of homemade ginger beer.

The one insoluble problem was (and is) abdominal distension. The methods used by the Famous Five actually *contribute* to each of its causes: fat, fluid, faeces, flatus, and fetus. If you think it far-fetched to implicate ginger-beer in the genesis of fetuses, note that because it was home-made, like the fun, there was no limit to its intoxicating powers in those long-gone vintage summers.

Enid Blyton did her best to minimize the risks of unwanted pregnancies by gender reassignment (George) and by making one of her characters a dog (Timmy)—but accidents *must* have happened. The point is to remember to ask 'when was your last period' *whenever* confronted by a distended abdomen.

1 Any intra-abdominal organ, eg colon, stomach, pancreas, liver, kidney.

Anaemia is haemoglobin concentration below the normal range (see p310). It ma be assessed from the conjunctivae and skin creases. Koilonychia and stomatit (p26) suggest iron deficiency. Anaemia with jaundice suggests haemolysis.

Athetosis This is due to a lesion in the putamen, causing slow sinuous writhir movements in the hands, which are present at rest. ***Pseudoathetosis*** refers athetoid movements in patients with severe proprioceptive loss.

Backache p528. **Blackouts** p452. **Breathlessness** (dyspnoea) p58.

Breast pain Often this is premenstrual (*cyclical mastalgia*, *OHCS* p254)—but th patient may be worried that she has breast cancer. So examine carefully (p61C and refer eg for mammography as appropriate. If there is no sign of brea pathology, and it is not cyclical, think of:

- Tietze's syndrome
- Gallstones
- Angina
- Oestrogens (HRT)
- Bornholm disease[1]
- Lung disease
- Thoracic outlet syndrome

If none of the above, *wearing a firm bra* all day may help, as may NSAIDs.

Cachexia Severe generalized muscle wasting implying malnutrition, neoplasia, cc Alzheimer's disease, prolonged inanition, or infection—eg TB, enteropathic AII ('slim disease', eg from *Cryptosporidium*, p380).

Carotid bruits may signify stenosis (>30%) caused by atheroma, often near th internal carotid origin. Heard best behind the angle of jaw. The key question is: *he/she symptomatic?* If symptomatic (ie has had a TIA or carotid artery territo stroke) and the disability is not too severe, do a doppler ultrasound of the carot arteries, and consider surgery if stenosis ≥70%, and *possibly* if ≥50% (p468 Surgery for asymptomatic patients is debatable.[3] In anyone with a carotid bru consider aspirin prophylaxis. Ask a neurologist's advice.

Chest deformity • ***Barrel chest:*** AP diameter↑, tracheal descent and che expansion↓, seen in chronic hyperinflation (eg asthma/COPD). • ***Pigeon che (pectus carinatum):*** Prominent sternum with a flat chest, seen with lur hyperinflation while bony thorax is still developing eg in chronic childhood asthm Often seen with ***Harrison's sulcus***, a groove deformity caused by indrawing of th lower ribs at the diaphragm attachment site. • ***Funnel chest (pectus excavatum*** Developmental defect involving local sternum depression (lower end). • ***Kyphosi*** 'Humpback' from ↑ AP thoracic spine curvature. • ***Scoliosis:*** Lateral curvature (*OH* p672); both of these may cause a restrictive ventilatory defect.

Chest pain See p80 & p772.

Cheyne–Stokes respiration Breathing becomes progressively deeper and the shallower (±episodic apnoea) in cycles. ***Causes:*** Brainstem lesions or compressic (stroke, ICP↑). If the cycle is long (eg 3min), the cause may be a long lung-to-bra circulation time (eg in chronic pulmonary oedema or poor cardiac output). It enhanced by opioids.

Chorea means dance—a continuous flow of jerky movements, flitting from o limb or part to another. Each movement looks like a fragment of a norm movement. It should be distinguished from athetosis/pseudoathetosis (above), a hemiballismus (see p460). ***Causes:*** Basal ganglia lesion: Huntington's disea (p694), post-infective: Sydenham's chorea (St Vitus' dance—p128), SLE (p54(Wilson's disease (p257), kernicterus, polycythaemia (p350), neuroacanthocyto (a familial association of acanthocytes in peripheral blood with chorea, oro-fac dyskinesia, and axonal neuropathy), hyperthyroidism (p202), drugs (L-dop contraceptive steroids, chlorpromazine). Early stages of chorea may be detected feeling fluctuations in muscle tension while the patient grips your finger. Treat wi dopamine antagonists, eg tetrabenazine 12.5mg/12h (/24h if elderly) PO; increas eg to 25mg/8h PO; max 200mg/d.

Chvostek's sign Tapping on the facial nerve over the parotid gland causes a fac twitch in hypocalcaemia, due to nerve hyperexcitability. See **Trousseau's sign**.

Signs and symptoms

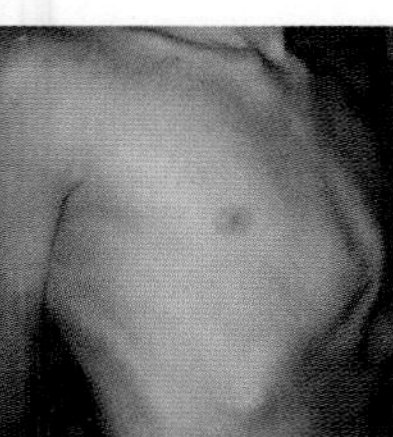

1. Pectus carinatum (pigeon chest).

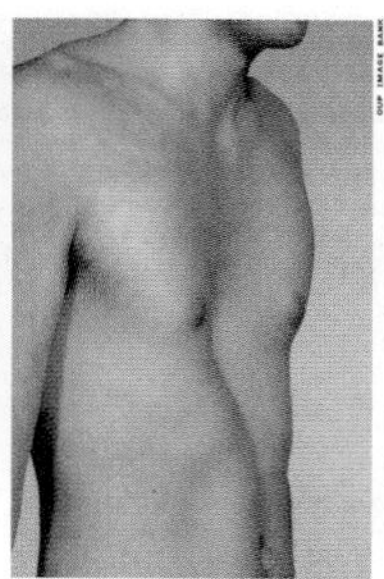

Fig 2. Pectus excavatum. The medical term for funnel or sunken chest. It is usually asymptomatic, but may cause displacement of the heart to the left, and restricted ventilatory capacity. Associations: Scoliosis, Marfan's, and Ehlers–Danlos syndromes.

ornholm disease (Devil's grip) is due eg to Coxsackie B virus, causing chest and abdominal pain which be mistaken for cardiac pain or an acute surgical abdomen. It resolves within ~2 weeks.
1% reduction in 5yr risk of stroke or surgical death if stenosis ≥70%; 5.7% reduction if 50–70% osis; below 50% stenosis surgery is unhelpful/harmful. See PM Rothwell 2003 *Stroke* **34** 514.
F Toole 2004 *BMJ* **329** 635.

Clubbing Finger nails (± toenails) have exaggerated curvature in all directior There is a loss of the angle between nail and nail-fold, and the nail-fold feels bogg There are changes in local blood flow, but the exact mechanism is unclear.

Thoracic causes:
- Bronchial carcinoma (usually *not* small cell)
- Chronic lung suppuration
  - empyema, abscess
  - bronchiectasis
  - cystic fibrosis
- Fibrosing alveolitis
- Mesothelioma

GI causes:
- Inflammatory bowel disease (especially Crohn's)
- Cirrhosis
- GI lymphoma
- Malabsorption, eg coeliac

Rare:
- Familial
- Thyroid acropachy (p546)
- Unilateral clubbing, from:
  - axillary artery aneurysm
  - brachial arteriovenous malformations

Cardiac causes:
- Cyanotic congenital heart disease
- Endocarditis
- Atrial myxoma

Confusion This common phenomenon is often multifactorial (p476). Rememb alcohol withdrawal as a cause, classically occurring 48 hours after admission wi vivid hallucinations.

Constipation See p240. **Cough** See p37. See also **Haemoptysis** (p63).

Cramp (Painful muscle spasm). Cramp in the legs is common, especially at night after exercise. It only occasionally indicates disease, in particular: salt depletic muscle ischaemia, or myopathy. Forearm cramps suggest motor neurone diseas Night cramps may respond to passive exercises or quinine bisulfate 300mg at nig PO. Writer's cramp is a focal dystonia causing difficulty with the motor act writing. The pen is gripped firmly, with excessive flexion of the thumb and ind finger (± tremor). There is normally no CNS deficit. Oral drugs or psychothera rarely work, but botulinum toxin (*OHCS* p460) often helps, sometimes dramatica (it has side-effects). Similar specific dystonias may apply to other muscle grou

Cyanosis Dusky blue skin (***peripheral***—of the fingers) or mucosae (***central***—of t tongue), representing ≥2.5g/dL of Hb in its reduced form, hence it occurs mo readily in polycythaemia than anaemia. ***Causes:***
- ***Lung disease*** with inadequate oxygen transfer eg luminal obstruction, asthn COPD, pneumonia, PE, pulmonary oedema—may be correctable by ↑ inspired
- ***Cyanotic congenital heart disease***, where there is shunting from pulmonary systemic circulation bypassing the lungs, eg patent ductus arterios transposition of the great arteries, VSD with right to left shunting (Eisenmenge syndrome, see p143)—cyanosis is *not* reversed by increasing inspired oxyge
- Rare cause: methaemoglobinaemia, a congenital or acquired red cell disorde

►Acute cyanosis is a sign of impending emergency. Is there asthma, an inhal foreign body, a pneumothorax (p735, fig 1) or pulmonary oedema? See p798.

Peripheral cyanosis will occur in causes of central cyanosis, but may also induced by changes in the peripheral and cutaneous vascular systems in patier with normal oxygen saturations. It occurs in the cold, in hypovolaemia, and arterial disease, and is therefore not a specific sign.

How to test for finger clubbing

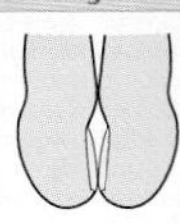

The dorsal aspect of 2 fingers, side by side with the nails touching. Normally, you should see a kite-shaped gap. If not, there is clubbing.

Fig. 1a

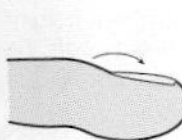

Fig. 1b

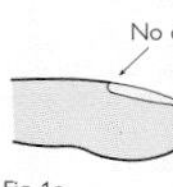

Fig. 1c

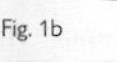

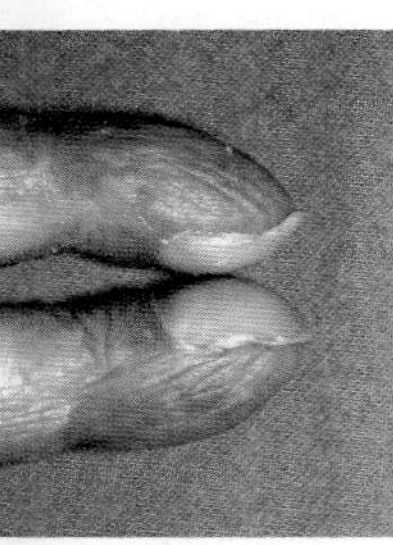

ig 1. Clubbing: increased curvature of he nail, with loss of angle between the ail and nail-fold.

Deafness See p456. **Dehydration** See p666. **Diarrhoea** See p238.

Dizziness is a loose term meaning: ***vertigo*** (p454), the illusion of rotation ± a unwilled need to cast oneself into any nearby abyss ***or imbalance***, a difficulty i walking straight, from peripheral nerve, posterior column, cerebellar, or other centra pathway failure ***or faintness***, ie 'light-headedness', seen in anaemia, ↓BP, postura hypotension, hypoglycaemia, carotid sinus hypersensitivity, and epilepsy. All may co exist: *'At the place where I stood, the hillside was cut away like a cliff, with the se groaning at its foot, blue and pure. There was no more than a moment to suffer. how terrible was the dizziness of that thought! Twice I threw myself forward, and do not know what power flung me back, still alive, on to the grass which I kissed.'*

Dysarthria See p46. **Dysdiadochokinesis** See p491.

Dyspepsia and **indigestion** See 234. These are broad terms, used often to signif epigastric or retrosternal pain (or discomfort), which may be related to meals. Fin out exactly what your patient is complaining of. 30% have no abnormality o endoscopy (p248).

Dysphasia See p46. **Dysphonia** See p46. **Dysphagia** See p232.

Dyspnoea (p770) is the subjective sensation of shortness of breath, ofte exacerbated by exertion. Try to quantify exercise tolerance (eg dressing, distanc walked, climbing stairs, NYHA classification—p121). May be due to:

- ***Cardiac***—eg mitral stenosis, ischaemic heart disease or left ventricular failur (LVF) of any cause. LVF is associated with ***orthopnoea*** (dyspnoea worse on lying 'how many pillows?') and ***paroxysmal nocturnal dyspnoea*** (PND; dyspnoe waking one up). Other features include ankle oedema, lung crepitations and ↑JV
- ***Lung***—both airway and interstitial disease. It may be hard to separate fro cardiac causes; asthma may also wake the patient, as well as cause earl morning dyspnoea and wheeze. Focus on the circumstances in which dyspnoe occurs (eg on exposure to an occupational allergen).
- ***Anatomical***—eg diseases of the chest wall, muscles, pleura. Ascites can caus breathlessness by splinting on the diaphragm, restricting its movement.
- ***Others*** ►Any patient who is shocked may also be dyspnoeic (p581)—and thi may be shock's presenting feature. Other causes: anaemia or metabolic acidosi causing respiratory compensation eg ketoacidosis, aspirin poisoning. Look fo other clues—dyspnoea at rest *unassociated with exertion* may be psychogeni prolonged hyperventilation causes respiratory alkalosis. This causes a fall i ionised calcium leading to an apparent hypocalcaemia. Symptoms and sign include peripheral and perioral paraesthesiae ± carpopedal spasm.

The speed of onset helps diagnosis:

Acute	Subacute	Chronic
Foreign body	Asthma	COPD and chronic
Pneumothorax (p735, fig 1)	Parenchymal disease	parenchymal diseases
Acute asthma	eg alveolitis	Non-respiratory causes
Pulmonary embolus	effusion	eg cardiac failure
Acute pulmonary oedema	pneumonia	anaemia

Dyspraxia See p46.

Dysuria is painful micturition from urethral or bladder inflammation, typically fro infection (see also urethral syndrome, p282). ***Strangury*** is pain in the urethr referred from the base of the bladder, associated with the constant distressin desire to urinate even when there is little urine to void. Causes include a stone, a indwelling catheter, cystitis, prostatitis, and bladder cancer.

Facial pain This can be neurological (eg trigeminal neuralgia, p449) or from ar other pain-sensitive structure in the head or neck (see BOX). ***Postherpet neuralgia:*** This nasty burning-and-stabbing pain involves dermatomal area previously affected by shingles (herpes zoster, p388); it may affect cranial nerve V and VII in the face. It all too often becomes chronic and intractable, and the sk affected is exquisitely sensitive. Treatment is difficult. Give strong psychologic support whatever else is tried. Transcutaneous nerve stimulation, capsaic ointment, and infiltration of local anaesthetic may be tried. Amitriptyline eg 1C 25mg/24h at night may help, as may carbamazepine (NNT ≈ 4). NB: Meta-analyse indicate that famciclovir and valaciclovir given in the acute stage may ↓duration neuralgia.

Faecal incontinence This is common in the elderly. Be sure to find out who doe the washing: they may be under severe stress (Social Services may help wit laundry). The cause may disappear if constipation (p240) is treated (='overflo incontinence'/diarrhoea). Do a PR to check for this. ***GI causes:*** Rectal prolaps tumour, sphincter laxity, severe piles, causes of diarrhoea (p238). Others: see BO

Faints, Collapse, Blackouts See p452.

Falls These are a common cause of admission in the elderly, and can lead to a spir of loss of confidence and dependence. Causes are often multifactorial and includ ***Intrinsic:*** CNS disease, visual impairment, cognitive impairment, depressio postural hypotension, peripheral neuropathy, medication (eg antihypertensive sedatives), pain eg arthritis, Parkinsonism (including medications: prochlorperazin neuroleptics, metoclopramide), muscle weakness, incontinence, alcohol. ***Enviror ment:*** Poor lighting, uneven walking surface. Treatment includes addressir injuries, reducing risk factors, and reducing the risk of injury eg treat osteoporos (p674). A multidisciplinary multifactorial approach alongside occupation therapists and physiotherapists is likely to be beneficial.

Fatigue This feeling is so common that it is a variant of normality. Only 1 in 40 episodes leads to a consultation with a doctor. ►Do not miss depression whic often presents in this way. Even if the patient is depressed, a screening history ar examination is important to rule out chronic disease. ***Tests*** to consider are FBC, ES U&E, plasma glucose, TFT ± CXR. Arrange follow-up to see what develops, and address any emotional problems that develop.

Fever and night sweats (see ***Sweating***) While some night sweating is common anxiety, drenching sweats requiring changes of night-clothes are a more omino symptom associated with infection (eg TB, brucellosis), lymphoproliferative diseas or mesothelioma. Patterns of fever may be relevant (see p376). See ***Rigors***.

Flatulence 400–1300mL of gas are expelled PR per day, and if this, coupled wi belching (eructation) and abdominal distension, seems excessive to the patient, may complain of flatulence. Eructation may occur in those with hiatus hernia—b most patients complaining of flatulence have no GI disease. The most likely cause air-swallowing (aerophagy).

Frequency (urinary) means ↑frequency of micturition. Aim to differentiate ↑uri production (eg diabetes mellitus, diabetes insipidus, polydipsia, diuretics, alcoh renal tubular disease, or adrenal insufficiency) from frequent passage of sm amounts of urine (eg in cystitis, urethritis, neurogenic bladder), or bladder con pression (eg from pregnancy, bladder tumour, or an enlarged prostate).

Gait disorders See p459.

Guarding Involuntary reflex contraction of abdominal muscles as you press on t abdomen (gently!), signifying local or general peritoneal inflammation (p580). It an imperfect sign of peritonism, but is one of the best we have; if you decide not operate on someone with RIF guarding, the risk of missing appendicitis is abo 25%. If you *do* operate, the chance of finding appendicitis is 50%. See **Rebour abdominal pain**.

Gynaecomastia p214. **Haematemesis** p244. **Haematuria** p278.

Non-neurological causes of facial pain

Neck	Cervical disc pathology
Sinuses	Sinusitis, neoplasia
Eye	Glaucoma, iritis, eye strain
Temporomandibular joint	Arthritis
Teeth	Caries, abscess, malocclusion
Ear	Otitis media, otitis externa
Vascular	Giant cell arteritis

NB: when all causes are excluded, a group which is mostly young and female remains ('atypical facial pain') who complain of unilateral pain deep in the face or at the angle of cheek and nose, which is constant, severe, and unresponsive to analgesia. Do not dismiss these as psychological: few meet criteria for hysteria or depression. Do not expose these patients to the risks of destructive surgery; while many are prescribed antidepressants, some neurologists advocate no treatment.

Non-gastrointestinal causes of faecal incontinence

Neurological	Spinal cord compression, Parkinson's disease, stroke, MS, spinal trauma (S2–S4), dementia.
Endocrinological	Diabetes mellitus (autonomic neuropathy), hypothyroidism.
Obstetric	Damage to puborectalis (or nerve roots) at childbirth.

Treatment is directed to the cause if possible. Avoid dehydration. Be sure to do a PR to exclude overflow incontinence. If all sensible measures fail, try the brake-and-accelerator approach: enemas to empty the rectum (eg twice weekly) and codeine phosphate eg 15mg/12h PO on non-enema days to constipate. This is not a cure, but makes the incontinence manageable.

Haemoptysis See BOX. Always think of TB or malignancy; don't confuse wit epistaxis or haematemesis. The blood is *coughed up*, eg frothy, alkaline, and brigh red, often in a context of known chest disease. NB: Melaena may occur if enoug blood is swallowed. Haematemesis is acidic and dark. Blood not mixed with sputur suggests lung infarction (pulmonary embolism, PE) or trauma. Haemoptysis rarel needs treating in its own right, but if massive (eg trauma, TB, hydatid cyst, cance AV malformation), call a chest physician/surgeon (the danger is drowning; lob resection, endobronchial tamponade, or arterial embolization may be needed). Se up IVI, do CXR, blood gases, FBC, INR/APTT, crossmatch. If distressing, conside *prompt* IV morphine, eg if inoperable malignancy.

Halitosis (fetor oris, oral malodour) results from gingivitis (Vincent's angina p704), metabolic activity of bacteria in plaque, or sulfide-yielding foo putrefaction. ***Contributory factors:*** Smoking, alcohol, drugs (disulfiram isosorbide); lung disease. Delusional halitosis is quite common. ***Treatment:*** Try t eliminate anaerobes: • Stand nearer the toothbrush • Dental floss • 0.2% aqueou chlorhexidine gluconate. See *Clinical Evidence* 2006, BMA.

Headache See p448 & p768.

Heartburn An intermittent, gripping, retrosternal pain usually worsened by stooping/lying, large meals and pregnancy. See oesophagitis, p236.

Hemiballismus This refers to the uncontrolled unilateral flailing movements c proximal limb joints caused by contralateral subthalamic lesions. See p460.

Hepatomegaly See BOX. **Hoarseness** See p36, and *OHCS* p568.

Hyperpigmentation See **Skin discolouration** (p70).

Hyperventilation is over-breathing; it may be *fast* (tachypnoea, ie >20breaths min) or *deep* (hyperpnoea, ie tidal volume ↑). Hyperpnoea is not troublesome t the patient (unlike dyspnoea). It may be enough to cause a respiratory alkalosis leading to paraesthesiae ± muscle spasm (plasma Ca^{2+}↓). The main cause is anxiety there is associated dizziness, chest tightness/pain, palpitations, and panic. Rare causes: response to metabolic acidosis and brainstem lesions.

- ***Kussmaul respiration*** is deep, sighing breathing that is principally seen in sever metabolic acidosis—eg diabetic ketoacidosis, renal failure.
- ***Neurogenic hyperventilation*** is produced by pontine lesions.
- The ***hyperventilation syndrome*** involves panic attacks associated with hyper ventilation, palpitations, dizziness, faintness, tinnitus, alarming chest pain/tight ness, perioral and peripheral tingling (plasma Ca^{2+}↓). Treatment: relaxatio techniques and breathing into a paper bag (↑ inspired CO_2 corrects the alkalosis

NB: The anxious patient in A&E with hyperventilation and a respiratory alkalosi may actually be presenting with an aspirin overdose (p828).

Insomnia When we are sleeping well this is a trivial and irritating complaint, but we suffer a few sleepless nights, sleep becomes the most desirable thin imaginable and the ability to bestow sleep the best thing we can do for a patien second only to relieving pain. As all *Sons and lovers know*, 'Sleep is most perfec when it is shared with a beloved.' Do not resort to drugs without asking: *What the cause? Can it be treated?* See BOX.

Management: 'Sleep hygiene' • Do not go to bed until you feel sleepy.

- Avoid daytime naps. Establish regular bedtime routines.
- If you can, reserve a room for sleep. Do not eat or study in it.
- Avoid caffeine, nicotine, alcohol—and late-evening hard exercise (sexual activit is the exception: it may produce excellent torpor).
- Consider monitoring with a sleep diary (quantifies sleep pattern and quality), bu this could feed insomnia by encouraging obsessions.

Prescribe hypnotics for a few weeks only: they are addictive and cause daytim somnolence ± rebound insomnia on stopping. Warn about driving/machine workin Example: zopiclone 3.75–7.5mg PO. ***Obstructive sleep apnoea:*** p186 ***parasomnia: sleep paralysis, & hypnopsychic states:*** *OHCS* p392. ***Narcolepsy:*** p692.

Causes of haemoptysis

1 ***Respiratory causes of haemoptysis***

Traumatic	Wounds, post-intubation, foreign body.
Infective	Bronchiectasis, acute bronchitis, pneumonia, lung abscess, TB, COPD, fungi, paragonimiasis (p433).
Neoplastic	Primary or secondary.
Vascular	Lung infarction (PE), vasculitis (pulmonary haemorrhage in Wegener's, RA, SLE, Osler–Weber–Rendu), AV malformation.
Parenchymal	Diffuse interstitial fibrosis, sarcoidosis, haemosiderosis, Goodpasture's syndrome, cystic fibrosis.

2 ***Cardiovascular (pulmonary hypertension)***	Pulmonary oedema, mitral stenosis, aortic aneurysm, Eisenmenger's syndrome (p143).

3 ***Bleeding diatheses***

The science of halitosis

Locally retained bacteria metabolize sulfur-containing amino acids to yield volatile hydrogen sulfide and methylmercaptane. Not only do these stink, but they also damage surrounding tissue, thereby perpetuating bacterial retention and periodontal disease.

At night and between meals conditions are optimal for odour production—so eating regularly may help. To supplement conventional oral hygienic measures, some people advise brushing of the tongue. Oral care products containing metal ions, especially Zn, inhibit odour formation, it is thought, because of affinity of the metal ion to sulfur.

It is possible to measure the level of volatile sulfur-containing compounds in the air in the mouth directly by means of a portable sulfide monitor (a great way to plague your friends).

Causes of hepatomegaly

- ***Malignancy:*** Metastatic or primary (usually craggy hepatomegaly).
- ***Hepatic congestion:*** Right heart failure—may be pulsatile in tricuspid incompetence, hepatic vein thrombosis (Budd–Chiari syndrome, p688).
- ***Anatomical:*** Riedel's lobe (normal variant).
- ***Infection:*** Infectious mononucleosis (glandular fever), hepatitis viruses, malaria, schistosomiasis, amoebic abscess, hydatid cyst.
- ***Haematological:*** Leukaemia, lymphoma, myeloproliferative disorders (eg myelofibrosis), sickle-cell disease, haemolytic anaemias.
- ***Others:*** Fatty liver, early cirrhosis, porphyria, storage disorders (eg amyloidosis, Gaucher's disease).

For causes of hepatosplenomegaly, see p624.

Examples of common causes of insomnia

- ***Self-limiting:*** Jet lag, depression, stress, shift work, in hospital.
- ***Psychological:*** Drugs, anxiety, mania, grief.
- ***Organic:*** Nocturia, alcoholism, pain, itch, tinnitus, asthma, dystonias, obstructive sleep apnoea (p186).

Internuclear ophthalmoplegia See BOX 1.

Itching (pruritus) is common and, if chronic, most unpleasant.

Local causes:	***Systemic:*** (Do FBC, ESR, glucose, LFT, U&E, ferritin, TFT)	
Eczema, atopy, urticaria	Liver disease (bile salts eg PBC)	Old age; pregnancy
Scabies	Chronic renal failure	Drugs (eg morphine)
Lichen planus	Malignancy (eg lymphoma)	Diabetes mellitus
Dermatitis herpetiformis	Polycythaemia rubra vera	Thyroid disease
	Iron deficiency anaemia	HIV infection

Questions: Is there itch with weals (urticaria); is itching worse at night and ar others affected (scabies); what provokes it? After a bath ≈ polycythaemia rubr vera (p350). Exposure, eg to animals (atopy?) or fibre glass (irritant eczema?) Loo for ***local causes:*** scabies burrows in the finger webs, lice on hair shafts, knee an elbow blisters (dermatitis herpetiformis). ***Systemic:*** splenomegaly, nodes, jaundic flushed face or thyroid signs? ***Treat*** primary diseases; try soothing blan emollients, eg E45®, ± emollient bath oils and sedative antihistamines at night, e chlorphenamine 4mg PO.

Jaundice See p242. **Jugular venous pulse and pressure** See p30.

Lid lag is lagging behind of the upper eyelid as the eye looks down (after firs looking upwards). **Lid retraction** is the static state of the upper eyelid traversin the eye *above* the iris, rather than over it, causing a 'staring' appearance. ***Caus*** (for both): hyperthyroidism (p202).

Lymphadenopathy may be localised or generalised (see BOX 2). A large le supraclavicular lymph node (Virchow's node) suggests carcinoma of the stomac (Troisier's sign, see p7).

Musculoskeletal symptoms Chiefly ***pain, deformity, reduced function.***

Pain: *Degenerative arthritis* generally produces an aching pain worse with exercis and relieved by rest. Discomfort may worsen with certain motions, and may b associated with 'gelling' of joints, so they get stuck in particular positions. Cervic or lumbar spine degeneration produces a subjective change in sensation no following a dermatomal distribution. Both inflammatory and degenerative joir disease produce *morning stiffness* in affected joints, but in the former th generally improves during the day, while in the latter the pain is worse at the en of the day. The pain of *bone erosion* due to tumour or aneurysm is deep, boring, an constant. The pain of *fracture* or *infection* of the bone is severe and throbbing an is increased by motion of the part. *Acute nerve compression* causes a sharp, seve pain radiating along the distribution of the nerve. Joint pain may be referred, e from a hip disorder to the anterior and lateral aspect of the thigh or the kne shoulder to the lateral aspect of the humerus; cervical spine to the interscapul area, medial border of scapulae or shoulder tip + lateral side of arms. (*Back pai* p528; *GALS locomotor test*, p527.) ***Reduced function:*** Causes include: pain, bone c joint instability, or ↓ joint movement (due to muscle weakness, contractures, bon fusion or mechanical block by intracapsular bony fragments or cartilage).

Nodules (subcutaneous) Rheumatoid nodules, PAN, xanthomata, tuberou sclerosis, neurofibromata, sarcoidosis, granuloma annulare, rheumatic fever.

Nystagmus See p44.

Obesity This is defined by the World Health Organisation as a BMI of over 30kg/m A higher waist to hip ratio, indicating central fat distribution, is commoner in and is associated with greater health risks, which include Type 2 diabetes mellitu IHD, dyslipidaemia, ↑BP, osteoarthritis of weight bearing joints, and cancer (breas and bowel). The majority of cases are not due to specific metabolic disorder Lifestyle change is key to treatment, to increase energy expenditure, and reduc intake (p228). Medication ± surgery may be considered if the patient fulfils stric criteria[1]. Conditions associated with obesity include: genetic (Prader–Wi syndrome, Lawrence-Moon syndrome), hypothyroidism, Cushing's syndrome ar hypothalamic damage (eg tumour or trauma → damage to satiety regions).

Internuclear ophthalmoplegia (INO) and its causes

To produce synchronous eye movements, cranial nerves III, IV, and VI communicate through the medial longitudinal fasciculus in the midbrain. In INO, a lesion disrupts this communication, causing weakness in adduction of the ipsilateral eye with nystagmus of the contralateral eye only when it is abducting. There may be incomplete or slow abduction of the ipsilateral eye during lateral gaze. Convergence is preserved. Chief causes: multiple sclerosis or vascular (more rarely: HIV; syphilis; Lyme disease; brainstem tumours; phenothiazine toxicity).

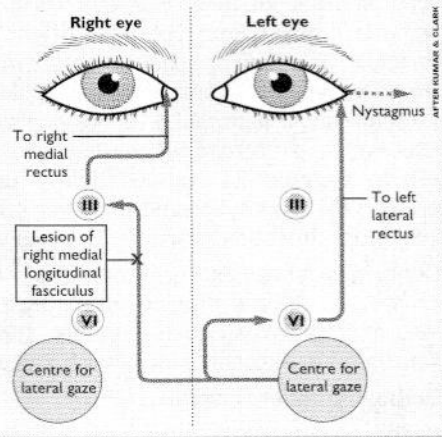

Causes of lymphadenopathy are either reactive or infiltrative

- **Reactive**
  - **Infective**
    - ***Bacterial:*** eg pyogenic, TB, brucella, syphilis.
    - ***Viral:*** EBV, HIV, CMV, infectious hepatitis.
    - ***Others:*** Toxoplasmosis, trypanosomiasis).
  - **Non-infective** Sarcoidosis, amyloidosis, berylliosis, connective tissue disease (eg rheumatoid, SLE), dermatological (eczema, psoriasis), drugs (eg phenytoin).
- **Infiltrative**
  - **Benign** Histiocytosis—*OHCS* p644, lipoidoses.
  - **Malignant**
    - ***Haematological:*** Lymphoma or leukaemia: ALL, CLL, AML (p340).
    - ***Metastatic carcinoma:*** From breast, lung, bowel, prostate, kidney or head and neck cancers.

See NICE guidance on orlistat, sibutramine (2001), and surgery for morbid obesity.

Oedema (p564). ***Causes:*** ↑*Local venous pressure* eg DVT or right-heart failure ↓*intravascular oncotic pressure:* ↓plasma proteins, eg in cirrhosis, nephrot syndrome, malnutrition, or protein-losing enteropathy: here water moves down tl osmotic gradient into the interstitium to dilute the solutes there—Starlinc principle. On standing, venous pressure at the ankle rises due to the height of bloc from the heart (~100mmHg). This is short-lived if leg movement pumps bloc through valved veins, but if venous pressure rises, or valves fail, capillary pressu rises and fluid is forced out causing oedema. ***Pitting oedema*** (fig 1 & p564). ***No pitting oedema:*** (ie non-indentible) ≈ poor lymph drainage (lymphoedema), e primary (Milroy's syndrome, p698) or secondary, due to radiotherapy, maligna infiltration, infection, filariasis. The mechanism is complex.

Oliguria is defined as a urine output of <400mL/24h. This occurs in renal failu causes are divided into pre-renal (hypovolaemia, severe dehydration, cardi failure), intrinsic causes or post-renal (urethral or bilateral ureteric obstructior **Anuria** means absent urine output. See p284 and p562. ARF: see p292.

Orthopnoea See **Dyspnoea** (p58).

Pallor is a non-specific sign and may be racial or familial. Pathology suggested l pallor includes anaemia, shock, Stokes–Adams attack, vasovagal faint, hypothyroi ism, hypopituitarism, and albinism.

Palmar erythema ***Causes:*** Pregnancy, hyperthyroidism, rheumatoid arthrit polycythaemia, drugs (eg 5-fluorouracil) or chronic liver disease—via ↓inactivati of vasoactive endotoxins by the liver.

Palpitations represent to the patient the sensation of feeling his heart beat; to tl doctor, the sensation of feeling his heart sink, as the symptom is notoriously elu ive. Have the patient tap out the rate and rhythm of the palpitations. • Irregul fast palpitations are likely to be paroxysmal AF, or atrial flutter with variable blo • Regular fast palpitations may reflect paroxysmal SVT or VT. • Dropped or miss beats related to rest, recumbency or eating are likely to be atrial or ventricul ectopics. • Regular pounding may be due to anxiety • Slow palpitations are like to be due to drugs such as β-blockers, or due to bigeminus. Ask about associat chest pain, dyspnoea, and faints, suggesting haemodynamic compromise. Ask *wh* symptoms occur: anxious people may be aware of their own heartbeat at nigh Reassurance is vital and can often be therapeutic. If the diagnosis is not simp heightened awareness, do TSH and a 24h ECG. (Holter monitor, p94) Transtelephon event recording, if available, is better than 24h ECGs which miss some attacks.

Paraesthesiae A sensation described as pins and needles, numbness or tinglin which can be intense and painful. ***Causes*** include: ↓Ca^{2+} (perioral), Raynaud syndrome or any sensory nerve lesion ie **1** Central—thalamic or parietal lesior **2** Spinal cord lesions or **3** Peripheral: *mononeuropathies* (p494): Carpal tunn syndrome, meralgia paraesthetica, lateral popliteal palsy, sciatica; *peripher neuropathy* (p496)—typically 'glove & stocking' in distribution.

Paraphimosis occurs when a tight foreskin is retracted and then becom irreplaceable as the glans swells. It can occur when a doctor/nurse fails to repla the foreskin after catheterization. ►►Treat by asking the patient to squeeze tl glans for half an hour. Or try soaking a swab in 50% dextrose, and applying it the oedematous area for an hour before trying to replace the foreskin—the oeder may follow the osmotic gradient.

Percussion pain Pain on percussing the abdomen is a sign of peritonitis, and often less painful for the patient than testing **Rebound abdominal pain** (p70).

Phimosis The foreskin occludes the meatus, obstructing urine. Tin (± trials of gentle retraction) usually obviates the need for circumcision.

Polyuria is an increase in urine volume eg >3L/24h. ***Causes:*** Diabetes mellit over-enthusiastic IVI treatment, diabetes insipidus (including ↑Ca^{2+}; see p224 psychogenic polydipsia, polyuric phase of renal failure.

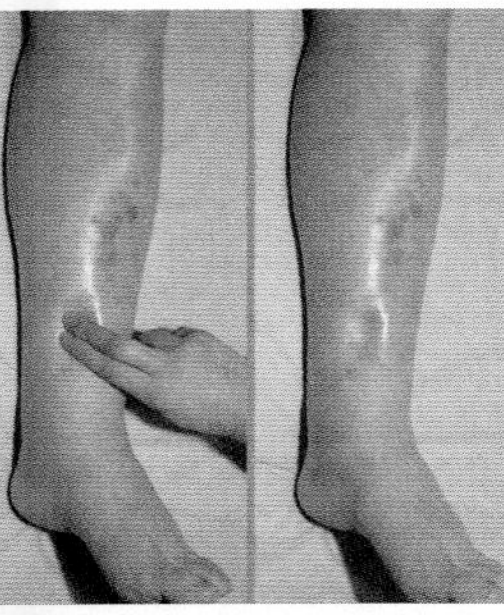

ig 1. Pitting oedema, detected by applying firm pressure for a few seconds.

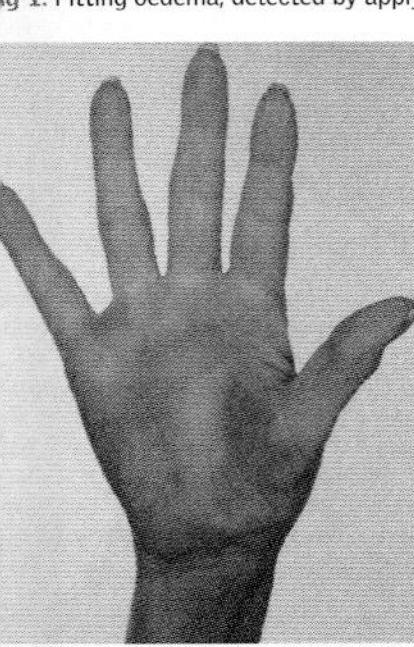

ig 2. Palmar erythema.

Palpitations, Russian roulette, and hypochondriasis

At night on my pillow the syncopated stagger
Of the pulse in my ear. Russian roulette:
Every heartbeat a fresh throw of the dice . . .
Hypochondria walked, holding my arm
Like a nurse, her fingers over my pulse . . .
The sudden lapping at my throat of loose blood . . . Ted Hughes, *Birthday Letters*. Faber & Faber, by kind permission.

Postural hypotension is defined as a drop in systolic BP >20mmHg or diastoli >10mmHg after standing for 3 minutes, compared with lying down. ***Causes*** Hypovolaemia (an early sign), drugs (eg nitrates, diuretics, antihypertensives Addison's disease (p210), hypopituitarism (↓ACTH), autonomic neuropathy (e diabetes, multisystem atrophy, p486), idiopathic orthostatic hypotension.

Prostatism (p40 and p602) Symptoms of prostate enlargement are often terme 'prostatism', but it is better to use the terms *irritative* or *obstructive* bladde symptoms. **1** ***Irritative bladder symptoms:*** Urgency, dysuria, frequency, noctur (the last two are also associated with causes of **Polyuria**). **2** ***Obstructiv symptoms***: Reduced size and force of urinary stream, hesitancy and interruption c stream during voiding and terminal dribbling—the usual cause is enlargement c the prostate (prostatic hypertrophy), but other causes include a urethral stricture tumour, urethral valves, or bladder neck contracture. The maximum flow rate c urine is normally ~18–30mL/s.

Pruritus See **Itching**, p64.

Ptosis is drooping of the upper eyelid. It is best observed with the patient sittin up, his head held by the examiner. The 3rd cranial nerve (oculomotor nerve, CNII innervates the main muscle concerned (levator palpebrae), but nerves from th cervical sympathetic chain innervate the superior tarsal muscle, and a lesion c these nerves will cause a mild ptosis which can be overcome on looking up. ***Causes*** **1** CNIII lesions (p45) cause a unilateral *complete* ptosis. Look for other evidence c a CNIII lesion: ophthalmoplegia with 'down and out' deviation of the eye, pup dilated and unreactive to light and accommodation. **2** Sympathetic paralysi usually causes a unilateral *partial* ptosis. Look for other evidence of a sympatheti lesion, as in Horner's syndrome (p694): constricted pupil = *miosis*, lack of sweatin on same side of the face (= *anhidrosis*). **3** Myopathy eg dystrophia myotonica myasthenia gravis. These cause a bilateral partial ptosis. **4** Congenital (preser since birth). May be unilateral or bilateral, is usually partial and is not associate with other neurological signs.

Pulses See p30.

Pupillary abnormalities The key questions are: • Are the pupils equal, centra circular, dilated, or constricted? • Do they react to light, directly and consensually • Do they constrict normally on convergence/accommodation?
Irregular pupils are caused by iritis, syphilis, or globe rupture. ***Dilated pupil*** Causes: 3rd cranial nerve (CNIII) lesions (▶including ↑ICP, p812) and mydriati drugs. But always ask: is this pupil dilated, or is it the other which is constricted ***Constricted pupils*** are associated with old age, sympathetic nerve damag (Horner's syndrome, p694, and see **Ptosis** above), opiates, miotics (eg pilocarpin eye-drops for glaucoma), and pontine damage. ***Unequal pupils (anisocoria)*** ma be due to a unilateral lesion, eye-drops, eye surgery, syphilis, or be a Holmes–Adi pupil (p70). Some inequality is normal.
Reaction to light: Test by covering one eye and shining light into the othe obliquely. Both pupils should constrict, one by the direct, and the other by th consensual or indirect light reflex. The lesion site may be deduced by knowing th pathway: from the retina the message passes up the optic nerve (cranial nerve I to the superior colliculus (midbrain) and thence to the CNIII nuclei bilaterally. CNII causes pupillary constriction. If a light in one eye causes only contralatera constriction, the defect is 'efferent', as the afferent pathways from the retina bein stimulated must be intact. Test for a *relative afferent pupillary defect* by movin the torch quickly from pupil to pupil. If there has been incomplete damage to th afferent pathway (eg due to optic neuritis in multiple sclerosis), the affected pup will paradoxically dilate when the light is moved from the normal eye to th abnormal eye. This is because, in the face of reduced afferent input from th affected eye, the consensual pupillary relaxation response from the normal ey predominates. This phenomenon is also known as the Marcus Gunn sign, and ma occur after apparent complete recovery from the initial lesion.

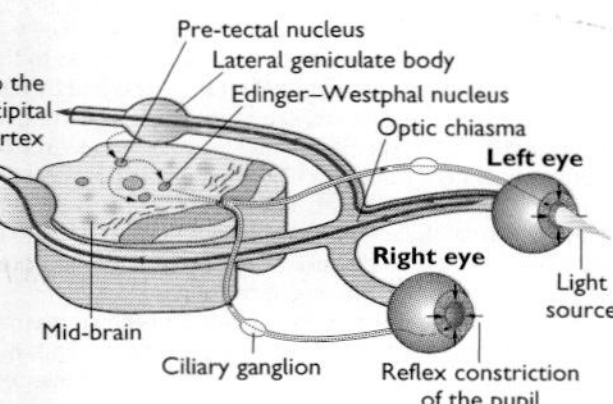

1. Light reflex. Action potentials are sent down the optic nerve (red arrow) ssing through the optic chiasma. These synapse at the pre-tectal nucleus and are t to the Edinger–Westphal nucleus of cranial nerve III, causing bilateral illary constriction.

Reaction to accommodation/convergence: If the patient first looks at a distan object and then at the examiner's finger held a few inches away, the eyes wi converge and the pupils constrict. Afferent fibres in each optic nerve pass to th lateral geniculate bodies. Impulses then pass to the pre-tectal nucleus and then t the parasympathetic nuclei of the 3rd cranial nerves, causing pupillary constrictior

- ***Holmes–Adie (myotonic) pupil:*** This is a benign condition, which occurs usuall in women and is unilateral in about 80% of cases. The affected pupil is normall moderately dilated and is poorly reactive to light, if at all. It is slowly reactive t accommodation; wait and watch carefully: it may eventually constrict more tha a normal pupil. It is often associated with diminished or absent ankle and kne reflexes, in which case the Holmes–Adie syndrome is present.
- ***Argyll Robertson pupil:*** This occurs in neurosyphilis; a similar phenomenon ma occur in diabetes mellitus. The pupil is constricted and unreactive to light, bu reacts to accommodation. The iris may be patchily atrophied and depigmentec Pseudo-Argyll Robertson pupils occur in Parinaud's syndrome (p700).
- ***Hutchinson pupil:*** This is the sequence of events resulting from rapidly risin unilateral intracranial pressure (eg in intracerebral haemorrhage). The pupil o the side of the lesion first constricts then widely dilates. The other pupil the goes through the same sequence. ►See p812.

Radio-femoral and radio-radial delay See p28.

Rebound abdominal pain is present if, on the sudden removal of pressure from th examiner's hand, the patient feels a *momentary increase* in pain. It signifies loca peritoneal inflammation, manifesting as pain as the peritoneum rebounds afte being gently displaced.

Rectal bleeding Ascertain details about • Pain on defecation? • Any mucus? • I it fresh or dark blood? • Is blood mixed with stool, or just on surface? • Is bloo just on toilet paper, or also in the pan? ***Causes & classical features:*** Diverticulit (painless, large volumes of blood in pan); colorectal cancer (blood mixed wit stool); haemorrhoids (bright red blood on paper and in pan); fissure-*in-ano* (painfu bright red blood on paper and stool surface); inflammatory bowel disease (bloo and mucus mixed with loose stool). Also seen with dysentery (gastroenteritis trauma, polyps, angiodysplasia, ischaemic colitis, iatrogenic (eg due to radiatio proctitis, post-polypectomy bleeding, aorto-enteric fistula after aortic surgery)

Regurgitation Gastric and oesophageal contents are regurgitated effortlessly int the mouth—without contraction of abdominal muscles and diaphragm (s distinguishing it from true vomiting). It may be worse on lying flat, and can caus cough and nocturnal asthma. Regurgitation is rarely preceded by nausea, and whe due to gastro-oesophageal reflux, it is often associated with heartburn. A oesophageal pouch may cause regurgitation. Very high GI obstructions (eg gastri volvulus, p595) cause non-productive retching rather than true regurgitation.

Rigors are uncontrolled, sometimes violent episodes of shivering, which occur as patient's temperature rises rapidly. See p376.

Skin discolouration Generalized hyperpigmentation may be genetic (racial), or du to radiation; ↑ACTH (cross reacts with melanin receptors, eg Addison's diseas p210, Nelson's syndrome p700, ectopic ACTH in bronchial carcinoma); chronic ren failure (↑urea, p294); malabsorption; chloasma (seen in pregnancy or with the or contraceptive pill); biliary cirrhosis; haemochromatosis ('bronzed diabetes' carotenaemia; or drugs (eg chlorpromazine, busulfan, amiodarone, gold).

Splenomegaly Abnormally large spleen. ***Causes:*** See p624. If massive, think c chronic myeloid leukaemia, myelofibrosis, leishmaniasis or malaria.

Sputum See p37.

Steatorrhoea These are pale stools that are difficult to flush, and are caused b malabsorption of fat in the small intestine and hence greater fat content in th stool. ***Causes:*** Ileal disease (eg Crohn's or ileal resection), pancreatic disease, ar obstructive jaundice (due to ↓excretion of bile salts from the gall bladder).

Stridor is an *inspiratory* sound due to partial obstruction of the upper airwa That obstruction may be due to something within the lumen (eg foreign bo tumour, bilateral vocal cord palsy), within the wall (eg oedema from anaphyla: laryngospasm, tumour, croup, acute epiglottitis), or extrinsic (eg goitre, lym adenopathy). It is a medical (or surgical) emergency (⊳⊳p760) if the airway compromised. NB: wheeze is an *expiratory* sound.

Surgical (subcutaneous) emphysema A crackling sensation felt on palpating skin over the chest or neck. It is caused by air tracking from the lungs, often due a pneumothorax (or, rarely, a pneumomediastinum, eg after oesophageal ruptu

Sweating excessively (hyperhidrosis) This may be **primary** (eg hidraden suppurativa may be very distressing to the patient who may shun soc encounters)—or be **secondary** to fever, pain or anxiety (cold & sweaty) o systemic condition: the menopause, hyperthyroidism (warm & sweaty), acromega malignancy, phaeochromocytoma, amyloidosis, or neuroleptic malignant syndro (+hyperthermia). Or it may reflect gabapentin or opiate **withdrawal**, or a **cholin gic** or **parasympathomimetic side-effect** (amitriptyline, bethanechol, distigmine also hormonal drugs, eg levothyroxine, gonadorelin or somatostatin analogu vasopressin, and ephedrine. Also amiodarone, ciprofloxacin, L-dopa, lisinop rivastigmine, ritonavir, pioglitazone, venlafaxine. ***At the bedside:*** Ask about drugs, examine *all over* for nodes; any signs of hyperthyroidism? Any sple megaly? Test the urine; do T°, ESR, TSH, FBC & blood culture. ***℞:*** Antiperspira (aluminium chloride 20%=Driclor®), sympathectomy, or iontophoresis may be tri

Syncope See p452. **Tactile vocal fremitus** See p38.

Tenesmus This is a sensation in the rectum of incomplete emptying *after* defec ion. It's common in irritable bowel syndrome (p268), but can be caused by a tumo

Terminal dribbling Dribbling at the end of urination, often seen in conjunction w incontinence following incomplete urination, associated with **prostatism** (p6

Tinnitus See p456. **Tiredness** See **Fatigue** p60.

Tremor is rhythmic oscillation of limbs, trunk, head, or tongue. 3 types:

1 ***Resting tremor***—worst at rest—eg from Parkinsonism (±bradykinesia a rigidity; tremor is more resistant to treatment than other symptoms). It usually a slow tremor (3–5Hz), typically 'pill-rolling' of the thumb over a fing
2 ***Postural tremor***—worst if arms are outstretched. Typically a rapid tren (frequency: 8–12Hz). May be exaggerated physiological tremor (eg anxie hyperthyroidism, alcohol, drugs), due to brain damage (eg Wilson's disea syphilis) or *benign essential tremor* (BET). This is usually a familial (autosor dominant) tremor of arms and head presenting at any age. It is suppressed large-ish amounts of alcohol. Rarely progressive. Propranolol (40–80mg/8–1 PO) helps in ~30% of patients.
3 ***Intention tremor***—worst on movement, seen in cerebellar disease, with pa pointing and dysdiadochokinesia (see p491). No effective drug has been fou

See also **chorea** (p54), **athetosis** (p460), and **hemiballismus** (p460).

Trousseau's sign Seen in hypocalcaemia (p670). This is elicited by inflating a blc pressure cuff on an arm/leg to above systolic pressure. The hands and feet go i spasm (carpopedal spasm). The metacarpophalangeal joints become flexed and interphalangeal joints are extended. See also **Chvostek's sign**.

Urinary changes ***Cloudy urine*** suggests pus (UTI) but is often normal phosph precipitation in an alkaline urine. ***Pneumaturia*** (bubbles in urine as it is pass occurs with UTI due to gas-forming organisms or may signal an enterovesi (bowel–bladder) fistula from diverticulitis, Crohn's disease or neoplastic diseas the bowel. ***Nocturia*** occurs with 'prostatism' (p68), diabetes mellitus, UTI, a reversed diurnal rhythm (seen in renal and cardiac failure). ***Haematuria*** (RBC urine) is due to neoplasia or glomerulonephritis (p288) until proven otherwis

Urinary frequency See **Frequency** p60. **Vaginal discharge** p406. **Vertigo** p4

Signs and symptoms

Visual loss ►Get ophthalmic help. See OHCS p434–p455 & BOX. ***If sudden, ask:***
- Is the eye red? (*glaucoma, iritis* p544)
- Is there pain?
  - *Giant cell arteritis*: severe temporal headache, jaw claudication, scal tenderness, ↑ESR: ►requires urgent steroids (p542).
  - *Optic neuritis*: eg as in multiple sclerosis.
- Any flashes/floaters? (*TIA, migraine, retinal detachment*?)
- Any past history of trauma, migraine, hypertension, cerebrovascular disease, M diabetes or connective tissue disease?

In the examination, consider:
- Is the eye red? See p545 for the *Red Eye*
- Is the cornea cloudy: *corneal ulcer* (OHCS p432), *glaucoma* (OHCS p430)?
- Is there a contact lens problem (*infection*)?
- Is there a visual field problem (*stroke, space-occupying lesion, glaucoma*)? Formal field testing requires ophthalmic help.
- Are there any focal CNS signs?
- Any valvular heart disease/carotid bruits (*emboli*)?; Hyperlipidaemia (p682)?
- Is there an afferent pupil defect (p68)?
- Any distant signs: eg *HIV* (causes retinitis), *SLE, sarcoidosis, Behçet's disease*?

Perform ophthalmoscopy, examine acuity, pupil reactions, red reflex, field loss.

Voice and disturbance of speech (p46) may be noted by the patient, relatives c the doctor. Assess if difficulty is with articulation (*dysarthria*, eg from musc problems), or of word command (*dysphasia*—always central).

Vocal resonance See p39 and p78.

Vomiting Causes of nausea/vomiting include (anti-emetic ℞: p233)

Gastrointestinal	CNS	Metabolic/Endocrine
Gastroenteritis	Meningitis/encephalitis	Uraemia
Peptic ulceration	Migraine	Hypercalcaemia
Pyloric stenosis	↑Intracranial pressure	Hyponatraemia
Intestinal obstruction	Brainstem lesions	Pregnancy
Paralytic ileus	Motion sickness	Diabetic ketoacidosis
Acute cholecystitis	Ménière's disease	Addison's disease
Acute pancreatitis	Labyrinthitis	Alcohol and drugs:
Other	Psychiatric:	• antibiotics
Myocardial infarction	• self-induced	• cytotoxics
Autonomic neuropathy	• psychogenic	• digoxin
UTI	• bulimia nervosa	• opiates

The history is vital: ask about timing, relationship to meals, amount, and conte (liquid, solid, bile, blood, 'coffee grounds'). Associated symptoms and previo medical history often indicate the cause. ***Signs:*** Look for signs of dehydratio Examine the abdomen for distension, tenderness, an abdominal mass, a succussic splash (pyloric stenosis), or tinkling bowel sounds (intestinal obstruction).

Walking difficulty ('Off my legs') In the elderly, this is a common and no specific presentation: the reason may not be ***local*** (typically osteo- or rheumato arthritis, but remember fractured neck of femur), and it may not even be ***system*** (eg UTI, pneumonia, anaemia, hypothyroidism, renal failure, drugs, hypothermia) but it may be a manifestation of depression or bereavement. *It is only rarely manipulative strategy.* See **Falls**, and gait disturbance, p459.

If there is ataxia, the cause is not always alcohol: other chemicals may b involved (eg cannabis or prescribed sedatives). There may be a metastatic or no metastatic manifestation of malignancy, or a cerebellar lesion.

►Bilateral weak legs may suggest a cord lesion: see p458. If there is associate urinary or faecal incontinence ± saddle anaesthesia or lower limb sensory los prompt imaging (MRI) and treatment for cord compression may well be needec

Causes of vision loss

Sudden
- Acute glaucoma
- Retinal detachment
- Vitreous haemorrhage (eg in diabetic proliferative retinopathy)
- Optic neuritis (eg MS)
- Temporal arteritis
- Central retinal artery or vein occlusion
- Migraine
- CNS: TIA (amaurosis fugax), stroke, space occupying lesion
- Drugs: quinine or methanol toxicity
- Pituitary apoplexy.

Gradual
- Optic atrophy
- Chronic glaucoma
- Cataracts
- Macular degeneration
- Tobacco amblyopia.

Non-gastrointestinal causes of vomiting

►Try not to forget these serious causes. The following *aide-mémoire* covers the most important non-gastrointestinal causes of vomiting: **ABCDEFGHI.**
- Acute renal failure/Addison's disease
- Brain (eg ↑ICP, p812)
- Cardiac (myocardial infarct)
- Diabetic ketoacidosis
- Ears (eg labyrinthitis, Ménière's disease)
- Foreign substances (alcohol, drugs eg opiates)
- Gravidity (eg hyperemesis gravidarum)
- Hypercalcaemia/Hyponatraemia
- Infection (eg UTI, meningitis).

Waterbrash refers to the excessive secretion of saliva, which suddenly fills the mouth. It typically occurs after meals, and may denote upper GI tract disease. It is suggested that this is an exaggeration of the oesophago-salivary reflex. It should not be confused with **regurgitation** (p70).

Weight loss is a feature of chronic disease and depression; also of malnutrition, malignancy, chronic infections (eg TB, HIV/enteropathic AIDS), diabetes mellitus and hyperthyroidism (typically in the presence of increased appetite). Severe generalized muscle wasting is also seen as part of a number of degenerative neurological diseases and in cardiac failure (cardiac cachexia), although in the latter, right heart failure may not make weight loss a major complaint. Do not forget anorexia nervosa (*OHCS* p348) as an underlying cause of weight loss.

Focus on treatable causes, eg diabetes is easy to diagnose—TB can be very hard. For example, the CXR may look like cancer, so you may forget to send bronchoscopy samples for ZN stain and TB culture (to the detriment not just of the patient, but to the entire ward).

Wheeze See p38.

Whispering pectoriloquy This refers to the increased transmission of a patient's whisper heard when auscultating over consolidated lung. It is a manifestation of increased vocal resonance. See p38–p39. ***Vocal resonance*** is sound vibration of the patient's spoken or whispered voice transmitted to the stethoscope. ***Tactile fremitus*** is the sound vibration of the spoken or whispered voice transmitted via the lung fields and detected by palpation over the back.

Xanthomata These are localized deposits of fat under the skin, occurring over joints, tendons, hands, and feet. They are a sign of dyslipidaemia (p682). ***Xanthelasma*** refers to xanthoma on the eyelid (p101, fig 1). ***Corneal arcus*** is a crescentic shaped opacity at the periphery of the cornea. It is common in the over 60yrs, and can be normal, but may represent hyperlipidaemia, especially in those under this age.

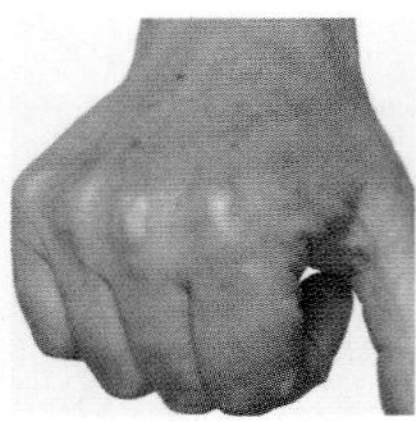

Fig 1. Tendon xanthomata.

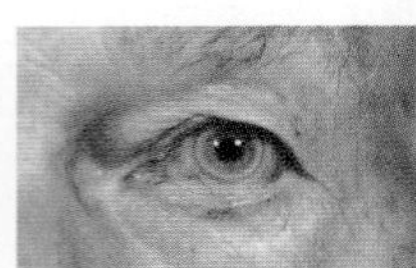

Fig 2. Corneal arcus.

Unexplained signs and symptoms: how to refer a patient for an opinion

►*When you don't know: ask.*

►*If you find yourself wondering if you should ask: ask.*

Frequently, the skills needed will lie beyond the firm you are working on, so, during ward rounds, agree who should be asked for an opinion. You will be left with the job of making the arrangements. This can be a daunting task, if you are very junior and have been asked to contact an intimidating registrar or consultant. Don't be intimidated: perhaps this may be an opportunity to learn something new. A few simple points can help the process go smoothly.

- Have the patient's notes, observations, and drug charts to hand.
- Be familiar with the history: you may be interrogated.
- Ask if it is a convenient time to talk.
- At the outset, state if you are just looking for advice or if you are asking if the patient could be seen. Make it clear exactly what the question is that you want addressed, 'We wonder why Mr Smith's legs have become weak today . . .' This helps the listener to focus their thoughts while you describe the story and will save you wasting time if the switchboard has put you through to the wrong specialist.
- Give the patient's age and occupation to give a snapshot of the person.
- Run through a brief history including relevant past medical history. Do not present the case as if you are in finals—it will take ages to get to the point and the listener will get more and more irritated.
- If you would like the patient to be seen, give warning if they will be going off the ward for a test at a particular time.
- It should not be necessary to write a long letter in the notes if you have given all the salient information available.
- The visiting doctor may be unfamiliar with your ward. When he or she arrives introduce yourself, get the notes and charts, and offer to introduce them to the patient. This will lead to all-round satisfaction and will make it easier to call the same doctor again.

We thank Martin Zeidler for providing the first draft of this page.

4 Cardiovascular medicine

Contents

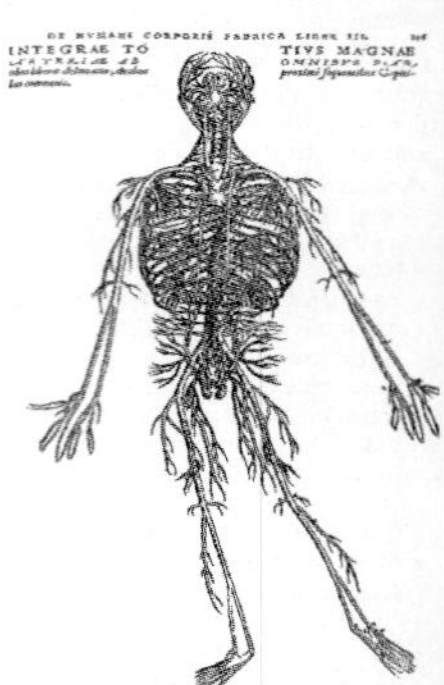

Fig 1. The vasculature, as depicted in Andreas Vesalius's, *De Humani Corporis Fabrica* (On the fabric of the human body). At the age of 23, the day after his finals, he dissected a body with such vivid brilliance that he was at once made Professor of Surgery at Padua. By general acclamation, modern medicine began that day: December 6th, 1537. Galen's infallibility was now and forever trumped by direct observation, experiment, and the painstaking accumulation of data.

Other relevant pages: Immediate management of MI (p782); cardiac shock (p788); CVS exam (p28); carotid bruit (p54); cyanosis (p56); dyspnoea (p58); haemoptysis (p62); oedema (p66); palpitations (p66); aneurysms (p586); dyslipidaemia (p682); risk factor analysis (p642); pulmonary oedema (p786); nuclear cardiology and other cardiac images (p726); broad & narrow complex tachycardias (p790 & p792); ***Cardiac arrest:*** see inside back cover.

We thank Dr Rajesh Kharbanda, our Specialist Reader for this chapter.

Cardiovascular health

Ischaemic heart disease (IHD) is the most common cause of death worldwide. Encouraging cardiovascular health is not *only* about preventing IHD: health entails the ability to *exercise*, and enjoying vigorous activity (within reason!) is one of the best ways of achieving health, not just because the heart likes it (BP↓, 'good' high-density lipoprotein, HDL↑)—it can prevent osteoporosis, improve glucose tolerance, and augment immune function (eg in cancer and if HIV+ve). People who improve *and maintain* their fitness live longer: ►*age-adjusted mortality from all causes is reduced by >40%*. Avoiding obesity helps too, but weight loss *per se* is only useful in reducing cardiovascular risk and the risk of developing diabetes when combined with regular exercise. Moderate alcohol drinking may also promote cardiovascular health. Alcohol also reduces gastric infection with *Helicobacter pylori*, a known risk marker for cardiovascular disease.

Smoking is the chief risk factor for cardiovascular mortality. You *can* help people give up, and giving up *does* undo much of the harm of smoking. *Simple advice works*. Most smokers want to give up (unlike the eaters of unhealthy diets who are mostly wedded to them by habit, and the pleasures of the palate). Just because smoking advice does *not always* work, do not stop giving it. Ask about smoking in consultations—especially those concerned with smoking-related diseases.

- Ensure advice is congruent with patient's beliefs about smoking.
- Concentrate on the benefits of giving up.
- Invite the patient to choose a date (when there will be few stresses) on which he or she will become a non-smoker.
- Suggest throwing away all accessories (cigarettes, pipes, ash trays, lighters, matches) in advance; inform friends of the new change; practise saying 'no' to their offers of 'just one little cigarette'.
- *Nicotine gum*, chewed intermittently to limit nicotine release: ≥ ten 2mg sticks may be needed/day. *Transdermal nicotine patches* may be easier. A dose increase at 1wk can help. Written advice offers no added benefit to advice from nurses. Always offer follow-up.
- *Bupropion* (=*amfebutamone*, p443) is said to ↑quit rate to 30% at 1yr *vs* 16% with patches and 15.6% for placebo (patches + bupropion: 35.5%): consider if the above fails. *Dose:* 150mg/24h PO (while still smoking; quit within 2wks); dose may be twice daily from day 7; stop after 7–9wks. ***Warn of SEs:*** Seizures (risk <1 : 1000), insomnia, headache. *CI:* Epilepsy; cirrhosis; pregnancy/lactation; bipolar depression; eating disorders; CNS tumours; on antimalarials etc; alcohol or benzodiazepine withdrawal, sedating antihistamines, systemic corticosteroids.

Lipids and BP (p682 & p124) are the other major modifiable risk factors (few can change their sex or genes).

To calculate how risk factors interact, see **risk equation**, p642.

►Apply preventive measures such as healthy eating (p228) *early* in life to maximize impact, when there are most years to save, and before bad habits get ingrained.

For an example of implementation of cardiovascular health strategies, see the UK NHS national service framework: www.doh.gov.uk/nsf/coronary.htm

Cardiovascular symptoms

Chest pain ►Cardiac-sounding chest pain may have no serious cause, but always think *'Could this be a myocardial infarction (MI), dissecting aortic aneurysm, pericarditis, or pulmonary embolism?'*

Nature: *Constricting* suggests angina, oesophageal spasm, or anxiety; a *sharp* pain may be from the pleura or pericardium. A prolonged (>½h), dull, central crushing pain or pressure suggests MI.

Radiation: To shoulder, either or both arms, or neck/jaw suggests cardiac ischaemia. The pain of aortic dissection is classically instantaneous, tearing, and interscapular, but may be retrosternal. Epigastric pain may be cardiac.

Precipitants: Pain associated with cold, exercise, palpitations, or emotion suggest cardiac pain or anxiety; if brought on by food, lying flat, hot drinks, or alcohol, consider oesophageal spasm (but meals *can* cause angina).

Relieving factors: If pain is relieved *within minutes* by rest or glyceryl trinitrate (GTN), suspect angina (GTN relieves oesophageal spasm more slowly). If antacids help, suspect GI causes. Pericarditic pain improves on leaning forward.

Associations: Dyspnoea occurs with cardiac pain, pulmonary emboli, pleurisy, or anxiety. MI may cause nausea, vomiting, or sweating. Angina is caused by coronary artery disease—and also by aortic stenosis, hypertrophic obstructive cardiomyopathy (HOCM), paroxysmal supraventricular tachycardia (SVT) and be exacerbated by anaemia. Chest pain with *tenderness* suggests self-limiting Tietze's syndrome.[1]

Pleuritic pain (ie exacerbated by inspiration) implies inflammation of the pleura from pulmonary infection, inflammation, or infarction. It causes us to 'catch our breath'. ΔΔ: Musculoskeletal pain;[1] fractured rib (pain on respiration, exacerbated by gentle pressure on the sternum); subdiaphragmatic pathology (eg gallstones).

Acutely ill patients: • Admit to hospital • Check pulse, BP in both arms, JVP, heart sounds; examine legs for DVT • Give O_2 by mask • IV line • Relieve pain (eg morphine 5–10mg IV slowly (2mg/min) + an antiemetic) • Cardiac monitor • 12-lead ECG • CXR • Arterial blood gas (ABG). ***Famous traps:*** Aortic dissection; zoster (p388); ruptured oesophagus; cardiac tamponade (shock with JVP↑); opiate addiction.

Dyspnoea may be from LVF, pulmonary embolism, any respiratory cause, or anxiety. ***Severity:*** ►►Emergency presentations: p770. Ask about shortness of breath at rest or on exertion, exercise tolerance, and in daily tasks. ***Associations:*** Specific symptoms associated with heart failure are orthopnoea (ask about number of pillows used at night), paroxysmal nocturnal dyspnoea (waking up at night gasping for breath), and peripheral oedema. Pulmonary embolism is associated with acute onset of dyspnoea and pleuritic chest pain; ask about risk factors for DVT.

Palpitation(s) may be due to ectopics, AF, SVT and ventricular tachycardia (VT), thyrotoxicosis, anxiety, and rarely phaeochromocytoma. See p66. ***History:*** Ask about previous episodes, precipitating/relieving factors, duration of symptoms, associated chest pain, dyspnoea, or dizziness. *Did the patient check his pulse?*

Syncope may reflect cardiac or CNS events. Vasovagal 'faints' are common (pulse↓, pupils dilated). The history from an observer is invaluable in diagnosis. ***Prodromal symptoms:*** Chest pain, palpitations, or dyspnoea point to a cardiac cause, eg arrhythmia. Aura, headache, dysarthria, and limb weakness indicate CNS causes. ***During the episode:*** Was there a pulse? Limb jerking, tongue biting, or urinary incontinence? **NB:** hypoxia from lack of cerebral perfusion may cause seizures. ***Recovery:*** Was this rapid (arrhythmia) or prolonged, with drowsiness (seizure)?

1 25% of non-cardiac chest pain is **musculoskeletal**: look for pain on specific postures or activity. Aim to reproduce the pain by movement and, sometimes, palpation over the structure causing it. Focal injection of local anaesthetic helps diagnostically and is therapeutic. **Tietze's syndrome:** self-limiting costochondritis ± costosternal joint swelling. Causes: idiopathic; microtrauma; infection; psoriatic/rheumatoid arthritis. **℞:** NSAIDs or steroid injections. Tenderness is also caused by: fibrositis, lymphoma, chondrosarcoma, myeloma, metastases, rib TB. Imaging: bone scintigraphy; CT.

ow patients communicate ischaemic cardiac sensations

n emergency wards we are always hearing questions such as 'is your pain harp or dull?', followed by an equivocal answer. The doctor goes on 'Sharp like a nife—or dull and crushing?' The doctor is getting irritated because the patient nust know the answer, but is not saying it. A true story paves the way to being ess inquisitorial, and having a more creative understanding of the nature of ymptoms. A patient came to one of us (JML) saying 'Last night I dreamed I had pain in my chest. Now I've woken up, and I'm not sure—have I got chest pain, octor? What do you think?' How odd it is to find oneself examining a patient to xclude a symptom, not a disease. (It turned out that she *did* have serious chest athology.) Odd, until one realizes that symptoms are often half-formed, and it is ur role to give them a local habitation and a name. Dialogue can transform a ymptom from 'airy nothingness' to a fact.[1] Patients often avoid using the word ain' to describe ischaemia: 'wind', 'tightening', 'pressure', 'burning', or 'a lump in ne throat' (angina means to choke) may be used. He may say 'sharp' to ommunicate severity, and not character. So be as vague in your questioning as our patient is in his answers. 'Tell me some more about what you are feeling ong pause) ... as if someone was doing *what* to you?' 'Sitting on me', or 'like a otness' might be the response (suggesting cardiac ischaemia). Do not ask 'Does go into your left arm'. Try 'Is there anything else about it?' (pause) ... 'Does it o anywhere?' Note down your patient's exact words.

Note also non-verbal clues: the clenched fist placed over the sternum is a elling feature of cardiac pain (Levine sign positive).

A good history, taking account of these features, is the best way to stratify atients likely to have cardiac pain. If the history is non-specific, and there are o risk factors for cardiovascular diseases, and ECG and plasma troponin T p104) are normal (<0.2µg/L) 6–12h after the onset of pain, discharge will robably be OK. When in doubt, get help. Features making cardiac pain unlikely:

- Stabbing, shooting pain
- Pain lasting <30s, however intense
- Well-localized, left sub-mammary pain ('in my heart, doctor')
- Pains of continually varying location
- Youth.

o not feel that you must diagnose every pain. ***Chest pain with no cause*** is ommon, even after extensive tests. Do not reject these patients: explain your ndings to them. Some have a 'chronic pain syndrome' which responds to a ricyclic, eg imipramine 50mg at night (this dose does not imply any depression). t is similar to post-herpetic neuralgia.

[1] Dialogue-transformed symptoms explain one of the junior doctor's main vexations: when patients ell symptoms to a consultant in the light of day, they bear no resemblance to what you originally ard. But do not be vexed: your dialogue may have helped the patient far more than any ward round.

ECG—a methodical approach

►First confirm the patient's name and age, and the ECG date. Then:

- ***Rate:*** At usual speed (25mm/s) each 'big square' is 0.2s; each 'small square' i 0.04s. To calculate the rate, divide 300 by the number of big squares per R–interval (p83).
- ***Rhythm:*** If the cycles are not clearly regular, use the 'card method': lay a car along ECG, marking positions of 3 successive R waves. Slide the card to and fro t check that all intervals are equal. If not, note if different rates are multiples o each other (ie varying block), or is it 100% irregular (atrial fibrillation (AF) o ventricular fibrillation, VF)? *Sinus rhythm* is characterized by a P wave (upright ir II, III, & aVF; inverted in aVR) followed by a QRS complex. AF has no discernible waves and the QRS complexes are irregularly irregular. *Atrial flutter* (p111) has a 'sawtooth' baseline of atrial depolarization (~300/min) and regular QRS complexes. *Nodal rhythm* has a normal QRS complex but P waves are absent o occur just before or within the QRS complex. *Ventricular rhythm* has QRS complexes >0.12s with P waves following them.
- ***Axis:*** The mean frontal axis is the sum of all the ventricular forces durin ventricular depolarization. The axis lies at 90° to the isoelectric comple (ie the one in which positive and negative deflections are equal). *Normal axis* i between −30° and +90°. As a simple rule of thumb, if the complexes in leads and II are both 'positive', the axis is normal. *Left axis deviation* (LAD) is −30° t −90°. Causes: left anterior hemiblock, inferior MI, VT from LV focus, Wolff-Parkinson–White (WPW) syndrome (some types). *Right axis deviation* (RAD) is +90° to +180°. Causes: RVH, PE, anterolateral MI, left posterior hemiblock (rare) WPW syndrome (some types).
- ***P wave:*** Normally precedes each QRS complex. *Absent P wave:* AF, sinoatrial block junctional (AV nodal) rhythm. Dissociation between P waves and QRS complexes indicates complete heart block. *P mitrale:* bifid P wave, indicates left atria hypertrophy. *P pulmonale:* peaked P wave, indicates right atrial hypertrophy Pseudo-P-pulmonale seen if $K^+\downarrow$.
- ***P–R interval:*** Measure from start of P wave to start of QRS. *Normal range:* 0.12-0.2s (3–5 small squares). A *prolonged P–R interval* implies delayed AV conduction (1st degree heart block). A *short P–R interval* implies unusually fast AV conduction down an accessory pathway, eg WPW p112 (ECG p117).
- ***QRS complex:*** *Normal duration:* <0.12s. If ≥0.12s suggests ventricula conduction defects, eg a bundle branch block (p86 & p111). Large QRS complexe suggest *ventricular hypertrophy* (p86). *Normal Q wave* <0.04s wide and <2mm deep. They are often seen in leads V_5 and V_6, aVL and I, and reflect normal septa depolarization, which usually occurs from left to right. *Pathological Q waves* ma occur within a few hours of an acute MI.
- ***QT interval:*** Measure from start of QRS to *end* of T wave. It varies with rate Calculate *corrected QT interval* (QT^c) by dividing the measured QT interval by the square root of the cycle length, ie $QT^c = QT/\sqrt{RR}$. Normal QT^c: 0.38–0.42s. *Prolonged QT interval:* acute myocardial ischaemia, myocarditis, bradycardia (eg AV block) head injury, hypothermia, U&E imbalance ($K^+\downarrow$—ECG p669, $Ca^{2+}\downarrow$, $Mg^{2+}\downarrow$) congenital (Romano–Ward and Jervell–Lange–Nielson syndromes); sotalol quinidine, antihistamines, macrolides (eg erythromycin), amiodarone phenothiazines, tricyclics.
- ***ST segment:*** Usually isoelectric. Planar elevation (>1mm) or depression (>0.5mm) usually implies infarction (p105) or ischaemia (p95), respectively.
- ***T wave:*** Normally inverted in aVR, V_1 and occasionally V_2. Abnormal if inverted in I, II, and V_4–V_6. Peaked in hyperkalaemia (ECG 13, p669) and flattened in hypokalaemia.

ECG nomenclature (ventricular activation time, VAT)

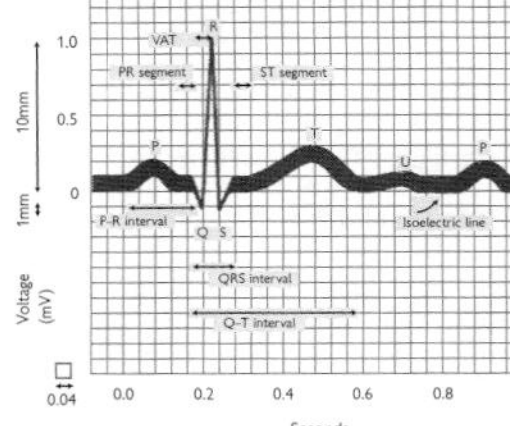

Calculating the R–R interval

To calculate the rate, divide 300 by the number of big squares per R–R interval—if the UK standard ECG speed of 25mm/s is used (elsewhere, 50mm/s may be used: don't be confused!)

R–R duration (s)	Big squares	Rate (per min)
0.2	1	300
0.4	2	150
0.6	3	100
0.8	4	75
1.0	5	60
1.2	6	50
1.4	7	43

Determining the ECG axis

- The axis lies at 90° to the isoelectric complex (the one in which positive and negative deflections are equal in size).
- If the complexes in I and II are both predominantly positive, the axis is normal.

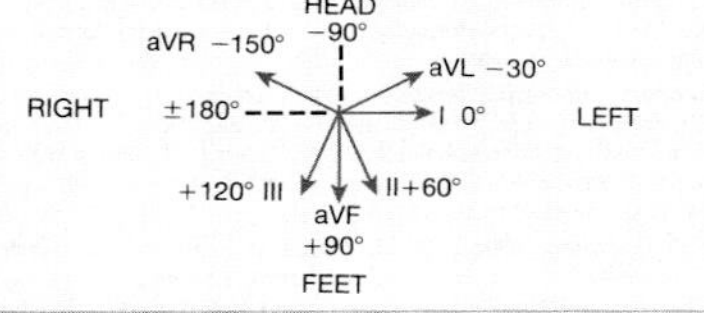

Causes of LAD (left axis deviation)	*Causes of RAD*
Left anterior hemiblock	RVH
Inferior MI	Pulmonary embolism
VT from LV focus	Anterolateral MI
WPW syndrome p112	Left posterior hemiblock (rare)
	WPW syndrome

Sinus tachycardia: Rate >100. Causes: Anaemia, anxiety, exercise, pain, ↑ sepsis, hypovolaemia, heart failure, pulmonary embolism, pregnancy, thy toxicosis, beri beri, CO_2 retention, autonomic neuropathy, sympathomimet eg caffeine, adrenaline, and nicotine (may produce abrupt changes in sinus r or other arrhythmia).

Sinus bradycardia: Rate <60. Causes: Physical fitness, vasovagal attacks, s sinus syndrome, acute MI (esp. inferior), drugs (β-blockers, digoxin, amiodarc verapamil), hypothyroidism, hypothermia, ↑intracranial pressure, cholestasis.

AF: (ECG p111) *Common causes:* IHD, thyrotoxicosis, hypertension. See p116.

1st and 2nd degree heart block: *Causes:* Normal variant, athletes, sick sir syndrome, IHD, acute carditis, drugs (digoxin, β-blockers).

3rd degree complete heart block: *Causes:* Idiopathic (fibrosis), congenital, I aortic valve calcification, cardiac surgery/trauma, digoxin toxicity, infiltrat (abscesses, granulomas, tumours, parasites).

Q waves: Pathological Q waves are usually >0.04s wide and >2mm deep. Usually sign of infarction, and may occur within a few hours of an acute MI.

ST elevation: Normal variant (high take-off), acute MI, Prinzmetal's angina (p70 acute pericarditis (saddle-shaped), left ventricular aneurysm.

ST depression: Normal variant (upward sloping), digoxin (downward slopin ischaemic (horizontal): angina, acute posterior MI.

T inversion: In V_1–V_3: normal (Blacks and children), right bundle branch blc (RBBB), pulmonary embolism. In V_2–V_5: subendocardial MI, HOCM, subarachn haemorrhage, lithium. In V_4–V_6 and aVL: ischaemia, LVH, associated with left bun branch block (LBBB).

NB: ST and T wave changes are often non-specific, and must be interpreted in light of the clinical context.

MI: (ECG p105.)

- Within hours, the T wave may become peaked and ST segments may begin to r
- Within 24h, the T wave inverts, as ST segment elevation begins to resolve. elevation rarely persists, unless a left ventricular aneurysm develo T wave inversion may or may not persist.
- Within a few days, pathological Q waves begin to form. Q waves usually pers but may resolve in 10%.

The leads affected reflect the site of the infarct: inferior (II, III, aVF), anterosep (V_{1-4}), anterolateral (V_{4-6}, I, aVL), posterior (tall R and ST↓ in V_{1-2}).

► 'Non-Q wave infarcts' (formerly called subendocardial infarcts) have ST an changes without Q waves.

Pulmonary embolism: Sinus tachycardia is commonest. There may be RAD, RE (p83), *right ventricular strain pattern* (R-axis deviation. Dominant R wave an wave inversion/ST depression in V_1 and V_2. Leads II, III and aVF may show simi changes). Rarely, the '$S_I Q_{III} T_{III}$' pattern occurs: deep S waves in I, pathologica waves in III, inverted T waves in III.

Metabolic abnormalities: Digoxin effect: ST depression and inverted T wave V_{5-6} (reversed tick). In *digoxin toxicity,* any arrhythmia may occur (ventricu ectopics and nodal bradycardia are common). *Hyperkalaemia:* Tall, tented T wa widened QRS, absent P waves, 'sine wave' appearance (ECG 13, p669). *Hypokalaem* Small T waves, prominent U waves. *Hypercalcaemia:* Short QT interv *Hypocalcaemia:* Long QT interval, small T waves.

ECG—additional points

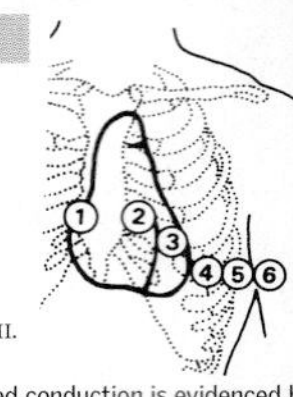

Where to place the chest leads

V_1: right sternal edge, 4th intercostal space
V_2: left sternal edge, 4th intercostal space
V_3: half-way between V_2 and V_4
V_4: the patient's apex beat (p64); all subsequent leads are in the same horizontal plane as V_4
V_5: anterior axillary line
V_6: mid-axillary line (V_7: posterior axillary line)
Finish 12-lead ECGs with a long rhythm strip in lead II.

Disorders of ventricular conduction

Bundle branch block (p87–p88, ECGS 1 & 2) Delayed conduction is evidenced by prolongation of QRS >0.12s. Abnormal conduction patterns lasting <0.12s are incomplete blocks. The area that would have been reached by the blocked bundle depolarizes slowly and late. Taking V_1 as an example, right ventricular depolarization is normally +ve and left ventricular depolarization is normally –ve.

In RBBB, the following pattern is seen: QRS >0.12s, 'RSR' pattern in V_1, dominant R in V_1, inverted T waves in V_1–V_3 or V_4, deep wide S wave in V_6. Causes: normal variant (isolated RBBB), pulmonary embolism, cor pulmonale.

In LBBB, the following pattern is seen: QRS >0.12s, 'M' pattern in V_5, no septal Q waves, inverted T waves in I, aVL, V_5–V_6. Causes: IHD, hypertension, cardiomyopathy, idiopathic fibrosis. ►NB: If there is LBBB, no comment can be made on the ST segment or T wave.

Bifascicular block is the combination of RBBB and left bundle hemiblock, manifest as an axis deviation, eg LAD in the case of left anterior hemiblock.

Trifascicular block is the combination of bifascicular block and 1st degree heart block.

Ventricular hypertrophy There is no single marker of ventricular hypertrophy: electrical axis, voltage, and ST wave changes should all be taken into consideration. Relying on a single marker such as voltage may be unreliable as a thin chest wall may result in large voltage whereas a thick chest wall may mask it.

Suspect ***left ventricular hypertrophy*** (LVH) if the R wave in V_6 >25mm or the sum of the S wave in V_1 and the R wave in V_6 is >35mm (ECG 8 on p127).

Suspect ***right ventricular hypertrophy*** (RVH) if dominant R wave in V_1, T wave inversion in V_1–V_3 or V_4, deep S wave in V_6, RAD.

Other causes of ***dominant R wave in V_1***: RBBB, posterior MI, some types of WPW syndrome (p112).

Causes of low voltage QRS complex: *(QRS <5mm in all limb leads)* Hypothyroidism, chronic obstructive pulmonary disease (COPD), ↑haematocrit (intra-cardiac blood resistivity is related to haematocrit), changes in chest wall impedance (eg in renal failure, subcutaneous emphysema but *not* obesity), pulmonary embolism, bundle branch block, carcinoid heart disease, myocarditis, cardiac amyloid, adriamycin cardiotoxicity, and other heart muscle diseases, pericardial effusion, pericarditis.

See http://homepages.enterprise.net/djenkins/ecghome.html for MRCP-ish examples of ECGs

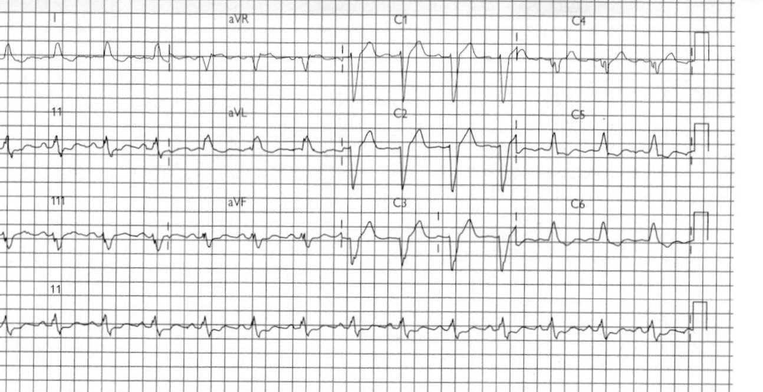

ECG 1—Left bundle branch block: note the W pattern in C1 (=V_1) and the M pattern in C6 (=V_6).

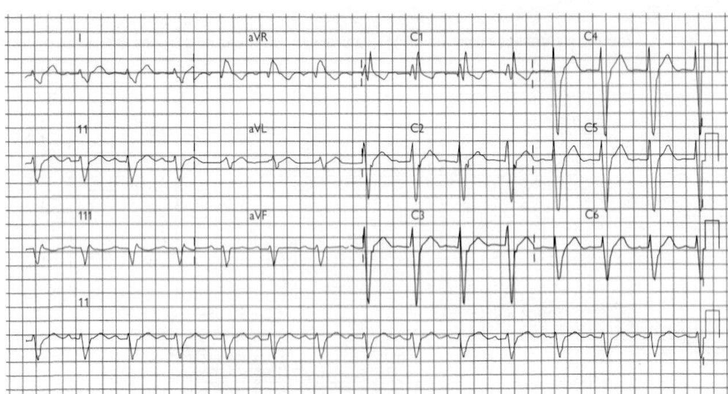

ECG 2—Right bundle branch block—note the M pattern in C1 and the W pattern in C5.

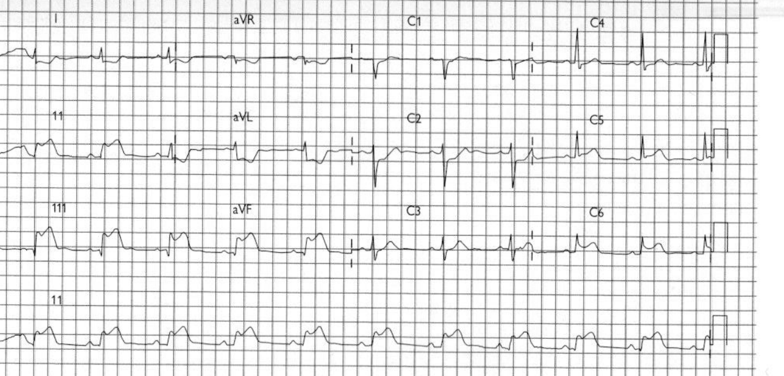

ECG 3—Acute infero-lateral myocardial infarction: note the marked ST elevation in the inferior leads (II, III, aVF), but also in C5 and C6, indicating lateral involvement as well. There is also 'reciprocal change' ie ST-segment depression in leads I and aVL. The latter is often seen with a large myocardial infarction.

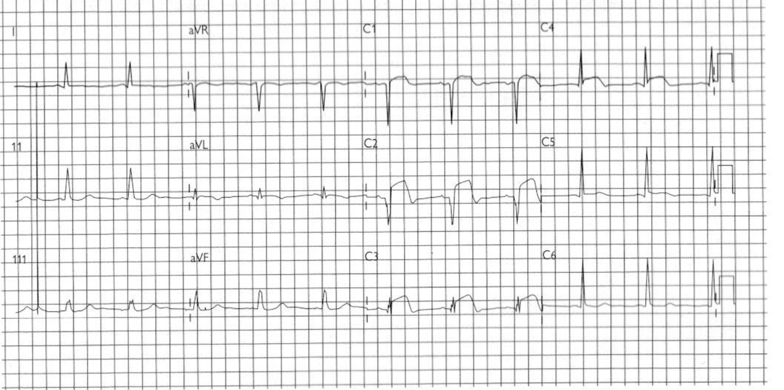

ECG 4—Acute anterior myocardial infarction—note the marked ST segment elevation and evolving Q waves in leads C1–C4.

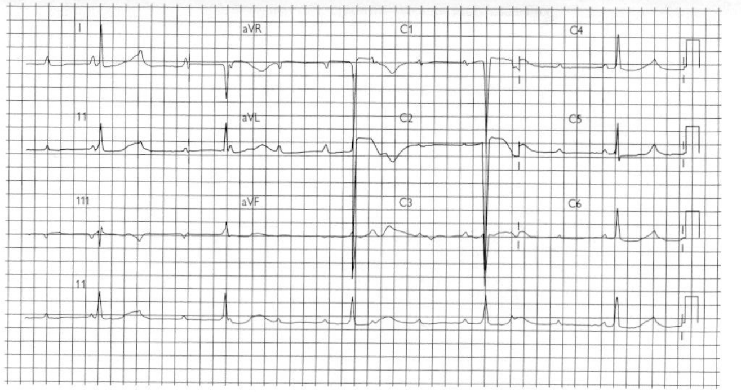

ECG 5—Complete heart block. Note the dissociation between the P waves and the QRS complexes. QRS complexes are relatively narrow, indicating that there is a ventricular rhythm originating from the conducting pathway.

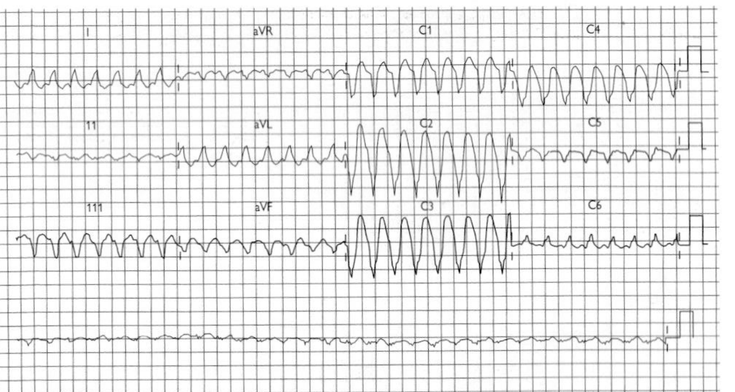

ECG 6—Ventricular tachycardia—note the broad complexes.

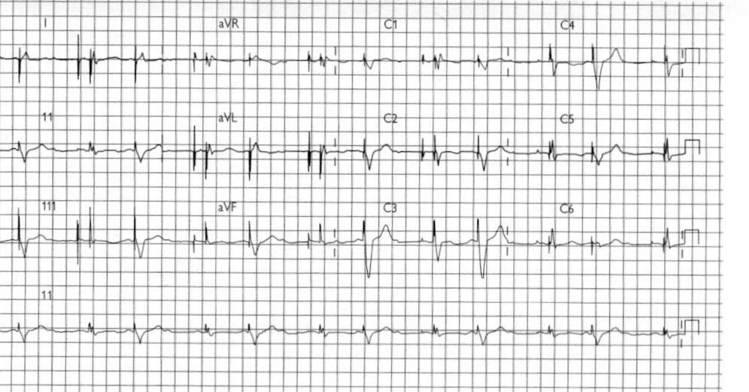

ECG 7—Dual chamber pacemaker. Note the pacing spikes which occur before some of the P waves, and the QRS complexes.

Exercise ECG testing

The patient undergoes a graduated, treadmill exercise test, with continuous 12-lead ECG and blood pressure monitoring. There are numerous treadmill protocols; the 'Bruce protocol' is the most widely used.

Indications:

- To help confirm a suspected diagnosis of IHD.
- Assessment of cardiac function and exercise tolerance.
- Prognosis following MI. Often done pre-discharge (if +ve, worse outcome).
- Evaluation of response to treatment (drugs, angioplasty, coronary artery bypass grafting, CABG).
- Assessment of exercise-induced arrhythmias.

Contraindications:

- Unstable angina
- Recent Q wave MI (<5 days ago)
- Severe AS
- Uncontrolled arrhythmia, hypertension, or heart failure.

Be cautious about arranging tests that will be hard to perform or interpret:

- Complete heart block, LBBB
- Pacemaker patients
- Osteoarthritis, COPD, stroke, or other limitations to exercise.

Stop the test if:

- Chest pain or dyspnoea occurs.
- The patient feels faint, exhausted, or is in danger of falling.
- ST segment elevation/depression >2mm (with or without chest pain).
- Atrial or ventricular arrhythmia (not just ectopics).
- Fall in blood pressure, failure of heart rate or blood pressure to rise with effort or excessive rise in blood pressure (systolic >230mmHg).
- Development of AV block or LBBB.
- Maximal or 90% maximal heart rate for age is achieved.

Interpreting the test: A positive test only allows one to assess the *probability* that the patient has IHD. 75% with significant coronary artery disease have a positive test, but so do 5% of people with normal arteries (the false positive rate is even higher in middle-aged women, eg 20%). The more positive the result, the higher the predictive accuracy. Down-sloping ST depression is much more significant than up-sloping, eg 1mm J-point depression with down-sloping ST segment is 99% predictive of 2–3 vessel disease.

Morbidity: 24 in 100,000. ***Mortality:*** 10 in 100,000.

Ambulatory ECG monitoring (Holter monitor)

Continuous ECG monitoring for 24h may be used to try and pick up paroxysmal arrhythmias. However, >70% of patients will not have symptoms during the period of monitoring. ~20% will have a normal ECG during symptoms and only up to 10% will have an arrhythmia coinciding with symptoms. Give these patients a recorder they can activate themselves during an episode. Recorders may be programmed to detect ST segment depression, either symptomatic (to prove angina), or to reveal 'silent' ischaemia (predictive of re-infarction or death soon after MI).

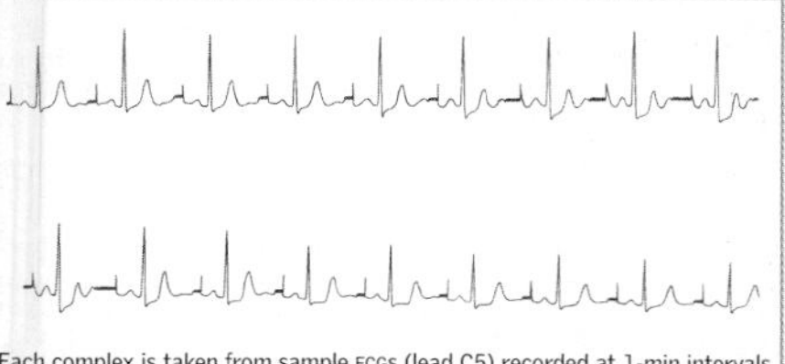

Each complex is taken from sample ECGS (lead C5) recorded at 1-min intervals during exercise (top line) and recovery (bottom line). At maximum ST depression, the ST segment is almost horizontal. This is a positive exercise test.

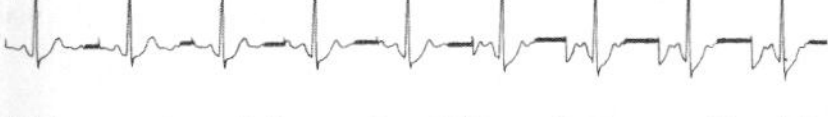

This is an exercise ECG in the same format. It is negative because although the J point is depressed, the ensuing ST segment is steeply up-sloping.

Cardiac catheterization

This involves the insertion of a catheter into the heart via the femoral (c radial/brachial) artery or vein. The catheter is manipulated within the heart an great vessels to measure pressures. Catheterization can also be used to:

- Sample blood to assess oxygen saturation.
- Inject radiopaque contrast medium to image the anatomy of the heart and flov in blood vessels.
- Perform angioplasty (± stenting), valvuloplasty, and cardiac biopsies.
- Perform intravascular ultrasound to quantify arterial narrowing.

During the procedure, ECG and arterial pressures are monitored continuously. In th UK, 40% of cardiac catheters are performed as day-case procedures (provided th patient can rest lying down for 4h).

Indications:

- *Coronary artery disease:* diagnostic (assessment of coronary vessels and gra patency); therapeutic (angioplasty, stent insertion).
- *Valvular disease:* diagnostic (to assess severity); therapeutic valvuloplasty (if th patient is too ill or declines valve surgery).
- *Congenital heart disease:* diagnostic (assessment of severity of lesions therapeutic (balloon dilatation or septostomy).
- *Other:* cardiomyopathy; pericardial disease; endomyocardial biopsy.

Pre-procedure checks:

- Brief history/examination; **NB:** peripheral pulses, bruits, aneurysms.
- Investigations: FBC, U&E, LFT, clotting screen, group & save, CXR, ECG.
- Consent for angiogram ± angioplasty ± stent ± CABG. Explain reason fc procedure and possible complications (below).
- IV access, ideally in the left hand.
- Patient should be nil by mouth (NBM) from 6h before the procedure.
- Patients should take all their morning drugs (and pre-medication if needed Withhold oral hypoglycaemics.

Post-procedure checks:

- Pulse, blood pressure, arterial puncture site (for bruising or swelling? fals aneurysm), peripheral pulses.
- Investigations: FBC and clotting (if suspected blood loss), ECG.

Complications:

- *Haemorrhage:* Apply firm pressure over puncture site. If you suspect a fals aneurysm, ultrasound the swelling and consider surgical repair.
- *Contrast reaction:* This is usually mild with modern contrast agents.
- *Loss of peripheral pulse:* May be due to dissection, thrombosis, or arterial spasr Occurs in <1% of brachial catheterizations. Rare with femoral catheterizatio
- *Angina:* May occur during or after cardiac catheterization. Usually responds t sublingual GTN; if not give analgesia and IV nitrates.
- *Arrhythmias:* Usually transient. Manage along standard lines.
- *Pericardial tamponade:* Rare, but should be suspected if the patient becom hypotensive and anuric.
- *Infection:* Post-catheter pyrexia is usually due to a contrast reaction. If persists for >24h, take blood cultures before giving antibiotics.

Mortality: <1 in 1000 patients, in most centres.

Intra-cardiac electrophysiology This catheter technique can determine types ar origins of arrhythmias, and locate (and ablate) aberrant pathways (eg causir atrial flutter or ventricular tachycardia). Arrhythmias may be induced, and th effectiveness of control by drugs assessed.

Normal values for intracardiac pressures and saturations

Location	Pressure (mmHg) Mean	Range	Saturation (%)
Inferior vena cava			76
Superior vena cava			70
Right atrium	4	0–8	74
Right ventricle			74
Systolic	25	15–30	
End-diastolic	4	0–8	
Pulmonary artery			74
Systolic	25	15–30	
Diastolic	10	5–15	
Mean	15	10–20	
Pulmonary artery	a	3–12	74
Wedge pressure	v	3–15	
Left ventricle			
Systolic	110	80–140	98
End-diastolic	70	60–90	
Aorta			
Systolic	110	80–140	98
Diastolic	70	60–90	
Mean	85	70–105	
Brachial			
Systolic	120	90–140	98
Diastolic	72	60–90	
Mean	83	70–105	

Gradients across stenotic valves

Valve	Normal gradient (mmHg)	Stenotic gradient (mmHg) Mild	Moderate	Severe
Aortic	0	<30	30–50	>50
Mitral	0	<5	5–15	>15
Prosthetic	5–10			

Coronary artery anatomy

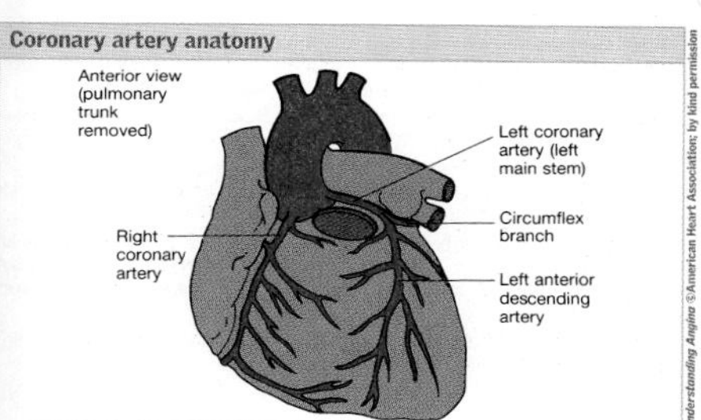

Understanding Angina ©American Heart Association; by kind permission

Echocardiography

This non-invasive technique uses the differing ability of various structures within the heart to reflect ultrasound waves. It not only demonstrates anatomy but provides a continuous display of the functioning heart throughout its cycle. There are various types of scan:

M-mode (motion mode): Scans are displayed on light-sensitive paper moving at constant speed to produce a permanent single dimension (time) image.

2-dimensional (real time): A 2-D, fan-shaped image of a segment of the heart is produced on the screen, which may be 'frozen' and hard-copied. Several views are possible and the 4 commonest are: long axis, short axis, 4-chamber, and subcostal. 2-D echocardiography is good for visualizing conditions such as: congenital heart disease, LV aneurysm, mural thrombus, LA myxoma, septal defects.

Doppler and colour-flow echocardiography: Different coloured jets illustrate flow and gradients across valves and septal defects (p142). (Doppler effect, p722)

Trans-oesophageal echocardiography (TOE) is more sensitive than transthoracic echocardiography (TTE) as the transducer is nearer to the heart. Indications: diagnosing aortic dissections; assessing prosthetic valves; finding cardiac source of emboli, and IE/SBE. Don't do if oesophageal disease or cervical spine instability.

Stress echocardiography is used to evaluate ventricular function, ejection fraction, myocardial thickening, and regional wall motion pre- and post-exercise. Dobutamine or dipyridamole may be used if the patient cannot exercise. Inexpensive and as sensitive/specific as a thallium scan (p726).

Cardiovascular medicine

Uses of echocardiography

Quantification of global LV function: Heart failure may be due to systolic or diastolic ventricular impairment (or both). Echo helps by measuring end-diastolic volume. If this is large, systolic dysfunction is the likely cause. If small, diastolic. Pure forms of diastolic dysfunction are rare. Differentiation is important, as vasodilators are less useful in diastolic dysfunction as a high ventricular filling pressure is required.

Echo is also useful for detecting focal and global hypokinesia, LV aneurysm, mural thrombus, and LVH (echo is 5–10 times more sensitive than ECG in detecting this).

Estimating right heart haemodynamics: Doppler studies of pulmonary artery flow allow evaluation of RV function and pressures.

Valve disease: Measurement of pressure gradients and valve orifice areas in stenotic lesions. Detecting valvular regurgitation and estimating its significance is less accurate. Evaluating function of prosthetic valves is another role.

Congenital heart disease: Establishing the presence of lesions and determining their functional significance.

Endocarditis: Vegetations may not be seen if <2mm in size. TTE with colour doppler is best for aortic regurgitation (AR). TOE is useful for visualizing mitral valve vegetations, leaflet perforation, or looking for an aortic root abscess.

Pericardial effusion is best diagnosed by echo. Fluid may first accumulate between the posterior pericardium and the left ventricle, then anterior to both ventricles and anterior and lateral to the right atrium. There may be paradoxical septal motion.

HOCM (p138): Echo features include asymmetrical septal hypertrophy, small LV cavity, dilated left atrium, and systolic anterior motion of the mitral valve.

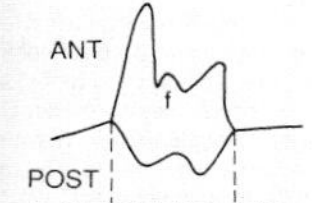

Chest wall
RV
AO
AV
LV
MV
LA
Chest wall
RV
RV outflow
IVS
AO
AV
LV
MV
LA
PW
e
ANT
f
POST
1. Normal mitral valve
CLOSED
OPEN
CLOSED
2. Mitral stenosis
• reduced e–f slope
a
b
3. Aortic regurgitation
• fluttering of ant. leaflet
4. (a) Systolic anterior leaflet movement (SAM) in HOCM
(b) Mitral valve prolapse (late systole)

Normal M-mode echocardiogram (RV=right ventricle; LV=left ventricle; AO= aorta; AV=aortic valve; LA=left atrium; MV=mitral valve; PW=posterior wall of LV; IVS=interventricular septum). After R Hall *Med International* 17 774.

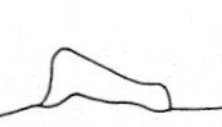

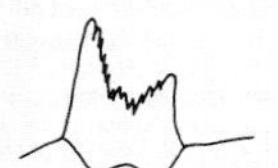

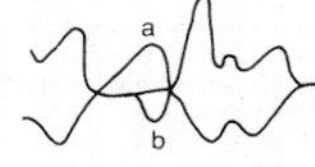

Cardiovascular drugs

Antiplatelet drugs Aspirin irreversibly acetylates cyclo-oxygenase, preventing production of thromboxane A_2, thereby inhibiting platelet aggregation. Used in low dose (eg 75mg/24h PO) for secondary prevention following MI, TIA/stroke, and for patients with angina or peripheral vascular disease. May have a role in primary prevention. ADP receptor antagonists (eg clopidogrel) also block platelet aggregation, but may cause less gastric irritation. They have a role if truly intolerant of aspirin, and post-coronary stent insertion.

β-blockers Block β-adrenoceptors, thus antagonizing the sympathetic nervous system. Blocking β_1-receptors is negatively inotropic and chronotropic (pulse↓ by ↓firing of sinoatrial node), and β_2-receptors induce peripheral vasoconstriction and bronchoconstriction. Drugs vary in their β_1/β_2 selectivity (eg propranolol is non-selective, and bisoprolol relatively β_1 selective), but this does not seem to alter their clinical efficacy. *Uses:* Angina, hypertension (2nd line), antidysrhythmic, post MI (↓mortality), heart failure (with caution). ***CI:*** Asthma/COPD, heart block. ***Caution:*** Peripheral vascular disease, heart failure/(but see carvedilol, p122). ***SE:*** Lethargy, erectile dysfunction, *joie de vivre*↓, nightmares, headache.

Diuretics Loop diuretics (eg *furosemide=frusemide*) are used in heart failure, and inhibit the Na/2Cl/K co-transporter. Thiazides are used in hypertension and inhibit Na/Cl co-transporter. ***SE:*** *Loop:* dehydration, ↓K^+, ↓Ca^{2+}, ototoxic; *thiazides:* ↓K^+, ↑Ca^{2+}, ↓Mg^{2+}, ↑urate (±gout), impotence (**NB:** small doses, eg bendroflumethiazide 2.5mg/24h rarely cause significant SEs); *Amiloride:* ↑K^+, GI upset.

Vasodilators used in heart failure, IHD, and hypertension. Nitrates preferentially dilate veins and the large arteries, ↓ filling pressure (pre-load), while hydralazine (often used with nitrates) primarily dilates the resistance vessels thus ↓ BP (after-load). Prazosin (an α-blocker) dilates arteries and veins.

Calcium antagonists These ↓cell entry of Ca^{2+} via voltage-sensitive channels on smooth muscle cells, thereby promoting coronary and peripheral vasodilatation and reducing myocardial oxygen consumption.

Pharmacology: All current drugs block L-type Ca^{2+} channels. However, their effects differ because of differential binding properties. The *dihydropyridines* eg nifedipine; amlodipine, are mainly peripheral vasodilators (also dilate coronary arteries) and cause a reflex tachycardia, so are often used with a β-blocker. They are used mainly in hypertension and angina. The *non*-dihydropyridines—verapamil and diltiazem—also slow conduction at the atrioventricular and sinoatrial nodes and may be used to treat hypertension, angina, and dysrhythmias. Don't give verapamil with β-blockers (risk of bradycardia ± LVF). ***SE:*** Flushes, headache, oedema (diuretic unresponsive), LV function↓, gingival hypertrophy. ***CI:*** heart block.

Digoxin Blocks the Na^+/K^+ pump. It is used to slow the pulse in fast AF (p116; aim for <100). As it is a weak +ve inotrope, its role in heart failure in sinus rhythm may be best reserved if symptomatic despite optimal ACE-i therapy (p123); here there is little benefit *vis-à-vis* mortality (but admissions for worsening CCF are ↓by ~25%). Old people are at ↑risk of toxicity: use lower doses. Do plasma levels >6h post-dose (p739). Typical dose: 500μg stat PO, repeated after 12h, then 125μg (if elderly) to 375μg/d PO (62.5μg/d is almost never enough). IV dose: 0.75–1mg in 0.9% NaCl over 2h. Toxicity risk↑ if: K^+↓, Mg^{2+}↓, or Ca^{2+}↑. t½ ≈ 36h. If on digoxin, use less energy in cardioversion (start at 5J). ►If on amiodarone, halve the dose of digoxin. ***SE:*** Any arrhythmia (supraventricular tachycardia with AV block is suggestive), nausea, appetite↓, yellow vision, confusion, gynaecomastia. In toxicity, stop digoxin; check K^+; treat arrhythmias; consider Digibind® by IVI (p826). ***CI:*** HOCM; WPW syndrome (p112 & p792).

ACE-inhibitors p123; **Nitrates** p102; **Antihypertensives** p142.

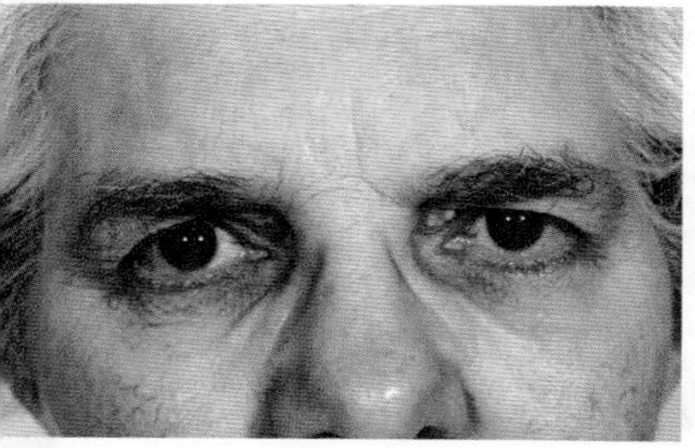

g 1. Xanthelasma. *Xanthos* is Greek for yellow, and *elasma* means plate. ınthelasma are lipid-laden yellow plaques congregating around the lids. They e typically a few mm wide, and signify hyperlipidaemia, p682

Statins

Statins (eg simvastatin, pravastatin, p682) inhibit the enzyme HMG-COA reductase, which is responsible for the *de novo* synthesis of cholesterol in the liver. This leads to an increase in LDL receptor expression by hepatocytes and ultimately reduced circulating LDL cholesterol. More effective if given at night, but optimum dose, and target cholesterol are unknown. SE: muscle aches, abdominal discomfort, ↑transaminases (eg ALT), ↑CK, myositis, rarely rhabdomyolysis (more common when used in combination with fibrates). Besides lowering LDL cholesterol, statins have other favourable or 'pleiotropic' effects:

- Anti-thrombotic.
- Anti-inflammatory (CRP↓).
- Plaque stabilization; high doses *may* even reverse plaque growth (note that recent trials have not shown that when this occurs there is ↓morbidity—and high doses of some statins may cause renal impairment and myopathy).
- Restoration of normal endothelial function.
- Reduction in cholesterol synthesis by within-vessel macrophages.
- Reduction of within-vessel macrophage proliferation and migration.

Angina pectoris

This is due to myocardial ischaemia and presents as a central chest tightness c heaviness, which is brought on by exertion and relieved by rest. It may radiate to or or both arms, the neck, jaw or teeth. ***Other precipitants:*** Emotion, cold weathe and heavy meals. ***Associated symptoms:*** Dyspnoea, nausea, sweatiness, faintnes

Causes Mostly atheroma. Rarely: anaemia, AS; tachyarrhythmias; HOCN arteritis/small vessel disease (microvascular angina/cardiac syndrome X).

Types of angina *Stable angina:* induced by effort, relieved by rest. *Unstab (crescendo) angina:* angina of increasing frequency or severity; occurs on minim exertion or at rest; associated with ↑↑risk of MI. *Decubitus angina:* precipitated b lying flat. *Variant (Prinzmetal's) angina:* caused by coronary artery spasm (rar may co-exist with fixed stenoses).

Tests ECG: usually normal, but may show ST depression; flat or inverted T wave signs of past MI. If resting ECG normal, consider exercise ECG (p94), thallium sca (p726), or coronary angiography. Exclude precipitating factors: anaemia, diabete hyperlipidaemia, thyrotoxicosis, giant cell arteritis.

Management *Alteration of lifestyle:* Stop smoking, encourage exercise, weight los *Modify risk factors:* Hypertension, diabetes, etc., p79.

- *Aspirin* (75–150mg/24h) reduces mortality by 34%.
- *β-blockers:* eg atenolol 50–100mg/24h PO, reduce symptoms unless contr indications (asthma, COPD, LVF, bradycardia, coronary artery spasm).
- *Nitrates:* for symptoms, give GTN spray or sublingual tabs, up to every ½ Prophylaxis: give regular oral nitrate, eg isosorbide mononitrate 10–30mg PO (e bd; an 8h nitrate-free period to prevent tolerance) or slow-release nitrate (e Imdur® 60mg/24h). Alternatives: adhesive nitrate skin patches or buccal pills. s headaches, BP↓.
- *Calcium antagonists:* amlodipine 10mg/24h; diltiazem-MR 90–180mg/12h P
- If total cholesterol >4mmol/L give a statin—see p682.
- Consider adding a *K⁺ channel activator*, eg nicorandil 10–30mg/12h PO.

►Unstable angina requires admission and urgent treatment: *emergencies*, p78

Indications for referral Diagnostic uncertainty; new angina of sudden onse recurrent angina if past MI or CABG; angina uncontrolled by drugs; unstable angin Some units routinely do exercise tolerance tests on those <70yrs old, but age alo is a poor way to stratify patients.

Percutaneous transluminal coronary angioplasty **(PTCA)** involves balloo dilatation of the stenotic vessel(s). *Indications:* poor response or intolerance medical therapy; refractory angina in patients not suitable for CABG; previous CAB post-thrombolysis in patients with severe stenoses, symptoms, or positive stre tests. Comparisons of PTCA vs drugs alone show that PTCA may control sympton better but with more frequent early cardiac events (eg MI and need for CABG and little effect on overall mortality. However, early intervention may bene high risk patients presenting with non-ST-segment elevation ACS (p104) *Complications:* Restenosis (20–30% within 6 months); emergency CABG (<3%); (<2%); death (<0.5%). Stenting reduces restenosis rates and the need for bail o CABG. NICE recommends that >70% of angioplasties should be accompanied stenting. Drug-coated stents reduce restenosis. Antiplatelet agents, eg clopidog reduce the risk of stent thrombosis. IV platelet glycoprotein IIb/IIIa-inhibitors (eptifibatide) can reduce procedure-related ischaemic events.

CABG: *Indications:* Left main stem disease, multi-vessel disease; multiple seve stenoses; distal vessel disease; patient unsuitable for angioplasty; failed angioplas refractory angina; MI; pre-operatively (valve or vascular surgery). Comparisons CABG *vs* PTCA have found that CABG results in better symptom control and lower intervention rate, but longer recovery time and length of inpatient stay.

Acute coronary syndromes (ACS)

Definitions ACS includes unstable angina and evolving MI, which share a commo underlying pathology—plaque rupture, thrombosis, and inflammation. However, AC may rarely be due to emboli or coronary spasm in normal coronary arteries, c vasculitis (p542). Usually divided into ***ACS with ST-segment elevation*** or new onse LBBB—what most of us mean by acute MI; and ***ACS without ST-segment elevation***— the ECG may show ST-depression, T-wave inversion, non-specific changes, or b normal (includes non-Q wave or subendocardial MI). The degree of irreversibl myocyte death varies, and significant necrosis can occur without ST-elevatio Cardiac troponins (T and I) are the most sensitive and specific markers c myocardial necrosis, and are the test of choice in patients with ACS (see below)

Risk factors *Non-modifiable:* age, ♂ gender, family history of IHD (MI in first degre relative <55yrs). *Modifiable:* smoking, hypertension, DM, hyperlipidaemia, obesit sedentary lifestyle. *Controversial* risk factors include: stress, type A personality, LV apoprotein A↑, fibrinogen↑, hyperinsulinaemia, homocysteine levels↑ (p79), AC genotype, and cocaine use.

Incidence 5/1000 per annum (UK) for ST-segment elevation.

Diagnosis is based on the presence of at least 2 out of 3 of: typical history, EC changes, and cardiac enzyme rise (WHO criteria).

Symptoms Acute central chest pain, lasting >20min, often associated with nause sweatiness, dyspnoea, palpitations. May present without chest pain ('silent' infarc eg in elderly or diabetics. In such patients, presentations may include: syncop pulmonary oedema, epigastric pain and vomiting, post-operative hypotension oliguria, acute confusional state, stroke, diabetic hyperglycaemic states.

Signs Distress, anxiety, pallor, sweatiness, pulse↑ or ↓, BP↑ or ↓, 4th heart soun There may be signs of heart failure (↑ JVP, 3rd heart sound and basal crepitation or a pansystolic murmur (papillary muscle dysfunction/rupture, VSD). A low-grac pyrexia may be present. Later, a pericardial friction rub or peripheral oedema m develop.

Tests ***ECG:*** Classically, hyperacute (tall) T waves, ST elevation or new LBBB occ within hours of acute Q wave (transmural infarction). T wave inversion and t development of pathological Q waves follow over hours to days (p84). In other AC ST-depression, T-wave inversion, non-specific changes, or normal. ►*In 20% of M the ECG may be normal initially.*

CXR: Look for cardiomegaly, pulmonary oedema, or a widened mediastinum (?aor dissection). Don't routinely delay ℞ whilst waiting for a CXR.

Blood: FBC, U&E, glucose↑, lipids↓, cardiac enzymes (CK, AST, LDH, troponin)↑, CK found in myocardial and skeletal muscle. It is raised in: MI; after trauma (fal seizures); prolonged exercise; myositis; Afro-Caribbeans; hypothermia; hyp thyroidism. Check CK-MB isoenzyme levels if there is doubt as to the source (norr CK-MB/CK ratio <5%). Troponin T better reflects myocardial damage (peaks at 1 24h; elevated for >1wk). If normal ≥6h after onset of pain, and ECG normal, risk missing MI is tiny (0.3%).[16] Peak post-MI levels also help risk stratification.[17]

Differential diagnosis (p80) Angina, pericarditis, myocarditis, aortic dissecti (p586), pulmonary embolism, and oesophageal reflux/spasm.

Management See *emergencies*, p782. The management of ACS with and withc ST-segment elevation varies. Likewise, if there is no ST-elevation, and sympto settle without a rise in cardiac troponin, then no myocardial damage has occurr the prognosis is good, and patients can be discharged. Therefore, the two k questions are: is there ST-segment elevation; and is there a rise in troponin?

Mortality 50% of deaths occur within 2h of onset of symptom.

Enzyme changes following acute MI

Cardiac enzymes

×50 ×5 ×4 ×3 ×2 ×1

Serum enzyme level

Trop CK CK–MB AST LDH

0 1 2 3 4 5 6 7 8 9 10

Days

CK Creatine kinase
CK–MB CK cardiac isoenzyme
AST Aspartate transaminase
LDH Lactate dehydrogenase
Trop Cardiac troponin

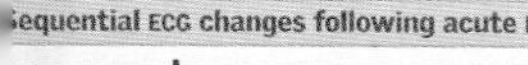

Sequential ECG changes following acute MI

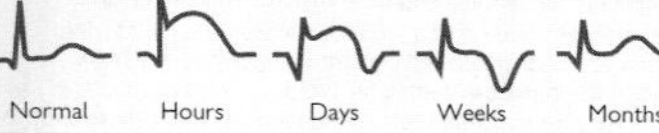

Management of acute coronary syndrome (ACS)

Pre-hospital Arrange emergency ambulance. Aspirin 300mg chewed (if *absolute* CI) and GTN sublingual. Analgesia, eg morphine 5–10mg IV metoclopramide 10mg IV (not IM because of risk of bleeding with thrombolysi

In hospital—O_2, IVI, morphine, aspirin ⇥p782

Then the key question for subsequent management of ACS is whether there is s segment elevation (includes new onset LBBB or a true posterior MI).

ST-segment elevation

- *Thrombolysis*, if no contraindication, or primary angioplasty ⇥ p782.
- *β-blocker*, eg atenolol 5mg IV unless contraindicated, eg asthma.
- *ACE-inhibitor*: Consider starting ACE-i (eg lisinopril 2.5mg) in all normotensi patients (systolic ≥120mm/Hg) within 24h of acute MI, especially if there clinical evidence of heart failure or echo evidence of LV dysfunction.

ACS without ST-segment elevation

- *β-blocker*, eg atenolol 5mg IV unless contraindicated.
- *Low molecular weight heparin* (eg enoxaparin 1mg/kg/12h SC for 2–8d).
- *Nitrates*, unless contraindication (usually given intravenously).
- High-risk patients (persistent or recurrent ischaemia, ST-depression, diabet ↑ troponin) require infusion of a *GPIIb/IIIa antagonist* (eg tirofiban), ar ideally, urgent angiography. *Clopidogrel*, in addition to aspirin, should considered for up to 12 months.
- Low-risk patients (no further pain, flat or inverted T waves, or normal ECG, a negative troponin) can be discharged if a repeat troponin is negative. Tre medically and arrange further investigation eg stress test, angiogram.

Subsequent management *Bed rest for 48h;* continuous ECG monitoring.

- Daily examination of heart, lungs, and legs for complications (p108).
- Daily 12-lead ECG, U&E, cardiac enzymes for 2–3d.
- *Prophylaxis against thromboembolism:* eg heparin 5000U/12h SC until fu mobile. If large anterior MI, consider warfarin anticoagulation for 3 months prophylaxis against systemic embolism from LV mural thrombus. Continue da *low-dose aspirin* (eg 75–150mg) indefinitely. Aspirin reduces vascular events (stroke, or vascular death) by 29%.
- Start oral β-*blocker* (eg metoprolol ~50mg/6h, enough to decrease the pulse ≤60; continue for at least 1yr). Long-term β-blockade reduces mortality from causes by ~25% in patients who have had a previous MI. If contraindicat consider verapamil or diltiazem as an alternative.
- *Continue* ACE-i in all patients. ACE-i in those with evidence of heart failure ↓ mortality by 25–30%.
- *Start a* statin. Cholesterol reduction post-MI has been shown to be of bene in patients with both elevated and normal cholesterol levels. Some treat patients, others only if total cholesterol >4.0mmol/L (p682).
- *Address modifiable risk factors:* Discourage smoking (p79). Encourage exerc Identify and treat diabetes mellitus, hypertension, and hyperlipidaemia.
- *Exercise ECG.* May be useful in risk stratification post-MI after 3–4wks, and subjects without ST-segment elevation or a troponin rise.
- *General advice.* If uncomplicated, discharge after 5–7d. *Work:* He may returr work after 2 months. A few occupations should not be restarted post-MI: airl pilots; air traffic controllers; divers. Drivers of public service or heavy goc vehicles may be permitted to return to work if they meet certain criteria Patients undertaking heavy manual labour should be advised to seek a ligh job. *Diet:* A diet high in oily fish, fruit, vegetables, and fibre, and low in satura fats should be encouraged. *Exercise:* Encourage regular daily exercise. S Intercourse is best avoided for 1 month. *Travel:* Avoid air travel for 2 mont

Review at 5wks post-MI to review symptoms: Angina? dyspnoea? palpitations angina recurs, treat conventionally, and consider coronary angiography.

Review at 3 months Check fasting lipids. Is there a need for a statin (p682)?

Acute postero-lateral MI

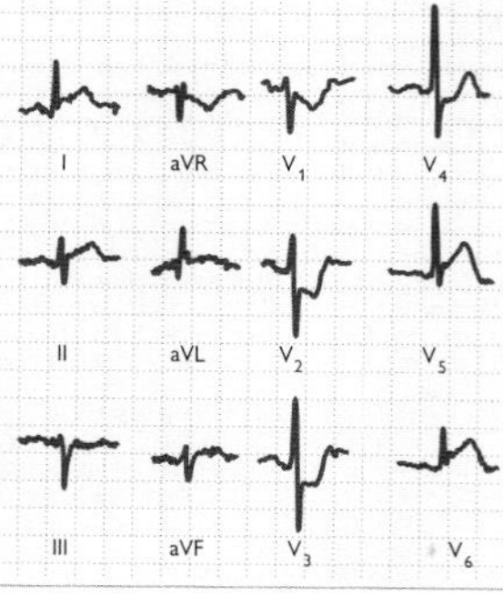

Complications of MI

- ***Cardiac arrest*** (inside backcover); ***cardiogenic shock*** (p788).
- ***Unstable angina:*** Manage along standard lines (p784) and refer to a card ologist for urgent investigation.
- ***Bradycardias or heart block:*** *Sinus bradycardia:* treat with atropine 0.6–1.2m IV. Consider temporary cardiac pacing if no response, or poorly tolerated by th patient. *1st degree AV block:* Observe closely as approximately 40% develc higher degrees of AV block. *Wenckebach (Mobitz type I) block:* Does not requi pacing unless poorly tolerated. *Mobitz type II block:* Carries a high risk developing complete AV block; should be paced. *Complete AV block:* inse pacemaker; may not be necessary after inferior MI if narrow QRS and reasonab stable and pulse ≥40–50. *Bundle branch block:* MI complicated by trifascicul block or non-adjacent bifascicular disease should be paced.
- ***Tachyarrhythmias:*** NB: K^+↓, hypoxia and acidosis all predispose to arrhythmi and should be corrected. Regular broad complex tachycardia after MI is almo always *VT*. If haemodynamically stable, treat with antidysrhythmic. Early (<24h): give lidocaine by infusion for 12–24h or amiodarone. Late VT (>24 amiodarone and start oral therapy (amiodarone or sotalol): if compromised gi DC shock. *SVT:* p112. *AF or flutter:* If compromised, DC cardioversion. Otherwis control rate with digoxin (load with 0.5mg/12h PO for 3 doses; maintenanc 0.125–0.25mg/24h) ± β-blocker. In atrial flutter or intermittent AF, try ami darone or sotalol (details p130).
- ***Left ventricular failure (LVF):*** p786.
- ***Right ventricular failure (RVF)/infarction:*** Presents with low cardiac outp and JVP↑. Consider a Swan–Ganz catheter to measure right-sided pressures a guide fluid replacement. If BP remains low, give inotropes.
- ***Pericarditis:*** Central chest pain, relieved by sitting forwards. ECG: saddle-shap ST elevation. Treatment: NSAIDs. Echo to check for effusion.
- ***DVT & PE:*** Patients are at risk of developing DVT & PE and should be pr phylactically heparinized (enoxaparin, p106) until fully mobile.
- ***Systemic embolism:*** May arise from a LV mural thrombus. After large anteri MIs, consider anticoagulation with warfarin for 3 months.
- ***Cardiac tamponade:*** (p788) Presents with low cardiac output, puls paradoxus, JVP↑, muffled heart sounds. Diagnosis: Echo. Treatment: Pericard aspiration (provides temporary relief ▸▸see p761 for technique), surgery.
- ***Mitral regurgitation:*** May be mild (minor papillary muscle dysfunction) severe (chordal or papillary muscle rupture or ischaemia). Presentati Pulmonary oedema. Treat LVF (p786) and consider valve replacement.
- ***Ventricular septal defect:*** Presents with pansystolic murmur, JVP↑, cardi failure. Diagnosis: Echo. Treatment: Surgery. 50% mortality in first week.
- ***Late malignant ventricular arrhythmias:*** Occur 1–3wks post-MI and are t cardiologist's nightmare. Avoid hypokalaemia, the most easily avoidable cau Consider 24h ECG monitoring prior to discharge if large MI.
- ***Dressler's syndrome:*** (p690) Recurrent pericarditis, pleural effusions, fev anaemia and ESR↑ 1–3wks post-MI. Treatment: NSAIDs; steroids if severe.
- ***Left ventricular aneurysm:*** This occurs late (4–6wks post-MI), and prese with LVF, angina, recurrent VT, or systemic embolism. ECG: Persistent ST segm elevation. Treatment: anticoagulate, consider excision.

Arrhythmias

(Emergency management: ▸▸p790 & p792

Disturbances of cardiac rhythm or arrhythmias are:

- Common
- Often benign (but may reflect underlying heart disease)
- Often intermittent, causing diagnostic difficulty
- Occasionally severe, causing cardiac compromise.

Causes *Cardiac:* MI, coronary artery disease, LV aneurysm, mitral valve diseas cardiomyopathy, pericarditis, myocarditis, aberrant conduction pathways. *No cardiac:* Caffeine, smoking, alcohol, pneumonia, drugs (β_2-agonists, digoxi L-dopa, tricyclics, adriamycin, doxorubicin), metabolic imbalance (K^+, Ca^{2+}, Mg hypoxia, hypercapnia, metabolic acidosis, thyroid disease), & phaeochromocytom

Presentation is with palpitation, chest pain, presyncope/syncope, hypotension, pulmonary oedema. Some arrhythmias may be asymptomatic and incidental, eg

History Take a detailed history of palpitations (p66). Ask about precipitati factors, onset, nature (fast or slow, regular or irregular) duration, associat symptoms (chest pain, dyspnoea, collapse). Review drug history. Ask about pa medical history or family history of cardiac disease.

Tests FBC, U&E, glucose, Ca^{2+}, Mg^{2+}, TSH. ECG: Look for signs of IHD, AF, short P interval (WPW syndrome), long QT interval (metabolic imbalance, drugs, congenita U waves (hypokalaemia). 24h ECG monitoring; several recordings may be neede Echo: Any structural heart disease, eg mitral stenosis, HOCM? Provocation tes Exercise ECG, cardiac catheterization ± electrophysiological studies may be need

Treatment If the ECG is normal during palpitations, reassure the patie Otherwise, treatment depends on the type of arrhythmia.

Bradycardia: (p111) If asymptomatic and rate >40bpm, no treatment required. Look for a cause (drugs, sick sinus syndrome, hypothyroidism) and st any drugs that may be contributing (β-blocker, digoxin). If rate <40bpm or patie is symptomatic, give atropine 0.6–1.2mg IV (up to maximum of 3mg). If response, insert a temporary pacing wire (p764). If necessary, start an isoprenali infusion or use external cardiac pacing.

Sick sinus syndrome: Sinus node dysfunction causes bradycardia ± arre sinoatrial block or SVT alternating with bradycardia/asystole (tachy–bra syndrome). AF and thromboembolism may occur. Pace if symptomatic.

SVT: (p112) Narrow complex tachycardia (rate >100bpm, QRS width <120m Acute management: Vagotonic manoeuvres followed by IV adenosine or verapa (if not on β-blocker); DC shock if compromised. Maintenance therapy: β-blockers verapamil.

AF/flutter: (p130) May be incidental finding. Control ventricular rate with digo loading dose (~500µg/12h × 2) followed by maintenance dc (0.125–0.25mg/24h). Alternatives: Verapamil, β-blocker, or amiodarone. Flecain for pre-excited AF. DC shock if compromised (p758).

VT: (p114) Broad complex tachycardia (rate >100bpm, QRS duration >120r Acute management: IV lidocaine (=lignocaine), or amiodarone IV, if no response o compromised DC shock. Oral therapy: amiodarone loading dose (200mg/8h PO 7d, then 200mg/12h for 7d) followed by maintenance therapy (200mg/24h). Corneal deposits, photosensitivity, hepatitis, pneumonitis, lung fibrosis, nightma INR↑ (warfarin potentiation), T4↑, T3↓. Monitor LFT and TFT.

►Finally, permanent pacing may be used to overdrive tachyarrhythmias, to tr bradyarrhythmias, or prophylactically in conduction disturbances (p11 Implanted automatic defibrillators can save lives.

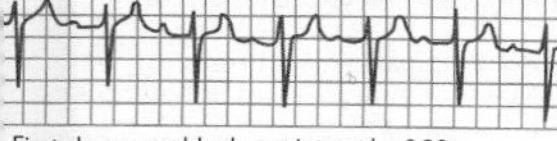

First degree AV block. P–R interval = 0.28s

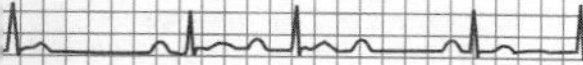

Mobitz type I (Wenckebach) AV block. With each succesive QRS, the P–R interval increases—until there is a non-conducted P wave.

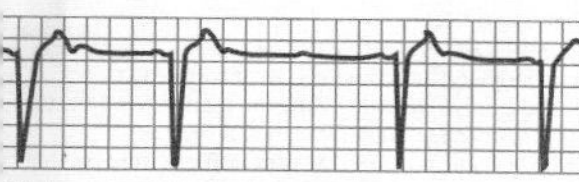

Mobitz type II AV block. Ratio of AV conduction varies from 2:1 to 3:1

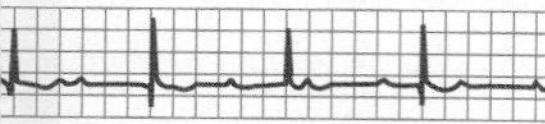

Complete AV block with narrow ventricular complexes. There is no relation between atrial and the slower ventricular activity.

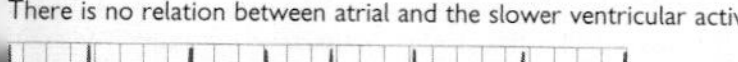

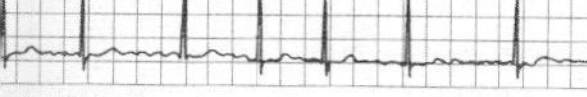

Atrial fibrillation

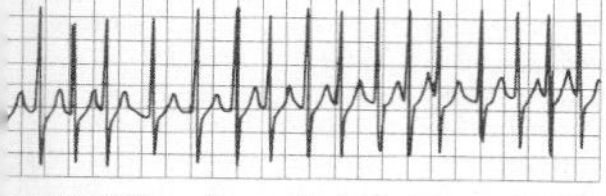

Atrial fibrillation with a rapid ventricular response. Diagnosis is based on the totally irregular ventricular rhythm.

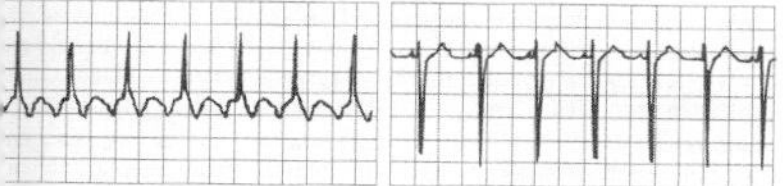

Atrial flutter with 2:1 AV block. Lead aVF (on left) shows the characteristic saw-tooth baseline whereas lead V1 (on right) shows discrete atrial activity, alternate 'F' waves being superimposed on ventricular T waves.

Narrow complex tachycardia

ECG shows rate of >100bpm and QRS complex duration of <120ms.

Differential diagnosis

- Sinus tachycardia: normal P wave followed by normal QRS.
- Supraventricular tachycardia (SVT): P wave absent or inverted after QRS.
- AF: absent P wave, irregular QRS complexes.
- Atrial flutter: atrial rate usually 300bpm giving 'flutter waves' or 'sawtoo baseline (p111), ventricular rate often 150bpm (2:1 block).
- Atrial tachycardia: abnormally shaped P waves, may outnumber QRS.
- Multifocal atrial tachycardia: 3 or more P wave morphologies, irregular Q complexes.
- Junctional tachycardia: rate 150–250bpm, P wave either buried in QRS compl or occurring after QRS complex.

Principles of management See p792.

- If the patient is compromised, use DC cardioversion (p758).
- Otherwise, identify the underlying rhythm and treat accordingly.
- Vagal manoeuvres (carotid sinus massage, Valsalva manoeuvre) transien increase AV block, and may unmask an underlying atrial rhythm.
- If unsuccessful, give adenosine which causes transient AV block. It has a short (10–15s) and works in 2 ways: by transiently slowing ventricles to sh underlying atrial rhythm; by cardioverting a junctional tachycardia to sin rhythm.

Adenosine dose: Give 6mg IV bolus into a big vein; follow by saline flush, wh recording a rhythm strip; if unsuccessful, after 1–2min, give 12mg, then 12 again, unless on dipyridamole or post cardiac transplantation (see *BNF*). Warn of transient chest tightness, dyspnoea, headache, flushing. CI: asthma, 2nd/3rd deg AV block, or sinoatrial disease (unless pacemaker). Drug interactions: potentiated dipyridamole, antagonized by theophylline. Transplanted hearts are very sensiti use a smaller dose.

Specific management ***Sinus tachycardia*** Identify and treat the cause (p84

SVT: If adenosine fails, use verapamil 2.5–5mg IV over 2min, or over 3min if elde (►not if already on β-blocker). If no response, give further dose of 5mg IV after 10min. Alternatives: atenolol 2.5mg IV at 1mg/min repeated at 5min intervals t maximum of 10mg or sotalol 20–60mg IV. If no good, use DC cardioversion.

AF/flutter: Manage along standard lines (p116).

Atrial tachycardia: Rare. If due to digoxin toxicity, stop digoxin; consic digoxin-specific antibody fragments (p826). Maintain K^+ at 4–5mmol/L.

Multifocal atrial tachycardia: Most commonly occurs in COPD. Corr hypoxia and hypercapnia. Consider verapamil if rate remains >110bpm.

Junctional tachycardia: There are 3 types of junctional tachycardia: AV nodal entry tachycardia (AVNRT), AV re-entry tachycardia (AVRT), and His bun tachycardia. Where anterograde conduction through the AV node occurs, va manoeuvres are worth trying. Adenosine will usually cardiovert a junctional rhyt to sinus rhythm. If it recurs, treat with a β-blocker or amiodarone. Radiofreque ablation is increasingly being used in AVRT and in some patients with AVNRT.

WPW syndrome (Wolff–Parkinson–White ECG p117) Caused by congen accessory conduction pathway between atria and ventricles. Resting ECG sho short P–R interval and wide QRS complex due to slurred upstroke or 'delta wa 2 types: WPW type A (+ve δ wave in V_1), WPW type B (–ve δ wave in V_1). Patie present with SVT which may be due to an AVRT, pre-excited AF, or pre-excited at flutter. Refer to cardiologist for electrophysiology and ablation of access pathway.

Broad complex tachycardia

ECG shows rate of >100 and QRS complexes >120ms (>3 small squares, p82). If no clear QRS complexes, it is VF or asystole, p766.

Principles of management
- Identify the underlying rhythm and treat accordingly.
- If in doubt, treat as ventricular tachycardia (VT)—the commonest cause.

Differential diagnosis
- VT; includes Torsade de pointes, below
- Supraventricular tachycardia (SVT) with aberrant conduction, eg AF, atrial flutter

(NB: Ventricular ectopics should not cause confusion when occurring singly; but if >3 together at rate of >120, this constitutes VT.)

Identification of the underlying rhythm (see OPPOSITE) may be difficult, seek expert help. Diagnosis is based on the history (IHD increases the likelihood of a ventricular arrhythmia), a 12-lead ECG, and the lack of response to IV adenosine (p112). ECG findings in favour of VT:
- Positive QRS concordance in chest leads
- Marked left axis deviation
- AV dissociation (occurs in 25%) or 2:1 or 3:1 AV block
- Fusion beats or capture beats; see OPPOSITE
- RSR complex in V_1 (with positive QRS in V_1)
- QS complex in V_6 (with negative QRS in V_1).

Concordance means QRS complexes are all +ve or −ve. ***A fusion beat*** is when a 'normal beat' fuses with a VT complex to create an unusual complex, and a ***capture beat*** is a normal QRS between abnormal beats (see OPPOSITE).

Management Connect to a cardiac monitor; have a defibrillator to hand.
- Give high-flow oxygen by face mask
- Obtain IV access and take blood for U&E, cardiac enzymes, Ca^{2+}, Mg^{2+}
- Obtain 12-lead ECG
- ABG (if evidence of pulmonary oedema, reduced conscious level, sepsis).

VT: Haemodynamically stable
- Correct hypokalaemia and hypomagnesaemia.
- Amiodarone 300mg IV over 20-60min, then 900mg over 24hr.
- OR lidocaine 50mg over 2min repeated every 5min to 200mg max.
- If this fails, or if cardiac arrest, use DC shock (p758 & inside backcover).
- After correction of VT, establish the cause from history/investigations.
- Maintenance antiarrhythmic therapy may be required. If VT occurs <24h after MI give IV amiodarone or IVI lidocaine for 12–24h. If VT occurs >24h after MI, give IV lidocaine infusion and start oral antiarrhythmic: eg amiodarone.
- Prevention of recurrent VT: Surgical isolation of the arrhythmogenic area or implantation of tiny automatic defibrillators may help.

Ventricular fibrillation (VF): (ECG, see OPPOSITE) ➡Use asynchronized DC shock (p758): see also the *European Resuscitation Guidelines* (see inside backcover).

Ventricular extrasystoles (ectopics) are the commonest post-MI arrhythmia but they are also seen in healthy people (≥10/h). Post-MI they suggest electrical instability, and there is a risk of VF if the 'R on T' pattern (ie no gap before the T wave) is seen. If frequent (>10/min), consider amiodarone IV as above. Otherwise just observe patient.

Torsade de pointes: Looks like VF but is VT with varying axis (ECG, see OPPOSITE). It is due ↑QT interval (a SE of anti-arrhythmics, so consider stopping). ℞: Mg sulfate 2g IV over 10 min ± overdrive pacing.

Fusion and capture beats

(a) A capture beat

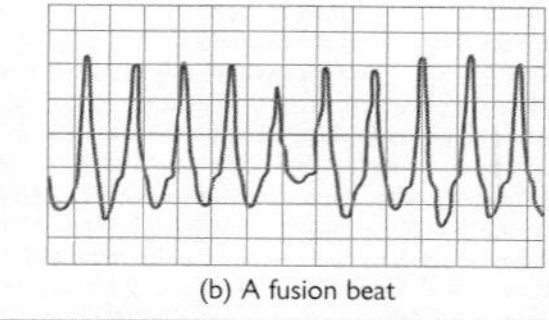

(b) A fusion beat

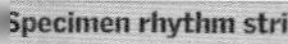

Specimen rhythm strips

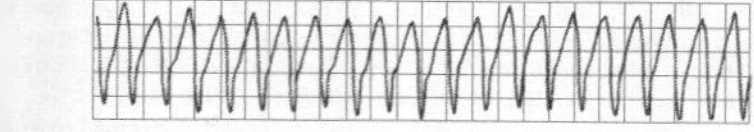

/T with a rate of 235/min.

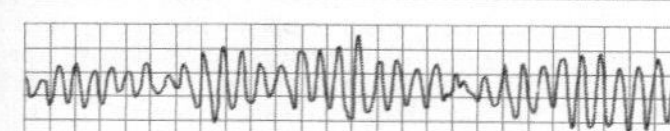

/F (p767).

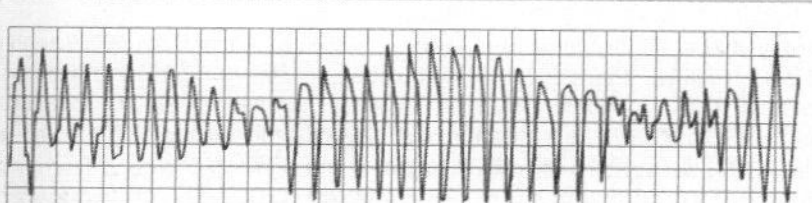

'*orsade de pointes* tachycardia.

Atrial fibrillation (AF) and flutter

ECG p111; NICE 200

AF is a chaotic, irregular atrial rhythm at 300–600bpm; the AV node responds inte mittently, hence an irregular ventricular rate. If the ventricles aren't primed reliab by the atria, cardiac output drops by 10–20%. AF is common in the elderly (≤9% The main risk is embolic stroke. Warfarin reduces this to 1%/yr from 4%. So, *do ECG on everyone with an irregular pulse* (±24h ECG if dizzy, faints, palpitations et

Causes Heart failure/ischaemia; hypertension; MI (seen in 22%);[25] PE; mitral val disease; pneumonia; hyperthyroidism; alcohol; post-op; K⁺↓; Mg^{2+}↓.[26] ***Rare cause*** Cardiomyopathy; constrictive pericarditis; sick sinus syndrome; lung cancer; atr myxoma; endocarditis; haemochromatosis; sarcoid. 'Lone' AF means no cause foun

Symptoms May be asymptomatic or cause chest pain, palpitations, dyspnoea, faintness. ***Signs:*** *Irregularly irregular pulse*, the apical pulse rate is greater than t radial rate and the 1st heart sound is of variable intensity; signs of LVF (p78 ►Examine the whole patient: AF is *often* associated with non-cardiac disease.

Tests *ECG* shows absent P waves, irregular QRS complexes. *Blood tests:* U&E, cardi enzymes, thyroid function tests. Consider echo to look for left atrial enlargeme mitral valve disease, poor LV function, and other structural abnormalities.

Acute AF (≤48h) Treat associated illnesses (eg MI, pneumonia). Control ventricu rate (as *below*) and start full anticoagulation with **heparin** 5000–10000U IV (p33 to keep options open for cardioversion even if the 48h time limit is running c (thrombi are now prevented).[27] If the 48h period has elapsed, cardioversion withc anticoagulation is OK if trans-oesophageal echo shows no intracardiac thromb *Cardioversion regimen:* ››O_2 ››ITU/CCU ››GA or IV sedation ››200J ››360J ››36 (monophasic; if 100J is tried 1st, it only works in <20%). Relapses back into AF a common, and *drug cardioversion* is often preferred: **amiodarone** IVI (5mg/kg over then ~900mg over 24h via a central line max 1.2g in 24h) or PO (200mg/8h for 1w 200mg/12h for 1wk, 100–200mg/24h maintenance). Alternative (if stable and known IHD or WPW): **flecainide** 2mg/kg IV over >25min, max 150mg (or 300mg stat); monitor ECG. Unfortunately, flecainide is a strong negative inotrope.

Chronic AF • **Control rate**, as below. Rate-control is as good as rhythm-contro decreasing morbidity & mortality in most people with chronic AF.[28][29] • Consic rhythm control if 1st episode or younger patient, as below. • Anticoagulate w **warfarin** (INR 2–3).[30] Less good alternative: **aspirin** ~300mg/d PO—eg if warfa contraindicated or at very low risk of emboli (<65yrs, and no hypertensi diabetes, LV dysfunction, ↑LA size, rheumatic valve disease, MI, or past TIA). ***CI warfarin in AF:***[31] Bleeding diathesis; platelets <50×10⁹/L; BP>160/ (consistently); compliance issues around dosing or INR monitoring; patient choi after risks discussed. Factors such as age ≥75–80yrs old, frequent falls, on NSAI past intracranial bleeds, Hb↓, and polypharmacy are CI according to so authorities,[32] but are less evidence-based.

Paroxysmal AF Pill-in-the-pocket may be appropriate (see box); if not, try a regu β-blocker (below). If fails and no LV dysfunction, **sotalol** 40mg/12h PO; after >4 gradually ↑dose to 80mg/12h, then 160mg/12h if needed; SE: ↑QT interval, monitor QT on ECG.[33] Alternative if LV dysfunction: **amiodarone** PO. Anticoagula

Controlling the ventricular rate In ***acute*** or ***paroxysmal*** AF, a good 1st choice **diltiazem** (60–120mg/8h PO) *or* **verapamil** (40–120mg/8h PO) *or* **metopro** (50mg/12h PO, or just 10mg/8h to start with if LV function poor). 2nd-line: **digo** and **amiodarone**. For ***chronic*** AF, a β-blocker or rate limiting Ca^{2+} blocker are choice. If this fails, add **digoxin** (p100), then consider **amiodarone**. **Digoxin** monotherapy in chronic AF is only OK in sedentary patients. ►*Don't give β-block with diltiazem or verapamil without expert advice (bradycardia risk).* NB: bad effe of rapid rates: greater irregularity of ventricular response, variable changes in au nomic output,[34] and tachycardia-mediated cardiomyopathy.[35][36] Don't get fixated a single figure to aim at: dialogue with patients tells what works best, and allo desired exercise levels, eg <90 at rest and on exertion 200–age (yrs) if ambulat

Managing various AF scenarios (NICE 2006)

When in doubt...get help.

If acute onset AF and **very ill** or **haemodynamically unstable:** ⇒O_2 ⇒U&E ⇒Emergency cardioversion; if unavailable try IV amiodarone. Do not delay emergency treatment in order to start anticoagulation. In other patients...

Try **rate control** 1st if: • >65yrs • Coronary artery disease • Contraindications to antiarrhythmics • Unsuitable for cardioversion, ie anticoagulants contra-indicated; left atrium >5cm across or mitral stenosis (maintaining *longterm* sinus rhythm is unlikely); AF has lasted >1yr; past attempts have failed (despite concurrent antiarrhythmics); an on-going *reversible* cause, eg thyrotoxicosis.

Try **rhythm control** 1st if: • Symptomatic or CCF • Younger • Presenting for 1st time with lone AF • AF is secondary to a corrected precipitant (eg U&E↑↓). If cardioversion is chosen, do pre-cardioversion echo; pre-treat for ≥4wks with **sotalol** or **amiodarone** if there is ↑risk of cardioversion failure (past failure, or past AF recurrence). In pharmacological cardioversion, **flecainide** is 1st-choice if no structural heart disease (IV **amiodarone** if structural heart disease).

In **paroxysmal AF** 'pill in the pocket' (eg flecainide PRN) may be tried if: infrequent AF, BP >100mmHg systolic, no past LV dysfunction. Anticoagulate (below).

If despite, the above, **AF continues to cause big problems,** AV node ablation, pacing, and pulmonary vein ablation are options to ask about.

Use **heparin** in acute AF until a full risk assessment for emboli (see below) is made—eg AF started <48h ago and elective cardioversion is being planned (if >48h, ensure ≥3wks of therapeutic anticoagulation before elective cardioversion; NB trans-oesophageal-guided cardioversion is also an option here).

Use **warfarin** (target INR: 2.5; range 2–3) if risk of emboli **high** (past ischaemic stroke, TIA or emboli; ≥75yrs with BP↑, DM; coronary or peripheral arterial disease; evidence of valve disease or ↓LV function/CCF (only do echo if unsure).

Use **aspirin** if warfarin contraindicated or <65 + no risk factors (?also if risk **moderate**, ie ≥65 + no high-risk factors or <75 + BP↑, DM or vascular disease. If 'warfarin or aspirin?' is equivocal, consider an echo (warfarin if abnormal).

Use **no anti-coagulation** if *stable* sinus rhythm has been restored **and** no risk factors for emboli, **and** AF recurrence unlikely (ie no failed cardioversions, no structural heart disease, no previous recurrences, no sustained AF for >1yr).

Note on atrial flutter

See p111 for ECGs.

ECG: continuous atrial depolarization (eg ~300/min, but very variable) produces a sawtooth baseline ± 2 : 1 AV block (as if SVT at, eg 150bpm). **Carotid sinus massage** and IV **adenosine** transiently block the AV node and may unmask flutter waves.

Treatment Cardioversion may be indicated (anticoagulate before, see opposite). Anti-AF drugs may not work—but consider amiodarone to restore sinus rhythm, and amiodarone or sotalol to maintain it. Cavotricuspid isthmus ablation (this flutter isthmus' is low in the right atrium) may be tried.

Wolff–Parkinson–White (WPW) syndrome

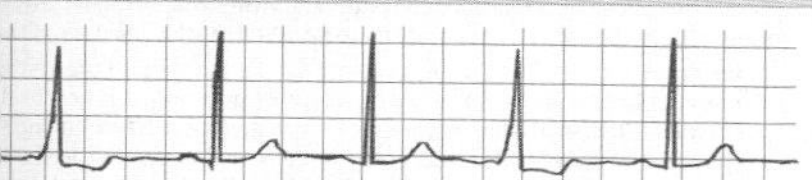

ECG of WPW syndrome (p112) in 1st & 4th beats; compared with the other beats, it can be seen how the delta wave both broadens the ventricular complex, and shortens the PR interval. ►If WPW is the underlying cause of AF, avoid AV node blockers such as diltiazem, verapamil and digoxin—but flecainide may be used.

Pacemakers

Pacemakers supply electrical initiation to myocardial contraction. The pacemal lies subcutaneously where it may be programmed through the skin as necessa Pacemakers usually last 7–15yrs.

Indications for temporary cardiac pacing

- Symptomatic bradycardia, unresponsive to atropine.
- After acute *anterior* MI, prophylactic pacing is required in:
  - Complete AV block
  - Mobitz type I AV block (Wenckebach)
  - Mobitz type II AV block
  - Non-adjacent bifascicular or trifascicular block (p86).
- After *inferior* MI, pacing may not be needed in complete AV block if reasona stable, and rate is >40–50, and QRS complexes are narrow.
- Suppression of drug-resistant tachyarrhythmias, eg SVT, VT.
- Special situations: During general anaesthesia; during cardiac surgery; dur electrophysiological studies; drug overdose (eg digoxin, β-blockers, verapam

►See p764 for further details and insertion technique.

Indications for a permanent pacemaker

- Complete AV block (Stokes–Adams attacks, asymptomatic, congenital)
- Mobitz type II AV block (p111)
- Persistent AV block after anterior MI
- Symptomatic bradycardias (eg sick sinus syndrome, p110)
- Drug-resistant tachyarrhythmias.

Some say persistent bifascicular block after MI requires a permanent system: t remains controversial.

Pre-operative assessment: FBC, clotting screen, hepatitis B status. Insert cannula. Consent for procedure under local anaesthetic. Consider pre-medicati Give antibiotic cover (eg flucloxacillin 500mg IM and benzylpenicillin 600mg 20min before, and 1 and 6h after.

Post-op assessment: Prior to discharge, check wound for bleeding or haemato check position on CXR; check pacemaker function. During 1st week, inspect wound haematoma or dehiscence. Count apical rate (p64): if this is ≥6 bpm be the rate quoted for the pacemaker, suspect malfunction. Other problems: le fracture; pacemaker interference (eg from patient's muscles). Driving rules: p1

3-letter codes These enable pacemaker identification: the **1**st letter indicates chamber paced (A =atria, V =ventricles, D =dual chamber); the **2**nd letter identifies chamber sensed (A =atria, V =ventricles, D =dual chamber, O =none), and the **3**rd let indicates the pacemaker response (T =triggered, I =inhibited, D =dual, R =revers VVI pacemakers are the most frequently used in the UK. DDD pacemakers are only pacemakers that sense and pace both chambers. ***5-letter codes*** In the letter, P =programmable; M =multiprogrammable. In the **5**th letter, P means tha tachycardia, the pacemaker will pace the patient. S means that in tachycardia pacemaker shocks the patient. D =dual ability to pace and shock. O =neither of the

ECG of paced rhythm: (ECG 7 p105, and OPPOSITE for rhythm strip) If the syste on 'demand' of 60bpm, a pacing spike will be seen only if the intrinsic heart ra <60bpm. If it is cutting in at a higher rate, its sensing mode is malfunctioning. is failing to cut in at slower rates, its pacing mode is malfunctioning, ie the l may be dislodged, the pacing threshold is too high, or the lead (or insulatior faulty. If you see spikes but no capture (ie no systole), suspect dislodgment.

ome confusing pacemaker terms

usion beat: Union of native depolarization and pacemaker impulse.

seudofusion: The pacemaker impulse occurs just after cardiac depolarization, ɔ it is ineffective, but it distorts the QRS morphology.

seudopseudofusion beat: If a DVI pacemaker gives an atrial spike within a ative QRS complex, the atrial output is non-contributory.

acemaker syndrome: In single-chamber pacing, retrograde conduction to the tria, which then contract during ventricular systole. This leads to retrograde ow in pulmonary veins, and ↓cardiac output.

acemaker tachycardia: In dual-chamber pacing, a short-circuit loop goes etween the electrodes, causing an artificial WPW-like syndrome. Solution: ingle-chamber pacing. For ECG images, see www.monroecc.edu./depts/pstc/ ackup/paracar6.htm

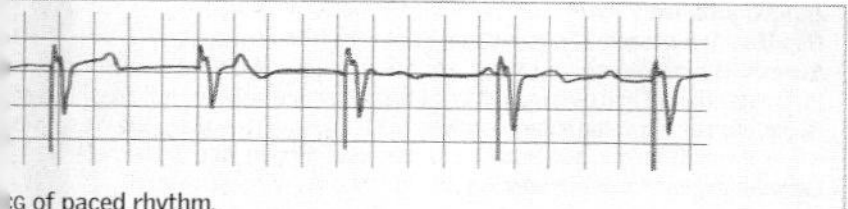

:G of paced rhythm.

Heart failure—basic concepts

Definition Cardiac output and BP are inadequate for the body's requiremen Prognosis is poor with 82% of patients dying within 6yrs of diagnosis.

Classification *LVF* and *RVF* may occur independently, or together as ***congesti cardiac failure (CCF)***. ***Low-output cardiac failure:*** The heart's output is inadequa (eg ejection fraction <35%), or is only adequate with high filling pressures. Caus Usually ischaemia, hypertension, valve disorders, or ↑alcohol use.

- ***Pump failure due to:***
  Heart muscle disease: IHD; cardiomyopathy (p138).
  Restricted filling: Constrictive pericarditis, tamponade, restrictive card myopathy. This may be the mechanism of action of fluid overload: an expandi right heart impinges on the LV, so filling is restricted by the ungiving pericardiu (the mechanism invoking a 'hump in the Starling curve' is now said to be an er based on an artefact).
  Inadequate heart rate: β-blockers, heart block, post MI.
  Negatively inotropic drugs: eg most antiarrhythmic agents.
- ***Excessive preload:*** eg mitral regurgitation or fluid overload (eg NSAID causi fluid retention). Fluid overload may cause LVF in a normal heart if renal excreti is impaired or big volumes are involved (eg IVI running too fast). More commo there is simultaneous compromise of cardiac function, and in the elderly.
- ***Chronic excessive afterload:*** eg aortic stenosis, hypertension.

NB: High-output failure is rare. Here, output is normal or increased in the face much increased needs. Failure occurs when cardiac output fails to meet the needs. It will occur with a normal heart, but even earlier if there is heart disea ***Causes:*** Heart disease with anaemia or pregnancy, hyperthyroidism, Page disease, arteriovenous malformation, beri beri. ***Consequences:*** Initially features RVF; later LVF becomes evident.

Symptoms Depend on which ventricle is more affected. *LVF:* Dyspnoea, pc exercise tolerance, fatigue, orthopnoea, paroxysmal nocturnal dyspnoea (PN nocturnal cough (±pink frothy sputum), wheeze (cardiac 'asthma'), nocturia, c peripheries, weight loss, muscle wasting. *RVF:* Peripheral oedema (up to thig sacrum, abdominal wall), abdominal distension (ascites), nausea, anorexia, fac engorgement, pulsation in neck and face (tricuspid regurgitation), epistaxis. addition, patients may be depressed or complain of drug-related side effects.

Signs Looks ill and exhausted, cool peripheries, peripheral cyanosis. Pulse: rest tachycardia, pulsus alternans. Systolic BP↓, narrow pulse pressure, raised J Praecordium: displaced apex (LV dilatation), RV heave (pulmonary hypertensic Auscultation: S_3 gallop (p32), murmurs of mitral or aortic valve disease. Che tachypnoea, bibasal end-inspiratory crackles, wheeze ('cardiac asthma'), pleu effusions. Abdomen: hepatomegaly (pulsatile in tricuspid regurgitation), ascit peripheral oedema.

Investigations According to NICE, if ECG and BNP (b-type natriuretic pept (BNP), p665) are normal, heart failure is unlikely, and an alternative diagnosis sho be considered; if either abnormal, then echocardiography (p98) is required.

Blood tests: FBC; U&E; BNP; ***CXR:*** Cardiomegaly (cardiothoracic ratio >50 prominent upper lobe veins (upper lobe diversion), peribronchial cuffing, diff interstitial or alveolar shadowing, classical perihilar 'bat's wing' shadowing, fluic the fissures, pleural effusions, Kerley B lines (variously attributed to intersti oedema and engorged peripheral lymphatics). ***ECG*** may indicate cause (look evidence of ischaemia, MI, or ventricular hypertrophy). It is rare to get a complet normal ECG in chronic heart failure. ***Echocardiography*** is the key investigation. may indicate the cause (MI, valvular heart disease) and can confirm the presence absence of LV dysfunction. ***Endomyocardial biopsy*** is rarely needed.

New York classification of heart failure: summary

- **I** Heart disease present, but no undue dyspnoea from ordinary activity.
- **II** Comfortable at rest; dyspnoea on ordinary activities.
- **III** Less than ordinary activity causes dyspnoea, which is limiting.
- **IV** Dyspnoea present at rest; all activity causes discomfort.

The CXR in left ventricular failure (see also fig 2 p714)

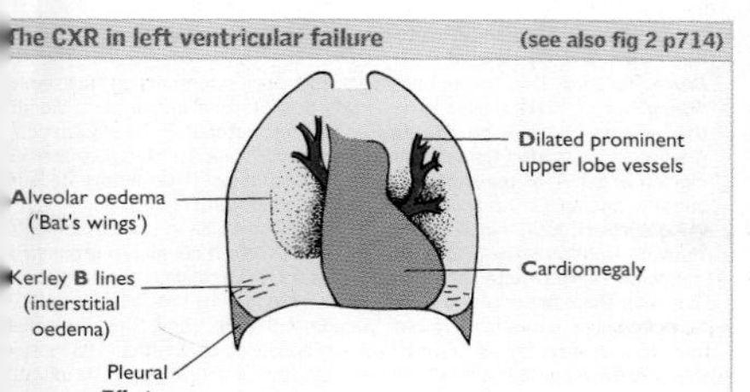

These features can be remembered as ABCDE.

Heart failure—management

Acute heart failure ⇒This is a medical emergency (p786).

Chronic heart failure Treat the cause (eg if dysrhythmias; valve disease).
- Treat exacerbating factors (anaemia, thyroid disease, infection, ↑BP).
- Avoid exacerbating factors, eg NSAIDs (cause fluid retention), and verapam (negative inotrope).
- Stop smoking. Eat less salt. Maintain optimal weight and nutrition.
- Drugs: the following are used:

1 ***Diuretics:*** Loop diuretics routinely used to relieve symptoms eg **furosemid** 40mg/24h PO; increase dose as necessary. SE: K^+↓, renal impairment. Monit U&E and add K^+ sparing diuretic (eg **spironolactone**) if K^+ <3.2mmol/ predisposition to arrhythmias, concurrent digoxin therapy (K^+↓ increases risk digoxin toxicity), or pre-existing K^+-losing conditions. If refractory oedem consider adding a thiazide eg **metolazone** 5–20mg/24h PO.

2 ***ACE-inhibitor:*** Consider in all patients with left ventricular systolic dysfunctio improves symptoms and prolongs life (see OPPOSITE). If cough is a problem a angiotensin receptor antagonist may be substituted (eg candesartan 4mg/d; ma 32mg PO). These are occasionally used in combination by specialists, SE ↑K^+.

3 ***β-blockers*** (eg **carvedilol**) Recent randomized trials show that β-blocke ↓mortality in heart failure. These benefits appear to be additional to those ACE-i in patients with heart failure due to LV dysfunction. Should be initiate after diuretic and ACE-i. Use with caution: 'start low and go slow'; if in doubt see specialist advice first (eg carvedilol 3.125mg/bd → 25–50mg/bd); wait ≥2wk between each dose increment.

4 ***Spironolactone:*** The RALES trial showed that spironolactone (25mg/24h P ↓mortality by 30% when added to conventional therapy. It should be initiated patients who remain symptomatic despite optimal therapy as listed above. improves endothelial dysfunction (↑nitric oxide bio-availability) and preven remodelling. Spironolactone is K^+-sparing, but there is little risk of significa hyperkalaemia, even when given with ACE-i.

5 ***Digoxin*** improves symptoms even in those with sinus rhythm (data from th RADIANCE and other trials). Use it if diuretics, ACE-i, and β-blocker do not contr symptoms, or in patients with AF. Dose: 0.125–0.25mg/24h PO. Monitor U&E an maintain K^+ at 4–5mmol/L. Other inotropes are unhelpful in terms of outcom

6 ***Vasodilators:*** The combination of **hydralazine** (SE: drug-induced lupus) an **isosorbide dinitrate** should be used in combination in people intolerant of an ACE or angiotensin receptor antagonist as it reduces mortality. It also reduce mortality when given in addition to standard therapy (including ACE-i) in Bla subjects with heart failure.

Intractable heart failure Reassess the cause. Are they taking the drugs?—a maximum dose? Admit to hospital for:
- Strict bed rest.
- Metolazone and IV frusemide (p786).
- IV opiates and nitrates may relieve symptoms (p786).
- Daily weight and frequent U&E (beware K^+↓).
- DVT prophylaxis: eg heparin 5000U/8h SC and TED (thromboembolic deterren stockings.
- *In extremis*, IV inotropes (p788) may be needed (it may be difficult to wea patients off them).
- Finally, consider a heart transplant. NB: reports of the Jarvik thumb-size titanium axial-flow impeller pump seem promising. It is implanted in to the L A graft takes the blood to the descending aorta—making surgery hazardous

How to start ACE-inhibitors

Check that there are no contraindications/cautions:

- Renal failure (serum creatinine >200µmol/L; but not an absolute CI)
- Hyperkalaemia: K^+ >5.5mmol/L
- Hyponatraemia: caution if <130mmol/L (relates to a poorer prognosis)
- Hypovolaemia
- Hypotension (systolic BP <90mmHg)
- Aortic stenosis or LV outflow tract obstruction
- Pregnancy or lactation
- Severe COPD or cor pulmonale (not an absolute CI)
- Renal artery stenosis[1] (Suspect if arteriopathic, eg cerebrovascular disease, IHD, peripheral vascular disease. ACE-inhibitors reduce GFR and may precipitate acute renal failure).

Warn the patient about possible side effects:

- Hypotension, especially with 1st dose (so lie down after swallowing)
- Dry cough (1:10)
- Taste disturbance
- Hyperkalaemia
- Renal impairment
- Urticaria and angioneurotic oedema (<1:1,000)
- Rarely: proteinuria, leucopenia, fatigue

Starting ACE-inhibitors:

Hypertensive patients can be safely started on ACE-inhibitors as outpatients. Warn them about SE (*note: postural hypotension is rare in pure hypertension*) and advise them to take the 1st dose on going to bed. Use a long-acting ACE-inhibitor, eg lisinopril 10mg PO per day, 2.5mg per day in the elderly.

Patients with CCF are best started on ACE-inhibitors under close medical supervision. Start with small dose and increase every 2wks until at target dose (equivalent of 30–40mg lisinopril a day) or side effects supervene (↓BP, ↑creatinine). Review in ~1wk for assessment; monitor U&E regularly. Patients on high doses of diuretics (>80mg furosemide a day) may need a reduction in their diuretic dose first—seek expert help.

1 If renovascular disease precludes the use of ACE-i and furosemide is providing no answer, consider maximal vasodilatation with nitrates and hydralazine: seek expert advice.

Hypertension

►Hypertension is a major risk factor for stroke and MI. It is usually asymptomati so screening is vital.

Defining hypertension Blood pressure has a skewed normal distribution (p73 within the population, and risk is continuously related to blood pressure. Therefore, it is impossible to define 'hypertension'. We choose to select a valu above which risk is significantly increased, and the benefit of treatment is clear cu see below. BP should be assessed over a period of time (don't rely on a sing reading). The 'observation' period depends on the BP and the presence of other ris factors or end-organ damage.

Whom to treat All patients with malignant hypertension or a sustaine pressure ≥160/100mmHg should be treated (see p125). For those ≥140/90, th decision depends on the risk of coronary events, presence of diabetes or end-orga damage; see the *Joint British Guidelines*, p125.

Systolic SBP or diastolic DBP pressure? For many years diastolic pressure wa considered to be more important than systolic pressure. However, evidence fro the Framingham and the MrFIT studies indicates that systolic pressure is the mo important determinant of cardiovascular risk in the over 50s.

Isolated systolic hypertension (ISH): The most common form of hypertension the UK—affects >50% of the over 60s, and results from stiffening of the larg arteries (arteriosclerosis). It is not benign: doubles risk of MI, triples risk of CV Treatment reduces this is excess risk, and is as, if not more effective than treatir moderate hypertension in middle-aged patients.

'Malignant' hypertension: This refers to severe hypertension (eg systolic >20 diastolic>130mmHg) in conjunction with bilateral retinal haemorrhages ar exudates; papilloedema may or may not be present. Symptoms are common, e headache ± visual disturbance. Alone it requires urgent treatment. However, it ma precipitate acute renal failure, heart failure, or encephalopathy, which a hypertensive emergencies. Untreated, 90% die in 1yr; treated, 70% survive 5yr Pathological hallmark is fibrinoid necrosis. It is more common in younger patien and in Blacks. Look hard for any underlying cause.

Essential hypertension (primary, cause unknown). ~95% of cases.

Secondary hypertension ~5% of cases. Causes include:

- ***Renal disease:*** The most common secondary cause. 75% are from *intrinsic ren disease:* glomerulonephritis, polyarteritis nodosa (PAN), systemic sclerosis, chron pyelonephritis, or polycystic kidneys. 25% are due to *renovascular disease,* mo frequently atheromatous (elderly ♂ cigarette smokers, eg with peripher vascular disease) or rarely fibromuscular dysplasia (young ♀), p300.
- ***Endocrine disease:*** Cushing's (p208) and Conn's syndromes (p212 phaeochromocytoma (p212), acromegaly, hyperparathyroidism.
- ***Others:*** Coarctation, pregnancy (*OHCS* p48), steroids, MAOI, 'the Pill'.

Signs & symptoms Usually asymptomatic (except malignant hypertension, above Headache is no more common than in the general population. Always examine th CVS system fully and check for retinopathy. Are there features of an underlyir cause (phaeochromocytoma, p212 etc.), signs of renal disease, radio-femoral dela or weak femoral pulses (coarctation), renal bruits, palpable kidneys, or Cushing syndrome? Look for end-organ damage: LVH, retinopathy and proteinuria—indicate severity and duration of hypertension and associated with a poorer prognosis.

Investigations *Basic:* U&E, creatinine, cholesterol, glucose, ECG, urine analysis (fo protein, blood). *Specific* (exclude a secondary cause): renal ultrasound, ren arteriography, 24h urinary VMA × 3 (p212), urinary free cortisol (p209), renin, ar aldosterone. ECHO and 24h ambulatory BP monitoring may be helpful in some case eg white coat or borderline hypertension. Ambulatory readings are always lowe add-on 12/7mmHg to 'convert' to clinic pressures for decision making).

Hypertensive retinopathy

Grade

I Tortuous arteries with thick shiny walls (silver or copper wiring, p544, fig 2)
II A–V nipping (narrowing where arteries cross veins, p544, fig 1)
III Flame haemorrhages and cotton wool spots
IV Papilloedema, p544, fig 3.

Measuring blood pressure

(see also p29)

- Use the correct size cuff. The cuff width should be >40% of the arm circumference. The bladder should be centred over the brachial artery, and the cuff applied snugly. Support the arm in a horizontal position at mid-sternal level.
- Inflate the cuff while palpating the brachial artery, until the pulse disappears. This provides an estimate of systolic pressure.
- Inflate the cuff until 30mmHg above systolic pressure, then place stethoscope over the brachial artery. Deflate the cuff at 2mmHg/s.
- *Systolic pressure:* The appearance of sustained repetitive tapping sounds (Korotkoff I).
- *Diastolic pressure:* Usually the disappearance of sounds (Korotkoff V). However, in some individuals (eg pregnant women) sounds are present until the zero-point. In this case, the muffling of sounds, Korotkoff IV, should be used. State which is used for a given reading. For children, see *OHCS* p156.

Joint British recommendation on preventing coronary heart disease[1]

www.bhsoc.org/latest_BHS_management_guidelines.htm

Measure BP and other risk factors (plasma lipids, glucose)

- SBP ≥160 and/or DBP ≥100 → Lifestyle change + drugs if BP sustained at these levels on repeated measurements
- SBP 140–159 and/or DBP 90–99
  - CHD + stroke risk* ≥20% over 10yrs or target organ damage or diabetes → Lifestyle and drug(s) if BP sustained on repeat measurements
  - CHD + stroke risk* <20% and no target organ damage → Lifestyle and reassess every year
- SBP <140 and DBP <90 → Reassess in 5yrs. Give advice on healthy lifestyle

All values are mmHg; SBP = systolic; DBP = diastolic.

Target pressure is <140/85mmHg, but in diabetes mellitus, aim for <130/80mmHg, and <125/75 if proteinuria).

*To quantify this, see www.hyp.ac.uk/bhs/resources/guidelines.htm. **NB:** most sources older than 2004 just tabulate CHD risk, not CHD + stroke. The new CHD + stroke threshold of 20% ≈ 15% for CHD alone.[1]

Examples of target (end-organ) damage:

- LVH
- PMH myocardial infarct or angina
- PMH stroke/TIA
- Peripheral vascular disease
- Renal failure.

1 See British Cardiac Society & British Hyperlipidaemia Association & British Hypertension Society (BHS) British Diabetic Association *Heart* 2005 **91** (1); see also USA Joint National Committee regimen (JNC 7) 3 *JAMA* **289** 2560-72; BHS-IV *2004 Guidelines, BMJ* 2004 **328** 634.

Hypertension—management

Look for and treat underlying causes (eg renal disease, alcohol↑: see p124). Dru therapy reduces the risk of cardiovascular disease and death. Almost any adult ove 50 would benefit from the antihypertensives below, *whatever their starting BP*. Treatment is especially important if: BP is persistently ≥160/100mmHg **or** cardi vascular risk ↑ (10yr risk of vascular disease ≥20%) **or** existing vascular disease target organ damage (eg brain, kidney, heart, retina) with BP >140/90mmHg.

Treatment goal <140/85mmHg (<130/80 in diabetes). Reduce blood pressu *slowly*; rapid reduction can be fatal, especially in the context of an acute stroke

Lifestyle changes ↓Concomitant risk factors: stop smoking; low-fat diet. Reduc alcohol and salt intake; increase exercise; reduce weight if obese.

Drugs Explain that long-term treatment is needed. Essential hypertension is no 'curable'. The ALLHAT study suggests that adequate BP reduction is more importa than the specific drug used; but ALLHAT did not include β-blockers, and new da cast doubt on their value, particularly atenolol, and especially if combined with thiazide. Conversely, ACE-i may provide added *renal* benefit in diabetics or if GFR

- If ≥55yrs, and in Black patients of any age, 1st choice is a Ca^{2+} channel blocker thiazide. If <55, 1st choice is ACE-i (or ARB if ACE–i intolerant, eg from cough)
- If initial ℞ was with a Ca^{2+} channel blocker or a thiazide, and a 2nd drug is neede add an ACE-i. If initial ℞ was with ACE-i, add a Ca^{2+} channel blocker or a thiazic
- If treatment with 3 drugs is needed, try ACE-i, Ca^{2+} channel blocker and thiazic
- If BP still uncontrolled on adequate doses of 3 drugs, add a 4th and get help.
- If a 4th drug is needed, consider: higher dose thiazide (unlikely to help) or a ne diuretic, eg spironolactone (monitor U&E), or β-blockers, or selective α-blocker
- β-blockers are not 1st-line for hypertension, but consider in younger peop particularly: if intolerance or contra-indication to ACE-i/ARB (angiotensin recept blockers) exists, or she is a women of child-bearing potential, or there ↑sympathetic drive. Here, if therapy is initiated with a β-blocker and a 2nd dru is needed, add a Ca^{2+} blocker not a thiazide to reduce risk of developing diabete

Dose examples ***Thiazides:*** eg chlortalidone 25–50mg/24h PO *mane*. SEs: K^+↓, Na^+ postural hypotension, impotence. CI: gout. ***Ca^{2+} channel blockers:*** eg nifedipine M 30–60mg/24h PO. SE: flushes, fatigue, gum hyperplasia, ankle oedema. Avo short-acting drugs. ***ACE-i:*** eg lisinopril 2.5–20mg/24h PO (max 40mg/d). ACE-i may 1st choice if co-existing LVF, or in diabetics (esp. if microalbuminuria, p301) proteinuria. SE: cough, K^+↑, renal failure, angio-oedema. CI bilateral renal arte or aortic valve stenosis; p123. ***ARB:*** losartan (50mg/d); caution if valve disease cardiomyopathy; monitor K^+. SE: diarrhoea, vertigo, urticaria, pruritus. ***β-blocker*** eg bisoprolol 2.5–5mg/24h PO. SE: bronchospasm, heart failure, cold peripherie lethargy, impotence. CI: asthma; caution in heart failure. Consider ***aspirin*** when controlled, if aged >55yrs. Add a ***statin*** (p682, esp. if other risk factors). ►Mo drugs take 4–8wks to gain maximum effect: don't assess efficacy with just one measurement.

Malignant hypertension In general, use oral therapy, unless there is enceph opathy or CCF. The aim is for a controlled reduction in blood pressure over days, n hours. Avoid sudden drops in BP as cerebral autoregulation is poor (so stroke risk

- Bed rest; there is no ideal hypotensive, but atenolol, or long-acting Ca^{2+} blocke may be used PO.
- Encephalopathy (headache, focal CNS signs, seizures, coma): aim to reduce BP ~110mmHg diastolic over 4h. Admit to monitored area. Insert intra-arterial li for pressure monitoring. Furosemide 40–80mg IV; then either IV labetalol (50mg IV over 1min, repeated every 5min, max 200mg), or sodium nitroprussi infusion (0.5μg/kg/min IVI titrated up to 8μg/kg/min, eg 50mg in 1L dextro 5%; expect to give 100–200mL/h for a few hours only, to avoid cyanide risk

►Never use sublingual nifedipine to reduce BP (∵ big drop in BP and stroke risk)

Cardiovascular medicine

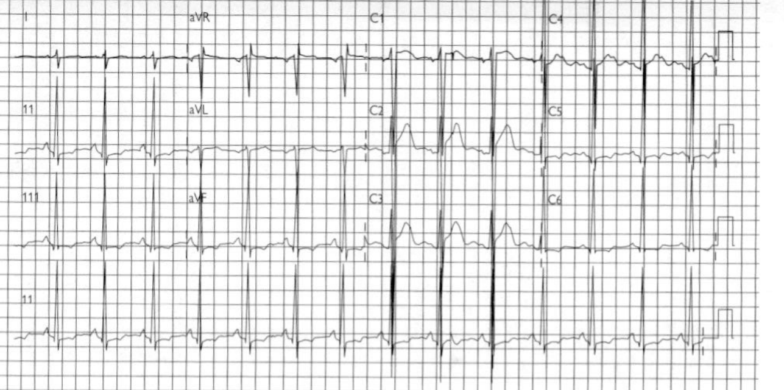

ECG 8—left ventricular hypertrophy—this is from a patient with malignant hypertension—note the sum of the S-wave in C2 and R-wave in C6 is greater than 35mm.

Rheumatic fever

This systemic infection is still common in developing countries but increasin rare in the West. Peak incidence: 5–15yrs. Tends to recur unless prevent Pharyngeal infection with Lancefield Group A β-haemolytic streptococci trigg rheumatic fever 2–4wks later, in the susceptible 2% of the population. An antibo to the carbohydrate cell wall of the streptococcus cross-reacts with valve tiss (antigenic mimicry) and may cause permanent damage to the heart valves.

Diagnosis Use the ***revised Jones criteria.*** There must be evidence of recent str infection plus 2 major criteria, or 1 major + 2 minor.

Evidence of streptococcal infection:
- Recent streptococcal infection
- History of scarlet fever
- Positive throat swab
- Increase in ASOT >200U/mL
- Increase in DNase B titre.

Major criteria:
- *Carditis:* Tachycardia, murmurs (mitral or aortic regurgitation, Carey Coom murmur, p34), pericardial rub, CCF, cardiomegaly, conduction defects (45–70 An apical systolic murmur may be the only sign.
- *Arthritis:* A migratory, 'flitting' polyarthritis; usually affects larger joints (75
- *Subcutaneous nodules:* Small, mobile painless nodules on extensor surfaces joints and spine (2–20%).
- *Erythema marginatum:* Geographical-type rash with red, raised edges and cle centre; occurs mainly on trunk, thighs, arms in 2–10% (p546).
- *Sydenham's chorea* (St Vitus' dance): Occurs late in 10%. Unilateral bilateral involuntary semi-purposeful movements. May be preceded by emotio lability and uncharacteristic behaviour.

Minor criteria:
- Fever
- Raised ESR or CRP
- Arthralgia (but not if arthritis is one of the major criteria)
- Prolonged P–R interval (but not if carditis is major criterion)
- Previous rheumatic fever.

Management
- Bed rest until CRP normal for 2wks (may be 3 months).
- Benzylpenicillin 0.6–1.2g IM stat then penicillin V 250mg/6h PO.
- Analgesia for carditis/arthritis: Aspirin 100mg/kg/d PO in divided doses (m 8g/d) for 2d, then 70mg/kg/d for 6wks. Monitor salicylate level. Toxicity cau tinnitus, hyperventilation, metabolic acidosis. Alternative: NSAIDs (p532).
- Steroids are thought not to have a major impact on sequelae, but they m improve symptoms.
- Immobilize joints in severe arthritis.
- Haloperidol (0.5mg/8h PO) or diazepam for the chorea.

Prognosis 60% with carditis develop chronic rheumatic heart disease. T correlates with the severity of the carditis. Acute attacks last an average o months. Recurrence may be precipitated by further streptococcal infectio pregnancy, or use of the Pill. Cardiac sequelae affect mitral (70%), aortic (40 tricuspid (10%), and pulmonary (2%) valves. Incompetent lesions develop dur the attack, stenoses years later.

Secondary prophylaxis Penicillin V 250mg/12h PO until no longer at risk (>30y Alternative: sulfadiazine 1g daily (0.5g if <30kg). Thereafter, give antibic prophylaxis for dental or other surgery (p136).

Mitral valve disease

Mitral stenosis ***Causes:*** Rheumatic; congenital, mucopolysaccharidoses, end cardial fibroelastosis, malignant carcinoid (p270), prosthetic valve.

Presentation: Dyspnoea; fatigue; palpitations; chest pain; systemic emb haemoptysis; chronic bronchitis-like picture ± complications (below).

Signs: Malar (ie cheek) flush; low-volume pulse; AF common; tapping, non-displac apex beat (palpable S_1). On auscultation: loud S_1; opening snap (pliable valv rumbling mid-diastolic murmur (heard best in expiration, with patient on left sic Graham Steell murmur (p34) may occur. *Severity:* The more severe the stenosis, longer the diastolic murmur, and the closer the opening snap is to S_2.

Tests: *ECG:* AF; P-mitrale if in sinus rhythm; RVH; progressive RAD. *CXR:* left at enlargement; pulmonary oedema; mitral valve calcification. *Echocardiography* diagnostic. Significant stenosis exists if the valve orifice is <1cm²/m² body surf area. Indications for *cardiac catheterization:* previous valvotomy; signs of ot valve disease; angina; severe pulmonary hypertension; calcified mitral valve.

Management: If in AF, *rate control (p116) is crucial*; anticoagulate with warfa (p334). Diuretics ↓preload and pulmonary venous congestion. If this fails to cont symptoms, balloon valvuloplasty (if pliable, non-calcified valve), open mit valvotomy or valve replacement. SBE/IE prophylaxis for dental or surgi procedures (p136). Oral penicillin as prophylaxis against recurrent rheumatic fe if <30yrs old (p128).

Complications: Pulmonary hypertension; emboli, pressure from large LA on lo structures, eg hoarseness (recurrent laryngeal nerve), dysphagia (oesophagu bronchial obstruction; infective endocarditis (rare).

Mitral regurgitation ***Causes:*** Functional (LV dilatation); annular calcificat (elderly); rheumatic fever, infective endocarditis, mitral valve prolapse, ruptu chordae tendinae; papillary muscle dysfunction/rupture; connective tissue disord (Ehlers–Danlos, Marfan's); cardiomyopathy; congenital (may be associated w other defects, eg ASD, AV canal); appetite suppressants (eg fenflurami phentermine).

Symptoms: Dyspnoea; fatigue; palpitations; infective endocarditis. ***Signs:*** displaced, hyperdynamic apex; RV heave; soft S_1; split S_2; loud P_2 (pulmon hypertension) pansystolic murmur at apex radiating to axilla. *Severity:* The m severe, the larger the left ventricle.

Tests: *ECG:* AF ± P-mitrale if in sinus rhythm (may mean left atrial size↑); LVH. C big LA & LV; mitral valve calcification; pulmonary oedema.

Echocardiogram to assess LV function (trans-oesophageal to assess severity a suitability for repair rather than replacement). *Doppler echo* to assess size and of regurgitant jet. *Cardiac catheterization* to confirm diagnosis, exclude other va disease, assess coronary artery disease.

Management: Control rate if fast AF. Anticoagulate if: AF; history of emboli prosthetic valve; additional mitral stenosis. Diuretics improve symptoms. Surg for deteriorating symptoms; aim to repair or replace the valve before LV irrevers impaired. Antibiotics to prevent endocarditis.

Mitral valve prolapse *Prevalence*: ~5%. Occurs alone or with: ASD, patent duc arteriosus, cardiomyopathy, Turner's syndrome, Marfan's syndrome, osteogen imperfecta, pseudoxanthoma elasticum, WPW (p112). ***Symptoms:*** Asymptomati or atypical chest pain and palpitations. ***Signs:*** Mid-systolic click and/or a systolic murmur. ***Complications:*** Mitral regurgitation, cerebral emboli, arrhythm sudden death. ***Tests:*** *Echocardiography* is diagnostic. *ECG* may show inferior T w inversion. ***R:*** β-blockers may help palpitations and chest pain. Give endocard prophylaxis (p136), if co-existing mitral regurgitation.

Aortic valve disease

Aortic stenosis (AS) ***Causes:*** Senile calcification is the commonest. Othe congenital (bicuspid valve, William's syndrome, p139).

Presentation: Angina; dyspnoea; dizziness; faints; systemic emboli if infecti endocarditis; CCF; sudden death. ***Signs:*** Slow rising pulse with narrow pul pressure (feel for diminished and delayed carotid upstroke—'*parvus et tardus* heaving, non-displaced apex beat; LV heave; aortic thrill; ejection systolic murm (heard at the base, left sternal edge and the aortic area, radiates to the carotid As stenosis worsens, A_2 is increasingly delayed, giving first a single S_2 and th reversed splitting. But this sign is rare. More common is a quiet A_2. In severe AS, may be inaudible (calcified valve). There may be an ejection click (pliable valve) an S_4 (said to occur more often with bicuspid valves, but not in all populations)

Tests: *ECG:* P-mitrale, LVH with strain pattern; LAD (left anterior hemiblock); poo wave progression; LBBB or complete AV block (calcified ring). *CXR:* LVH; calcifi aortic valve; post-stenotic dilatation of ascending aorta. *Echo:* diagnostic (p9 *Doppler echo* can estimate the gradient across valves: severe stenosis if gradie ≥50mmHg and valve area <0.5cm². If the aortic jet velocity is >4m/s (or increasing by >0.3m/s per yr) risk of complications is increased. *Cardiac cathe* can assess: valve gradient; LV function; coronary artery disease; the aortic roo

Differential diagnosis: Hypertrophic obstructive cardiomyopathy (HOCM, p13

Management: If symptomatic, prognosis is poor: 2–3yr survival if angina/synco 1–2yr if cardiac failure. Prompt valve replacement (p134) is recommended. asymptomatic patients with severe AS and a deteriorating ECG, valve replacemen also recommended. If the patient is not medically fit for surgery, percutanec valvuloplasty may be attempted. Endocarditis prophylaxis (p136).

Aortic sclerosis is senile degeneration of the valve. There is an ejection systc murmur, no carotid radiation, and a normal pulse and S_2.

Aortic regurgitation (AR) ***Causes:*** *Congenital valve disease:* rheumatic fev infective endocarditis, rheumatoid arthritis; SLE; pseudoxanthoma elasticu appetite suppressants (eg fenfluramine, phentermine). *Aortic root disease:* hyp tension; trauma; aortic dissection; seronegative arthritides (ankylosing spondyli Reiter's syndrome, psoriatic arthropathy); Marfan's syndrome; osteogene imperfecta; syphilitic aortitis.

Symptoms: Dyspnoea; palpitations; cardiac failure. ***Signs:*** Collapsing (wat hammer) pulse—see p31; wide pulse pressure; displaced, hyperdynamic apex be high pitched early diastolic murmur (heard best in expiration, with patient sitt forward). Eponyms: **Corrigan's sign** (carotid pulsation); **de Musset's sign** (he nodding); **Quincke's sign** (capillary pulsations in nail beds); **Duroziez's sign** (femc diastolic murmur as blood flows *backwards* in diastole); **Traube's sign** ('pistol sh sound over femoral arteries). In severe AR, an **Austin Flint** murmur may be hea (p34).

Tests: *ECG:* LVH. *CXR:* cardiomegaly; dilated ascending aorta; pulmonary oeden *Echocardiography* is diagnostic. *Cardiac catheterization* to assess: severity of lesi anatomy of aortic root; LV function; coronary artery disease; other valve disea

Management: Indications for surgery: increasing symptoms; enlarging heart CXR/echo; ECG deterioration (T wave inversion in lateral leads); infective endocard refractory to medical therapy. Aim to replace the valve before significant dysfunction occurs. Endocarditis prophylaxis (p136).

Right heart valve disease

Tricuspid regurgitation ***Causes:*** Functional (pulmonary hypertension); rheumat fever; infective endocarditis (IV drug abusers); carcinoid syndrome; congenital (e ASD, AV canal, Ebstein's anomaly ie downward displacement of the tricuspid valve see *OHCS* p642). ***Symptoms:*** Fatigue; hepatic pain on exertion; ascites; oedem ***Signs:*** Giant *v* waves and prominent *y* descent in JVP (p30); RV heave; pansystol murmur, heard best at lower sternal edge in inspiration; pulsatile hepatomega jaundice; ascites. ***Management:*** Treat underlying cause. Drugs: diuretics, digoxi ACE-inhibitors. Valve replacement (20% operative mortality).

Tricuspid stenosis ***Cause:*** Rheumatic fever; almost always occurs with mitral aortic valve disease. ***Symptoms:*** Fatigue, ascites, oedema. ***Signs:*** Giant *a* wave ar slow *y* descent in JVP (p30); opening snap, early diastolic murmur heard at the le sternal edge in inspiration. ***Diagnosis:*** Doppler echo. ***Treatment:*** Diuretics; surgic repair.

Pulmonary stenosis ***Causes:*** Usually congenital (Turner's syndrome, Noonar syndrome, William's syndrome, Fallot's tetralogy, rubella). Acquired cause rheumatic fever, carcinoid syndrome. ***Symptoms:*** Dyspnoea; fatigue; oedem ascites. ***Signs:*** Dysmorphic facies (congenital causes); prominent *a* wave in JVP; R heave. In mild stenosis, there is an ejection click, ejection systolic murmur (whi radiates to the left shoulder); widely split S_2. In severe stenosis, the murm becomes longer and obscures A_2. P_2 becomes softer and may be inaudible. ***Test*** ECG: RAD, P-pulmonale, RVH, RBBB. CXR: post-stenotic dilatation of pulmonary arte oligaemic lung fields; RV hypertrophy; right atrial hypertrophy. Cardi catheterization is diagnostic. ***Treatment:*** Pulmonary valvuloplasty or valvotor

Pulmonary regurgitation is caused by any cause of pulmonary hypertensi (p186). A decrescendo murmur is heard in early diastole at the left sternal ed (the Graham Steell murmur).

Cardiac surgery

Valvuloplasty can be used in mitral or pulmonary stenosis (pliable, non-calcifi valve, no regurgitation). A balloon catheter is inserted across the valve and inflate

Valvotomy Closed valvotomy is rarely performed now. Open valvotomy performed under cardiopulmonary bypass through a median sternotomy.

Valve replacements *Mechanical valves* may be of the ball-cage (Starr–Edward tilting disc (Bjork–Shiley), or double tilting disc (St Jude) type. These valves a very durable but the risk of thromboembolism is high; patients require lifelo anticoagulation. *Xenografts* are made from porcine valves or pericardium. The valves are less durable and may require replacement at 8–10yrs. Anticoagulation not required unless there is AF. *Homografts* are cadaveric valves. They a particularly useful in young patients and in the replacement of infected valve *Complications of prosthetic valves:* systemic embolism, infective endocardit haemolysis, structural valve failure, arrhythmias.

CABG See OPPOSITE.

Cardiac transplantation Consider this when cardiac disease is *severely* curtaili quality of life, and survival is not expected beyond 6–12 months. Refer to specialist centre.

Coronary artery bypass grafts (CABG)

Indications for CABG: to improve survival
- Left mainstem disease
- Triple vessel disease involving proximal part of the left anterior descending

To relieve symptoms
- Angina unresponsive to drugs
- Unstable angina (sometimes)
- If angioplasty is unsuccessful

NB: When CABG and percutaneous coronary intervention (PCI, eg angioplasty) are both clinically valid options, NICE recommends that the availability of new stent technology should push the decision towards PCI.

Procedure: Surgery is planned in the light of angiograms. Not all stenoses are bypassable. The heart is stopped and blood pumped artificially by a machine outside the body (cardiac bypass). (Minimally invasive thoracotomies not requiring this are well-described, but have not yet been validated in randomized trials.) The patient's own saphenous vein or internal mammary artery is used as the graft. Several grafts may be placed. >50% of vein grafts close in 10yrs (low-dose aspirin helps prevent this). Internal mammary artery grafts last longer (but may cause chest-wall numbness).

After CABG: If angina persists or recurs (from poor run-off from the graft, distal disease, new atheroma, or graft occlusion) restart anti-anginal drugs, and consider angioplasty (repeat surgery is dangerous). Mood, sex, and intellectual problems are common early. Rehabilitation helps:
- Exercise: walk→cycle→swim→jog
- Drive at 1 month: no need to tell DVLA if non-HGV licences, p144
- Get back to work eg at 3 months
- Attend to: smoking; BP; lipids
- Aspirin 75mg/24h PO forever; consider clopidogrel if aspirin CI.

Infective endocarditis (IE)

►*Fever + new murmur = endocarditis until proven otherwise.*

Classification

- 50% of all endocarditis occurs on *normal valves*. It follows an *acute course*, ar presents with acute heart failure.
- Endocarditis on *abnormal valves* tends to run a *subacute course*. Predisposir cardiac lesions: aortic or mitral valve disease; tricuspid valves in IV drug user coarctation; patent ductus arteriosus; VSD; prosthetic valves. Endocarditis c prosthetic valves may be 'early' (acquired at the time of surgery, poor prognosi or 'late' (acquired haematogenously).

Causes ***Bacteria:*** Any cause of bacteraemia exposes valves to the risk of bacteri colonization (dentistry; UTI; urinary catheterization; cystoscopy; respiratory infec ion; endoscopy (); colon cancer; gall bladder disease; skin disease; IV cannulatio surgery; abortion; fractures). Quite often, no cause is found. *Strep viridans* is th commonest (35–50%). Others: enterococci; *Staph aureus* or *epidermid* diphtheroids and icroaerophilic streptococci. Rarely: **HACEK** group of Gram –v bacteria (*Haemophilus–Actinobacillus–Cardiobacterium–Eikenella–Kingella Coxiella burnetii*; *Chlamydia*. ***Fungi:*** These include *Candida*, *Aspergillus*, ar *Histoplasma*. ***Other causes:*** SLE (Libman–Sacks endocarditis); malignancy.

Clinical features The patient may present with any of the followin ***Septic signs:*** Fever, rigors, night sweats, malaise, weight loss, anaemia, splenome aly, and clubbing. ***Cardiac lesions:*** Any new murmur, or a change in the nature of pre-existing murmur, should raise the suspicion of endocarditis. Vegetations ma cause valve destruction, and severe regurgitation, or valve obstruction. An aort root abscess causes prolongation of the P–R interval, and may lead to complete A block. LVF is a common cause of death. ***Immune complex deposition:*** Vasculit (p542) may affect any vessel. Microscopic haematuria is commo glomerulonephritis and acute renal failure may occur. Roth spots (boat-shape retinal haemorrhage with pale centre; fig 1, p376); splinter haemorrhages (c finger or toe nails); Osler's nodes (painful pulp infarcts in fingers or toes) ar Janeway lesions (painless palmar or plantar macules) are pathognomonic. ***Embol phenomena:*** Emboli may cause abscesses in the relevant organ, eg brain, hear kidney, spleen, GI tract. In right-sided endocarditis, pulmonary abscesses may occu

Diagnosis The *Duke* criteria for definitive diagnosis of endocarditis are give OPPOSITE. ***Blood cultures:*** Take 3 sets at different times and from different sites a peak fever. 85–90% are diagnosed from the first two sets; 10% are culture negative. ***Blood tests:*** Normochromic, normocytic anaemia, neutrophil leucocytosi high ESR/CRP. Also check U&E, Mg^{2+}, LFT. ***Urinalysis*** for microscopic haematuria. *CX* (cardiomegaly) and ***ECG*** (prolonged P–R interval) at regular interval ***Echocardiography*** TTE (p98) may show vegetations, but only if >2mm. TOE (p98) more sensitive, and better for visualizing mitral lesions and possible development aortic root abscess.

Management Liaise early with a microbiologist and a cardiologist.

- Antibiotics: see BOX.
- Consider surgery if: heart failure, valvular obstruction; repeated emboli; fung endocarditis; persistent bacteraemia; myocardial abscess; unstable infecte prosthetic valve.

Prognosis 30% mortality with staphylococci; 14% with bowel organisms; 6% wi sensitive streptococci.

Prevention ►See BNF 5.1. Example: amoxicillin 3g PO 1h before dentistry. This suitable for those who have not received penicillin in the last month, includir those with prosthetic valves. (If penicillin allergic, clindamycin 600mg PO 1h pr op). If past endocarditis, IV gentamicin and amoxicillin (see *BNF*).

Duke criteria for infective endocarditis

Major criteria:

- Positive blood culture:
  - typical organism in 2 separate cultures or
  - persistently +ve blood cultures, eg 3, >12h apart (or majority if ≥4)
- Endocardium involved:
  - positive echocardiogram (vegetation, abscess, dehiscence of prosthetic valve) or
  - new valvular regurgitation (change in murmur not sufficient).

Minor criteria:

- Predisposition (cardiac lesion; IV drug abuse)
- Fever >38°C
- Vascular/immunological signs
- Positive blood culture that do not meet major criteria
- Positive echocardiogram that does not meet major criteria.

How to diagnose: Definite infective endocarditis: 2 major **or** 1 major and 3 minor **or** all 5 minor criteria (if no major criterion is met).

Antibiotic therapy for infective endocarditis

- Consult a microbiologist early. The following are guidelines only:
- *Empirical therapy:* **benzylpenicillin**[1] 1.2g/4h IV + **gentamicin**, eg 1mg/kg/8h IV for 4wks. Do gentamicin levels (p738; in IE/SBE, the *BNF* recommends a serum peak of 3–5mg/L & a pre-dose trough of <1mg/L; see p738). If acute, add **flucloxacillin** 2g/6h IV to cover staphylococci.
- *Enterococci:* **amoxicillin**[1] 1g/6h IV + gentamicin as above.
- *Streptococci:* **benzylpenicillin**[1] 1.2g/4h IV for 2–4wks; then **amoxicillin** 1g/8h PO for 2wks. Monitor minimum inhibitory concentration (MIC). Add gentamicin.
- *Staphylococci:* **flucloxacillin**[1] 2g/6h IV + **gentamicin** as above IV. Treat for 6–8wks; stop gentamicin after 1wk. If prosthetic valve or MRSA suspected, substitute flucloxacillin with vancomycin plus rifampicin.
- *Coxiella:* **doxycycline** 100mg/12h PO indefinitely + **co-trimoxazole**, **rifampicin**, or **ciprofloxacin**.
- *Fungi:* **flucytosine** 50mg/kg/6h IVI over 30 minutes followed by **fluconazole** 50mg/24h PO (higher doses may be needed). **Amphotericin** (p160) if flucytosine resistance or *Aspergillus*. **Miconazole** if renal function is poor.

1 For penicillin allergy, use vancomycin 1g/12h IV.

Diseases of heart muscle

Acute myocarditis ***Causes:*** Inflamed myocardium from viruses (coxsackie, po HIV, Lassa fever); bacteria (Clostridia, diphtheria, Meningococcus, Mycoplasn psittacosis); spirochaetes (Leptospirosis, syphilis, Lyme disease); protozoa (Chag disease p426); drugs; toxins; vasculitis, p542.

Signs & symptoms: Fatigue, dyspnoea, chest pain, palpitations, tachycardia, s S_1, S_4 gallop (p32).

Tests: ECG: ST segment elevation/depression, T wave inversion, atrial arrhythmi transient AV block. Serology may be helpful.

Management: Treat the underlying cause. Supportive measures. Patients m recover or get intractable heart failure (p122).

Dilated cardiomyopathy A dilated, flabby heart of unknown cause. Associatio alcohol, ↑BP, haemochromatosis, viral infection, autoimmune, peri- or postpartu thyrotoxicosis, congenital (x-linked). ***Prevalence:*** 0.2%. ***Presentation:*** Fatig dyspnoea, pulmonary oedema, RVF, emboli, AF, VT. ***Signs:*** ↑Pulse, ↓BP, ↑JVP, displac diffuse apex, S_3 gallop, mitral or tricuspid regurgitation (MR/TR), pleural effusi oedema, jaundice, hepatomegaly, ascites. ***Tests:*** CXR: cardiomegaly, pulmon oedema. *ECG:* tachycardia, non-specific T wave changes, poor R wave progressi *Echo:* globally dilated hypokinetic heart and low ejection fraction. Look for MR, TR mural thrombus. ***Management:*** Bed rest, diuretics, digoxin, ACE-inhibitor, antico ulation. Consider cardiac transplantation. ***Mortality:*** Variable, eg 40% in 2yrs

Hypertrophic cardiomyopathy *HOCM≈LV* outflow tract (LVOT) obstruction fr asymmetric septal hypertrophy.

Prevalence: 0.2%. Autosomal dominant inheritance, but 50% are sporadic. 70 have mutations in genes encoding β-myosin, α-tropomyosin, and troponin T. M present at any age. Ask about family history or sudden death.

Symptoms & signs: Angina; dyspnoea; palpitation; syncope; sudden death (v amenable to implantable defibrillators). Jerky pulse; *a* wave in JVP; double ap beat; systolic thrill at lower left sternal edge; harsh ejection systolic murmur.

Tests: *ECG:* LVH; progressive T wave inversion; deep Q waves (inferior + lateral lead AF; WPW syndrome (p112); ventricular ectopics; VT. *Echo:* asymmetrical sep hypertrophy; small LV cavity with hypercontractile posterior wall; midsyst closure of aortic valve; systolic anterior movement of mitral valve. *Card catheterization* may provoke VT. It helps assess: severity of gradient; coron artery disease or mitral regurgitation. Electrophysiological studies may be need (eg if WPW, p112). Exercise test (p94) ± Holter monitor (p66) to risk stratify.

Management: β-blockers or verapamil for symptoms (p100). Amiodarone (p1 for arrhythmias (AF, VT). Anticoagulate for paroxysmal AF or systemic emboli. Du chamber pacing (p118) is used if symptomatic despite drugs. Septal myomecto (surgical, or chemical, with alcohol, to ↓LV outflow tract gradient) is reserved those with severe symptoms. Consider implantable defibrillator.

Mortality: 5.9%/yr if <14yrs; 2.5%/yr if >14yrs. *Poor prognostic factors:* a <14yrs or syncope at presentation; family history of HOCM/sudden death.

Restrictive cardiomyopathy ***Causes:*** Amyloidosis; haemochromatosis; sarco osis; scleroderma; Löffler's eosinophilic endocarditis, endomyocardial fibrosis.

Presentation is like constrictive pericarditis (p140). Features of RVF predomina ↑JVP, with prominent *x* and *y* descents; hepatomegaly; oedema; ascites.

Diagnosis: Cardiac catheterization.

Cardiac myxoma Rare benign cardiac tumour. Prevalence ≤5/10,000, ♀:♂≈2 Usually sporadic, may be familial (autosomal-dominant). It may mimic infect endocarditis (fever, weight loss, clubbing, ↑ESR), or mitral stenosis (left at obstruction, systemic emboli, AF). A 'tumour plop' may be heard, and signs may va according to posture. ***Tests:*** Echocardiography. ***Treatment:*** Excision.

The heart in various, mostly rare, systemic diseases

This list reminds us to look at the heart *and* the whole patient, not just in exams (where those with odd syndromes congregate), but always.

Acromegaly: (p222) BP↑; LVH; hypertrophic cardiomyopathy; high output cardiac failure; coronary artery disease.

Amyloidosis: (p354) Restrictive cardiomyopathy.

Ankylosing spondylitis: Conduction defects; AV block; AR.

Behçet's disease: (p686) Aortic regurgitation; arterial ± venous thrombi.

Cushing's syndrome: (p208) Hypertension.

Down's syndrome: (*OHCS* p152) ASD; VSD; mitral regurgitation.

Ehlers–Danlos syndrome: (*OHCS* p642) Mitral valve prolapse + hyperelastic skin ± aneurysms and GI bleeds. Joints are loose and hypermobile; mutations exist, eg in genes for procollagen (COL3A1); there are 6 types.

Friedreich's ataxia: (p690) Hypertrophic cardiomyopathy.

Haemochromatosis: (p254) AF; cardiomyopathy.

Holt–Oram syndrome: ASD or VSD with upper limb defects.

Human immunodeficiency virus: (p396) Myocarditis; dilated cardiomyopathy; effusion; ventricular arrhythmias; SBE/IE; non-infective thrombotic (marantic) endocarditis; RVF (pulmonary hypertension); metastatic Kaposi's sarcoma.

Hypothyroidism: (p204) Sinus bradycardia; low pulse pressure; pericardial effusion; coronary artery disease; low voltage ECG.

Kawasaki disease: (*OHCS* p646) Coronary arteritis similar to PAN; commoner than *rheumatic fever* (p128) as a cause of acquired heart disease.

Klinefelter's syndrome:♂ (*OHCS* p646) ASD. Psychopathy; learning difficulties; libido↓; gynaecomastia; sparse facial hair and small firm testes. XXY.

Marfan's syndrome: (p698) Mitral valve prolapse; AR; aortic dissection. Look for long fingers and a high-arched palate.

Noonan's syndrome: (*OHCS* p650) ASD; pulmonary stenosis ± low-set ears.

PAN: (p543) Small and medium vessel vasculitis + angina; MI; arrhythmias; CCF; pericarditis and conduction defects.

Rheumatoid nodules: Conduction defects; pericarditis; LV dysfunction; aortic regurgitation; coronary arteritis. Look for arthritis signs, p532.

Sarcoidosis: (p178) Infiltrating granulomas may cause complete AV block; ventricular or supraventricular tachycardia; myocarditis; CCF; restrictive cardiomyopathy. ECG may show Q waves.

Syphilis: (p419) Myocarditis; ascending aortic aneurysm.

Systemic lupus erythematosus: (p540) Pericarditis/effusion; myocarditis; Libman–Sacks endocarditis; mitral valve prolapse; coronary arteritis.

Systemic sclerosis: (p538) Pericarditis; pericardial effusion; myocardial fibrosis; myocardial ischaemia; conduction defects; cardiomyopathy.

Thyrotoxicosis: (p202) Pulse↑; AF ± emboli; wide pulse pressure; hyperdynamic apex; loud heart sounds; ejection systolic murmur; pleuropericardial rub; angina; high output cardiac failure.

Turner's syndrome:♀ Coarctation of aorta. Look for webbed neck. XO.

William's syndrome: Supravalvular aortic stenosis (visuo-spatial IQ↓).

Pericardial diseases

Acute pericarditis Inflammation of the pericardium which may be primary • secondary to systemic disease.

Causes:
- Viruses (coxsackie, 'flu, Epstein–Barr, mumps, varicella, HIV)
- Bacteria (pneumonia, rheumatic fever, TB)
- Fungi
- Myocardial infarction, Dressler's (p690)
- Others: uraemia, Rheumatoid arthritis, SLE, myxoedema, trauma, surger malignancy, radiotherapy, procainamide, hydralazine.

Clinical features: Central chest pain worse on inspiration or lying flat ± relief t sitting forward. A pericardial friction rub may be heard. Look for evidence of pericardial effusion or cardiac tamponade (see below). Fever may occur.

Tests: *ECG* classically shows concave (saddle-shaped) ST segment elevation, but ma be normal or non-specific (10%). *Blood tests:* FBC, ESR, U&E, cardiac enzymes (*N troponin may be raised*), viral serology, blood cultures, and, if indicate autoantibodies (p539), fungal precipitins, thyroid function tests. Cardiomegaly c CXR may indicate a pericardial effusion. *Echo* (if suspected pericardial effusion).

Treatment: Analgesia, eg ibuprofen 400mg/8h PO with food. Treat the caus Consider colchicine before steroids/immunosuppressants if relapse or continuir symptoms occur. 15–40% *do* recur.

Pericardial effusion Accumulation of fluid in the pericardial sac.

Causes: Any cause of pericarditis (see above).

Clinical features: Dyspnoea, raised JVP (with prominent x descent, p31), bronchi breathing at left base (Ewart's sign: large effusion compressing left lower lobe Look for signs of cardiac tamponade (see below).

Diagnosis: *CXR* shows an enlarged, globular heart. *ECG* shows low voltage QR complexes and alternating QRS morphologies (electrical alternans). *Echocarc iography* shows an echo-free zone surrounding the heart.

Management: Treat the cause. Pericardiocentesis may be *diagnostic* (suspecte bacterial pericarditis) or *therapeutic* (cardiac tamponade). See p761. Sen pericardial fluid for culture, ZN stain/TB culture, and cytology.

Constrictive pericarditis The heart is encased in a rigid pericardium.

Causes: Often unknown (UK); elsewhere TB, or after *any* pericarditis.

Clinical features: These are mainly of right heart failure with ↑JVP (wit prominent x and y descents, p30); Kussmaul's sign (JVP rising paradoxically wit inspiration); soft, diffuse apex beat; quiet heart sounds; S_3; diastolic pericardi knock, hepatosplenomegaly, ascites, and oedema.

Tests: CXR: small heart ± pericardial calcification (if none, CT/MRI helps distinguis from other cardiomyopathies). *Echo*; cardiac catheterization.

Management: Surgical excision.

Cardiac tamponade Accumulation of pericardial fluid raises intra-pericardi pressure, hence poor ventricular filling and fall in cardiac output.

Causes: Any pericarditis (above); aortic dissection; haemodialysis; warfarin; trans septal puncture at cardiac catheterization; post cardiac biopsy.

Signs: Pulse↑, BP↓, pulsus paradoxus, JVP↑, Kussmaul's sign, muffled S_1 & S_2.

Diagnosis: *Beck's triad:* falling BP; rising JVP; small, quiet heart. *CXR*: big globula heart (if >250mL fluid). *ECG*: low voltage QRS ± electrical alternans. *Echo* i diagnostic: echo-free zone (>2cm, or >1cm if acute) around the heart ± diastoli collapse of right atrium and right ventricle.

Management: Seek expert help. The pericardial effusion needs urgen drainage (p761). Send fluid for culture, ZN stain/TB culture and cytology.

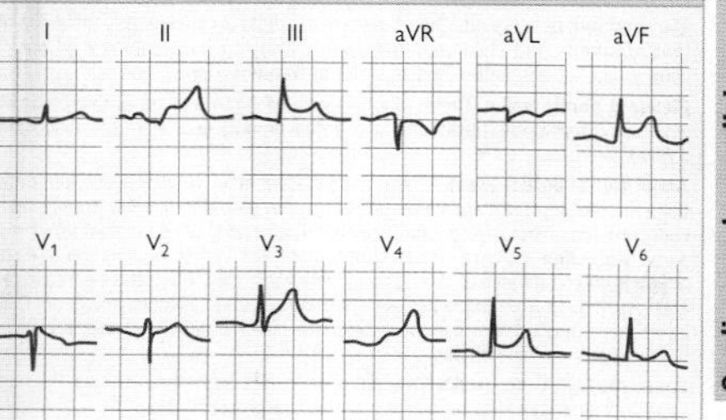
Pericarditis
I
II
III
aVR
aVL
aVF
V1
V2
V3
V4
V5
V6

Congenital heart disease

The spectrum of congenital heart disease in adults is considerably different fro that in infants and children; adults are unlikely to have complex lesions. T commonest lesions, in descending order of frequency, are:

Bicuspid aortic valve These function well at birth and go undetected. Mo eventually develop AS (requiring valve replacement) and/or AR (predisposing IE/SBE). See p132.

Atrial septal defect (ASD) A hole connects the atria. *Ostium secundum* defec (high in the septum) are commonest; *ostium primum* defects (opposing t endocardial cushions) are associated with AV valve anomalies. Primum ASDs prese early. Secundum ASDs are often asymptomatic until adulthood, as the L→R shu depends on compliance of the right and left ventricles. The latter decreases wi age (esp. if BP↑). This augments L→R shunting causing dyspnoea and heart failu eg at age 40–60. There may be pulmonary hypertension, cyanosis, arrhythm haemoptysis, and chest pain.

Signs: AF; ↑JVP; wide, fixed split S_2; pulmonary ejection systolic murmur. Pulmona hypertension may cause pulmonary or tricuspid regurgitation.

Complications: Reversal of left to right shunt (Eisenmenger's complex, s OPPOSITE), paradoxical embolism (rare).

Tests: ECG: RBBB with LAD and prolonged P–R interval (primum defect) or R (secundum defect). CXR: small aortic knuckle, pulmonary plethora, progressive atr enlargement. Echocardiography is diagnostic. Cardiac catheterization shows st up in O_2 saturation in the right atrium.

Treatment: In children, surgical closure is recommended before age 10yrs. adults, closure is recommended if symptomatic, or if asymptomatic but havi pulmonary to systemic blood flow ratios of ≥1.5:1.

Ventricular septal defect (VSD) A hole connecting the two ventricles.

Causes: congenital (prevalence 2:1000 births); acquired (post-MI).

Symptoms: May present with severe heart failure in infancy, or rem asymptomatic and be detected incidentally in later life.

Signs: These depend upon the VSD's size and site: smaller holes, which are haem dynamically less significant, give louder murmurs. Classically, a harsh pansysto murmur is heard at the left sternal edge, with a systolic thrill, ± left paraster heave. Larger holes are associated with signs of pulmonary hypertension.

Complications: AR, infundibular stenosis, infective endocarditis, pulmon hypertension, Eisenmenger's complex (OPPOSITE).

Tests: ECG: normal (small VSD), LAD + LVH (moderate VSD) or LVH + RVH (large VS CXR: normal heart size ± mild pulmonary plethora (small VSD) or cardiomegaly, la pulmonary arteries and marked pulmonary plethora (large VSD). Cardiac cathe step up in O_2 saturation in right ventricle.

Treatment: This is medical, at first, as many VSDs close spontaneously. Indicati for surgical closure: failed medical therapy, symptomatic VSD, shunt >3 : 1, SBE, Give SBE/IE prophylaxis for untreated defects (p136).

Coarctation of the aorta Congenital narrowing of the descending aorta; usu occurs just distal to the origin of the left subclavian artery. More common in bo ***Associations:*** Bicuspid aortic valve, Turner's syndrome. ***Signs:*** Radio-femoral de weak femoral pulse, BP↑, scapular bruit, systolic murmur (best heard over the scapula). ***Complications:*** Heart failure, infective endocarditis. ***Tests:*** CXR shows notching. ***Treatment:*** Surgery.

Pulmonary stenosis may occur alone or with other lesions (p134).

Cardiovascular medicine

isenmenger's syndrome

congenital heart defect which is at first associated with a left to right shunt ıay lead to pulmonary hypertension and shunt reversal. If so, cyanosis develops : heart failure and respiratory infections), and Eisenmenger's syndrome is resent.

Driving and the heart[1] (Ordinary UK licences onl

UK licences are inscribed 'You are required by law to inform Drivers Medical Bran DVLA, Swansea SA99 1AT at once if you have any disability (physical or medica which is, or may become likely to affect your fitness as a driver, unless you do r expect it to last more than 3 months'. It is the responsibility of drivers to infor the DVLA, and that of their doctors to advise patients that medical conditions (a drugs) may affect their ability to drive and for which conditions patients sho inform the DVLA. Drivers should also inform their insurance company of a condition disclosed to the DVLA. If in doubt, ask your defence union. The followi are examples of the guidance for holders of standard licences. **Different rules ap for group 2 vehicle licence-holders (eg lorries, buses).**

Angina Driving must cease when symptoms occur at rest or at the wheel. Driv may recommence when satisfactory symptom control is achieved. DVLA need not notified.

Angioplasty Driving must cease for 1wk, and may recommence thereaf provided no other disqualifying condition. DVLA need not be notified.

MI/CABG Driving must cease for >4wks. Driving may recommence thereaf provided there is no other disqualifying condition. DVLA need not be notified.

Arrhythmias ***Sinoatrial:*** Driving may recommence 4 weeks after success control provided there is no other disqualifying condition.

Significant atrioventricular conduction defects: Driving may be permitted wh underlying cause has been identified and controlled for >4wks.

AF/flutter: DVLA need not be notified unless there are distracting/disabl symptoms.

Pacemaker implant Stop driving for 1wk.

Implanted cardioverter/defibrillator The licence is subject to annual revie Driving may occur when these criteria can be met:

- The 1st device has been implanted for at least 6 months.
- The device has not administered therapy (shock and/or symptoma antitachycardia pacing) within the last 6 months (except during testing).
- Any previous therapy has not been accompanied by *incapacity* (whether caus by the device or arrhythmia).
- A period of 1 month off driving must occur following any revision of the dev (generator and/or electrode) or alteration of antiarrhythmics.
- The device is subject to regular review with interrogation.
- There is no other disqualifying condition.

Syncope ***Simple faint:*** no restriction. ***Unexplained syncope*** with low risk recurrence 4wks off driving, high risk of recurrence 4wks off driving if ca identified and treated otherwise, 6 months off. See driving and epilepsy, OPPOS Patients who have had a single episode of loss of consciousness (no cause fou still need to have at least 1yr off driving.

Hypertension Driving may continue unless treatment causes unacceptable s effects. DVLA need not be notified.

1 See www.dvla.gov.uk/at_a_glance/content.htm

Other conditions: UK DVLA[1] state they must be informed if:

- An epileptic event. A person who has suffered an epileptic attack while awake must not drive for 1yr from the date of the attack. A person who has suffered an attack while asleep must also refrain from driving for 1yr from the date of the attack, unless they have had an attack while asleep >3yrs ago and have not had any awake attacks since that asleep attack. In any event, they should not drive if they are likely to cause danger to the public or themselves.
- Patients with TIA or stroke should not drive for at least 1 month. There is no need to inform the DVLA unless there is residual neurological defect after 1 month eg visual field defect. If TIAs have been recurrent and frequent, a 3-month period free of attacks may be required.
- Sudden attacks or disabling giddiness, fainting, or blackouts. Multiple sclerosis, Parkinson's (any 'freezing' or on–off effects), motor neurone diseases are relevant here.
- Severe mental handicap. Those with dementia should only drive if the condition is mild (do not rely on armchair judgements: on-the-road trials are better). Encourage relatives to contact DVLA if a dementing relative should not be driving. GPs may desire to breach confidentiality (the GMC approves) and inform DVLA of demented or psychotic patients (tel. 01792 783686). Many elderly drivers (~1 in 3) who die in accidents are found to have Alzheimer's.
- A pacemaker, defibrillator, or anti-ventricular tachycardia device fitted.
- Diabetes controlled by insulin or tablets.
- Angina while driving.
- Parkinson's disease.
- Any other chronic neurological condition.
- A serious problem with memory.
- A major or minor stroke with deficit continuing for >1 month.
- Any type of brain surgery, brain tumour. Severe head injury involving inpatient treatment at hospital.
- Any severe psychiatric illness or mental disorder.
- Continuing/permanent difficulty in the use of arms or legs which affects ability to control a vehicle.
- Dependence on or misuse of alcohol, illicit drugs, or chemical substances in the past 3yrs (do not include drink/driving offences).
- Any visual disability which affects *both* eyes (do not declare short/long sight or colour blindness).

Vision (new drivers) should be 6/9 on Snellen's scale in the better eye and 6/12 on the Snellen scale in the other eye and (wearing glasses or contact lenses if needed) and 3/60 in each eye without glasses or contact lenses.

1 DVLA is the UK Driving and Vehicle Licensing Authority.

5 Chest medicine

Contents

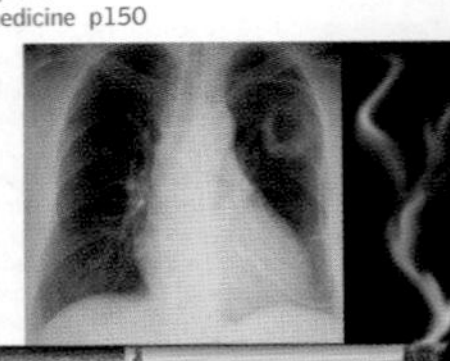

Fig 1. Smoke ring sign: cavitating lung carcinoma (OTM)

Relevant pages in other sections:

Symptoms and signs: The respiratory history & examination (p36–38); che[st] deformities (p54); chest pain (p80); clubbing (p56); cough (p37); cyanosis (p56); dyspnoea (p58); haemoptysis (p62); sputum (p37); stridor (p72).

Radiology: CXR (p714); chest CT (p718); V̇/Q̇ scan (p724).

Procedures: Aspirating pleural effusions (p752); pleural biopsy (p752); che[st] drains (p754); pneumothorax aspiration (p755); arterial blood gas sampli[ng] (p759).

▸▸***Emergencies:*** Asthma (p794); COPD (p796); tension pneumothorax (p79[8]); pneumonia (p800); pulmonary embolism (p802).

Others: Sickle-cell acute chest (p327); acid–base balance (p658); tuberculo[sis] (p386).

We thank Dr Phillippa Lawson, who is our Specialist Reader for this chapter.

Bedside tests in chest medicine

Sputum examination Collect a good sample; if necessary ask a physiotherapi to help. Note the appearance: clear and colourless (chronic bronchitis), yellow-gree (pulmonary infection), red (haemoptysis), black (smoke, coal dust), or frothy whit pink (pulmonary oedema). Send the sample to the laboratory for microscopy (Gra stain and auramine/ZN stain, if indicated), culture, and cytology.

Peak expiratory flow (PEF) is measured by a maximal forced expiration througl peak flow meter. It correlates well with the forced expiratory volume in 1 secor (FEV_1) and is used as an estimate of airway calibre. Peak flow rates should measured regularly in asthmatics to monitor response to therapy and disea control.

Pulse oximetry allows non-invasive assessment of peripheral O_2 saturation (SpO It provides a useful tool for monitoring those who are acutely ill or at risk deterioration. On most pulse oximeters, the alarm is set at 90%. An oxyg saturation of ≤80% is clearly abnormal and action is required (unless this is norr for the patient, eg in COPD). Here, check arterial blood gases (ABG) as P_aCO_2 may rising despite a normal P_aO_2). Erroneous readings may be caused by: poor perfusic motion, excess light, skin pigmentation, nail varnish, dyshaemoglobinaemias, a carbon monoxide poisoning. As with any bedside test, be sceptical, and check AE whenever indicated (p173).

Arterial blood gas (ABG) analysis Heparinized blood is taken from the radi brachial, or femoral artery (see p759), and pH, P_aO_2, and P_aCO_2 are measured usi an automated analyser. Remember to note the FiO_2 (fraction or percent of inspir O_2).

- ***Acid–base balance:*** Normal pH is 7.35–7.45. A pH <7.35 indicates *acidosis* anc pH >7.45 indicates *alkalosis*. For interpretation of abnormalities, see p658.
- ***Oxygenation:*** Normal P_aO_2 is 10.5–13.5kPa. Hypoxia is caused by one or more the following reasons: ventilation/perfusion ($\dot{V}/\dot{Q}$) mismatch, hypoventilatic abnormal diffusion, right to left cardiac shunts. Of these, $\dot{V}/\dot{Q}$ mismatch is t commonest cause. Severe hypoxia is defined as a P_aO_2 <8kPa (see p172).
- ***Ventilatory efficiency:*** Normal P_aCO_2 is 4.5–6.0kPa. P_aCO_2 is directly related alveolar ventilation. A P_aCO_2 <4.5kPa indicates *hyperventilation* and P_aCO_2 >6.0kPa indicates *hypoventilation*. Type I respiratory failure is defined P_aO_2 <8kPa and P_aCO_2 <6.0kPa, whereas type II respiratory failure is defined P_aO_2 <8kPa and P_aCO_2 >6.0kPa.

Alveolar-arterial O_2 concentration gradient may be calculated from the Fi(P_aO_2, and P_aCO_2: see OPPOSITE.

Spirometry measures functional lung volumes. Forced expiratory volume in (FEV_1) and forced vital capacity (FVC) are measured from a full forced expirati into spirometer (Vitalograph®); exhalation continues until no more breath can exhaled. FEV_1 is less effort-dependent than PEF. The FEV_1/FVC ratio gives a go estimate of the severity of airflow obstruction; normal ratio is 75–80%.

- ***Obstructive defect*** (eg asthma, COPD) FEV_1 is reduced more than the FVC and t FEV_1/FVC ratio is <75%.
- ***Restrictive defect*** (eg lung fibrosis) FVC is ↓ and the FEV_1/FVC ratio is ↔ or ↑. Oth causes: sarcoidosis; pneumoconiosis, interstitial pneumonias; connective tiss diseases; pleural effusion; obesity; kyphoscoliosis; neuromuscular problems.

Aa)PO_2: the Alveolar-arterial (Aa) oxygen gradient

his is the difference in the O_2 partial pressures between the alveolar and rterial sides. In type II respiratory failure it helps tell if hypoventilation is rom lung disease or poor respiratory effort. (Aa)$PO_2 = P_AO_2 - P_aO_2$. How o we find P_AO_2, the partial pressure of oxygen in the alveoli? Respiratory hysiology teaches that this depends on **R**, the respiratory quotient (≈0.8, nearer o 1 if eating all carbohydrates); barometric pressure ($P_B \approx$ 101kPa at sea level), nd P_{H_2O}, the water saturation of airway gas ($P_{H_2O} \approx$ 6.2kPa as inspired air is sually fully saturated by the time it gets to the carina). P_AO_2 clearly depends on $_iO_2$, the fractional concentration of O_2 in inspired air (eg F_iO_2 is 0.5 if breathing 0% O_2, and 0.21 if breathing room air). So...

$_AO_2 = (P_B - P_{H_2O}) \times F_iO_2 - (P_aCO_2/R)$

$= (101 - 6.2) \times F_iO_2 - (P_aCO_2/0.8)$ (at sea level)

$= (94.8 \times F_iO_2) - (1.25 \times P_aCO_2)$ See A Williams *BMJ* 1998 **317** 1213

reathing air and having a P_aCO_2 of 8kPa.

n this case, $P_AO_2 = 94.8 \times 0.21 - (1.25 \times 8) = 10$kPa. *Aa normal ranges breathing ir:* 0.2–1.5kPa at 25yrs old; increasing with age to 1.5–3.0 at 75yrs.

Examples of expected Aa gradients: 6.65 at an F_iO_2 of 0.5 ($P_AO_2 - P_aO_2 =$ 4.6 − 37.95 = 6.65) and 16 for an F_iO_2 of 1.0 ($P_AO_2 - P_aO_2 = 89 - 73 = 16$).

ormal peak expiratory flow (PEF)

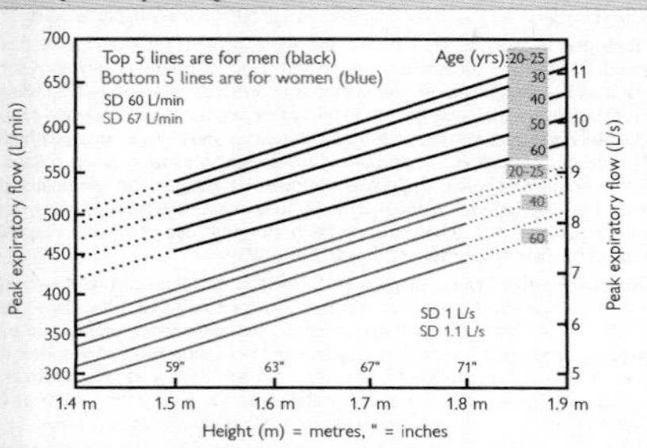

xamples of spirograms

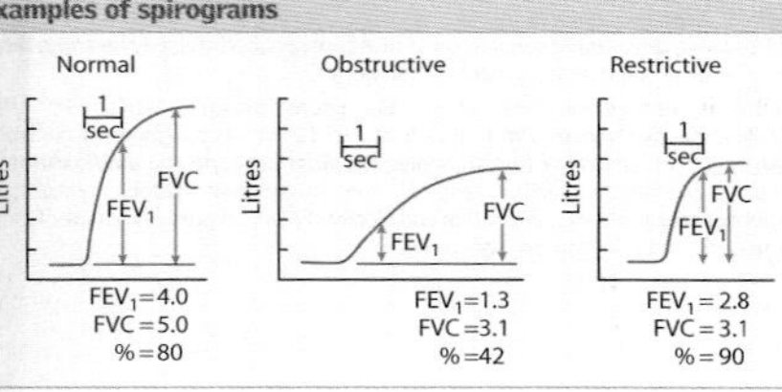

Further investigations in chest medicine

Lung function tests PEF, FEV_1, FVC (see p148). ***Total lung capacity*** (TLC) a ***residual volume*** (RV) are useful in distinguishing obstructive and restrict diseases. TLC and RV are increased in obstructive airways disease and reduced restrictive lung diseases and musculoskeletal abnormalities. The ***gas transfer*** efficient (KCO) across alveoli is calculated by measuring carbon monoxide upta from a single inspiration in a standard time (usually 10s). Low in emphysema a interstitial lung disease, high in alveolar haemorrhage. KCO represents the carb monoxide diffusing capacity (DLCO) corrected for alveolar volume. ***Flow volu loop*** measures flow at various lung volumes. Characteristic patterns are seen w intra-thoracic airways obstruction (asthma, emphysema) and extra-thora airways obstruction (tracheal stenosis).

Radiology *Chest x-ray* see p714. ***Ultrasound*** is used in the diagnosis and draina of pleural effusions (particularly loculated effusions) and empyema. ***Radionucl scans*** *Ventilation/perfusion ($\dot{V}/\dot{Q}$, p724) scans* are used to diagnose pulmona embolism (PE) (unmatched perfusion defects are seen). *Bone scans* are used diagnose bone metastases. ***Computed tomography*** (CT, p718) of the thorax is us for diagnosing and staging lung cancer, imaging the hila, mediastinum and pleu and guiding biopsies. Thin (1–1.5mm) section high resolution CT (HRCT) is used in t diagnosis of interstitial lung disease and bronchiectasis. Spiral CT pulmon angiography (CTPA, p725) is used increasingly in the diagnosis of PE. ***Pulmona angiography*** is also used for diagnosing PE and pulmonary hypertension.

Fibreoptic bronchoscopy is performed under local anaesthetic via the nose mouth. *Diagnostic indications:* suspected lung carcinoma, slowly resolv pneumonia, pneumonia in the immunosuppressed, interstitial lung disea Bronchial lavage fluid may be sent to the lab for microscopy, culture, and cytolo Mucosal abnormalities may be brushed (cytology) and biopsied (histopatholog *Therapeutic indications:* aspiration of mucus plugs causing lobar collapse removal of foreign bodies. *Pre-procedure investigations:* FBC, CXR, spirometry, pu oximetry and arterial blood gases (if indicated). Check clotting if rec anticoagulation and a biopsy may be performed. *Complications:* respirat depression, bleeding, pneumothorax (fig 1, p785).

Bronchoalveolar lavage (BAL) is performed at the time of bronchoscopy instilling and aspirating a known volume of warmed, buffered 0.9% saline into distal airway. *Diagnostic indications:* suspected malignancy, pneumonia in immunosuppressed (especially HIV), suspected TB (if sputum negative), intersti lung diseases (eg sarcoidosis, extrinsic allergic alveolitis, histiocytosis *Therapeutic indications:* alveolar proteinosis. *Complications:* hypoxia (g supplemental O_2), transient fever, transient CXR shadow, infection (rare).

Lung biopsy may be performed in several ways. ***Percutaneous needle biopsy*** performed under radiological guidance and is useful for peripheral lung and pleu lesions. ***Transbronchial biopsy*** performed at bronchoscopy may help in diagnos diffuse lung diseases, eg sarcoidosis. If these are unsuccessful, an ***open lung biop*** may be performed under general anaesthetic.

Surgical procedures are performed under general anaesthetic. ***Ri bronchoscopy*** provides a wide lumen, enables larger mucosal biopsies, controll bleeding, and removal of foreign bodies. ***Mediastinoscopy*** and ***mediastinoto*** enable examination and biopsy of the mediastinal lymph nodes/lesio ***Thoracoscopy*** allows examination and biopsy of pleural lesions, drainage of pleu effusions, and talc pleurodesis.

ung volumes: physiological and pathological

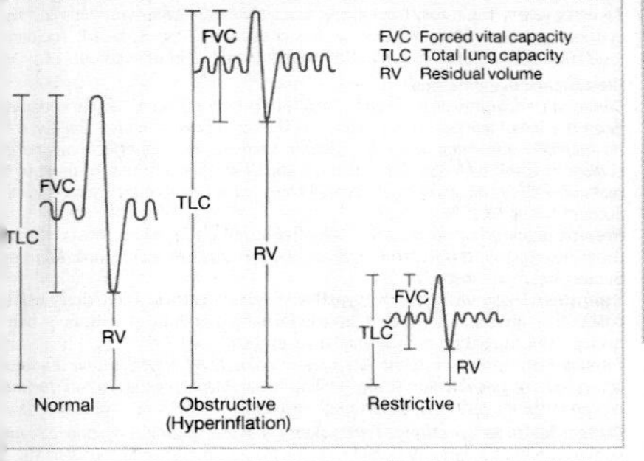

low volume loops

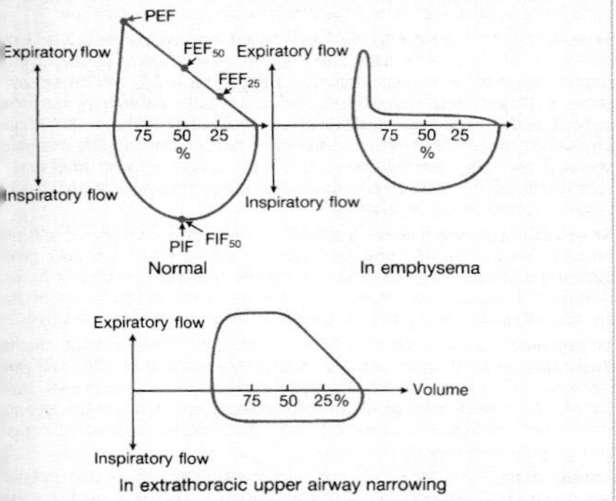

PEF

Expiratory flow

FEF50

FEF25

75 50 25 %

Inspiratory flow

PIF FIF50

Normal

Expiratory flow

75 50 25 %

Inspiratory flow

In emphysema

Expiratory flow

75 50 25%

Volume

Inspiratory flow

In extrathoracic upper airway narrowing

EF=peak expiratory flow; FEF_{50}=forced expiratory flow at 50% TLC; FEF_{25}=forced xpiratory flow at 25% TLC; PIF=peak inspiratory flow; FIF_{50}=forced inspiratory ow at 50% TLC.

Pneumonia

»Emergency treatment: p80

An acute lower respiratory tract illness associated with fever, symptoms and sig in the chest, and abnormalities on the chest x-ray—fig 1, p714. Inciden 1–3/1000 population. Mortality: 10% (patients admitted to hospital).

Classification and causes

Community-acquired pneumonia (CAP) may be primary or secondary to underlyi disease. *Streptococcus pneumoniae* is the commonest cause, followed *Haemophilus influenzae* and *Mycoplasma pneumoniae*. *Staphylococcus aure Legionella* species, *Moraxella catarrhalis*, and *Chlamydia* account for most of t remainder. Gram negative bacilli, *Coxiella burnetii* and anaerobes are rare. Virus account for up to 15%.

Hospital acquired (nosocomial) (>48h after hospital admission). Most commo Gram negative enterobacteria or *Staph. aureus*. Also *Pseudomonas*, *Klebsie Bacteroides*, and *Clostridia*.

Aspiration Those with stroke, myasthenia, bulbar palsies, ↓consciousness (postictal or drunk), oesophageal disease (achalasia, reflux), or with poor den hygiene, risk aspirating oropharyngeal anaerobes.

Immunocompromised patient *Strep. pneumoniae*, *H. influenzae*, *Staph. aureus*, *catarrhalis*, *M. pneumoniae*, Gram –ve bacilli and *Pneumocystis jiroveci* (forme named *P. carinii*, p398–9). Other fungi, viruses (CMV, HSV), and mycobacteria.

Clinical features ***Symptoms:*** Fever, rigors, malaise, anorexia, dyspnoea, cou purulent sputum, haemoptysis, and pleuritic pain. ***Signs:*** Fever, cyanosis, confusi (may be the only sign in the elderly), tachypnoea, tachycardia, hyp tension, signs of consolidation (diminished expansion, dull percussion note, ↑tact vocal fremitus/vocal resonance, bronchial breathing), and a pleural rub.

Tests aim to establish diagnosis, identify pathogen, and assess severity (see belo *CXR* (fig 1, p714): lobar or multilobar infiltrates, cavitation or pleural effusi ***Assess oxygenation:*** oxygen saturation, p148 (ABGs if S_aO_2 <92% or seve pneumonia). ***Blood tests:*** FBC, U&E, LFT, CRP, blood cultures. ***Sputum*** for microsco and culture. In severe cases, check for *Legionella* (sputum culture, urine antige atypical organism/viral serology (complement fixation tests acutely and pair serology) and check for pneumococcal antigen in urine. ***Pleural fluid*** may aspirated for culture. Consider ***bronchoscopy*** and bronchoalveolar lavage if patie is immunocompromized or on ITU.

Severity Core adverse features: 'CURB-65' score: Confusion (abbreviated men test ≤8); Urea >7mmol/L; Respiratory rate ≥30/min; BP <90 systolic and 60mmHg diastolic); age ≥65. Score: 0–1 home treatment possible; 2 hospi therapy; ≥3 indicates severe pneumonia. Other features increasing the risk of dea are: co-existing disease; bilateral/ multilobar involvement; P_aO_2 <8kPa/S_aO_2<92

Management »p800. ***Antibiotics*** (p153), orally if not severe and not vomitir severe give by IV. ***Oxygen*** keep P_aO_2 >8.0 and/or saturation ≥92%. ***IV flui*** (anorexia, dehydration, shock). ***Analgesia*** if pleurisy—eg paracetamol 1g/ Consider ITU if shock, hypercapnia, or uncorrected hypoxia. If failure to improve, CRP remains high, repeat CXR and look for progression/complications. All patier need 6week follow-up with repeat CXR.

Complications (p156) Pleural effusion, empyema, lung abscess, respiratory failu septicaemia, brain abscess, pericarditis, myocarditis, cholestatic jaundice. Repe CRP and CXR in patients not progressing satisfactorily.

Pneumococcal vaccine (eg 23-valent Pneumovax II®, 0.5mL SC) Offer to at-r groups: • ≥65yrs old • Chronic heart, liver (eg cirrhosis), renal (eg renal failu nephrosis*, post-transplant*) or lung conditions • Diabetes mellitus • Immunosu pression, eg spleen function↓ (eg splenectomy, asplenia*, sickle cell* or coel disease), AIDS, or on chemotherapy or prednisolone >20mg/d). CI: pregnan lactation, fever. If at ↑risk of fatal pneumococcal infection (* above), re-vaccina after 6yrs (3–5yrs in children >2yrs old), unless past severe vaccine reaction.

Empirical treatment of pneumonia

Clinical setting	Organisms	Antibiotic (further dosage details: p368 & p369)
Community acquired		
Mild not previously Rx	*Streptococcus pneumoniae* *Haemophilus influenzae*	Amoxicillin 500mg–1.0g/8h or erythromycin[1] 500mg/6h PO
Mild	*Streptococcus pneumoniae* *Haemophilus influenzae* *Mycoplasma pneumoniae*	Amoxicillin 500mg–1.0g/8h PO + erythromycin[1] 500mg/6h PO or fluoroquinolone; if IV required: ampicillin 500mg/6h + erythromycin[1] 500mg/6h IVI
Severe	As above	Co-amoxiclav IV or cephalosporin IV (eg cefuroxime 1.5g/8h IV) AND erythromycin[1] 1g/6h IVI
Atypical	*Legionella pneumophilia*	Clarithromycin 500mg/12h PO/IVI ± rifampicin
	Chlamydia species	Tetracycline
	Pneumocystis jiroveci	High-dose co-trimoxazole (p398–9)
Hospital acquired		
	Gram negative bacilli Pseudomonas Anaerobes	Aminoglycoside IV + antipseudomonal penicillin IV or 3rd gen. cephalosporin IV (p369)
Aspiration		
	Streptococcus pneumoniae Anaerobes	Cefuroxime 1.5g/8h IV + metronidazole 500mg/8h IV
Neutropenic patients		
	Gram positive cocci Gram negative bacilli	Aminoglycoside IV + antipseudomonal penicillin IV or 3rd gen. cephalosporin IV
	Fungi (p160)	Consider antifungals after 48h

3rd gen=3rd generation, eg cefotaxime, p369; gentamicin is an example of an aminoglycoside (p371).

1 Clarithromycin 500mg/12h PO/IVI may be used in place of erythromycin throughout the above.

Specific pneumonias

For antibiotic doses, see p368 & p370. TB: ►see p386.

Pneumococcal pneumonia is the commonest bacterial pneumonia. It affects a ages, but is commoner in the elderly, alcoholics, post-splenectomy, immun suppressed, and patients with chronic heart failure or pre-existing lung diseas Clinical features: fever, pleurisy, herpes labialis. CXR shows lobar consolidatio Treatment: amoxicillin, benzylpenicillin, or cephalosporin.

Staphylococcal pneumonia may complicate influenza infection or occur in th young, elderly, intravenous drug users, or patients with underlying disea (eg leukaemia, lymphoma, cystic fibrosis, (CF). It causes a bilateral cavitatir bronchopneumonia. Treatment: flucloxacillin. MRSA: contact lab; conside vancomycin.

Klebsiella pneumonia is rare. Occurs in elderly, diabetics and alcoholics. Causes cavitating pneumonia, particularly of the upper lobes. Treatment: cefuroxime.

Pseudomonas is a common pathogen in bronchiectasis and CF. It also cause hospital acquired infections, particularly on ITU or after surgery. Treatment: ant pseudomonal penicillin, ceftazidime, meropenem, or ciprofloxacin.

Mycoplasma pneumoniae occurs in epidemics about every 4yrs. It present insidiously with 'flu-like symptoms (headache, myalgia, arthralgia) followed by dry cough. CXR shows bilateral patchy consolidation. Diagnosis: mycoplasm serology. Cold agglutinins may cause an autoimmune haemolytic anaemi Complications: skin rash (erythema multiforme, fig 3, p546), Stevens–Johnsc syndrome), meningoencephalitis or myelitis; Guillain–Barré syndrome. Treatmer erythromycin/clarithromycin or tetracycline.

Legionella pneumophilia colonizes water tanks kept at <60°C (eg hotel ai conditioning and hot water systems) causing outbreaks of Legionnaire's diseas 'Flu-like symptoms (fever, malaise, myalgia) precede a dry cough and dyspnoe Extra-pulmonary features include anorexia, D&V, hepatitis, renal failure, confusio and coma. CXR shows bi-basal consolidation. Blood tests may show lymphopeni hyponatraemia, and deranged LFTs. Urinalysis may show haematuria. Diagnosi *Legionella* serology/urine antigen. Treatment: clarithromycin ± rifampicin c fluoroquinolone. 10% mortality.

Chlamydia pneumoniae is the commonest chlamydial infection. Person-t person spread occurs causing a biphasic illness: pharyngitis, hoarseness, otiti followed by pneumonia. Diagnosis: *Chlamydia* serology (non-specific). Treatmer tetracycline.

Chlamydia psittaci causes psittacosis, an ornithosis acquired from infected birc (typically parrots). Symptoms include headache, fever, dry cough, letharg arthralgia, anorexia, and D&V. Extra-pulmonary features are legion but rare, e meningoencephalitis, infective endocarditis, hepatitis, nephritis, rash, splenomega CXR shows patchy consolidation. Diagnosis: *Chlamydia* serology. Treatmer tetracycline.

Viral pneumonia The commonest cause is influenza (p390 and BOX). Other virus that can affect the lung are: measles, CMV, and varicella zoster.

Pneumocystis pneumonia (PCP) causes pneumonia in the immunosuppressed (e HIV). The organism responsible was previously called *pneumocystis carinii*, and no called *pneumocystis jiroveci*. It presents with a dry cough, exertional dyspnoe fever, bilateral crepitations. CXR may be normal or show bilateral perihil interstitial shadowing. Diagnosis: visualization of the organism in induced sputur bronchoalveolar lavage, or in a lung biopsy specimen. Drugs: high-dose c trimoxazole (p398–9), or pentamidine by slow IVI for 2–3 weeks (p399). Steroi are beneficial if severe hypoxaemia. Prophylaxis is indicated if the CD4 count <200×10^6/L or after the 1st attack.

Avian influenza

Avian-to-human transmission of the H5N1 strain of influenza A causes serious infection in humans with a ≥50% mortality. Human-to-human transmission is reported but is unusual. Oseltamivir (Tamiflu®) can reduce morbidity from influenza A by 1–2 days (see p390; note that oseltamivir-resistant H5N1 has been reported).[14] A vaccine is under development, but the most likely cause of a pandemic of 'flu is a new mutant developing between human and avian influenza virus (genetic reassortment, p390) which may require a different vaccine.

►Suspect avian 'flu if undiagnosed fever and dyspnoea/pneumonia rapidly progresses to acute respiratory distress syndrome, especially if there is lymphopenia or thrombocytopenia.[15] There may also be a history of close contact with poultry. NB: D&V, abdominal pain, pleuritic pain, and bleeding from the nose and gums are reported to be an early feature in some patients.[16]

Diagnosis: Viral culture ± reverse transcriptase-PCR with H5 & N1 specific primers.[17]

Management: Get help. O_2; ventilatory support; antivirals. Contain the outbreak (p390). Nebulizers and high-air flow O_2 masks are implicated in nosocomial spread (so use only with meticulous precautions).[18]

SARS [19]

Severe acute respiratory syndrome (SARS) is caused by SARS-COV virus—a coronavirus. Major features are persistent fever >38°centigrade, chills, rigors, myalgia, dry cough, headache, diarrhoea, and dyspnoea—with an abnormal CXR and WCC↓. Respiratory failure is the big complication; >50% need supplemental O_2; ~20% progress to acute respiratory distress syndrome requiring invasive ventilation.[20]

Mortality is 1–50%, depending on age. Close contact with an index case, or travel to an area with known cases should raise suspicion. The mechanism of transmission of SARS-COV is only by close contact with other patients.

Management is supportive. No drugs have convincing efficacy (experts may advise on antivirals). Rapid diagnosis, early isolation, and good infection control measures are vital. Communicate with your consultant in infectious diseases.[21]

Complications of pneumonia

Respiratory failure (See p172.) Type 1 respiratory failure (P_aO_2 <8kPa) relatively common. Treatment is with high-flow (60%) oxygen. *Transfer the patie to ITU if hypoxia does not improve with O_2 therapy or P_aCO_2 rises to >6kPa.* careful with O_2 in COPD patients; check ABGs frequently, and consider elect ventilation if rising P_aCO_2 or worsening acidosis. Aim to keep SaO_2 at 90–94%

Hypotension may be due to a combination of dehydration and vasodilatation d to sepsis. If systolic BP is <90mmHg, give an intravenous fluid challenge of 250n colloid/crystalloid over 15min. If BP does not rise, insert a central line and g intravenous fluids to maintain the systolic BP >90mmHg. If systolic BP remai <90mmHg despite fluid therapy, request ITU assessment for inotropic suppc (adrenaline, noradrenaline).

Atrial fibrillation (p116) is quite common, particularly in the elderly. It usua resolves with treatment of the pneumonia. Digoxin may be required to slow t ventricular response rate in the short term.

Pleural effusion Inflammation of the pleura by adjacent pneumonia may cau fluid exudation into the pleural space. If this accumulates in the pleural spa faster than it is reabsorbed, a pleural effusion develops (fig 1, p714). If this is sm it may be of no consequence. If it becomes large and symptomatic, or infect (empyema), drainage is required (p176 & p754).

Empyema is pus in the pleural space. It should be suspected if a patient wit resolving pneumonia develops a recurrent fever. Clinical features and the c indicate a pleural effusion. The aspirated pleural fluid is typically yellow and turk with a pH <7.2, glucose↓, and LDH↑. The empyema should be drained using a che drain, preferably inserted under radiological guidance. Although intra-pleu streptokinase has been used to break down the adhesions (p176) the latest da indicate no benefit, and its routine use is not recommended.

Lung abscess is a cavitating area of localized, suppurative infection within the lun ***Causes:*** • Inadequately treated pneumonia • Aspiration (eg alcoholism, oesop ageal obstruction, bulbar palsy) • Bronchial obstruction (tumour, foreign boc • Pulmonary infarction • Septic emboli (septicaemia, right heart endocardit IV drug use) • Subphrenic or hepatic abscess.

Clinical features: Swinging fever; cough; purulent, foul-smelling sputu pleuritic chest pain; haemoptysis; malaise; weight loss. Look for: finger clubbir anaemia; crepitations. Empyema develops in 20–30%.

Tests: *Blood:* FBC (anaemia, neutrophilia), ESR, CRP, blood cultures. *Sputu* microscopy, culture, and cytology. *CXR:* walled cavity, often with a fluid lev Consider CT scan to exclude obstruction, and bronchoscopy to obtain diagnos specimens.

Treatment: Antibiotics as indicated by sensitivities; continue until heal (4–6 wks). Postural drainage. Repeated aspiration, antibiotic instillation, or surgic excision may be required.

Septicaemia may occur as a result of bacterial spread from the lung parenchyr into the bloodstream. This may cause metastatic infection, eg infective endocardit meningitis. Treatment with IV antibiotic according to sensitivities.

Pericarditis and myocarditis may also complicate pneumonia.

Jaundice This is usually cholestatic, and may be due to sepsis or secondary antibiotic therapy (particularly flucloxacillin and co-amoxiclav).

Bronchiectasis

Pathology Chronic infection of the bronchi and bronchioles leading to permane dilatation of these airways. Main organisms: *H. influenzae*; *Strep. pneumoni* *Staph. aureus; Pseudomonas aeruginosa.*

Causes ***Congenital:*** CF; Young's syndrome; primary ciliary dyskinesia; Kartagene syndrome. ***Post-infection:*** measles; pertussis; bronchiolitis; pneumonia; TB; H ***Other:*** Bronchial obstruction (tumour, foreign body); allergic bronchopulmona aspergillosis (ABPA p160); hypogammaglobulinaemia; rheumatoid arthri ulcerative colitis; idiopathic.

Clinical features ***Symptoms:*** persistent cough; copious purulent sputu intermittent haemoptysis. ***Signs:*** finger clubbing; coarse inspiratory crepitatio wheeze (asthma, COPD, ABPA). ***Complications:*** pneumonia, pleural effusi pneumothorax; haemoptysis; cerebral abscess; amyloidosis.

Tests *Sputum* culture. *CXR:* cystic shadows, thickened bronchial walls (tramline a ring shadows). *HRCT chest:* (p150) to assess extent and distribution of disea *Spirometry* often shows an obstructive pattern; reversibility should be assess *Bronchoscopy* to locate site of haemoptysis or exclude obstruction. *Other te* serum immunoglobulins; CF sweat test; *Aspergillus* precipitins or skin-prick te

Management • ***Postural drainage*** should be performed twice daily. Ch physiotherapy may aid sputum expectoration and mucous drainage. • ***Antibio*** should be prescribed according to bacterial sensitivities. Patients known to cult *Pseudomonas* will require either oral ciprofloxacin or IV antibiot • ***Bronchodilators*** (eg nebulized salbutamol) may be useful in patients w asthma, COPD, CF, ABPA (p160). • ***Corticosteroids*** (eg prednisolone) for AE • ***Surgery*** may be indicated in localized disease or to control severe haemopty

Cystic fibrosis (CF)

See OHCS (*Paediatrics*, p16

One of the commonest life-threatening autosomal recessive conditi (1:2000 live births) affecting Caucasians. Caused by mutations in the transmembrane conductance regulator (CFTR) gene on chromosome 7 (>8 mutations have now been identified). This leads to a combination of defec chloride secretion and increased sodium absorption across airway epithelium. changes in the composition of airway surface liquid predisposes the lung to chr pulmonary infections and bronchiectasis.

Clinical features ***Neonate:*** Failure to thrive; meconium ileus; rectal prolapse

Children and young adults: *Respiratory:* cough; wheeze; recurrent infecti bronchiectasis; pneumothorax; haemoptysis; respiratory failure; cor pulmor *Gastrointestinal:* pancreatic insufficiency (diabetes mellitus, steatorrhoea); d intestinal obstruction syndrome (meconium ileus equivalent); gallstones; cirrh *Other:* male infertility; osteoporosis; arthritis; vasculitis (p542); nasal po sinusitis; and hypertrophic pulmonary osteoarthropathy (HPOA). ***Signs:*** Cyan finger clubbing; bilateral coarse crackles.

Diagnosis *Sweat test:* sweat sodium and chloride >60mmol/L; chlo usually > sodium. *Genetics:* screening for known common CF mutations shoul considered. *Faecal elastase* is a simple and useful screening test for exo pancreatic dysfunction.

Tests *Blood:* FBC, U&E, LFTs; clotting; vitamin A, D, E levels; annual glucose tolera test (p190). *Bacteriology:* cough swab, sputum culture. *Radiology:* CXR; hy inflation; bronchiectasis. *Abdominal ultrasound:* fatty liver; cirrhosis; chr pancreatitis; *Spirometry:* obstructive defect. *Aspergillus serology/skin test* (2 develop ABPA, p160). *Biochemistry:* faecal fat analysis.

Chest medicine

Management of cystic fibrosis

Patients with cystic fibrosis are best managed by a multidisciplinary team, eg physician, physiotherapist, specialist nurse, and dietician with attention to psychosocial as well as physical well-being. Gene therapy (transfer of CFTR gene using liposome or adenovirus vectors) is not yet possible.

Chest: Physiotherapy regularly (postural drainage, active cycle techniques or forced expiratory techniques). Antibiotics are given for acute infective exacerbations (PO for *Staph. aureus*, IV for *P. aeruginosa*) and prophylactically PO (flucloxacillin) or nebulized (colomycin or tobramycin). Mucolytics may be useful (eg DNase, ie Dornase alfa, 2.5mg daily nebulized, *OHCS* p163). Bronchodilators.

Gastrointestinal: Pancreatic enzyme replacement; fat soluble vitamin supplements (A, D, E, K); ursodeoxycholic acid for impaired liver function; cirrhosis may require liver transplantation.

Other: Treatment of CF-related diabetes; screening for and treatment of osteoporosis; treatment of arthritis, sinusitis, and vasculitis; fertility and genetic counselling.

Advanced lung disease: Oxygen, diuretics (cor pulmonale); non-invasive ventilation; lung or heart/lung transplantation.

Prognosis: Median survival is now over 30yrs.

Fungi and the lung

Aspergillus This group of fungi affects the lung in 5 ways:

1 ***Asthma:*** Type I hypersensitivity (atopic) reaction to fungal spores, p164.

2 ***Allergic bronchopulmonary aspergillosis (ABPA):*** This results from a Type and III hypersensitivity reaction to *Aspergillus fumigatus*. Early on, the allerg response causes bronchoconstriction, but as the inflammation persis permanent damage occurs, causing bronchiectasis. *Symptoms:* wheeze, coug sputum (plugs of mucus containing fungal hyphae), dyspnoea, and 'recurre pneumonia'. *Investigations:* CXR (transient segmental collapse or consolidatic bronchiectasis); *Aspergillus* in sputum; positive aspergillus skin test and/ aspergillus-specific IgE RAST (radioallergosorbent test); positive serum pr cipitins; eosinophilia; raised serum IgE. *Treatment:* Prednisolone 30–40mg/2 PO for acute attacks; maintenance dose 5–10mg/d. Sometimes itraconazole used in combination with corticosteroids. Bronchodilators for asthm Sometimes bronchoscopic aspiration of mucous plugs is needed.

3 ***Aspergilloma (mycetoma):*** A fungus ball within a pre-existing cavity (oft caused by TB, sarcoidosis). It is usually asymptomatic but may cause coug haemoptysis (may be torrential), lethargy ± weight loss. *Investigations:* C (round opacity within a cavity, usually apical); sputum culture; strongly positi serum precipitins; *Aspergillus* skin test (30% +ve). *Treatment* (only symptomatic). Consider surgical excision for solitary symptomatic lesions severe haemoptysis. Oral itraconazole and other antifungals have been tri with limited success. Local instillation of amphotericin paste under CT-guidan yields partial success in carefully selected patients, eg in massive haemoptys

4 ***Invasive aspergillosis:*** *Risk factors:* immunocompromise, eg HIV, leukaem burns, Wegener's (p707), and SLE, or after broad-spectrum antibiotic thera *Investigations:* sputum culture; serum precipitins; CXR (consolidation, absces Early chest CT and serial serum measurements of galactomannan (*Aspergillus* antigen) can be very helpful. Diagnosis may only be made at lu biopsy or autopsy. *Treatment:* IV amphotericin B (see below). Alternatives: miconazole or ketoconazole (less effective). *Prognosis:* very poor.

5 ***Extrinsic allergic alveolitis (EAA)*** is caused by sensitivity to *Aspergillus cl atus* ('malt worker's lung'). Clinical features and treatment are as for ot causes of EAA (p180). Diagnosis is based on a history of exposure and prese of serum precipitins to *A. clavatus*. Pulmonary fibrosis may occur if untreat

Using amphotericin B Test dose: 1mg in 20mL 5% dextrose IV over 20–30 Observe closely for the next ½h for signs of anaphylaxis (shock, swelling, whe etc). There are various formulations. Consult *BNF*. *Do not give any other drug in same IVI.* SE: anaphylaxis; serious nephrotoxicity; fever; rash; anorexia; nausea; D headache; myalgia; arthralgia; anaemia; ↓K^+; ↓Mg^{2+}; hepatotoxicity; arrhythmi hearing loss; diplopia; seizures; neuropathy; phlebitis. *Monitor* U&E *daily*. **AmBison** (liposomal amphotericin) has fewer SEs, but is expensive; it is indicated in systemic deep mycoses where nephrotoxicity precludes conventional amphotericin; IV ini test dose: 1mg over 10min, then 1mg/kg/d, as a single IVI dose; gradually↑ if need to 3mg/kg/d (max 5mg/kg/d). Alternatives: ***Abelcet®*** and ***Amphocil®***.

Other fungal infections ***Candida*** and ***Cryptococcus*** may cause pneumonia in immunosuppressed (see p428).

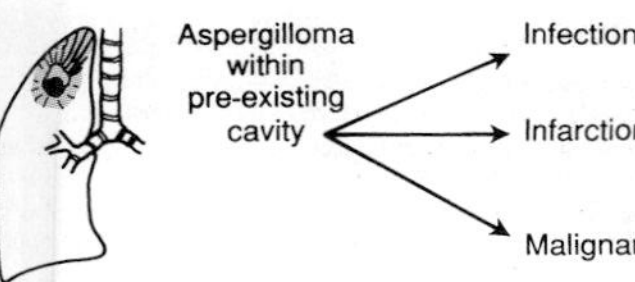

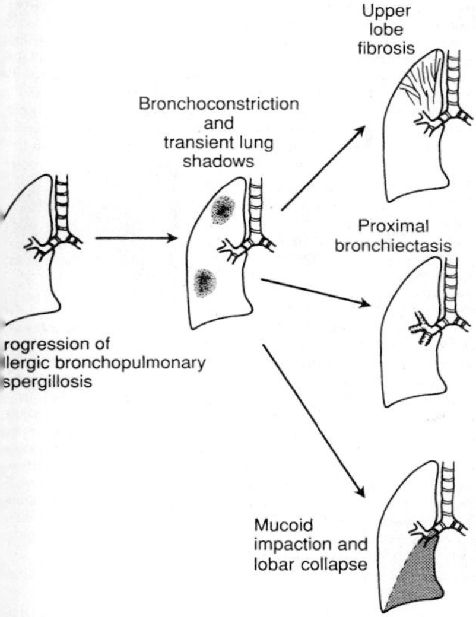

Upper
lobe
fibrosis

Bronchoconstriction
and
transient lung
shadows

Proximal
bronchiectasis

rogression of
llergic bronchopulmonary
spergillosis

Mucoid
impaction and
lobar collapse

AFTER PJ KUMAR AND ML CLARK CLINICAL MEDICINE, BAILLIÈRE TINDALL

Lung tumours

Carcinoma of the bronchus Accounts for ≈19% of all cancers and 27% of can deaths (40,000 cases/yr in UK). Incidence is increasing in women.

Risk factors: Cigarette smoking is the major risk factor. Others: asbes chromium, arsenic, iron oxides, and radiation (radon gas).

Histology: Squamous (30%); adenocarcinoma (30%); small (oat) cell (25%); la cell (15%); alveolar cell carcinoma (rare, <1%). Clinically the most import division is between small cell and non-small cell (NSCLC).

Symptoms: Cough (80%); haemoptysis (70%); dyspnoea (60%); chest pain (40 recurrent or slowly resolving pneumonia; anorexia; weight loss. ***Signs:*** Cache anaemia; clubbing; HPOA (hypertrophic pulmonary osteoarthropathy, causing w pain); supraclavicular or axillary nodes. *Chest signs:* none, or: consolidation; colla pleural effusion. *Metastases:* bone tenderness; hepatomegaly; confusion; fits; fo CNS signs; cerebellar syndrome; proximal myopathy; peripheral neuropathy.

Complications: *Local:* recurrent laryngeal nerve palsy; phrenic nerve palsy; obstruction; Horner's syndrome (Pancoast's tumour); rib erosion; pericarditis; *Metastatic:* brain; bone (bone pain, anaemia, ↑Ca^{2+}); liver; adrenals (Addiso *Endocrine:* ectopic hormone secretion, eg SIADH (↓Na^+ and ↑ADH, p666) and A (Cushing's) by small cell tumours; PTH (↑Ca^{2+}) by squamous cell tumours. N *metastatic neurological:* confusion; fits; cerebellar syndrome; proximal myopa neuropathy; polymyositis; Eaton–Lambert syndrome (p504). *Other:* clubbing, H dermatomyositis; acanthosis nigricans (p546); thrombophlebitis migrans (p2

Tests: *Cytology:* sputum & pleural fluid (send at least 20mL). *CXR:* peripheral circular opacity; hilar enlargement; consolidation; lung collapse; pleural effusion; bony secondaries. Peripheral lesions and superficial lymph nodes may be amenable to *percutaneous fine needle aspiration* or *biopsy*. *Bronchoscopy:* to give histology and assess operability. *CT* to stage the tumour (BOX). *¹⁸F-deoxyglucose PET scan* to help in staging (PET= positron emission tomography). *Radionuclide bone scan:* if suspected metastases. *Lung function tests.*

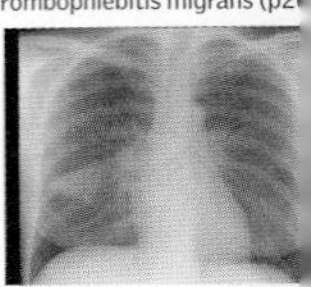

Fig 1. Name 3 abnormalities.[1]

Treatment: Non-small cell tumours: *Excision* is the treatment of choice for peripl tumours, with no metastatic spread: stage I/II (~25%). *Curative radiotherapy* i alternative if respiratory reserve is poor. *Chemotherapy ± radiotherapy* for r advanced disease. ***Small cell tumours*** are nearly always disseminated at presenta They may respond to *chemotherapy* (cyclophosphamide + doxorubicin + vinc ine + etoposide; **or** cisplatin ± *radiotherapy* if limited disease). ***Palliation:*** *Radiothe* is used for bronchial obstruction, SVC obstruction, haemoptysis, bone pain, and cere metastases. *SVC stent* + radiotherapy and dexamethasone for SVC obstruction. *E bronchial therapy:* tracheal stenting, cryotherapy, laser, brachytherapy radioactive source is placed close to the tumour). *Pleural drainage/pleurodesi* symptomatic pleural effusions. *Drugs:* analgesia; steroids; antiemetics; cough lin (codeine); bronchodilators; anti-depressants.

Prognosis: *Non-small cell:* 50% 2yr survival without spread; 10% with spr *Small cell:* median survival is 3 months if untreated; 1–1½yrs if treated.

Prevention: Quit smoking, p79. Prevent occupational exposure to carcinoge

Other lung tumours ***Bronchial adenoma:*** Rare, slow-growing. 90% are carci tumours; 10% cylindromas. ℞: surgery. ***Hamartoma:*** Rare, benign; CT: lobul mass ± flecks of calcification; ?excise to exclude malignancy. ***Mesothelioma*** (p1

1 A wedge-shaped density in the right middle lobe (a secondary). Also note a coin lesion at the costophrenic angle. The sharp upper boundary of the right middle lobe triangular mass is the right m lobe fissure. The right hilar structures are enlarged from metastases within the hilar lymph node

oin lesions of the lung on a CXR

Malignancy (1° or 2°)	• Arterio–venous malformation
Abscesses (p156)	• Encysted effusion (fluid, blood, pus)
Granuloma	• Cyst
Carcinoid tumour	• Foreign body
Pulmonary hamartoma	• Skin tumour (eg seborrhoeic wart)

IM staging for non-small cell lung cancer

imary tumour (T)	TX	Malignant cells in bronchial secretions, no other evidence of tumour
	Tis	Carcinoma *in situ*
	T0	None evident
	T1	≤3cm, in lobar or more distal airway
	T2	>3cm and >2cm distal to carina *or* any size if pleural involvement *or* obstructive pneumonitis extending to hilum, but not all the lung
	T3	Involves the chest wall, diaphragm, mediastinal pleura, pericardium, or <2cm from, but not at, carina
	T4	Involves the mediastinum, heart, great vessels, trachea, oesophagus, vertebral body, carina, *or* a malignant effusion is present
gional nodes (N)	N0	None involved (after mediastinoscopy)
	N1	Peribronchial and/or ipsilateral hilum
	N2	Ipsilateral mediastinum or subcarinal
	N3	Contralateral mediastinum or hilum, scalene, or supraclavicular
stant metastasis (M)	M0	None
	M1	Distant metastases present

age	**Tumour**	**Lymph nodes**	**Metastasis**
cult	TX	N0	M0
	Tis, T1, or T2	N0	M0
	T1 or T2	N1	M0
	T3	N0	M0
a	T3	N1	M0
	T1–T3	N2	M0
b	T1–T4	N3	M0
	T4	N0–N2	M0
	T1–T4	N0–N3	M1

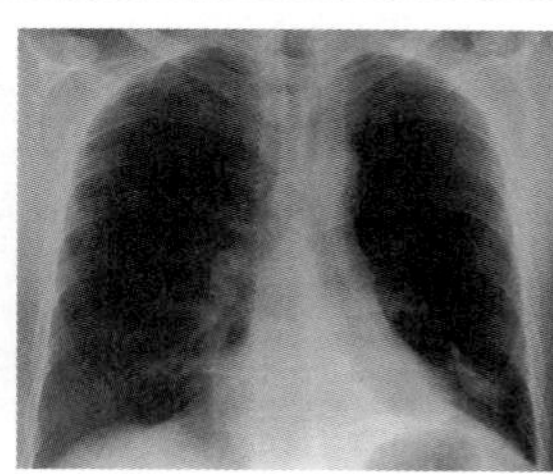

1. **Lungs:** Normal volume fewer markings in left g except at the base. **ura:** Observe loss of clarity the left hemidiaphragm. **diastinum:** Left main nchus is pulled down and re is a triangular opacity ind the left heart. This is a apsed left lower lobe. It resses the left **hilum**. **es:** Ask yourself: are there metastases—as the left er bronchus may be tructed by a neoplasm. **t tissues:** unremarkable.

Asthma

Asthma affects 5–8% of the population. It is characterized by recurre episodes of dyspnoea, cough, and wheeze caused by reversible airwa obstruction. Three factors contribute to airway narrowing: *bronchial mus contraction*, triggered by a variety of stimuli; *mucosal swelling/inflammati* caused by mast cell and basophil degranulation resulting in the release inflammatory mediators; *increased mucus production*.

Symptoms Intermittent dyspnoea, wheeze, cough (often nocturnal) and sputu Ask specifically about:

- ***Precipitants:*** Cold air, exercise, emotion, allergens (house dust mite, poll animal fur), infection, drugs (eg aspirin, NSAIDs, β-blockers).
- ***Diurnal variation*** in symptoms or peak flow. Marked morning dipping of pe flow is common and can tip the balance into a serious attack, despite havi normal peak flow at other times.
- ***Exercise:*** Quantify the exercise tolerance.
- ***Disturbed sleep:*** Quantify as nights per week (a sign of severe asthma).
- ***Acid reflux:*** This has a known association with asthma.
- ***Other atopic disease:*** Eczema, hay fever, allergy, or family history?
- ***The home (especially the bedroom):*** Pets? Carpet? Feather pillows or duv Floor cushions and other 'soft furnishings'?
- ***Occupation:*** If symptoms remit at weekends or holidays, something at w may be a trigger. Ask the patient to measure his peak flow at intervals at w and at home (at the same time of day) to confirm this.
- ***Days per week off work or school.***

Signs Tachypnoea; audible wheeze; hyperinflated chest; hyperresonant percuss note; diminished air entry; widespread, polyphonic wheeze. ***Severe attack:*** inabi to complete sentences; pulse >110bpm; respiratory rate >25/min; PEF 33–50% predicted. ***Life-threatening attack:*** silent chest; cyanosis; bradycardia; exhausti PEF <33% of predicted; confusion; feeble respiratory effort.

Tests ***Acute attack:*** PEF, sputum culture, FBC, U&E, CRP, blood cultures. ABG analy usually shows a normal or slightly reduced P_aO_2 and low P_aCO_2 (hyperventilatic If P_aO_2 normal but the patient is hyperventilating, watch carefully and repeat ABG a little later. ►*If P_aCO_2 is raised, transfer to high dependency unit or ITU ventilation*, as this signifies failing respiratory effort. CXR (to exclude infection pneumothorax). ***Chronic asthma:*** PEF monitoring (p148): a diurnal variation >20% on ≥3d a wk for 2wks. Spirometry: obstructive defect (↓FEV$_1$/FVC, p148); usually ≥15% improvement in FEV$_1$ following β_2 agonists or steroid tr CXR: hyperinflation. Skin-prick tests may help to identify allergens. Histamine methacholine challenge. *Aspergillus* serology.

Treatment Chronic asthma (p166). Emergency treatment (p794).

Differential diagnosis Pulmonary oedema ('cardiac asthma'); COPD (often exists); large airway obstruction (eg foreign body, tumour); SVC obstruct (wheeze/dyspnoea not episodic); pneumothorax; PE; bronchiectasis; obliterat bronchiolitis (suspect in elderly).

Associated diseases Acid reflux; polyarteritis nodosa (PAN, p543); Churg–Stra syndrome (p688); ABPA (p160).

Natural history Most childhood asthmatics (see *OHCS* p164) either grow out asthma in adolescence, or suffer much less as adults. A significant number people develop chronic asthma late in life.

Mortality Death certificates give a figure of 2000/yr (UK): more care surveys more than halve this figure. 50% are >65yrs old.

xamples of serial peak flow charts

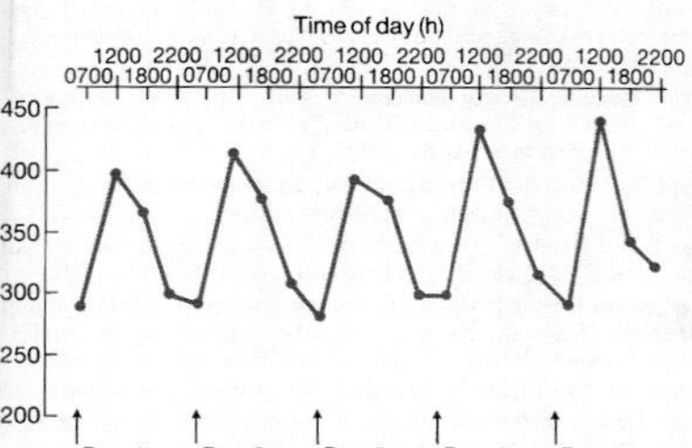

Classical diurnal variation of asthma
Arrows point to morning 'dips'

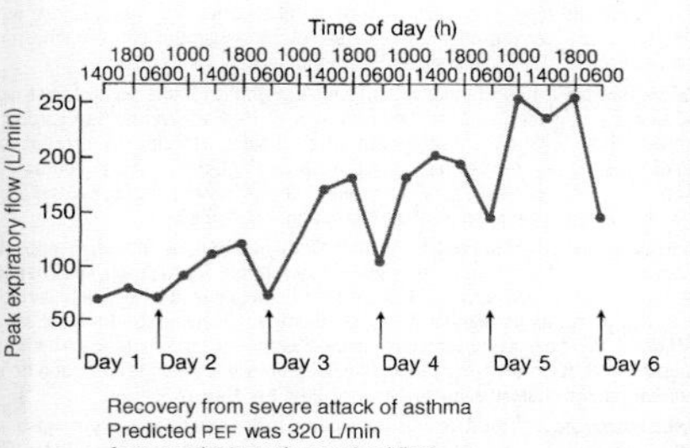

Recovery from severe attack of asthma
Predicted PEF was 320 L/min
Arrows point to early morning 'dips'

After B Harrison Thoracic Medicine, ed P Emerson, Butterworth, London

Management of chronic asthma

Behaviour Stop smoking and avoid precipitants. Check inhaler technique. Tea patients to use a peak flow meter to monitor PEF twice a day. Educate patients manage their disease by altering their medication in response to changes symptoms or PEF. Give specific advice about what to do in an emergency; provide written action plan.

British Thoracic Society guidelines Start at the step most appropriate severity; moving up if needed, or down if control is good for >3 months. Resc courses of prednisolone may be used at any time.

Step 1 Occasional short-acting inhaled **β2-agonist** as required for symptom reli If used more than once daily, or night-time symptoms, go to Step 2.

Step 2 Add standard-dose inhaled steroid: eg **beclometasone** 200µg/12h **fluticasone** 50–250µg/12h. Titrate to lowest dose needed for effective contr

Step 3 Add long-acting β_2-agonist (eg **salmeterol** 50µg/12h or formote 12µg/12h). If benefit—but still inadequate control—continue and ↑dose **beclometasone** to 400µg/12h. If no effect of long acting β_2-agonist stop it.

Step 4 Consider trials of: **beclometasone** up to 1000µg/12h; modified-release o **theophylline**; modified-release oral **β_2-agonist**; or oral leukotriene recept antagonist (see below), in conjunction with previous therapy.

Step 5 Add regular oral prednisolone (1 dose daily, at the lowest possible dos Refer to asthma clinic.

Chest medicine

Drugs ***β_2-adrenoceptor agonists*** relax bronchial smooth muscle (↑cAMP), acti within minutes. Salbutamol is best given by inhalation (aerosol, powder, nebulize but may also be given PO or IV. SE: tachyarrhythmias, ↓K^+, tremor, anxiety. Lon acting inhaled β_2-agonist (eg salmeterol, formoterol) can help nocturnal symptor and reduce morning dips. They may be an alternative to ↑steroid dose wh symptoms are uncontrolled. SE: as salbutamol, paradoxical bronchospas (salmeterol). Also: tolerance and arrhythmias may be a problem.

Corticosteroids are best inhaled to minimize systemic effects, eg beclometaso via spacer (or powder), but may be given PO or IV. They act over days to ↓bronch mucosal inflammation. Rinse mouth after inhaled steroids to prevent o candidiasis. Oral steroids are used acutely (high-dose, short courses, prednisolone 40mg/24h PO for 7d) and longer term in lower dose (eg 5–10mg/24 if control is not optimal on inhalers. Warn about SEs: p361.

Aminophylline (metabolized to theophylline) may act by inhibiting phosph diesterase, thus ↓bronchoconstriction by ↑cAMP levels. Try as prophylaxis, at nig PO, to prevent morning dipping. Stick with one brand name (bioavailability variab It is also useful as an adjunct if inhaled therapy is inadequate. In acute seve asthma, it may be given IVI. It has a narrow therapeutic ratio, causing arrhythmi GI upset, and fits in the toxic range. Check theophylline levels (p739), and do E monitoring and check plasma levels after 24h if IV therapy is used.

Anticholinergics (eg ipratropium, tiotropium) may ↓muscle spasm synergistica with β_2-agonists but are not recommended in current guidelines for asthma. Th may be of more benefit in COPD.

Cromoglicate May be used as prophylaxis in mild and exercise-induced asthr (always inhaled), especially in children. It may precipitate asthma.

Leukotriene receptor antagonists (eg montelukast, zafirlukast) block the effec of cysteinyl leukotrienes in the airways.

Anti-IgE monoclonal antibody Omalizumab be of use in highly selected patier with persistent allergic asthma.

)oses of some inhaled drugs used in bronchoconstriction

	Inhaled aerosol	Inhaled powder	Nebulized (supervised)
Salbutamol			
Dose example: Airomir® is a CFC-free example of a breath-actuated inhaler	100–200µg/6h	200–400µg/6h	2.5–5mg/6h
Terbutaline			
Single dose		500µg[1]	2.5mg/mL
Recommended regimen		500µg/6h	5–10mg/6–12h
Salmeterol			
Dose/puff	25µg	50µg	—
Recommended regimen	50–100µg/12h	50–100µg/12h	—
Ipratropium bromide (COPD)			
Dose/puff	20µg	40µg	250µg/mL
Recommended regimen	20–40µg/6h	40–80µg/6h	250–500µg/6h
Steroids			
(Becotide®=beclometasone; Pulmicort®=budesonide;[1] Flixotide®=fluticasone)			
Fluticasone (Flixotide®)			
Doses available/puff	50, 100µg & 250µg & 500µg	As for aerosol	250µg/mL
Recommended regimen	100–250µg/12h	100–250µg/12h max 1mg/12h	½–2mg/12h
Becotide 50 & 100®			
Doses available/puff	50 & 100µg Becloforte®=250µg	—	—
Recommended regimen	100µg/12h ↓ 200µg/12h ↓ 250µg/12h ↓ 500–1000µg/12h		

▶Prescribe beclometasone by brand name, and state that a CFC-free inhaler should be dispensed. This is because, dose for dose, Qvar® is twice as potent as the other available CFC-free brand (Clenil Modulite®) and older CFC-containing inhalers such as Becotide®.

Any dose ≥250µg ≈ significant steroid absorption: carry a steroid card; this recommendation is being widened, and lower doses (beclomethasone) are now said to merit a steroid card (manufacturer's information).

1 Available as a Turbohaler®; Autohalers® are an alternative (breath-actuated) and don't need breathing coordination eg Airomir (salbutamol) & Aerobec® & Qvar® (both beclometasone). Accuhalers deliver dry powders (eg Flixotide®, Serevent®).

Systemic absorption (via the throat) is less if inhalation is through a **large-volume device**, eg Volumatic® AeroChamber Plus® (for Airomir & Qvar) devices. The latter is more compact. Static charge on some devices reduces dose delivery, so wash in water before dose; leave to dry (don't rub). It is pointless to squirt many puffs into a device: it is best to repeat single doses, and be sure to inhale *as soon as the drug is in the spacer*. SE: local (oral) candidiasis (p230); ↑rate of cataract if lifetime dose ≥2g beclometasone.

Chronic obstructive pulmonary disease (COPD)

Definitions COPD is a common progressive disorder of airway obstruction (FEV_1 <8C predicted; FEV_1/FVC <0.7) with little or no reversibility. COPD includes chronic bronchi and emphysema. Usually patients have *either* COPD *or* asthma, not both: COPD is favour by: • Age of onset >35yrs • Smoking related • Chronic dyspnoea • Sputum producti • No marked diurnal or day-to-day FEV_1 variation. ***Chronic bronchitis*** is defined *clinicc* as cough, sputum production on most days for 3 months of 2 successive years. The is no excess mortality if lung function is normal. Symptoms improve in 90% if th stop smoking. ***Emphysema*** is defined *histologically* as enlarged air spaces distal to t terminal bronchioles, with destruction of the alveolar walls.

Prevalence ~1 million. ***COPD mortality:*** 23,000 deaths/yr in England & Wales.

Pink puffers and blue bloaters (Ends of a spectrum) ***Pink puffers*** have ↑alveol ventilation, a near normal P_aO_2 and a normal or low P_aCO_2. They are breathless but a not cyanosed. They may progress to type 1 respiratory failure (p172). *Blue bloate* have ↓alveolar ventilation, with a low P_aO_2 and a high P_aCO_2. They are cyanosed b not breathless and may go on to develop cor pulmonale. Their respiratory centr are relatively insensitive to CO_2 and they rely on hypoxic drive to mainta respiratory effort (p172)—►*supplemental oxygen should be given with care.*

Clinical features ***Symptoms:*** Cough, sputum, dyspnoea, and wheeze. ***Sig*** Tachypnoea; use of accessory muscles of respiration; hyperinflation; ↓cricostern distance (<3cm); ↓expansion; resonant or hyperresonant percussion note; qu breath sounds (eg over bullae); wheeze; cyanosis; cor pulmonale. ***Complicatio*** Acute exacerbations ± infection; polycythaemia; respiratory failure; cor pulmon (oedema; JVP↑); pneumothorax (ruptured bullae); lung carcinoma.

Tests ***FBC:*** ***PCV***↑. ***CXR:*** Hyperinflation (>6 anterior ribs seen above diaphragm mid-clavicular line); flat hemidiaphragms; large central pulmonary arteri ↓peripheral vascular markings; bullae. ***ECG:*** Right atrial and ventricular hypertrop (cor pulmonale). ***ABG:*** P_aO_2 ↓ ± hypercapnia. ***Lung function*** (p148–151): obstructi + air trapping (FEV_1 <80% of predicted—see p148, FEV_1:FVC ratio <70%, TLC↑, R DLCO↓ in emphysema). Learn how to do spirometry from an experienced pers ensure *maximal* expiration of the full breath (it takes ≥4sec; it's *not* a quick p out). ***Trial of steroids:*** See BOX.

Treatment ***Chronic stable:*** see BOX; ►***Emergency*** ℞: p796. Offer ***smoki cessation advice*** with cordial vigour (p79). BMI is often low: ***diet advice supplements*** *may* help, p572. ***Mucolytics*** (*BNF* 3.7) may help chronic producti cough (NICE). Disabilities may cause serious, treatable ***depression;*** screen for t (p13). ***Respiratory failure:*** p172. ***'Flu and pneumococcal vaccinations:*** p390

Long-term O_2 therapy (LTOT): An MRC trial showed that if P_aO_2 was maintain ≥8.0kPa for 15h a day, 3yr survival improved by 50%. UK DOH guidelines sugg LTOT should be given for: **1** clinically stable non-smokers with P_aO_2 <7.3kPa despite maximal ℞. These values should be stable on two occasions >3 wks apa
2 If P_aO_2 7.3–8.0 ***and*** pulmonary hypertension (eg RVH; loud S_2) + cor pulmona
3 O_2 can also be prescribed for terminally ill patients.

Predicted FEV_1 (Caucasian males; litres, ↓level in other races)[1]											♀									
Height cm	150	155	160	165	170	175	180	185	190	195	145150	155	160	165	170	175	180	185	1	
♂ *Age (yr)* 10	2.5	2.8	3.0	3.2	3.5	3.7	3.9	4.1	4.4	4.6	2.1	2.2	2.3	2.5	2.6	2.7	2.9	3.0	3.1	
25	2.9	3.2	3.4	3.7	4.0	4.2	4.3	4.7	5.0	5.3	2.6	2.7	2.9	3.0	3.1	3.3	3.4	3.5	3.7	
30	2.8	3.1	3.3	3.6	3.8	4.1	4.3	4.6	4.9	5.1	2.5	2.6	2.8	2.9	3.0	3.2	3.3	3.4	3.6	
40	2.5	2.8	3.0	3.3	3.6	3.8	4.1	4.3	4.6	4.9	2.3	2.4	2.5	2.7	2.8	3.0	3.0	3.2	3.3	
50	2.2	2.5	2.8	3.0	3.3	3.5	3.8	4.0	4.3	4.6	2.1	2.2	2.3	2.5	2.6	2.7	2.9	3.0	3.1	
60	2.0	2.2	2.5	2.8	3.0	3.3	3.5	3.8	4.0	4.3	1.7	2.0	2.1	2.3	2.4	2.5	2.7	2.8	2.9	
70	1.7	2.0	2.2	2.5	2.7	3.0	3.3	3.5	3.8	4.0	1.6	1.8	1.9	2.1	2.2	2.3	2.5	2.6	2.7	
80	1.4	1.7	2.0	2.2	2.5	2.7	3.0	3.3	3.5	3.8	1.4	1.6	1.7	1.9	2.0	2.1	2.2	2.4	2.5	

www.nationalasthma.org.au/publications/spiro/appc.html#M

1 African FEV_1 is 10–15% lower; Chinese: 20% lower; Indian: 10% lower; NB: PEF varies little betw groups.

[B]ritish Thoracic Society (BTS)/NICE COPD guidelines

[A]ssessment of COPD Spirometry
Bronchodilator response
Trial of oral steroids;[1] look for >15% ↑ in FEV_1
CXR: ?bullae ?other pathology
ABG: ?hypoxia ?hypercapnia

[S]everity of COPD
Mild FEV_1 50–80% predicted
Moderate FEV_1 30–49% predicted
Severe FEV_1 <30% predicted

[T]reating stable COPD NB: air travel is risky if FEV_1 <50% or P_aO_2 <6.7kPa

[N]on-pharmacological Stop smoking, encourage exercise, treat poor nutrition or obesity, influenza and pneumococcal vaccination, pulmonary rehabilitation/palliative care.[2] NIPPV p797

[P]harmacological: For inhaler regimens, see p167

Mild Antimuscarinic eg ipratropium or β_2 agonist inhaled PRN.

Moderate Regular ipratropium[3] or long-acting inhaled β_2 agonist (salmeterol) ± inhaled steroid (fluticasone) if FEV_1<50% and ≥2 exacerbations/yr. Seretide® combines these. Symbicort® is budesonide + formoterol; there is conflicting evidence on whether this ↑quality of life and symptom scores; but it *may* ↑time to 1st exacerbation. Oral theophylline.

Severe Combination therapy with regular short-acting β_2-agonist and anticholinergic. Refer to specialist. Consider steroid trial;[1] assess for home nebulizers.

Pulmonary hypertension Assess the need for LTOT (see opposite) Treat oedema with diuretics.

[M]ore advanced COPD
Consider pulmonary rehabilitation[2] ± theophylline (monitor blood levels).
Consider LTOT if P_aO_2 <7.3kPa (see OPPOSITE).
Indications for surgery: recurrent pneumothoraces; isolated bullous disease; lung volume reduction surgery (selected patients).
Assess home set-up and support needed. Treat depression (p13).

[I]ndications for specialist referral
Uncertain diagnosis.
Suspected severe COPD or a rapid decline in FEV_1.
Onset of cor pulmonale.
Assessment for oral corticosteroids, nebulizer therapy, or LTOT.
Bullous lung disease (to assess for surgery).
<10 pack-years smoking (=PYS=the number of packs/day × number of years of smoking). Smokers have an excess loss of FEV_1 of 7.4–12.6mL/PYS for men and 4.4–7.2mL per pack year for women.
Symptoms disproportionate to lung function tests.
Frequent infections (to exclude bronchiectasis).
COPD in patient <40yrs (eg is the cause α_1-antitrypsin deficiency? p256).

[1 S]teroid trial: 30mg prednisolone/24h PO for 2wks. If FEV_1 rises by >15%, the COPD is 'steroid [resp]onsive' and benefit may be had by using longterm inhaled corticosteroids (p167). If this doesn't [achi]eve the post-prednisolone FEV_1, do not simply give longterm oral prednisolone (side-effects may be [fat]al, p361); instead, request expert help. (BTS advice). NB: NICE says that 'reversibility testing is not [nec]essary as a part of the diagnostic process or to plan initial therapy with bronchodilators or [cort]icosteroids. It may be unhelpful or misleading because: (1) repeated FEV_1 measurements can show [sma]ll spontaneous fluctuations; (2) results of a reversibility tests on different occasions can be [i]nconsistent and not reproducible; (3) Over-reliance on a single reversibility test may be misleading unless [the] change in FEV_1 is >400 mL. (4) Definition of a significant change is arbitrary; (5) Response to long[-ter]m therapy is not predicted by acute reversibility testing.'

[2 P]alliative care involves referral to a multidisciplinary team ± use of benzodiazepines, antidepressants, [opia]tes, major tranquillizers, and O_2 with a view to diminish symptoms in end-stage COPD.

[3 T]iotroprium is like ipratropium, but longer acting: better in some trials.

Acute respiratory distress syndrome (ARDS)

ARDS, or acute lung injury, may be caused by direct lung injury or occur second to severe systemic illness. Lung damage and release of inflammatory mediat cause increased capillary permeability and non-cardiogenic pulmonary oeder often accompanied by multiorgan failure.

Causes ***Pulmonary:*** Pneumonia; gastric aspiration; inhalation; injury; vascu (p542); contusion. ***Other:*** Shock; septicaemia; haemorrhage; multiple transfusic DIC (p336); pancreatitis; acute liver failure; trauma; head injury; malaria; embolism; burns; obstetric events (eclampsia; amniotic fluid embolus); drugs/to (aspirin, heroin, paraquat).

Clinical features Cyanosis; tachypnoea; tachycardia; peripheral vasodilatati bilateral fine inspiratory crackles.

Investigations FBC, U&E, LFT, amylase, clotting, CRP, blood cultures, ABG. CXR sho bilateral pulmonary infiltrates. Pulmonary artery catheter to measure pulmon capillary wedge pressure (PCWP).

Diagnostic criteria One consensus requires these 4 to exist: **(1)** Acute onset. CXR: bilateral infiltrates. **(3)** PCWP <19mmHg or a lack of clinical congestive he failure. **(4)** Refractory hypoxaemia with $P_aO_2 : FiO_2$ <200 for ARDS. Others incl total thoracic compliance <30mL/cm H_2O.

Management Admit to ITU; give supportive therapy; treat the underlying ca

- ***Respiratory support*** In early ARDS, continuous positive airway pressure (CP with 40–60% oxygen may be adequate to maintain oxygenation. But m patients need mechanical ventilation. Indications for ventilation: P_aO_2: <8.3 despite 60% O_2; P_aCO_2: >6kPa. The large tidal volumes (10–15mL/kg) produ by conventional ventilation plus reduced lung compliance in ARDS may lea high peak airway pressures ± pneumothorax. A low-tidal-volume, press limited approach, with either low or moderate high positive end-expirat pressure (PEEP) improves outcome.
- ***Circulatory support*** Invasive haemodynamic monitoring with an arterial and Swan–Ganz catheter aids the diagnosis and may be helpful in monito PCWP and cardiac output. A conservative fluid management approach impro outcome. Maintain cardiac output and O_2 delivery with inotropes (eg dobutan 2.5–10μg/kg/min IVI), vasodilators, and blood transfusion. Consider trea pulmonary hypertension with low-dose (20–120 parts per million) nitric oxid pulmonary vasodilator. Haemofiltration may be needed in renal failure an achieve a negative fluid balance.
- ***Sepsis*** Identify organism(s) and treat accordingly. If clinically septic, but organisms cultured, use empirical broad-spectrum antibiotics (p153). A nephrotoxic antibiotics.
- ***Other:*** Nutritional support: enteral is best: p572 & p574, with high antioxidant formulations. Steroids protect those at risk of fat embolization with pneumocystosis and may improve outcome in subacute ARDS.

Prognosis Overall mortality is 50%–75%. Prognosis varies with age patient, cause of ARDS (pneumonia 86%, trauma 38%), and number of org involved (3 organs involved for >1wk is 'invariably' fatal).

Chest medicine

isk factors for ARDS

- Sepsis
- Hypovolaemic shock
- Trauma
- Pneumonia
- Diabetic ketoacidosis
- Gastric aspiration
- Pregnancy
- Eclampsia
- Amniotic fluid embolus
- Drugs/toxins
- Paraquat, heroin, aspirin
- Pulmonary contusion
- Massive transfusion
- Burns (p830)
- Smoke inhalation (p831)
- Near drowning
- Acute pancreatitis
- DIC (p336)
- Head injury
- ICP↑
- Fat embolus
- Heart/lung bypass
- Tumour lysis syndrome (p514)
- Malaria

Respiratory failure

Respiratory failure occurs when gas exchange is inadequate, resulting in hypoxia is defined as a P_aO_2 <8kPa and subdivided into 2 types according to P_aCO_2 lev

Type I respiratory failure is defined as hypoxia (P_aO_2 <8kPa) with normal or low P_aCO_2. It is caused primarily by ventilation/perfusion (V/ mismatch. Causes include:

- Pneumonia
- Pulmonary oedema
- PE
- Asthma
- Emphysema
- Fibrosing alveolitis
- ARDS (p170).

Type II respiratory failure is defined as hypoxia (P_aO_2 <8kPa) with hypercap (P_aCO_2 is >6.0kPa). This is caused by alveolar hypoventilation, w or without $\dot{V}/\dot{Q}$ mismatch. Causes include:

- *Pulmonary disease:* asthma, COPD, pneumonia, pulmonary fibrosis, obstruct sleep apnoea (OSA, p186).
- *Reduced respiratory drive:* sedative drugs, CNS tumour, or trauma.
- *Neuromuscular disease:* cervical cord lesion, diaphragmatic paraly poliomyelitis, myasthenia gravis, Guillain–Barré syndrome.
- *Thoracic wall disease:* flail chest, kyphoscoliosis.

Clinical features are those of the underlying cause together with symptoms signs of hypoxia, with or without hypercapnia.

Hypoxia: Dyspnoea; restlessness; agitation; confusion; central cyanosis. longstanding hypoxia: polycythaemia; pulmonary hypertension; cor pulmonale.

Hypercapnia: Headache; peripheral vasodilatation; tachycardia; bounding pu tremor/flap; papilloedema; confusion; drowsiness; coma.

Investigations are aimed at determining the underlying cause:

- Blood tests: FBC, U&E, CRP, ABG
- Radiology: CXR
- Microbiology: sputum and blood cultures (if febrile)
- Spirometry (COPD, neuromuscular disease, Guillain–Barré syndrome).

Management depends on the cause:

Type I respiratory failure

- Treat underlying cause.
- Give oxygen (35–60%) by face mask to correct hypoxia.
- Assisted ventilation if P_aO_2 <8kPa despite 60% O_2.

Type II respiratory failure the respiratory centre may be relatively insensitiv CO_2 and respiration could be driven by hypoxia. ►*Oxygen therapy should be gi with care.* Nevertheless, don't leave the hypoxia untreated.

- Treat underlying cause.
- Controlled oxygen therapy: start at 24% O_2.
- Recheck ABG after 20min. If P_aCO_2 is steady or lower, increase O_2 concentratio 28%. If P_aCO_2 has risen >1.5kPa and the patient is still hypoxic, conside respiratory stimulant (eg doxapram 1.5–4mg/min IVI) or assisted ventilation NIPPV, p797, ie non-invasive positive pressure ventilation).
- If this fails, consider intubation and ventilation, if appropriate.

'hen to consider ABG (arterial blood gas) measurement

these clinical scenarios:

ıy unexpected deterioration in an ill patient.
ıyone with an acute exacerbation of a chronic chest condition.
ıyone with impaired consciousness.
ıyone with impaired respiratory effort.

if any of these signs or symptoms are present:

ɔunding pulse, drowsy, tremor (flapping), headache, pink palms, papilloedema (signs of CO_2 retention).
ʼanosis, confusion, visual hallucinations (signs of hypoxia).

to monitor the progress of a critically ill patient:

ɔnitoring the treatment of known respiratory failure.
ıyone ventilated on ITU.
'ter major surgery.
'ter major trauma.

validate measurements from transcutaneous pulse oximetry:

lse oximetry (p148) *sometimes* suffices when it is not critical to know P_aCO_2. Even so, it is wise to do periodic blood gas checks.
arn arterial puncture from an expert (local anaesthesia *does* ↓pain) see p759.

Pulmonary embolism (PE)

Causes PEs usually arise from a venous thrombosis in the pelvis or legs. Clots br off and pass through the venous system and the right side of the heart bef lodging in the pulmonary circulation. Rare causes include: right ventricu thrombus (post-MI); septic emboli (right-sided endocarditis); fat, air, or amnic fluid embolism; neoplastic cells; parasites. ***Risk factors:*** Any cause of immobility hyper-coagulability:

- Recent surgery
- Recent stroke or MI
- Disseminated malignancy
- Thrombophilia/antiphospholipid syn. (p358)
- Prolonged bed rest
- Pregnancy; postpartum; the Pill/HRT

Clinical features These depend on the number, size, and distribution of the emb small emboli may be asymptomatic, whereas large emboli are often fa ***Symptoms:*** Acute breathlessness, pleuritic chest pain, haemoptysis; dizzin syncope. Ask about risk factors (above), past history or family history thromboembolism. ***Signs:*** Pyrexia; cyanosis; tachypnoea; tachycardia; hypotens raised JVP, pleural rub; pleural effusion. Look for signs of a cause, eg deep v thrombosis; scar from recent surgery.

Tests

- FBC, U&E, baseline clotting, D-dimers (BOX).
- ***ABG*** may show a low P_aO_2 and a low P_aCO_2.
- ***CXR*** may be normal, or may show oligaemia of affected segment, dila pulmonary artery, linear atelectasis, small pleural effusion, wedge-sha opacities or cavitation (rare).
- ***ECG*** may be normal, or show tachycardia, right bundle branch block, right ve ricular strain (inverted T in V_1 to V_4). The classical $S_I Q_{III} T_{III}$ pattern (p84) is r

►Further investigations are shown on p802; see also BOX, p725.

Treatment ►►See p802. Anticoagulate with low molecular weight heparin dalteparin 200U/kg/24h SC, max dose 18,000U/24h) and start oral warfarin 1((p334). Stop heparin when INR is >2 and continue warfarin for a minimum months (see p335); aim for an INR of 2–3. Consider placement of a ***vena caval f*** in patients who develop emboli despite adequate anticoagulation (NB increased if placed without concomitant anticoagulation).

Prevention Give heparin (eg dalteparin 2500U/24h SC) to all immobile patie Prescribe compression stockings and encourage early mobilization. Stop HRT the Pill pre-op (if reliable with another form of contraception). If past or fa history of thromboembolism, consider investigation for thrombophilia (p358

Pneumothorax

Management ►►p7

Causes Often spontaneous (especially in young thin men) due to rupture subpleural bulla. Other causes: asthma; COPD; TB; pneumonia; lung absc carcinoma; cystic fibrosis; lung fibrosis; sarcoidosis; connective tissue disor (Marfan's syndrome, Ehlers–Danlos syndrome), trauma; iatrogenic (subclaviar line insertion, pleural aspiration or biopsy, transbronchial biopsy, percutaneous biopsy, positive pressure ventilation).

Clinical features ***Symptoms:*** There may be no symptoms (especially if fit, young small pneumothorax) or there may be sudden onset of dyspnoea and/or pleuritic pain. Patients with asthma or COPD may present with a sudden deteriora Mechanically ventilated patients may present with hypoxia or an increas ventilation pressures. ***Signs:*** Reduced expansion, hyper-resonance to percussion diminished breath sounds on the affected side. *With a tension pneumothorax trachea will be deviated away from the affected side.* See x-ray p735.

►►**Managing a tension pneumothorax** See p798. Placing a chest drain, ►►p

ıvestigating suspected PE

iagnosis of PE is improved by adopting a stepwise approach, combining ı objective probability score, with subsequent investigations, as follows.

Assess the clinical probability of a PE: many systems exist and are usually based around elements drawn from the history and clinical examination

Scoring system for investigation of suspected DVT*

Feature	Score
Active cancer, or treatment within 6 months	1
Paralysis, paresis, or recent plaster immobilization of lower limbs	1
Recently bed-ridden (>3 days) or major surgery (< 4weeks)	1
Localized tenderness along venous system	1
Entire leg swollen	1
Calf circumference >3cm more than other side, 10cm below tibial tuberosity	1
Pitting oedema > than in asymptomatic leg	1
Collateral superficial veins	1
Alternative diagnosis as, or more, likely than DVT	−2
Total score: 0=low probability; 1-2 moderate probability; ≥3 high probability	

*Adapted from Wells et al. *Lancet* 1997 350 1795

D-dimers: only perform in those patients **without** a high probability of a PE. A negative D-dimer test excludes a PE in those with a low or intermediate clinical probability, and imaging is NOT required. However, a positive test does not prove a diagnosis of a PE, and imaging is required.

Imaging: The conventional 1st-line, if the CXR is normal, is a $\dot{V}/\dot{Q}$ ***scan*** (p150, p724 & p802; look for perfusion defects with no corresponding ventilation defects). If 'normal', a PE is reliably excluded. If non-diagnostic, further imaging is required, but may give some false positives. The recommended 1st-line imaging modality is now CT pulmonary angiography (**CTPA**), which can show clots down to 5th-order pulmonary arteries (after the 4th branching). This may also be useful for subjects with indeterminant isotope scans. Bilateral leg ultrasound (or rarely venograms) may also be sufficient to **confirm**, but not exclude, a PE in patients with a co-existing clinical DVT.

ajor risk factors for PE

- Surgery:
  - Major abdominal/pelvic
  - Hip/knee replacement
- Obstetrics:
  - Late pregnancy; post-partum
  - Caesarean section
- Lower limb problems:
  - Fracture
  - Varicose veins
- Malignancy
- Reduced mobility
- Previous PE

Pleural effusion

Definitions A pleural effusion is fluid in the pleural space. Effusions can be divid by their protein concentration into *transudates* (<25g/L) and *exudates* (>35g/ see OPPOSITE. Blood in the pleural space is a *haemothorax*; pus in the pleural spa is an *empyema*, and chyle (lymph with fat) is a *chylothorax*. Both blood and air the pleural space is called a *haemopneumothorax*.

Causes *Transudates* may be due to ↑venous pressure (cardiac failure, constrict pericarditis, fluid overload), or hypoproteinaemia (cirrhosis, nephrotic syndror malabsorption). Also occur in hypothyroidism and Meigs' syndrome (right pleu effusion and ovarian fibroma). ***Exudates*** are mostly due to increased leakiness pleural capillaries secondary to infection, inflammation, or malignancy. Caus pneumonia; TB; pulmonary infarction; rheumatoid arthritis; SLE; bronchogenic carc oma; malignant metastases; lymphoma; mesothelioma; lymphangitis carcinomato

Symptoms Asymptomatic—or dyspnoea, pleuritic chest pain.

Signs *Decreased expansion; stony dull percussion note; diminished breath sour* occur on the affected side. Tactile vocal fremitus and vocal resonance are (inconstant and unreliable). Above the effusion, where lung is compressed, th may be *bronchial breathing* and *aegophony* (bleating vocal resonance). With la effusions there may be *tracheal deviation* away from the effusion. Look aspiration marks and signs of associated disease: malignancy (cachexia, clubbi lymphadenopathy, radiation marks, mastectomy scar); stigmata of chronic li disease; cardiac failure; hypothyroidism; rheumatoid arthritis; butterfly rash of s

Tests *CXR:* Small effusions blunt the costophrenic angles, larger ones are seer water-dense shadows with concave upper borders. A completely horizontal up border implies that there is also a pneumothorax. (See figs 1&2, p714)

Ultrasound is useful in identifying the presence of pleural fluid and in guid diagnostic or therapeutic aspiration.

Diagnostic aspiration: Percuss the upper border of the pleural effusion a choose a site 1 or 2 intercostal spaces below it (don't go too low or you'll be in abdomen!). Infiltrate down to the pleura with 5–10mL of 1% lidocaine. Attac 21G needle to a syringe and insert it just above the upper border of an appropri rib (avoids neurovascular bundle). Draw off 10–30mL of pleural fluid and send i the lab for *clinical chemistry* (protein, glucose, pH, LDH, amylase); *bacteriol* (microscopy and culture, auramine stain, TB culture); *cytology* and, if indica *immunology* (rheumatoid factor, ANA, complement).

Pleural biopsy: If pleural fluid analysis is inconclusive, consider parietal pleu biopsy with an Abrams' needle. See p752 for details. Thoracoscopic or CT-gui pleural biopsy increases diagnostic yield (by enabling direct visualization of pleural cavity and biopsy of suspicious areas).

Management is of the underlying cause.

- ***Drainage*** If the effusion is symptomatic, drain it, repeatedly if necessary. Flui best removed slowly (≤2L/24h). It may be aspirated in the same way a diagnostic tap, or using an intercostal drain (see p754).
- ***Pleurodesis*** with tetracycline, bleomycin, or talc may be helpful for recurr effusions. Thoracoscopic talc pleurodesis is most effective for malignant effusi Empyemas (p156) are best drained using a chest drain, inserted under ultraso or CT guidance.
- ***Intra-pleural streptokinase*** Of no benefit.
- ***Surgery:*** Persistent collections and increasing pleural thickness (on ultrasou requires surgery.

Pleural fluid analysis

Gross appearance	*Cause*
Clear, straw-coloured	Transudate, exudate
Turbid, yellow	Empyema, parapneumonic effusion[1]
Haemorrhagic	Trauma, malignancy, pulmonary infarction
Cytology	
Neutrophils ++	Parapneumonic effusion, PE
Lymphocytes ++	Malignancy, TB, RA, SLE, sarcoidosis
Mesothelial cells ++	Pulmonary infarction
Abnormal mesothelial cells	Mesothelioma
Multinucleated giant cells	RA
Lupus erythematosus cells	SLE
Clinical chemistry	
Protein <25g/L	Transudate
>35g/L	Exudate
25–35g/L	If pleural fluid protein/serum protein >0.5, effusion is an exudate
Glucose <3.3mmol/L	Empyema, malignancy, TB, RA, SLE
pH <7.2	Empyema, malignancy, TB, RA, SLE
LDH↑ (pleural:serum >0.6)	Empyema, malignancy, TB, RA, SLE
Amylase↑	Pancreatitis, carcinoma, bacterial pneumonia, oesophageal rupture
Immunology	
Rheumatoid factor	RA
Antinuclear antibody	SLE
Complement levels↓	RA, SLE, malignancy, infection

Chest medicine

1 Inflammation of the pleura caused by pneumonia may lead to infected pleural fluid (empyema); if it is uninfected, the term parapneumonic effusion is used.

Sarcoidosis

A multisystem granulomatous disorder of unknown cause. Prevalence UK: 10–20/10^5 population. Commonly affects adults aged 20–40yrs. Afr Caribbeans are affected more frequently and more severely than Caucasiar particularly by extrathoracic disease.

Clinical features *Asymptomatic* In 20–40%, the disease is discover incidentally, after a routine CXR. ***Acute sarcoidosis*** often presents with erythen nodosum (fig 1, p547)[1] ± polyarthralgia. It usually resolves spontaneously.

Pulmonary disease 90% have abnormal CXRs with bilateral hilar lymphadenopat (BHL) ± pulmonary infiltrates or fibrosis; see below for staging. *Symptoms:* D cough, progressive dyspnoea, ↓exercise tolerance and chest pain. In 10–20 symptoms progress, with concurrent deterioration in lung function.

Non-pulmonary manifestations are legion: lymphadenopathy; hepatomega splenomegaly; uveitis; conjunctivitis; keratoconjunctivitis sicca; glaucoma; termir phalangeal bone cysts; enlargement of lacrimal and parotid glands (fig 4 on p33 Bell's palsy; neuropathy; meningitis; brainstem and spinal syndromes; space-occupyi lesion; erythema nodosum (fig 1, p547); lupus pernio; subcutaneous nodules; cardi myopathy; arrhythmias; hypercalcaemia; hypercalciuria; renal stones; pituita dysfunction.

Tests *Blood:* ↑ESR, lymphopenia, LFT↑, ↑serum ACE, ↑Ca^{2+}, ↑immunoglobuli *24h urine:* Ca^{2+}↑. ***Tuberculin skin test*** is –ve in two-thirds; *CXR* is abnormal in 90 *Stage 0:* normal. *Stage 1:* BHL. *Stage 2:* BHL + peripheral pulmonary infiltrat *Stage 3:* peripheral pulmonary infiltrates alone. *Stage 4:* progressive pulmona fibrosis; bulla formation (honeycombing); pleural involvement. *ECG* may sho arrhythmias or bundle branch block. ***Lung function tests*** may be normal or sho reduced lung volumes, impaired gas transfer, and a restrictive ventilatory defe ***Tissue biopsy*** (lung, liver, lymph nodes, skin nodules, or lacrimal glands) diagnostic and shows non-caseating granulomata.

Bronchoalveolar lavage (BAL) shows ↑lymphocytes in active disease; ↑neutrop with pulmonary fibrosis.

Ultrasound may show nephrocalcinosis or hepatosplenomegaly.

Bone x-rays show 'punched out' lesions in terminal phalanges.

CT/MRI may be useful in assessing severity of pulmonary disease or diagnosi neurosarcoidosis. ***Ophthalmology assessment*** (slit lamp examination, fluoresc angiography) is indicated in ocular disease. ***Kveim tests*** are obsolete.

Management ►*Patients with BHL alone do not require treatment since the major recover spontaneously.* ***Acute sarcoidosis:*** Bed rest, NSAIDs.

Indications for corticosteroid therapy:

- Parenchymal lung disease (symptomatic, static, or progressive)
- Uveitis
- Hypercalcaemia
- Neurological or cardiac involvement.

Prednisolone (40mg/24h) PO for 4–6 wks, then ↓dose over 1yr accordi to clinical status. A few patients relapse and may need a further course or lor term therapy. In severe illness, IV methylprednisolone or immunosuppressar (methotrexate, ciclosporin, cyclophosphamide) may be needed.

Prognosis 60% of patients with thoracic sarcoidosis show spontaneous resoluti within 2yrs. 20% of patients respond to steroid therapy. In the remaind improvement is unlikely despite therapy.

1 A detailed history and exam (including for synovitis) + CXR, 2 ASO-titres & a tuberculin skin tes usually enough to diagnose erythema nodosum: R Pugol 2000 *Arthr Rheu* **43** 584

Causes of BHL (bilateral hilar lymphadenopathy)	
Sarcoidosis	
Infection	TB
	Mycoplasma
Malignancy	Lymphoma
	Carcinoma
	Mediastinal tumours
Organic dust disease	Silicosis
	Berylliosis
Extrinsic allergic alveolitis	

ifferential diagnosis of granulomatous diseases		
nfections	Bacteria	TB
		Leprosy
		Syphilis
		Cat scratch fever
	Fungi	*Cryptococcus neoformans*
		Coccidioides immitis
	Protozoa	Schistosomiasis
Autoimmune	Primary biliary cirrhosis	
	Granulomatous orchitis	
Vasculitis (p542)	Giant cell arteritis	
	Polyarteritis nodosa	
	Takayasu's arteritis	
	Wegener's granulomatosis	
Organic dust disease	Silicosis	
	Berylliosis	
Idiopathic	Crohn's disease	
	de Quervain's thyroiditis	
	Sarcoidosis	
xtrinsic allergic alveolitis		
istiocytosis X		

Interstitial lung disease (ILD)

This is the generic term used to describe a number of conditions that primar affect the lung parenchyma in a diffuse manner. They are characterized by chro inflammation and/or progressive interstitial fibrosis, and share a number of clini and pathological features.

Clinical features Dyspnoea on exertion; non-productive paroxysmal cou abnormal breath sounds; abnormal CXR or high resolution CT; restrictive pulmona spirometry with a reduced DLCO (p150).

Pathological features Fibrosis and remodelling of the interstitium; chro inflammation; hyperplasia of type II epithelial cells or type II pneumocytes.

Classification The ILDs can be broadly grouped into three categories:

- ***Those with known aetiology eg***
  - Occupational/environmental eg asbestosis, berylliosis, silicosis
  - Drugs eg nitrofurantoin, bleomycin, amiodarone, sulfasalazine, busulfan
  - Hypersensitivity reactions eg extrinsic allergic alveolitis
  - Infections eg TB, fungi, viral
- ***Those associated with systemic disorders eg***
  - Sarcoidosis
  - Rheumatoid arthritis
  - SLE, systemic sclerosis, mixed connective tissue disease, Sjögren's syndror
  - Ulcerative colitis, renal tubular acidosis, autoimmune thyroid disease
- ***Idiopathic eg***
  - Idiopathic pulmonary fibrosis (IPF)/cryptogenic fibrosing alveolitis (p182)
  - Cryptogenic organizing pneumonia
  - Lymphocytic interstitial pneumonia

Extrinsic allergic alveolitis (EAA)

In sensitized individuals, inhalation of allergens (fungal spores or avian protei provokes a hypersensitivity reaction. In the acute phase, the alveoli are infiltra with acute inflammatory cells. With chronic exposure, granuloma formation a obliterative bronchiolitis occur.

Causes

- Bird fancier's and pigeon fancier's lung (proteins in bird droppings).
- Farmer's and mushroom worker's lung (*Micropolyspora faeni, Thermoacti myces vulgaris*).
- Malt worker's lung (*Aspergillus clavatus*).
- Bagassosis (*Thermoactinomyces sacchari*).

Clinical features *4–6h post-exposure:* Fever, rigors, myalgia, dry cough, dyspnc crackles (no wheeze). ***Chronic:*** Increasing dyspnoea, weight↓, exertional dyspnc Type I respiratory failure, cor pulmonale.

Tests *Acute:* Blood: FBC (neutrophilia); ESR↑; ABGs; positive serum precipit (indicate exposure only). *CXR:* mid-zone mottling/consolidation; hilar lym adenopathy (rare). *Lung function tests:* reversible restrictive defect; reduced transfer during acute attacks. ***Chronic:*** *Blood tests:* positive serum precipitins. c upper-zone fibrosis; honeycomb lung. *Lung function tests:* persistent changes (above). Bronchoalveolar lavage (BAL) fluid shows ↑ lymphocytes and mast ce

Management

Acute attack: Remove allergen and give O_2 (35–60%), then:

- Oral prednisolone (40mg/24h PO), followed by reducing dose.

Chronic: Avoid exposure to allergens, or wear a face mask or +ve pressure helr Long-term steroids often achieve CXR and physiological improvement. Comp sation (UK Industrial Injuries Act) may be payable.

Idiopathic pulmonary fibrosis

Inflammatory cell infiltrate and pulmonary fibrosis of unknown cause (also know as cryptogenic fibrosing alveolitis). The commonest cause of interstitial lung disea

Symptoms Dry cough; exertional dyspnoea; malaise; weight↓; arthralgia.

Signs Cyanosis; finger clubbing; fine end-inspiratory crepitations.

Complications Type 1 respiratory failure; increased risk of lung cancer.

Tests ***Blood:*** ABG (P_aO_2↓; P_aCO_2↑); CRP↑; immunoglobulins↑; ANA (30% +v rheumatoid factor (10% +ve). ***CXR:*** (fig 1) Lung volume↓; bilateral lower zo reticulo-nodular shadows; honeycomb lung (advanced disease). Magnetic resonan scan/CT show similar changes to the CXR but is more sensitive and is an essent tool for diagnosis. ***Spirometry:*** Restrictive (p148); ↓transfer factor. ***BAL*** (bronch alveolar lavage) may indicate activity of alveolitis: lymphocytes↑ (go response/prognosis) or neutrophils and eosinophils↑ (poor response/prognos ***$^{99}Tc^m$-DTPA scan:*** (diethylene-triamine-penta-acetic acid) may reflect disea activity. ***Lung biopsy*** may be needed for diagnosis.[39]

Management A large proportion of patients have chronic irreversible disea unresponsive to treatment. Prednisolone 0.5mg/kg/24h PO for 4 wks, then 0.25m kg/24h PO for 48 wks, then taper (~20% respond). Alternative: cyclophosphami 100–120mg/24h PO + prednisolone 20mg PO on alternate days. Monitor respor with symptom enquiry, CXR, and lung function tests. The patient may be suitable lung transplantation.[40] **Prognosis** 50% 5yr survival rate (range 1–20yrs).

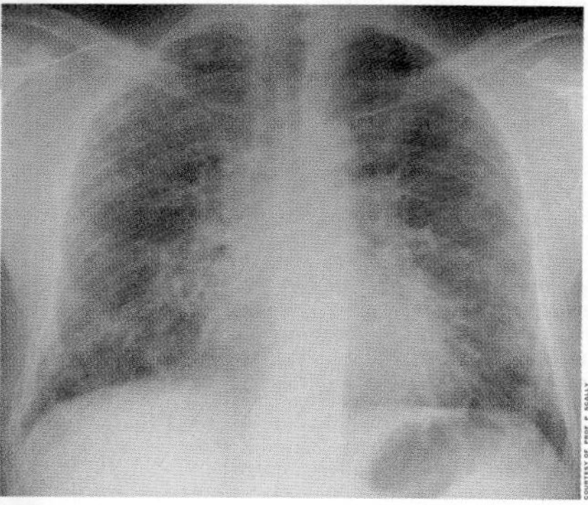

Fig 1. Systematic approach: **Lungs:** Lung volumes are normal, but the parenchyma shows increased markings extending to the chest wall. Normally arteries and veins are only seen for 80% of the distance from hilum to pleura. Bronchi should barely be visible.

Pleura: Following the pleura demonstrates that the heart borders are poorly defined, reflecting interstitial disease in the lung, adjacent to the heart.

Mediastinum: The mediastinal structures are normal.

Hila: The hila are difficult to interpret. So what? It is not unusual to be missing a piece of information when making a clinical decision. No need for wringing of hands. Either go ahead without it, or, if it is essential, find it (look at old films; do CT).

Bones and soft tissue: These appear normal.

Comment: This is interstitial lung disease (a similar appearance to the interstitial oedema of moderate left heart failure, but without a big heart). Check the previous films to see if it is acute. It is not. The diagnosis here is fibrosing alveolitis.

Industrial dust diseases

Coal worker's pneumoconiosis (CWP) is the commonest dust disease in the UK. results from inhalation of coal dust particles (1–3μm in diameter) over 15–20yr These are ingested by macrophages which die, releasing their enzymes and causir fibrosis.

Clinical features: Asymptomatic, but co-existing chronic bronchitis is commo CXR: many round opacities (1–10mm), especially upper zone.

Management: Avoid exposure to coal dust; treat co-existing chronic bronchiti claim compensation (in the UK, *via* the Industrial Injuries Act).

Progressive massive fibrosis (PMF) is due to progression of CWP, which cause progressive dyspnoea, fibrosis, and eventually, cor pulmonale. CXR: upper-zor fibrotic masses (1–10cm).

Management: Avoid exposure to coal dust; claim compensation (as above).

Caplan's syndrome is the association between rheumatoid arthritis, pneum coniosis, and pulmonary rheumatoid nodules.

Silicosis is caused by inhalation of silica particles, which are very fibrogenic. number of jobs may be associated with exposure, eg metal mining, stone quarryin sandblasting, and pottery/ceramic manufacture.

Clinical features: Progressive dyspnoea, ↑incidence of TB, CXR shows diffu miliary or nodular pattern in upper and mid-zones and egg-shell calcification hilar nodes. Spirometry: restrictive ventilatory defect.

Management: Avoid exposure to silica; claim compensation (as above).

Asbestosis is caused by inhalation of asbestos fibres. Chrysotile (white asbestos) the least fibrogenic—crocidolite (blue asbestos) is the most fibrogenic. Amosi (brown asbestos) is the least common and has intermediate fibrogenicity. Asbest was commonly used in the building trade for fire proofing, pipe lagging, electric wire insulation, and roofing felt. Degree of asbestos exposure is related to degree pulmonary fibrosis.

Clinical features: Similar to other fibrotic lung diseases with progressi dyspnoea, clubbing, and fine end-inspiratory crackles. Also causes pleural plaque ↑risk of bronchial adenocarcinoma and mesothelioma.

Management: Symptomatic. Patients are often eligible for compensation throu the UK Industrial Injuries Act.

Malignant mesothelioma is a tumour of mesothelial cells which usually occurs the pleura, and rarely in the peritoneum or other organs. It is associated wi occupational exposure to asbestos but the relationship is complex. 90% repo previous exposure to asbestos, but only 20% of patients have pulmona asbestosis. The latent period between exposure and development of the tumo may be up to 45yrs.

Clinical features include chest pain, dyspnoea, weight loss, finger clubbir recurrent pleural effusions. If the tumour has metastasized there may lymphadenopathy, hepatomegaly, bone pain/tenderness, abdominal pain/obst uction (peritoneal malignant mesothelioma).

Tests: CXR/CT: pleural thickening/effusion. Bloody pleural fluid.

Diagnosis is made on histology, following a pleural biopsy—Abrams' needle (p75 thoracoscopy. Often the diagnosis is only made post-mortem.

Management: Symptomatic, with industrial compensation, as above.

Prognosis is very poor (<2yrs, >650 deaths/yr in the UK).

Obstructive sleep apnoea syndrome

This disorder is characterized by intermittent closure/collapse of the pharynge airway which causes apnoeic episodes during sleep. These are terminated by part arousal.

Clinical features The typical patient is a obese, middle-aged man (or a po menopausal woman) who presents because of snoring or daytime somnolence. I partner often describes apnoeic episodes during sleep.

- Snorts loudly in sleep
- Daytime somnolence
- Poor sleep quality
- Morning headache
- Decreased libido
- Cognitive performance↓

Complications Pulmonary hypertension; Type II respiratory failure (p172). Sle apnoea is also reported as an independent risk factor for hypertension.

Investigations Simple studies (eg pulse oximetry, video recordings) may be that are required for diagnosis. Polysomnography (which monitors oxyg saturation, airflow at the nose and mouth, ECG, EMG chest and abdominal w movement during sleep) is diagnostic. The occurrence of 15 or more episodes apnoea or hypopnoea during 1h of sleep indicates significant sleep apnoea.

Management

- Weight reduction
- Avoidance of tobacco and alcohol
- CPAP via a nasal mask during sleep is effective
- Surgical procedures to relieve pharyngeal obstruction (tonsillector uvulopalatopharyngoplasty, or tracheostomy) are occasionally needed, but o after seeing a chest physician.

Cor pulmonale

Cor pulmonale is right heart failure caused by chronic pulmonary hypertensi Causes include chronic lung disease, pulmonary vascular disorders, a neuromuscular and skeletal diseases (see p187).

Clinical features Symptoms include dyspnoea, fatigue, or syncope. Signs: cyano tachycardia; raised JVP with prominent *a* and *v* waves; RV heave; loud P_2, pansyst murmur (tricuspid regurgitation); early diastolic Graham Steell murm hepatomegaly and oedema.

Investigations *FBC:* Hb and haematocrit↑ (secondary polycythaemia). *A* hypoxia, with or without hypercapnia. *CXR:* enlarged right atrium and ventri prominent pulmonary arteries. *ECG:* P pulmonale; right axis deviation; ri ventricular hypertrophy/strain.

Management

- ***Treat underlying cause***—eg COPD and pulmonary infections.
- ***Treat respiratory failure***—in the acute situation give 24% oxygen if P_aO_2 <8k Monitor ABG and gradually increase oxygen concentration if P_aCO_2 is sta (p172). In COPD patients, long-term oxygen therapy (LTOT) for 15h/d increa survival (see p168). Patients with chronic hypoxia when clinically stable sho be assessed for LTOT.
- ***Treat cardiac failure*** with diuretics such as furosemide, eg 40–160mg/24h Monitor U&E and give amiloride or potassium supplements if necess Alternative: spironolactone.
- Consider ***venesection*** if the haematocrit is >55%.
- Consider ***heart-lung transplantation*** in young patients.

Prognosis Poor. 50% die within 5yrs.

Causes of cor pulmonale

- ***Lung disease***
  Asthma (severe, chronic)
  COPD
  Bronchiectasis
  Pulmonary fibrosis
  Lung resection
- ***Pulmonary vascular disease***
  Pulmonary emboli
  Pulmonary vasculitis
  Primary pulmonary hypertension
  ARDS (p170)
  Sickle-cell disease
  Parasite infestation
- ***Thoracic cage abnormality***
  Kyphosis
  Scoliosis
  Thoracoplasty
- **Neuromuscular disease**
  Myasthenia gravis
  Poliomyelitis
  Motor neurone disease
- ***Hypoventilation***
  Sleep apnoea
  Enlarged adenoids in children
  Cerebrovascular disease

6 Endocrinology

Contents

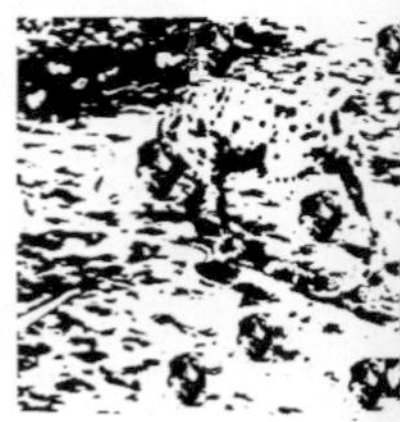

Fig 1. In German, *Gestalt* means bo[th] *the whole* form (as being more than t[he] sum of its parts) and *the pattern.* gestalt has come to mean (in WH Aude[n's] words) the place where indiscr[e]... perceptions and extensions meet and n[ew] meanings are created. The ideal endocr[in]ologist is a master of gestalt patte[rn] recognition (myxoedema, acromegaly, a[nd] the rest—see opposite). On viewing t[he] above, he or she sees the dots and t[he] dog, but does not get *too* carried away filling in the gaps: he detects t[he] amputated hind-leg—postulating diabe[tes] mellitus (autoimmune, if this Dalmati[an] has vitiligo).

Nor is he or she put off by missing paradoxical data (eg *increase* in weight [in] thyrotoxicosis, seen in up to 30%). Knowing when to stand back and lo[ok] *holistically*, when to go for *detail*, a[nd] when to *count* (how many heads are th[ere] in the image?) is a key skill in all medicine, not just endocrinology.

With inverse *gestalt* we deconstruc[t a] familiar picture into its component do[ts] to see what new forms emerge: a use[ful] technique for our most difficult patien[ts].

Relevant pages in other chapters: Diabetic ketoacidosis (➧p814); hypoglycaem[ia] (➧p816); the diabetic patient undergoing surgery (p576); the eye in diabetes (*OH*[*CS*] p446); thyroid emergencies (➧p816); thyroid lumps (p622); Addison's disea[se,] thyroid disease, and surgery (p579); Addisonian crisis & hypopituitary co[ma] (➧p818); phaeochromocytoma emergencies (➧p818).

In pregnancy: Thyroid disease (*OHCS* p25) and diabetes in pregnancy (*OHCS* p2...)

In childhood: Childhood diabetes (*OHCS* p186) and thyroid problems (*OHCS* p18...)

We thank Dr. Stephen Gilbey who is our Specialist Reader for this chapter.

The essence of endocrinology—for scientists

- Define a clinical syndrome, and match it to a gland malfunction.
- Measure the gland's output in the peripheral blood. Define clinical syndromes associated with too much or too little secretion (*hyper*- and *hypo*-syndromes, respectively; *eu*- means normal, neither ↑ nor ↓, as in *euthyroid*). Note factors that may make measurement variable eg diurnal release of cortisol.
- If suspecting hormone deficiency, test by stimulating the gland that produces it (eg Short ACTH stimulation test or *Synacthen*® test in Addison's disease). If the gland is not functioning normally, there will be a blunted response to stimulation.
- If suspecting hormone excess, test by inhibiting the gland that produces it (eg Dexamethasone suppression test in Cushing's). If there is a hormone secreting tumour then this will fail to suppress via normal feedback mechanisms.
- Find a radiological technique to image the gland. NB: non-functioning tumours or "incidentalomas" may be found in normal subjects, see p208. Imaging alone does not make the diagnosis.
- Aim to halt disease progression. An example is diet and exercise advice which can reduce progression of 'impaired fasting glucose (IFG)' to frank diabetes by 50%. For other glands, halting progression will depend on understanding autoimmunity, and the interaction of endogenous (genetic) and environmental factors. In the case of thyroid autoimmunity (an archetypal autoimmune disease), it is possible to track interactions between genetic and environmental factors (eg smoking and stress) via expression of immunologically active molecules (HLA class I & II, adhesion molecules, cytokines, CD40, and complement regulatory proteins).

The essence of endocrinology—for those doing exams

'What's wrong with *him*?' your examiner asks, baldly. While you apologise to the patient for this rudeness by asking: 'Is it alright if we speak about you as if you weren't there?' think to yourself that if you were a betting man or woman you would wager that the diagnosis will be endocrinological. In no other discipline are *gestalt* impressions so characteristic. To get good at recognizing these conditions, spend time in endocrinology out-patients and looking at collections of clinical photographs. Also, specific cutaneous signs are important, as follows.

Thyrotoxicosis: Hair loss; pretibial myxoedema (p202); onycholysis (nail separation from the nailbed); bulging eyes (exophthalmos).

Hypothyroidism: Hair loss; eyebrow loss; cold, pale skin; characteristic face. You might, perhaps *should*, fail your exam if you blurt out 'Toad-like face'.)

Cushing's syndrome: Central obesity and wasted limbs (='lemon on sticks'); moon facies; buffalo hump; supraclavicular fat pads; purple abdominal striae.

Addison's disease: Hyperpigmentation (face, neck, palmar creases).

Acromegaly: Acral (distal) and soft tissue overgrowth; big jaws (macrognathia), hands and feet; the skin is thick; facial features are coarse.

Hyperandrogenism (♀): Hirsutism; temporal balding; acne.

Hypopituitarism: Pale or yellow tinged thinned skin, resulting in fine wrinkling around the eyes and mouth, making the patient look older.

Hypoparathyroidism: Dry, scaly, puffy skin; brittle nails; coarse, sparse hair.

Pseudohypoparathyroidism: Short stature, short neck & short 4th & 5th metacarpals

DM signs: (There is no gestalt picture). Necrobiosis lipoidica; diabetic dermopathy; acanthosis nigricans (dark patches eg in axillae, neck).

Diabetes mellitus: classification and diagnosis

Essence Diabetes mellitus (DM) results from a lack (or diminished effectiveness) endogenous insulin. Hyperglycaemia is just one aspect of a far-reaching metabo derangement, which may cause serious microvascular (retinopathy, nephropatl neuropathy) or macrovascular complications (cardiovascular—coronary arte disease, cerebrovascular—stroke, and peripheral vascular disease).

Type 1 DM (formerly insulin-dependent DM, IDDM): usually juvenile onset but m occur at *any* age. ***Cause*** Insulin deficiency due to selective destruction of insuli secreting pancreatic β cells. Patients *always* need insulin, and are prone ketoacidosis and weight loss. It is associated with other autoimmune diseas (>90% carry HLA DR3 ± DR4; see index). Concordance is only ~30% in identic twins, indicating environmental influence. 4 genes are important—one (6 determines islet sensitivity to damage (eg from viruses or cross-reactivity fro cows' milk-induced antibodies). Latent autoimmune diabetes of adults (LADA) is form of Type 1 DM, with slower progression to insulin dependence in later life.

Type 2 DM (formerly non-insulin dependent DM, NIDDM) appears to be prevalent 'epidemic' levels in many places, mainly due to changes in lifestyle, but also becau of better diagnosis and improved longevity. Higher prevalence occurs in Asiar men, and the elderly (18% in men over 80 in Liverpool). Most are over 40yrs, b teenagers are increasingly getting type 2 DM. ***Cause*** ↓Insulin secretion and insu resistance. It is associated with obesity, lack of exercise and calorie excess. ≥80 concordance in identical twins, indicating stronger genetic influence than in Type DM. Typically progresses from a preliminary phase of impaired glucose toleran (IGT) or impaired fasting glucose (IFG), see BOX. (►This a unique window opportunity for lifestyle intervention.) Maturity onset diabetes of the young (MOL is a rare autosomal dominant form of Type 2 DM affecting young people witl positive family history.

Endocrinology

Diagnosis of diabetes mellitus (WHO criteria)

- Symptoms of hyperglycaemia (eg polyuria, polydipsia, unexplained weigh loss, visual blurring, genital thrush, lethargy) AND raised venous glucos detected once—fasting ≥7mmol/L or random ≥11.1mmol/L OR
- Raised venous glucose on 2 separate occasions—fasting ≥7mmol/L, randor ≥11.1mmol/L or oral glucose tolerance test—2h value ≥11.1mmol/L.

If there is doubt, use the oral glucose tolerance test (OGTT): look for a 2h le >11.1mmol/L. ***How to do a 2h OGTT:***

- Fast overnight. Give 75g of glucose in 300mL water to drink in the morning
- Measure venous plasma glucose before and 2h after the drink.

Hb_{A1c} or capillary glucose levels should not be used to diagnose diabetes. Glycosu detected on urine dipstick can be a normal finding.

Occasionally it may be difficult to differentiate whether a patient has Type 1 o DM. Features that suggest Type 1 DM include weight loss; persiste hyperglycaemia despite diet and medications; presence of autoantibodies: islet c antibodies (ICA) and anti-glutamic acid decarboxylase (GAD) antibodies; ketonu on urine dipstick.

Other causes of diabetes mellitus

- Drug induced: steroids, thiazides.
- Pancreatic: pancreatitis; surgery (where >90% pancreas is removed); traur pancreatic destruction (haemochromatosis, cystic fibrosis); pancreatic canc
- Endocrine: Cushing's disease; acromegaly; phaeochromocytoma; hyperthyroidisr
- Others: acanthosis nigricans; congenital lipodystrophy with insulin recep antibodies; glycogen storage diseases.

ther categories of diabetes mellitus

mpaired glucose tolerance (IGT) Fasting plasma glucose < 7mmol/L and OGTT h glucose ≥ 7.8mmol/L but <11.1 mmol/L.

mpaired fasting glucose (IFG) Fasting plasma glucose ≥ 6.1mmol/L but 7mmol/L. Should have an OGTT to exclude DM.

hese denote different abnormalities of glucose regulation (post-prandial and asting). There may be lower risk of progression to DM in IFG than IGT. Both are nanaged with lifestyle advice (exercise and diet, p79), and regular review. iving those with heart failure and IFG ACE-i drugs can prevent progression to DM 3% *vs* 48% over 3yrs).

estational diabetes (*OHCS* p24) This term includes gestational impaired lucose tolerance (GIGT) and gestational diabetes mellitus (GDM). Use the same iagnostic values as IGT and diabetes above. Glucose tolerance changes during regnancy. At ≥ 6wks post-partum, do a further 75g OGTT whether she still has iabetes or IGT/IFG. Regardless of this result, these women are at ↑risk of later eveloping diabetes, with an approximate 50% lifetime risk.

ype 1 versus Type 2 diabetes mellitus

	Type 1 DM	Type 2 DM
pidemiology	Younger patients	Older patients
enetics	HLA D3 and D4 linked	No HLA association
etiology	Autoimmune β cell destruction	Insulin resistance, β cell dysfunction
resentation	Polydipsia, polyuria, weight loss, ketoacidosis	Often asymptomatic; presents with micro- or macrovascular complications

auses of insulin resistance

- Obesity • Pregnancy • Renal failure • Polycystic ovarian syndrome
- Asians[1] • Acromegaly • Cystic fibrosis • Werner's syndrome (*OHCS* p655)
- TB drugs • Cushing's
- Metabolic syndrome (syndrome X—see p197): central obesity, hyperglycaemia, hypertension, dyslipidaemia (↑triglycerides, ↓HDL cholesterol).

Mechanisms: • Obesity may cause insulin resistance by ↑ rate of release of non-sterified fatty acids causing post-receptor defects in insulin's action • Mutation f genes encoding insulin receptors • Circulating autoantibodies to the xtracellular domain of the insulin receptor. ***℞ for Syndrome X:*** Exercise more; ontrol individual vascular risk factors ie weight↓, statins, antihypertensives, ypoglycaemics (eg glitazones).

[1] Especially Indians (Gujaratis; Punjabis), Sri Lankans, Pakistanis, Bangladeshis. ►Have a lower threshold diagnosing obesity (BMI >23) and for vigorous intervention in this group. *BMJ* 2003 327 1059

Treatment of diabetes mellitus

Enabling patients to manage their own condition, by education and motivati from a multi-disciplinary team of doctors, specialist nurses and dieticia chiropodists, podiatrists, and patient groups is central to successful treatment. T aim is to maintain near normal glucose control while avoiding hypoglycaemia.

Educate and negotiate on: Monitoring capillary glucose measurements ('BM regular exercise, diet: p228—saturated fats↓, sugar↓, starch-carbohydrat moderate protein. Give smoking cessation, foot-care (p196), & pre-concepti advice (*OHCS* p2). Care during pregnancy should be shared with an interest obstetrician (*OHCS* p24). Advise to inform the driving licence authority and not drive if hypoglycaemic (p145). Loss of awareness of hypoglycaemia may lead t loss of driving licence (permanent if HGV license)—see below.

Medication Type 1 DM patients invariably need insulin (see BOX). Type 2 DM patie may be managed initially on diet and exercise alone, but may progress to needi oral hypoglycaemic agents then insulin depending on glycaemic control.

Oral hypoglycaemics Generally, in Type 2 DM patients, start with metformir BMI>25. If BMI<25, use either a sulfonylurea or metformin. If this fails to cont combine metformin + sulfonylurea (some, but not NICE, say a glitazone[1] is mc appropriate as the 2nd add-in drug). Insulin may be needed if this still does r work (p193). ***Biguanides*** eg **metformin:** ↑ insulin sensitivity and maintains weig loss. *SE:* nausea and diarrhoea often transient; *not* hypoglycaemia. Avoid if creatin ≥150µmol/L due to risk of lactic acidosis. *Dose:* 0.5–1g/12h (o.d. MR form may ha fewer SE). Stop if tissue hypoxia (eg MI, sepsis), morning before GA and contr medium containing iodine (restart when renal function is OK). ***Sulfonylure*** ↑insulin secretion. *SE:* hypoglycaemia, weight gain. **Tolbutamide:** Short-acti (hypoglycaemia is rare); 0.5–1.5g/d in 2–3 doses. **Gliclazide:** Medium-acti 40–160mg PO, max 160mg/12h). **Glibenclamide:** Long-acting; 2.5–15mg/24h (rarely used as risk of hypoglycaemia). ***Thiazolidinediones*** ↑ insulin sensitivity. hypoglycaemia, fluid retention (caution in CCF), hepatotoxicity: do LFT every 2 mon for 1yr, stop if ALT up >3-fold. **Rosiglitazone** 4mg (max 8mg)/24h. **Pioglitazo** 15–30mg/24h. Use if metformin + sulfonylurea combination is problematic: glitazone replaces whichever is contraindicated or not tolerated.

Other treatments: Acarbose (***α-glucosidase inhibitor***) decreases breakdown starch to sugar. Use as an add-on drug, eg 50mg chewed at start of each me Start with a once daily dose, max 200mg/8h. SE: wind (often poorly tolerated; le if *slow* dose build-up), abdominal distension/pain, diarrhoea. **Nateglini** (***sulfonylurea receptor binder***): ↑β-cell insulin release. 60mg ½h before fo increased as needed. Alternative: **repaglinide**. They target post-prandial hypergl aemia ($t_{½}$ is short—metformin works mostly on fasting glucose). They may ha a role in those with irregular mealtimes if glycaemic control is poor.

Monitoring glycaemic control: 1 Patients with Type 1 DM (and selected patie with Type 2 DM) should keep a diary of home fingerstick glucose records, enabl detection of patterns of hypo/hyperglycaemia. **2** Glycated haemoglobin (= Hb levels relate to mean glucose level over previous 8 wks (ie RBC half-life). The tar level is <7.5%, or <6.5% if at increased arterial risk, eg previous MI or stroke (N advice). In patients at risk from the effects of hypoglycaemia, eg elderly patie prone to falls, it may be sensible to opt for less tight control. Complicati increase with increasing Hb_{A1c}, therefore advise any improvement is beneficial, e if targets are not reached. *Fructosamine* (glycated plasma protein) levels refl control over 2–3 wks: may be used in pregnancy to assess shorter term cont and in patients with haemoglobinopathies which interfere with Hb_{A1c} te **3** History of hypoglycaemic attacks (and whether symptomatic). Hypoglycae awareness may diminish if control is too tight, or with time in Type 1 DM, due ↓glucagon secretion. It may return if control is loosened ie avoiding hypoglycaem

1 Glitazones *may* preserve β-cells and control glycaemia for longer than sulphonylureas or biguanide

▸▸Ketoacidosis p814; HONK p816

Educating patients to self-adjust their insulin dose in the light of exercise and calorie intake to achieve normoglycaemia is vital for optimal control.

Subcutaneous insulin Strength: 100U/mL. There are many types, falling into 6 groups. Delivery devices used to inject the insulin also vary.

1. Ultra-fast acting, eg Humalog® and Novorapid®; inject at start of meal (or immediately after).
2. Soluble insulin eg Humulin S® or Actrapid: inject 15–30min before meals.
3. Intermediate Humulin I® or Insulatard®.
4. Long-acting ('lente'), eg Ultratard®.
5. Long-acting analogue, eg Lantus/insulin glargine, see below.
6. Pre-mixed insulins, eg with ultra-fast component (eg NovoMix® 30); or with soluble insulin (eg Humulin® M3 or Mixtard® 30).

Insulin glargine is a long-acting recombinant human insulin analogue used once daily at bedtime in type 1 or 2 DM; however, it is not recommended for routine use in type 2 DM (see *BNF*; NICE guidance).[18] Molecular modification has made an insulin that is soluble at acid pH, but precipitates in subcutaneous tissue and is slowly released from a depot. Given once daily, insulin glargine has comparable efficacy to insulin used twice daily. Its rate of hypoglycaemia is less than that of standard insulins, and there is evidence of less nocturnal hypoglycemia. It may be combined with ultra-short acting insulins given at the times of meals. In type 2 DM, if oral agents are failing, it can be used if a twice-daily dosing is problematic (NICE guidance).[19] ***Insulin detemir*** has similar characteristics.

Some commonly used subcutaneous insulin regimens

- Design the insulin regimen to suit your patient's lifestyle (not *vice versa*).
- 'BD regime': Twice daily premixed insulins by pen injector—useful in type 2 DM or type 1 with regular lifestyle.
- 'QDS regime': Before meals ultra-fast or soluble insulin, with bedtime intermediate- or long-acting analogue: useful in type 1 DM for achieving a flexible life-style (eg for adjusting doses with size of meals, or exercise).
- Once daily before bed intermediate- or long-acting insulin—good initial insulin regimen when switching from tablets in type 2 DM.
- Begin with at least a total daily dose of 1 unit of insulin for every unit of body mass index in adults.

Dose adjustment for normal eating (DAFNE): One way to optimize control is to use multi-disciplinary teams to fully engage people in self-management, promoting autonomy and independence. The randomized DAFNE study found that training in flexible, intensive insulin dosing improved glycaemic control as well as well-being/quality of life.[20] It is resource-intensive.

Subcutaneous insulin dosing during intercurrent illnesses (eg influenza)

- Illness often increases insulin requirements despite reduced food intake.
- Maintain calorie intake using milk or soft drinks containing sugar.
- Check blood glucose ≥ 4 times a day. Increase insulin doses if glucose rising. Patients should seek advice from a specialist diabetes nurse or GP if concerned, especially if glucose levels are rising or there is ketonuria.
- Admit if the patient is vomiting, dehydrated, or ketotic (see p576).
- Admit early if a child or pregnant.

Inhaled insulin is being developed: Exubera® is a rapid-acting (before meals) form. It is licensed in Type 2 DM for those poorly controlled on oral drugs, and in adults with Type 1 DM. It has similar efficacy to injected insulin, and improved patient compliance and satisfaction.[21] It is only suitable for non-smokers, and spirometry must be monitored. The inhaler device is bulky and needs careful explanation. Long term safety of inhaled insulin on lung function is unknown.

Helping people with established diabetes

Two prospective studies showed that tight control of hyperglycaemia is key delaying and preventing complications in Type 1 and 2 DM.[22] Diabetes should n be treated in isolation: do a *global* assessment of vascular risk, eg: BP, cholestero obesity and smoking. ►*Focus on education and lifestyle advice.* Promote exercis (to ↑insulin sensitivity), healthy eating and weight reduction—p228; NI comments that drugs such as orlistat have a role here if weight loss of >2.5kg h been achieved by lifestyle advice and BMI >28kg/m². ►*Find out what problems a being experienced* (eg glycaemic control, morale, erectile dysfunction—p214).

Assess vascular risk: ***BP*** (BOX). Target is <140/<80mmHg (or <125/<75 wi renal disease: ↑creatinine, microalbuminuria—see below, or dipstick proteinuria). control is critical for preventing macrovascular disease and mortality.[23] Discu ***smoking*** and offer referral to cessation services. Check ***cholesterol*** (see below

Look for complications • Check injection sites for infection or lipohypertrop (fatty change): advise on rotating sites of injection if present.

- ***Vascular disease*** Commonest cause of death. MI is 3–5 times commoner in D and is more likely to be 'silent' (without classic symptoms). Stroke is ~ twice common. Women are at high risk—DM removes the cardiovascular advanta conferred by the female gender. Address other risk factors—diet, smokir hypertension (p79). Consider statin therapy, eg simvastatin 40mg nocte esp evidence of IHD, peripheral or cerebrovascular disease, or if microalbuminu (indicates ↑vascular risk). Fibrates are useful for ↑triglycerides and ↓HDL (p68 Aspirin 75mg reduces cardiovascular risk and is recommended as statin c therapy (safe to use in diabetic retinopathy).
- ***Nephropathy*** (p301) Microalbuminuria is when urine dipstick is –ve for prot but the urine albumin:creatinine ratio is raised (p306). This reflects early rer disease and is a marker for ↑vascular risk. If microalbuminuria or proteinuria present, inhibiting the renin-angiotensin system, regardless of BP, protec against worsening renal failure. Use ACE-i (p123) or AT-2 blocker (p301).
- ***Diabetic retinopathy*** Blindness is uncommon and *preventable. Arrange annu fundoscopy or retinal photography for all patients.* Refer to an ophthalmologis pre-proliferative changes or if any uncertainty at or near the macula (the or place capable of 6/6 vision). ►Pre-symptomatic screening enables las photocoagulation to be used, aimed to stop production of angiogenic fact from the ischaemic retina. Indications: maculopathy or proliferative retinopat
  Background retinopathy: Microaneurysms (dots), haemorrhages (blots), and ha exudates (lipid deposits). Refer to a specialist if changes are near the macul
  Pre-proliferative retinopathy: Cotton wool spots (infarcts), haemorrhages, venc beading. These are signs of retinal ischaemia. Refer to a specialist.
  Proliferative retinopathy: New vessels form. Needs *urgent* referral.
  Maculopathy: This is often not visible at an early stage. Suspect if visual acuit
  Pathogenesis: Capillary endothelial change → vascular leak → microaneurysms capillary occlusion → local hypoxia + ischaemia → new vessel formation. High reti blood flow caused by hyperglycaemia (& BP↑ & pregnancy) triggers this, caus capillary pericyte damage. Microvascular occlusion causes ***cotton-wool spots blot haemorrhages*** at interfaces with perfused retina). ***New vessels*** form on disc or ischaemic areas, proliferate, bleed, fibrose, and can detach the reti Aspirin[1] (2mg/kg/d) may prevent it: there is no evidence that it ↑ bleeding.
- ***Cataracts:*** May be juvenile 'snowflake' form, or 'senile'—which occur earlie diabetic subjects. Osmotic changes in the lens induced in acute hyperglycae reverse with normoglycaemia (so wait before buying glasses).
- ***Rubeosis iridis:*** New vessels on iris: occurs late and may lead to glaucoma.
- ***Metabolic complications:*** p814. ***Diabetic feet:*** p196. ***Neuropathy:*** p196.

1 As DM has so many vascular events, give a statin (p706) if LDL >3mmol/L **or** BP >140. Even cons a statin *whatever* the pre-treatment cholesterol; discuss with your patient. Lindholm 2003 *Lancet* **361** 20

Starting insulin in those with type 2 DM

This is indicated when control with oral agents is suboptimal (eg HbA_{1c} >7.5–8.0% on maximum oral therapy). Transfer is supervised by a diabetes nurse specialist and dietician. Insulin (p193) may be given initially once or twice a day. Continue metformin to limit weight gain. NICE has commented that long-acting insulin glargine (p193) is not normally needed in this context, unless there is recurrent symptomatic hypoglycaemia or it is necessary to avoid twice daily insulin doses (eg if assistance is needed to inject).

Controlling BP in those with diabetes—3 typical scenarios

1 BP <145/80 and no microalbuminuria and 10yr coronary event risk (CER10, p642) ≤15%, simply check BP every 6 months, or more often.
2 BP ≥ 140/80 and <160/100 and CER10 >15%, but no microalbuminuria, start an antihypertensive (NICE recommends ACE-i, A2A, β-blocker, or a thiazide). Target BP <140/80. For doses and discussion, see p126.
3 BP ≥ 140/80 and microalbuminuria is present: ensure ACE-i or A2A are part of the approach (unless CI, p123). Target BP: <125/75.

• Aspirin prophylaxis (75mg/d PO) is indicated, eg if CER10 >15%.[1]

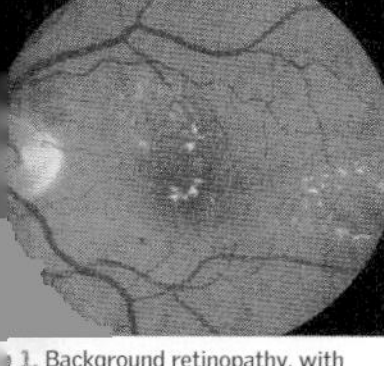

Fig 1. Background retinopathy, with microaneurysms and hard exudates.

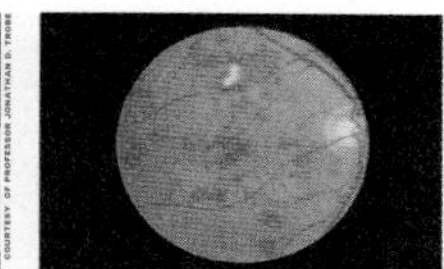

Fig 2. Pre-proliferative retinopathy, with haemorrhages and a cotton-wool spot.

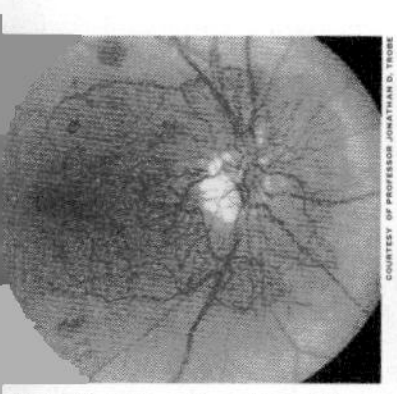

Fig 3. Proliferative retinopathy, with new vessel formation and haemorrhages.

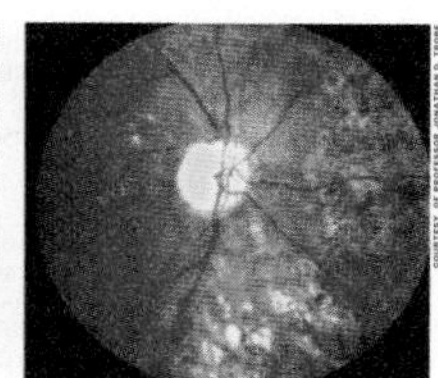

Fig 4. Scars from previous laser photocoagulation.

1 Aspirin is known to ↓ leucocyte adhesion in diabetic retinal capillaries. It ↓expression of integrins on the surface of leucocytes and it ↓nitric oxide synthetase (eNOS) levels and ↓production of the vasoactive cytokine, tumour necrosis factor, known to be raised in diabetic retinopathy. BMJ 2003 **327** 1060.

Diabetic neuropathy and diabetic foot care

►*Amputation is preventable: good care saves legs.* Examine feet regular[ly] Distinguish between ischaemia (critical toes ± absent dorsalis pedis pulses) a[nd] peripheral neuropathy (injury or infection over pressure points, eg the metatars[al] heads). In practice, many have both.

Signs *Neuropathy:* Sensation↓ (especially vibration) in 'stocking' distributio[n;] absent ankle jerks, neuropathic deformity: pes cavus, claw toes, loss of transver[se] arch, rocker-bottom sole. Sensory loss is patchy, so examine all areas using [a] monofilament. *Ischaemia:* If the foot pulses cannot be felt, do Doppler pressu[re] measurements. Any evidence of neuropathy or vascular disease puts the patient [at] high risk of foot ulceration. Educate (daily foot inspection; comfortable shoes— very soft leather, increased depth, cushioning insoles; weight-distributing cradle[s;] no barefoot walking, no corn-plasters). Regular chiropody to remove callus, [as] haemorrhage and tissue necrosis may occur below, leading to ulceration. Tre[at] fungal infections (p428).

Foot ulceration Usually painless, punched-out ulcer in an area of thi[ck] callus ± superadded infection. Can lead to cellulitis, abscess and osteomyelitis.

Assess degree of **1** Neuropathy (clinical). **2** Ischaemia (clinical and Doppler[;] consider angiography). **3** Bony deformity, eg Charcot joint (clinical, x-ray[).] **4** Infection (swabs, blood culture, XR for osteomyelitis, probe ulcer to asse[ss] depth).

Management Regular chiropody to remove callus. Relieve high-pressure areas wi[th] bedrest ± therapeutic shoes (Pressure Relief Walkers® and similar shoes may be [as] good as total contact casts); metatarsal head surgery may be needed. If there [is] cellulitis, admit for IV antibiotics. Common organisms are *staphylococ[ci,] streptococci* and occasionally anaerobes. Start with benzylpenicillin 1.2g/6h IV a[nd] flucloxacillin 1g/6h IV ± metronidazole 500mg/8h IV, refined when microbiolo[gy] results are known. Normoglycaemia improves healing—treat with IV insulin [if] needed. Get surgical help.

Absolute indications for surgery

- Abscess or deep infection
- Severe ischaemia—gangrene/rest pain
- Spreading anaerobic infection
- Suppurative arthritis

The degree of peripheral vascular disease, patient's general health, and patie[nt] request will determine whether local excision and drainage, vascul[ar] reconstruction, and/or amputation (and how much) is appropriate.

Types of neuropathy in diabetes

Sensory neuropathy Symmetric sensory polyneuropathy—distal numbness ('glo[ve] and stocking' distribution), tingling, and pain, often worse at night. *Order of dru[gs] to try:* aspirin/paracetamol → tricyclic (amitriptyline 10–25mg nocte; gradually [to] max 150mg) → gabapentin. *Alternatives:* carbamazepine (p484); lamotrigine; 0.075% capsaicin cream (a counter-irritant). Decompression may help.

Mononeuritis multiplex Especially III & VI cranial nerves. Treatment is difficult. [If] sudden and severe, immunosuppression with corticosteroids, IV immunoglobuli[n] and ciclosporin has been tried.

Amyotrophy Painful wasting of quadriceps and other pelvifemoral muscles. U[se] electrophysiology to show eg lumbosacral radiculopathy, plexopathy, or proxim[al] crural neuropathy. Natural course: variable with gradual but often incomple[te] improvement. IV immunoglobulins have been used.

Autonomic neuropathy (p494) Postural BP drop; ↓cerebrovascular autoregulati[on;] gastroparesis; urine retention; erectile dysfunction (ED); diarrhoea. The latter m[ay] respond to codeine phosphate (the lowest dose to control symptoms, eg 15mg/[8h] PO). Gastroparesis (early satiety, post-prandial bloating, nausea/vomiting) [is] diagnosed by gastric scintigraphy with a ^{99}technetium-labelled meal. It m[ay] respond to anti-emetics, or tetracycline if there is bacterial overgrowth. Postu[ral] hypotension may respond to fludrocortisone 100–300μg/24h PO (SE: oedema, ↑B[P)]

Preventing loss of limbs: primary or secondary prevention?

Traditionally prevention involves foot care advice in diabetic clinics (eg 'don't go bare-foot ...'), and maintaining good glycaemic and BP control.[1] But despite this, the sight of a diabetic patient minus one limb is not rare: whenever we see such patients we should redouble our commitment to primary prevention—ie stopping those at risk from ever getting diabetes. In one randomized prospective study of those with impaired glucose tolerance (IGT) and other risk factors, after 3 yrs, the incidence of diabetes per 100 person-years was 5 in those receiving simple exercise and diet advice, 8 in a group given metformin, and 11 in the placebo group. Advice and metformin decreased incidence of diabetes by 58% (NNT ≈7) and 31% (NNT ≈14), respectively, compared with placebo. One vital group to focus on are those with the metabolic syndrome.[2]

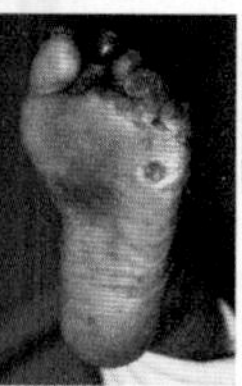

g 1. Diabetic foot: a typical punched-it neuropathic ulcer on the lateral le, with gangrene of toes 2, 4, and 5.

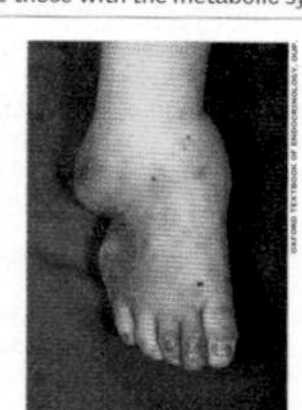

Fig 2. Charcot (neuropathic) joint, caused by loss of pain sensation, leading to ↑mechanical stress (unimpeded by pain) and repeated joint injury. Swelling, instability and, eventually, deformity, may develop, as seen here. ►Early recognition is essential. Treatment: rest (bed rest or non-weight bearing crutches) and immobilisation by a total contact cast until oedema and local warmth reduce and bony repair is complete (~2–3 months). The role of bisphosphonates is under investigation. Charcot joints are also seen in tabes dorsalis, syringomyelia, and leprosy. For an X-ray, see p526.

Hb_{A1c} ≤7.5% & BP ≤145/85 are current UK GP targets (GPs get a substantial quality payment if % have an Hb_{A1c} ≤7.4% and 60% have BP ≤145/85 (≤140/85 if eGFR <50); for non-diabetic pertensives, the target BP is ≤150/90mmHg in 70%. Targets exist for cholesterol, smoking, etc; see *CS* p471 for details of the largest public health results-driven intervention ever.

Metabolic syndrome is central obesity or BMI >30 s any 2 of: • Triglycerides ≥1.7mmol/L • HDL <1.03 P ≥130/85mmHg • Fasting glucose ≥5.6mmol/L or pe 2 DM. There is also insulin resistance, but it is rd to measure, and is not part of the operational finition (nor is a glucose tolerance test essential). e K Alberti 2006 *Diabetic Medicine* 23 469–80

Waist circumference for central obesity	
Europeans	♂ ≥94cm; ♀ ≥80cm
South (S) Asians	♂ ≥90cm; ♀ ≥80cm
Chinese	♂ ≥90cm; ♀ ≥80cm
Japanese	♂ ≥85cm; ♀ ≥90cm
S & Central Americans	use S Asian *pro tem*
Africans + Middle East	use European *pro tem*

Hypoglycaemia

►This is the commonest endocrine emergency—see p816. Prompt diagnosis an treatment is essential—brain damage & death can occur in severe prolonged case

Definition Plasma glucose <3mmol/L. Individual threshold for symptoms varie

Symptoms • ***Autonomic***—Sweating, anxiety, hunger, tremor, palpitations. • ***Neuroglycopenic***—Confusion, drowsiness, seizures, coma. Rarely foc symptoms, eg transient hemiplegia. Mutism, personality change, restlessness an incoherence may lead to misdiagnosis of alcohol intoxication or even psychosis.[36]

Two types:

Fasting hypoglycaemia (requires full investigation if documented).

Causes: By far the commonest cause is insulin or sulfonylurea treatment in known diabetic eg with ↑activity, missed meal, accidental or non-accident overdose. In the *non-diabetic* subject with fasting hypoglycaemia, the followin mnemonic is useful: EXPLAIN

- **E**xogenous drugs, eg *insulin, oral hypoglycaemics* (p192). Does he/she hav access to these (diabetic in the family)? Body-builders may misuse insulin t improve stamina.[37] *Alcohol*, eg alcoholic on binge with no food. Also: *aspiri poisoning; pentamidine; quinine sulfate; aminoglutethamide.*
- **P**ituitary insufficiency.
- **L**iver failure, plus some rare inherited enzyme defects.
- **A**ddison's disease.
- **I**slet cell tumours (insulinoma, see below) and immune hypoglycaemia (eg ant insulin receptor antibodies in Hodgkin's disease).
- **N**on-pancreatic neoplasms (especially retroperitoneal fibrosarcomas an haemangiopericytomas, typically due to IGF-1 secretion).

Diagnosis and investigations

- Document hypoglycaemia by taking finger-prick (on filter-paper at home fo later analysis) during attack and lab glucose if in hospital (monitors are ofte not reliable at low readings). • Take a drug history and exclude liver failure
- Admit for 72h fast. Take blood samples for glucose, insulin, C-peptide an plasma ketones if symptomatic.

Interpreting results

- Hypoglycaemia with high or normal insulin and no elevated ketone *Causes:* Insulinoma, sulfonylureas, insulin administration (no detectable c peptide—only released with endogenous insulin).
- Insulin low or undetectable, no excess ketones. *Causes:* Non-pancreati neoplasm; anti-insulin receptor antibodies.
- Insulin↓, ketones↑. *Causes:* Alcohol, pituitary insufficiency, Addison's diseas

Post-prandial hypoglycaemia May occur after gastric surgery ('dumping', p636 and in type 2 diabetes. ***Investigation:*** Prolonged OGTT (5h, p190).

Treatment ►►See p816. Treat with oral sugar, and a long-acting starch (eg toast If cannot swallow, 25–50ml 50% glucose IV (via large vein with 0.9% saline flus to prevent phlebitis) or glucagon 1mg IM if no IV access (short duration of effect s repeat after 20min and *follow with oral carbohydrate*). If episodes are ofte advise many small high-starch meals. If post-prandial glucose↓, give slow absorbed carbohydrate (high fibre). In diabetics, rationalise insulin therapy (p193

Insulinoma This pancreatic islet cell tumour is associated with MEN-1 (p207), an is usually benign. It presents as fasting hypoglycaemia, with Whipple's triad: **1** Symptoms associated with fasting or exercise **2** Recorded hypoglycaemia wit symptoms **3** Symptoms relieved with glucose. ***Screening test:*** Hypoglycaemia plasma insulin↑ during a long fast. ***Suppressive tests:*** Give IV insulin and measur C-peptide. Normally exogenous insulin suppresses C-peptide production, but th does not occur in insulinoma. ***Imaging:*** CT/MRI ± endoscopic pancreatic US (a fallible, so don't waste too much time before proceeding to intra-operativ visualization[38] ± intra-operative ultrasound).[39] ***Treatment:*** Surgical excision.

Thyroid function tests (TFTs)

Physiology The hypothalamus secretes thyrotrophin releasing hormone (TRH) tripeptide, which stimulates production of thyroid stimulating hormone (TSH) glycoprotein, from the anterior pituitary. TSH ↑production and release of thyroxi (T4) and triiodothyronine (T3) from the thyroid, which exert negative feedback TSH production. The thyroid produces mainly T4, which is 5-fold less active than T 85% of T3 is formed from peripheral conversion of T4. Most T3 and T4 in plasr is protein bound, mainly to thyroxine-binding globulin (TBG). The *unbound* portion the active part. T3 and T4 ↑cell metabolism, via nuclear receptors, and are th vital for growth and mental development. They also ↑catecholamine effects.

Thyroid hormone abnormalities are usually due to problems in the thyroid gla itself, and rarely caused by the hypothalamus or the anterior pituitary.

Basic tests Measurement of free T4 and T3 levels is more useful than total T4 a T3 levels as the latter are affected by TBG. Total T4 and T3 are ↑ when TBG is ↑ a vice versa. Free T3 and T4 levels are unaffected. TBG is ↑ in pregnancy, oestrog therapy (HRT, oral contraceptive pill) and hepatitis. TBG is ↓ in nephrotic syndror and malnutrition (protein loss), drugs (eg androgens, corticosteroids, phenytoi chronic liver disease and acromegaly.

- ***Hyperthyroidism suspected:*** Ask for T3, T4, and TSH. In hyperthyroidism, will have ↓TSH (except for the rare phenomenon of a TSH-secreting pituita adenoma). Most have raised T4, but ~1% have only raised T3.
- ***Hypothyroidism suspected or monitoring replacement treatment:*** Ask f only T4, and TSH. Measuring T3 does not add any extra information.

↑TSH, ↓T4	Hypothyroidism
↑TSH, normal T4	Treated hypothyroidism or subclinical hypothyroidism
↑TSH, ↑T4	TSH secreting tumour or thyroid hormone resistance
↓TSH, ↑T4 or ↑T3	Hyperthyroidism
↓TSH, normal T4 & T3	Subclinical hyperthyroidism
↓TSH, ↓T4 and ↓T3	Sick euthyroidism (below) or pituitary disease
Normal TSH, abnormal T4	Consider changes in thyroid-binding globulin, assay interference, amiodarone or pituitary TSH tumour

Sick euthyroidism In any systemic illness, TFTs may become deranged. The typi pattern is for 'everything to be low'. The test should be repeated after recove ***Assay interference*** is caused by antibodies in the serum, interfering with the te

Other tests

- ***Thyroid autoantibodies:*** Antithyroid peroxidase (TPO) antibodies or antithy globulin antibodies may be increased in autoimmune thyroid disease: Hashimot or Graves' disease. If +ve in Graves', there is an increased risk of developi hypothyroidism at a later stage.
- ***TSH receptor antibody:*** May be ↑ in Graves' disease (useful in pregnancy).
- ***Serum thyroglobulin:*** Useful in monitoring the treatment of carcinoma (p62 and in detection of factitious (self-medicated) hyperthyroidism, where it is lc
- ***Ultrasound:*** This distinguishes cystic (usually, but not always, benign) from sc (possibly malignant) nodules. If there is a solitary large nodule, or domina nodule in a multinodular goitre, a fine needle aspiration should be performed look for thyroid carcinoma. See fig 2, p623.
- ***Isotope scan:*** (^{123}Iodine or ^{99}Technetium pertechnetate). Useful for determini the cause of hyperthyroidism. Also used to detect retrosternal goitre, ecto thyroid tissue or thyroid metastases (using whole body CT scan). If there a suspicious nodules, the main question is: does the area have increased (hc decreased (cold), or the same (neutral) uptake of isotope as the remaini thyroid? 20% of 'cold' nodules are malignant. Few neutral and almost no h nodules are malignant. See also p724.

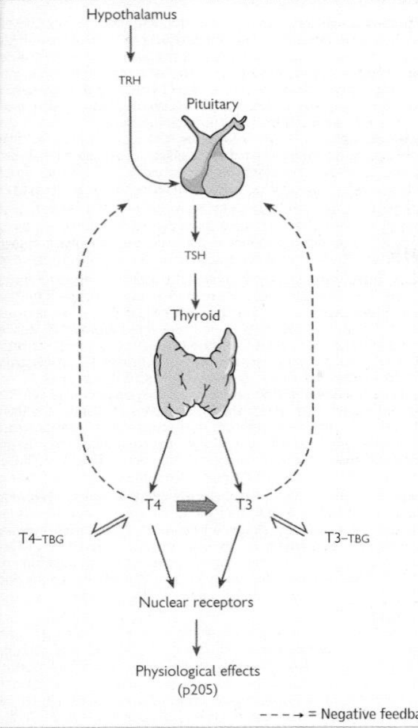

creening thyroid function

ne following should be screened for abnormalities in thyroid function:

- Patients with atrial fibrillation.
- Patients with hyperlipidaemia (4–14% have hypothyroidism).
- Diabetes mellitus—on annual review.
- Women with Type 1 DM during 1st trimester and post delivery (3-fold rise in incidence of postpartum thyroid dysfunction).
- Patients on amiodarone or lithium (6 monthly).
- Patients with Down's or Turner's syndrome, or Addison's disease (yearly).

Thyrotoxicosis

Symptoms Weight loss despite increased appetite (NB: paradoxical weight ga 10–30%), heat intolerance, sweating, diarrhoea, tremor, irritability, frer activity, emotional lability, psychosis, itch, oligomenorrhoea—may cause infert
Signs Pulse↑, AF, warm peripheries, fine tremor, palmar erythema, hair thinnin lag (eyelid lags behind eye's descent as patient watches your finger descend slo lid retraction (exposure of sclera above iris, causing 'stare'). There may be go (fig 2), thyroid nodules or bruit depending on the cause.
Graves' disease only: **1** *Eye disease* (see BOX): exophthalmos, ophthalmopl **2** *Pretibial myxoedema*: oedematous swellings above lateral malleoli: the t *myxoedema* is confusing here **3** *Thyroid acropachy*: extreme manifestation, clubbing, painful finger and toe swelling, and periosteal reaction in limb bone

Tests TSH↓ (suppressed), T4 and T3↑. There may be mild normocytic anaemia, leucopenia, ESR↑, Ca^{2+}↑, LFT↑. ***Also:*** Check thyroid autoantibodies. Isotope sc the cause is unclear, to detect nodular disease or subacute thyroiditi ophthalmopathy, test visual fields, acuity, and eye movements (see BOX).

Causes Thyrotoxicosis is the clinical and biochemical effect of excess thy hormone. This is usually due to hyperthyroidism, hyperfunction of the thyroid it
• ***Graves' disease:*** ♀:♂≈9:1. Common between 30–50 yrs. This is an autoimm disease caused by stimulatory TSH-receptor antibodies (which also react orbital autoantigens.) There is diffuse thyroid enlargement. Patients are o hyperthyroid but may be, or become, hypo- or euthyroid. It is associated with o autoimmune diseases: vitiligo, type 1 DM, Addison's disease, p210.
• ***Toxic multinodular goitre:*** Seen in the elderly and in iodine-deficient are There are nodules that secrete thyroid hormones. **℞:** Control the thyrotoxic first with medication, then follow with radioiodine. Surgery is indicated if there compressive symptoms from the enlarged thyroid (dysphagia or dyspnoea).
• ***Toxic adenoma:*** There is a solitary nodule producing T3 and T4. On isotope s the nodule is 'hot' (p200), and the rest of the gland is suppressed. **℞:** Radioioc

Others (not hyperthyroidism) • ***Subacute (de Quervain's) thyroiditis:*** A s limiting viral infection with painful goitre, fever and ↑ESR. There is low iso uptake on scan. **℞:** NSAIDs. • ***Drugs:*** Amiodarone (p204), lithium (hypothyroidis commoner.) • ***Exogenous:*** Thyroxine intoxication causes ↑T4, ↓T3 and ↓th globulin. Rarely seen with iodine excess eg contrast media, food contaminatic
• ***Ectopic thyroid tissue:*** Metastatic follicular thyroid cancer, choriocarcin or struma ovarii: ovarian teratoma containing thyroid tissue.

Treatment

1 ***Drugs:*** β-blockers (eg propranolol 40mg/6h) for rapid control of symptom ***Anti-thyroid medication:*** 2 strategies: **1** *Titration* eg carbimazole 40mg/24h PO for 4wks, reduce according to TFTs every 1–2 months. **2** *Bl replace:* Give carbimazole and thyroxine simultaneously (less risk of iatrog hypothyroidism). In Graves', maintain on either regime for 12–18 months withdraw. ~50% will relapse, requiring radioiodine or surgery. Carbimazole agranulocytosis (↓↓neutrophils, can lead to life-threatening sepsis; rare (0.C of patients) but serious—warn to stop and get an urgent FBC if signs of infec eg fever, sore throat or mouth ulcers. Alternative: propylthiouracil.
2 ***Radioiodine (^{131}I):*** Most become hypothyroid post-treatment. There is evidence for ↑cancer, birth defects or infertility in women. CI: pregna lactation. Caution in active hyperthyroidism as risk of thyroid storm (p817
3 ***Thyroidectomy:*** Carries a risk of damage to recurrent laryngeal nerve (ho voice) and hypoparathyroidism. Patients may become hypo- or hyperthyro
4 ***In pregnancy and infancy:*** Get expert help. See *OHCS* p25.

Complications Heart failure (thyrotoxic cardiomyopathy, ↑ in elderly), angin (seen in 10–25%: control hyperthyroidism and warfarinize if no contraindicati osteoporosis, ophthalmopathy, gynaecomastia. ››Thyroid storm (p817).

yroid eye disease

yroid eye disease is associated with Graves' disease in 25–50% of people with condition. The main known risk factor is smoking. The eye disease may not relate with thyroid disease and the patient can be euthyroid, hypothyroid, or perthyroid at presentation. Eye disease may be the first presenting sign of aves' disease, and can also be worsened by treatment, typically with lioiodine (usually a transient effect). Retro-orbital inflammation and nphocyte infiltration results in swelling of the orbit.

mptoms Eye discomfort, grittiness, excess tear production, photophobia. plopia, decreased acuity or an afferent pupillary defect (p68) may mean optic rve compression: ►*Seek expert advice immediately as decompression may be eded.* Nerve damage does not necessarily go hand-in-hand with protrusion. deed, if the eye cannot protrude for anatomical reasons, optic nerve npression is more likely—a paradox!

gns Exophthalmos—appearance of protruding eye; proptosis—eyes otrude beyond the orbit (look from above in the same plane as the forehead); njunctival oedema; corneal ulceration; papilloedema; loss of colour vision. Ophth-noplegia (especially of upward gaze) occurs due to muscle swelling and fibrosis.

sts Diagnosis is clinical. CT/MRI of the orbits may reveal enlarged eye muscles.

anagement Eye disease should be managed by a specialist. Treat hyper- or pothyroidism. Advise to stop smoking as this worsens prognosis. Most have ld disease which can be treated symptomatically ie artificial tears, sunglasses, oid dust, elevate bed when sleeping to reduce periorbital oedema. Diplopia ay be managed with a Fresnel prism stuck to one lens of a spectacle, so owing for easy changing as the exophthalmos changes.

minority experience more severe disease with ophthalmoplegia or gross dema, and are treated with steroids, started at high dose (prednisolone mg/day PO), decreased gradually according to symptoms. Surgical decomp-ssion is used for severe sight-threatening disease, or for cosmetic reasons ce the activity of eye disease has reduced. This is usually done by an inferior bital approach, using space in the ethmoidal, sphenoidal, and maxillary sinuses. elid surgery may improve cosmesis and function. Orbital radiotherapy can be ed to treat ophthalmoplegia but has little effect on proptosis.

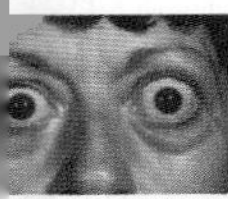

1. Thyroid eye disease: traction causing a ing' appearance.

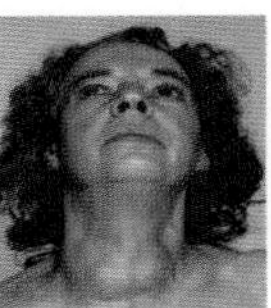

Fig 2. Goitre

Causes of goitre

Diffuse
- Physiological
- Graves' disease
- Hashimoto's thyroiditis
- Subacute (de Quervain's) thyroiditis (painful)

Nodular
- Multinodular goitre
- Adenoma
- Carcinoma

Hypothyroidism (myxoedema)

This is common and easy to treat. ►*As it is insidious, both the patient and doctor may not realize anything is wrong*, so be alert to subtle and non-spe symptoms, particularly in women over 40yrs old.

Symptoms Tiredness, lethargy, depression, dislike of cold, weight gain, cons ation, menorrhagia, hoarse voice, poor cognition/dementia, myalgia.

Signs Bradycardia, dry skin and hair, non-pitting oedema (eyelids, hands, fe cerebellar ataxia, slow relaxing reflexes, peripheral neuropathy, 'toad-like fa There may be goitre depending on the cause, or signs of CCF or pericardial effus

Diagnosis TSH↑, T4↓ (in secondary hypothyroidism: T4↓ and ↓ or normal TSH to lack from the pituitary, p216). Cholesterol and triglyceride may be Occasionally normochromic macrocytic anaemia. See also p200.

Causes of primary hypothyroidism

(1) Autoimmune

- ***Primary atrophic hypothyroidism:*** ♀:♂≈6:1. Common. Diffuse lymphoc infiltration of the thyroid, leading to atrophy, hence no goitre.
- ***Hashimoto's thyroiditis:*** Autoimmune disease as above plus goitre due lymphocytic and plasma cell infiltration. Commoner in older women, aged 70yrs. May be hypothyroid or euthyroid—occasionally initial period hyperthyroidism ('Hashitoxicosis'). Autoantibody titres are very high.

Both are associated with other autoimmune diseases: Type 1 DM, Addison's dise pernicious anaemia (p320).

(2) Acquired

- ***Iodine deficiency:*** Poor intake, commonest cause world-wide.
- ***Post-thyroidectomy or radioiodine treatment.***
- ***Drug-induced:*** Antithyroid drugs, amiodarone, lithium, iodine.
- ***Subacute thyroiditis:*** Temporary hypothyroidism after hyperthyroid phas

Secondary hypothyroidism (from hypopituitarism, p216) is very rare.

Associations with hypothyroidism: Turner's syndrome, Down's syndrome, cy fibrosis, primary biliary cirrhosis, POEMs syndrome (**p**olyneuropathy, **o**rganomeg **e**ndocrinopathy, **m**-protein band from a plasmacytoma + **s**kin pigmentati tethering). ***Genetic***: Dyshormonogenesis: genetic (mostly autosomal recess defect in hormone synthesis. One form is Pendred's syndrome (with deafne there is ↑uptake on isotope scan, which is displaced by potassium perchlorat

Treatment

- ***If healthy and young:*** Levothyroxine (T4), 50–100μg/24h PO; review at 12w Adjust 6 weekly by clinical state and to normalize but not suppress Thyroxine's $t_{½}$ is ~7 days, so any change in dosage will take ~4 weeks to assessed accurately by checking TSH. Once normal, check TSH yea Metabolism of levothyroxine is increased by enzyme-inducers (p681).
- ***If elderly or ischaemic heart disease:*** Start with 25μg/24h; ↑dose by 25 4wks according to TSH (►cautiously, as thyroxine may precipitate angina or
- ***If diagnosis is in question and T4 already given:*** Stop T4; recheck TSH in 6w

The effects of amiodarone on the thyroid are complex: it can cause both hy and hyperthyroidism. Effects are due both to the drug and the iodine contai within it. Hypothyroidism is caused by iodine excess, inhibiting thyroid horm synthesis and release. Thyrotoxicosis is caused either by iodine excess, resultin increased hormone synthesis, or by direct toxic effect causing thyroiditis release of hormones. 2% of patients on amiodarone have clinically detecta thyroid abnormalities. Seek expert help. The $t_{½}$ of amiodarone is long (40–10 so problems persist after withdrawal. If on amiodarone, check TFTs 6 monthl

Thyroid disease in pregnancy and neonates See *OHCS* p25.

hy are symptoms of thyroid disease so many, so various, d so subtle?

most all our cell nuclei have receptors showing a high affinity for T3: at known as TRα-1 is abundant in muscle and fat; TRα-2 is abundant in brain; d TRβ-1 is abundant in brain, liver, and kidney. These receptors, via their luence on various enzymes, affect the following processes:

The metabolism of substrates, vitamins, and minerals.
Modulation of all other hormones and their target-tissue responses.
Stimulation of O_2 consumption and generation of metabolic heat.
Regulation of protein synthesis, and carbohydrate and lipid metabolism.
Stimulation of demand for co-enzymes and related vitamins.

bclinical thyroid disease

bclinical hypothyroidism suspect if TSH↑, with normal T4 and T3, and no vious symptoms. It is common: ~10% of those >55yrs old have a raised TSH. e risk of progression to frank hypothyroidism is ~2%, and increases as TSH↑; k doubles if thyroid autoantibodies are present, and is also increased in men.

nagement:

Confirm that raised TSH is persistent (recheck in 2–4 months).
Recheck the history: if any non-specific features (eg depression), discuss benefits of treating (p204) with the patient: they may simply feel better, without realizing that they were not functioning optimally.
One approach is to treat (with thyroxine) those with a TSH >10, positive thyroid autoantibodies, previously treated Graves' disease, or other organ-specific autoimmunity (Type 1 DM, myasthenia, pernicious anaemia, vitiligo), as these patients are more likely to progress to clinical hypothyroidism. If the patient does not fall into any of these categories, monitor TSH annually.
Risks from well-monitored treatment of subclinical hypothyroidism are small (but there is an ↑risk of atrial fibrillation and osteoporosis if over-treated).

bclinical hyperthyroidism occurs when TSH↓, with normal T4 and T3. Again, ere is no consensus regarding management, with ongoing trials to assess ether treatment prevents subsequent complications of clinical hyper-roidism (especially AF and osteoporosis).

nagement:

Confirm that suppressed TSH is persistent (recheck in 2–4 months).
Check for a non-thyroidal cause: illness, pregnancy, pituitary or hypothalamic nsufficiency (suspect if T4 or T3 are in the lower end of the reference range), use of TSH suppressing medication eg thyroxine, steroids.
If TSH <0.1, treat on an individual basis eg with symptoms of hyperthyroidism, AF, unexplained weight loss, osteoporosis, goitre.
Options are antithyroid medication (carbimazole or propylthiouracil) or radioiodine therapy.
If no symptoms, recheck 6 monthly.

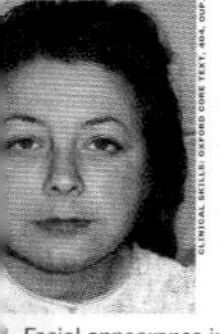

1. Facial appearance in hypothyroidism.

Parathyroid hormone and hyperparathyroidism

Parathyroid hormone (PTH) is normally secreted in response to low ionised levels, by 4 parathyroid glands situated posterior to the thyroid (p670). The gl are controlled by –ve feedback via Ca^{2+} levels. PTH acts by: • ↑ osteoclast act releasing Ca^{2+} & PO_4^{3-} from bones; • ↑Ca^{2+} & ↓PO_4^{3-} reabsorption in the kic • Active 1,25dihydroxy-vitamin D_3 production is ↑. Overall effect is ↑Ca^{2+} & ↓

Primary hyperparathyroidism ***Causes:*** ~80–85% solitary adenoma, ~15– hyperplasia of all glands, <0.5% parathyroid carcinoma.

Presentation: Often asymptomatic, with ↑Ca^{2+} on routine tests. Symptoms re to ↑Ca^{2+} (p672): weakness, tiredness, depression, dehydration, polyuria polydipsia, renal stones, abdominal pain, pancreatitis, ulcers (duodenal: gastric ≈ MEN1 can cause ↑PTH and Zollinger–Ellison syndrome). Bone resorption effec PTH can cause pain, fractures and osteopenia/osteoporosis. Also, there may be and if untreated, long-term ↑cardiovascular risk and ↑mortality.

Associations with multiple endocrine neoplasia (MEN): See BOX.

Tests: Ca^{2+}↑ & PTH↑ (or inappropriately normal). Differentials with these t thiazide diuretics, lithium, familial hypocalciuric hypercalcaemia, ter hyperparathyroidism. Also PO_4^{3-}↓ (unless there is renal failure), alk phos↑ from activity, 24h urinary Ca^{2+}↑. ***DEXA bone scan*** to assess for osteoporosis (p **Osteitis fibrosa cystica** is bone marrow fibrosis and cyst formation, due to se resorption (seen rarely now). *Appearances:* brown tumours, subperiosteal eros of distal phalanges on hand x-ray, pepper-pot skull on skull x-ray.

Treatment: Surgical excision, of the adenoma or of all 4 hyperplastic gl prevents fractures and peptic ulcers. *Indications:* high serum or urinary Ca^{2+}, disease, osteoporosis, renal calculi, ↓renal function, age ≤50y. *Complicat* Hypoparathyroidism, recurrent laryngeal nerve damage (hoarse voice), pos symptomatic Ca^{2+}↓ (hungry bones syndrome; check Ca^{2+} daily ≥14d post-op). op ultrasound & MIBI (methoxyisobutyl isonitrile) isotope scan may localis adenoma; intra-operative PTH sampling is used to confirm removal. *Recurre* ~8% of patients in 10yrs. Mild symptoms may not merit surgery: advise ↑flu take to prevent stones, avoid thiazides or high Ca^{2+} & vit D intake, review 6 mo Cinacalcet is a new drug, which ↑sensitivity of the parathyroid cell to Ca^{2+} (∴ secretion); monitor Ca^{2+} within 1wk of any dose change; SE: myalgia; testoster

Secondary hyperparathyroidism Ca^{2+}↓, PTH↑ (appropriately). *Causes:* A hypocalcaemia (p670), eg low vitamin D intake, chronic renal failure (p294)

Tertiary hyperparathyroidism Ca^{2+}↑, ↑↑PTH (inappropriately). Occurs prolonged secondary hyperparathyroidism, causing glands to act autonomo having undergone hyperplastic or adenomatous change. This causes Ca^{2+}↑ ↑↑secretion of PTH unlimited by feedback control. Seen in chronic renal failure

Malignant hyperparathyroidism Parathyroid-related protein (PTHrP) is prod by some squamous cell lung cancers, breast and renal cell carcinomas. This mi PTH resulting in Ca^{2+}↑ (PTH is ↓, as PTHrP is not detected in the assay).

Hypoparathyroidism

Primary hypoparathyroidism PTH secretion is ↓ due to gland failure. *T* Ca^{2+}↓, PO_4^{3-}↑ or normal, alk phos normal. ***Symptoms:*** As in hypocalcaemia (p ***Causes:*** Autoimmune (associated with other autoimmune disorders—BOX 2), congenital: Di George syndrome (*OHCS* p642). ***R:*** Alfacalcidol.

Secondary hypoparathyroidism Radiation, surgery (thyroidectomy, parathy ectomy), hypomagnesaemia (magnesium is required for PTH secretion).

Pseudohypoparathyroidism Failure of target cell response to PTH. ***Signs:*** S metacarpals (esp 4th and 5th), round face, short stature, mental retardation. *T* Ca^{2+}↓, ↑PTH, alk phos ↔ or ↑. ***Treatment:*** As for 1° hypoparathyroidism.

Pseudopseudohypoparathyroidism The morphological features of pseudoh parathyroidism, but with normal biochemistry. The cause for both is genetic

ıltiple endocrine neoplasia (MEN)

ɜ MEN syndromes are a group of genetic syndromes inherited in an *autosomal minant* manner, where there are functioning hormone-producing tumours in ıltiple organs. They comprise of:
MEN1 & 2 • Neurofibromatosis (p506) • Von Hippel Lindau syndrome (p704).
'eutz–Jeghers' syndrome (p700).
arney complex: This consists of spotty skin pigmentation, schwannomas, xoma of skin, mucosa or heart (especially atrial myxoma), and endocrine nours: eg pituitary adenoma, adrenal hyperplasia, testicular tumour.

N type-1 (=MEN1): Parathyroid hyperplasia/adenoma (~95%; most ↑Ca^{2+}).
Pancreatic endocrine tumours (~70%)—usually gastrinoma (p708) or insulinoma (p198), rarely, somatostatinoma,[1] glucagonomas or VIPoma (p238).
Pituitary adenoma (~50%)—usually prolactinoma or GH secreting tumour (acromegaly: p218).
Also, adrenal and carcinoid tumours are associated.

ɜ MEN1 gene is a tumour suppressor gene. Menin, its protein, alters nscription activation. Many are sporadic, presenting in the 3rd–5th decades.

N2a: Thyroid: Medullary thyroid carcinoma (seen in ~100%, p622)
Adrenal: Phaeochromocytoma (~50%, usually benign and bilateral)
Parathyroid hyperplasia (~80%, but less than 20% have ↑Ca^{2+}).

N2b has similar features to MEN2a plus mucosal neuromas and Marfanoid ɔearance (p698), but no hyperparathyroidism. Mucosal neuromas consist of mps' on: lips, cheeks, tongue, glottis, eyelids, and visible corneal nerves.
The gene involved in MEN2a and b is the *ret* proto-oncogene, a receptor osine kinase. Tests for *ret* mutations are revolutionizing MEN2 treatment by ıbling a prophylactic thyroidectomy to be performed before neoplasia occurs, ıally done before 3 yrs of age. **NB:** *ret* mutations rarely contribute to ɔradic parathyroid tumours.

ıtoimmune polyendocrine syndromes

toimmune disorders cluster into two defined syndromes:
ɔe 1: Autosomal recessive, rare.
use: Mutations of AIRE (Auto ImmuneREgulator) gene on chromosome 21.
ıtures: • Addison's disease • Chronic mucocutaneous candidiasis
ypoparathyroidism.
o associated with primary hypogonadism, pernicious anaemia, autoimmune nary hypothyroidism, chronic active hepatitis, vitiligo, alopecia.

ɔe 2: HLA D3 and D4 linked, common.
use: Polygenic.
ıtures: • Addison's disease • Type 1 diabetes mellitus (in 20%).
ʌutoimmune thyroid disease—hypothyroidism or Graves' disease.
o associated with primary hypogonadism, vitiligo, alopecia, pernicious ıemia, chronic atrophic gastritis, coeliac disease, dermatitis herpetiformis.

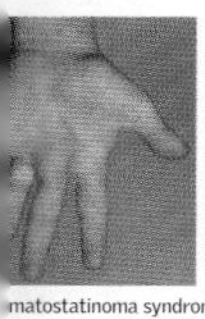

Fig 1. Pseudohypoparathyroidism: short 4th & 5th metacarpals. (Other signs include ectopic calcification, eg in basal ganglia)

[1] matostatinoma syndrome = DM + steatorrhoea + cholelithiasis ± relapsing cholangitis.

Adrenal cortex and Cushing's syndrome

Physiology The adrenal cortex produces steroids: **1** *Glucocorticoids* (eg corti which affect carbohydrate, lipid and protein metabolism, **2** *Mineralocortic* which control sodium and potassium balance (eg aldosterone, p664), **3** *Androgens*, sex hormones which have weak effect until peripheral conversio testosterone and dihydrotestosterone. Corticotrophin-releasing factor (CRF) f the hypothalamus stimulates ACTH secretion from the pituitary, which in stimulates cortisol and androgen production by the adrenal cortex. Cortis excreted as urinary free cortisol and various 17-oxogenic steroids.

Cushing's syndrome This is chronic glucocorticoid excess. The commonest cau steroid treatment. Endogenous causes are much rarer: 85% are due to ↑ACT these a pituitary adenoma (Cushing's disease) is the commonest cause.

1 **ACTH-dependent causes: (↑*ACTH*)**

- ***Cushing's disease*** Bilateral adrenal hyperplasia due to an ACTH secre pituitary adenoma (usually a microadenoma, p218). ♀:♂>1. Peak age: 30–5C
- ***Ectopic ACTH production*** Especially small cell lung cancer and carci tumours, p270. Specific features: pigmentation (due to ↑↑ACTH), hypokala metabolic alkalosis (↑↑cortisol leads to mineralocorticoid activity), weight hyperglycaemia. Classical features of Cushing's are often absent.
- **Rare: *Ectopic CRF production***—reported with medullary thyroid carcinoma prostate carcinoma. ***Iatrogenic*** ACTH administration.

2 **ACTH-independent causes: (↓*ACTH* due to –ve feedback)**

- ***Iatrogenic*** Pharmacological doses of steroids (common).
- ***Adrenal adenoma*** or ***carcinoma*** Carcinoma may be associated with abdor pain and virilization in women (p214).
- ***Adrenal nodular hyperplasia***
- **Rare: *Carney complex*** p207. ***McCune Albright syndrome*** *OHCS* p650.

The patient ***Symptoms:*** Weight↑, mood change (depression, lethargy, irritabi proximal weakness, gonadal dysfunction: ♂: impotence. ♀: irregular mer hirsutism, acne. ***Signs:*** Central obesity, moon face, neck (buffalo hump) supraclavicular fat distribution, thin skin, bruising, purple abdominal st osteoporosis (±fractures), hypertension, impaired glucose tolerance or o diabetes mellitus (30%), predisposition to infection, slow wound healing.

Tests See BOX. *Pitfalls:* (1) Random cortisol measurements are of no value, as le are affected by diurnal variation, stress (including venepuncture), and illness Imaging cannot be relied on alone to localise the cause: Non-functio 'incidentalomas' occur in ~5% on adrenal CT and ~10% on pituitary MRI. Also, detects only ~70% of pituitary tumours causing Cushing's, as they may be too sn

Treatment Depends on the cause. • ***Iatrogenic:*** Stop medications if possibl

- ***Cushing's disease:*** Selective removal of pituitary adenoma via a tr sphenoidal approach. Bilateral adrenalectomy if the source cannot be locate recurrence post-surgery (complications include *Nelson's syndrome*: adrenalectomy development of a locally aggressive pituitary tumour (c cotrophinoma) due to lack of –ve feedback, p700). Pituitary radiothera effective in children, and is used in adults to prevent Nelson's syndrome.
- ***Adrenal adenoma or carcinoma:*** Adrenalectomy: curative for adenoma, ra for carcinoma. Radiotherapy & adrenolytic drugs (mitotane) follow if carcin
- ***Ectopic ACTH:*** Surgery if the tumour can be located and has not spread.
- Medical treatment, eg metyrapone or ketoconazole, are used to reduce cor secretion pre-surgery or while awaiting radiation to become effective.

Prognosis Untreated Cushing's syndrome has an increased mortality rate, du cardiovascular complications. Treated Cushing's syndrome has a good progr usually with resolution of physical features and psychological disorders. Howe osteoporosis, hypertension, obesity, subtle mood changes, glucose intoleranc diabetes mellitus may persist, which require follow up and addressing individu

nvestigation of suspected Cushing's syndrome

'irst, confirm the diagnosis (a raised cortisol), then localize the source on the asis of laboratory testing. Use imaging studies to confirm the likely source.

1) 1st line screening tests

- The ***overnight dexamethasone suppression test*** is a useful outpatient test. Give dexamethasone 1mg PO at midnight; check serum cortisol before, and at 8AM. In normal patients, this high dose of steroid causes –ve feedback, ↓ACTH and ↓cortisol secretion to <50nmol/L. In Cushing's syndrome, there is a failure to suppress cortisol secretion. False –ve rate: <2%; **False +ves**: 2% normal, 13% obese and 23% of hospital inpatients.
- ***24h urinary free cortisol*** (normal: <280nmol/24 h) is an alternative.

NB: False +ves ('Pseudocushing's') are seen in depression, obesity, alcohol excess, nd inducers of liver enzymes which ↑ the rate of dexamethasone metabolism eg phenytoin, phenobarbital, and rifampicin, p681).

2) 2nd line screening tests, if above abnormal:

- The ***48h dexamethasone suppression test:*** Give dexamethasone 0.5mg/6h PO for 2d. Measure cortisol at 0 and 48h (last test at 6h after last dose). Again, in Cushing's syndrome, there is a failure to suppress cortisol secretion.
- ***Midnight cortisol:*** Requires admission. Often inaccurate due to difficulties in measurement. Normal circadian rhythm (cortisol *lowest* at midnight, *highest* early in the morning) is lost in Cushing's syndrome. Cortisol level is taken at midnight, via a cannula whilst the patient is asleep, and is ↑ in Cushing's.

3) Localization tests (where is the lesion?)—If the above are positive.

- ***Plasma ACTH:*** If ACTH is undetectable, an adrenal tumour is likely → CT adrenal glands. If no mass is seen, proceed to adrenal vein sampling or adrenal scintigraphy (radiolabelled cholesterol derivative). If ACTH is detectable, distinguish a pituitary cause from ectopic ACTH production by the following:
  - ***High-dose dexamethasone suppression test:*** Give dexamethasone 2mg/6h PO for 2d. Measure plasma and urinary cortisol at 0 and 48h. Complete or partial suppression indicates Cushing's disease as the pituitary retains some feedback control. An ectopic source is not under feedback control.
  - Or ***corticotrophin releasing hormone test:*** 100μg ovine or human CRH IV. Measure cortisol at 120min. Cortisol rises with pituitary disease but not with ectopic ACTH production. CRH is corticotrophin-releasing hormone.

f tests indicate that cortisol responds to manipulation, Cushing's disease is ikely. Image the pituitary (MRI). If no mass is seen, ***bilateral inferior petrosal sinus sampling*** may help in confirming a pituitary adenoma, where the sinuses re sampled for ACTH release from the pituitary.

f tests indicate that cortisol does not respond to manipulation, hunt for the ource of ectopic ACTH production. CT ± MRI of neck, thorax and abdomen should e performed to detect small ACTH secreting carcinoid tumours.

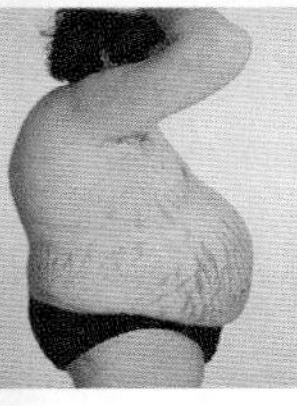

Fig 1. Signs of Cushing's include central obesity and purple abdominal striae.

Addison's disease (adrenal insufficiency)

»Anyone on prednisolone for long enough to suppress the pituitary–adrenal axis c has overwhelming sepsis, or has metastatic cancer may suddenly develop adrena insufficiency with deadly hypovolaemic shock. »See p818.

Primary adrenocortical insufficiency (Addison's disease) is rare (~0.8 /100,000 but can be fatal. Destruction of the adrenal cortex leads to glucocorticoid (cortiso and mineralocorticoid (aldosterone) deficiency. Signs are capricious: it is *'th unforgiving master of non-specificity and disguise'.* You may diagnose a vira infection or anorexia nervosa in error (K^+ is ↓ in the latter but ↑ in Addison's).

Cause 80% are due to an autoimmune cause in the UK. *Other causes:* T (commonest cause worldwide), adrenal metastases (eg from lung, breast, renal Ca lymphoma, opportunistic infections in HIV (eg CMV, *Mycobacterium avium*, p399 adrenal haemorrhage (»Waterhouse–Friederichsen syndrome p706; antiphospho lipid syndrome; SLE), congenital (late-onset congenital adrenal hyperplasia).

Symptoms Often diagnosed late: Fatigue, weakness, anorexia, weight loss dizziness, fainting, myalgia, arthralgia. *Mood:* depression, psychosis, low self esteem.[1] *GI:* nausea or vomiting, abdominal pain, diarrhoea or constipation. *Think c Addison's in all those with unexplained abdominal symptoms.* **Signs** Hyper pigmentation due to ↑ACTH (cross-reacts with melanin receptors): palmar creases buccal mucosa. Postural hypotension. Vitiligo may be associated.
»*Signs of critical deterioration* (p818): Shock (↓BP, tachycardia), fever, coma.

Tests Na^+↓ & K^+↑ (due to ↓mineralocorticoid), glucose ↓ (due to ↓cortisol). Also uraemia, Ca^{2+}↑, eosinophilia, anaemia. ***Diagnosis*** *Short ACTH stimulation tes (Synacthen® test):* Do plasma cortisol before and 30 minutes after tetracosactid (=Synacthen®) 250μg IM. Addison's is excluded if 2nd cortisol >550nmol/L. Steroi drugs may interfere with this assay—check with lab. NB: in pregnancy or the ora contraceptive pill, cortisol levels may be reassuring but falsely↑, due to ↑cortisol binding globulin. ***Also*** • *ACTH:* In Addison's disease, 9 a.m. ACTH is raised (>300ng/ inappropriately high). It is low in secondary causes (see below). • *21-Hydroxylas adrenal autoantibodies:* +ve in autoimmune disease in >80%. • *Plasma renin an aldosterone:* To assess mineralocortocoid status. ***AXR/CXR:*** Any signs of past T eg upper zone fibrosis or calcification of adrenals? If autoantibodies are negative consider further tests (eg adrenal CT) to look for TB or metastatic disease.

Treatment Replace steroids: ~15–25mg *hydrocortisone* daily, in 2–3 divided dose eg 10mg on waking, 5mg lunchtime. Avoid giving late in the day, as it can caus insomnia. Mineralocorticoid replacement may be needed eg if postural hypotension Na^+↓, K^+↑ or plasma renin↑: *fludrocortisone* PO from 50–200μg daily. Adjust bot on clinical grounds. If there is a poor response to treatment, suspect an associate autoimmune disease (check thyroid, do coeliac serology: p272).

Steroids Warn against abruptly stopping steroids. Emphasize that prescribin doctors/dentists/surgeons *must* know of steroid use: give *steroid card,* advis wearing a bracelet declaring steroid use. Add 5–10mg hydrocortisone to dai intake before strenuous activity/exercise. Double steroids in febrile illness, injury c stress. Patients should be given syringes and in-date IM hydrocortisone, and show how to inject themselves in case vomiting prevents oral intake. If vomiting, tak hydrocortisone 100mg IM, and seek medical help; admit for IV fluids if dehydratec

Follow-up Yearly (BP, U&E). Prognosis is good: watch for autoimmune diseases.

Secondary adrenal insufficiency The commonest cause is iatrogenic, due to lon term steroid therapy leading to suppression of the pituitary-adrenal axis. This onl becomes apparent on withdrawal of the steroids. Other causes are rare and includ hypothalamic-pituitary disease leading to ↓ACTH production. Mineralocorticoi production remains intact, and there is no hyperpigmentation as ↓ACTH.

1 Adrenal destruction also causes depletion of adrenal androgens. These may have an effect o quality of life. However, studies on replacement of dehydroepiandosterone (DHEA), a precursor of se hormone synthesis, in adrenal failure have been inconclusive. Løvas K. Lancet 2005; **365**: 2058-61.

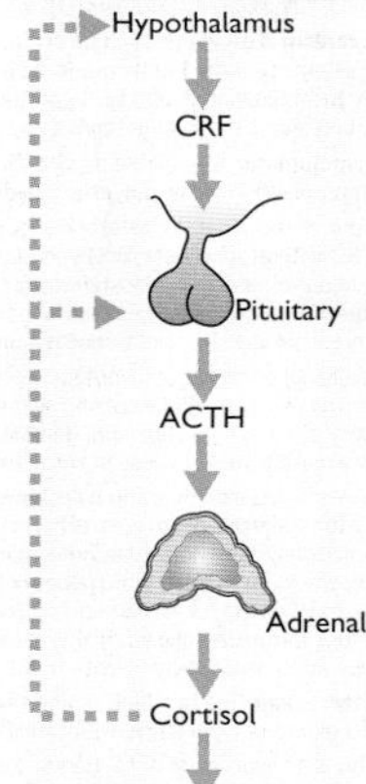
Hypothalamus
CRF
Pituitary
ACTH
Adrenal
Cortisol
Physiological effects
= Negative feedback
CRF = Corticotrophin-releasing factor
ACTH= Adrenocorticotrophic hormone

Hyperaldosteronism

Primary hyperaldosteronism is excess production of aldosterone, independent of the renin-angiotensin system, causing ↑sodium and water retention, and ↓renin release. Consider with the following features: hypertension, hypokalaemia or alkalosis in someone not on diuretics. Sodium tends to be mildly raised or normal.

Symptoms Usually asymptomatic. May present with features of hypokalaemia (p668): weakness, cramps, paraesthesiae, polyuria, polydipsia.

Causes Around ⅔ are due to a solitary aldosterone-producing adenoma (***Conn's syndrome***). ~⅓ are due to bilateral adrenocortical hyperplasia. Rare causes: adrenal carcinoma or glucocorticoid-remediable aldosteronism (GRA). In GRA, the ACTH regulatory element of the 11β-hydroxylase gene fuses to the aldosterone synthase gene, increasing aldosterone production, and bringing it under the control of ACTH.

Tests (see BOX) U&E (ideally not on diuretics, hypotensives, steroids, K^+, or laxatives for 4 wks). Do not rely on a low K^+, as >20% are normokalaemic. For GRA (suspect if there is a family history of early hypertension), genetic testing is available. NB: Renal artery stenosis is a more common cause of refractory ↑BP and ↓K^+ (p30...

Treatment • *Conn's:* Surgery—laparoscopic adrenalectomy. Spironolactone is used up to 300mg per 24h PO for 4wks pre-op, to control hypertension and to treat ↓K. • *Hyperplasia:* Treated medically: spironolactone, amiloride, or eplerenone: a new selective aldosterone receptor antagonist, which does not cause gynaecomastia. • *GRA:* dexamethasone 1mg/24h PO for 4wks, normalizes biochemistry but not always BP. If BP is still ↑, use spironolactone as an alternative. • *Adrenal carcinoma:* Surgery ± post-operative adrenolytic therapy with mitotane—prognosis is poor.

Secondary hyperaldosteronism Due to a high renin from ↓renal perfusion eg renal artery stenosis, accelerated hypertension, diuretics, CCF or hepatic failure.

Bartter's syndrome This is a major cause of congenital (autosomal recessive) salt wasting—via a sodium and chloride leak in the loop of Henle via a defective channel. Presents in childhood with failure to thrive, polyuria and polydipsia. BP *normal.* Sodium loss leads to volume depletion, causing ↑renin and aldosterone production, leading to hypokalaemia and metabolic alkalosis, ↑urinary K^+ and C... ***Treatment:*** K^+ replacement, NSAIDs (to inhibit prostaglandins), and ACE-inhibitors.

Phaeochromocytoma

These are rare catecholamine-producing tumours. They arise from sympathetic paraganglia cells (=phaeochrome bodies), which are collections of adrenalin-secreting chromaffin cells. They are usually found within the adrenal medulla. Extra-adrenal tumours (paragangliomas) are rarer, often found by the aortic bifurcation (the organs of Zuckerkandl). Phaeochromocytomas *roughly* follow the 10% rule: 10% are malignant, 10% are extra-adrenal, 10% are bilateral, and 10% are familial. They are a dangerous but treatable cause of hypertension (in <0.1%...

Associations ~90% are sporadic. 10% are part of a hereditary cancer syndrome (p207) eg MEN2a and 2b, neurofibromatosis, von Hippel–Lindau syndrome.[84]

The patient Episodic hypertension, anxiety, chest tightness, etc.—see BOX.

Tests • *Screening:* 3 x 24h urinary collections for free catecholamines. A clonidine suppression test is done in some centres for borderline cases. • *Localisation:* Abdominal CT/MRI, or meta-iodobenzylguanidine (MIBG—chromaffin-seeking isotope) scan: useful for detection of extra-adrenal tumours, see p725.

Treatment Surgery, α- & β-blockade pre-op: phenoxybenzamine (α-blocker) is used *before* β-blocker to avoid crisis from unopposed α-adrenergic stimulation. ►Consult the anaesthetist. *Post-op:* Do 24h urine catecholamines 2wks post-op, monitor BP (risk of BP↓↓). ►►Emergency ℞: p818. In malignant disease, chemotherapy may be used.[85] **Follow-up** Lifelong: malignant recurrence may present late.[86]

Endocrinology

ypertension: a common context for hyperaldosteronism tests

hink of Conn's in these contexts: • Hypertension associated with hypokalaemia
Refractory hypertension eg despite three antihypertensive drugs
Hypertension occurring before 40yrs of age (especially in women).

he approach to investigation remains controversial. The **aldosterone/renin atio** (ARR) is a good initial screening test. It is ideally measured when the atient has been upright or sitting for 2h, as posture affects results. Anti-ypertensives should be withheld for 2 weeks (spironolactone for 6 weeks) if ossible. α-blockers can be used to control hypertension, as they do not affect ne test. A raised ratio ie ↑aldosterone and ↓renin, indicates hyperaldosteronism. dditional **suppression tests** are done in some centres with fludrocortisone or aline, to test their ability to suppress aldosterone production.

urther investigation is needed to differentiate the cause of hyperaldosteronism. ne method is to assess the effect of posture. Renin, aldosterone and cortisol e measured after the patient has been lying overnight, then repeated after eing upright for 4 hours. Renin production increases on standing, causing aldosterone production. This is exaggerated in bilateral hyperplasia, but there is o effect in Conn's, as aldosterone production is autonomous.

T or MRI of the adrenals is done to localise the cause. This should be done after yperaldosteronism is proven, due to the high number of adrenal incidentalomas. imaging shows a unilateral adenoma, surgical excision is indicated. If no odules or bilateral nodules are seen, a **trial of glucocorticoids** (eg examethasone) may be used to test for GRA. In GRA, dexamethasone causes ACTH production by negative feedback, and therefore ↓aldosterone production.

the above are inconclusive, **adrenal vein sampling** may then be performed, here venous blood is sampled from both adrenals. If one side demonstrates creased aldosterone production compared to the other, an adenoma is likely. **drenal scintigraphy** is an alternative, where increased unilateral uptake of the otope indicates adenoma.

he clinical features of phaeochromocytoma

haeochromocytomas present with sustained or episodic hypertension, not ontrolled by treatment, or vague *episodic* features eg:

General features, such as sweating, heat intolerance, pallor, flushing, a feeling of apprehension, or pyrexia.
Neurological: Headaches, visual disturbances, seizures
Cardiovascular: Palpitations, chest tightness, dyspnoea, faints (postural BP drop), pulmonary oedema.
Gastrointestinal: Abdominal pain, nausea, constipation.

ymptoms may be precipitated by straining, exercise, stress, pressure on the odomen, surgery, or parturition—or by agents such as β-blockers, IV contrast gents, or the tricyclic you so kindly prescribed, thinking that the patient's zarre symptoms were only explicable by psychopathology, such as depression. ne site of the phaeochromocytoma may determine precipitants, eg if pelvic, recipitants include sexual intercouse, parturition, and micturition. These crises ay last minutes to days. Suddenly patients feel 'as if about to die'—and then et better, or go on to develop a stroke or cardiovascular collapse. On xamination, there may be no signs, or hypertension (± signs of cardiomyopathy heart failure), thyroid swelling (episodic), glycosuria during attacks, or rminal haematuria from a bladder phaeochromocytoma.

omplications: Heart failure, dilated cardiomyopathy, arrhythmias, stroke and eath due to hypertensive crisis.

Hirsutism is common (10% of women) and usually benign. It implies hair grc in women, in the male pattern. Causes are familial, idiopathic or are due androgen secretion by the *ovary* (eg polycystic ovarian syndrome, ovarian car OHCS p252), the *adrenal gland* (eg late-onset congenital adrenal hyperpla OHCS p134, Cushing's syndrome, adrenal cancer), or *drugs* (eg steroids).

Polycystic ovarian syndrome (PCOS) causes secondary oligo- or amenorrh infertility, obesity, acne and hirsutism (OHCS p252). ***Tests:*** Ultrasound sh bilateral polycystic ovaries. Blood tests: ↑testosterone, ↓sex-hormone bin globulin, ↑LH:FSH ratio (not consistent). ℞: Metformin may restore regular cy and fertility in some, as it counteracts insulin resistance found in this conditi

Management: ►Be supportive.

- Local measures: Shaving; depilation: wax, creams (eg eflornithine), or electro (expensive and time-consuming, but *effective*); bleach (1:10 hydrogen peroxi
- Oestrogens help by ↑serum sex hormone-binding globulin and therefore ↓ androgens; but always combine with a progesterone (eg as in contraceptive to prevent an excess risk of uterine neoplasia. An alternative is cyprote acetate, an anti-androgen and progestogen, eg up to 100mg on days 1–11, v oestrogen on days 1–21. It is teratogenic so advise contraception. Cyprotero also present in Dianette® (but this is now not licensed as a contraceptive p
- Clomifene is used for infertility (a fertility expert should prescribe).

Virilism is rare but is associated with androgen-secreting adrenal and ova tumours and therefore needs investigation. It is the development of r secondary sexual characteristics in the female, characterized by a rapid onse amenorrhoea, clitoromegaly, deep voice, temporal hair recession, and hirsuti

Gynaecomastia implies an abnormal amount of breast tissue in males, but occur in normal puberty. It is unrelated to galactorrhoea (which is due ↑prolactin). There is an increase in the oestrogen/androgen ratio. ***Cau*** Hypogonadism (see BOX), liver cirrhosis (oestrogens↑), hyperthyroidism, dr oestrogens, spironolactone, digoxin, cimetidine, testosterone, marijuana; tumc *oestrogen-producing* eg testicular, adrenal; *hCG-producing* eg testicular, bronc

Erectile dysfunction (ED = impotence—the inability of an adult male to sustai adequate erection for penetration.) It is common in old age, and is often m factorial. A psychological element is common and is more likely if ED occurs on some situations, if there is a clear stress to account for its onset, and if e morning 'incidental' erections still occur (these also persist at the onset of org disease). Psychological causes may exacerbate organic causes.

- ***Organic causes:*** The major causes are smoking, alcohol, and diabetes. A *Endocrine*: hypogonadism, hyperthyroidism, ↑prolactin; *Neurological*: spinal lesions, MS, autonomic neuropathy (eg in DM); *Pelvic surgery* eg bladder-n prostate surgery; *radiotherapy*; *peripheral vascular disease*; *renal* or *hep failure*; *prostatic hypertrophy*; *penile abnormalities* eg post-priapism, Peyror
- ***Drug causes:*** Antihypertensives (especially β-blockers and diuretics), digo major tranquillizers, alcohol, oestrogens, antidepressants, cimetidine, sterc

Tests: U&E, LFT, glucose, TFT, LH, FSH, cholesterol, testosterone, prolactin. Noctu tumescence studies are not usually needed. Doppler may show ↓blood flow, b rarely needed as vascular reconstruction is difficult.

Treatment: • Treat causes • Counselling • Oral phosphodiesterase (PDE5) inhibi act by ↑ cyclic guanosine monophosphate (GMP). Erection isn't automatic (depe on stimuli). **Sildenafil** (Viagra®) 25–100mg ½–1h pre-sex (food & alcohol upset orption). 88 89 ***SE:*** headache (16%); flushing (10%); dyspepsia (7%); nasal conges (4%); transient blue-green tingeing of vision (inhibition of retinal PDE6). 90 ***CI:*** See **Tadalafil** (Cialis®; long $t_{½}$) 10–20mg ½–36h pre-sex. Don't use >once daily. SE: he ache, dyspepsia, myalgia; ?no visual SEs. **Vardenafil** (Levitra® 5–20mg). 91 Vac aids, intracavernosal injections, transurethral pellets, and implants are used

ɔntraindications[ci]/cautions to Viagra® and other oral ED agents

- Concurrent use of nitrates[ci]
- BP↑↑ or ≤90/50mmHg;[ci] arrhythmias
- Myocardial infarction <90d ago[ci]
- Degenerative retinal disorders,[ci] eg retinitis pigmentosa (for sildenafil)
- Unstable angina[ci]
- Stroke in last 6 months[ci]
- Bleeding disorders (sildenafil)
- Active peptic ulceration (sildenafil)
- Marked renal or hepatic impairment

:her cautions

- Angina (especially if during intercourse).
- Peyronie's disease or cavernosal fibrosis.
- Risk of priapism (sickle-cell anaemia, myeloma, leukaemia).
- Concurrent complex antihypertensive regimens.
- Dyspnoea on minimal effort (sexual activity may be unsupportable).

;e in coronary disease has been a question, but in one good study, no adverse rdiovascular effects were detected even in severe coronary artery disease.[92]

teractions: Processed by the cytochrome p450 system: Macrolides, anti-HIV ɹgs, theophylline, ketoconazole, rifampicin, phenytoin, carbamazepine, phenorbital, grapefruit juice (↑bioavailability).

hen does a lifestyle malcontent become a disease?

'hen should health providers pay for erectile treatment?' In the UK, the NHS ll pay (write 'SLS'/selected list substances on the prescription) if ED is causing *vere* distress,[1] or there has been:

- Prostatectomy
- Prostate cancer
- Dialysis or a renal transplant
- Spinal cord or pelvic injury
- Radical pelvic surgery[2]
- Diabetes mellitus
- Multiple sclerosis
- Parkinson's disease
- Spina bifida
- Single gene neurological disease
- Poliomyelitis and its after-effects

is easy to criticise politicians who produce these rather arbitrary-looking iteria by recourse to clever counter-examples, but they really need our ɒpport because they are making rationing (which is an inescapable fact of nical life) *overt, open, available to scrutiny*, and *rational modification*. All too :en rationing is covert, and no source takes responsibility for it.

uses of hypogonadism

pogonadism is the failure of testes to produce testosterone, spermatozoa or th. The testes are small, with symptoms of reduced libido, impotence and loss secondary sexual hair. There are many causes which are divided into:

imary hypogonadism: Due to testicular failure. *Causes*: • Local trauma, 'sion, chemotherapy or irradiation • Post-orchitis eg mumps, HIV, brucellosis, ɹrosy • Renal failure, liver cirrhosis or alcohol excess (toxic to Leydig cells). :hromosomal abnormalities eg Klinefelter's syndrome (47XXY)—delayed sexual velopment, small testes and gynaecomastia.

condary hypogonadism: Due to ↓gonadotrophins (LH and FSH). *Causes*: Hypopituitarism • Kallman's syndrome—isolated gonadotrophin releasing ɾmone deficiency, often with anosmia and colour blindness • Systemic illness Also: Laurence–Moon–Biedl syndrome, Prader–Willi syndrome.

'iteria include marked disruption to relationships or mood, as judged by any prescriber with ɪaser-certified special skill in this area, usually a GP specialist or staff at clinics for ED.
ɹccess for reversing ED post-op is only 43% *vs* 85% in those with neurological conditions.

Hypopituitarism

Hypopituitarism is the diminished secretion of the anterior pituitary hormon[es]. They are affected in the following order: growth hormone (GH), gonadotrophi[ns:] follicle-stimulating hormone (FSH) and luteinizing hormone (LH), prolactin (PR[L],) thyroid-stimulating hormone (TSH), and adrenocorticotrophic hormone (ACT[H]). Panhypopituitarism is deficiency of all anterior hormones, usually caused [by] irradiation, surgery or pituitary tumour.

Causes are from 3 levels **1** *Hypothalamus:* Kallman's syndrome (p215), tumo[ur,] inflammation, infection (eg meningitis, TB), ischaemia. **2** *Pituitary stalk:* Traum[a,] surgery, mass lesion (eg craniopharyngioma—p218), meningioma, carotid arte[ry] aneurysm. **3** *Pituitary:* Tumour, irradiation, inflammation, infiltration (haem[o]chromatosis, amyloidosis, metastatic ca), ischaemia (pituitary apoplexy: p2[..]; Sheehan's syndrome[1]).

Features are due to **1↓ Hormone:** • ***GH lack:*** Central obesity, atherosclerosis, [dry] wrinkly skin, strength↓, balance↓, well-being↓, exercise ability↓, cardiac outpu[t↓,] osteoporosis, glucose↓. • ***Gonadotrophin (FSH; LH) lack:*** ♀: Few, scant, or [no] menses (oligomenorrhoea or amenorrhoea), fertility↓, libido↓, osteoporosis, bre[ast] atrophy, dyspareunia. ♂: Erectile dysfunction, libido↓, muscle bulk↓, hypogonadi[sm] (↓hair, all over; small testes; ejaculate volume↓; spermatogenesis↓). • ***Thyr[oid] lack:*** As for hypothyroidism (p204). • ***Corticotrophin lack:*** As for adre[nal] insufficiency (p210). NB: no ↑skin pigmentation as ↓ACTH. • ***Prolactin lack:*** Rar[e;] failure of lactation.

2 Cause: eg pituitary tumour (p218), causing mass effect, or hormone secret[ion] with ↓secretion of other hormones—eg prolactinoma, acromegaly, rarely Cushin[g's].

Tests (The triple stimulation test is now rarely done.)

- ***Basal:*** LH & FSH (↓ or ↔), **testosterone** or **oestradiol** (↓); TSH (↓ or ↔), **T4** [↓,] **prolactin** (may be ↑, due to loss of dopamine from the hypothalamus wh[ich] normally inhibits its release), **insulin-like growth factor-1** (IGF-1; ↓—used [as] measure of GH axis, see p222), **cortisol** (↓). Thyroid, gonadotrophin and prolac[tin] hormone secretion are adequately assessed on basal tests. Also U&E (Na⁺↓ [...] dilution), Hb↓ (normochromic, normocytic).
- ***Dynamic tests:*** **1 Short Synacthen® test:** (p210) to assess the adrenal axi[s.] **2 Insulin tolerance test (ITT):** Done in specialist centres to assess the adre[nal] and GH axes. *CI:* epilepsy, heart disease, adrenal failure. Consult lab first. [It] involves IV insulin to induce hypoglycaemia, causing stress to ↑cortisol and [GH] secretion. It is done in the morning (water only taken from 22:00h the ni[ght] before). Have 50% glucose & hydrocortisone to hand and IV access. Gluc[ose] must fall below 2.2mmol/L and the patient should become symptomatic wh[en] cortisol and GH are taken. Normal: GH >20mu/L, and peak cortisol >550mmol[/L.] **3 Arginine + growth hormone releasing hormone test** and **4 Glucag[on] stimulation test** are alternatives when ITT is contraindicated.
- ***Investigate cause:*** MRI scan to look for a hypothalamic or pituitary lesion.

Treatment involves hormone replacement and treatment of underlying cause.

- *Hydrocortisone* for secondary adrenal failure (p210).
- *Thyroxine* if hypothyroid (p204, but TSH is useless for monitoring).
- Hypogonadism (for symptoms and to prevent osteoporosis). ♂: Options incl[ude] testosterone enanthate 250mg IM every 3 weeks, daily topical gels or buc[cal] mucoadhesive tablets. Patches or tablets are used less often. ♀: (*premenopaus[al]*) *Oestrogen:* Transdermal oestradiol patches, oestradiol implants or oral thera[py.] The oral contraceptive pill exceeds replacement requirement. Gonadotrop[hin] therapy is needed to induce fertility in both men and women.
- The importance of GH deficiency in adults has been increasingly recognised, w[ith] effects on protein and fat metabolism. GH deficiency impairs physical fitn[ess,] quality of life, promotes insulin resistance and dyslipidaemia. If GH deficienc[y is] suspected, refer to an endocrinologist for insulin tolerance testing. See BOX[.]

1 Sheehan's syndrome is pituitary necrosis after post-partum haemorrhage.

Endocrinology

NICE guidelines on giving somatropin (GH) in those >25yrs old

Somatropin is produced by DNA technology; it has the same sequence as human GH. It should only be used if all the following criteria are fulfilled:

1 There is severe GH deficiency, defined by peak GH response of <9mU/L (3ng/mL) during an ITT (or equivalent).
2 There is impaired quality of life (QOL), as measured by QOL-AGHDA questionnaires (assessment of hormone deficiency in adults score ≥ 11 points).[1]
3 The person is already receiving treatment for other pituitary hormone deficiencies, as required.

Achieving adult bone mass is a valid indication for somatropin in adults <25yrs old who fulfil criteria 1 but not 2. (Maximum GH secretion is during adolescence; then secretion normally falls by ~14% per decade.)

Self-injection 0.15–0.3mg/d; needs decrease with age. Dose titration (1st 3 months of therapy) is done by an endocrinologist. *SE:* dose related fluid retention may cause oedema, carpal tunnel syndrome, myalgia, congestive heart failure, BP↑, ICP↑ (rare). IGF-1 levels increase with GH replacement. High IGF-1 levels have been linked with an increased risk of colon, breast and prostate cancer, but an increase in rates of cancer in adults on GH replacement has not been proven—long term data is lacking. *CI:* malignancy, pregnancy, renal transplant, closed epiphyses.

Somatropin should be stopped after 9 months if QoL-AGHDA does not improve by 7 points or more.[1] ***Using GH in children:*** See *OHCS* p180.

1 Relying on improvement in QoL scores during GH replacement has to be viewed with scepticism. This can be dispelled only by randomized trials. Barkan A 2003 *J Clin Endocrinol* **86** 1905.

Pituitary tumours

Pituitary tumours (almost always benign adenomas) account for 10% o[f] intracranial tumours. They may be divided by size: a microadenoma is a tumou[r] <1cm, and a macroadenoma is >1cm. There are 3 histological types.

1 ***Chromophobe***—70%. Some are non-secretory, but cause hypopituitarism. Hal[f] produce prolactin (PRL); a few produce ACTH or GH. Local pressure effect in 30%
2 ***Acidophil***—15%. Secrete GH or PRL. Local pressure effect in 10%.
3 ***Basophil***—15%. Secrete ACTH. Local pressure effect rare.

Classification by hormone secreted (may be revealed by immunohistology)

PRL only (→prolactinoma)	35%	ACTH (→Cushing's disease)	7%
GH only (→acromegaly)	20%	LH/FSH/TSH	≥1%[1]
PRL and GH	7%	No obvious hormone	30%[2]

Symptoms are caused by local pressure, hormone secretion, or hypopituitarism (p216). FSH secreting tumours can cause macro-orchidism in men, but are rare.

Features of local pressure Headache, visual field defects (bilateral tempora[l] hemianopia, due to compression of the optic chiasm), palsy of cranial nerves III, IV, VI (pressure or invasion of the cavernous sinus). Also, diabetes insipidus (DI) (p224, more likely from hypothalamic disease); disturbance of hypothalamic centres of T°, sleep, and appetite; erosion through floor of sella leading to CSF rhinorrhoea.

Investigations Pituitary MRI (defines intra- and supra-sellar extension); accurat[e] assessment of visual fields; screening tests: PRL, IGF-1 (p222), ACTH, cortisol, TFTs, LH/FSH, testosterone in ♂, short Synacthen® test. Glucose tolerance test i[f] acromegaly suspected (p222). If Cushing's disease suspected, see p209. Wate[r] deprivation test if DI is suspected (p224).

Treatment Start hormone replacement as needed. Ensure steroids are give[n] before thyroxine, as thyroxine may precipitate an adrenal crisis. For Cushing's disease see p209, prolactinoma p220, acromegaly p222.

- ***Surgery:*** Most pituitary surgery is trans-sphenoidal, but if there is supra-sella[r] extension, a trans-frontal approach may be required. NB: for prolactinoma, firs[t] line treatment is medical with a dopamine agonist, see p220. *Pre-op:* Ensur[e] hydrocortisone 100mg IV/IM pre-op. Subsequent cortisol replacement and reass[-]essment varies with local protocols—ask advice. *Post-op:* Retest pituitary functio[n] (p216) to assess replacement needs. Wait 6–8 weeks post-op before repeatin[g] dynamic tests for adrenal function.
- ***Radiotherapy:*** Post-op if complete removal of the tumour has not been possible.

Post-op Recurrence may occur late after surgery, so life-long follow up is required. Fertility should be discussed: this may be reduced post-op due to ↓ gonadotrophins.

Pituitary apoplexy Rapid pituitary enlargement due to haemorrhage into [a] tumour may cause sudden mass effects, cardiovascular collapse due to acut[e] hypopituitarism, and death. Suspect if acute onset of headache, meningism, ↓GCS, ophthalmoplegia and visual field defects, especially in someone with a known tumou[r] (may present like subarachnoid haemorrhage). ***Treatment:*** Urgent steroid[s] (hydrocortisone 100mg IV) and surgery.

Craniopharyngioma Not strictly a pituitary tumour: it originates from Rathke's pouch so is situated between pituitary and the 3rd ventricle floor. They are rare, bu[t] are the commonest childhood intracranial tumour. Over 50% present in childhoo[d] with growth failure; adults may present with amenorrhoea, ↓libido, hypothalami[c] symptoms (eg diabetes insipidus, hyperphagia, sleep disturbance) or tumour mas[s] effect, see above. ***Tests:*** CT/MRI (calcification in 50%, may also be seen on sku[ll] XR). ***Treatment:*** Surgery ± post-op radiation; test pituitary function post-op.

1 Sensitive methods of TSH measurement have improved recognition of TSH-secreting tumours. Thes[e] are now more frequently found at microadenoma stage, medially located, and *without* associate[d] hormone hypersecretion. In these tumours, somatostatin analogues (p222) are very helpful.
2 Many produce an alpha-subunit which may serve as a tumour marker.

Endocrinology

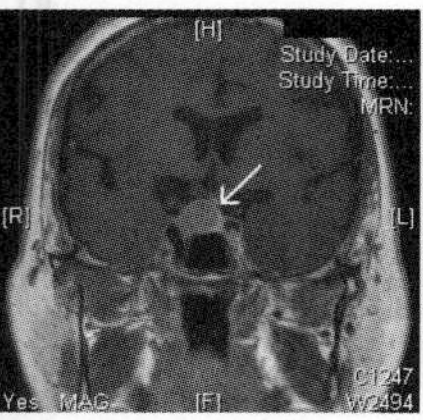

Fig 1. Coronal T1 weighted MRI of the brain post IV gadolinium showing a pituitary adenoma.

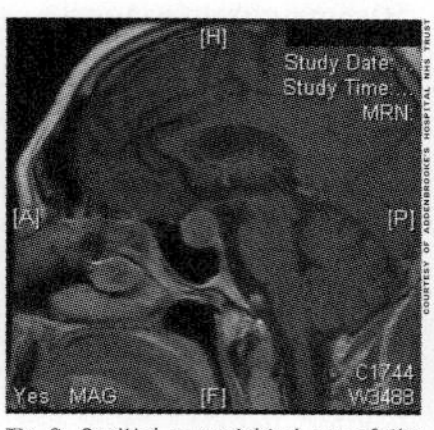

Fig 2. Sagittal T1 weighted MRI of the brain post IV gadolinium showing a pituitary adenoma.

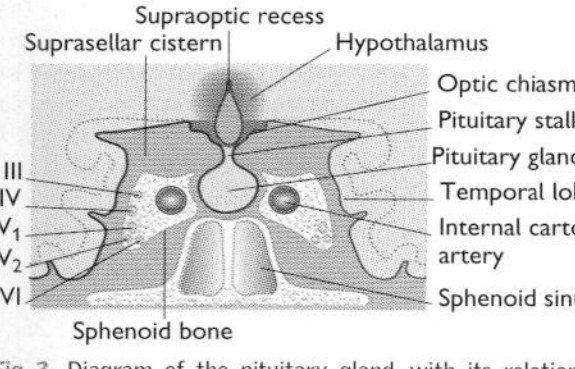

Fig 3. Diagram of the pituitary gland, with its relation to surrounding structures and cranial nerves III, IV, V, and VI.

Hyperprolactinaemia

This is the most common biochemical disturbance of the pituitary. It present earlier in women (due to menstrual disturbance) but late in men. Prolacti stimulates lactation. Raised levels lead to secondary hypogonadism, and therefor infertility and osteoporosis, by inhibiting secretion of gonadotrophin releasin hormone, resulting in low LH/FSH and low testosterone or oestrogen levels.

Causes of raised basal plasma prolactin (PRL) (>390mU/L) PRL is secreted fror the anterior pituitary and release is inhibited by dopamine produced in th hypothalamus. Hyperprolactinaemia may result from 1 Excess production from th pituitary, eg prolactinoma. 2 Disinhibition, by compression of the pituitary stall reducing local dopamine levels or 3 Administration of a dopamine antagonis A PRL of 1000–5000mU/L may result from any, but >5000 is likely to be du to a prolactinoma, with macroadenomas (>10mm) having the highest level eg 10,000–100,000.

- ***Physiological:*** Pregnancy; breast-feeding; stress eg post-seizure.
- ***Drugs (most common cause):*** Phenothiazines; metoclopramide; haloperidc α-methyldopa; oestrogens.
- ***Diseases:*** *Prolactinoma:* micro- or macroadenoma; *Stalk damage:* pituitar adenomas, surgery, trauma; *Hypothalamic disease:* craniopharyngioma, othe tumours; *Other:* hypothyroidism (due to ↑TRH), chronic renal failure (↓excretion

Symptoms ♀: Amenorrhoea or oligomenorrhoea; infertility; galactorrhoea. Alsc libido↓, weight↑, dry vagina. ♂: Impotence, reduced facial hair, galactorrhoea. Ma present late with osteoporosis or local pressure effects from the tumour (p218

Tests Basal PRL: non-stressful venepuncture between 09.00 and 16.00h. Do pregnancy test, TFT, U&E. MRI pituitary if other causes are ruled out.

Management Dopamine agonists (bromocriptine or cabergoline) are 1st line.

Microprolactinomas: A tumour <10mm on MRI (NB: ~25% of the population hav asymptomatic microprolactinomas). Bromocriptine, a dopamine agonist, ↓PF secretion, restores menstrual cycles and ↓tumour size. Dose is titrated up:1.25m PO; increase weekly by 1.25–2.5mg/d until ~2.5mg/12h. SE: Nausea, depressio postural hypotension (minimise by giving at night). If pregnancy is planned in patients, use barrier contraception until two periods have occurred. If subsequer pregnancy occurs, bromocriptine should be stopped after the first missed period. An alternative dopamine agonist is cabergoline: more effective and less SE, bu there is less data on safety during pregnancy.

Trans-sphenoidal surgery may be considered if intolerant of dopamine agonists. has a high success rate, but there are risks of permanent hormone deficiency ar prolactinoma recurrence, and so is usually reserved as a second-line treatment

Macroprolactinomas: A tumour >10mm diameter on MRI. Macroprolactinoma should be initially treated with a dopamine agonist (bromocriptine if fertility is th goal). Surgery is indicated if there are visual symptoms or pressure effects whic fail to respond quickly to medical treatment, or if pregnancy is contemplated a ~25% of macroadenomas will expand during pregnancy. Bromocriptine, and some cases radiation therapy, may be required post-op as complete surgic resection is uncommon. Pre-op assessment is often difficult: familiarize yourse with case-histories to show complexities of this aspect of endocrinology.[1]

Follow up: Monitor PRL levels. If headache or visual loss occur, check fields ar consider MRI. Medication can be decreased after 2 years of treatment, althouc recurrence of hyperprolactinaemia and expansion of the tumour may occur, and these patients should be monitored carefully.

1 Harms E 2003 *Dtsch Med Wochenschr* **128** 667. A 46yr-old lady had galactorrhoea for 7y and a ↑prolactin (3133mU/L) and intact pituitary function with no eye signs. MRI showed a 1.9c pituitary tumour with extrasellar extension. Is trans-sphenoidal resection needed for a presume macroadenoma with functional hyperprolactinaemia, or should there be a dopamine-agonist tria *One possible answer:* try drugs, and monitor MRI if initial prolactin ≥2000mU/L.

Acromegaly

This disease is due to hypersecretion of GH (growth hormone) from a pituitar tumour in >99% of cases, and is rarely associated with ectopic production of GH-releasing hormone eg from a carcinoid tumour. ♀:♂=1:1. It mainly present between 30–50yrs old. Prevalence is ~40–60 per million. ~5% are associated wit MEN1. GH stimulates soft tissue and skeletal growth through ↑secretion of insulin like growth factor-1 (IGF-1), and its secretion is inhibited by somatostatin.

Clinical features Onset is insidious.

- ***Excessive soft tissue growth:*** Growth of hands and feet: ie ↑ring size, thic spade-like hands and ↑shoe size; coarsening of facial features: prominen supraorbital ridge, prognathism, wide-spaced teeth; large tongue (macroglossia headache; excess sweating; hoarse voice and obstructive sleep apnoea (sof tissue swelling in the larynx); arthralgia, osteoarthritis, proximal muscl weakness; carpal tunnel syndrome (p495).
- ***Features of a pituitary tumour:*** Hypopituitarism ± local mass effect (p218)

Complications

- Impaired glucose tolerance (40%), DM (20%), as GH is counter-regulatory to insulir
- Vascular: BP↑, left ventricular hypertrophy, cardiomyopathy. There is ↑risk c ischaemic heart disease and stroke, due to ↑BP and insulin resistance.
- Malignancy: Controversy exists over the extent of ↑risk of colonic polyps an development of colon cancer; guidelines suggest colonoscopy at 50yr.
- Mortality is increased (2–3 fold), mainly due to cardiovascular risk.

Investigations

- Random GH measurements are not helpful as GH is secreted in a markedl pulsatile manner. During peaks, levels can overlap between normal subjects an acromegalic patients. GH is ↑ in stress, sleep, and puberty, and ↓ in pregnanc
- Serum IGF-1 (p216) is used as a screening test for acromegaly. Levels correlat with GH secretion over the preceding 24h, and so are ↑ with excessive G secretion. But in up to 25% of cases, IGF-1 remains normal with ↑GH secretio
- The definitive test is the oral glucose tolerance test (OGTT) with GH measuremen as described on p190. The test is done at 09.00, with fasting from midnigh Collect samples for GH and glucose at: 0, 30, 60, 90, 120, 150min. *Interpretatio* normally GH secretion is inhibited by a rise in glucose, and GH should b undetectable (<0.5mU/L—check with lab for reference level). In acromega there is failure to suppress GH release. False +ves for this test are seen in pubert pregnancy, hepatic and renal disease, anorexia nervosa and DM.
- MRI scan of pituitary fossa. • Test pituitary function (p216)—hypopituitarism
- Visual fields and acuity. • ECG, echocardiogram. Obtain old photos if possible.

Treatment • ***Trans-sphenoidal surgery:*** Usually the treatment of choice. Cu rate ~80% microadenomas, and ~40% macroadenomas. At 3 months post-o measure GH day curve (4–5 samples during day, aim for mean GH <5mU/L) or repe OGTT, measure IGF-1, and do pituitary function tests (p216) to check for hyp pituitarism. If GH remains high, adjuvant medical or radiotherapy may be neede

- ***Medical:*** Somatostatin analogues eg *octreotide* (Sandostatin LAR®, give monthly IM), and *lanreotide* (Somatuline LA®) are replacing dopamine agonists. include: pain at the injection site; gastrointestinal: abdominal cramps, flatulenc loose stools, ↑gallstones; impaired glucose tolerance. Control of GH and IGF levels occurs in up to 60%. Pegvisomant, a recombinant GH analogue, acts as GH receptor antagonist. It suppresses IGF-1 to normal in 90%, but GH levels ris Occasionally tumour size increases, so monitor closely. We await long term dat
- ***Radiotherapy:*** If surgery inappropriate or as adjuvant; may take years to wo

Follow-up: Yearly, GH and IGF-1 measurement ± OGTT; visual fields; clinical photo cardiovascular assessment. Aim serum GH <5mU/L to reverse mortality risk.

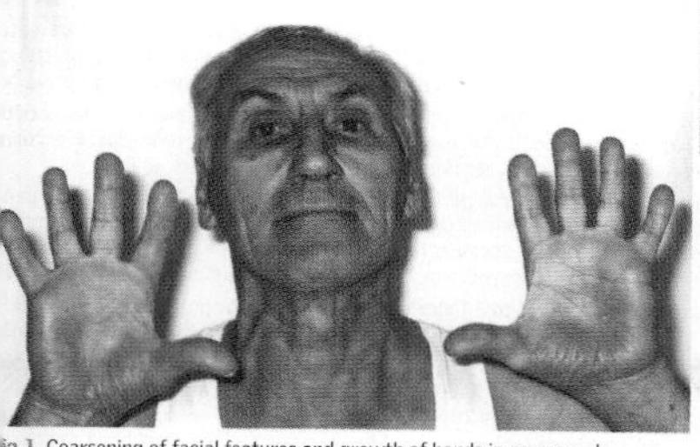

ig 1. Coarsening of facial features and growth of hands in acromegaly.

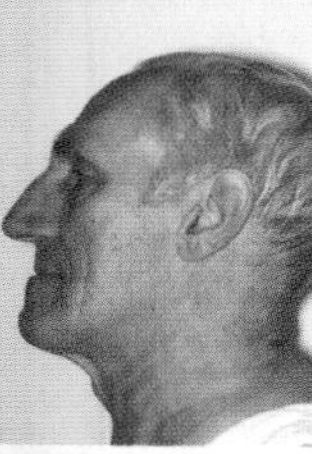

g 2. Prognathism: abnormal
'otrusion of the jaw, due to
creased growth of the
andible.

Diabetes insipidus (DI)

This is the passage of big volumes (>3L/day) of dilute urine due to impaired wate resorption by the kidney, because of reduced ADH secretion from the posterio pituitary (cranial DI), or impaired response of the kidney to ADH (nephrogenic DI)

Symptoms Polyuria; polydipsia; dehydration; symptoms of hypernatraemia (p666 Polydipsia can be uncontrollable, with the patient drinking anything *and everythin* to hand: in such cases, if beer is on tap, disaster will ensue.[103]

Causes of cranial DI • *Idiopathic* (≤50%) • *Congenital:* defects in ADH gen DIDMOAD syndrome[1] • *Tumour:* craniopharyngioma, metastases, pituitary tumou (rare) • *Trauma:* hypophysectomy, head injury • *Infiltration:* histiocytosis, sarcoid sis[2] • *Vascular:* Sheehan's syndrome,[3] haemorrhage • *Infection:* meningoencephaliti

Causes of nephrogenic DI • Inherited • *Metabolic:* Low potassium, high calciu • *Drugs:* lithium, demeclocycline • Chronic renal disease • Post-obstructive uropath

Tests U&E, Ca^{2+}, glucose (exclude DM), serum and urine osmolalities. Serum osm olality estimate≈2×(Na^+ + K^+) + urea + glucose (all in mmol/L). It is normal tightly controlled between 285–295mOsmol/kg. In DI, urine osmolality is lo (usually <400mOsmol/kg) as it cannot be concentrated and so plasma osmolali rises. Serum sodium rises, due to fluid loss. In primary polydipsia there may b dilutional hyponatraemia—and as hyponatraemia may itself cause mania,[104] b cautious in using terms such as 'water intoxication from psychogenic polydipsi

Diagnosis The ***water deprivation test*** aims to test the ability of kidneys t concentrate urine for diagnosis of DI, and then to localise the cause. See BOX. NB: it is often difficult to differentiate primary polydipsia from partial DI. OTM4 3.207

ΔΔ: DM; diuretics or lithium use; ***primary polydipsia***—this causes symptoms polydipsia & polyuria with dilute urine. Its cause is poorly understood;[4] it may b associated with schizophrenia or mania (±Li^+ therapy[105]), or, rarely, hypothalam disease (neurosarcoid; tumour; encephalitis; brain injury; HIV encephalopathy). As part of this syndrome, the kidneys may lose their ability to fully concentra urine, due to a wash-out of the normal concentrating gradient in the renal medull

Treatment

Cranial DI: Find the cause—MRI (head); test anterior pituitary function (p216). Gi desmopressin, a synthetic analogue of ADH. Dose: 10–20µg/12–24h intranasa (smallest dose that controls polyuria: higher doses ↑risk of hyponatraemia). An o formulation is available but dosing is difficult due to differences in bioavailabili ***Nephrogenic:*** Treat the cause. If it persists, try bendroflumethiazide 5mg PO/24 NSAIDs lower urine volume and plasma Na^+ by inhibiting prostaglandin synthas prostaglandins locally inhibit the action of ADH.[107]

➡Emergency management • Do urgent plasma U&E, and serum and uri osmolalities. Monitor urine output carefully and check U&E twice a day initially

- IVI to keep up with urine output. If severe hypernatraemia, do not lower N rapidly as this may cause cerebral oedema and brain injury. If Na^+ is ≥170, u 0.9% saline initially—this contains 150mmol/L of sodium. Aim to reduce Na^+ a rate of less than 12mmol/L per day. Use of 0.45% saline can be dangerous.
- Desmopressin 2µg IM (lasts 12–24h) may be used as a therapeutic trial.

1 DIDMOAD is a rare autosomal recessive disorder: Diabetes Insipidus, Diabetes Mellitus, O Atrophy and Deafness (also known as Wolfram's syndrome).
2 Suspect neurosarcoidosis if CSF protein↑ (seen in 34%), facial nerve palsy (25%), CSF pleocyt (23%), diabetes insipidus (21%), hemiparesis (17%), psychosis (17%), papilloedema (15%), ata (13%), seizures (12%), optic atrophy (12%), hearing loss (12%), or nystagmus (9%).
3 This is pituitary infarction after severe hypotension, eg postpartum haemorrhage. It's rare.
4 Most of us could drink 20L/d and not get hyponatraemic; some get hyponatraemic drinking 5L/ they may have the Psychosis, Intermittent hyponatraemia, and Polydipsia (PIP syndrome, ?f ↑intravascular volume leading to ↑atrial natriuretic peptide, hence natriuresis & hyponatraemia).

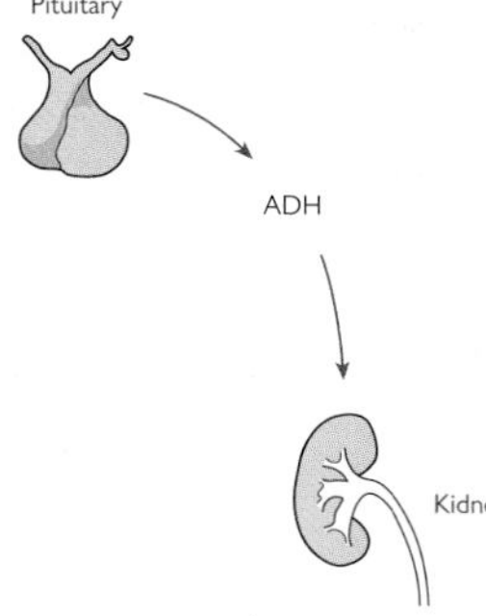

Vater deprivation test

he purpose of this test is to see if the kidneys persist in producing dilute urine espite dehydration, and then to localise the cause. Do not do the test before stablishing that urine volume >3L/d (output less than this with normal plasma a+ and osmolality excludes significant disturbance of water balance).

Stop test if urine osmolality >600mOsmol/kg in Stage 1 (DI is excluded).

Free fluids until 07.30. Light breakfast at 06.30, no tea, no coffee, no smoking.

tage 1 Fluid deprivation (0–8h): For diagnosis of DI. Start at 08.00.

Empty bladder, then no drinks and only dry food.

Weigh hourly. If >3% weight lost during test, order urgent serum osmolality. If >300mOsmol/kg, proceed to Stage 2. If <300, continue test.

Collect urine every 2 hours; measure its volume and osmolality.

Venous sample for osmolality every 4 hours.

Stop test after 8h (16.00) if urine osmolality >600mOsmol/kg (ie normal).

tage 2 Differentiate cranial from nephrogenic DI.

Proceed if urine still dilute—ie urine osmolality <600mOsmol/kg.

Give desmopressin 20μg intranasally (or 2μg IM). Water can be drunk now.

Measure urine osmolality hourly for the next 4 hours.

nterpreting the water deprivation test	
• Normal	Urine osmolality >600mOsmol/kg in Stage 1 (normal concentrating ability).
• Primary polydipsia	Urine concentrates, but less than normal, eg >400–600mOsmol/kg.
• Cranial DI	Urine osmolality increases to >600mOsmol/kg *after* desmopressin.
• Nephrogenic DI	No increase in urine osmolality after desmopressin.

7 Gastroenterology

Contents

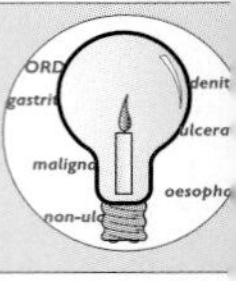

Fig 1. What shall be guiding light through twists and turns of tunnelous GI tract? Perh more so than in any field symptoms can be vague nonspecific (eg dyspe p234), often leaving us little choice but turn invasive procedures, w we know are not with risk (p248). Yet if we le pathology in the dark, b benign or malignant, we be doing a disservice. not every symptom n illuminating by a scan gadget: ►get used listening to patients' sto ►get good at dealing uncertainty, and ►know in time you will learn right level of illuminatio use to reveal the su nuances and shades of g rointestinal phenomena.

Relevant pages in other chapters: ***Signs & symptoms:*** Abdominal disten (p52); epigastric pain (p52); flatulence (p60); guarding (p60); heartburn (p hepatomegaly (p63); LIF and LUQ pain (p52); palmar erythema (p66); rebo tenderness (p70); regurgitation (p70); RIF pain (p52); RUQ pain (p52); discolouration (p70); splenomegaly (p624); tenesmus (p72); vomiting (p waterbrash (p76); weight loss (p76). ***Surgical topics:*** Contents to **Surgery** (p5 ***Haematology:*** Iron-deficiency anaemia (p312). ***Infections:*** Viral hepatitis (p3 ***Radiology:*** The plain abdominal film (AXR) (p716); radiological GI procedures (p7 ***Emergencies:*** Upper GI bleeding (p804); acute liver failure (p806).

We thank Dr Simon Campbell who is our Specialist Reader for this chapter.

e learn about gastroenterological diseases as if they were separate entities, dependent species collected by naturalists, each kept in its own dark atchbox—collectors' items collecting dust in a desiccated world on a library elf. But this is not how illness works. Otto had diabetes, but refused to see a ctor until it was far advanced, and an amputation was needed. He needed oking after by his wife Aurelia. But she had her children Warren and Sylvia to ok after too. And when Otto was no longer the bread-winner, she forced rself to work as a teacher, an accountant, and at any other job she could get. to's illness manifested in Aurelia's duodenum—as an ulcer. The gut often bears e brunt of other people's worries. Inside every piece of a gut is a lumen[1]—the orld is in the gut, and the gut is in the world. But the light does not always ine. So when the lumen filled with Aurelia's blood, we can expect the illness to pact on the whole family. Her daughter knows where blood comes from traight from the heart... pink fizz'). After Otto died, Sylvia needed long-term ychiatric care, and Aurelia moved to be near her daughter. The bleeding odenal ulcer got worse when Sylvia needed electroconvulsive therapy. The erapy worked and now, briefly, Sylvia, before her own premature death, is able look after Aurelia, as she prepares for a gastrectomy.

The story of each illness told separately misses something; but even taken in its cial context, this story is missing something vital—the poetry, in most of our tients lived rather than written—tragic, comic, human, and usually obscure—t in the case of this family not so obscure. Welling up, as unstoppable as the eding from her mother's ulcer, came the poetry of Sylvia Plath.[2]

Gastroenterology

men is Latin for light (hence its medical meaning of a tubular cavity open to the world at both ends), ell as being the SI unit of light flux falling on an object—ie the power to transilluminate. All doctors this power, whether by insightfully interpreting patients' lives and illnesses to them, or by acts of ess—even something so simple as bringing a cup of tea.

And here you come, with a cup of tea
Wreathed in steam.
The blood jet is poetry,
There is no stopping it.
You hand me two children, two roses.

Sylvia Plath, *Kindness*, Collected Poems, 1981, Faber
Historical source: www.katemoses.com/books/w_chronology.html

Healthy, enjoyable eating

'There's a lot of people in this world who spend so much time watching their health that they haven't the time to enjoy it.' Josh Billings (1818–85).

There are no good or bad **foods**, and no universally good or bad **diets**. We must consider diet out of context with a desired lifestyle, and nor should we assume t everyone wants to be thin, healthy, and live for ever. If we are walking to the So Pole, our bodies need a diet as full of energy-rich fat as possible: taking any ot food would be a waste of space. But if we live a sedentary life, the converse is necessarily true. After decades of research, we still do not know who should what, or when. Are 3 meals a day healthier than 1? Is fat bad if weight is norm Is a balanced diet (see BOX) best? Should we eat 3, 5, 7, or 9 fruits per d The latter is one recommendation for men, but recent studies find no ben beyond 3.[2] The traditional answer to these questions is 'Yes'—and the more f the better—but evidence is far from complete, not just because of the paucity randomized trials, but because of complex interactions between eating and hea All diets have unintended consequences: eg the 'good' antioxidant epicatechi flavonoid) in dark chocolate is annulled by taking milk at the same tim Randomized trials show how an Atkins-type diet (low in carbohydrate ∴ ↑fa ↑protein) can improve lipid profiles and insulin resistance, but with possible SE renal problems and excessive calcium excretion.[RCT 4][5] To complicate matters fut diet is also confounded by lifestyle—whilst some studies have shown t vegetarians may be less likely to die from ischaemic heart disease,[RCT 6] is this eff because vegetarians in the UK are more likely to be non-smokers?[7]

Current recommendations must take into account 3 facts:

- Obesity is an escalating epidemic costing health services as much as smoking in 4 adults in the UK are now classified as obese.[8]
- Diabetes mellitus is burgeoning: in some places prevalence is >7% (p190).
- Past advice has not changed eating habits in large sections of the populatic

Advice is likely to focus on the following

- ***Body mass index (BMI):*** see TABLE; aim for 20–25; ie **eat less**. Control quantity may be more important than quality. In hypertension, eating the 'ri things lowered BP by 0.6mmHg, but controlling weight (*OHCS* p529) cause 3.7mmHg reduction in 6 months in 1 RCT.[RCT 9]
- ***Oily fish:*** Rich in omega-3 fatty acid (eg mackerel, herring, pilchards, salmc but benefits are not fully substantiated).[10] If tinned fish, avoid thos unspecified oils. Nuts are also valuable: walnuts lower total cholesterol and h one of the highest ratios of polyunsaturates to saturates (7:1). Soya pro lowers cholesterol, low-density lipoproteins, and triglycerides.
- ***Refined sugar:*** (See BOX for its deleterious effects.) Use fruit to add sweetr Have low-sugar drinks: a 330mL can of non-diet carbonated soft drink can h up to 10 teaspoons (40g) of refined sugar. Don't add sugar to drinks or cere (In a thin, active, elderly, normoglycaemic person, sugar may be no great e
- ***Eat enough fruit and fibre:*** See BOX and ***reduce salt intake.***
- ***Enjoy moderate alcohol use (adults):*** ♀:<15U/wk; ♂:<20U/wk (higher le are controversial)—taken regularly, not in binges. Alcohol inhibits plat aggregation and is an antioxidant (∴ cardioprotective). There is no evidence spirit or beer drinkers should switch to wine. There is evidence that the ber accrues **only** to those whose LDL cholesterol is ≥5.25mmol/L.[11]

►***Avoid this diet if:*** • <5yrs old • Need for low residue (eg Crohn's, UC, p266 special diet (coeliac disaese, p272) • Weight loss is expected. ***Emphasis may different in:*** Dyslipidaemia (p682); DM (p190); obesity; constipation (p240); failure (p250); chronic pancreatitis (p272); renal failure (less protein); BP↑.[12]

Difficulties It is an imposition to ask us to change our diet (children often re point-blank); a more subtle approach is to take a meal we enjoy (eg Coke® crisps) and make it healthier (eg fresh fruit juice, low-salt crisps made from ja potatoes, and fried in sunflower oil).

aditional low-fat nutritional advice: *the balance of good health*

low-fat diet may not only be for the sake of good health, as it can can also help ntrol symptoms, eg as in gallstone disease, and while it is unrealistic to expect all ır patients' troubles to drift away as the weight comes off, we **can** offer the centive of an improvement in both symptoms and health as encouragement.

tarchy foods: Bread, rice, pasta, potatoes, etc. form the main energy source specially wholemeal). ↑Fluid intake with a diet high in non-starch polyccharide (NSP)—eg 8 cups (1–2½ pints) daily. Warn about bulky stools. NSP calcium and iron absorption, so restrict main intake to 1 meal a day.

uit, vegetables: eg >6 different pieces of fruit (ideally with skins) or rtions of pulses, beans, or lightly cooked greens per day. This probably cardiovascular and cancer mortality. The term **fibre** is imprecise. Most is P—the preferred term.

eat and alternatives: Meat should be cooked without additional fat. Lower t alternatives, such as white meat (poultry, without skin), white fish, and getable protein sources (eg pulses, soya) are encouraged.

airy foods: Low-fat semi-skimmed milk/yoghurt; edam or cottage cheese.

t and sugary foods: Avoiding extra fat in cooking is advised ('grill, boil, steam, bake, but don't fry'). Fatty spreads (eg butter) are kept to a minimum and ack foods (crisps, sweets, biscuits, or cake) are avoided.

osing weight—why and how?

e risks of too much sugar Excess sugar causes caries, diabetes, obesity—nich itself contributes to osteoarthritis, cancer, hypertension, and xidative stress—(so raising cardiovascular mortality) and much more.

osing weight Consider referral to a dietician—a needs-specific diet may be ore effective. In conjunction with exercise and diet strategies, targeted eight-loss can also be achieved successfully with psychotherapy.

ugs for obesity? The most desirable treatment for obesity is still primary evention, but pharmacotherapy does work. ***Orlistat*** lowers fat absorption ence SE of oily faecal incontinence). ***Sibutramine*** increases post-ingestive tiety (SE hypertension and tachycardia)—see *OHCS* p529.[1]

rgery for obesity? See p579.

lculating BMI

II is calculated as (weight in kg)/(height in m)^2

II	State	Some implications within the categories
.8.5	Underweight	<17.5 is one of the criteria for anorexia nervosa
.5–25	Target	
–30	Overweight	Weight loss should be considered
–40	Obesity	>32 is unsuitable for day-case general surgery
'0	Extreme/morbid obesity	>40 is an indication for bariatric surgery

aveats: BMI does not take into account the distribution of body fat, and is harder to erpret for children and adolescents. **Waist circumference** >94cm in men and >80cm women reflects omental fat and correlates better with risk than does BMI. For ethnic iations, see p197.

1 esearch continues into the hormones involved in obesity—eg the satiety-inducing **leptin** and the er-inducing **ghrelin**.

White intra-oral lesi
• Idiopathic keratosis
• Carcinoma
• Leucoplakia
• Hairy oral leucoplak
• Lichen planus
• Lupus erythematosu
• Poor dental hygiene
• Smoking
• Candidiasis
• Aphthous stomatitis
• Squamous papilloma
• Secondary syphilis

Leucoplakia White thickening of the tongue or oral mucosa of unknown cause (fig 1). It is premalignant. Oral hairy leucoplakia is a shaggy white patch on the side of the tongue seen in HIV, caused by EBV. ►When in doubt, refer all intra-oral white lesions (see MINIBOX).

Aphthous ulcers (fig 2) 20% of us get these shallow, painful ulcers on the tongue or oral mucosa that heal without scarring. ***Causes of severe ulcers:*** Crohn's & coeliac disease; Behçet's (p686); trauma; erythema multiforme; lichen planus; pemphigus; pemphigoid; infections (herpes simplex, syphilis, Vincent's angina, p704). ***Treatment*** is difficult: ***hydrocortisone*** lozenges held on the ulcer may help, as may ***tetracycline*** mouthwash. ►Biopsy any ulcer healing after 3 weeks to exclude malignancy; refer to an oral surgeon if uncert

Candidiasis (thrush) (fig 3) causes white patches or erythema of the buccal muc Patches may be hard to remove and bleed if scraped. ***Risk factors:*** extremes of a DM; antibiotics; immunosuppression (long-term corticosteroids, including inhal cytotoxics; malignancy; HIV). ►Oropharyngeal candidiasis in an apparently patient may suggest underlying HIV infection. ***Treatment: Nystatin*** suspensior ***amphotericin*** lozenges. ***Fluconazole*** for oropharyngeal candidiasis.

Cheilitis (angular stomatitis) Fissuring of the mouth's corners is caused denture problems, candidiasis (above), or deficiency of iron or riboflavin (vitamin

Gingivitis Gum inflammation ± hypertrophy occurs with poor oral hygiene, dr (phenytoin, ciclosporin, nifedipine), pregnancy, vitamin C deficiency (scurvy, p27 acute myeloid leukaemia (p340), or Vincent's angina (p704).

Microstomia (fig 4) The mouth is too small, eg from thickening and tightenin the perioral skin after burns or in epidermolysis bullosa (destructive skin mucous membrane blisters ± ankyloglossia) or systemic sclerosis (p538).

Oral pigmentation Perioral brown spots characterize Peutz–Jeghers' (p7(Pigmentation anywhere in the mouth suggests Addison's disease or drugs (eg a malarials). Consider malignant melanoma. ***Telangiectasia:*** Systemic sclerc Osler–Weber–Rendu syndrome (p700). ***Fordyce glands*** (creamy yellow spots at border of the oral mucosa and the lip vermillion) are sebaceous cysts, comr and benign. *Aspergillus niger* colonisation may cause a black tongue.

Teeth A blue line at the gum–tooth margin suggests lead poisoning. Prenata childhood tetracycline exposure causes a yellow–brown discolouration.

Tongue This may be furred or dry (xerostomia) in dehydration, if on tricyclics, e after radiotherapy, in Crohn's disease, Sjögren's (p702) and Mikulicz's syndrom

- ***Glossitis*** means a smooth, red, sore tongue, eg caused by iron, folate, or B_{12} deficie (fig 1, p321). If local loss of papillae leads to ulcer-like lesions that change in co and size, use the term **geographic tongue** (harmless migratory glossitis).
- ***Macroglossia:*** The tongue is too big. Causes: myxoedema; acromegaly; amyloi *ranula* is a bluish salivary retention cyst to one side of the frenulum, named a the bulging vocal pouch of frogs' throats (genus *Rana*).
- ***Tongue cancer*** typically appears on its edge as a raised ulcer with firm ed and environs. Main risk factors are smoking and alcohol.[2] Examine under tongue and ask patient to deviate his extended tongue sideways. Spread: ante ⅓ of the tongue drains to the submental nodes; middle ⅓ to the submandib nodes; posterior ⅓ to the deep cervical nodes (see BOX, p621). ***Treatme*** Surgery or radiotherapy. 5yr survival (early disease): 80%. ►When in doubt, r a tongue ulcer.

1 Drugs causing xerostomia: ACE-i, antidepressants; antihistamines; antipsychotics; antimuscari anticholinergics; bromocriptine; diuretics; loperamide; nifedipine; opiates; prazocin; prochlorperazine

2 Betel nut (*Areca catechu*) chewing, common in South Asia, may be an independent risk factor.

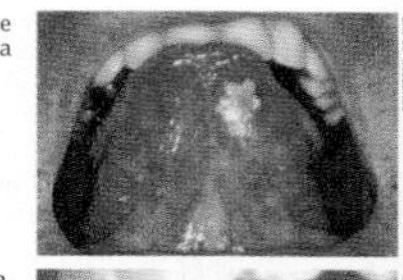

1. Leucoplakia on the underside of the ıgue. It is important to refer leucoplakia :ause it is a premalignant.

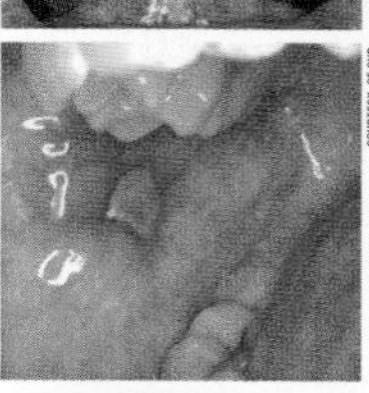

2. An aphthous ulcer in the buccal mucosa. e name is tautological, literally meaning an er-like ulcer—the adjective aphthous comes m the latinised Greek noun *aphtha*, meaning eration. This is a fine example of the metimes unnessecary) complexity of language ıt has historically pervaded medicine. A light ısp of the classical languages can help but it is no means prerequisite!

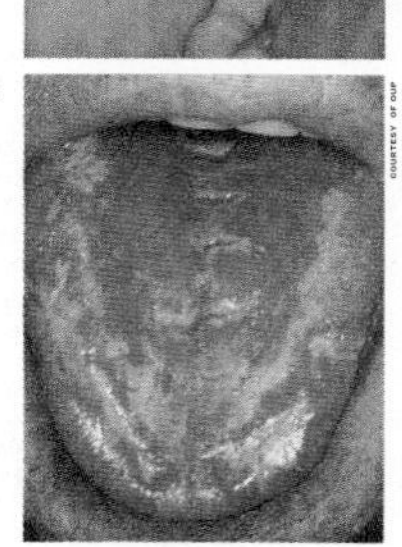

3. White fur on an erythematous tongue ısed by oral candidiasis.

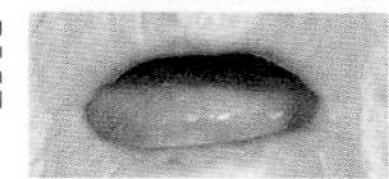

4. Microstomia (small, narrow moth), eg m hardening of the skin around the mouth ich causes the oral opening to close in eroderma. It can be both cosmetically and ıctionally disabling.

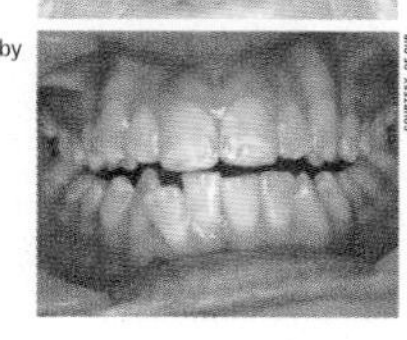

5. White bands on the teeth can be caused by :essive fluoride intake.

Dysphagia

Dysphagia is difficulty in swallowing and always needs investigating to excl malignancy. If symptoms are progressive or prolonged then **urgent** investigatic required.

Causes Oral, pharyngeal, or oesophageal? Mechanical or motility related (see BO

Clinical features There are a number of key questions to ask:

1 Was there difficulty swallowing solids **and** liquids from the start?
  Yes: Motility disorder (achalasia, neurological), or pharyngeal causes.
  No: Solids **then** liquids: suspect a stricture (benign or malignant).
2 Is it difficult to make the swallowing movement?
  Yes: Suspect bulbar palsy, especially if he coughs on swallowing.
3 Is swallowing painful (odynophagia)?
  Yes: Suspect cancer, severe oesophagitis, achalasia, or oesophageal spa
4 Is the dysphagia intermittent or is it constant and getting worse?
  Intermittent: Suspect oesophageal spasm.
  Constant and worsening: Suspect malignant stricture.
5 Does the neck bulge or gurgle on drinking?
  Yes: Suspect a pharyngeal pouch (see fig 1, p621).

Gastroenterology

Signs Is the patient cachectic or anaemic? Examine the mouth; feel for supracla ular nodes (left supraclavicular node = Virchow's node—suggests intra-abdon malignancy); look for signs of systemic disease, eg systemic sclerosis, CNS disea

Investigations FBC (anaemia); U&E (dehydration); CXR (mediastinal fluid le absent gastric bubble, aspiration); barium swallow (fig 1) +/– video fluorosc upper GI endoscopy and biopsy. Further investigations: oesophageal manometr normal barium swallow); ENT opinion if suspected pharyngeal cause.

Specific conditions ***Oesophagitis*** p236. ***Diffuse oesophageal spasm*** ca intermittent dysphagia ± chest pain. Barium swallow: abnormal contractions corkscrew oesophagus.[1] ***Achalasia:*** Failure of relaxation of the lower oesopha sphincter (due to degeneration of the myenteric plexus) causes dyspha regurgitation, substernal cramps, and ↓weight. Barium swallow: dilated tape oesophagus. Treatment: endoscopic balloon dilatation, or Heller's cardiomyoton then proton pump inhibitors (PPIs, p236). Botulinum toxin injection is an alterna if unsuitable for an invasive procedure. ***Benign oesophageal stricture:*** Cause gastro-oesophageal reflux disease (GORD, p236), corrosives, surgery, or radiother Treatment: endoscopic balloon dilatation. ***Oesophageal cancer:*** (p614) Associat ♂; GORD, tobacco, alcohol, Barrett's oesophagus (p686), achalasia, tylosis (pal hyperkeratosis), Paterson–Brown–Kelly syndrome. ***Paterson–Brown–K (Plummer–Vinson) syndrome:*** Post-cricoid web + iron-deficiency.

Nausea and vomiting

Causes: p

Tests ***Bloods:*** FBC, U&E, LFT, Ca^{2+}, glucose, and amylase. ***ABG:*** A metal (hypochloraemic) alkalosis from loss of gastric contents (pH >7.45, ↑HC indicates severe vomiting. Request a plain ***AXR*** if suspected bowel obstruction— p716 for AXR findings in obstruction. Consider upper GI endoscopy (p248 persistent vomiting. Identify and **treat the underlying cause** if possible.

Treatment See TABLE. Try to use pre-emptive therapy, eg pre-operatively for p operative symptoms. When possible try the oral route first. Roughly ⅓ of pati with nausea will require a second-line anti-emetic, so be prepared to presc more than one on occasions, but avoid drugs in pregnancy and children. Giv fluids with K^+ replacement if severely dehydrated or nil by mouth and mor electrolytes and fluid balance.

1 Non-propulsive contractions manifest as tertiary contractions or **'corkscrew oesophagus'** and su a motility disorder and may lead to impaired acid clearance. Symptoms and radiology do not neces correlate. ***Nutcracker oesophagus*** denotes distal peristaltic contractions >180mmHg. It can pain, eg relieved by nitrates, sublingual ***nifedipine***, or the smooth muscle relaxant ***sildenafil*** (p3

auses of dysphagia

lechanical block
Malignant stricture (fig 1)
- Oesophageal cancer
- Gastric cancer
- Pharyngeal cancer

Benign strictures
- Oesophageal web or ring p232
- Peptic stricture

Extrinsic pressure
- Lung cancer
- Mediastinal lymph nodes
- Retrosternal goitre
- Aortic aneurysm
- Left atrial enlargement

Pharyngeal pouch

Motility disorders
- Achalasia
- Diffuse oesophageal spasm
- Systemic sclerosis (p538)
- Myasthenia gravis (p504)
- Bulbar palsy (p498)
- Pseudobulbar palsy (p498)
- Syringobulbia (p508)
- Bulbar poliomyelitis (p420)
- Chagas' disease (p426)

Others
- Oesophagitis (p236)
  - Infection (*Candida*, HSV)
  - Reflux oesophagitis
- Globus hystericus

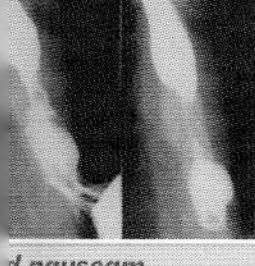

Fig 1. A malignant lower oesophageal stricture shown on barium swallow. The shouldered edges of the stricture produce an 'apple core' effect with an irregular mucosal pattern. On video fluoroscopy there would be no peristalsis visible in this segment. A benign stricture would have a more funnelled appearance with a normal mucosal pattern. Note the normal but similar appearance of the gastro-oesophageal junction inferiorly.

d nauseam...

mping into the sea is a certain cure for seasickness. John Ruskin (1819-1900)

ausea is often described by patients as their most intolerable symptom when ey are unwell (especially by those enduring palliative care). It can be an ually difficult symptom to help control. Not all anti-emetics will work for eryone, so it is worthwhile persevering with your options to help alleviate such disparaging and sometimes intractable symptom, since not everyone is able to mp ship so easily.

emembering your anti-emetics

ne way of recalling anti-emetics involves using (simplified) pharmacology.

eceptor	Antagonist	Dose	Notes
	Cyclizine	50mg/8h PO/IV/IM	GI causes
	Cinnarizine	30mg/8h PO	Vestibular disorders
	Metoclopramide	10mg/8h PO/IV/IM	GI causes; also prokinetic
	Domperidone	60mg/12h PR 20mg/6h PO	Also prokinetic
	Prochlorperazine	12.5mg stat IM 25mg stat PR 5mg/8h PO	Vestibular/GI causes
	Haloperidol	1.5mg bd PO	Chemical causes eg opioids
T_3	***Ondansetron***	4mg/8h IV	Doses can be much higher for eg emetogenic chemotherapy
hers	***Hyoscine butylbromide***	20mg stat IM/IV	Antimuscarinic ∴ also antispasmodic and antisecretory (don't prescribe with a prokinetic)
	Dexamethasone	6–10mg/d PO/SC	Unknown mode of action; as adjuvant therapy
	Midazolam	2–4mg/d IV	Unknown action; anti-emetic effect outlasts sedative effect[RCT 25]

All anti-dopaminergics can cause dystonias and oculogyric crisis, especially in younger patients.

Dyspepsia (indigestion) & peptic ulcer disease (PUD

Dyspepsia is a non-specific group of symptoms related to the upper GI tract.

ΔΔ of dyspepsia
• Non-ulcer dyspepsi
• Duodenal ulcer
• Duodenitis
• Gastritis/gastric ul
• Gastric malignancy
• GORD (reflux, p236)
• Oesophagitis

Non-specific symptoms Epigastric pain eg related to hunger, eating specific foods, or time of day; may be associated with bloating ± fullness after meals; heartburn (retrosternal pain with demonstrable acid reflux). **Alarm symptoms:** Anaemia (iron deficiency); loss of weight; anorexia; recent-onset of progressive symptoms; melaena or haematemesis; swallowing difficulty. **Signs** Tender epigastrium (non-specific). Any abdominal mass; supraclavicular nodes ± hepatomega

Managing new dyspepsia See FLOWCHART/NICE advice. ***If ≤55yrs old:*** test *Helicobacter pylori*; treat if +ve.[1] 'Test and treat' is more effective at reduci symptoms and recurrence than acid suppression alone (eg with ***lansopraz*** 30mg/24h PO for 4 weeks; SE: D&V, oedema, bronchospasm, Stevens–Johns syndrome, toxic epidermal necrolysis, alopecia, photosensitivity, intersti nephritis, LFT↑, agranulocytosis).[26] When choosing anti-acid therapy, PPIs are bet than H_2-receptor antagonists (H_2RA) at controlling symptoms in those w uninvestigated dyspepsia. The most accurate non-invasive test for *H. pylori* is t ^{13}C breath test (see TABLE). ►***If ≥55*** (and **new** dyspepsia not accounted for NSAID use and persisting for >4–6 weeks) **or *alarm symptoms***, refer for urg endoscopy (p248). Platelets↑, ESR↑ ± LFT↑ suggest organic causes.[27]

Duodenal ulcers (DU) are 4-fold commoner than GU. ***Major risk factors:*** *H. py* (~90%); drugs (aspirin; NSAIDs; steroids). ***Minor:*** ↑Gastric acid secretion; ↑gast emptying (↓duodenal pH); blood group O; smoking. The role of stress is cont versial. ***Symptoms:*** Epigastric pain typically before meals or at night, relieved eating, or drinking milk. 50% are asymptomatic; others experience recurr episodes. ***Signs:*** Epigastric tenderness. ***Diagnosis:*** Upper GI endoscopy (stop PF weeks before), see fig 1, p245. Test for *H. pylori*. Measure gastrin concentratio whilst off PPIs if Zollinger–Ellison syndrome (p709) is suspected. ***ΔΔ:*** Non-ul dyspepsia; duodenal Crohn's; TB; lymphoma; pancreatic cancer (p268).

Gastric ulcers (GU) occur mainly in the elderly, on the lesser curve. Ulc elsewhere are more often malignant. ***Risk factors:*** *H. pylori* (~80%); smoki NSAIDs; reflux of duodenal contents; delayed gastric emptying; stress, neurosurgery (Cushing's ulcers) or burns (Curling's ulcers). ***Symptoms:*** Asymp matic or epigastric pain (related to meals ± relieved by antacids) ± weight↓. ***Te*** Upper GI endoscopy to exclude malignancy (stop PPI 2weeks before); take mult biopsies from the ulcer's rim & base (histology, *H. pylori*) and brushings (cytolo

Treating peptic ulcers *Lifestyle* Avoid food that worsens symptoms; stop smok (smoking slows healing in GU and ↑relapse rates in DU). ***H. pylori eradication:*** Tr therapy is 80–85% effective at eradication.[1] ***Drugs to reduce acid:*** PPIs are most effective, eg ***lansoprazole*** 30mg/24h PO for 4 (DU) or 8 (GU) weeks. H_2 may have a place for individual responders, eg ***ranitidine*** 300mg *nocte* PO ***cimetidine*** 800mg *nocte* PO for 8 weeks. ***NSAID-associated ulcers:*** Stop NSAI possible (if not, use H_2RA, PPI, or ***misoprostol*** for prevention). If symptoms pers re-endoscope, recheck for *H. pylori*, and reconsider the differential diagno ***Surgery:*** p638.

Complications Bleeding, ↠(p244), perforation, ↠(p580), malignancy, gas outflow obstruction, (p638).

Treatment of non-ulcer dyspepsia *H. pylori eradication* may be beneficia relieving symptoms and preventing ulcers,[MET 28] but we do not know enough about long-term effects of such a strategy (SE include ↑reflux) for authoritative adv and so we start eradication therapy for *H. pylori* only after a +ve result. ***Med therapy:*** Prokinetic agents (eg ***metoclopramide*** 10mg/8h PO) may reli symptoms. PPIs or H_2RAs are unlikely to be beneficial.[29]

Managing new dyspepsia

If ≥55yrs old or ALARM symptoms (opposite) refer for urgent endoscopy. If on NSAIDs, stop. In all other cases, consider the following management plan.

See www.nice.org.uk

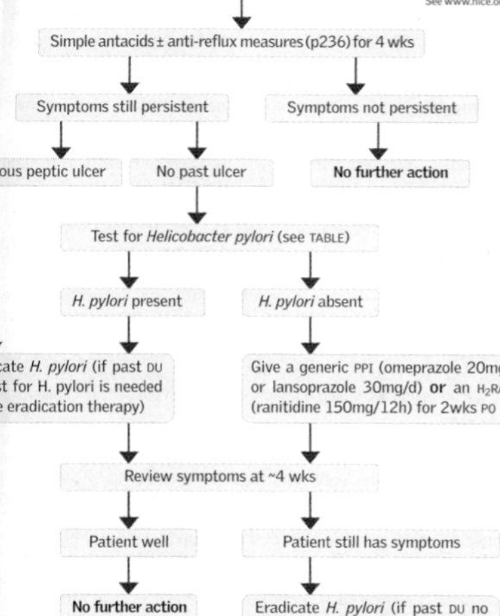

'hy do we use the ^{13}C breath test to detect *Helicobacter pylori*?

' all the non-invasive tests, the ^{13}C breath test is the most accurate.

st	Sensitivity	Specificity
vasive		
CLO test	95%	95%
Histology	95%	95%
Culture	90%	100%
n-invasive		
^{13}C breath test	95%	96%
Stool antigen	95%	94%
Serology	92%	83%

: Stop PPI 2 weeks before ^{13}C breath and stool antigen testing, as well 2 weeks before endoscopy.

'.pylori eradication (NICE/*BNF*): **either** PAC$_{500}$ regimen (full dose ***PPI***, ***amoxicillin*** 1g, ***clarithromycin*** mg) bd **or** PMC$_{250}$ (full dose ***PPI***, ***metronidazole*** 400mg, ***clarithromycin*** 250mg) bd for 7d. PPIs: ***prazole*** 20mg/12h; ***lansoprazole:*** 30mg/12h; PPI alternative: ***ranitidine bismuth citrate*** 400mg/12h. **stant cases:** ***tripotassium dicitratobismuthate*** (De Noltab® 2 bd ½h ac) + PPI + 2 antibiotics for 14d. nuth causes black stools: warn the patient!

Gastro-oesophageal reflux disease (GORD)

Dysfunction of the lower oesophageal sphincter predisposes to the gast oesophageal reflux of acid. If reflux is prolonged or excessive, it may ca oesophagitis, benign oesophageal stricture, or Barrett's oesophagus (p686).

Associations Smoking; alcohol; hiatus hernia (see below); pregnancy; obesity; meals; surgery in achalasia; drugs (tricyclics, anticholinergics, nitrates); syste sclerosis; *Helicobacter pylori?*[1] GORD can also contribute to asthma.

Symptoms Heartburn (burning, retrosternal discomfort related to meals, ly down, stooping, and straining, relieved by antacids); belching; acid brash (acid bile regurgitation); waterbrash (excessive salivation); odynophagia (pair swallowing, eg from oesophagitis or ulceration); nocturnal asthma (cough/whe with apparently minimal inhalation of gastric contents).

Complications Oesophagitis, ulcers, benign stricture, Barrett's oesophag oesophageal adenocarcinoma, and rarely iron deficiency anaemia.

ΔΔ: Oesophagitis (corrosives, NSAID); infection (CMV, herpes, *Candida*); DU; gast ulcers or cancers; non-ulcer dyspepsia.

Tests Isolated symptoms do not require investigation. ***Indications for uppe endoscopy:*** Age >55yrs; symptoms >4 wks; dysphagia; persistent sympto despite treatment; relapsing symptoms; weight↓. ***Endoscopic classification:*** BOX. At endoscopy, record complications of GORD (above) as *present* or *abs* Barium swallow may show hiatus hernia. 24h oesophageal pH monitoring oesophageal manometry help diagnose GORD when endoscopy is normal.

Treatment

- ***Lifestyle:*** **Encourage:** Weight loss; smoking cessation; raise the bed head; sm regular meals. **Avoid:** Hot drinks, alcohol, and eating <3h before bed. Avoid dr affecting oesophageal motility (nitrates, anticholinergics, tricyclic antidepre sants, calcium channel blockers—relax the lower oesophageal sphincter) or t damage the mucosa (NSAIDs, K^+ salts, bisphosphonates).
- ***Drugs:*** Antacids eg ***magnesium trisilicate mixture*** (10mL/8h) or alginates ***Gaviscon®*** (10–20mL/8h PO) relieve symptoms. If symptoms persist >4 weeks (or weight↓; dysphagia; excessive vomiting; GI bleeding), refer fo endoscopy. If oesophagitis confirmed, try a PPI (the most effective and m expensive drug option) eg ***lansoprazole*** 30mg/24h PO. Prokinetic drugs: Th help gastric emptying (eg ***metoclopramide*** 10mg/8h PO; dystonias can b serious side-effect). ***Cisapride*** is no longer licensed in the UK.
- ***Surgery:*** (eg Nissen fundoplication, p638) is not indicated unless symptoms severe, refractory to medical therapy **and** there is pH-monitoring evidence severe reflux. Laparoscopic repairs are gaining favour.

Hiatus hernia

The proximal stomach herniates through the diaphragm into the thorax. See fi

Sliding hiatus hernia (80%) is where the gastro-oesophageal junction slides into the chest—see BOX. ***Rolling hiatus hernia*** (20%) is where the gast oesophageal junction remains in the abdomen but a bulge of stomach herniates into the chest alongside the oesophagus—see BOX and fig 3.

Clinical features Common: 30% of patients >50yrs, especially obese women. 5 have symptomatic gastro-oesophageal reflux.

Imaging Barium swallow is the best diagnostic test; upper GI endoscopy allows ualization of the mucosa (?oesophagitis) but cannot reliably exclude a hiatus her

Management Lose weight. Treat reflux symptoms (see above). Indications surgery (eg Nissen, see above): intractable symptoms; recurrent stricture.

1 The role of *H. pylori* in GORD is still not yet established, with the evidence pointing both ways...

Gastroenterology

he Los Angeles (LA) classification of GORD

inor diffuse changes (erythema, oedema; friability) are not included, and the erm **mucosal break** (a well-demarcated area of slough/erythema) is used to ncompass the old terms erosion and ulceration. There are 4 grades:

One or more mucosal breaks <5mm long, not extending beyond 2 mucosal fold tops.

Mucosal break >5mm long limited to the space between 2 mucosal fold tops.

Mucosal break continuous between the tops of 2 or more mucosal folds but which involves less than 75% of the oesophageal circumference.

Mucosal break involving ≥75% of the oesophageal circumference. Useful though the grading is, it is still important to document the actual findings at endoscopy.

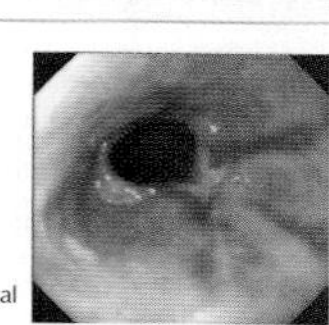

1. Upper GI endoscopy showing longitudinal mucosal aks in severe oesophagitis.

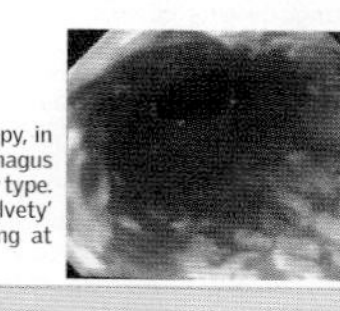

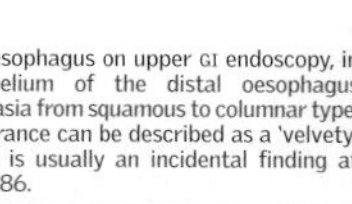

2. Barrett's oesophagus on upper GI endoscopy, in ich the epithelium of the distal oesophagus ergoes metaplasia from squamous to columnar type. loscopic appearance can be described as a 'velvety' thelium, and it is usually an incidental finding at loscopy. See p686.

atus hernia—sliding and rolling

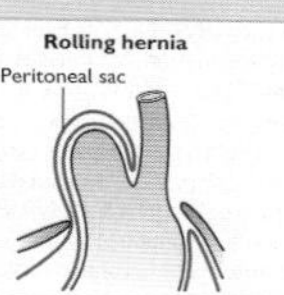

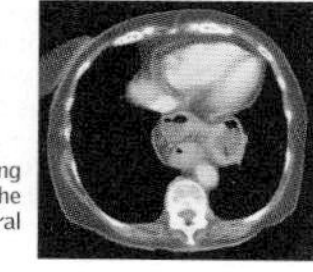

3. CT chest with IV contrast showing the rolling ponents of a hiatus hernia anterior to the phagus. Between the oesophagus and the vertebral umn on the left hand side, is the aorta.

Diarrhoea

Traveller's diarrhoea p3

Diarrhoea means increased stool water (hence ↑stool volume, eg >200mL daily), and this increases stool frequency and the passage of liquid stool. If it is the stool's fat content which is increased, use the term **steatorrhoea** (=pale, malodorous stool that is difficult to flush away, p272). Distinguish both from faecal urgency (which suggests rectal pathology eg cancer, UC).

Clinical features Take a detailed history:

- ***Acute or chronic?*** If acute suspect gastroenteritis. Ask about travel, change in diet, and contact history. Chronic diarrhoea alternating with constipation suggests irritable bowel (p248). Anorexia, weight↓, nocturnal diarrhoea & anaemia suggest an organic cause.
- ***Bloody diarrhoea:*** *Campylobacter, Shigella, Salmonella, E. Coli*, amoebiasis, UC, Crohn's disease, colorectal cancer (p612), colonic polyps, pseudomembranous colitis, ischaemic colitis (p488).
- ***Fresh PR bleeding:*** See p594.
- ***Mucus*** occurs in IBS, colorectal cancer, and polyps.
- ***Pus*** suggests IBD (inflammatory bowel disease), diverticulitis, or a fistula/abscess.
- ***Large bowel symptoms:*** Watery stool ± blood or mucus; pelvic pain relieved by defecation; tenesmus; urgency.
- ***Small bowel symptoms:*** periumbilical (or RIF) pain not relieved by defecation; watery stool or steatorrhoea.
- ***Non-GI causes:*** Antibiotics; PPIs; cimetidine; propranolol, cytotoxics; NSAIDs; digoxin; alcohol; laxative abuse); **medical conditions:** thyrotoxicosis; autonomic neuropathy; Addison's disease; carcinoid syndrome.

Common causes
• Gastroenteritis · Viral · Bacterial · Parasites/protozoa • IBS (p268) • Drugs (see below) • Colorectal cancer • Ulcerative colitis (UC • Crohn's disease • Coeliac disease
Uncommon causes
• Microscopic colitis[1] • Chronic pancreatitis • Bile salt malabsorptio • Thyrotoxicosis • Laxative abuse • Lactose intolerance • Ileal/gastric resectio • Overflow diarrhoea • Bacterial overgrow • Pseudomembranous colitis[2]
Rare causes
• Autonomic neuropathy • Addison's disease • Ischaemic colitis • Amyloidosis • Tropical sprue • Gastrinoma • VIPoma[3] • Carcinoid syndrome • Medullary thyroid c • Pellagra

Examination Look for weight↓, clubbing, anaemia, oral ulcers (p230), rashes and abdominal scars. Assess severity of dehydration (dry mucous membranes, ↓skin turgour and capillary refill >2s). **Feel** for an enlarged thyroid or an abdominal m Do a rectal examination for masses (eg rectal carcinoma), or impacted fa (overflow diarrhoea). Test for faecal occult blood.

Tests *Bloods:* FBC (iron deficiency; MCV↑ in coeliac disease, ↑alcohol use, Crohn's); U&E (K^+↓); ESR↑ (cancer, IBD); CRP↑ (infection, IBD). TSH↓ (thyrotoxico coeliac serology (p272 ± duodenal biopsy).

- ***Stool*** Test for pathogens & *C. difficile* toxin (pseudomembranous colitis).[2] Fa fat excretion or ^{13}C-hiolein (highly labelled triolein) breath test (nicer and able) if symptoms of chronic pancreatitis, malabsorption, or steatorrhoea.
- ***Rigid sigmoidoscopy*** with biopsy of normal and abnormal looking muc ~15% of patients with Crohn's disease have macroscopically normal muco
- ***Colonoscopy/Barium enema:*** To exclude malignancy and in colitis (►but during an acute episode). If normal, consider small bowel radiology (eg Cro disease) ± ERCP (eg chronic pancreatitis).

Management Treat causes. ***Oral rehydration*** is better than IV rehydratio impossible, give 0.9% saline + 20mmol K^+/L IVI. ***Codeine phosphate*** 30mg/6 or ***loperamide*** 2mg PO after each loose stool (max 16mg/day) reduce s frequency. Avoid antibiotics except in infective diarrhoea causing systemic ill (see p239 CHART)—because of the risk of developing antibiotic resistance.

1 Think of this in any chronic diarrhoea; do biopsy (may be +ve on normal looking colonic muc reported as 'lymphocytic' or 'collagenous' colitis). Prognosis: good. ***Budesonide*** is first-line th followed by a 5-aminosalycilic acid, ***bismuth subsalicylate*** (eg Pepto-Bismol®), or ***loperamide***.

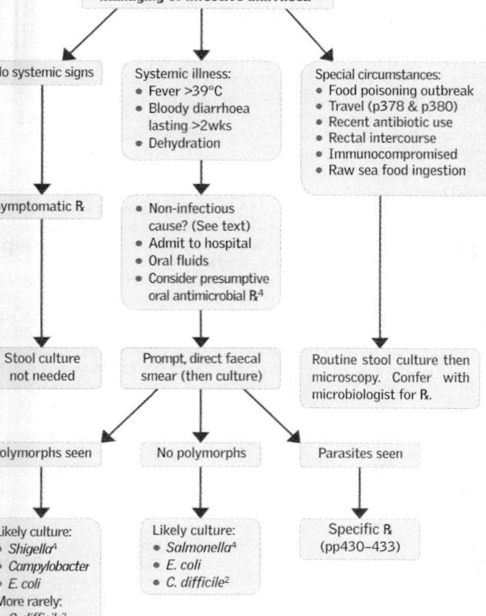

Be aware of your local pathogens, and be prepared to close wards and hospitals if contagion is afoot.
Pseudomembranous colitis is caused by overgrowth of *Clostridium difficile*. Risk factors: increasing ; any antibiotic therapy (especially IV); a stay in hospital. PCR is used to defect *C. difficite* toxins (CDT). atment: ***metronidazole*** 400mg/8h PO (cheaper and more palateable than the alternative ***vancomycin*** 5mg/6h PO). Most labs use ELISA to test for the enteropathic toxins A and B (sensitivity and specificity h >95%), though beware that mortality in test -ve cases have been reported—when in doubt liaise h a microbiologist about commencing therapy, especially in the elderly.
Vasoactive intestinal polypeptide-secreting tumour—suspect if hypokalaemic acidosis; $Ca^{2+}\uparrow$; $Mg^{2+}\downarrow$.
Prompt, specific treatment (eg ***ciprofloxacin***, p556) may be needed before sensitivities are known. guided by likely diagnosis following microscopy.

Constipation

Always ask the patient exactly what he means by 'constipation'—bowel habit var greatly between individuals and according to diet. There are various formal a different definitions of constipation but the infrequent passage of stool (<3 tir weekly) or difficulty in defecation, with straining or discomfort, is a reasonal practical working definition. The causes of constipation are numerous (see BOX

Clinical features Ask about frequency, nature, and consistency of the stool. there blood or mucus in/on the stools? Is there diarrhoea alternating w constipation? Has there been a recent change in bowel habit? Ask about diet a drugs. ►PR **examination** is essential.

Tests Most do not need investigation, especially young, mildly affected patien Indications for investigation: age >40yrs; change in bowel habit; associat symptoms (weight↓, PR mucus or blood, tenesmus). ***Blood tests:*** FBC, U&E, Ca^{2+}, T ***Sigmoidoscopy*** and biopsy of abnormal mucosa. ***Barium enema*** or ***colonoscop*** suspected colorectal malignancy. Special investigations (eg transit studi anorectal physiology) are occasionally needed.

Treatment Treat causes (BOX). Advise exercise and a good fluid intake (a high-fib diet is often advised, but may cause bloating without helping constipation). ►Co sider drugs only if these measures fail, and try to use them for short periods onl Often, a stimulant such as ***senna*** ± a bulking agent is more effective and cheap than agents such as ***lactulose***. ***Bulking agents*** ↑Faecal mass, so stimulati peristalsis. They must be taken with plenty of fluid and may take a few days to a CI: difficulty in swallowing; intestinal obstruction; colonic atony; faecal impacti ***Bran*** powder 3.5g 2–3 times/d with food (may hinder absorption of dietary tra elements if taken with every meal). ***Ispaghula husk***, eg 1 Fybogel® 3.5g sach after a meal, mixed in water and swallowed promptly (or else it becomes unpleasant sludge). ***Methylcellulose***, eg Celevac® 3–6 500mg tablets/12h w ≥300mL water. ***Sterculia***, eg Normacol® granules, 10mL sprinkled on food da

Stimulant laxatives increase intestinal motility, so do not use in intesti obstruction or acute colitis. Avoid prolonged use as it **may** cause colonic atony a hypokalaemia (but there are no good long-term data). Abdominal cramps are important SE. Pure stimulant laxatives are ***bisacodyl*** tablets (5–10mg at night) suppositories (10mg in the mornings) and ***senna*** (2–4 tablets at night). ***Docusa sodium*** and ***danthron***[2] (=dantron) have stimulant and softening actions. ***Glyce*** suppositories act as a rectal stimulant. ***Sodium picosulfate*** (5–10mg up to 1 beforehand) is useful for rapid bowel evacuation prior to procedures.

Stool softeners are particularly useful when managing painful anal conditions fissure. ***Arachis oil*** enemas lubricate and soften impacted faeces. ***Liquid paraf*** should not be used for a prolonged period (SE: anal seepage, lipoid pneumor malabsorption of fat-soluble vitamins).

Osmotic laxatives retain fluid in the bowel. ***Lactulose***, a semisynthetic disacchari produces osmotic diarrhoea of low faecal pH that discourages growth of ammor producing organisms. It is useful in hepatic encephalopathy (initial dose: 3 50mL/12h). SE: bloating ∴ it has a limited role in the treatment of constipati ***Magnesium salts*** (eg magnesium hydroxide; magnesium sulfate) are useful wh rapid bowel evacuation is required. ***Sodium salts*** (eg Microlette® and Micrala enemas) should be avoided as they may cause sodium and water retenti ***Phosphate enemas*** are useful for rapid bowel evacuation prior to procedures.

What if laxatives don't help? A multi-disciplinary approach with behavic therapy, psychological support, habit training ± sphincter-action biofeedback m help. $5HT_4$ agonists, which induce peristalsis by systemic rather than luminal mea are under trial (***tegaserod*** and ***prucalopride***: neither currently licensed in UK).

1 Risks of laxative abuse are overemphasized ('cathartic colon' is a questionable entity); stimu laxatives may be used chronically on those who do not respond to bulk or osmotic laxatives alone.
2 ***Danthron*** causes colon & liver tumours in animals, so reserve use for the very elderly or terminall

auses of constipation

eneral
- Poor diet
- Inadequate fluid intake or dehydration
- Immobility (or lack of exercise)
- Irritable bowel syndrome (p268)
- Old age
- Post-operative pain
- Hospital environment (lack of privacy, having to use a bed pan)
- Distant, squalid, or otherwise unsatisfactory toilets

norectal disease
- Anal fissure (p626)
- Anal stricture
- Rectal prolapse

testinal obstruction
- Colorectal carcinoma (p612)
- Strictures (eg Crohn's disease)
- Pelvic mass (eg fetus, fibroids)
- Diverticulosis (rectal bleeding is a commoner presentation)
- Pseudo-obstruction (p598)

etabolic/endocrine
- Hypercalcaemia (p672)
- Hypothyroidism (can cause constipation, but rare in those presenting with constipation—p204)
- Hypokalaemia (p668)
- Porphyria
- Lead poisoning

ugs (anticipate the potential effect and give dietary advice)
- Opiate analgesics (eg morphine, codeine)
- Anticholinergics (tricyclics, phenothiazines)
- Iron

uromuscular (slow transit with ↓propulsive activity)
- Spinal or pelvic nerve injury (eg trauma, surgery)
- Aganglionosis (Chagas' disease, Hirschsprung's disease)
- Systemic sclerosis
- Diabetic neuropathy

her causes
- Chronic laxative abuse (rare—diarrhoea is commoner)
- Idiopathic slow transit
- Idiopathic megarectum/colon
- Psychological (eg associated with depression or abuse as a child).

Constipation alone is unlikely to be a symptom of serious organic disease and erefore can be met with reassurance.

Jaundice

Jaundice (**icterus**) refers to yellow pigmentation of skin, sclerae, and mucosae to ↑plasma bilirubin (visible at >35μmol/L—not always easy to spot when mi Jaundice is classified by the site of the problem (pre-hepatic, hepatocellular, cholestatic/obstructive) or by the type of circulating bilirubin (conjugated or unc ugated). **Kernicterus** is seen in infants with unconjugated hyperbilirubinaemia involves deposition of jaundice in the basal ganglia, which can cause **opisthotor**

Bilirubin metabolism (see BOX) Bilirubin is formed from the breakdowr haemoglobin. It is conjugated with glucuronic acid by hepatocytes, making it wa soluble. Conjugated bilirubin is secreted into the bile and passes out into the g Some is taken up again by the liver (via the enterohepatic circulation) and the is converted to urobilinogen by gut bacteria. Urobilinogen is either reabsorbed excreted by the kidneys, or converted to stercobilin, which colours faeces bro

Pre-hepatic jaundice If there is ↑bilirubin production (haemolysis), ↓liver upt or ↓conjugation, unconjugated bilirubin enters the blood. As it is water insolubl does not enter urine resulting in **unconjugated (acholuric) hyperbilirubinaer** ***Causes:*** Physiological (neonatal); haemolysis; dyserythropoiesis; glucurc transferase deficiency (Gilbert's, p692, & Crigler–Najjar syndromes, p688).

Hepatocellular jaundice There is hepatocyte damage, usually with some ch stasis. ***Causes:*** Viruses: hepatitis (p394, eg A, B, C, etc.), CMV (p392), EBV (p3 drugs (see TABLE); alcoholic hepatitis; cirrhosis; liver metastases/abscess; hae chromatosis; autoimmune hepatitis (AIH); septicaemia; leptospirosis; α_1-antitry deficiency (p256); Budd–Chiari (p688); Wilson's disease (p257); failure to exc conjugated bilirubin (Dubin–Johnson, p690, and Rotor syndromes, p702); right he failure; toxins, eg carbon tetrachloride; fungi (*Amanita phalloides*, fig 1).

Cholestatic (obstructive) jaundice If the common bile duct is blocked, conjuga bilirubin overspills into the blood causing a **conjugated hyperbilirubinaemia**. Be water soluble, it is excreted in urine, making it dark. Less conjugated bilirubin ent the bowel and the faeces become pale. When severe, it can be associated with intractable pruritus which is best treated by relief of the obstruction. ***Caus*** Common bile duct gallstones; pancreatic cancer; lymph nodes at the porta hepa drugs (see BOX); cholangiocarcinoma; primary sclerosing cholangitis; primary bil cirrhosis; choledochal cyst; biliary atresia; Mirrizi's syndrome (obstructive jaun secondary to compression of the common hepatic duct by a gallstone impacte the cystic duct, often associated with cholangitis).

Clinical features ***Ask*** about blood transfusions, intravenous drug use, b piercing, tattoos, sexual activity, travel abroad, jaundiced contacts, family hist alcohol consumption, and **all** medications (eg old drug charts; GP records). ***Exam*** for signs of chronic liver disease (p252), hepatic encephalopathy (p250), lym adenopathy, hepatomegaly, splenomegaly, ascites and a palpable gall blac (which in conjunction with painless jaundice suggests a cause other t gallstones—Courvoisier's 'law'). Pale stools with dark urine ≈ obstructive jaunc

Tests See BOX (p257) for screening tests in suspected liver disease. ***Urine:*** Bilir is absent in pre-hepatic causes, hence 'acholuric' jaundice; urobilinogen is abse obstructive jaundice. ***Haematology:*** FBC, clotting, blood film, reticulocyte co Coombs' test. ***Biochemistry:*** U&E, LFT[1] (bilirubin, ALT, AST, alk phos, γ-GT, total pro albumin). ***Ultrasound:*** Are the bile ducts dilated >6mm (obstruction—see fi p723)? Are there gallstones, hepatic metastases or a pancreatic mass? E (p728) if bile ducts are dilated and LFT not improving. ***MRCP*** (p729) or endosc ultrasound (EUS) if conventional ultrasound shows gallstones but no definite c mon bile duct stones. Perform a ***liver biopsy*** (p248) if the bile ducts are nor Consider abdominal ***CT*** or ***MRI*** if abdominal malignancy is suspected clinically

1 Albumin and INR are the best indicators of hepatic synthetic function. ↑Transaminases (ALT, AST) inc hepatocyte damage. ↑Alk phos is typical of obstructive jaundice, but also occurs in hepatocellular jau malignant infiltration, pregnancy (placental isoenzyme), Paget's disease and childhood (bone isoenzy

he pathway of bilirubin metabolism

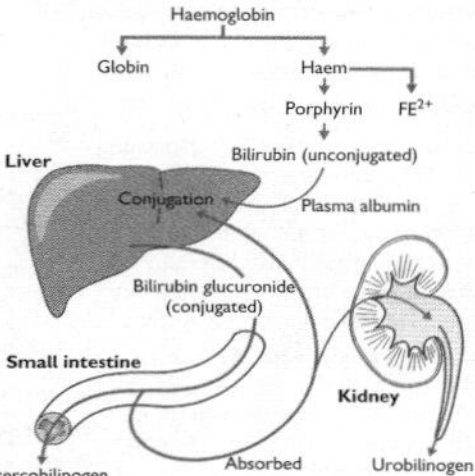

auses of jaundice in a previously stable patient with cirrhosis

Sepsis: especially emanating from UTI, pneumonia, or SBP (see p252).
Alcohol
Drugs: see TABLE
Malignancy: eg hepatocellular carcinoma
GI bleeding
ook for signs of decompensation: ascites; dilated abdominal veins; neurological nset; peripheral oedema.

rug-induced jaundice

Haemolysis	• Antimalarials • Dapscine
Hepatitis	• ***Paracetamol*** overdose (p828) • Anti-TB (***isoniazid, rifampicin, pyrazinamide***) • Statins (BOX, p101) • ***Sodium valproate*** • Monoamine oxidase inhibitors • ***Halothane*** (any recent anaesthetics?)
Cholestasis	• Antibiotics (***flucloxacillin***—may occur weeks after treatment, ***fusidic acid, co-amoxiclav, nitrofurantoin***) • Anabolic steroids • Oral contraceptives • ***Chlorpromazine*** • ***Prochlorperazine*** • Sulfonylureas • ***Gold***

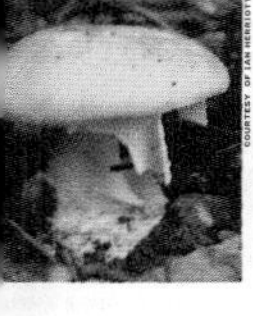

Fig 1. *Amanita phalloides*, or the 'death cap', is a lethal cause of jaundice—it is, in fact, the most lethal mushroom in the world. Its hepatotoxic effects are mediated by amatoxins that induce hepatic necrosis. Ingestion (usually as a result of misidentification from its benign appearance) can result in death through acute liver failure, though cases have been treated successfully with liver transplantation. NB: Not to be used for identification purposes.

Upper gastrointestinal bleeding: 1

Haematemesis is vomiting of blood. It may be bright red or look like coffee grou **Melaena** (from the Greek *melas* = black) means black motions, often like tar, has a characteristic smell of altered blood. Both indicate upper GI bleeding.

►Take a brief history and examine to assess severity.

History Ask about previous GI bleeds; dyspepsia or known ulcers (p234); known liver disease or oesophageal varices (p246); dysphagia; vomiting; weight loss. Check drugs (see MINIBOX) and alcohol consumption. Is there serious co-morbidity (bad for prognosis) eg cardiovascular disease, respiratory disease, hepatic or renal impairment, or malignancy?

Examination Look for signs of chronic liver disease (p252) and do a PR to check for melaena. Is the patient shocked? "Do you feel faint when you sit up?"

- Peripherally shut down (cool and clammy); capillary refilling (CR) time >2s.
- ↓GCS (may be tricky to assess in decompensated liver disease) or signs of encephalopathy (p251).
- Poor urine output, eg <25mL/h or <½mL/kg/h.
- Tachycardic (pulse >100bpm, and JVP not raised).
- Hypotensive (systolic BP <100mmHg)
- Postural drop in BP (>20mmHg systolic).

Calculate the ***Rockall risk score*** (see TABLE).

Common causes

- Mallory–Weiss tear
- Oesophagitis
- Oesophageal varices
- Peptic ulcers
- Gastritis/gastric erosic
- Duodenitis
- Malignancy
- Drugs (NSAIDs, aspirin, steroids, thrombolytics anticoagulants)
- No obvious cause

Rare causes

- Bleeding disorders
- Portal hypertensive gastropathy
- Aorto-enteric fistula[1]
- Angiodysplasia
- Haemobilia
- Dieulafoy lesion[2]
- Meckel's diverticulum
- Peutz–Jeghers' syndro
- Osler–Weber–Rendu s

Acute management (see p778). In summary:

- ►► Protect airway and give high-flow oxygen.
- ►► Insert 2 large-bore (14–16G) IV cannulae and take blood for FBC (an early may be normal because haemodilution has not yet taken place), U&E (↑urea of proportion to creatinine is indicative of a massive blood meal), LFT, clott and cross-match 4–6 units (give 1 unit per g/dL <14g/dL).
- ►► Give IV crystalloid to restore intravascular volume while waiting for blood t crossmatched.[MET 44] In a dire emergency—ie haemodynamically deteriora despite fluid resuscitation measures—give group O Rh-ve blood.
- ►► Insert a urinary catheter and monitor hourly urine output.
- ►► Organize a CXR, ECG, and check ABG.
- ►► Consider a CVP line to monitor and guide fluid replacement.
- ►► Transfuse (with crossmatched blood) until haemodynamically stable.
- ►► Correct clotting abnormalities (***vitamin K***, FFP, platelets).
- ►► Monitor pulse, BP, and CVP (keep >5cm H_2O) at least hourly until stable.
- ►► Arrange an urgent ***endoscopy***, preferably at a dedicated endoscopy unit.[45]
- ►► Inform surgeons of all severe bleeds on admission.

Further management

- Re-examine after 4h and give FFP if >4 units transfused.
- Monitor pulse, BP, CVP, and urine output hourly; ↓frequency to 4hrl haemodynamically stable.
- Transfuse to keep Hb >10g/dL; always keep 2 units of blood in reserve.
- Give ***omeprazole*** 40 mg IV **after** endoscopy (reduces risk of rebleeding and r for surgery, but not mortality, in peptic ulcer bleeding).[MET 46]
- Check FBC, U&E, LFT, and clotting daily.
- Keep nil by mouth for 24h. Allow clear fluids after 24h and light diet after as long as there is no evidence of rebleeding (p246).

►►See p246 for additional management in suspected variceal beeding.

1 A patient with an aortic graft repair and upper GI bleeding is considered to have an aorto-ent fistula until proven otherwise: CT abdomen is usually required as well as endoscopy.
2 A Dieulafoy lesion is the rupture of an unusually big arteriole, eg in the fundus of the stomach.

ʀockall risk-scoring for upper GI bleeds

	0 pts	1 pt	2 pts	3 pts
ʀre-endoscopy				
ʌge[I]	<60yrs	60–79yrs	≥80yrs	
ʃhock: systolic ʀ pulse rate[I]	BP >100mmHg <100/min	BP >100mmHg Pulse >100/min	BP <100mmHg	
ɔo-morbidity[I]	Nil major	Cardiac failure Ischaemic heart disease	Renal failure Liver failure	Metastases
ʼost-endoscopy				
ɪiagnosis[F]	Mallory–Weiss tear; no lesion; no sign of recent bleeding	All other diagnoses	Upper GI malignancy	
ɪigns of recent aemorrhage on ndoscopy[F]	None, or dark red spot		Blood in upper GI tract; adherent clot; visible vessel	

These criteria make up the initial Rockall score, which is a more reliable predictor of mortality in ɛptic ulcer bleeding than the final score.
Added to the initial score, these criteria make up the final Rockall score.

ʀediction of rebleeding and mortality from the Rockall score

ɔckall scores help predict risk of rebleeding and mortality after upper GI bleedɡ. An initial score >6 is said to be an indication for surgery, but decisions lating to surgery are rarely taken on the basis of Rockall scores alone (p246).

Score	Mortality: Initial score	Mortality: Final score (after endoscopy)
0	0.2%	0%
1	2.4%	0%
2	5.6%	0.2%
3	11.0%	2.9%
4	24.6%	5.3%
5	39.6%	10.8%
6	48.9%	17.3%
7	50.0%	27.0%
8+	-	41.1%

ɔle adapted from *Mangement Guidelines of Haematemesis and/or Malaena 2004*, at p://static.oxfordradcliffe.net/med/gems/HMGuidelines04.pdf.

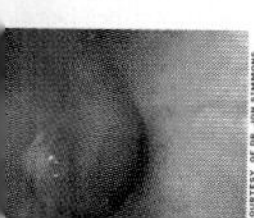

Fig 1. Upper GI endoscopy image of a duodenal ulcer. See p234 for the topic of peptic ulceration and 'Lumen' BOX, p227, for possible enlightenment.

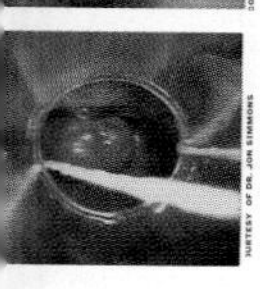

Fig 2. Upper GI endoscopy image of variceal banding. The technique involves sucking up a varix into the transparent banding chamber, then placing an elastic band around the varix. After a few days the banded varix starts to slough, leaving behind scar tissue in a shallow ulcer. See also p246.

Upper GI bleeding: 2 and ➤➤bleeding varices

Endoscopy should be arranged after resuscitation, within 4h of a suspec variceal haemorrhage, or when bleeding is ongoing within 24h of admission. It c identify the site of bleeding, be used to estimate the risk of rebleeding, and administer treatment, preferably 2 of: eg *adrenaline*, sclerotherapy, varic banding (fig 2, p245) or argon plasma coagulation (for superficial lesions *Endoscopic signs associated with risk of rebleeding:* active arterial bleed (80% risk); visible vessel (50% risk); adherent clot/black dots (30% risk).

Rebleeding 40% of rebleeders die of complications. Identify high-risk patie (TABLE, p245) and monitor closely for signs of rebleeding. IV *omeprazole* ha preventive role. Get help; **inform a surgeon at once if:** • Haematemesis w melaena • ↑pulse rate; • ↓CVP (assess via JVP or CVP line) • ↓BP; • ↓urine outp

Indications for surgery (p638) ►Contact the surgical team at the onset
- Severe bleeding or bleeding despite transfusing 6U if >60yrs (8U if <60yrs)
- Rebleeding
- Active or uncontrollable bleeding at endoscopy
- Initial Rockall score ≥3 or final Rockall score >6 (but see TABLE, p245).

Varices Portal hypertension causes dilated collateral veins (varices) at sites portosystemic anastomosis. Varices most commonly occur in the lower oesophag but may also be found in the stomach around the umbilicus (*caput medusae* is ra and in the rectum. Varices develop in patients with cirrhosis once portal press (measured by hepatic venous pressure gradient) is >10mmHg; if >12mmHg vari bleeding may develop—associated with a mortality of 30–50% per episode.[50]

Other causes of portal hypertension ***Pre-hepatic:*** Portal vein thrombosis; sple vein thrombosis. ***Intrahepatic:*** Cirrhosis (80% in UK); schistosomiasis (commor worldwide); sarcoidosis; myeloproliferative diseases; congenital hepatic fibro ***Post-hepatic:*** Budd–Chiari syndrome (p688); right heart failure; constric pericarditis; veno-occlusive disease. ***Risk factors for variceal haemorrha*** ↑Portal pressure, variceal size, endoscopic features of the variceal wall haematocystic spots) and Child–Pugh score ≥8 (see TABLE, P253).[51]

Suspect varices as a cause of GI bleeding if there is alcohol abuse or cirrho Look for signs of chronic liver disease, encephalopathy, splenomegaly, asc hyponatraemia, coagulopathy and thrombocytopaenia.

Prophylaxis ***Primary*** Without treatment ~30% of cirrhotic patients with var bleed—reducible to 15% by: **1** non-selective β-blockade (***propranolol*** 40–80mg/ PO) **2** Repeat endoscopic banding ligation. One recent study showed that ban had significantly better outcome than β-blocker therapy in patients with cirrhosi Endoscopic sclerotherapy is not used as complications (eg stricturing) may outw benefits.[53] ***Secondary*** After an initial variceal bleed, risk of further bleedir high—80% will rebleed within 2 years. Options are **1** and **2** as above + transjuc intrahepatic portosystemic shunting (TIPSS)[1] for varices resistant to bandin surgical shunts if TIPSS is impossible for technical reasons. Endoscopic banding be better than sclerotherapy (lower bleeding rates & fewer complications).[MET 54]

Acute variceal bleeding Get help at the bedside from your senior.
- ➤➤Resuscitate until haemodynamically stable (do not give 0.9% saline).
- ➤➤Correct clotting abnormalities with ***vitamin K*** and FFP.
- ➤➤Start IVI of ***terlipressin*** 2mg bolus, then 2mg/4h for ≤3d; relative risk of dea by 34%).[55] Somatostatin analogues are no longer used in the UK.[MET 56]
- ➤➤Endoscopic banding (p245, fig 2) or sclerotherapy should be tried (banding be impossible because of limited visualization).
- ➤➤If bleeding uncontrolled, a Minnesota tube or Sengstaken–Blakemore tube BOX) should be placed by someone with experience; get anaesthetist's help

1 TIPSS works by shunting blood away from the portal circulation through an artificial side-t portosystemic anastamosis created in the liver; also used in uncontrolled variceal haemorrhage.

alloon tamponade with a Sengstaken–Blakemore tube

ı life-threatening variceal bleeding, this can buy time to arrange transfer ɔ a specialist liver centre or for surgical decompression. It uses balloons to ɔmpress gastric and oesophageal varices. Before insertion, inflate balloons with measured volume (120–300mL) of air giving pressures of 60mmHg (check ɪith a sphygmomanometer).

- Deflate, and clamp exits.
- Pass the lubricated tube (try to avoid sedation) and inflate the gastric balloon with the predetermined volume of air. Cooling the tube beforehand probably doesn't make it any easier to pass.
- Check position with a portable x-ray before inflating the oesophageal balloon. Check pressures (should be 20–30mmHg greater than on the trial run). This phase of the procedure is dangerous: do not over inflate the balloon because of the risk of oesophageal necrosis or rupture.
- Tape to patient's forehead to ensure the gastric balloon impacts gently on the gastro-oesophageal junction.
- Place the oesophageal aspiration channel on continuous low suction and arrange for the gastric channel to drain freely.
- Leave *in situ* until bleeding stops. Remove after <24h.

ɜrious other techniques of insertion may be used, and tubes vary in ructure. ►**Do not try to pass one yourself if you have no or little experience:** ɪk an expert; if unavailable, transfer urgently to a specialist liver centre.

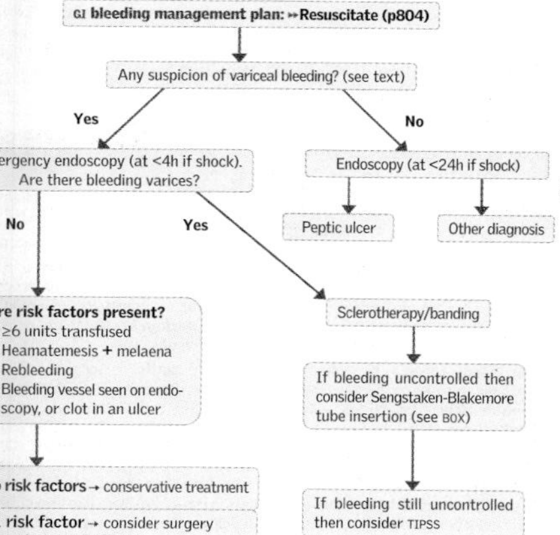

Endoscopy and biopsy

►**Consent** is required for all these interventions and procedures—see p554.

Upper GI endoscopy ***Indications:*** See TABLE. ***Pre-procedure:*** Stop anti-ac therapy for 2 weeks beforehand if possible—these mask diagnosis of up to ~30% adenocarcinomas. Nil by mouth for 8h (but water up to 4h pre-op may be o Advise the patient not to drive for 24h if sedation is being given. Arrange follo up. ***Procedure:*** Sedation may be given (eg ***midazolam*** 1–5mg IV; monitor saturation with a pulse oximeter). The pharynx is sprayed with local anaesthe and a flexible endoscope is passed. Continuous suction must be available to preve aspiration. ***Complications:*** Transient sore throat; amnesia following sedati perforation (<0.1%); cardiorespiratory arrest (<0.1%).

Duodenal biopsy is the gold standard for diagnosing coeliac disease (p272). It also useful in investigating unusual causes of malabsorption, eg giardias lymphoma, Whipple's disease, amyloid, or microscopic colitis (p238).

Sigmoidoscopy views the rectum; rigid or flexible sigmoidoscopy should prece barium enema in suspected colorectal cancer. Flexible sigmoidoscopes gain bet access than rigid ones (→splenic flexure), but ~25% of colon cancers are still c of reach. It can be used therapeutically (±insertion of a flatus tube) decompression of sigmoid volvulus (Box, p599). ***Preparation:*** Give 2 ***phospho enemas.*** ***Procedure:*** PR examination is performed first. Do biopsies—macrosco appearances may be normal in some diseases, eg IBD, amyloidosis, microscopic coli

Colonoscopy ***Indications:*** See TABLE. ***Preparation:*** Prescribe ***sodium picosulfa*** (Picolax®) 1 sachet for the morning and afternoon of the day before the procedu ***Procedure:*** PR examination is performed first. Sedation (monitor O_2 saturation w a pulse oximeter) and analgesia are given before a flexible colonoscope is pass and guided around the colon. ***Complications:*** Abdominal discomfort; incompl examination; perforation (0.1%); haemorrhage after biopsy or polypectomy.

Capsule endoscopy ***Indications:*** Assessment of small bowel disease, especially in Crohn's (after exclusion of strictures with a small bowel contrast study) or obscure/occult GI bleeding. Also now able to image the oesophagus, despite quick transit time. ***Pre-procedure:*** Clear fluids only the evening before and then nil by mouth from 10pm. ***Procedure:*** A pill-sized capsule (fig 1) transmits video images via radiowaves to pads on the skin. Information is stored in a device worn on the b Normal activity can take place during the examination. ***Complications:*** Caps retention (occurs in 1%: endoscopic or surgical removal is required); obstruct (usually in the terminal ileum or site of a stricture); incomplete examination battery failure, slow transit, achalasia). ***Disadvantages:*** Unable to perfo therapeutic intervention and gives poor localisation of lesions.

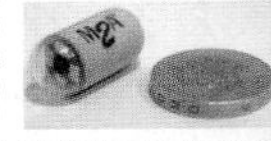

Fig 1. The size of a capsu in comparison to a £1 coin.

Liver biopsy This may be done percutaneously (if clotting is normal) or via transjugular route with FFP cover. ***Indications:*** Abnormal LFT, chronic v hepatitis; alcoholic hepatitis; autoimmune hepatitis (AIH); suspected cirrho suspected carcinoma; biopsy of hepatic lesions; investigation of PUO. Now usu performed with US/CT guidance. ***Pre-procedure:*** Nil by mouth for 8h. Ch clotting (INR <1.5) and platelet count (>100 × 10^9/L). Prescribe analge ***Procedure:*** Sedation may be given. If not done under US guidance, the liver bord are percussed out and where there is dullness in the mid-axillary line in expirat local anaesthetic (***lidocaine*** 2%) is infiltrated down to the liver capsule. Breath is rehearsed and a needle biopsy is taken with the breath held in expirat Afterwards the patient lies on the right side for 2h, then in bed for 6h wi regular pulse and BP observations are taken. ***Complications:*** Local p pneumothorax; bleeding (<0.5%); death (<0.1%).

[I]ndications for upper GI endoscopy

[D]iagnostic indications	Therapeutic indication
• Haematemesis • Dyspepsia (>55yrs old p234) • Gastric biopsy (?cancer) • Duodenal biopsy • Persistent vomiting • Iron deficiency anaemia	• Treatment of bleeding lesions • Variceal banding and sclerotherapy • Stricture dilatation • Palliation eg stent insertion, laser therapy • Argon plasma coagulation for suspected vascular abnormality

[I]ndications for colonoscopy

[D]iagnostic indications	Therapeutic indication
• Rectal bleeding—when settled, if acute • Iron deficiency anaemia • Persistent diarrhoea • Biopsy of lesion seen on barium enema • Assessment or suspicion of IBD • Colon cancer surveillance • *Streptococcus bovis* endocarditis.[1]	• Polypectomy • Angiodysplasia (argon plasma photocoagulation) • Decompression • Pseudo-obstruction • Volvulus

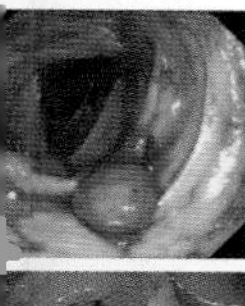

Fig 1. Colonoscopy image of a large colonic polyp. An advantage of colonoscopy over barium enema is the ability to perform biopsy or intervention at the same time—in this case, polypectomy.

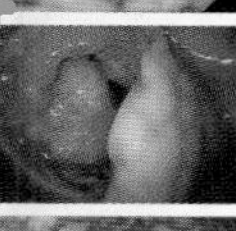

Fig 2. Colonoscopy image of a colonic adenocarcinoma—see p612. Compared to a colonic polyp (fig 1), the carcinoma is irregular in shape and colour, larger and more aggressive.

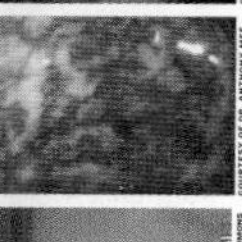

Fig 3. Colonoscopy image of the colonic mucosa in active ulcerative colitis (UC). The mucosa is red, inflamed and can be friable (bleed on touching). In more severe disease there may also be endoscopic findings of mucopurulent exudate, mucosal ulceration, and spontaneous bleeding. In quiescent disease there may only be a distorted or absent mucosal vascular pattern. See p264 for the topic of UC.

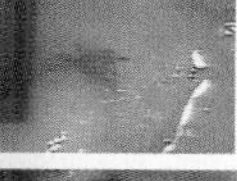

Fig 4. Colonoscopy image of a small angiodyplasia lesion in the colonic mucosa. Argon plasma coagulation is a common treatment for this condition—see p588.

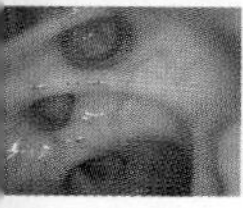

Fig 5. Colonoscopy image showing diverticulosis of the colon. Navigating safely through the colon, avoiding the false lumina of the diverticula can be a challenge. Endoscopy is avoided if the diverticula are acutely inflamed in an attack of diverticulitis because of the risk of perforation. See p588 for the topic of diverticular disease.

[O]ther endoscopy images: See www.gastrosource.com/kisweb/atlas.htm

[1] [T]he cancer is the portal of entry: think of this whenever *Strep. bovis* is cultured from the blood.

Liver failure

Definitions Liver failure may occur suddenly in the previously healthy liver: **acu hepatic failure**. More commonly it occurs as a result of decompensation of chro liver disease = **acute-on-chronic hepatic failure**. **Fulminant hepatic failure** is clinical syndrome resulting from massive necrosis of liver cells leading to seve impairment of liver function: **hyperacute** = encephalopathy within 7d of onset jaundice; **acute** = within 8–28d; **subacute** = within 5–26 weeks. There is decreas risk of cerebral oedema as the onset of encephalopathy is increasingly delayed.

Causes ***Infections:*** Viral hepatitis, yellow fever, leptospirosis. ***Drugs:*** Paraceta overdose, halothane, isoniazid. ***Toxins:*** *Amanita phalloides* mushroom (fig 1, p24 carbon tetrachloride. ***Vascular:*** Budd–Chiari syndrome (p688), veno-occlus disease. ***Others:*** Alcohol hepatitis, primary biliary cirrhosis, haemochromato autoimmune hepatitis, α_1-antitrypsin deficiency, Wilson's disease, fatty liver pregnancy (*OHCS* p26), malignancy.

Signs Jaundice, hepatic encephalopathy (see TABLE), *fetor hepaticus* (smells li pear drops), asterixis, constructional apraxia (ask the patient to draw a 5-point star). Signs of chronic liver disease (p252) suggest acute-on-chronic hepatic failu

Tests ***Blood:*** FBC (?infection,[1] ?GI bleed), U&E,[2] LFT, clotting (↑PT/INR), glucose, pa cetamol level, hepatitis, CMV & EBV serology, ferritin, α_1-antitrypsin, caeruloplasm autoantibodies (p539). ***Microbiology:*** Blood culture; urine culture; ascitic tap M,C+S of ascites—neutrophils >250/mm^3 indicates spontaneous bacter peritonitis (p252). ***Radiology:*** CXR; abdominal ultrasound; Doppler flow studies the portal vein (& hepatic vein in suspected Budd–Chiari syndrome, p688). ***Neu physiology:*** EEG, evoked potentials (and neuroimaging) have a limited role.

Management ⇒Beware **sepsis**, **hypoglycaemia**, and **encephalopathy**:
- Nurse with a 20° head-up tilt in ITU. Protect the airway with intubation a insert an NG tube to avoid aspiration and remove any blood from stomach.
- Insert urinary and central venous catheters to assess fluid status.
- Monitor T°, respirations, pulse, BP, pupils, urine output hourly. Daily weights
- Check FBC, U&E, LFT, and INR daily.
- 10% dextrose IV, 1L/12h to avoid hypoglycaemia. Do blood glucose every 1–
- Treat the cause, if known (eg paracetamol poisoning, p828). N-acetylcyste probably does not help in non-paracetamol liver failure.
- If malnourished, get dietary help because good nutrition ↓ mortality (eg diet r in carbohydrate- and protein-derived calories, preferably orally). Give thiam and folate supplements.
- Haemofiltration or haemodialysis, if renal failure develops (see BOX).
- Avoid sedatives or other drugs with hepatic metabolism (see BOX and *BNF*), t treat seizures with ***lorazepam***.
- Consider PPI as prophylaxis against stress ulceration eg ***omeprazole*** 40mg/d
- Liaise early with nearest transplant centre regarding appropriateness—see B

Treat complications ***Bleeding:*** ***Vitamin K*** 10mg/d IV for 3d, platelets, FFP + bl as needed. ***Infection:*** Until sensitivities are known, give ***ceftriaxone*** 1–2g/24h ►Avoid ***gentamicin*** (↑risk of renal failure). ***Ascites:*** Fluid restriction, low-salt d daily weights, diuretics (see p252). ***Hypoglycaemia:*** Check blood glucose regul and give 50mL of 50% glucose IV if levels fall below 2mmol/L or symptoma ***Encephalopathy:*** Avoid sedatives; 20° head-up tilt in ITU; ***lactulose*** 30–50mls, PO + regular enemas to ↓numbers of nitrogen-forming bowel organisms. Aim 2–4 soft stools/d. ***Cerebral oedema:*** Give 20% ***mannitol*** IV; hyperventilate.

Prognosis Poor prognostic factors: Grade III or IV encephalopathy, age >40 albumin <30g/L, ↑INR, drug-induced liver failure, late-onset hepatic failure wo than fulminant failure. 65% survival post-transplantation.

1 Neutrophilic leucocytosis need not mean a secondary infection: alcoholic hepatitis may be the cause i
2 As urea is synthesized in the liver, it is a poor test of renal function in liver failure, so use creatinine inste

Hepatic encephalopathy

As the liver fails, nitrogenous waste (as ammonia) builds up in the circulation and passes to the brain, where astrocytes clear it (by processes involving the conversion of glutamate to glutamine). This excess glutamine causes an osmotic imbalance and a shift of fluid into these cells—hence cerebral oedema.[65]

Grade I	Altered mood/behaviour; sleep disturbance (eg reversed sleep pattern)
Grade II	Increasing drowsiness; confusion, slurred speech
Grade III	Stupor; incoherence; restlessness, significant confusion
Grade IV	Coma

►Other causes of reduced conscious level should always be ruled out when considering hepatic encephalopathy—eg sepsis, trauma, hypoglycaemia or seizure activity.

What is hepatorenal syndrome (HRS)?

HRS is not well understood. It occurs in ~18% of cirrhotic patients with ascites, showing splanchnic arterial vasodilatation, ↓effective circulatory volume, (↓venous return and cardiac output),[66] intense renal vasoconstriction, ↓glomerular filtration rate, and **normal** renal histology. Raised neuropeptide Y (NPY) and activation of the renin-angiotensin-aldosterone axis occur, further worsening renal vasoconstriction. ADH levels also ↑ in an attempt to restore intravascular volume. ►It is important to make the diagnosis only after other causes of renal impairment have been excluded. Two types of HRS have been described: ***HRS 1*** is a rapidly progressive deterioration in circulatory and renal function (median survival <2weeks); ***HRS 2*** is a more steady deterioration (median survival ~6 months). Other factors in cirrhosis may contribute to poor renal function (p253).

Treatment is IV ***albumin*** + arterial vasocontrictors eg ***terlipressin*** to replenish the depleted volume. Haemodialysis (as supportive therapy) and TIPSS (p246) may be required. Liver transplantation remains treatment of choice, even after improvement in renal function, since prognosis is so poor.[67]

Prescribing in liver failure

Avoid opiates, diuretics (↑risk of encephalopathy), oral hypoglycaemics, and saline-containing IVIs. ***Warfarin*** effects are enhanced. ***Hepatotoxic drugs include:*** Paracetamol, methotrexate, phenothiazines, isoniazid, azathioprine, oestrogen, 6-mercaptopurine, salicylates, tetracycline, mitomycin.

King's College Hospital[UK] criteria for liver transplantation

Paracetamol liver failure	• Arterial pH <7.3 24h after ingestion **Or all of the following:** • Prothrombin time (PT) >100s • Creatinine >300µmol/L • Grade III or IV encephalopathy
Non-paracetamol liver failure	• PT >100s **Or 3 out of 5 of the following:** 1 Drug-induced liver failure 2 Age <10 or >40 yrs old 3 >1wk between onset of jaundice and encephalopathy 4 PT >50s 5 Bilirubin >300µmol/L

Fulfilment of the criteria is a good predictor of poor outcome in acute liver failure, but failure to meet the criteria does not predict survival. Transplantation is either **cadaveric** (heart-beating or non-heart-beating)[1] or from **live donors** (right lobe)—may cause a biliary fistula. Gaining **valid consent** from the donor is difficult (see BOX, p555). See also BOX, p255 for indications in chronic disease.

1 There has been a recent renewed interest and ↑ in the number of non-heart-beating cadaveric donors.

Cirrhosis

Cirrhosis (Greek *kirrhos* = yellow) implies irreversible liver damage. Histological there is loss of normal hepatic architecture with fibrosis and nodular regeneratic

Causes Most commonly chronic alcohol abuse, HBV, and HCV infection. Others: see BC

Signs May be none (just ↑LFT) or decompensated end-stage liver disease. ***Chron liver disease:*** Leuconychia: white nails with lunulae undemarcated, from hyp albuminaemia; Terry's nails—white proximally but distal ⅓ reddened by telanc ectasias; clubbing; palmar erythema; hyperdynamic circulation; Dupuytrer contracture; spider naevi (fig. 1); xanthelasmata; gynaecomastia; atrophic teste loss of body hair; parotid enlargement; hepatomegaly, or small liver in late diseas

Complications ***Hepatic failure:*** Coagulopathy (↓factors II, VII, IX, & X causes ↑INF encephalopathy—ie liver flap (asterixis) + confusion/coma; hypoalbuminaem (oedema, leuconychia); sepsis (pneumonia; septicaemia); spontaneous bacteri peritonitis (SBP); hypoglycaemia. ***Portal hypertension:*** Ascites (fig 2); splenomega portosystemic shunt including oesophageal varices (± life-threatening upper bleed) and *caput medusae* (enlarged superficial periumbilical veins). ***HCC:*** ↑risk

Tests ***Blood:*** LFT: ↔ or ↑bilirubin, ↑AST, ↑ALT, ↑alk phos and ↑γGT. Later, with loss synthetic function, look for ↓albumin ± ↑PT/INR. ↓WCC and ↓platelets indica hypersplenism. ***Find the cause:*** Ferritin, iron/total iron-binding capacity (p254 hepatitis serology; immunoglobulins (p258); autoantibodies (ANA, AMA, SMA, p539 α-fetoprotein (p262); caeruloplasmin in patients <40yrs old (p257); α_1-antitryps (p256). ***Liver ultrasound + duplex*** may show a small liver or hepatomega splenomegaly, focal liver lesion(s), hepatic vein thrombus, reversed flow in t portal vein, or ascites. ***MRI:*** Caudate lobe size↑, smaller islands of regenerati nodules, and the presence of the right posterior hepatic notch are more frequent alcoholic cirrhosis than in virus-induced cirrhosis. MRI scoring systems based spleen volume, liver volume, and presence of ascites or varices/collaterals c quantify severity of cirrhosis in a way that correlates well with Child grades (s BOX). ***Ascitic tap*** should be performed and fluid sent for urgent MC+S neutrophils >250/mm³ indicates spontaneous bacterial peritonitis (see below f treatment). ***Liver biopsy*** (p248) confirms the clinical diagnosis.

Management ***General:*** Good nutrition is vital; low-salt diet (if ascites). Alcoh abstinence. Avoid NSAIDs, sedatives, and opiates. ***Colestyramine*** may help prurit (4g/12h PO, 1h after other drugs). Consider ultrasound and α-fetoprotein eve 3–6 months to screen for HCC, p262. ***Specific: Interferon-α*** (± ***ribavirin***) improv LFT and may slow development to HCC in HCV-induced cirrhosis (p394). There may some benefit of high dose ***ursodeoxycholic acid*** in PBC (see p258)—it can normali LFT, though may have no effect on longterm disease progression. ***Penicillamine*** f Wilson's disease (p257). ***Ascites:*** Bedrest, fluid restriction (<1.5L/d), low-salt di (40–100mmol/d). Give ***spironolactone*** 100mg/24h PO; ↑dose every 48h, 400mg/24h—it counters the deranged renin-angiotensin-aldosterone (RAA) ax Chart daily weight and aim for weight loss of ≤½kg/d. If response is poor, add ***furosemide*** ≤120mg/24h PO; do U&E often. Therapeutic paracentesis wi concomitant albumin infusion (6–8g/L fluid removed) may be tried. ***Spontaneo bacterial peritonitis (SBP):*** ►Must considered in any patient with ascites w deteriorates suddenly (may be asymptomatic). Common organisms are *E. cc Klebsiella*, and *Streptococcus*. Treatment: eg ***cefotaxime*** 2g/6h or ***tazocin*** 4.5g/ (consult the datasheet) for 5 days or until sensitivities known (+ ***metronidazc*** 500mg/8h IV if there has been instrumentation to the ascites). Give prophylaxis f high risk patients (↓albumin, ↑PT/INR, low ascitic albumin) or those who have had previous episode: eg ***norfloxacin*** 400mg PO daily.

Prognosis Overall 5yr survival is ~50%. Poor prognostic indicators: encephalopatl serum Na⁺ <110mmol/L; serum albumin <25g/L; ↑INR.

Liver transplantation is the only definitive treatment for cirrhosis (p255). Tl increases 5yr survival from ~20% in end-stage disease to ~70%.

Fig 1. Spider naevi. These consist of a central arteriole, from which numerous vessels radiate (like the legs of a spider). These fill from the centre as opposed to telangiectasias that fill from the edge. They occur most commonly in skin drained by the superior vena cava. Up to 5 are said to be normal (they are common in young ♀). Causes include liver disease, contraceptive steroids, and pregnancy (ie changes in oestrogen metabolism).

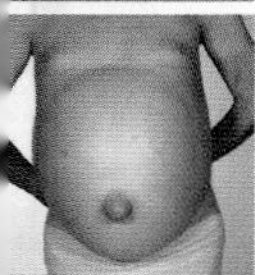

Fig 2. Gross ascites. Note the umbilical hernia (see p631) and a mild degree of gynaecomastia. There are veins visible on the anterior abdominal wall, though they are not in the pattern of caput medusae.

Causes of cirrhosis

- Chronic alcohol abuse.
- Chronic HBV or HCV infection[1]
- Autoimmune disease: PBC (p258); PSC (p259); AIH (p260).
- Genetic disorders: Haemachromatosis (p254); α_1-antitrypsin deficiency (p256); Wilson's disease (p257).
- Others: can be cryptogenic in up to 20%; Budd–Chiari syndrome (p688, hepatic vein thrombosis).
- Drugs: eg amiodarone, methyldopa, methotrexate.

Child–Pugh grading and risk of variceal bleeding

The severity of cirrhosis can be graded according to the score. Grade A = 5–6, grade B = 7–9, grade C >10, with the risk of variceal bleeding ↑↑ if score is >8. The grading can also be used to predict mortality and quantify the need for liver transplantation (see p255).

	1 point	2 points	3 points
Bilirubin (μmol/L)	<34	34-51	>51
Albumin (g/L)	>35	28-35	<28
Prothrombin time (seconds > normal)	1-3	4-6	>6
Ascites	none	slight	moderate
Encephalopathy (p251)	none	1-2	3-4

Cirrhosis and deteriorating renal function

In cirrhosis reduced hepatic clearance of immune complexes leads to their trapping in the kidney (∴ IgA nephropathy ± hepatic glomerulosclerosis). HCV can cause cryoglobulinaemia and membranoproliferative glomerulonephritis, HBV may cause membranous nephropathy and PAN and membranoproliferative glomerulonephritis can occur in α_1-antitrypsin deficiency. See p251 for hepatorenal syndrome (HRS).

1 Clues as to which patients with chronic HCV will get cirrhosis: platelet count ≤140 x 10^9/L, globulin/albumin ratio ≥1, and AST/ALT ratio ≥1—100% +ve predictive value but lower sensitivity (30%).

Hereditary haemochromatosis (HH)

This is an inherited disorder of iron metabolism in which increased intestinal iro absorption leads to deposition in multiple organs (joints, liver, heart, pancrea pituitary, adrenals and skin). Middle-aged males are more frequently and severe affected than women, in whom the disease tends to present ~10yrs late (menstrual blood loss is protective).

Genetics HH is one of the commonest inherited disease in those of Northern Europea (especially Celtic) ancestry (carrier rate of ~1 in 10 and a frequency of homozygosi of ~1: 200–400). The gene responsible for most HH is called HFE, found on the sho arm of chromosome 6. The 2 major mutations are termed C282Y and H63D. C282 accounts for 60–90% of HH, and H63D accounts for 3–7%, with compour heterozygotes accounting for 1–4%. Penetrance is unknown but is <100%.

Clinical features Asymptomatic early on—then tiredness and arthralgia (MCP ar large joints). Later, look for: slate-grey skin pigmentation; diabetes mellitus ('bron diabetes'); signs of chronic liver disease (p252); hepatomegaly; cirrhosis; cardia failure (dilated cardiomyopathy); hypogonadism (p216) from pituitar dysfunction↓ or via cirrhosis (not from testicular iron deposition); associate osteoporosis. Other endocrinopathies include hyporeninaemic hypoaldosteronism.

Tests ***Blood:*** LFT↑, ↑serum ferritin; ↑serum iron; ↓TIBC; transferrin saturatic >80%.[1] HFE genotyping. Blood glucose (?DM). ***Joint x-rays*** may show chondr calcinosis. ***Liver biopsy:*** Perl's stain quantifies iron loading (hepatic iron index (HII >1.9μmol/kg/yr) and assesses disease severity. ***MRI*** can be used to estimate hepat iron loading—haemosiderin and ferritin have a paramagnetic quality that affects T and T2 relaxation times (p720). Do ***ECG*** & ***ECHO*** if you suspect cardiomyopathy

Management ***Venesect*** ~1 unit/wk, until mildly iron-deficient. Iron will continue t accumulate, so maintenance venesection is needed for life (1U every 2–3 months Aim to maintain haematocrit <0.5, serum ferritin <100micrograms/L, TIB >50μmol/L, and transferrin saturation <40%. ***Other monitoring:*** Diabetes (p190 HbA_{1c} levels may be falsely low as venesection reduces the time available for H glycosylation. ***Over-the-counter self-medication:*** Make sure that vitami preparations etc. contain no iron. ***Dietary intake:*** Maintaining a well-balanced low iron diet may help. Drinking tea, coffee or red wine with meals reduces iro absorption, but fruit and fruit juice (high in vitamin C) and white wine increas absorption. ***Screening:*** Test serum ferritin and genotype in 1st-degree relative Prevalence of iron overload in asymptomatic C282Y homozygotes is ≤4.5 per 100 persons screened. How many will go on to develop iron overload is unknown.

Prognosis Venesection returns life expectancy to normal if non-cirrhotic and no diabetic. Arthropathy may improve or worsen. Gonadal failure is irreversible. In no cirrhotic patients, venesection may improve liver histology. ►Cirrhotic patients hav >10% chance of developing HCC. Sources vary on the exact risk: some authoriti quote 30%, others 22%. One cause of variability is varying co-factors: age ove 50yrs ↑risk by 13-fold; being HBsAg +ve by 5-fold and alcohol abuse by 2-fold.

Secondary haemochromatosis may occur in any haematological condition whe many transfusions (~40L in total) have been given. To reduce need fo transfusions, find out if the haematological condition responds to erythropoietin o marrow transplantation before irreversible effects of iron overload become to great. See iron management in thalassaemia, p328.

1 In heterozygotes, biochemical tests may be normal or show mild ↑ in transferrin saturation or ferriti

2 The HII aims to separate HH from other causes of hepatic siderosis (eg HBV; alcoholic cirrhosis). It less used now that genotyping is available. HII in μmol iron/gram liver/year = [Iron concentration (μg iro per gram dry weight of liver)/55.846 (atomic weight of Fe)]/patient's age. HII >1.9 in a non-cirrhotic live strongly suggests HH. ►*Caveats*: • ~7% of those with HH have a HII <1.9. Using a threshold hepatic ir concentration of 71μmol/g as well as HII can detect most of these. • Cirrhotic livers can rapid accumulate iron in non-HH liver disease making HII >1.9. Some say that an HII cut-off of ~4.2 is best diagnosing HH in cirrhotics. • Iron is not uniformly distributed in the liver (sampling variatio • Correlation among HII, phenotypic HH, & genotypic HH is not 100%.

A bit about iron metabolism

The average daily diet contains ~180–270μmol (~3–4g) of iron, with red meats, liver, seafoods, enriched breakfast cereals and pulses and even some spices (eg paprika) being particularly iron-rich. Most dietary iron is Fe^{3+}, which is reduced by low gastric pH and ascorbic acid (vitamin C) to better-absorbed Fe^{2+}. Absorption occurs mainly in the duodenum and jejunum, though very small amounts are absorbed in the stomach and ileum. Regulation of iron levels (by an unknown mechanism) is based mainly on absorption, while iron excretion is in the form of uncontrolled shedding of the gut lining.[85] The majority (60–70%) of body iron circulates in haemoglobin, though it is also found in myoglobin, bound to enzymes and proteins (such as the β-globulin, transferrin), in mitochondria, and in hepatocytes—as ferritin and haemosiderin. Iron requirements are greater for women (menstrual loss), when growing, in pregnancy and in chronic infection.

In HH the total body iron is up to 10-fold that of a normal person, with loading found particularly in the liver and pancreas (×100). Hepatic disease classically starts with fibrosis, progressing to cirrhosis as a late feature.

Liver transplantation in chronic liver disease

The first ever liver transplantation was performed by Starzl in Denver, USA, in 1963. The first in the UK was in 1968 at Addenbrooke's Hospital, Cambridge.[86] Between 1996 and 2000 there were ~3,400 liver transplants performed in the UK and Ireland and the limiting step for the procedure is now the waiting-list for a donor organ (live or cadeveric—see p251). The indications for transplantation in chronic disease (see TABLE) are generally because of advanced cirrhosis (p252), the grading of which has been used as a selection criterion.[1]

Indications	Contraindications
• Advanced cirrhosis secondary to:	• Extrahepatic malignancy
· Alcoholic liver disease	• Multiple primary or secondary tumours
· Hepatitis B & C	• Severe cardiorespiratory disease
· PBC (p258)	• Systemic sepsis
· AIH (p260)	• HIV infection
· Wilson's disease	• Non-compliance with drug therapy
· α_1-antitrypsin deficiency	
· PSC (p259)	
• HCC (1 nodule <5cm or 2–3 nodules <3cm)	

The post-operative period involves 12-24h on ITU, with enteral feeding starting as soon as possible and close monitoring of LFT. Immunosuppressant protocols usually involve a combination of ***ciclosporin*** or ***tacrolimus*** together with ***azathioprine*** or ***mycophenolate mofetil*** and ***prednisolone***. Hyperacute rejection is a result of ABO incompatabilty. Acute rejection (T-cell mediated) occurs in about 50% at 5–10 days, with the patient feeling unwell and developing pyrexia and tender hepatomegaly—it can usually be managed by increasing or altering the immunosuppressant regime. Other complications include sepsis (especially gram –ve), hepatic artery thrombosis, CMV infection, chronic rejection (at 6–9 months), disease recurrence,[87] and very rarely, graft-versus-host disease.[88] The average patient survival at 1yr is ~80% and at 5yrs is 60–90%, though this varies between different patients with different diseases. Poor pre-transplant renal function has been identified as a predictor of poor outcome.[89] (See also BOX, Indications for transplantation in acute liver failure, p251.)

1 The incredibly difficult selection of patients for liver transplantation can also be made according to the Model for End-stage Liver Disease (MELD).

α_1-antitrypsin deficiency

The glycoprotein α_1-antitrypsin is one of a family of serine protease inhibitc (deficiency is termed a 'serpinopathy') controlling inflammatory cascades. It synthesized in the liver, making up 90% of serum α_1-globulin on electrophore (p679). α_1-antitrypsin deficiency is the chief genetic cause of liver disease children. In adults, its lack causes emphysema in ~75% (p168),[1] chronic liv disease in and HCC (p262). ***Other associations:*** Asthma, pancreatitis, gallston Wegener's (p706). ***Prevalence:*** 1:2000-7000

Genetics The gene for this autosomal recessive disorder is found on chromosor 14; carrier frequency of 1:10. Genetic variants are typed by electrophore mobility as **medium** (M), **slow** (S), or **very slow** (Z). S and Z types are due to sinc amino acid substitutions at positions 264 and 342, respectively. These result ↓production of α_1-antitrypsin (S=60%, Z=15%). The normal genotype is PiMM, t homozygote is PiZZ; heterozygotes are PiMZ & PiSZ (at low risk of developing liv disease).

Clinical features Symptomatic patients usually have the PiZZ genotype: dyspno from emphysema; cirrhosis; cholestatic jaundice. NB: cholestasis often remits adolescence.

Tests Serum α_1-antitrypsin levels↓. ***Liver biopsy:*** (p248) Periodic acid Schiff (PA +ve; diastase-resistant globules. ***Phenotyping*** by isoelectric focusing requir expertise to distinguish SZ and ZZ phenotypes. ***Prenatal diagnosis*** is possible DNA analysis of chorionic villus samples obtained at 11–13wks' gestation. DNA tes are likely to find greater use in the future. Measuring lung density with *CT* may better than lung function tests at predicting disease progression and mortality

Management Mostly supportive for emphysema and liver complications. Qu smoking. Consider **augmentation therapy** with ***α_1-antitrypsin*** pooled from hum plasma if FEV_1<80% of predicted and if not smoking (it is very expensive!).[2] Plasr levels of >0.7g/L are considered protective. ***Liver transplantation*** (p251) treatment of choice in decompensated cirrhosis.

Prognosis Male gender and obesity may predispose to advanced liver disease Emphysema is the cause of death in most, liver disease in ~5%. In adults, cirrhos ± HCC affect 25% of α_1-antitrypsin-deficient adults >50yrs.

Gastroenterology

1 The role of α_1-antitrypsin in the lung is to protect against tissue damage from neutrophil elastase—a process that is also induced by cigarette smoking.
2 120mg/kg IV every 2wks is conveniently self-given via SC intravenous injection port systems.

Wilson's disease/hepatolenticular degeneration

A rare inherited disorder with toxic accumulation of copper (Cu) in the liver and CNS (especially basal ganglia, eg globus pallidus hypodensity ± putamen cavitation) due to failure of biliary copper excretion. It is treatable, so screen all young patients with cirrhosis. ***Prevalence:*** 3:100,000.

Genetics It is an autosomal recessive disorder of a gene on chromosome 13 that codes for a copper transporting ATPase, ATP7B. Many mutations are known (>200) with HIS1069GLU being the commonest in European populations.

Clinical features Children usually present with ***liver disease*** (hepatitis, cirrhosis, fulminant liver failure); young adults often start with ***CNS signs:*** tremor; dysarthria, dysphagia; dyskinesias; dystonias; purposeless stereotyped movements (eg hand clapping); dementia; parkinsonism; micrographia; ataxia/clumsiness. ***Affective features:*** Depression/mania; labile emotions; libido↑↓; personality change. ►Ignoring these may cause years of needless misery. ***Cognitive/behavioural:*** Memory↓; quick to anger; slow to solve problems; IQ↓; delusions; mutism. ***Kayser–Fleischer rings:*** Cu deposits in iris (Descemet's membrane), pathognomonic but not invariable; may need slit lamp to see. ***Also:*** Haemolysis; blue lunulae (nails); polyarthritis; hypermobile joints; grey skin; abortions; hypoparathyroidism.

Tests Serum copper and caeruloplasmin usually↓. 24h urinary copper excretion↑ (>100μg/24h, normal <40μg). Molecular genetic testing can confirm the diagnosis. ***Liver biopsy:*** ↑hepatic copper content. ***MRI:*** Basal ganglia degeneration (± fronto-temporal, cerebellar, and brain stem atrophy).

Management ***Chelation:*** Lifelong ***penicillamine*** (500mg/6–8h PO for 1yr, maintenance: 0.75–1g/d). SE: nausea, rash, WCC↓, Hb↓, platelets↓ haematuria, nephrosis, lupus. Monitor FBC & urinary Cu (and protein) excretion. Say 'report sore throat, T°↑, or bruising at once' in case WCC/platelets↓↓. Stop if WCC <2.5×10^9/L or platelets falling (or <120×10^9/L). Alternative: ***Trientine dihydrochloride*** 600mg/6–12h PO (SE: rash; sideroblastic anaemia). ***Liver transplantation*** (p255) if severe liver disease. ***Screen siblings*** as asymptomatic homozygotes need treatment.

Prognosis Pre-cirrhotic liver disease is reversible, though neurological damage is less so. There are no clear clinical prognostic indicators. Death occurs from liver failure, variceal haemorrhage (p246), or infection.

Screening tests for suspected liver disease

- EBV, CMV, HAV, HBV, & HCV serologies—see p394.
- Iron studies for haemochromatosis: ↑ferritin, ↑iron, ↓TIBC—see p254.
- α_1-antitrypsin deficiency (plasma for genetics)—see opposite.
- Wilson's disease: ↓serum copper, ↓caeruloplasmin—see above.
- PBC: ↑AMA—see p258.
- PSC: ANA, AMA & ANCA may be +ve—see p259.
- AIH: ↑ANA + ↑ASMA; ↑IgG—see p260.
- Check all immunoglobulins: IgA (↑ in alcoholic liver disease); IgG (↑ in AIH) & IgM (↑ in PBC).
- HCC: ↑α-fetoprotein—see p262.
- Conjugated and unconjugated bilirubin.

Primary biliary cirrhosis (PBC)

Interlobular bile ducts are damaged by chronic granulomatous inflammation causing progressive cholestasis, cirrhosis, and portal hypertension. ***Cause:*** Possibly an autoimmune response triggered by environmental factors, with genetic predisposition thought to be of importance. ♀:♂ ≈ 9:1. ***Prevalence:*** ≤4/100,000. ***Peak presentation:*** ~50yrs old.

Associations with PB
- Thyroid disease
- Rheumatoid arthritis
- Sjögren's syndrome
- Keratoconjunctivitis sicca
- Systemic sclerosis
- Renal tubular acidosi
- Membranous glomerulonephritis

Clinical features Often asymptomatic and diagnosed after finding ↑alk phos on routine LFT. Lethargy and pruritus may occur, and can precede jaundice by months to years. ***Signs:*** Jaundice; skin pigmentation; xanthelasma (p682); xan omata; hepatomegaly; and splenomegaly. ***Complications:*** Osteoporosis is comm Malabsorption of fat-soluble vitamins (A, D & K) results in osteomalacia and coa ulopathy. Other complications include: portal hypertension; ascites; varic haemorrhage; hepatic encephalopathy; HCC (p262). See MINIBOX for associatio

Tests ***Blood tests:*** ↑Alk phos, ↑γGT, and mildly ↑AST and ALT; late disea ↑bilirubin, ↓albumin, ↑prothrombin time. 98% are antimitochondrial antibc (AMA) M_2 subtype +ve (highly specific). Other autoantibodies (p539) may occur low titres (see BOX). Immunoglobulins are ↑ (especially IgM). TSH and choleste may be ↑. ***Radiology:*** US & ERCP (p728) to exclude extrahepatic cholesta ***Liver biopsy:*** Granulomas around the bile ducts, progressing to cirrhosis.[1]

Treatment ***Symptomatic:*** Pruritus: try ***colestyramine*** 4–8g/24h PO; ***naltrexo*** and ***rifampicin*** may also help. Diarrhoea: ***codeine phosphate***, eg 30mg/8h Osteoporosis prevention: p674. ***Specific:*** Fat-soluble vitamin prophylaxis: vitar A, D, and K. Consider high dose ***ursodeoxycholic acid (UDCA)***, 10–15mg/kg/d in 2 divided doses. One review claimed that it had a marginal therapeutic effect w improvement of ascites, jaundice and LFT, but no long term effect on mortality need for liver transplantation, though others have suggested a trend towa improved survival and a lower transplantation rate... A main benefit was t paucity of SE. ***Liver transplantation*** (p251) is the last recourse for patients w end-stage disease (eg bilirubin >100μmol/L) or intractable pruritus. Recurrence in t graft has been histologically estimated at 17% after ~5 years, and although gr failure can occur as a result of recurrence, this is rare and not predictable. 96

Prognosis Once jaundice develops, survival is <2yrs. In one study, at 2yrs po transplant, predicted survival without transplant was 55% and actual survival w 79%. At 7yrs, these figures were 22% and 68%, respectively. 97

Testing for autoantibodies—entering a minefield?

The conditions in the next few pages all include the measurement autoantibodies—with their varying sensitivities and specificities—as part of a investigative work-up. But dare we tread our way precariously through th dangerous minefield scattered with duds and tripwires, just to reach the othe side in some degree of greater diagnostic certainty? Although we do measur some autoantibodies in the routine screen for suspected liver disease (p257), ju how far should we go into this minefield with our patients before we think abou the consequences? The best approach is most likely a combination of experienc close attention to the latest medical evidence, and individual circumstances.

1 Hepatic granulomas are not specific to PBC as they are also found in sarcoidosis, tuberculosis, schistosomiasis, brucellosis, parasitic infection and drug reactions.

rimary sclerosing cholangitis (PSC)

SC is a disorder of unknown cause characterized by nflammation, fibrosis, and strictures of the intra- and xtrahepatic bile ducts. Immunological mechanisms ave been implicated.

Associations with PSC
- Ulcerative colitis[1]
- HLA-A1, B8, & DR3
- Crohn's disease (much rarer)
- HIV infection

he Patient Chronic biliary obstruction and secondry biliary cirrhosis lead to liver failure and death (or ransplantation) over ~10yrs. ***Symptoms:*** Patients may be asymptomatic and ound incidentally after finding alk phos↑ on LFT; or else symptoms may fluctuate, g: jaundice; pruritus; abdominal pain; fatigue. ***Signs:*** Jaundice; hepatomegaly; ortal hypertension. ***Complications:*** Bacterial cholangitis; cholangiocarcinoma 20–30%); ↑risk of colorectal cancer. 30% of patients in some series had an verlap syndrome with type 1 AIH (p260).[2] See MINIBOX for associations.

ests ***Blood:*** ↑Alk phos initially followed by ↑bilirubin; hypergammalobulinaemia; AMA negative, but ANA, SMA, & ANCA may be +ve, see p539. ***ERCP*** see fig 1) shows multiple strictures of the biliary tree with a characteristic eaded' appearance. ***MRCP*** (see fig 2) is cost effective and accurate in diagnosis n comparison to ERCP. ***Liver biopsy*** shows a fibrous, obliterative cholangitis.

lanagement ***Drugs: Colestyramine*** 4–8g/24h PO for pruritus (***naltrexone*** and ***ifampicin*** may also help). ***Ursodeoxycholic acid*** improves cholestasis but has no lear clinical effects. Antibiotics for bacterial cholangitis. ***Endoscopic stenting*** elps symptomatic dominant strictures. Yearly ***ultrasound*** screening may help etect cholangiocarcinoma, with cholecystectomy advocated for gallbladder olyps. ***Liver transplantation*** (p251) is indicated in end-stage disease. ecurrence occurs in up to 30%; 5yr graft survival is >60%. Prognosis is worse or those with concomitant IBD, as 5–10% develop colorectal cancer postransplant. ***Colonoscopy screening*** should be performed yearly for patients vith UC to because of the increased risk of colorectal carcinoma.

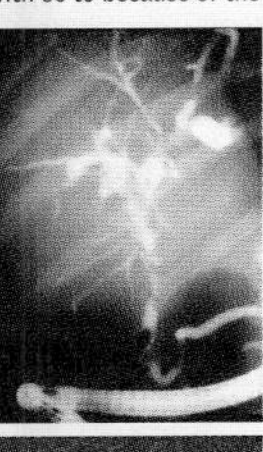

Fig 1. ERCP showing the features of PSC.

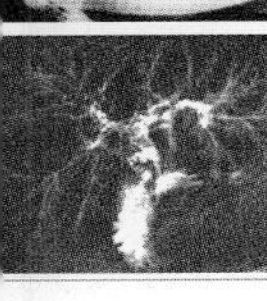

Fig 2. MRCP showing features of PSC. The intra- and extrahepatic ducts show extensive multifocal strictures. MRCP = magnetic resonance choleangiopancreatography.

3% of those with UC have PSC, but 80% of those with PSC have UC/Crohn's associated with PSC has igher rate of backwash ileitis and rectal sparing—it may be a distinct IBD-phenotype.

Do anti-mitochondrial, anti-nuclear, anti-smooth muscle, anti-liver kidney microsomal type 1, anti-liver osol type 1, perinuclear anti-neutrophil nuclear, & anti-soluble liver antigen antibodies.

Autoimmune hepatitis (AIH)

An inflammatory liver disease of unknown cause[1] characterized by suppressor T-cell defects with autoantibodies directed against hepatocyte surface antigens. Two types have been distinguished by the presence of circulating autoantibodies (see TABLE).

Associations
- Pernicious anaemia
- AI haemolysis
- Ulcerative colitis
- Diabetes mellitus
- Glomerulonephritis
- PSC
- AI thyroiditis
- HLA A1, B8, & DR3 haplotype

Clinical features Predominantly affects young and middle-aged women. 25% present with acute hepatitis and features of an autoimmune disease, eg fever, malaise, urticarial rash, polyarthritis, pleurisy, pulmonary infiltration, or glomerulonephritis. The remainder present insidiously are asymptomatic and diagnosed incidentally with signs of chronic liver disea Amenorrhoea is common and disease tends to attenuate during pregnan ***Complications:*** those associated with cirrhosis (p252) and drug therapy. S MINIBOX for associations.

Tests Abnormal LFT (AST↑), hypergammaglobulinaemia (especially IgG), + autoantibodies (ANA, SMA, or LKM1). Other autoantibodies, eg anti-soluble liv antigen (SLA) and antimeasles virus may be seen. Anaemia, WCC↓, and platelet indicate hypersplenism. ***Liver biopsy*** (p248) shows mononuclear infiltrate of por and periportal areas + piecemeal necrosis, fibrosis, or cirrhosis. ***MRCP*** (p729) hel exclude PSC if alk phos disproportionately↑.

Diagnosis depends on excluding other diseases as there is no pathognomonic si or laboratory test. There is genuine overlap with other chronic liver disease: eg P (p258), PSC (p259) and chronic viral hepatitis. 100 Diagnostic criteria exist but a not fully validated (eg the revised IAHG system).[2]

Management
- ***Immunosuppressant therapy: Prednisolone*** 30mg/d PO for 1 month; ↓by 5r a month to a maintenance dose of 5–10mg/d PO. Corticosteroids can sometim be stopped after 2yrs but relapse occurs in 50–86%. ***Azathioprine*** (5(100mg/d PO) may be used as a steroid sparing agent. Remission is achievable 80% of patients within 3yrs. 10- and 20yr survival rates are >80%. 101
- ***Non-standard proposed therapies*** to avoid steroid SE: ***Ciclosporin, budesonic tacrolimus, mycophenolate mofetil, ursodeoxycholic acid, methotrexat cyclophosphamide, mercaptopurine,*** and free radical scavengers. 102
- ***Liver transplantation*** (p251) is indicated for decompensated cirrhosis or the is if failure to respond to medical therapy, but recurrence may occur. It effective (actuarial 10yr survival is 75%).

Prognosis appears not to matter whether symptomatic or asymptomatic presentation (10yr survival ~80% for both). The presence of cirrhosis presentation reduces 10yr survival from 94% to 62%. 103

1 Hepatotropic viruses (eg measles, herpes viruses) and some drugs appear to trigger AIH in genetica predisposed individuals exposed to a hepatotoxic *milieu intérieur*. Viral interferon can inactiva cytochrome P-450 enzymes (∴ ↓ metabolism of ex- or endogenous hepatotoxins). Putative examples exogenous agents: monosodium glutamate (MSG; E621) and aspartame (E951), which, if regula consumed in excess, may promote formation of salt bridges between amino acids. These compoun then act as autoantigens causing CD4 T-helper cell activation.

2 International Autoimmune Hepatitis Group (revised) 1999.

Types of autoimmune hepatitis

Type I

- Affects adults or children (bimodal distribution)
- Anti-smooth muscle antibodies (SMA) +ve in 80% 104
- Antinuclear antibody (ANA) +ve in 10%.

Type II

- Affects children
- More commonly progresses to cirrhosis
- Anti-liver/kidney microsomal type 1 (LKM1) antibodies.

Liver tumours

The commonest (90%) liver tumours are secondary (metastatic) tumours eg fro breast, bronchus, or the gastrointestinal tract (see TABLE). Primary hepatic tumou are much less common and may be benign or malignant (see TABLE).

Symptoms Fever, malaise, anorexia, weight↓, RUQ pain (∵ liver capsule stretch Jaundice is late, except with cholangiocarcinoma. Benign tumours are oft asymptomatic. Tumours may rupture causing intraperitoneal haemorrhage.

Signs Hepatomegaly (smooth, or hard and irregular, eg metastases, cirrhosis, HC Look for signs of chronic liver disease (p252) and evidence of decompensati (jaundice, ascites). Feel for an abdominal mass. Listen for a bruit over the liver (HC

Tests ***Blood:*** FBC, clotting, LFT, hepatitis serology, α-fetoprotein (↑ in 80% of HC though it is a poor prognostic indicator,[105] and may be normal if tumour <3cm ***Imaging:*** US (fig 1) or CT to identify lesions and guide diagnostic biopsies. MRI better for distinguishing benign from malignant lesions. ERCP (p728) and biop should be performed for suspected cholangiocarcinoma. ***Liver biopsy*** (p248) m achieve a histological diagnosis; ►careful multidisciplinary discussion is required potentially resectable, as seeding along the biopsy tract can occur. Oth investigations for metastases (eg CXR, mammography, endoscopy, colonoscopy, MRI, marrow biopsy) are tailored according to the suspected primary.

Liver metastases signify advanced disease. Treatment and prognosis vary with t type and extent of primary tumour. Chemotherapy may be effective (eg lymphom germ cell tumours). Small, solitary metastases may be amenable to resection (colorectal carcinoma).[106] In most, treatment is palliative. ***Prognosis:*** <6 months

Hepatocellular carcinoma (HCC) A malignant tumour of hepatocytes, accounti for 90% of primary liver cancers. Common in China & sub-Saharan Africa (40% cancers), rare in the West (~2% of cancers). ***Causes:*** Viral hepatitis (persistent H or HBV, especially if >2.3×10⁴ virions/mL);[1] cirrhosis (alcohol, haemochromatos PBC); aflatoxin; parasites (*Clonorchis sinensis*); anabolic and contraceptive steroi ***Management:*** Resection of solitary tumours <3cm diameter improves 3yr surviv rate (59% from 13%), though ~50% have recurrence by 3yrs. Applying the Mil criteria for liver transplantation gives a 5yr survival rate of 70%.[2] Chemothera percutaneous ablation, and tumour embolization are also options.[107] ***Prognos*** Often <6 months, with a 95% 5yr mortality. Fibrolamellar HCC, which occurs children/young adults, has a better prognosis (60% 5yr survival). ***Prevention*** vital. ►Ensure HBV vaccination (see BOX). ►Don't reuse needles. ►Screen blo products. ►Reduce exposure to aflatoxins (anti-humidity measures such as su drying to ↓spread of this common fungal contaminant in stored maize); this is mo important for those who harbour HBV (risk is highly synergistic).[108] ***Screening*** usi ultrasound and α-fetoprotein levels needs further evaluation.[109]

Cholangiocarcinoma = biliary tree malignancy; ~10% of liver primaries. ***Caus*** Flukes (*Clonorchis*, p433) in the East; PSC (p259); congenital biliary cysts; biliar enteric drainage surgery;[110] N-nitroso toxins.[111] ***The patient:*** Fever, abdominal p (±ascites), malaise, ↑bilirubin; ↑↑alk phos. ***Pathology:*** Usually slow-growing. Mo are distal extrahepatic or perihilar. ***Management:*** 70% are unsuitable for surgi resection. Of those that are, 76% recur. **Surgery:** eg major hepatectomy extrahepatic bile duct excision + caudate lobe resection. 5yr survival is ~30% Specific post-op complications include liver failure, bile leak and GI bleeding **Palliative stenting** of an obstructed extrahepatic biliary tree, percutaneously or ERCP (p728), improves quality of life. ***Prognosis:*** ~5 months.

Benign tumours ***Haemangiomas*** are the commonest benign liver tumours. Th are often an incidental finding on ultrasound or CT scan and do not requ treatment. Biopsy should be avoided! ***Adenomas*** are common. Causes: Anab steroids, the oral contraceptive pill; pregnancy. Only treat if symptomatic.

1 2.3×10^4 virions/mL by PCR is a low level, so almost all are at risk.
2 Milan criteria for liver transplantation in HCC: 1 nodule <5cm or 2–3 nodules <3cm.

Primary liver tumours

Malignant	Benign
• HCC	• Cysts
• Cholangiocarcinoma	• Haemangioma
• Angiosarcoma	• Adenoma
• Hepatoblastoma	• Focal nodular hyperplasia
• Fibrosarcoma	• Fibroma
• Leiomyosarcoma	• Leiomyoma

Origins of secondary liver tumours

Common in ♂	Common in ♀	Less common (either sex)
• Stomach	• Breast	• Pancreas
• Lung	• Colon	• Leukaemia
• Colon	• Stomach	• Lymphoma
	• Uterus	• Carcinoid tumours

Preventing of hepatitis B, hepatitis B-associated cirrhosis, chronic hepatitis, and hepatic neoplasia

Use hepatitis B vaccine, Engerix B®, 1mL into deltoid; repeat at 1 & 6 months (child: 0.5mL × 3 into the anterolateral thigh). ***Indications:*** Everyone (WHO advice, even in areas of 'low' endemicity). This strategy is expensive, but not as expensive as trying to rely on the ultimately unsuccessful strategy of vaccinating at-risk groups—health workers (eg GPs, dentists, nurses, etc.), IV drug users, sexual adventurers, male or immigrant prostitutes (homo- or heterosexual), those on haemodialysis, and the sexual partners of known HB_e antigen +ve carriers. The immunocompromised and others may need further doses. Serology helps time boosters and finds poor or non-responders (correlates with older age, smoking, and ♂ sex). ►**Know your own antibody level!**

Anti-HBs (IU/L)	Actions and comments: (UK advice: USA advice is different)
>1000	Good level of immunity; retest in ~4yrs.
100–1000	Good level of immunity; if level approaches 100, retest in 1yr.
<100	Inadequate; give booster and retest.
<10	Non-responder; give booster and retest; if <10 get consent to check hepatitis B status: HBsAg +ve means chronic infection; anti-HB core +ve represents past infection and immunity.

NB: Protective immunity begins about 6 weeks after the 1st immunizing dose, so it is inappropriate if exposure is recent; here, specific anti-hepatitis B immunoglobulin is the best option if not already immunized.

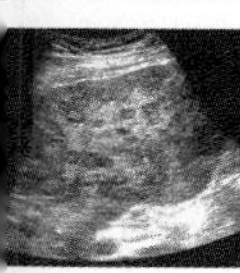

Fig 1. Ultrasound of the liver showing multiple heterogeneous lesions suggestive of hepatic metastasis.

Ulcerative colitis (UC)

UC is a relapsing and remitting inflammatory disorder of the colonic mucosa. It m affect just the rectum (proctitis, as in ~50%) or extend proximally to involve pa of the colon (left-sided colitis, in ~30%) or all of the colon (pancolitis, in ~20%). 'never' spreads proximally to the ileocaecal valve (except for backwash ileit **Cause:** Unknown;[1] there is some genetic susceptibility. **Pathology:** Hyperaem haemorrhagic granular colonic mucosa ± pseudopolyps formed by inflammati Punctate ulcers may extend deep into the lamina propria—inflammation is nor ally not transmural. **Histology:** See biopsy, below. **Prevalence:** 100–200/100,00 **Incidence:** 10–20/100,000/yr. ♀/♂ >1. Most present aged 15–30yrs. UC is 3-f as common in non-smokers (the opposite is true for Crohn's disease)—sympto may relapse on stopping smoking.

Symptoms Gradual onset of diarrhoea ± blood & mucus. Crampy abdominal c comfort is common; bowel frequency is related to severity of disease (see TABL Systemic symptoms are common during attacks, eg fever, malaise, anore weight↓. Urgency and tenesmus occur with rectal disease.

Signs May be none. In acute, severe UC there may be fever, tachycardia, an tender, distended abdomen. ***Extraintestinal signs:*** Clubbing; aphthous oral ulce erythema nodosum (p267); pyoderma gangrenosum; conjunctivitis; episcleri iritis; large joint arthritis; sacroiliitis; ankylosing spondylitis; fatty liver; PSC (p25 cholangiocarcinoma; renal stones; osteomalacia; nutritional deficits; amyloidosis

Tests *Blood:* FBC, ESR, CRP, U&E, LFT, and blood cultures. ***Stool MC+S*** and ***CDT*** (p238) exclude infections (*C. difficile, Salmonella, Shigella, Campylobacter, E. coli, amoebc* ***AXR:*** No faecal shadows; mucosal thickening/islands (fig 4, p716); colonic dilatat (below). ***Erect CXR:*** Perforation. ***Sigmoidoscopy:*** Inflamed, friable mucosa. ***Rec biopsy:*** Inflammatory infiltrate; goblet cell depletion; glandular distortion; muco ulcers; crypt abscesses. ***Barium enema:*** Loss of *haustra*; granular muco shortened colon. ►**Never do a barium enema during a severe acute attack or a diagnostic test.** ***Colonoscopy*** shows disease extent and allows biopsy (fig 3, p24

Assessing severity in UC: the Truelove and Witts criteria

Parameter	Mild	Moderate	Severe
Motions/day	<4	4–6	>6
Rectal bleeding	Small	Moderate	Large
Temperature at 6am (p26)	Apyrexial	37.1–37.8°C	>37.8°C
Pulse rate (beats/min)	<70	70–90	>90
Haemoglobin	>11g/dL	10.5–11g/dL	<10.5g/dL
ESR	<30mm/h		>30mm/h

Complications ►Perforation and bleeding are 2 serious dangers, also:

- Toxic dilatation of colon (mucosal islands, colonic diameter >6cm).
- Venous thrombosis—consider prophylaxis (p334) during hospital admissior
- Colonic cancer: risk ≈15% with pancolitis for 20yrs; surveillance colonosc may be used (eg 2–4yearly), but proving this saves lives has been difficult.

Inducing remission *Mild UC:* If <4 motions/d and the patient is well, give ***pr nisolone*** (eg 20–40mg/d PO) + ***mesalazine***, eg Pentasa® (modified-release 500 tabs; up to 1g/6h) or Asacol MR® (400mg tabs; in an acute attack 2tabs/8h). mild distal disease use twice-daily steroid foams PR (eg ***hydrocortisone*** Colifoam®), or ***prednisolone*** 20mg **retention enemas** (Predsol®). If symptc improve, ↓steroids gradually. If no improvement after 2wks, treat as moderate

Moderate UC: If 4–6 motions/d, but otherwise well, give oral ***prednisolone*** 40m for 1wk, then 30mg/d for 1wk, then 20mg for 4 more weeks + a 5-aminosaly acid (5-ASA) + and twice-daily steroid enemas.[2] If improving, ↓steroids gradua If no improvement after 2 weeks, treat as a severe UC.

1 UC & Crohn's *may* involve adhesin-expressing strains of *E. coli* capable of inducing interleuk production and transepithelial migration of WBCs—see OTM 2.613.

2 *Budesonide* (Entocort) enemas, 1 *nocte*, may have fewer SEs ∵ ↓suppression of plasma cortisol

Gastroenterology

vere UC: If systemically unwell and passing >6 motions/d, admit for:
lil by mouth and IV maintenance hydration (eg 1L of 0.9% saline + 2L dextrose-aline/24h, + 20mmol K^+/L; less if elderly).
lydrocortisone 100mg/6h IV.
lectal steroids, eg ***hydrocortisone*** 100mg in 100mL 0.9% saline/12h PR.
Aonitor T°, pulse, and BP—and record stool frequency/character on a stool chart.
wice-daily exam: document distension, bowel sounds and tenderness.
)aily FBC, ESR, CRP, U&E ± AXR.
:onsider the need for blood transfusion (if Hb <10g/dL). Parenteral nutrition is nly very rarely required (eg if severely malnourished).
f improving in 5d, transfer to ***prednisolone*** PO (40mg/24h) with a 5-ASA (below, g ***sulfasalazine*** 500mg/6h) to maintain remission.
f on day 3 CRP >45 or stool frequency >6, consider ***ciclosporin/infliximab***/surgery.

ical therapies: Proctitis may respond to ***suppositories*** (***prednisolone*** 5mg or *salazine*, eg Asacol® 250mg/8h or Pentasa® 1g at bedtime). Topical 5-ASAs rk better than topical steroids.[MET 120] Procto-sigmoiditis may respond to ***foams*** PR mg Predfoam®/12–24h or 5-ASA, eg Asacol® 1g/d); disposable applicators aid urate delivery. Retention enemas may be needed in left-sided colitis.

Indications for surgery
• Perforation
• Massive haemorrhage
• Toxic dilatation
• Failure to respond to medical therapy

gery: ~20% will require surgery at some stage. ***cedures:*** Proctocolectomy + terminal ileostomy ay be possible to retain the ileocecal valve, and hence uce liquid loss);[121] colectomy with later ileo-anal ich. ***Surgical mortality:*** 2–7%, ↑ to 50% if perf-tion. Pouchitis can be successfully treated with anti-tics (eg ***metronidazole*** + ***ciprofloxacin*** for 2wks) and immunosuppressants.[122]

vel therapies: A short course of ***ciclosporin*** (eg 2mg/kg IV per day) may help ain remission quickly in patients with steroid-refractory UC, although it is rkedly nephrotoxic and not suitable for long courses (►monitor levels, do U&E, and BP often—stop if raised and get expert help).[123] Oral ***tacrolimus*** may also) in steroid-refractory disease. ***Infliximab*** (see p267) may be effective as :ue therapy in UC, though evidence is scarce.[RCT 124] Transdermal ***nicotine*** is superior lacebo for induction of remission, but SEs are common (eg dizziness, nausea).[MET 125]

intaining remission: All ***5-ASAs*** ↓relapse rate from 80% to 20% at 1yr—mples are ***sulfasalazine***, ***mesalazine***, and ***olsalazine***.[1] Maintenance is continued life. ***Sulfasalazine*** (500mg/6h PO) remains 1st-line. SEs related to sulfapyridine lerance include headache, nausea, anorexia, and malaise. Other SEs: fever, rash, molysis (►monitor FBC), hepatitis, pancreatitis, paradoxical worsening of colitis, reversible oligospemia.[126] ***Newer 5-ASAs*** (eg ***Mesalazine*** 400–800mg/8h PO or *lazine* 500mg/12h PO) are just as effective at maintaining remission, have er SEs, but are more expensive. They are indicated in ***sulfasalazine*** intolerance young men in whom fertility is a concern (less effect on sperm).[127] ***thioprine*** (2–2.5mg/kg/d PO after food) is indicated as a steroid-sparing agent iose with steroid side-effects or those who relapse quickly when steroids are iced. Treat for several months, and monitor FBC every 4–6 weeks.

determinate colitis

is is a diagnosis reserved for cases of IBD that have been fully investigated and nnot be definitely recognised as either UC or Crohn's disease. It tends to semble UC more than Crohn's disease, and some cases may be due to lack of cognition of unusual variants of UC that involve transmural inflammation or p lesions. Regarding surgical management, it is probably appropriate to rform colectomy + pouch formation, if indicated (see MINIBOX), though pouch lure rate is higher than in UC.[128]

1 *ulfasalazine* is a 5-aminosalicylic acid (5-ASA—the active ingredient) + sulfapyridine (carries 5-ASA to :olon, where it is cleaved off), ***mesalazine*** is 5-ASA and ***olsalazine*** is a dimer of 5-ASA that is also ed in the colon. Rare hypersensitivity reactions: worsening colitis, pancreatitis, pericarditis, nephritis.

Gastroenterology

Crohn's disease

Crohn's disease[1] is a chronic inflammatory GI disease characterized by transmu granulomatous inflammation. It may affect any part of the gut, but favours terminal ileum (in 50%) and proximal colon. Unlike UC, there is unaffected bo between areas of active disease (skip lesions). ***Cause:*** Unknown.[2] Mutations of NOD2/CARD15 gene ↑risk. ***Prevalence:*** 50–100/100,000. ***Incidence:*** 5–10 100,000/yr. ***Associations:*** High sugar, low-fibre diet; anaerobes; mucins; alte cell-mediated immunity. Smoking ↑risk ×3–4 and NSAIDs may exacerbate disea

Symptoms Diarrhoea, abdominal pain, and weight loss are common (failure thrive in children). Fever, malaise, anorexia occur with active disease.

Signs Aphthous ulceration; abdominal tenderness; right iliac fossa mass; peria abscesses/fistulae/skin tags; anal/rectal strictures. ***Extraintestinal sig*** Clubbing, erythema nodosum (fig 1), pyoderma gangrenosum, conjunctiv episcleritis, iritis, large joint arthritis, sacroiliitis, ankylosing spondylitis, fatty li PSC, cholangiocarcinoma, renal stones,[3] osteomalacia, malnutrition, amyloidos

Complications Small bowel obstruction; toxic dilatation (colonic diameter >6c abscess formation (abdominal, pelvic, or ischiorectal); fistulae (present in ~1C eg colovesical (bladder), colovaginal, perianal, enterocutaneous; perforation; re haemorrhage; colonic carcinoma (rarer than in UC).

Gastroenterology

Tests ***Blood:*** FBC, ESR, CRP, U&E, LFT, blood culture. Serum iron, B_{12}, and red cell fo if anaemia. ***Markers of activity:*** Hb↓; ↑ESR; ↑CRP; ↑WCC; ↓albumin. ***Stool M*** and ***CDT*** (p238) to exclude infectious diarrhoea (*C. difficile, Salmonella, Shig Campylobacter, E. coli*). Do ***sigmoidoscopy*** + ***rectal biopsy*** if the mucosa lo normal (20% have microscopic granulomas). ***Small bowel enema*** detects i disease (strictures, proximal dilatation, inflammatory mass; fistulae). ***Caps endoscopy*** (p248) also has an important and growing role in assessing sm bowel disease. ***Barium enema*** may show cobblestoning, 'rose thorn' ulcers, colon strictures with rectal sparing. ***Colonoscopy*** is preferred to barium enem assess disease extent and enables biopsies to be taken. ***MRI*** assesses pelvic dise

Management Severity is harder to assess than in UC, but T°↑; pulse↑; ↑ESR; ↑ ↑WCC; ↓albumin reflect severity and merit admission. ***Mild attacks:*** Patients symptommatic but systemically well. ***Prednisolone*** 30mg/d PO for 1wk, t 20mg/d for 1 month. See in clinic every 2–4 weeks. If symptoms resolve, ↓pr nisolone by 5mg every 2–4 weeks; stop steroids when parameters are norma

Severe attacks: Admit for IV steroids, nil by mouth, and IV hydration (eg 1L 0 saline + 2L dextrose-saline/24h, + 20mmol K^+/L, less if elderly). Then:

- ***Hydrocortisone*** 100mg/6h IV.
- Treat rectal disease with topical steroids (eg ***hydrocortisone*** 100mg in 10(0.9% saline/12h PR).
- ***Metronidazole*** 400mg/8h PO, or 500mg/8h IV, helps (esp. in perianal diseas superadded infection). SEs: alcohol intolerance; irreversible neuropathy.
- Monitor T°, pulse, BP, and record stool frequency/character on a stool char
- Physical examination twice daily. Daily FBC, ESR, CRP, U&E, and plain AXR.
- Consider need for blood transfusion (if Hb <10g/dL) and parenteral nutriti
- If improving after 5d, transfer on to oral ***prednisolone*** (40mg/d).
- If no response (or deterioration) during IV therapy, seek surgical advice.

Perianal disease occurs in about 50%. MRI and examination under anaesth (EUA) are an important part of assessment. Treatment includes oral antibio immunosuppressant therapy ± ***infliximab***, and local surgery ± seton insertio

1 Burrill B. Crohn was a US gastroenterologist (1884–1983). The original paper was penned in 193
2 **Environmental agents** are implicated. **Genetics:** Colon involvement goes with ↑CARD15 gene expr in macrophages & intestinal epithelial cells. **Dysregulated immune responses** might be primary or fro ecting gut commensals, eg *Mycobacterium avium paratuberculosis*; *E. coli* adhesins, p264, may have
3 Malabsorption of fat → Ca^{2+} binds fat left in lumen (saponification) → oxalate free to be absorbed mally binds Ca^{2+} in lumen & excreted in stool) → renal excretion of oxalate → hyperoxaluria & renal sto

dditional therapies in Crohn's disease

zathioprine (2–2.5mg/kg/d PO) is effective therapy and useful as a steroid-paring agent, eg for those with steroid SEs or if experiencing multiple/rapid lapses. It takes 6–10 weeks to work.[130]

ulfasalazine other 5-ASAs (p264) are not regarded as useful for the aintenance of remission in Crohn's disease.[131]

lemental diets (eg E028®) are made by mixing single amino acids and are ntigen free. They are not as good as steroids at inducing remission in active sease but do have a beneficial effect.[132] A **low residue diet** may help control sease activity, though diet alone is not effective at inducing remission.

lethotrexate A Cochrane review found good evidence from a single large RCT 1 which to recommend 25mg IM weekly for induction of remission and omplete withdrawal from steroids in patients with refractory Crohn's disease. NT ≈ 5—see p650. There was no evidence for lower doses, and no substantial SE ere reported.[133]

urgery 50–80% need ≥1 operation in their life. In the severely affected, it can ecome a devastating cycle of deterioration. Indications for surgery:

Failure to respond to drugs (most commonly)
Intestinal obstruction from strictures
Intestinal perforation
Local complications (fistulae, abscesses).

urgery is never curative. The aims are **1** to defunction (rest) distal disease eg ith a temporary ileostomy or **2** limited resection of the worst areas—short owel syndrome can be a complication (p566).[134] <1m of small bowel in the sence of a colon may require regular parenteral nutrition (p574). Bypass and ouch surgery is **not** done in Crohn's (∵ ↑risk of recurrence).

nfliximab This is an anti-tumour necrosis factor monoclonal antibody which can Crohn's disease activity. It counters neutrophil accumulation and granuloma rmation, activates complement, and causes cytotoxicity to CD4+ T-cells, thus earing cells driving the immune response. A single dose (5mg/kg) of ***infliximab*** ven by IVI over 2h is effective at inducing remission.[135] NNT ≈ 3–4 (see p650). esponse may be short-lived, but it may be repeated at 8 weeks. Some trials have so shown it to be effective as maintenance therapy.[136] CI: Sepsis, ↑LFT >3-fold oove top end of normal, concurrent ***ciclosporin*** or ***tacrolimus***. SE: rash. It should avoided in people with known underlying malignancy.[137] Cost per QALY: (see 12) £6700 (higher in fistulizing Crohn's).[138]

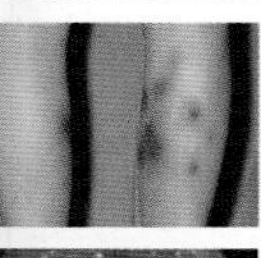

Fig 1. Erythema nodosum is an extraintestinal manifestation of Crohn's disease and UC, presenting as painful purplish nodules usually over the shins. They regress after a few weeks, leaving behind a bruised appearance. Other causes include sarcoidosis, drugs, streptococcal infection, and TB.[139]

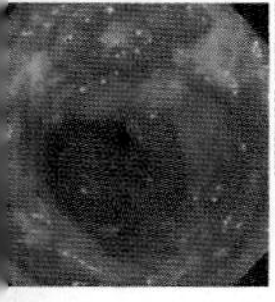

Fig 2. Colonscopy image showing deep fissured ulcers of the colonic mucosa in Crohn's disease.

Irritable bowel syndrome (IBS)

IBS is used to describe a heterogeneous group of abdominal symptoms for which organic cause can be found. Most are probably due to disorders of intesti motility or enhanced visceral perception (the 'brain–gut' axis: see BOX). Seve diagnostic criteria exist that evaluate symptoms and their duration (eg Manni Rome II), but they are not always helpful in clinical practice.

Clinical features Patients are usually 20–40yrs; ♀>♂.[1] ***Symptoms:*** Central lower abdominal pain (relieved by defecation); abdominal bloating; altered bov habit (constipation alternating with diarrhoea); tenesmus; mucus PR. Le commonly: nausea; dyspareunia; pain in the back, thigh, or chest; urinary frequen depression. Symptoms are chronic (>6 months), and exacerbated by stress, me struation, or gastroenteritis. ***Signs:*** Examination is often normal, but generaliz abdominal tenderness is common. Insufflation of air during sigmoidoscopy m reproduce the pain. ***Markers suggesting a disease other than IBS:*** Age >40y history <6 months; anorexia; weight↓; waking at night with pain/diarrhoea; mou ulcers; abnormal investigations (eg ↑CRP, ↓Hb); ►Investigate PR bleeding urgen

Management see BOX.

Carcinoma of the pancreas

Epidemiology: ≤2% of all malignancy; ~6500 deaths/yr (UK). UK incidence is risi ***Typical patient:*** ♂ >60yrs old. ***Risk factors:*** Smoking, alcohol, diabetes, chro pancreatitis. ***Pathology:*** Mostly ductal adenocarcinoma (metastasize early; prese late). 60% arise in the pancreas head, 25% in the body, 15% the tail. A few arise the Ampulla of Vater (ampullary tumour) or pancreatic islet cells (insulinon gastrinoma, glucagonomas, somatostatinomas (p207), VIPomas); both have better prognosis. ***Genetics:*** ~95% have mutations in the KRAS2 gene.

Symptoms & signs Tumours in the head of the pancreas present with **painle obstructive jaundice**. 75% of tumours in the body and tail present with epigast pain (radiates to back and relieved by sitting forward). Either may cause anore weight loss, diabetes or acute pancreatitis. ***Rarer features:*** Thrombophlebi migrans (eg an arm vein becomes swollen and red, then a leg vein); Ca^{2+}↑; maran endocarditis; portal hypertension (splenic vein thrombosis); nephrosis (renal v metastases). ***Signs:*** Jaundice + palpable gall bladder (Courvoisier's 'law': s p242); epigastric mass; hepatomegaly; splenomegaly; lymphadenopathy; ascit

Tests ***Blood:*** Cholestatic jaundice. CA 19-9↑ (p680) is non-specific, but may h assess prognosis. ***Imaging:*** US or CT can show a pancreatic mass[2] ± dilated bili tree ± hepatic metastases. They are also used to guide biopsy and provide stag prior to surgery/stent insertion. MRI & MRCP have an increasing role in diagnosis ERCP (p728) shows the biliary tree anatomy and may localize the site of obstructi

Treatment Most ductal carcinomas present with metastatic disease; <1C are suitable for radical surgery. ***Surgery:*** Consider pancreatoduodenectomy (Wh ple's, p271) if fit and the tumour <3cm with no metastases. Post-op morbidit high (mortality <5% in experienced hands) and non-curative resections confer survival benefit. ***Post-op chemotherapy*** delays disease progression. ***Palliation jaundice:*** Endoscopic or percutaneous stent insertion may help jaundice a anorexia. Rarely, palliative bypass surgery is done for duodenal obstruction unsuccessful ERCP. ***Pain relief:*** Disabling pain may require opiates in large dos p560, or radiotherapy. Coeliac plexus infiltration with alcohol may be done at t time of surgery, or percutaneously. Referral to a palliative care team is essent

Prognosis Dismal. Mean survival <6 months. 5yr survival: <2%. Overall 5 survival after Whipples' procedure 5–14%. Prognosis is better if: tumour <3cm; nodes involved; –ve resection margins at surgery; ampullary or islet cell tumou

1 IBS is common: ~16% of the population are estimated to be affected.
2 Endoscopic US is the most accurate diagnostic tool available for pancreatic tumours.

Management of IBS

The 1st step is to exclude other diagnoses, so:

- If young, with a classic history, FBC, ESR, LFT, coeliac serology (p272), and urinalysis ± sigmoidoscopy with rectal biopsy is sufficient investigation.
- If the patient is aged ≥45yrs or has **any** marker or organic disease, request colonoscopy (barium enema if unavailable).
- If diarrhoea is prominent, do: LFT; stool culture; B_{12}/folate; antiendomysial antibodies (p272); TSH; consider referral ± barium follow-through (if symptoms suggest small bowel disease) ± rectal biopsy.
- Further investigation should be guided by symptoms and include:
  - Upper GI endoscopy (dyspepsia, reflux)
  - Duodenal biopsy (coeliac disease), eg if antiendomysial antibodies +ve
  - Giardia tests, p424 (it often triggers IBS; anti-parasitic ℞ may not help)
  - Small bowel radiology (Crohn's disease)
  - ERCP (p728, eg chronic pancreatitis) or MRCP, p259 if active pancreatitis.
  - Transit studies and anorectal physiological studies—rarely used.

Refer: 1 If equivocal diagnosis. 2 If changing symptoms in 'known IBS'. 3 ***To surgeon*** if rectal mucosal prolapse. 4 ***To dietician*** if food intolerance. 5 ***To psychiatrists*** if stress/depression is pronounced.[1] 6 ***To gynaecologist*** if cyclical pain (endometriosis, *OHCS* p288) or if difficult pelvic infection, p406.

Treatment Rarely 100% successful (especially medical therapy) so be pragmatic. Careful explanation and reassurance are vital, as is developing a good relationship with your patient.

- ***Food intolerance:*** Try exclusion diets (difficult; may lead to obsessions).
- ***Constipation:*** See p240; ↑fibre intake gradually (can paradoxically worsen flatulence/bloating). Fybogel® (***ispaghula***) or Celevac® (***methylcellulose***; start with 3–6 tabs night and morning with >300mL fluid) have non-fermentable fibre—and are better than ***lactulose*** which ferments (↑gas production is hard to distinguish from bloating). A recent RCT showed that the $5HT_4$ agonist ***tegaserod*** was successful at relieving constipation in women and was tolerated well (SE: ↑diarrhoea)—it is not yet licensed in the UK.
- ***Diarrhoea:*** Bulking agent ± ***loperamide*** 2mg after each loose stool; max 16mg/d; SEs: colic, nausea, dizziness, constipation, bloating, ileus.
- ***Colic and bloating:*** Antispasmodics may help (eg ***mebeverine*** 135mg/8h PO (available over the counter); ***alverine citrate*** 60–120mg/8h PO; ***dicycloverine*** 10–20mg/8h PO).
- ***Dyspeptic symptoms:*** May respond to ***metoclopramide*** or antacids.
- ***Psychological therapy:*** Emphasize positive aspects and prognosis: in 50% symptoms go or improve after 1yr; <5% worsen. Symptoms are still troublesome in the rest at 5yrs. Tricyclic antidepressants (low dose) are often helpful, eg ***amitriptyline*** 10–50mg at night (SEs: constipation, dry mouth, etc., *OHCS* p340). Psychotherapy (*OHCS* p370), cognitive-behavioural therapy (*OHCS* p372), and gut-focused hypnotherapy[2] all have roles. Explain that all forms of stress (sexual, physical, or verbal abuse) perpetuate IBS.

The future Much interest is being expressed in modulating the 'brain–gut' axis by neurotransmitter manipulation. ***Visceral hypersensitivity:*** Those with IBS have lower visceral pain thresholds, and since 5HT antagonists increase pain tolerance, highly selective $5HT_3$-receptor antagonists (eg ***alosetron***) are under trial. ***Alosetron*** 1mg/12h PO can ↓symptoms in non-constipated IBS female patients, but its efficacy is unclear in males. SE: ~25% may get constipated; ►it may be associated with ischaemic colitis, which has raised questions on its place in practice. It is not currently available in the UK.

A remarkable 50–90% of patients with IBS seeking medical care have psychiatric co-morbidity.
12wks of hypnosis helps abnormal sensory perception: ►Do not think of hypnosis as dubious; it is a neat way to influence the brain–gut axis, reducing doctor dependency and stopping patients from being patients (passive recipients of suffering). Benefits may last ≥5yrs.

Nutritional disorders

(also see TABLE, p27

►Always consider that more than one nutritional disorder is likely to be prese

Scurvy This is due to lack of vitamin C in the diet.[1] Is the patient poor, pregna or on an odd diet? ***Signs:*** 1 Listlessness, anorexia, cachexia (p54). 2 Gingivitis, lo teeth, and foul-smelling breath (halitosis). 3 Bleeding from gums, nose, hair follic or into joints, bladder, gut. ***Diagnosis:*** No test is completely satisfactory. v ascorbic acid↓. ***Treatment:*** Dietary education; ***ascorbic acid*** ≥250mg/24h PC

Beriberi There is heart failure with general oedema (wet beriberi) or neuropat (dry beriberi) due to lack of vitamin B_1 (thiamine). For treatment and diagnos tests, see Wernicke's encephalopathy (p706).

Pellagra = lack of nicotinic acid. Classical triad: diarrhoea, dementia, dermatitis neuropathy, depression, insomnia, tremor, rigidity, ataxia, fits). It may occur carcinoid syndrome and anti-TB drugs (isoniazid). It is endemic in China and Afr ***Treatment:*** Education, electrolyte replacement, ***nicotinamide*** 100mg/4h PO.

Xerophthalmia This vitamin A deficiency syndrome is a major cause of blindnes the Tropics. Conjunctivae become dry and develop oval or triangular spots (Bitó spots). Corneas become cloudy and soft. See *OHCS* p450. Give ***vitamin A*** 200,000 stat PO, repeat in 24h and a week later (halve dose if <1yr old; quarter if months old); ►get special help if pregnant: vitamin A embryopathy must avoided. Re-educate and monitor diet.

Gastroenterology

Carcinoid tumours

A diverse group of tumours of enterochromaffin cell (neural crest) origin, definition capable of producing 5HT. Common sites: appendix (45%), ileum (30 or rectum (20%).[2] They also occur elsewhere in the GI tract, ovary, testis, a bronchi. 80% of tumours >2cm across will metastasize (ie consider all malignant). ***Symptoms & signs:*** Initially few. GI tumours can cause appendicit intussusception, or obstruction. Hepatic metastases may cause RUQ pain. Tumou may secrete bradykinin, tachykinin, substance P, VIP, gastrin, insulin, glucagon, AC (∴ Cushing's syndrome), parathyroid, and thyroid hormones. 10% are part of ME syndrome (p207) and 10% occur with other neurendocrine tumours.[148]

Carcinoid syndrome occurs in ~5% and implies hepatic involvement. ***Symptor and signs:*** Bronchoconstriction; paroxysmal flushing especially in upper body migrating weals); diarrhoea; CCF (tricuspid incompetence and pulmonary stenos from 5HT-induced fibrosis). ***CNS effects:*** Many, eg **enhanced** ability to learn ne stimulus–response associations.[149] ►***Carcinoid crisis:*** (see EMERGENCY BOX).

Diagnosis 24h urine 5-hydroxyindoleacetic acid↑ (5HIAA, a 5HT metabolite; leve change with drugs and diet: discuss with lab). If liver metastases are not found, t to find the primary (CXR; chest/pelvis MRI/CT). ***New tests:*** Plasma chromogranin (reflects tumour mass);[150] ^{111}Indium octreotide scintigraphy (octreoscan); positron emission tomography (p472) techniques are alse being developed.

Treatment ***Carcinoid syndrome: Octreotide*** (somatostatin analogue) bloc release of tumour mediators and counters peripheral effects. Effects lessen ov time. Other options: ***loperamide*** or ***cyproheptadine*** for diarrhoea;[152] ***interferon-α*** add-in therapy with ***octreotide***.[153] ***Tumour therapy:*** Curative resection is possib so it is important to identify the primary (see above); at surgery the tumours ha an intense yellow appearance. Surgical debulking (eg enucleating), embolization, radiofrequency ablation of hepatic metastases can ↓symptoms. These requi ***octreotide*** cover to avoid precipitating a massive carcinoid crisis. ***Medi survival:*** 5–8yrs; 38 months if metastases are present, but may be **much long** (~20 yrs); so beware of giving up too easily, even if metastases are present.[154]

1 The link of diet (oranges and lemons) with the symptoms of 'the scurvy' is accredited to t naval surgeon James Lind, as described in his *Treatise* of 1753.

2 Some are never clinically detected: 1 in 300 autopsies have a small bowel carcinoid tumour.

ood mountains, the pellagra paradox, and the sorrow that eeping cannot symbolize[1]

'he sweet smell is a great sorrow on the land. Men who can graft the trees and ake the seed fertile and big can find no way to let the hungry people eat their oduce ... The works of the roots of the vines, of the trees, must be destroyed to eep up the price ...

There is a crime here that goes beyond denunciation. There is a sorrow here 1at weeping cannot symbolize. There is a failure here that topples all our iccess. The fertile earth, the straight tree rows, the sturdy trunks, and the ripe uit. And children dying of pellagra must die because a profit cannot be taken om an orange. And coroners must fill in the certificates—died of alnutrition—because the food must rot, must be forced to rot.

The people come with nets to fish for potatoes in the river, and the guards old them back; they come in rattling cars to get the dumped oranges, but the erosene is sprayed. And they stand still and watch the potatoes float by, listen the screaming pigs being killed in a ditch and covered with quicklime, watch ne mountains of oranges slop down to a putrefying ooze; and in the eyes of the eople there is a failure; and in the eyes of the hungry there is a growing wrath. 1 the souls of the people the grapes of wrath are filling and growing heavy, rowing heavy for the vintage.'

ow do John Steinbeck's grapes grow in our 21st century soil? Too well; a ouble harvest, it turns out, as not only is much of the world starving, amid lenty (for those who can pay) but there is a new 'sorrow in our land that veeping cannot symbolize': pathological 'voluntary' **self-starvation**, again amid lenty, in pursuit of the body-beautiful according to images laid down by media ods. If gastroenterologists had one wish it might not be the ending of all their iseases, but that human-kind stand in a right-relationship with Steinbeck's ertile earth, his straight trees, his sturdy trunks, and his ripe fruit.

Vhipple's procedure

a) Areas of reflection of different parts (b) Post-operation

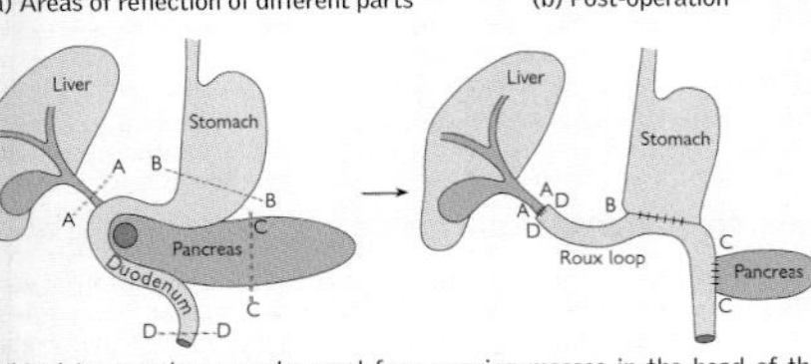

Vhipple's procedure may be used for removing masses in the head of the ancreas—typically from pancreatic carcinoma, or rarely, a carcinoid tumour.

Carcinoid crisis

Vhen a tumour outgrows its blood supply or is handled too much during surgery, nediators flood out. There is life-threatening vasodilatation, hypotension, achycardia, bronchoconstriction and hyperglycaemia. It is treated with high-lose ***octreotide***, supportive measures and careful management of fluid balance ie a central line is needed—see p762 for insertion technique).

1 J Steinbeck *The Grapes of Wrath*, chapter 25.

Gastrointestinal malabsorption

Causes—see B

Symptoms Diarrhoea; ↓weight; lethargy; steatorrhoea (fatty stools, hard to flush aw… **Deficiency signs** Anaemia (↓Fe, B_{12}, folate); bleeding disorders (↓vit K); oede… (↓protein); metabolic bone disease (↓vit D); neurological features, eg neuropath…

Tests FBC (↓ or ↑MCV); ↓Ca^{2+}; ↓Fe; ↓B_{12} + folate; ↑INR; lipid profile; coeliac serol… (below). ***Stool:*** Sudan stain for fat globules; stool microscopy for infestati… ***Barium follow-through:*** Diverticula; Crohn's; radiation enteritis. ***Breath hydrog… analysis:*** for bacterial overgrowth. Take samples of end-expired air; give gluco… take more samples at ½h intervals; ↑exhaled hydrogen = overgrowth. ***Endoscop… small bowel biopsy. ERCP:*** (p728) biliary obstruction; chronic pancreatitis.

Tropical malabsorption ***Typical causes:*** *Giardia intestinalis, Cryptosporidi… parvum, Isospora belli, Cyclospora cayetanensis,* and the microsporidia. ***Tropi… sprue:*** Villous atrophy and malabsorption occurring in the Far and Middle East a… Caribbean (it is rarer in Africa)—the cause is unknown. ***Tetracycline*** 250mg/… PO + ***folic acid*** 15mg/24h PO + optimum nutrition may help.

Coeliac disease

Gastroenterology

This is a T-cell mediated autoimmune disease of the small bowel in which prolam… (alcohol-soluble proteins in wheat, barley, rye ± oats) intolerance causes villo… atrophy and malabsorption.[1] ***Associations:*** HLA DQ2 in 95%; the rest are D… autoimmune disease; dermatitis herpetiformis. ***Prevalence:*** 1 in 300–1500 (mo… common in Irish). Occurs at any age (peaks in infancy and 50–60yrs). ♀>♂. There… a 10% prevalence in 1st degree relatives and a 30% relative risk for siblings.

Presentation: Steatorrhoea; abdominal pain; bloating; nausea + vomiting; aphtho… ulcers, angular stomatitis; weight↓; fatigue; weakness; incidental iron-deficien… anaemia; osteomalacia; failure to thrive (children). ⅓ are asymptomatic.

Diagnosis Antibodies: α-gliadin, transglutaminase & anti-endomysial—an IgA an… body, 95% specific unless the patient is IgA-deficient. Duodenal biopsy done… endoscopy (p248—as good as jejunal biopsy if ≥4 taken): subtotal villous atrophy… crypt hyperplasia, **reversing** on gluten-free diet (along with ↓symptoms & antibodie…

Treatment **Lifelong gluten-free diet** (ie no prolamins)—patients become expert… Rice, maize, soya, potatoes, oats (≤50g/d), and sugar are OK. Gluten-free biscui… flour, bread, & pasta are prescribable. Verify diet by endomysial antibody tests.

Complications Anaemia; 2° lactose-intolerance; GI T-cell lymphoma (rare; suspect… refractory symptoms or ↓weight); ↑risk of malignancy (gastric, oesophage… bladder, breast, brain); myopathies; neuropathies; hyposplenism; osteoporosis.

Chronic pancreatitis

Epigastric pain 'bores' through to back, eg relieved by sitting forward or hot wat… bottles on epigastrium/back (look for *erythema ab igne*'s mottled dusky greynes… bloating; steatorrhoea; ↓weight; brittle diabetes. Symptoms relapse and worse…

Causes: Alcohol; *rarely:* familial; cystic fibrosis; haemochromatosis; pancreatic du… obstruction (stones/tumour); ↑PTH; congenital (*pancreas divisum*).

Tests ***Ultrasound*** (eg pseudocyst) (p259) ± ***CT, MRCP*** + ***ERCP*** (risks acute attack… ***AXR:*** speckled pancreatic calcification; ↑glucose; breath tests eg ^{13}C-hiolien.

Treatment: ***Drugs:*** Give analgesia (± coeliac-plexus block); ***lipase***, eg Creon®; fa… soluble vitamins (eg Multivite®). Insulin requirements may be greater than… idiopathic diabetes and hypoglycaemia is a risk. ***Diet:*** No alcohol; low fat may hel… Medium-chain triglycerides (MCT oil®) may be tried (no lipase needed for absor… tion, but diarrhoea may be worsened). ***Surgery:*** For unremitting pain; narcot… abuse (beware of this); weight↓: eg pancreatectomy or pancreaticojejunostom…

Complications Pseudocyst; diabetes; biliary obstruction; local arterial aneurysm… splenic vein thrombosis; gastric varices.

Causes of gastrointestinal malabsorption

Common in the UK:
- Coeliac disease.
- Chronic pancreatitis.
- Crohn's disease.

Rarer:
- ***↓Bile:*** PBC; ileal resection; biliary obstruction; colestyramine.
- ***Pancreatic insufficiency:*** Pancreatic cancer; cystic fibrosis.
- ***Small bowel mucosa:*** Whipple's diseases (p708); tropical sprue; radiation enteritis; small bowel resection; brush border enzyme deficiencies (eg lactase insufficiency); drugs (metformin, neomycin, alcohol); amyloid (p354).
- ***Bacterial overgrowth:*** Spontaneous (especially in elderly); in jejunal diverticula; post-op blind loops. Try ***metronidazole*** 400mg/8h PO or ***oxytetracycline*** 250mg/6h.
- ***Infection:*** Giardiasis; diphyllobothriasis (B_{12} malabsorption); strongyloidiasis.
- ***Intestinal hurry:*** Post-gastrectomy dumping; post-vagotomy; gastro-jejunostomy.

Deficiency syndromes and the sites of nutrient absorption

Nutrient	Site of absorption	Deficiency syndrome
Vitamin		
A^F	Small intestine	Xerophthalmia (p270)
B_1 (thiamine)	Small intestine	Beriberi (p270); Wernicke's encephalopathy (p706)
B_2 (riboflavin)	Proximal small intestine	Angular stomatis; cheilitis (p230)
B_6 (pyridoxine)	Small intestine	Polyneuropathy
B_{12}	Terminal ileum	Macrocytic anaemia (p318); neuropathy; glossitis
C	Proximal ileum	Scurvy (p270)
D^F	Jejunum as free vitamin	Rickets (p670); osteomalacia (p670)
E^F	Small intestine	Haemolysis; neurological deficit
K^F	Small intestine	Bleeding disorders (p330)
Folic acid	Jejunum	Macrocytic anaemia (p318)
Nicotinamide	Jejunum	Pellagra (p270)
Mineral		
Calcium	Duodenum + jejunum	p670
Copper	Stomach + Jejunum	Menkes' kinky hair syndrome
Fluoride	Stomach	Dental caries
Iodide	Small intestine	Goitre (p622); cretinism
Iron	Duodenum + jejunum	Microcytic anaemia (p312)
Magnesium	Small intestine	p672
Phosphate	Small intestine	Osteoporosis; anorexia; weakness
Selenium	Small intestine	Cardiomyopathy
Zinc	Jejunum	Acrodermatitis enteropathica; poor wound healing

F = fat-soluble vitamin, thus deficiency is likely if there is fat malabsorption.

Infectious aetiological agents have been implicated: eg *Candida albicans* could be one trigger. HWP1 has amino acid sequences identical to coeliac disease-related α-gliadin T-cell epitopes.

Alcoholism

An alcoholic is one whose repeated drinking leads to harm in his work or social li
It is common (~25%), ranging from binge drinking to heavy daily intake, and is us
ally tied in with other life or health issues. Other addictions may also be involve
►Denial is a leading feature of alcoholism, so be sure to question relatives. Alcoh
can do you good in low doses, eg <20U/wk in men, <15U/wk in women (see p228

CAGE questions Ever felt you ought to cut down on your drinking? Have peop annoyed you by criticizing your drinking? Ever felt bad or guilty about yo drinking? Ever had an eye-opener to steady nerves in the morning? CAGE (yes to ≥ is quite good at detecting alcohol abuse and dependence (sensitivity 43–94 specificity 70–97%),[MET 160] but accuracy does change according to backgrou population. There are several other screening methods: eg TWEAK (see BOX); AUDIT.

Organs affected (►Don't forget the risk of trauma whilst intoxicated.)[162]

- ***The liver:*** Normal in 50% of alcoholics; γGT↑ or ↑↑, but is non-specific (may be in any condition that causes liver inflammation, eg AIH (p260), HBV). ***Fatty live*** Acute and reversible, but may progress to cirrhosis if drinking continues (also see in obesity, DM, and with amiodarone). ***Alcoholic hepatitis:*** see BOX. 80% progre to cirrhosis (hepatic failure in 10%). ***Cirrhosis*** (p252): 5yr survival is 48% drinking continues (if not, 77%). ***Biopsy:*** Mallory bodies ± neutrophil infiltrat
- ***CNS:*** Poor memory/cognition: multiple high-potency vitamins IM may reverse i cortical atrophy; retrobulbar neuropathy; fits; falls; wide-based gait neuropath confabulation; Korsakoff's (p696) ± Wernicke's encephalopathy (p706).
- ***GI tract:*** Obesity; diarrhoea; gastric erosions; peptic ulcers; varices (p246 pancreatitis (acute and chronic); carcinoma; oral mucosal lesions.
- ***Blood:*** MCV↑; anaemia from: marrow depression, GI bleeding, alcoholism associated folate deficiency, haemolysis; sideroblastic anaemia. See p318.
- ***Heart:*** Arrhythmias; BP↑; cardiomyopathy; sudden death in binge drinkers.

Withdrawal starts 10–72h after last drink. ***Signs:*** Pulse↑; BP↓; tremor; confusio fits; hallucinations (*delirium tremens*)—may be visual or tactile, eg animals crawlin all over skin. Consider it in any new (≤3d) ward patient with acute confusion.

Alcohol contraindications Driving; hepatitis; cirrhosis; peptic ulcer; drugs (e antihistamines, metronidazole); carcinoid; pregnancy (fetal alcohol syndrome—IQ↓ short palpebral fissure, absent philtrum, and small eyes).

Management ***Alcohol withdrawal:*** Admit; do BP + TPR/4h. Beware BP↓. For th 1st 3d give generous ***chlordiazepoxide***, eg 10–50mg/6h PO, weaning over 7–14 (see TABLE); alternative: ***diazepam***; the once-preferred ***clomethiazole*** readily cause addiction. Vitamins may be needed (p706). ***Prevention:*** (*OHCS* p513): Alcohol-fre beers; low-risk drinking (see below), remembering that there are no absolutes an that risk is a continuum. *1U≈9g ethanol≈1 spirits measure ≈1 glass wine ≈½ pint bee* ***Treating established alcoholics*** may be rewarding, particularly if they really wan to change. If so, **group therapy** or **self-help** (eg 'Alcoholics Anonymous') may b useful—especially if self-initiated and determined. Encourage the will to change ***Suggest:*** 1 Graceful ways of declining a drink, eg 'I'm seeing what it's like to g without for a bit'; 2 not buying him- or herself a drink when it is his/her turn 3 'Don't lift your glass to your lips until after the slowest drinker in your grou takes a drink'; 4 'Sip, don't gulp'. Give follow-up and encouragement.

Relapse 50% will relapse soon after starting treatment. ***Acamprosate*** (p443)[163] may help intense anxiety, insomnia, and craving. CI: pregnancy, severe liver failure creatinine >120µmol/L. SE: D&V, libido ↑ or ↓; dose example: 666mg/8h PO if >60kg and <65yrs old.[164] It should be started as soon as acute withdrawal is complete and continued for ~1yr. ***Disulfiram*** can be used to treat chronic alcoho dependence. It causes acetaldehyde build-up (like metronidazole) with extremely unpleasant effects to **any** alcohol ingestion—eg flushing, throbbing headache palpitations. Care must be taken to avoid alcohol (eg toiletries, food, medicines since severe reactions can occur. ►Confer with experts if drugs are to be used.

TWEAK screening questions

- Have you an increased tolerance of alcohol? 2pts
- Do you worry about your drinking? 2pts
- Have you ever had alcohol as an eye-opener in the morning? 1pt
- Do you ever get amnesia after drinking alcohol? 1pt
- Have you ever felt the need to c(k)ut down on your drinking? 1pt

A score of ≥2 suggests an alcohol problem. It may be more sensitive than the CAGE questionnaire in some populations (eg pregnant women).

Patterns of lab tests in alcoholic and other liver disease

	AST	ALT	AST : ALT	MCV
Alcoholic liver disease	↑↑	↑	>2	↑↑
Hepatitis C (HCV)	↑ or ↔	↑↑	<1*	↔
Non-alcoholic fatty liver disease	↑	↑↑	<1	↑ or ↔

*ratio may reverse if cirrhosis develops. See p742 for reference intervals.

Managing alcoholic hepatitis

Clinical picture TPR↑; anorexia; D&V; tender hepatomegaly ±jaundice; bleeding; ascites. ***Bloods:*** WCC↑; INR↓; AST↑; MCV↑; urea↑. ►Severe hepatitis is indicated by **jaundice**, **encephalopathy** and **coagulopathy**.

- Stop alcohol consumption: for withdrawal symptoms, if ***chlordiazepoxide*** by the oral route is impossible, try ***lorazepam*** IM.
- High-dose B vitamins IV as ***Pabrinex***®—1 pair of ampoules in 50mL 0.9% saline IVI over ½h; (see Datasheet)—have resuscitation equipment to hand.
- Optimize nutrition (35–40kcal/kg/d non-protein energy) + 1.5g/kg/d of protein (use ideal body weight for calculations eg if malnourished). This prevents encephalopathy, sepsis, and some deaths.
- Daily weight; LFT; U&E; INR. If creatinine↑, get help with this HRS (p251). Na^+↓ is common, but water restriction may make matters worse. See p250.
- Culture ascites fluid and treat for SBP, if suspected (p252).
- Work out the Maddrey Discriminant Factor (DF) = (4.6 × PT-control time) + [bilirubin] (in µmol/L). If >32 (ie severe disease) then start steroid therapy ►provided sepsis has been excluded: eg ***prednisolone*** 40mg/d for 5d tapered off over 3 weeks. Mortality roughly equivilates to the DF score—see below.

Prognosis: Mild episodes often resolve with no affect on mortality. Severe hepatitis can have a 30d mortality of 50%, reduced to 5% if only mild. ►At 1 year after an admission for alcoholic hepatitis, 40% are dead—a sobering thought.

An example of a chlordiazepoxide reducing regime

Day	am	noon	pm	nocte	total/d
1	20mg	20mg	20mg	20mg	80mg
2	20mg	15mg	15mg	20mg	70mg
3	15mg	15mg	15mg	15mg	60mg
4	15mg	10mg	10mg	15mg	50mg
5	10mg	10mg	10mg	10mg	40mg
6	10mg	5mg	5mg	10mg	30mg
7	5mg	5mg	5mg	5mg	20mg
8	5mg	-	-	5mg	10mg
9	-	-	-	5mg	5mg
10	-	-	-	-	discontinue

►***Caveats:*** doses may need to be higher for the 1st few days for severe withdrawal; there may still be mild withdrawal symptoms at day 3. Have a 5mg dose written for PRN use.

8 Renal medicine

Contents

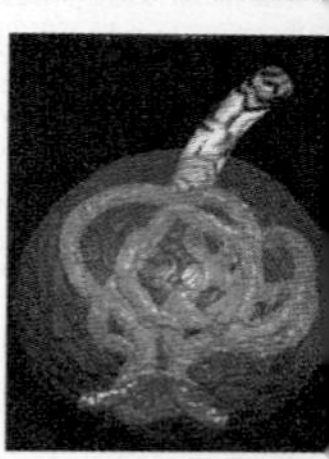

Fig 1. Electron microscopy imag of arterioles in a glomerulus.

Relevant pages in other chapters: Symptoms and signs: Frequency (p60); lo pain (p76); oedema (p66); oliguria (p66); polyuria (p66).

Surgery: Renal and urological malignancies (p606); urinary retention (p602 incontinence (p604).

Emergencies: Management of acute renal failure: p820.

Also: Vasculitis (p542); polyarteritis nodosa (p543); urological cancers (p60(genitourinary TB (p564); immunosuppressives (p360); biochemistry of ren function (p660); electrolyte physiology (p664); sodium (p664 & p666); potassiu (p668); calcium (p694); urate and the kidney (p686); osteomalacia (p676); urina tract imaging (p730); catheters (p750).

In OHCS: Gynaecological urology (*OHCS* p306); bacteriuria and pyelonephritis pregnancy (*OHCS* p28); obstetric causes of acute tubular necrosis (*OHCS* p28 chronic renal disease in pregnancy (*OHCS* p28); UTI in children (*OHCS* p174); urethr valves (*OHCS* p132); horseshoe kidney (*OHCS* p132); ectopic kidney (*OHCS* p132 hypospadias (*OHCS* p132); Wilms' nephroblastoma (*OHCS* p133); acute and chron renal failure in children (*OHCS* p176); nephritis and nephrosis in children (*OHC* p178); Potter's syndrome (*OHCS* p120).

Calculating creatinine clearance (CrCl) and the eGFR: See p661.

We thank Dr. Andrew Mooney who is our Specialist Reader for this chapter.

Renal disease typically presents with one or more of rather a short list of clinical syndromes—listed from 1 to 7 below. One underlying pathology may have a variety of clinical presentations.

roteinuria and nephrotic syndrome: Normal protein excretion is <150mg/d. This may rise to ~300mg/d—eg orthostatic proteinuria (related to posture), luring fever, or after exercise. *Proteinuria* (excessive protein excretion) is a sign of glomerular or tubular disease. *Nephrotic syndrome* (p290) is the triad of proteinuria (>3g/d), hypoalbuminaemia (albumin <30g/L) and oedema.

Haematuria and nephritic syndrome: Blood in the urine may arise from anywhere in the renal tract. It may be *macroscopic* (visible to the naked eye) or *microscopic* (found on dipstick testing and microscopy). **Haematuria with dysuria** is usually from a UTI. **Painless haematuria** is more ominous, eg bladder or other GU cancer (eg if >40yrs old, esp if a smoker) or glomerulonephritis. **Nephritic syndrome** comprises haematuria and proteinuria—often with hypertension, pulmonary and peripheral oedema, oliguria (urine output <400mL/d), and a rising plasma urea and creatinine. The question of who to refer haematuria patients to (urologist or nephrologist) is answered on p278.

Renal pain and dysuria: **Renal pain** is usually a dull and constant and in the loin. It may be due to renal obstruction (look for swelling ± tenderness), pyelonephritis, acute nephritic syndrome, polycystic kidneys, or renal infarction. **Renal (ureteric) colic** is severe waxing and waning loin pain radiating to groin or thigh eg with fever and vomiting. It is caused by a renal stone, clot, or a sloughed papilla. **Urinary frequency** with **dysuria** (pain on voiding) suggests a UTI.

Oliguria and polyuria: **Oliguria** is a urine output of <400mL/d—a normal response to hot climates or fluid restriction. *Pathological causes*: renal perfusion↓, renal parenchymal disease, renal tract obstruction. **Polyuria** is the voiding of abnormally high volumes of urine, usually from high fluid intake—or diabetes mellitus, diabetes insipidus (p224), hypercalcaemia, renal medulla disorders (urine concentration is impaired), and SVT (p112).

Acute renal failure (ARF) is significant decline in renal function occurring over hours or days, detected by a rising plasma creatinine (± oliguria). ARF usually occurs secondary to a circulatory dysfunction (hypotension, hypovolaemia, sepsis) or urinary obstruction. Primary renal disease is a less common cause.

Chronic renal failure (CRF) or chronic kidney disease (CKD) is defined as irreversible, substantial, and long-standing loss of renal function. It is classified according to glomerular filtration rate (GFR): see p661. There is often a poor correlation between symptoms and severity of CRF. Progression may be so insidious that patients attribute symptoms to age or a minor illnesses. **Current guidelines advise nephrology referral if CKD stage ≥3** (p661), ie GFR <60mL/min, ***if other features are present:*** • GFR is falling progressively
• Microscopic haematuria • Urine protein:creatinine ratio (PCR)↑, p301
• Unexplained anaemia, hyperkalaemia, or calcium or phosphate imbalance
• Suspected systemic illness (eg SLE) • BP uncontrolled despite taking 3 drugs.
Refer ***urgently*** if GFR 15–29 (same-day if <15) even if ***no*** other features present.

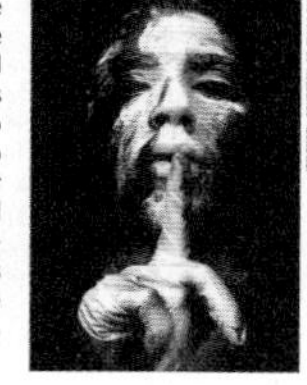
'SILENCE'—COURTESY OF TIAGO-PHELIPE

Silence: Serious renal failure may cause **no symptoms at all**. This is why we do U&Es before surgery and other major interventions. The silence of renal disease creeps up on us (doctors and patients)—with uncanny stealth which is as alarming as the image opposite—'Silence', by Tiago Phelipe. This picture serves to remind us not to dismiss odd chronic symptoms such as fatigue or 'not being quite with it'—without doing a blood test. ***Microalbuminuria*** is a famously silent harbinger of serious renal and cardiovascular risk. It is described on p306. In one study, 30% of those with type 2 diabetes mellitus died within ~5 years of developing microalbuminuria.

Urine

Examine mid-stream urine (MSU) whenever you suspect renal disease. **Dipsti**

- ***Haematuria:*** *Renal causes:* Neoplasia, glomerulonephritis (often nephropathy, p288), tubulointerstitial nephritis, polycystic kidney, papi necrosis, infection (pyelonephritis), trauma. *Extrarenal:* Calculi, infection (cys prostatitis, urethritis), neoplasia (bladder, prostate, urethra), trauma (eg f catheter). ***Tests:*** Urine MC&S, FBC, ESR, CRP, U&E, clotting. *Others:* AXR/KUB, p (stones), urine cytology, estimation of proteinuria (see below), renal ultrasou renal biopsy. ***Management:*** Usually refer first to a urologist, and do ultraso Only refer initially to renal physician if the risk of urothelial malignancy is and risk of glomerulonephritis is not negligible (eg <40yrs old, creatinine↑, proteinuria, systemic symptoms, family history of renal disease). Not all wo with recurrent UTI + haematuria need cystoscopy, but have a good reason *n* do cystoscopy (Reynard's rule). ***False +ve dipstick haematuria:*** Hae globinuria, myoglobin (eg in rhabdomyolysis), beetroot, porphyria, alkapton rifampicin, phenindione, phenolphthalein.
- ***Proteinuria:*** Normal protein excretion is <150mg/d, consisting of <30g/ albumin. *Renal causes of proteinuria:* UTI, orthostatic proteinuria, glomerulonepl (GN), ↑BP, DM, myeloma, amyloid. *Extrarenal:* Fever, exercise, pregnancy, CCF, va mucus, recent ejaculation. *Tests:* BP, urine MC&S. *Estimation of proteinuria:* 24h collection for protein and creatinine quantifies proteinuria *if* collected accura spot tests for urine albumin:creatinine ratio or urine protein:creatinine inde much easier and provide reasonably accurate information; renal ultraso autoantibodies eg immunoglobulins, serum electrophoresis, urinary Bence J protein (p288); consider a renal biopsy if renal function is deteriora ***Microalbuminuria*** is undetectable on dipstick, with albuminuria of 30–300mg on lab tests. ***Causes:*** DM, ↑BP, minimal change GN.
- ***Other substances—Glucose:*** Low renal threshold (eg chronic renal failure) pregnancy, sepsis, renal tubular damage. ***Ketones:*** Starvation, ketoacid ***Leucocytes:*** UTI, vaginal discharge. ***Nitrites:*** UTI, high-protein meal. ***Bilir*** Obstructive jaundice. ***Urobilinogen:*** Pre-hepatic jaundice. ***Specific gra*** Normal range: 1.000–1.030 (useful to assess degree of proteinuri haematuria). ***pH:*** Normal range: 4.5–8 (acid–base balance: p658).

Microscopy Put a drop of fresh urine (MSU or suprapubic aspirate) c microscope slide, cover with a coverslip and examine under low (×100) and (×400) power for leucocytes, red cells, bacteria, casts and crystals. If renal dis is suspected, a centrifuged urine should be examined.

Leucocytes: $>10/mm^3$ in an unspun urine specimen is abnormal. Usually due UTI, see p283 for causes of sterile pyuria (when no bacteria are found).

Red cells: $>2/mm^3$ in unspun urine is abnormal. *Causes:* See haematuria.

Casts are cylindrical bodies formed in the lumen of distal tubules.

- ***Finely granular*** and ***hyaline casts*** (clear, colourless) are found in no concentrated urine. They are increased in fever, exercise or loop diuretics.
- ***Densely granular:*** Glomerular or tubular disease eg GN, interstitial nephri
- ***Fatty casts:*** Moderate–heavy proteinuria. Don't mistake fat globules for R
- ***Red cell casts*** are a diagnostic marvel, as they *prove* that haematuria is g erular, allowing you to start an interesting dialogue with a nephrologist: 'is t vasculitis (p542), glomerulonephritis, or malignant hypertension?'
- ***White cell casts*** occur in pyelonephritis.
- ***Tubular cell casts*** occur in acute tubular necrosis.

Crystals are common in old or cold urine and may not signify pathology. The important in stone formers: cystine crystals are diagnostic of cystinuria, oxalate crystals in fresh urine may indicate a predisposition to form calculi.

24h urine for Na^+, K^+, Ca^{2+}, urea, creatinine ± protein excretion. Take b simultaneously for creatinine to calculate creatinine clearance (p661).

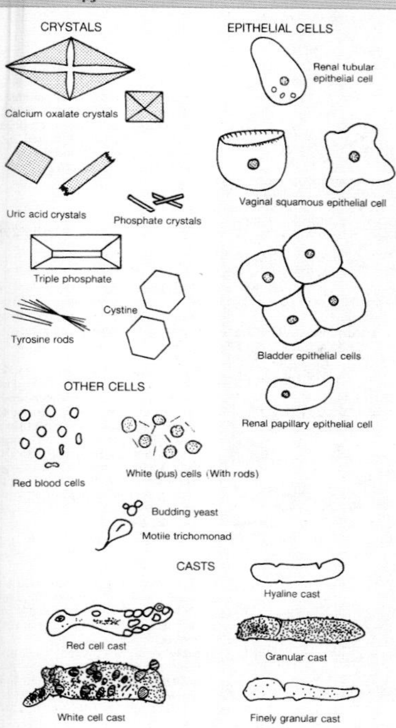

Principal source: *Atlas of Bedside Microscopy* ©JM Longmore; RCGP

hen you find red cells, consider their morphology to understand where in the GU t they come from. If >10% of RBCs are dysmorphic G1 cells, suspect glomerular ding, and look hard for red cell casts. G1 cells have doughnut shapes, target igurations, and membrane protrusions or blebs. NB: identifying dysmorphic red is subjective and often difficult.

nthocyturia ≈ RBCs with spicules.

ell images (stained urine cytology): www.uninet.edu/cin2003/conf/nguyen/nguyen.html

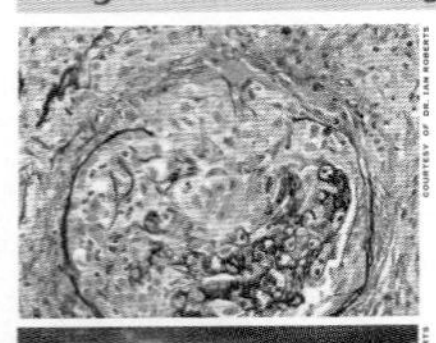

Fig 1. Crescentic glomerulonephritis: a liferation of epithelial cells macrophages with rupture of Bowm capsule, in this patient caused by a glomerular basement membrane (Gc pasture's) disease, see p692.

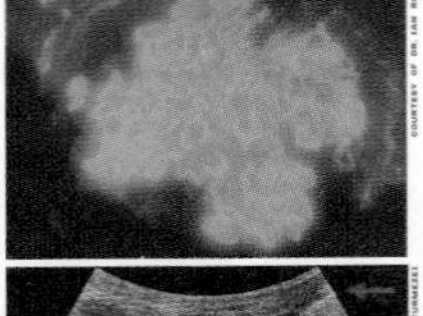

Fig 2. Immunofluorescence for IgG, sh ing linear staining for glomerular basem characteristic of anti-glomerular basem membrane (Goodpasture's) disease.

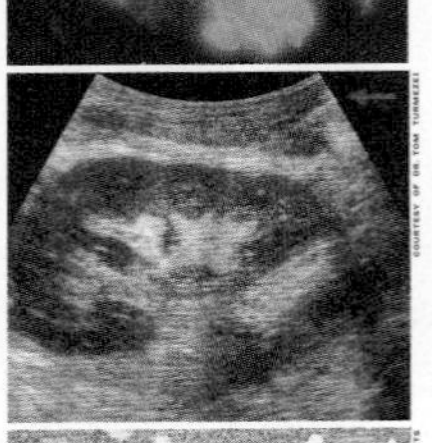

Fig 3. US-guided biopsy of a transplant kidn this reduces the risk of damaging the r vessels and pelvis, as well as any nearby b (although the graft is usually extra-peritor The red arrow is point of entry of the bi needle. The hypoechoic tissue around needle is from the infiltration of local ar thetic. 3 separate 'shots' of the biopsy 'gur usually enough to get a good sample, the let the patient know what a 'shot' sounds before starting, so that they don't start down the ward!

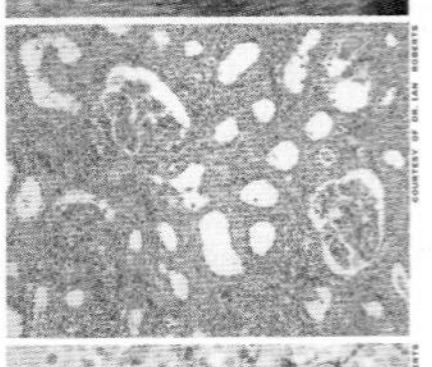

Fig 4. Renal allograft rejection: Cellular ection, showing a tubulointerstitial infilt of lymphocytes—this is usually gra according to the *Banff* criteria. Altho 'rejection' may sound fierce, it is usu easily and well-treated by increa immunosuppression eg with a pulse methylprednisolone. ►Watch for infec (eg CMV).

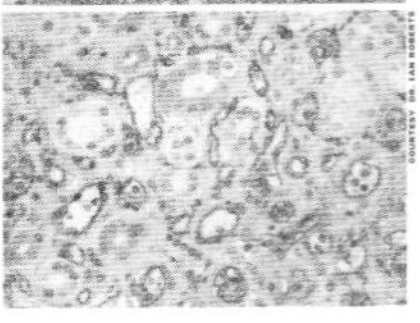

Fig 5. Renal allograft rejection: Antib mediated rejection, with diffuse p tubular capillary staining for complement. Humoral (antibody-media rejection is more problematic than mediated rejection (above); it may r immunoglobulin therapy with plas pheresis in an attempt to clear the sys of donor-specific antibodies.

enal biopsy

lost acute renal failure is due to pre-renal causes or acute tubular necrosis, and covery of renal function typically occurs over the course of a few weeks. Renal opsy should be performed only if knowing histology will influence management. Once chronic renal failure is established, the kidneys are small, there is a gher risk of bleeding from biopsy, and the results are usually unhelpful.

dications for renal biopsy:

What is the cause of this acute renal failure (p292)?

Investigating glomerulonephritis, eg is persistent haematuria from IgA nephropathy, thin basement membrane disease, or hereditary nephropathy?

What is the cause of this heavy proteinuria (eg >1g/d, when you know that diabetes mellitus is not the cause).

Renal dysfunction post-transplantation (p297): is the cause rejection, acute tubular necrosis, drug toxicity, or recurrence of renal disease?

e-procedure: Check FBC, clotting, group & save. Obtain written informed nsent. Ultrasound (if only 1 kidney, risk is magnified). Stop aspirin 1 week and arfarin at least 2 days in advance.

ntraindications: • Abnormal clotting • Hypertension >160/>90 • Single dney • Chronic renal failure with small kidneys (<9cm) • Uncooperative patient

ocedure: Biopsy is done under ultrasound guidance with the patient lying in e prone position and the breath held. Samples should be sent to histology. A ear indication on the request form of why the test has been done, eg exclude nyloidosis, will help in the selection of special stains, immunofluorescence and e of electron microscopy.

st procedure: Bed rest for a minimum of 6hrs. Monitor pulse, BP, symptoms, d urine colour. Bleeding is the main complication; most occurs within 8 hrs, though it may be delayed by up to 72hrs. Macroscopic haematuria occurs in 0%, although blood transfusion is only needed in ~1-2%. Aspirin or warfarin n be restarted the next day if uncomplicated.

Urinary tract infection (UTI)

Childhood UTI: *OHCS* p17

Definitions **Bacteriuria:** Bacteria in the urine, may be asymptomatic symptomatic. **UTI:** The presence of a pure growth of $>10^5$ organisms per mL fresh MSU. UTI sites: urethra (**urethritis**), bladder (**cystitis**), prostate (**prostatiti** or renal pelvis (**pyelonephritis**). Up to ⅓ of women with symptoms have bacte uria; (=**abacterial cystitis** or the **urethral syndrome**). ***Classification:*** UTIs may **uncomplicated** (normal renal tract and function) or **complicated** (abnorm renal/GU tract, ↓renal function, impaired host defences, or virulent organism *Staph. aureus*). Assume that UTI in men without risk factors (below) is complicat until proved otherwise. A **recurrent** UTI is a further infection with a new organis A **relapse** is a further infection with the same organism. For urethritis, see p40

Risk factors ♀, sexual intercourse, exposure to spermicide in ♀ (by diaphragm condoms), pregnancy, menopause; ↓*host defence*: immunosuppression, DM; *urin tract*: obstruction (p286), stones, catheter, malformation. **NB:** in pregnancy, UT common and often asymptomatic, until serious pyelonephritis, premature delive (± fetal death) supervenes, so do routine dipstix in pregnancy. Urine in catheteriz bladders is almost always infected—it is pointless sending samples or treati unless the patient is ill.

Organisms *E. coli* is the main organism (>70% in the community but ≤41% hospital). Also *Staphylococcus saprophyticus, Proteus mirabilis*. Rarer: *Ente coccus faecalis, Klebsiella, Enterobacter* and *Acinetobacter* species, *Pseudomo aeruginosa, Serratia marascens, Candida albicans,* and *Staph. aureus*.

Symptoms ***Cystitis:*** Frequency, dysuria, urgency, strangury, haematuria, sup pubic pain. ***Acute pyelonephritis:*** High fever, rigors, vomiting, loin pain a tenderness, oliguria (if acute renal failure). ***Prostatitis:*** Flu-like symptoms, l backache, few urinary symptoms, swollen or tender prostate on PR.

Signs Fever, abdominal or loin tenderness, foul-smelling urine. Occasiona distended bladder, enlarged prostate. **NB:** see *Vaginal discharge*, p406.

Tests If symptoms are present, dipstick the urine and treat empirically if nitrites leucocytes are positive. If they are negative, consider sending an MSU for lab MC to confirm this. Send a lab MSU anyway if male, a child (*OHCS* p174), pregna immunosuppressed or ill, or if symptoms don't resolve after one course of empiri treatment. A pure growth of $>10^5$ organisms per mL is diagnostic. If <1 organisms/mL and pyuria (eg >20 WBCs/mm³), the result may still be significa Cultured organisms are tested for sensitivity to a range of antibiotics (p368).

Blood tests: FBC, U&E, CRP, and blood cultures eg if systemically unwell.

Ultrasound or IVU/cystoscopy: Consider for UTI in children; men; if failure respond to treatment; recurrent UTI (>2/year); pyelonephritis; unusual organis persistent haematuria. In one study on men, ultrasound combined with plain XR kidneys, ureters and bladder (KUB) was as effective as IVU in detecting urinary tr abnormalities, and avoided exposure to IV contrast.[5]

Treatment ►Drink plenty of fluids; urinate often (don't 'hold on'). In pregnancy, expert help. *Know your local pattern of resistance.* Until the organism is know

- ***Cystitis:*** Trimethoprim 200mg/12h PO (3d course in ♀, 7d in ♂). Alternat cefalexin 1g/12h. 2nd line: ciprofloxacin or co-amoxiclav PO (7d course).
- ***Acute pyelonephritis:*** Cefuroxime 1.5g/8h IV then oral × 7d course.
- ***Prostatitis:*** Ciprofloxacin 500mg/12h PO for ~4wks.

Prevention Antibiotic prophylaxis, continuously or post-coital, ↓infection rate women with recurrent UTIs. Self-treatment with a single antibiotic dose symptoms start is an option. Drinking 200–750ml of cranberry or lingonberry ju a day, or taking cranberry concentrate tablets, reduces the risk of symptoma recurrent infection in women by 10–20%,[6] may be by inhibiting adherence bacteria to bladder uroepithelial cells. There is no evidence that postcoital void or advice on wiping patterns in females is of benefit.[7]

Causes of sterile pyuria

Always remember renal TB (do 3 early morning urines). Other causes:

- Treated UTI <2 weeks prior
- Inadequately treated UTI
- Appendicitis
- Calculi
- Prostatitis
- Bladder tumour
- UTI with fastidious culture requirement
- Papillary necrosis (eg DM or analgesic excess)
- Tubulointerstitial nephritis
- Polycystic kidney
- Chemical cystitis (eg cyclophosphamide).

What is the predictive value of urinary symptoms and dipstick for diagnosing UTI?

This is a controversial area, with a meta-analysis on 70 studies concluding that in the general population, a combination of negative nitrite and leucocyte tests on dipstick was sufficient to rule out UTI.[MET 8]

However, a recent small prospective study (n=59) showed that although a negative dipstick test accurately predicted the absence of UTI according to urine culture, treating these patients with trimethoprim still reduced symptoms of dysuria, suggesting that the cause in these patients may be infection not detected by current urine dipstick or culture techniques.[9]

Renal calculi (nephrolithiasis)

Renal stones (calculi) consist of crystal aggregates. Stones form in collecting du and may be deposited anywhere from the renal pelvis to the urethra.

Prevalence Common: lifetime incidence up to 15%. *Peak age:* 20–40yr. ♂:♀≈:

Types of stone • Calcium oxalate: 75%.
• Magnesium ammonium phosphate (struvite, triple phosphate): 10–20%.
• Others: urate (5%), hydroxyapatite (5%), brushite, cystine (1%), mixed.

The patient may be asymptomatic or present with a variety of symptoms. *Pc* Stones in the kidney cause loin pain. Stones in the ureter cause renal (urete colic. This occurs in spasms, classically radiates from the 'loin to the groin', an associated with nausea and vomiting. Patients often cannot lie still, differentiat this from peritonitis. Bladder or urethral stones cause pain on micturiti strangury or interruption of urine flow. ***Infection*** can co-exist with renal stor presenting with cystitis (frequency, dysuria), pyelonephritis (fever, rigors, loin p nausea, vomiting), or pyonephrosis (infected hydronephrosis). ***Others:*** Haematu proteinuria, sterile pyuria, anuria.

Tests: FBC, U&E, Ca^{2+}, PO_4^{3-}, glucose, bicarbonate, urate. ***Urine dipstick:*** Usually + for blood. ***MSU:*** MC&S. ***Further tests for cause:*** Urine pH (on dipstick); 24h ur for: calcium, oxalate, urate, citrate, sodium, creatinine; stone biochemistry. ***Imaging:*** KUB XR (kidneys+ureters+bladder). Look along the ureters for cal ication, over the transverse processes of the vertebral bodies: 80% of stones visible (99% on CT). Ultrasound to look for hydronephrosis or hydroureter. C superior to IVU for imaging stones, and helps exclude differential causes of an ac abdomen. ►A ruptured abdominal aortic aneurysm may present similarly.

Management Give prompt analgesia, ideally an NSAID: eg diclofenac 75mg IV or or 100mg suppository. If contraindicated: morphine 5–10mg IV w metoclopramide 10mg IV. Give IV fluids if unable to tolerate orally; antibiotics cefuroxime 1.5g/8h IV) if infection. After imaging ►*seek urological help urgent, evidence of obstruction,* delay may lead to infection and permanent loss of re function. Procedures include extracorporeal shockwave lithotripsy (ESWL) us ultrasonic waves to shatter the stone, percutaneous nephrostomy to reli obstruction, ureteroscopy ± laser, or percutaneous nephrolithotomy (PCNL), us keyhole techniques to remove stones. Open surgery is rarely done.

Stones not causing obstruction between attacks of renal colic may be mana conservatively. Advise to increase fluid intake and sieve the urine to catch the st for biochemical analysis. Most pass within 48h, although some take ≥30d. Sto <5mm in diameter pass spontaneously in ~90% and so are treated conservativ with their progress monitored on serial abdominal films every 1-2 weeks. remainder may require intervention to remove the stone. Ureteric stones <1cm suitable for ESWL, with ureteroscopy preferred if >1cm, (although there is sc debate over the preferred approach in distal stones). For renal stones, ESW preferred if <2cm; PCNL is reserved for larger stones.

Prevention ***General:*** Drink plenty of fluid, especially in the summer or wa weather (aim for 2-3L/day of colourless urine). A *normal* calcium intake is r recommended, as low calcium diets increase oxalate excretion. ***Specific*** • *Calcium stones:* if there is hypercalciuria, a thiazide diuretic (eg bendro methiazide) is used to ↓calcium excretion • *Oxalate:* ↓oxalate intake (less chocolate, nuts, strawberries, rhubarb, spinach, beans, beetroot); pyridoxine ma used (p304) • *Magnesium aluminium phosphate:* treat infection promptly • *Ur* allopurinol (100–300mg/24h PO) to ↓uric acid. Urine alkalinization may also recommended, as urate is more soluble at pH>6 (eg with potassium citrate sodium bicarbonate) • *Cystine:* vigorous hydration to keep urine output >3L/ and urinary alkalinization (as above). D-penicillamine is used to chelate cyst given with pyridoxine to prevent Vitamin B6 deficiency.

uestions to address when confronted by a stone

What is its composition?

Type	Causative factors	Appearance on XR
Calcium oxalate	Metabolic or idiopathic	Spiky, radiopaque
Calcium phosphate	Metabolic or idiopathic	Smooth, may be large, radiopaque
Magnesium ammonium phosphate (struvite)	UTI	Large, horny, 'staghorn' radiopaque
Urate	Hyperuricaemia	Smooth, brown, radiolucent
Cystine	Renal tubular defect	Yellow, crystalline, semi-opaque

Why has he or she got this stone now?

'*What do you eat?*' Chocolate, tea, rhubarb and spinach ↑oxalate levels.
'*Is it summer?*' Seasonal variations in calcium and oxalate levels are thought to be mediated by vitamin D synthesis via sunlight on skin.
'*What's your job?*' Can he/she drink freely? Is there dehydration?
'*Are there any precipitating drugs?*' These include:
Loop diuretics, antacids, acetazolamide, corticosteroids, theophylline, aspirin, thiazides, allopurinol, vitamin C & D, indinavir.
'*Are there any predisposing factors?*' eg:
Recurrent UTIs (in magnesium aluminium phosphate calculi).
Metabolic abnormalities:
- Hypercalciuria/hypercalcaemia (p672): hyperparathyroidism, neoplasia, sarcoidosis, hyperthyroidism, Addison's, Cushing's, lithium, vit D excess.
- Hyperuricosuria/↑plasma urate: on its own, or with gout.
- Hyperoxaluria (p304).
- Cystinuria (p304).
- Renal tubular acidosis (p302).

Urinary tract abnormalities: eg pelviureteric junction obstruction, hydronephrosis (renal pelvis or calyces), calyceal diverticulum, horseshoe kidney, ureterocele, vesicoureteric reflux, ureteral stricture, medullary sponge kidney.[1]

Is there a family history? ↑risk of stones x 3-fold. Specific diseases include X-linked nephrolithiasis and Dent's disease: proteinuria, hypercalciuria and nephrocalcinosis.

Is there infection above the stone? eg fever, loin tender, pyuria? This needs urgent intervention.

Medullary sponge kidney is a typically asymptomatic developmental anomaly of the kidney mostly seen adult females, where there is dilatation of the collecting ducts, which if severe leads to a sponge-like pearance of the renal medulla. *Complications/associations:* UTIs, nephrolithiasis, haematuria and ercalciuria, hyperparathyroidism (if present, look for genetic markers of MEN type 2A, see p207).

Urinary tract obstruction

►*Urinary tract obstruction is common and should be considered in any patient wi impaired renal function.* Damage can be permanent if the obstruction is not treat promptly. It occurs anywhere from the renal calyces to the urethral meatus, a may be *partial* or *complete, unilateral* or *bilateral*. Obstructing lesions are *lumir* (stones, blood clot, sloughed papilla, tumour: renal, ureteric, or bladder), *mural* (congenital or acquired stricture, neuromuscular dysfunction, schistosomiasis), *extra-mural* (abdominal or pelvic mass/tumour, retroperitoneal fibrosis). Unilate obstruction may be clinically silent (normal urine output and U&E), if the oth kidney is functioning. ►Bilateral obstruction or obstruction with infection requir urgent treatment. See emergency box 603.

Clinical features • ***Acute upper tract obstruction:*** Loin pain radiating to the gro There may be superimposed infection ± loin tenderness, or an enlarged kidney.
• ***Chronic upper tract obstruction:*** Flank pain, renal failure, superimpos infection. Polyuria may occur owing to impaired urinary concentration.
• ***Acute lower tract obstruction:*** Acute urinary retention typically presents w severe suprapubic pain, often preceded by symptoms of bladder outflc obstruction (as below). Clinically: distended, palpable bladder, dull to percussic
• ***Chronic lower tract obstruction:*** *Symptoms:* urinary frequency, hesitancy, po stream, terminal dribbling, overflow incontinence. *Signs:* distended, palpak bladder ± large prostate on PR. *Complications:* UTI, urinary retention.

Tests *Blood:* U&E, creatinine. ***Urine:*** MC&S. ***Ultrasound*** (p730) is the imagi modality of choice. If there is hydronephrosis or hydroureter (distension of t renal pelvis and calyces or ureter), the next test is ***antegrade or retrogra ureterograms*** (p730): it offers a therapeutic option of drainage. **NB:** In ~5% cases of obstruction, no distension is seen on ultrasound. ***Radionuclide imagi*** enables functional assessment of the kidneys. ***CT & MRI*** also have a role.

Treatment *Upper tract obstruction:* Nephrostomy or ureteric stent. Pyeloplas to widen the PUJ, may be performed if obstruction is at this level.

Lower tract obstruction: Urethral or suprapubic catheter (p750). Treat t underlying cause if possible. Beware of a large diuresis after relief of obstruction temporary salt-losing nephropathy may occur resulting in the loss of several litr of fluid a day. Monitor weight, fluid balance, and U&E closely.

Renal medicine

Peri-aortitis (retroperitoneal fibrosis *et al*)

Causes include idiopathic retroperitoneal fibrosis (RPF), inflammatory aneurysms the abdominal aorta, and perianeurysmal RPF. Idiopathic RPF is an autoimmu disorder, where there is B-cell and CD4(+) T-cell associated vasculitis. This results fibrinoid necrosis of the vasa vasorum, affecting the aorta and small and mediu retroperitoneal vessels. The ureters get embedded in dense, fibrous tissue resulti in progressive bilateral ureteric obstruction. Secondary causes of RPF inclu malignancy, typically lymphoma.

Associations: Drugs (eg β-blockers, bromocriptine, methysergide, methyldopa autoimmune disease (eg thyroiditis, SLE, ANCA+ve vasculitis), smoking, asbesto

Typical patient: Middle-aged ♂ with vague loin, back or abdominal pain, BP↑.

Tests: • *Blood:* ↑urea and creatinine; ↑ESR; ↑CRP; anaemia.
• *Ultrasound/IVU:* dilated ureters (hydronephrosis) + medial deviation of urete
• *CT/MRI:* peri-aortic mass (this allows biopsy, to rule out malignancy).

Treatment: Retrograde stent placement to relieve obstruction ± ureterolys (dissection of the ureters from the retroperitoneal tissue). Immunosuppressi with steroids or other agents is controversial, but some studies show benefit.

'roblems of ureteric stenting (depend on site)

Common	*Rare*
Trigonal irritation	Obstruction
Haematuria	Kinking
Fever	Ureteric rupture
Infection	Stent misplacement
Tissue inflammation	Stent migration (especially if made of silicone)
Encrustation	Tissue hyperplasia
Biofilm formation	

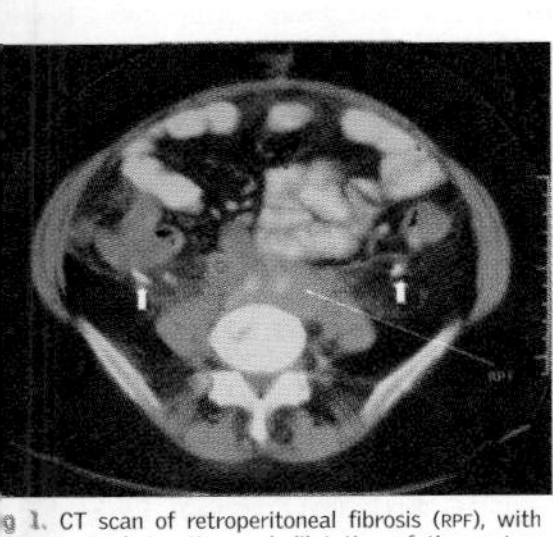

g 1. CT scan of retroperitoneal fibrosis (RPF), with ıbsequent obstruction and dilatation of the ureters hick arrows).

Glomerulonephritis (GN)

(images: p28

Features GN is a common cause of ESRF[1] in adults in the UK, along with diabetes a hypertension. They are a group of disorders where there is damage to t glomerular filtrating apparatus. This causes a leak of protein ± blood into the uri depending on the disease. Patients may be asymptomatic or present w haematuria (may be microscopic, ± red cell casts, p278), proteinuria, nephro syndrome, nephritic syndrome, renal failure, or hypertension.

Tests ***Blood:*** FBC, U&E, LFT, ESR, CRP; immunoglobulins, electrophoresis, compleme (C3, C4); autoantibodies (p539): ANA, ANCA, anti-dsDNA, anti-GBM; blood culture, AS HBsAg, anti-HCV (p394). ***Urine:*** RBC casts, MC&S, Bence-Jones protein. ***24h urin*** protein. ***CXR, renal ultrasound ± renal biopsy*** (p280).

General management ►Refer to a nephrologist. Keep BP ≤130/80, or ≤125/7 proteinuria >1g/d. Include an ACE-i or A2A; in a recent study, a combination of bo was better in preventing progression to renal failure in proteinuria.

Thin basement membrane nephropathy Genetic cause, autosomal domina **persistent microscopic haematuria**, rarely minor proteinuria. ***Diagnosis:*** Re biopsy: thin glomerular BM on electron microscopy (EM). ***Prognosis:*** Usually beni Small risk of CRF, preceded by ↑BP and proteinuria—monitor 1–2 yearly.

Minimal change glomerulonephritis (MCGN) Commonest cause of **nephro syndrome** in children (76%, and 20% of nephrotic adults), and is thought to be lymphocyte mediated. May also present with haematuria or ↑BP. ***Associatio*** Hodgkin's lymphoma, drugs. ***Tests:*** *Selective* proteinuria: only smaller protei leaked eg albumin. ***Renal biopsy:*** Normal on light microscopy (hence the nam EM: fusion of podocytes. ***℞:*** 95% of children and 70% of adults undergo remissi with corticosteroids, but are prone to relapse. Cyclophosphamide or ciclosporin a used if frequent relapses or steroid SE/dependence. ***Prognosis:*** ~1% → ESRF.

Membranous nephropathy Accounts for 20–30% of nephrotic syndrome adults; 2–5% in children. Unknown cause. ***Associations:*** Malignancy, drugs (go penicillamine, captopril), autoimmune (RA, SLE, thyroid disease), infections (HE syphilis, leprosy, filiariasis). ***Presentations:*** Usually **nephrotic syndrome**. Risk renal vein thrombosis (p290). ***Diagnosis:*** Biopsy shows diffuse thicken glomerular BM: IF shows IgG and C3 subepithelial deposits. ***℞:*** Corticosteroids wi cyclophosphamide or chlorambucil are used if renal function deteriorate ***Prognosis:*** If untreated ~40% have spontaneous remission—treatment is based poor prognostic factors: ie deteriorating renal function, heavy proteinuria.

Focal segmental glomerulosclerosis (FSGS) may be primary (idiopathic) secondary (reflux or IgA nephropathy, Alport's syndrome, vasculitis (p542), sickl cell disease, heroin use). HIV is associated with a subtype. ***Presentations:*** Usua **nephrotic syndrome** or **proteinuria**. ~50% have impaired renal function. ***Ren biopsy:*** Some glomeruli have scarring of certain segments (ie *focal sclerosis*). (immunofluorescence): IgM and C3 deposits in affected areas. ***℞:*** Responds corticosteroids in ~30%. Cyclophosphamide or ciclosporin are considered if steroi resistant. ***Prognosis:*** 30–50% → ESRF. There is a risk of recurrence post-ren transplant in 20–50%, which may respond to plasma exchange.

IgA nephropathy (Berger's disease) Commonest GN in the developed world. Mo present with **macro-** or **microscopic haematuria**; occasionally nephritic syndrom ***Typical patient:*** Young ♂ with episodic macroscopic haematuria, occurring a fe days after URTI eg pharyngitis. Recovery is often rapid between attacks. There overproduction of IgA, possibly due to infection, which forms immune complex and deposits in mesangial cells. ***Renal biopsy:*** Mesangial proliferation, IF sho deposits of IgA and C3. ***℞:*** General measures. With renal impairme immunosuppression (eg cyclophosphamide, mycophenolate) may be used, althou

1 ***Abbreviations:*** ANA=antinuclear antibody; ASOT=anti-streptolysin O titre; BM=baseme membrane (glomerular); EM=electron microscope; ESRF=end-stage renal failure; HCV=hepatitis virus; IF=immunofluorescence. Commonest presentations are in **bold**.

nefit is unclear. ***Prognosis:*** Worse if ↑BP, male, proteinuria or renal failure at esentation. 20% of adults develop ESRF over ~20yrs.

noch-Schönlein purpura (HSP) is a systemic variant of IgA nephropathy, using a small vessel vasculitis. ***Features:*** Purpuric rash on extensor surfaces pically on the legs), flitting polyarthritis, abdominal colic and GN. ***Diagnosis:*** ually clinical. Confirmed with positive IF for IgA and C3 in skin or renal biopsy entical to IgA nephropathy). ***R:*** As IgA nephropathy. ***Prognosis:*** 15% nephritic tients → ESRF; if both nephritic & nephrotic syndrome, 50% →ESRF.

oliferative GN is classified histologically: focal, diffuse, or mesangiocapillary GN. e chief cause is post-streptococcal GN (a diffuse proliferative GN), occurring 1–12 eks after a sore throat or skin infection. A streptococcal antigen is deposited on e glomerulus, causing a host reaction and immune complex formation. ***esentation:*** Usually **nephritic syndrome**. ***Renal biopsy:*** Inflammatory reaction ecting mesangial and endothelial cells, IF: IgG and C3 deposits. ***Serology:*** ↑ASOT; 3. ***R:*** Supportive: >95% recover renal function.

esangiocapillary GN A rare GN, often presenting with **nephrotic syndrome**, 0% nephritic syndrome. ***Diagnosis:*** Biopsy shows large glomeruli: mesangial oliferation and thickened capillary walls → 'tramline' appearance of a double BM. ypes: ***Type I*** (subendothelial immune deposits): Idiopathic or seen with HCV, o endocarditis, visceral abscess, infected arteriovenous shunts, HBV. ↓C4 levels *assical* complement activation); ***Type II*** (intramembranous deposits): sometimes th partial lipodystrophy (gaunt facial appearance). ↓serum C3 and +ve C3 phritic factor (*alternative* complement activation) ***Treatment:*** None proven of nefit so far; steroids are used in children, and use of anti-CD20 (Rituximab) erapy has been reported. ***Prognosis:*** 50% develop ESRF.

pidly progressive GN (RPGN) The most aggressive GN, with potential to cause RF over days. There are different causes, all have the biopsy finding of crescents ecting most glomeruli (a proliferation of parietal epithelial cells and acrophages in Bowman's capsule). ***Causes:*** Often microscopic polyangiitis (CANCA e), Wegener's granulomatosis (PANCA +ve, p706) or anti-GBM disease oodpasture's disease, p692). Also seen with other causes of GN (eg IgA phropathy), infections (eg endocarditis, shunt nephritis), or with multi-system sease (eg SLE). ***Clinically:*** Signs of **renal failure**. There may be features of the dividual systemic disease (eg fever, malaise, myalgia, weight loss, haemoptysis). ***eatment:*** Aggressive immunosuppression with high-dose corticosteroids and clophosphamide, with plasma exchange to remove existing antibodies. ***ognosis:*** Poor if initial serum creatinine >600μmol/L. Below this, ~80% have me improvement of renal function with treatment.

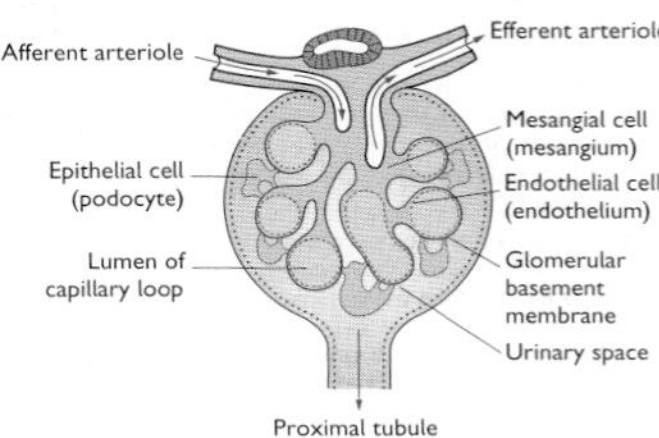

g. 1 A normal glomerulus. Blood is filtered from the capillary lumen, through the nestrated endothelial layer, glomerular basement membrane and the epithelial cell layer.

The nephrotic syndrome

►*If there is oedema, dipstick an* MSU *for protein to avoid missing this diagnos*

Definition Nephrotic syndrome is a triad of proteinuria (>3g/24h), hy albuminaemia (albumin <30g/L), and oedema. It was thought that protein caused ↓serum albumin, resulting in ↓plasma oncotic pressure and oede However, plasma oncotic pressure remains unchanged in nephrotic syndrome, oedema is now thought to result from sodium retention in the extracell compartment and molecular changes in the capillary barrier.

Causes >80% are due to glomerulonephritis (GN, p288), especially minimal cha GN (commonest cause in children), focal segmental glomerulosclerosis, membran GN (commonest cause in adults), mesangiocapillary GN or proliferative GN. Also s with DM, amyloidosis, SLE, drugs and allergies.

Clinical features Ask about acute or chronic infections, drugs, allergies, syste symptoms (vasculitis, p542; malignancy). ***Signs:*** Oedema: typically pitting dependent (↑ with gravity). It occurs periorbitally (tissue resistance is low he and peripherally in limbs—genital oedema, ascites and anasarca[1] develop la Hypertension may be present. ***Differentials:*** Cardiac failure (↑JVP, pulmon oedema, *mild* proteinuria) or liver disease (↓albumin).

Complications • ↑***susceptibility to infection***, due in part to loss of immu globulin in urine and also to immunosuppressive treatments. Patients are pron cellulitis, *Streptococcus* infections and spontaneous bacterial peritonitis.

- ***Thromboembolism*** (up to 40%): eg DVT/PE, renal vein thrombosis. This hyp coagulable state is partly due to ↑clotting factors & platelet abnormalities.
- ***Hyperlipidaemia:*** ↑cholesterol and triglycerides, thought to be due to hepa lipoprotein synthesis in response to low oncotic pressure.

Tests As for GN (p288). Also check cholesterol. ***Renal biopsy:*** Do in all adults children, the majority of cases are due to minimal change GN, so a course of sterc is usually tried initially. Biopsy is reserved for those whose proteinuria has reduced after 1 month, or if features suggest another cause eg age<1yr, fan history, extrarenal disease (eg arthritis, rash, anaemia), renal failure, haematu

General measures ►Monitor U&E, BP, fluid balance and weight regularly. T individual disease should be treated as appropriate (eg GN, see p288).

- Salt intake should be restricted. A normal protein intake is advised.
- In adults, diuretics are often used, eg furosemide 80–250mg/24h PO metolazone or spironolactone, with monitoring of U&E. Aim ~1kg/day loss.
- In chronic nephrotic syndrome, ACE-i are proven to ↓proteinuria and sl progression of renal impairment. Some advocate combination with an A2A.
- Treat infections promptly. Pneumococcal vaccinations are recommended.
- Prophylactic heparin if immobile (adjust dose if renal impairment eg enoxapa 20mg SC daily). Avoid prolonged bed rest.
- Treat hypertension (p126). Proteinuria is an independent risk factor cardiovascular disease: if >1g/24h, target BP is 125/75. ACE-i or A2A should used 1st line. Address other risk factors such as smoking, exercise, diet. Persist hyperlipidaemia should be treated with a statin (p682).

Renal vein thrombosis The hypercoagulable state in nephrotic syndro predisposes to renal vein thrombosis, with an increased incidence noted in patie with membranous nephropathy. *Other causes*: Invasion by renal cell carcino thrombophilia. ***Clinically:*** Often asymptomatic, but may present with loin pa haematuria, palpable kidney, sudden deterioration in renal function (eg in kno GN), or with pulmonary embolism. ***Diagnosis:*** Doppler ultrasound, CT, MRI or re angiography (venous phase). ***Treatment:*** Anticoagulate with warfarin for 3 months (or until albumin >25g/L) if no contraindications. Target INR is 2–3.

1 ↑Fluid in organs and cavities with severe oedema (+ tissue hardening). Anasarca is also seen in: CCF, l failure, protein-losing enteropathy, fetal hydrops, capillary leak syndrome with monoclonal gammopa

Acute renal failure (ARF): diagnosis

Definition A significant deterioration in renal function occurring over hour days. Clinically, there may be no symptoms or signs, but oliguria (urine vol <400mL/24h) is common. Biochemically, ARF is detected by rising plasma urea creatinine. ARF may arise as an isolated problem; more commonly it occurs in setting of circulatory disturbance, eg severe illness, sepsis, trauma, or surgery in the context of nephrotoxic drugs.

Causes NB: Pre-renal failure and ATN accounts for >80%. 1 ***Pre-renal:*** Due to r hypoperfusion eg hypovolaemia, sepsis (causing systemic vasodilatat congestive cardiac failure, liver cirrhosis, renal artery stenosis, NSAIDs or A (these interfere with renal blood flow). 2 ***Intrinsic:*** acute tubular necrosis (A this is damage to the renal tubular cells, caused by *ischaemia* (with causes of re hypoperfusion as above) or *nephrotoxins* (see p299 for fuller list): often du drugs (aminoglycosides, amphotericin B, tetracyclines), radiological cont agents, uric acid crystals, haemoglobinuria (in rhabdomyolysis), or myelo Recovery of renal function usually occurs within weeks, although mortality rem ~50%. Others: *Vascular:* vasculitis, malignant hypertension, cholesterol em haemolytic uraemic syndrome, thrombotic thrombocytopenic purpura (p3 glomerulonephritis; interstitial nephritis (p298); hepatorenal syndrome. 3 ***Po renal:*** Due to urinary tract obstruction.

Renal medicine

Assessment ►Make sure you know about the renal effects of *all* drugs taker

1 ***Is the renal failure acute or chronic?*** Suspect chronic renal failure if:
- History of co-morbidity eg diabetes, ↑BP, signs of chronic renal failure.
- Previously abnormal blood tests (GP records, laboratory results).
- Small kidneys on ultrasound (<9cm), with increased echogenicity.

The *presence* of anaemia, Ca^{2+}↓ or PO_4^{3-}↑ may not help to distinguish ARF fr CRF, as these can occur within days, but their *absence* suggests ARF.

2 ***Is there urinary tract obstruction?*** Obstruction should always be conside as a cause of ARF because it is reversible and prompt treatment preve permanent renal damage. Obstruction should be suspected in patients wit single functioning kidney, or in those with history of renal stones, anu prostatism, or previous pelvic/retroperitoneal surgery. Examine for a palpa bladder, pelvic or abdominal masses, or an enlarged prostate.

3 ***Is there a rare cause of ARF?***—eg glomerulonephritis. These are usu associated with haematuria or proteinuria, and warrant urgent renal referral consideration of a renal biopsy and treatment.

Tests • ***Blood tests:*** U&E (►►beware K^+↑), FBC, LFT, clotting, CK, ESR, CRP. Consi ABG, blood cultures, and also hepatitis serology if dialysis is considered. If the ca is unclear, consider: serum immunoglobulins, electrophoresis, complement lev (C3/C4), autoantibodies (ANA, ANCA, anti-dsDNA, anti-GBM—p288 & p539) and AS • ***Urine:*** *Dipstick* for leucocytes, nitrite, blood, protein, glucose. *Microscopy* for R WBC, crystals, casts. *Culture* and *sensitivity*. *Chemistry:* it U&E, creatini osmolality, Bence-Jones protein. • ***CXR:*** Pulmonary oedema? • ***ECG:*** Signs hyperkalaemia? • ***Renal ultrasound:*** Renal size or obstruction?

Distinguishing pre-renal failure and ATN

	Pre-renal	*ATN*
Urine Na (mmol/L)	<20	>40
Urine osmolarity (mosm/L)	>500	<350
Urine/plasma urea	>8	<3
Urine/plasma creatinine	>40	<20
Fractional Na excretion (%)	<1	>2

In pre-renal failure, urine is concentrated and sodium is reabsorbed by workin tubular cells. This fails to happen in ATN. NB: Values are influenced by diuretics an pre-existing disease, and they do not predict prognosis.

cute renal failure (ARF): management

Enlist specialist help. While awaiting this, make sure that recent U&E and urine icroscopy results are to hand. Treat the treatable:

If shock is the cause (↓intravascular volume, *below*), use protocol on p779. Urgent US scan (today); you *must* check for a palpable bladder, but its absence does not rule out obstruction.

Stop nephrotoxic drugs—eg NSAIDs, ACE-i, gentamicin, vancomycin, amphotericin. Stop metformin if creatinine is >150mmol/L, see p192.

Signs of vasculitis? Nosebleed, haematuria, rash, ESR/CRP↑? do autoantibodies.

Find and treat exacerbating factors: eg hypovolaemia, sepsis, BP↑↑.

: Assessing signs of ↓intravascular volume can be difficult: look for ↓urine lume, invisible JVP, poor tissue turgor, ↓BP, ↑pulse. When in doubt, insert a CVP e to measure the venous pressure. Signs of fluid overload: gallop rhythm on rdiac auscultation, ↑BP, ↑JVP, lung crepitations, peripheral oedema.

onitoring Consider transfer to HDU or ICU. Pulse, BP, CVP, & urine output hourly sert a urinary catheter). Daily fluid balance + weight chart. Match input to ss (urine, vomit, diarrhoea, drains) + 500mL for insensible loss (more if T°↑).

Correct volume depletion with intravenous fluid—colloid, saline, or blood (only if hyperkalaemia is not a problem) as appropriate.

If the patient is septic, take appropriate cultures and treat empirically with antibiotics (p372). Remove any potential sources of sepsis when no longer required, eg IV or urinary catheters.

Re-check if any nephrotoxic drugs; adjust doses of renally excreted drugs (p295).

Nutrition is vital: aim for normal calorie intake (more if catabolism↑↑, eg burns, sepsis) and protein ~0.5/kg/d. If oral intake is poor, consider nasogastric nutrition early (parenteral if NGT impossible, p574).

eat complications ***Hyperkalaemia*** may cause arrhythmias or cardiac arrest. ***G changes*** (in order): Tall 'tented' T waves; small or absent P wave; increased R interval; widened QRS complex; 'sine wave' pattern; asystole. ECG p786. ***R̷:***

ntravenous calcium: 10mL of 10% calcium gluconate IV via a big vein over 2min, repeated as necessary until ECG improves. This is cardioprotective.

ntravenous insulin + glucose: 10U Actrapid® insulin + 50mL 50% glucose IV over 30min. Insulin stimulates intracellular uptake of K^+, lowering serum K^+ by 1–2mmol/L over ~60min. Check capillary glucose ~30 minutes after giving nsulin.

Salbutamol 5mg nebulizer. ►►Consider calcium resonium, 15g/8h, p821, PO or PR to bind K^+ in the gut. This works over a longer period. SE: constipation.

Haemodialysis or haemofiltration is usually required if anuric.

lmonary oedema (p786): ►►Sit up and give high-flow oxygen by face mask.

Venous vasodilator, eg morphine 2.5mg IV (+metoclopramide 10mg IV).

Furosemide 120–250mg IV over 1 hour (larger doses are needed in renal failure).

f no response, urgent haemodialysis or haemofiltration is necessary.

Consider continuous positive airways pressure ventilation (CPAP) therapy.

Consider venesection (100–200mL) if the patient is *in extremis*.

ntravenous nitrates also have a role (see p786).

eeding: Impaired haemostasis due to ↑urea may be compounded by the ecipitating cause. In patients with ARF who are actively bleeding, give:

Fresh frozen plasma & platelets as needed—if there are clotting problems.

Blood transfusion to maintain Hb >10g/dL and haematocrit >30%.

Desmopressin (p330) to ↑factor VIII activity, normalizing bleeding time.

dications for acute dialysis • Refractory pulmonary oedema • Persistent perkalaemia (K^+ >7mmol/L) • Severe metabolic acidosis (pH<7.2 or base cess <10) • Uraemic encephalopathy • Uraemic pericarditis (pericardial rub).

ognosis Worse if oliguric. Mortality depends on the cause: burns (80%); uma/surgery (60%); medical illness (30%); obstetric/poisoning (10%).

Chronic renal failure (CRF)

Chronic renal failure (or chronic kidney disease, CKD) is classified into 5 sta (p661). Symptoms usually only occur once stage 4 is reached (GFR <30). Endst renal failure (ESRF) occurs when dialysis or transplant is required to prolong li

Causes ***Common:*** Glomerulonephritis, DM, renovascular disease, BP↑, pyelonephr polycystic disease. Also prostatic hypertrophy, interstitial nephritis, analge nephropathy, nephrolithiasis. ***Rarer:*** Myeloma, amyloidosis, SLE, sclerode vasculitis (p542), haemolytic uraemic syndrome, nephrocalcinosis, gout, re tumour, cystinosis, oxalosis, Alport's syndrome, Fabry's disease (p690).

History Ask about: past UTI, known ↑BP, DM, family history. Take a careful d history. Any fatigue, weakness, anorexia, vomiting, metallic taste, pruritus, rest legs, bone pain, impotence/infertility? Symptoms are common when ure >40mmol/L. Dyspnoea, ankle swelling (fluid overload?) Urine output?

Signs: Pallor, yellow skin pigmentation, brown nails, purpura, bruising, excoriat BP↑, cardiomegaly, pericardial rub, pleural effusion, pulmonary or periph oedema, proximal myopathy (+ cause eg DM: peripheral neuropathy, retinopat Later if untreated: arrhythmias, encephalopathy, seizures, and coma.

Tests • ***Blood:*** Hb↓ (normochromic, normocytic), ESR, U&E (↑urea, ↑creatini glucose (DM); ↓Ca^{2+}, ↑PO_4^{3-}, ↑alk phos (renal osteodystrophy); ↑PTH (hyperp thyroidism, p206). • ***Urine:*** MC&S, dipstick, urine PCI or 24h urinary prot • ***Imaging: Renal ultrasound*** to exclude obstruction and look at renal size (usu small, eg <9cm, but may be normal or large with CRF in DM, polycystic kid disease, amyloidosis, myeloma, systemic sclerosis, asymmetric renal vasc disease). Consider ***DTPA scan. CXR:*** Cardiomegaly, pleural/pericardial effusion pulmonary oedema. ***Bone x-rays*** may show renal osteodystrophy. • ***Renal bio*** should be considered if the cause is unclear and there are normal-sized kidne

Treatment ►*Refer early to a nephrologist.* Treat reversible causes: relieve ob uction, stop nephrotoxic drugs, deal with Ca^{2+}↑ and cardiovascular risk: in stages 1 & 2, risk from cardiovascular death is higher than the risk of reaching E

- ***Hypertension:*** Even a small BP drop may save significant renal function. A or A2A can ↓rate of loss of function even if BP is normal, if proteinuric, aim fo of <130/80 (<125/75 if >1g proteinuria/d). ***Hyperlipidaemia:*** Statins (p6
- ***Oedema:*** This may require high doses of loop diuretics (eg furosemide 250 2g/24h ± metolazone 5–10mg/24h PO mane), and restriction on fluid intak
- ***Anaemia:*** Exclude iron deficiency & chronic infection; consider erythropoie
- ***Renal bone disease (osteodystrophy):*** Treat if ↑PTH. PO_4 rises in CRF, which ↑ further, and also precipitates in the kidney and vasculature. Restrict dietary (milk, cheese, eggs). Give binders (eg Calcichew®)[2] to bind PO_4^{3-} in the gut to ↓ absorption. Vit. D analogues (eg alfacalcidol=1α-hydroxycholecalciferol)[3] & C supplements ↓bone disease and hyperparathyroidism (2° & 3°, p206).
- ***Diet:*** Match dietary and fluid intake with excretion. Na^+ restriction: helps co BP and prevent oedema. A moderate protein diet is recommended. K^+ restric only if hyperkalaemia; HCO_3^- supplements to correct acidosis.
- ***Restless legs:*** Clonazepam (0.5mg–2mg daily) or gabapentin (p496) may h
- ***Prepare for dialysis/transplantation:*** See p296.

1 *Recombinant human erythropoietin (r-HuEPO):* darbepoetin alfa (Aranesp®) dose **if not on dial** 0.75μg/kg SC every 2wks initially, then ↑ by ~25% if Hb rises by <1g/dL in 4 wks (↓by 25–50% if by >2.5g/dL in 4wks). Once target Hb is reached (eg 10g/dL), give twice the 2-weekly dose month. **If on dialysis:** Give injections every 2wks, once target Hb has been reached on the renal Monitor BP, Hb, Fe & K^+. SureClick® prefilled 0.3mL pens contain 30, 60 or 150μg; 0.4mL pens give 80μg; 0.6mL gives 300μg. If Hb falls despite adequate Fe, B_{12} & folate (and no infection, haemolys blood loss etc), suspect red cell aplasia (∵ EPO antibodies)⟶**stop *at once***; get help.

2 Aluminium-containing agents are toxic so are rarely used now. Ca^{2+}-containing agents hypercalcaemia and soft tissue calcification. Sevelamer is a newer alternative, and doesn't ↑calc

3 Alfacalcidol & calcitriol (=1,25-dihydroxycholecalciferol) help by ↓parathyroid hormone, but gr ↑ intestinal Ca^{2+} & PO_4^{3-} absorption and bone mineral mobilization, leading to PO_4^{3-}↑ & Ca^{2+}↑ (risks ular calcification). New vit. D analogues (eg paricalcitol weekly IV) retain suppressive action on gland growth, but have less effect on Ca^{2+} & PO_4 absorption, and help cardiovascular status.

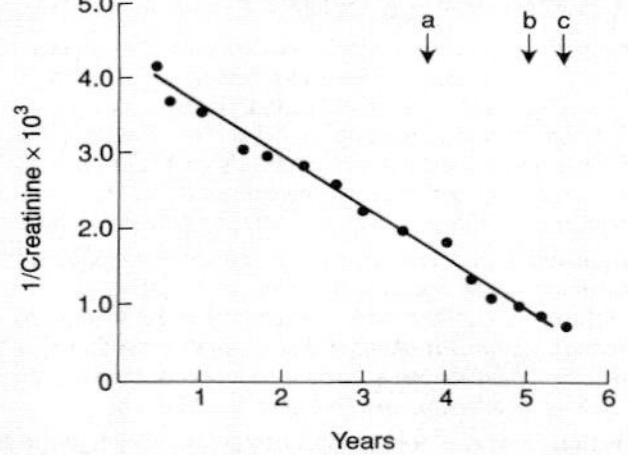

ig 1. Plot of reciprocal plasma creatinine (µmol/L) against time in a patient ith adult polycystic kidney disease. The letters represent life events: (a) work romotion, (b) arterio-venous fistula, and (c) haemodialysis.

Some patients with CRF lose renal function at a constant rate. Creatinine is ade at a fairly constant rate and rises on a hyperbolic curve as renal function eclines, so the reciprocal creatinine plot is a straight line, parallel to the fall in FR. This is used to monitor renal function and to predict need for dialysis—but ere is much individual variation in progression, so the plot is of limited use.[20] apid decline in renal function greater than that expected may be due to: fection, dehydration, uncontrolled ↑BP, metabolic disturbance (eg Ca^{2+}↑), ostruction, nephrotoxins (eg drugs). Intervention at this point may delay ESRF.

Background decline may be retardable by using ACE-i ± A2A (angiotensin-II ntagonists). In the COOPERATE randomized prospective trial (over 3yrs) in non-abetic renal disease, the NNT was ~9 for preventing one case of ESRF (or a oubling of plasma creatinine) by adding losartan (100mg/d) to trandolapril mg/d)—ie 11% progressed rather than 23% on ACE-i alone.[21]

rescribing in renal failure

elate dose modification to GFR, and the extent to which a drug is renally creted. This is significant for aminoglycosides (gentamicin, p738), cephalo-orins, and a few other antibiotics (p368–71), heparin, lithium, opiates, and goxin. ►Never prescribe in renal failure before checking how its administration ould be altered. Loading doses (eg digoxin) should not be changed. If the tient is on dialysis (peritoneal or haemodialysis), dose modification depends on w well it is eliminated by dialysis. Consult the drug's *Data Sheet* or the armacist. Dosing should be timed around dialysis.

ephrotoxic drugs: Reduce the dose (the dose adjustment factor, DAF, reflects e fraction excreted unchanged in the urine—*F*). DAF = $1/(F(kf-1)+1)$, where e kf is the relative kidney function = creatinine clearance/120. The usual dose ut not the loading dose) should be *divided* by the DAF. In only a few drugs is *F* g enough to be important, as below.

minoglycosides	0.9	Cephalosporins	1.0
ithium	1.0	Sulfamethoxazole	0.3–0.5
igoxin	0.75	Procainamide	0.6
thambutol	0.7	Tetracycline	0.4–0.6

Renal replacement therapy

Optimal timing to start dialysis is widely debated; guidelines suggest starting w GFR <15mL/min with symptoms. *Early* psychological preparation is vital. Mec preparation involves Hep B vaccination and creating an arteriovenous fis (p307) for haemodialysis, or inserting a Tenchkoff catheter for peritoneal dial Choice of haemo- *vs* peritoneal dialysis depends on medical, social,[1] and psy logical factors. Mortality was higher in peritoneal *vs* haemodialysis in one st more are needed. **NB:** Kidney function is only *partly* replaced by dialysis.

Haemodialysis (HD) Blood flows on one side of a semi-permeable membrane w dialysis fluid flows in the opposite direction on the other side. Solute tran occurs by diffusion. Ultrafiltration is the removal of excess fluid by creating transmembrane pressure. ***Problems:*** • Disequilibration syndrome[2] • BP↓/arrh mias • Time consuming • Access: *fistula:* thrombosis, stenosis, aneurysm, s syndrome, ischaemia or *temporary line:* infection, blockage.

Haemofiltration Blood is filtered continuously across a highly permeable synth membrane, allowing removal of waste products by a process of convection diffusion). The ultrafiltrate is substituted with an equal volume of replacen fluid. It is more expensive and takes longer than HD, but there is haemodynamic instability and so is used for critically ill patients.

Peritoneal dialysis (PD) is simple to perform, requires less complex equipn than haemodialysis and is easier at home. It is useful in children, the elderly, ar those with cardiovascular disease. PD fluid is introduced into the peritoneal ca via a Tenchkoff catheter and uraemic solutes diffuse into it across the perito membrane. Ultrafiltration is achieved by adding osmotic agents, eg glucose to dialysis fluid. ***Problems:*** • Peritonitis (60% *Staphylococci*, 20% Gram organisms, <5% fungi) • Exit-site infection • Catheter malfunction • Los membrane function. • Obesity (glucose in dialysis fluid) • Hernias • Back pai
Continuous ambulatory peritoneal dialysis (CAPD) uses the smallest daily vol of dialysate fluid to prevent uraemia. 2L bags are changed 3–5 times a da produce, with ultrafiltration, a total dialysate of 10L.
Automated peritoneal dialysis uses a cycler machine to enhance solute and removal. Techniques include continuous cyclic peritoneal dialysis (cc intermittent peritoneal dialysis (IPD), night intermittent peritoneal dialysis (N and tidal intermittent peritoneal dialysis (TIPD).

Complications of dialysis ***Cardiovascular disease***, eg IHD, cardiac failure and st are much more common in dialysis patients and are a major cause of mort ***Hypertension*** persists in 25–30% of patients on haemodialysis. ***Anaemia*** is com and is treated with erythropoietin (± haematinic supplements). ***Bleeding tenden*** due to platelet dysfunction. Acute bleeding is treated with desmopressin transfusion, as necessary. ***Renal bone disease*** is treated with dietary modifica alfacalcidol, Ca^{2+} supplements, and phosphate binders (p294). ***Infection*** ma due to non-sterility in peritoneal dialysis or intravascular lines in haemodialysis ***microglobulin amyloidosis*** is due to amyloid which accumulates in long–t dialysis patients: it may cause carpal tunnel syndrome, arthralgia, and fract ***Acquired renal cysts*** occur years after dialysis and may present with haema or malignant transformation. ***Malignancy*** is commoner in dialysis patients; may be related to the cause, eg urothelial tumours in analgesic nephropathy

Stopping dialysis Dialysis exerts a big toll on quality of life, and it may all bec too much for patients, eg if very old or there is co-morbidity (eg psychiatr mobility issues).[1] 8–20% of deaths in dialysis patients are due to its withdraw ►Good palliation allows a good death and mitigates discomfort caused by urae • Respiratory distress: morphine • Myoclonic jerks: clonazepam • Hallucinat haloperidol ± midazolam • Secretions: hyoscine. *Doses:* p438. Good communic in the renal team, well-rehearsed protocols, and advance directives (living w help the big ethical dilemma.

›nal transplantation

›is is the treatment of choice for end stage renal failure (ESRF). Each patient ›quires careful assessment and consideration of the advantages and ›sadvantages of dialysis vs transplantation.

›sessment ***Note the following:*** Virology status: CMV, Hepatitis B & C, HIV: these ›ay cause severe disease while immunocompromised. Note if there is existing ›ne output, and cardiovascular disease. Previous TB may reactivate so isoniazid ›d pyridoxine prophylaxis is given to proven cases and high risk groups. ›ABO blood group and tissue typing for HLA is required. ›Make sure pre-op potassium is ≤5. If above, dialysis may be needed.

›ntraindications Active infection, Ca, severe heart disease or co-morbidity.

›pes of graft >6000 are waiting in the UK, often in vain, for a transplant. ***Cad-›eric donor*** grafts are obtained from a brainstem dead donor with supported ›culation and ventilation. ***Non-heart beating donor*** grafts are retrieved from ›tients without an active circulation, and hence rapid retrieval is needed to ›nimise ischaemia. Success rates from these is approaching that of cadaveric ›afts. ***Living related donor*** (LRD) grafts offer the advantages of an optimally ›ned surgical procedure, HLA haplotype matching, and improved graft survival. ***›ve unrelated donation*** has become increasingly common, between spouses or ›ends who satisfy the complex rules of ULTRA.[3] Consent is problematic: p251.

›mmunosuppressants Most regimes involve 1 ciclosporin or tacrolimus, ›azathioprine or mycophenolate ± 3 prednisolone. Pre-op anti-interleukin ›eceptor antibodies (eg basiliximab) reduce rates of early rejection.[MET 27]

›mplications ***Post-op:*** Bleed, thrombosis, infection, urinary leaks, oliguria.

›ute rejection: (<6 months) This is characterized by rising serum creatinine ± ›ver and graft pain. Graft biopsy shows an immune cell infiltrate and tubular ›mage. ***℞:*** High-dose IV methylprednisolone. Resistant cases require anti-›ymocyte globulin (ATG).

›ronic rejection: (>6 months) Presents with a gradual rise in serum creatinine ›d proteinuria. Graft biopsy shows vascular changes, fibrosis, and tubular ›ophy. It is not responsive to ↑immunosuppression.

›losporin/tacrolimus toxicity: *Acute:* afferent arteriole vasoconstriction, ›using ↓renal blood flow and ↓GFR. *Chronic:* tubular atrophy and fibrosis.

›fection: Often community acquired infections or those related to ›-cell immunity (∵ immunosuppression), eg skin infections (fungi, warts, HSV, ›ster) and opportunists (TB, fungi, *Pneumocystis carinii* pneumonia, CMV).

›alignancy: Immunosuppression causes ↑risk of neoplasia 5-fold and ↑ ›ection with viruses of malignant potential (EBV, HBV, HHV-8: p694). Typical ›mours: skin (basal & squamous) Ca, lymphoma (EBV-related), anogenital Ca.

›heromatous vascular disease: This is commoner in transplant patients than ›the general population and is a leading cause of death.

›pertension: This occurs in >50% of transplant patients and may be due to ›eased native kidneys, immunosuppressant drugs or dysfunction in the graft. ›anagement is along standard lines (p126).

›ognosis 1yr graft survival: HLA identical 95%; 1 mismatch 90–95%; ›mplete mismatch 75–80%. Average *half-life* of cadaveric grafts is ~10yrs, ›yrs for HLA-identical living related donor grafts—this is increasing.

›me haemodialysis gets over some problems with dialysis. Consider in all needing dialysis if: • Willing ›arn • Stable on dialysis • Space for the equipment • No precluding concomitant disease • Good ›ilar access ie fistula • There is a carer to assist (get their *informed* consent).

›aracterised by nausea, vomiting, headache, altered consciousness, and rarely seizures or coma, ›g to rapid changes in plasma osmolality and cerebral oedema, occurring on initial dialysis.

›e Unrelated Live Transplant Regulatory Authority: http://www.advisorybodies.doh.gov.uk/ultra.

Interstitial nephritides and nephrotoxins

Tubulointerstitial nephritis: Inflammation of the renal interstitium may be a or chronic. ***Acute tubulointerstitial nephritis*** is mediated by an immune reac to medications, infections and other causes. **Drugs:** NSAIDs, *antibiotics:* ceph sporins, penicillins, sulphonamides, rifampicin; *diuretics:* furosemide, thiazides; allopurinol, cimetidine, amphotericin; **infections:** *Staphylococci*, *Streptoc Brucella*, *Leptospira*, hantaviruses; **immune disorders** eg SLE, glomerulonephrit or *no* obvious cause. *Features:* May present with renal impairment, hypertensio acute renal failure. Systemic symptoms eg fever, rash, arthralgia, with eosinopl uveitis, and ↑IgE. *Diagnosis:* Renal biopsy: infiltration of the renal interstitium tubules with T lymphocytes, macrophages, and plasma cells. Urinary eosinop may be seen. *Treatment:* Stop any cause. ARF: p293. Prednisolone 1mg/kg is u but has not been studied in a randomised trial. *Prognosis:* Most have full reco of renal function. ***Chronic tubulointerstitial nephritis*** results from m disorders, leading to extensive fibrosis and tubular loss on renal biopsy. Pati present with chronic renal failure. *Causes:* chronic pyelonephritis often with re nephropathy, sickle cell disease, lead or cadmium intoxication.

Balkan nephropathy is a form of chronic tubulointerstitial nephritis cau progressive renal impairment to ESRF. It is endemic in areas along the R Danube. Environmental and genetic factors are thought to be important. ***Featu*** coppery-yellow pigmentation of the palms and soles, β_2-microglobinuria. The an ↑ risk of urothelial tumours, reported in up to 40%.

Analgesic nephropathy is associated with the prolonged, heavy ingestio compound analgesics, especially those containing caffeine (as it lead habituation), NSAIDs, paracetamol, and phenacetin (now withdrawn), leadin interstitial nephritis and papillary necrosis. There is often a history of chronic ***Signs:*** Presents with sterile pyuria, UTI, or symptoms of chronic renal failur hypertension. Renal colic and haematuria can result from a sloughed papilla. ***Te*** IVU demonstrates papillary necrosis. CT may also be used. Biopsy shows chr interstitial nephritis. ***Treatment:*** Stop analgesics, antibiotics for infection. Suc flank pain should prompt an ultrasound or IVU to look for obstruction fro sloughed papilla. There is an ↑ risk of urothelial tumours.

Urate nephropathy ***Acute crystal nephropathy*** occurs when insoluble uric crystals deposit causing blockage of the tubules. It is mainly caused by excess acid released during cell lysis in chemotherapy eg in myeloid tumours. The r parenchyma appears bright on ultrasound. Plasma urate is often markedly rais urinary birefringent crystals on microscopy (p351, fig 1). *Treatment:* p336: well hydrated, allopurinol pre-chemotherapy, urinary alkalinization with soc bicarbonate (as uric acid is more soluble in alkaline urine). ***Chronic u nephropathy:*** Whether chronic hyperuricaemia (eg with gout) leads to r failure is debated. This does, however, occur in Lesch–Nyhan syndro *Treatment:* allopurinol (↓dose in renal impairment). ***Uric acid calculi***, see p2

Hypercalcaemia is associated with the following renal diseases: nephrog diabetes insipidus (p224), renal calculi (p284) and nephrocalcinosis: diffuse r parenchymal calcification, often asymptomatic, causing progressive r impairment. Nephrocalcinosis is seen in hypercalcaemia (eg malignancy, hy parathyroidism, myeloma, sarcoidosis, vitamin D intoxication) or type 1 r tubular acidosis. ***Tests:*** AXR for renal calculi/nephrocalcinosis. ***℞:*** Treat caus

Radiation nephritis is renal impairment following radiotherapy and occurs ac (<1 year) or chronic (years later). *Signs:* Hypertension, proteinuria, progressi chronic renal failure. Biopsy shows interstitial fibrosis. ***℞:*** Strict BP contro specific. *Prevention:* Exclusion of renal areas during radiotherapy.

1 An X-linked disorder due to hypoxanthine-guanine phosphoribosyltransferase deficiency, lead ↑uric acid, and mental retardation, involuntary movement, self-mutilation, gout and renal failure

phrotoxins

ıny agents may be toxic to the kidneys and cause acute renal failure (ARF), ıally by direct acute tubular necrosis, or by causing interstitial nephritis.

ogenous nephrotoxins include:
Analgesics (NSAIDs).
Antimicrobials (gentamicin, sulphonamides, tetracycline, vancomycin, amphoːericin, aciclovir).
Radio-contrast media (see below).
Anaesthetic agents (methoxyflurane, enflurane).
Chemotherapeutic agents (cisplatin).
ACE-i and A2As (angiotensin II receptor antagonists).
Immunosuppressants (ciclosporin, methotrexate).
Heavy metal poisoning (mercury, lead, cadmium, arsenic, bismuth).
Organic solvents (ethylene glycol, carbon tetrachloride).
Insecticides, herbicides, *Amanita* mushrooms, snake venom.

dogenous nephrotoxins include:
Pigments: eg *haemoglobinuria* in haemolysis: p322, *myoglobin*—see below.
Crystals: eg urate. • Proteins: eg immunoglobulin light chains in myeloma.

ıinoglycosides (gentamicin, amikacin, kanamycin and streptomycin) are wellːognized nephrotoxins. The typical picture is of mild non-oliguric renal failure, 2wks into therapy. Risk is increased by old age, renal hypoperfusion, presting renal impairment, high dosage or prolonged treatment, and coministration of other nephrotoxic drugs. Recovery may be delayed or omplete. Single bolus doses of aminoglycosides can be as effective as multiple ses in treating infection and less nephrotoxic.

diocontrast nephropathy is a very common cause of iatrogenic ARF with IV ıtrast radiological studies. Risk factors are diabetes mellitus, high doses of ıtrast medium, hypovolaemia, other nephrotoxic agents, and pre-existing al impairment. Prevention is key: stop nephrotoxic agents peri-procedure, and -hydrate with IV 0.9% sodium chloride in patients with risk factors. etylcysteine or IV sodium bicarbonate may be used ►follow local protocols, l inform radiology, who may use less nephrotoxic contrast.

abdomyolysis This results from skeletal muscle breakdown, with release of contents into the circulation, including myoglobin, potassium, phosphate, te and creatinine kinase (CK). Complications include hyperkalaemia and ARF: oglobin is filtered by the glomeruli and precipitates, obstructing renal tubules. ***uses:*** Many, including *trauma:* prolonged immobilisation (eg after falling), ns, crush injury, excessive exercise, uncontrolled seizures; *drugs and toxins:* tins, fibrates, alcohol, ecstasy, heroin, snake bite, carbon monoxide, neuroleptic lignant syndrome (p827); *infections:* coxsackie, EBV, influenza; *metabolic:* K^+↓, $_4^{3-}$↓, myositis, malignant hyperpyrexia (p558); *inherited muscle disorders:* Ardle's disease (p696), Duchenne's muscular dystrophy (p502). ***Clinical tures:*** Often of the cause, with muscle pain, swelling, tenderness, and redwn urine. ***Tests:*** Blood tests show a raised CK >1000iu/L (often >10000iu/L). k urine is +ve for blood on dipstick but *without* RBCs on microscopy. Confirm by +ve urinary myoglobin. Others: K^+↑, PO_4^{3-}↑↑, Ca^{2+}↓ (enters muscle), urate↑. occurs 12–24 hours later, and disseminated intravascular coagulation is ociated (p336). Compartment syndrome can result from muscle injury. ***atment:*** Urgent treatment for hyperkalaemia (p821). IV fluid rehydration is a ority to prevent ARF: maintain urine output at 300mL/h until myoglobinuria ceased, initially up to 1.5L fluid/h may be needed. If oliguric, CVP monitoring seful to prevent fluid overload. IV sodium bicarbonate is used to alkalinize e to pH >6.5, to stabilise a less toxic form of myoglobin. Dialysis may be ded, but full renal recovery is likely.

Renal vascular disease

Hypertension may be a cause or consequence of renal disease. ***Esser hypertension*** (p124) The extent to which renal impairment develops in m moderate hypertension is debated. ***Accelerated (malignant) hypertensio*** characterized by a severe increase in BP, grade III or IV hypertensive retinop (p544) and renal failure. ℞: p124. ***Pre-eclampsia:*** *OHCS* p48. ↑BP + proteinur oedema in 2nd/3rd trimester. Proteinuria is due to glomerular endothelial swelling. ARF may result. **Renal diseases causing hypertension** are the commo cause of secondary hypertension. Most renal diseases are associated with commonly: diabetic nephropathy, glomerulonephritis, chronic interstitial neph polycystic kidneys or renovascular disease.

Renovascular disease This is stenosis of the renal artery or one of its branc ***Causes:*** Atherosclerosis (in 80%: >50yrs, arteriopaths: often co-existent stroke or PVD), fibromuscular dysplasia (10%, younger ♀). Rarer: Takaya arteritis, antiphospholipid syndrome, post-renal transplant, thromboembol external mass compression. ***Clinically:*** ↑BP resistant to treatment; worsening r function after ACE-i/A2A; 'flash' pulmonary oedema: sudden onset, withou impairment on cardiac echo. Abdominal ± carotid or femoral bruits, and weal pulses may be found. ***Tests:*** Ultrasound: renal size asymmetry (affected sic smaller), disturbance in renal blood flow on Doppler ultrasound. CT/MR angiogr are more sensitive. Renal angiography is 'gold standard', but done after C as it is invasive. See p731. ***℞:*** Percutaneous renal angioplasty ± stent revascularisation surgery. Long-term benefits of each are under study.

Haemolytic uraemic syndrome (HUS) is characterised by microangiopa haemolytic anaemia (MAHA): intravascular haemolysis + red cell fragmenta Endothelial damage triggers thrombosis, platelet consumption and fibrin st deposition, mainly in the renal microvasculature. The strands cause mechar destruction of passing red blood cells. Thrombocytopenia and ARF result. ***Cau*** 90% due to *E. coli* 0157: produces a verotoxin which attacks endothelial c This affects young children most, often occurring in outbreaks due to consump of undercooked contaminated meat, with abdominal pain, bloody diarrhoea ARF. Rarely sporadic. ***Tests:*** Blood film: fragmented RBC (schistocytes, p3 ↓platelets, ↓Hb. Clotting tests are normal. There may be haematuria/protein ***℞:*** Seek expert advice. Often resolves spontaneously. Dialysis for ARF ma needed. Plasma exchange is used in severe persistent disease. ***Prognosis:*** Wor non-*E. Coli* cases. Mortality 3–5%.

Thrombotic thrombocytopenic purpura (TTP) is a pentad of: **1** Fever **2** F uating CNS signs (eg fits, hemiparesis, ↓consciousness, ↓vision) **3** MAHA (se often with jaundice) **4** Thrombocytopenia (severe, often mucosal bleeding) **5** R failure. Also: haematuria or proteinuria. Adult ♀ are chiefly affected, mortali higher than HUS. There is a genetic or acquired deficiency of a protease w normally cleaves multimers of von Willebrand factor (vWf). Large vWf multir form, causing platelet aggregation and fibrin deposition in small vessels, leadir microthrombi. ***Causes:*** Often unknown: drugs (eg clopidogrel, ciclospo pregnancy, HIV, SLE. ►*It is a haematological emergency: get expert help.* ***Test*** HUS. ***℞:*** Urgent plasma exchange may be life-saving. Steroids,[29] IV vincristine[30] splenectomy have roles in non-responders.[31]

Cholesterol emboli may be released from atheromatous plaques (often ac which lodge in the distal microcirculation (eg renal vessels, peripheral circula GIT) to cause ischaemia. An inflammatory response leads to fever, myalgia ↑eosinophils. ***Risks:*** Atheroma, ↑cholesterol, aortic aneurysm, thrombo arterial catheterisation eg during interventional radiological procedures. ***S*** Livedo reticularis (p542), gangrene, GI bleeds, renal failure. ***℞:*** Statins are (p682); avoid anticoagulants and instrumentation. ***Prognosis:*** Often progre and fatal; some regain renal function after dialysis.

abetes mellitus (type 2) and the kidney

abetes is best viewed as a vascular disease—with the kidney as one of its chief rgets for end-organ damage. The single most important intervention in the g-term care of DM is the control of BP, to protect the heart, the brain, and the ney. Renal damage may be preventable. ►Everyone with type 2 DM should be sted regularly (6-monthly) for microalbuminuria (30–300mg albumin excreted r day). A convenient way to do this test is to look for an early-morning urine MU) albumin:creatinine ratio of >3 (using EMUs improves consistency).

Microalbuminuria gives early warning of impending renal problems and is also strong independent risk factor for cardiovascular disease. Those who are sitive should be started on an ACE-i (p123) or angiotensin-2 receptor tagonists (A2A), *irrespective* of blood pressure. ***Examples of A2A doses:*** esartan 150–300mg/24h PO or losartan 50mg/d PO; increase after 1 month 100mg daily. ***SE:*** U&E↑ (monitor K^+ & creatinine periodically, stop if there is a e in creatinine of >20%), flushing, myalgia, headaches, dyspepsia, cough though commoner with ACE-i). Usually, ACE-i are first-line and ARAs for ACE-i olerant individuals. Increasingly they may be combined.

xample of target BP in DM ***if no proteinuria:*** 140/80 (negotiate with tient; ensure he/she is well informed); ***if microalbuminuria/proteinuria*** is esent, aim: 125/75mmHg.

targets work? Target-driven, long-term, intense therapy (including ophylactic aspirin) revolving around microalbuminuria and other risk factors n halve risk of macro- and microvascular events (MI etc.). 33 Steno-2 N=180; 2003

microalbuminuria reversible? Answer: sometimes—and more likely if: ecent onset • Hb_{A1c} <8% • Systolic <115mmHg • Cholesterol <5mmol/L.[1]

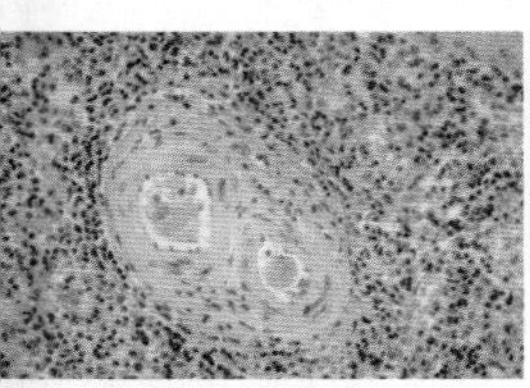

1. Thrombi in small arterioles due to fibrin and platelet osition, characteristic of TTP. 34

Renal medicine

rkins B 2003 *NEJM* **348** 2285 *n*=386; Regression of microalbuminuria had a 6yr cumulative ence of 58%. This could not be linked specifically to use of ACE-i.

Renal tubular disease

Renal tubular acidosis (RTA) is a metabolic acidosis, due to impaired secretion by the kidney. There is a hyperchloraemic metabolic acidosis with no anion gap (p658). Type 3 RTA is a rare combination of Types 1 & 2.

- **Type 1 (distal)** RTA is due to an inability to excrete H^+ and generate acidic u in the *distal* tubule, even in states of metabolic acidosis. It may complicate m renal disorders. ***Features*** include rickets (+ growth failure) or osteomalacia to buffering of H^+ with calcium in bone. Nephrocalcinosis with renal ca leading to recurrent UTIs, is due to a combination of hypercalciuria (from bo ↓urinary citrate (reabsorbed as a buffer for H^+) and alkaline urine: all fa calcium phosphate stone formation. ***Diagnosis:*** Acid load: oral ammon chloride load is given—there is failure to lower urine pH <5.5. ***Treatment:*** sodium bicarbonate or citrate. Complications are from renal calculi—end-s renal failure may result from unrecognised obstruction.
- **Type 2 (proximal)** RTA is due to a 'bicarbonate leak': a defect in reabsorption in the *proximal* tubule resulting in excess HCO_3 in the urine. tubules are able to reabsorb some HCO_3, so urine can acidify during syste acidosis. Type 2 RTA is often associated with a more generalised tubular de (Fanconi syndrome, below), and is rarer than Type 1. Hypokalaemia is comr due to the osmotic diuretic effect of ↓HCO_3 reabsorption, causing ↑flow ra distal tubule ∴ ↑K^+ excretion. ***Diagnosis:*** IV sodium bicarbonate load: there high fractional excretion of HCO_3 (>15%). ***Treatment:*** High doses of bicarbo (≥10mmol/kg/d) are required (this is often intolerable).
- **Type 4 (hyperkalaemic)** RTA is due to "hyporeninaemic hypoaldosteroni Hypoaldosteronism causes hyperkalaemia and acidosis (↓K^+ and H^+ excret ***Causes:*** Mild renal impairment (eg with tubulointerstitial disease or hypoadrenalism or drugs (K^+ sparing diuretics, NSAIDs, ACE-i/A2A). ***Treatm*** Remove any cause. Fludrocortisone 0.1mg PO, furosemide or calcium resor are used to control hyperkalaemia.

Fanconi syndrome The proximal tubule is responsible for reabsorption of m solutes, including 50% of filtered sodium, most bicarbonate and all filtered glu and amino acids. Fanconi syndrome is a disturbance of proximal tubule func with defective reabsorption of amino acids, K^+, phosphate (leading to hypop phataemic rickets and osteomalacia), glucose (glycosuria) and bicarbonate (Ty RTA: above). Also, there is polyuria (due to osmotic diuresis), and hypokalae (↑Na delivery to distal tubules leads to ↑exchange). **Causes:** ***Idiopathic Fan syndrome:*** No identifiable cause. Mostly sporadic, some inherited. *Features*: de ration, failure to thrive. Vitamin D resistant rickets is typical. There may progressive renal failure in early adulthood. ***Inherited:*** Errors of metabolisr cystinosis (below), fructose intolerance, galactosaemia, glycogen storage dise Wilson's disease (p257), Lowe's syndrome,[1] tyrosinaemia. ***Acquired:*** Tu damage eg heavy metals (lead, mercury, cadmium, platinum, uranium), drugs (of-date tetracycline, iphosphamide), light chains (myeloma, amyloidosis), imm logical (interstitial nephritis, transplant rejection). ***℞:*** Remove any cause replace losses. K^+, sodium bicarbonate, PO_4^{3-} and vitamin D supplements are u

Cystinosis There is accumulation of cystine in lysosomes due to an autosc recessive defect. Cystine deposits cause Fanconi syndrome, visual impairment hypothyroidism, with progression to ESRF <10yrs. ***℞:*** As Fanconi syndrome. cysteamine ↓intralysosomal cystine and delays ESRF, but is poorly tolerated. R cystinosis does not recur after transplant; extra-renal disease progresses.

Hereditary hypokalaemic tubulopathies ***Bartter's syndrome:*** p212; ***Gitel syndrome:*** ↓Na^+Cl reabsorption at the distal tubule due to an autosomal reces mutation, causing ↑solute loss, and ↑K^+ loss due to 2° hyperaldosteronism. hypocalciuria and hypomagnesaemia.

Nephrogenic diabetes insipidus p224.

...auses of renal tubular acidosis

...pe 1 (distal)

- Idiopathic.
- Genetic (eg Marfan's, Ehlers-Danlos syndrome).
- Autoimmune disease (eg SLE, Sjögren's, autoimmune hepatitis).
- Nephrocalcinosis (eg hypercalcaemia, medullary sponge kidney).
- Tubulointerstitial disease (eg chronic pyelonephritis, chronic interstitial nephritis, obstructive uropathy, renal transplant rejection).
- Drugs (eg lithium, amphotericin).

...pe 2 (proximal)

- Idiopathic.
- Fanconi syndrome.
- Tubulointerstitial disease (eg myeloma, interstitial nephritis).
- Drugs (eg lead or other heavy metals, acetazolamide, out of date tetracycline).

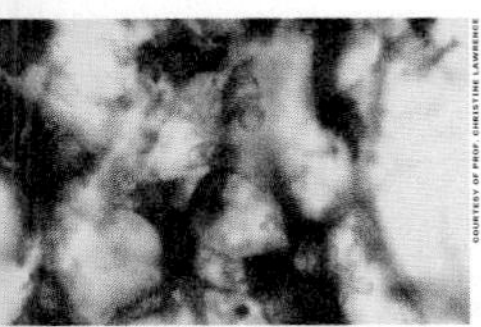
COURTESY OF PROF. CHRISTINE LAWRENCE

...1. Cystine crystals in the bone marrow, found in ...tinosis. Crystals accumulate in most tissues, ...ecially the kidneys.

An X-linked inherited disorder affecting ♂ with aminoaciduria, mental retardation, hypotonia, ...aracts, abnormal skull shape and progressive renal failure (oculocerebrorenal syndrome).

Inherited kidney diseases

Autosomal dominant polycystic kidney disease (ADPKD) ***Prevalence:*** 1:10 Genes on chromosomes 16 (PKD1) and 4 (PKD2). ***Signs:*** Renal enlargement w cysts, abdominal pain ± haematuria (haemorrhage into a cyst), cyst infection, re calculi, BP↑, progressive renal failure. *Extrarenal*: liver cysts, intracra aneurysm→subarachnoid haemorrhage (SAH), mitral valve prolapse. ***Treatme*** Monitor U&E. Treating ↑BP is important to prevent cardiovascular complicati and SAH. Treat infections, dialysis or transplantation for ESRF, genetic counselli Pain may be helped by laparoscopic cyst removal or nephrectomy. ***Screening SAH*** with magnetic resonance angiography may be done in 1st-degree relatives those with SAH + ADPKD. Some screen with no family history.

Autosomal recessive polycystic kidney disease *OHCS* p132. Prevalence 1:40,0 chromosome 6. *Signs*: Infancy: renal cysts, congenital hepatic fibrosis.

Medullary cystic disease Inherited disorder with tubular loss and medullary c formation. The juvenile (autosomal recessive) form accounts for 10–20% of ESR children. The adult form (autosomal dominant; restricted to the kidney) is ra ***Signs:*** Polyuria, polydipsia, enuresis (↓urine concentrating ability), failure to thr renal impairment → ESRF. *Extrarenal:* include retinal degeneration, retinitis pigme osa, skeletal changes, cerebellar ataxia, liver fibrosis.

Renal phakomatoses (neuroectodermal syndromes). ***Tuberous sclerosis:*** *O* p638. A complex autosomal dominant disorder with hamartoma formation in s brain, eye, kidney, and heart caused by genes on chromosomes 9 (TSC1) & (TSC2). *Signs* are variable: • Skin: adenoma sebaceum, angiofibromas, 'ash le hypomelanic macules, shagreen patches (sacral plaques of shark-like sk periungual fibroma • IQ↓ • Epilepsy. ***Von Hippel–Lindau syndrome*** (p704) is chief cause of inherited renal cancers. ***Cause:*** Germline mutations of the tumour-suppressor gene (also inactivated in most sporadic renal cell cancers)

Alport's syndrome *OHCS* p638. ***Prevalence:*** 1:5000. Variable inheritance (ma expressed in ♂: 85% are X-linked). The affected genes code for type IV collag molecules. ***Pathology:*** Thickened GBM with 'splitting'. The Goodpasture's antig is missing (hence risk of anti-GBM glomerulonephritis post-renal transplant). ***Sig*** Haematuric nephritis, sensorineural deafness, and progressive renal failure. So have lenticonus: bulging of lens capsule seen on slit-lamp examination. ***℞:*** No specific, as for renal failure.

Fabry's disease See p690.

Hyperoxaluria ***Primary hyperoxaluria*** is an autosomal recessive inherited erro metabolism due to an enzyme defect. ***Secondary hyperoxaluria*** is due to • ↑int eg rhubarb, spinach, tea • ↑intestinal reabsorption due to ileal disease (Croh ileal bypass), short bowel syndrome, low Ca^{2+} intake. ***Signs:*** Oxalate renal sto (p284), nephrocalcinosis, progressive renal failure, cardiac conduction defec arterial disease (oxalate crystallisation), osteodystrophy. ***Treatment:*** High fl intake to prevent calculi (keep urine output ~3L/day), ↓dietary oxalate, calci supplements (binds oxalate in the gut so ↓absorption). If these do not wo pyridoxine (vitamin B_6) is used to ↓endogenous oxalate production (SE: periphe neuropathy in high doses). Magnesium or cholestyramine are also used to ↓oxal absorption. Hepatic transplantation may be curative in primary hyperoxaluria, a may be combined with renal transplant.

Cystinuria The commonest aminoaciduria, causing ↓tubular reabsorption of dibasic amino acids **COAL** Cystine, Ornithine, Arginine and Lysine, due to autosomal recessive defect. ***Features:*** Manifests with cystine renal stones (p28 ***Treatment:*** ↑Fluid intake to keep urine output ~3L/day; urine alkalinization w potassium citrate (↑solubility of cystine). Penicillamine is used, which binds cyst in soluble complexes. **NB:** Do not confuse this condition with cystinosis where th are no stones (p302).

[Ge]netics: triumphs and disasters

[A]s soon as genetics solves one problem, others appear. You might think that the [a]pplication of science to medicine is an undisputed boon. Petty has provided a [co]mpelling counter-example. A man with adult polycystic kidney disease due [to] a PKD1 mutation is in end-stage renal failure. A transplant from a matched, [livi]ng, related, unaffected donor is highly desired. There are problems in his [fa]mily, but he persuades his adult children to have genetic testing to see if there [ar]e eligible donors. Each is apparently happy to donate a kidney to his/her [fa]ther.

A can of worms is opened when one son realizes that he is the only child who [ca]n offer a good match—and that his brother is carrying the same mutation as [hi]s estranged father (there is a 50:50 chance of passing on the PKD gene). The [eli]gible son would rather save his kidney to help his brother than his father. Old [an]imosities resurface, and the family is in turmoil. How will you feel if the father [di]es of a complication of dialysis, and both his sons feel guilty forever? We [sh]ould not be too surprised at all this: often in medicine bad comes out of our [go]od intentions. How can we make good come out of bad? By remembering this [ex]ample, and not doing tests lightly, and by making genetic counselling as [pr]ofessional as possible, so complications can be foreseen and disasters pre-[e]mpted. Furthermore, do not have unreasonable expectations about what [ge]netic counselling can do. The number of diseases being found to have a [si]gnificant genetic component is increasing faster than geneticists can formulate [ra]tional guidelines for screening.[1]

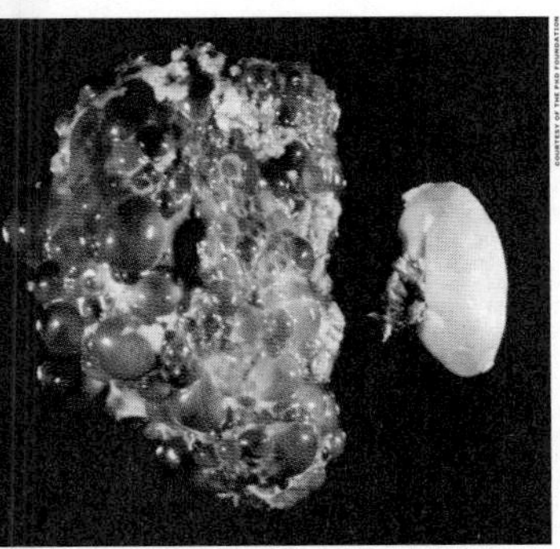

[Fig] 1. A polycystic kidney (left) compared to a normal sized kidney (right). [Th]e progressive increase in size often leads to abdominal discomfort, and [the]re may be haemorrhage into a cyst causing haematuria, or infection.

1 [H]emminki K 2004 Data for clinical counselling & cancer genetics. *Int J Cancer* **108** 109

Renal manifestations of systemic disease

Amyloidosis (p354) can cause proteinuria, nephrotic syndrome or progress renal failure. ***Diagnosis:*** US: large kidneys; biopsy: see p354. ***Treatment*** p354.

Diabetes This is one of the commonest causes of ESRF in the UK, accounting ~18%. ***Pathology:*** Hyperglycaemia causes renal hyperperfusion, increasing G This causes hypertrophy and ↑renal size. Mesangial hypertrophy and fo glomerulosclerosis (Kimmelstiel–Wilson lesion) occur later due to ↑glomeru pressure. This initially causes ***microalbuminuria*** (detectable on laboratory te but not on dipstick: albuminuria 30–300mg/d), a sign of early diabetic nephropa and a strong independent predictor of cardiovascular mortality. This progresses proteinuria (albuminuria >300mg/d): ESRF usually occurs within 5–10 yea Diabetic retinopathy usually co-exists, and hypertension is common. It occurs ~30%, partly due to genetic predisposition.

- ***Type 1 DM nephropathy*** occurs typically 20–40yrs post-diagnosis.
- ***Type 2 DM ('maturity onset') nephropathy:*** ►See p301 (BOX). >10–30% ha nephropathy at diagnosis, and prevalence increases linearly with time.

Treatment: Good glycaemic control delays onset and progression of nephropat If microalbuminuria is present, additional important interventions to sl progression of renal disease are • BP target <125/<75 • Use of ACE-i or A2A, eve normotensive (these ↓intraglomerular pressure, p301) • Smoking cessation. Or ESRF has been reached, combined pancreas and renal transplant is possible *selected* patients.

Infection associated nephropathies are common causes of renal disease. ***Glomerulonephritis*** occurs with many bacterial, viral and parasitic infections, includ post-streptococcal, hepatitis B or C, HIV, SBE/IE, shunt nephritis, visceral absce syphilis, malaria, schistosomiasis and filiariasis. ***Vasculitis*** (p542) may occur w hepatitis B or C, post-streptococcal or staphylococcal septicaemia. ***Interstit nephritis:*** Seen with bacterial pyelonephritis, viral (CMV, HIV, hepatitis hantavirus), fungal and parasitic (leishmaniasis, toxoplasmosis) infections.

Malignancy ***Direct effects:*** Renal infiltration (leukaemia, lymphoma), obstructi (pelvic tumours), metastases. ***Indirect:*** Hypercalcaemia, nephrotic syndrome, acu renal failure, amyloidosis, glomerulonephritis. ***Treatment associated:*** Nephroto drugs, tumour lysis syndrome, radiation nephritis.

Myeloma (p352) is characterized by excess production of monoclonal antibody light chains, which are excreted and detected in ⅔ of cases as Bence-Jor proteinuria. Myeloma kidney is due to blockage of tubules by casts, consisting light chains. The light chains have a direct toxic effects on tubular cells, causi ATN. ***Features:*** ARF, CRF, amyloidosis (may cause proteinuria and nephro syndrome), hypercalcaemic nephropathy. ***Treatment:*** Ensure fluid intake of 3L/d to prevent further impairment. Dialysis may be required in ARF.

Rheumatological diseases ***Rheumatoid arthritis (RA)*** NSAIDs may cau interstitial nephritis. Penicillamine and gold can cause membranous nephropat AA amyloidosis (p354) occurs in ~15% of RA (often asymptomatic). ***SLE*** involves t glomerulus in 40–60% of adults, causing acute or chronic disease. Proteinuria a ↑BP are common. Histological patterns range from minimal change to crescentic Consider a renal biopsy if nephritic syndrome or deteriorating renal function. ACE-i if proteinuria. Corticosteroids and immunosuppressants (cyclophosphamide mycophenolate) are used if biopsy shows aggressive GN (p540). ***Systemic scleros*** (p538) may affect the kidney, especially in diffuse disease. 'Renal crisis' preser with ARF + accelerated hypertension. ***℞:*** ACE-i if ↑BP or in renal crisis. Dialysis transplant may be required.

Hyperparathyroidism Clinical features are from hypercalcaemia: p298.

Sarcoidosis may involve the kidney, often by abnormal calcium metabolis (p178). Interstitial nephritis and rarely glomerulonephritis are also associated

pilogue: the man in a red canoe who saved a million lives

ostly we commute to work each day driven by motives we would rather not ok at too deeply. But one renal physician used a red canoe to commute each ay from his houseboat to the hospital. He could have been a very rich man but stead Belding Scribner gave his invention away, and continued his modest xistence. He invented the Scribner shunt—a **U** of teflon connecting an artery to vein, so allowing haemodialysis to be something which could be repeated as ften as needed. Before Scribner, glass tubes had to be painfully inserted into ood vessels, which would be damaged by the procedure and haemodialysis ould only be done for a few cycles. Clyde Shields was his first patient with ronic renal failure to receive the shunt—on 9 March 1960, and said that his rst treatment 'took so much of the waste I'd stored up out of me that it was st like turning on the light from darkness'.[40] Scribner took something that was 00% fatal and overnight turned it into a condition with a 90% survival. In so oing he founded a branch of bioethics because not everyone could have the eatment immediately. This is the branch of ethics that is to do with who gets hat—ie distributive justice. In Scribner's day, this was decided by the famous ife and Death Committee' which had the unenviable job of choosing who would urvive by placing people in order precedence.

Scribner has said that his inventions sprang from his empathy for patients, cluding himself. 'I was a sickly child' he said, and at various times he needed a eart-lung machine, a new hip, and donated corneas. He was the sort of man hose patients would inspire him to worry away at their problems during the ay—and then to awake at night with a brilliant solution.

On 19 June 2003, his canoe was found afloat but empty—and like those ncient Indian burial canoes found at Wiskam which have been polished to an nimaginable lustre by the action of the shifting sands around the Island of the ead, so we polish and cherish the image of this man who gave everything away.

9 Haematology

Contents

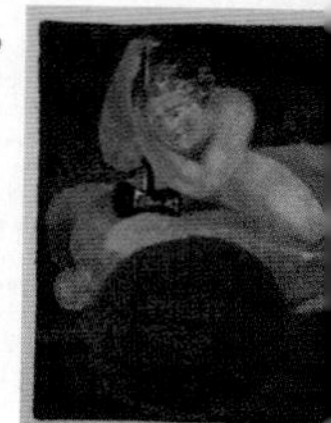

Fig 1. The **old** methodology naked haematologist works al hammering a red cell into sha "Every space larger than a globule of man's blood visionary, and it is created by Hammer of Los." Image from *Song of Los,* William Blake.

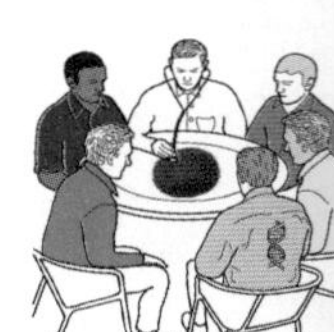

Fig 2. The **new** methodology: tea work in action, as haematologi geneticist, and lab staff deal w a troublesome spherocyte. (×30

Relevant pages elsewhere: Haemolytic uraemic syndrome p300; Thrombo thrombocytopenic purpura p300; Transfusion (p570); normal values (p741).

Further reading: D Nathan *Genes, Blood, and Courage,* Harvard University Pre ISBN 0-674-34473-L. Dayem Saif, introduced as a 6-year-old with a stature of 2-year-old, has an Hb of 1.5g/dL, as low as his chance of survival with thala aemia. This story about laboratory medicine and its stormy application at t bedside is definitely worth reading when feeling hemmed in by difficult patients, it demonstrates that there are no difficult patients, only difficult times. The bo portrays the vital nature of the doctor–patient relationship, and warns us agai labelling people, unless the label is a poem: Dayem is Arabic for *Immortal Swo*

We thank Dr Drew Provan who is our Specialist Reader for this chapter.

n the taking of blood and of holidays

is is not one of those pages about how you should be kind to the patient, plain in full what you are going to do, talk him or her through venepuncture, bel the bottles carefully, and make a plan for communicating the results. Be all is as it may, there is something else which needs communicating about the *act* taking blood. It is partly to do with the fact that as blood is life, and, because, Ruskin taught us, 'there is no wealth but life', we are led to the conclusion that hat is special about taking blood is that for once *we* are being given something luable by the patient. What is this wealth? The answer is *time*. For while the ood is flowing into our tube we cannot be disturbed. We are excused from swering our bleeps, and from making polite conversation (a few grunts in ply to patients' enquires about the colour of their blood is quite sufficient)— d we can indulge in that almost unimaginable luxury, at least as far as life on e wards is concerned, of *being alone with our own thoughts*. Thinking of this cred time as a sort of hypnotic holiday is excellent. For however many nights have been awoken, and through however many wards we have traipsed to is bedside, this little holiday will be worth an hour's sleep—if our mind is rnished and ready to empty itself of all objectivity. The best sight in ematological practice is, during venepuncture, to watch for those occasions hen, owing to some chance characteristic of flow, the jet of blood streaming to our tube breaks up into countless globules, and before coalescing again, ese globules jostle together like the overcrowded chain of events which led us this bedside. During this time, allow your own thoughts to coalesce into a ore peaceful order if you can, and let William Blake help you in the task of rnishing your mind to banish objectivity, for he knew some truths about ematology unknown to strictly rational practitioners of this art:

he Microscope knows not of this nor the Telescope: they alter
he ratio of the Spectators Organs but leave Objects untouch'd
or every space larger than a red globule of Mans blood
s visionary, and it is created by the Hammer of Los:[1]
And every space smaller than a Globule of Mans blood opens
nto eternity of which this vegetable Earth is but a shadow.
he red Globule is the unwearied Sun by Los created
o measure Time and Space to mortal Men ...

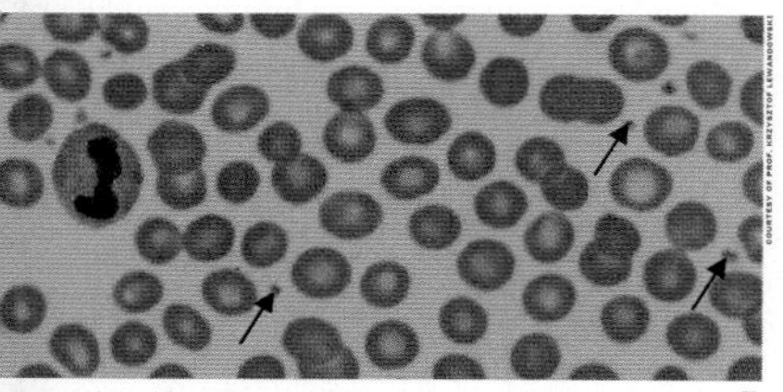

1. A normal blood film, with a neutrophil, normal red cells, and platelets (arrows).

os, the *globe of fire*, is a symbol used by Blake to encompass the exultant energy of creation, the c imagination, and the burning brightness where all his noble images were pounded out of ity and compounded into the most compressed verse and art we have (*see* P Ackroyd 1996 , Minerva). These lines are from his poem *Milton*, section 29, lines 17–24, page 516 in OUP's e: *Complete Writings*, edited (1925–1969) by Geoffrey Keynes, the surgeon, who, incidentally, e way to lumpectomy for breast cancer, in preference to the much-hated radical mastectomy.

Anaemia

Anaemia is defined as a low haemoglobin (Hb) concentration, and may be eit due to a low red cell mass, or increased plasma volume (eg in pregnancy). A low (at sea level) is <13.5g/dL for men and <11.5g/dL for women. Anaemia may be to reduced production or increased loss of RBC and has many causes. These often be distinguishable by history, examination, and inspection of the blood f

Symptoms Due to the underlying cause or to the anaemia itself: fatigue, dyspn faintness, palpitations, headache, tinnitus, anorexia—and angina if there is p existing coronary artery disease.

Signs May be absent even in severe anaemia. There may be pallor (eg conjuncti although this is not a reliable sign). In severe anaemia (Hb <8g/dL), there may signs of a hyperdynamic circulation, eg tachycardia, flow murmurs (ejecti systolic loudest over apex), and cardiac enlargement; or retinal haemorrha (rarely). Later, heart failure may occur: here, rapid blood transfusion may be fa

Types of anaemia The first step in diagnosis is to look at the mean cell volu (MCV, *normal* MCV is 76–96 femtolitres, 10^{15} fL = 1L).

Low MCV (microcytic anaemia)

- Iron-deficiency anaemia (IDA, most common cause): p312.
- Thalassaemia (suspect if the MCV is 'too low' for the level of anaemia and the cell count is raised): p328.
- Sideroblastic anaemia (very rare): p312.

NB: The last two are conditions where there is an accumulation of iron, and so t will show serum iron↑, ferritin↑, and a low total iron-binding capacity (TIBC).

Normal MCV (normocytic anaemia)

- Acute blood loss
- Anaemia of chronic disease (or ↓MCV)
- Bone marrow failure
- Renal failure
- Hypothyroidism (or ↑MCV)
- Haemolysis (or ↑MCV)
- Pregnancy

If WCC↓ or platelet↓, suspect marrow failure: see p348.

High MCV (macrocytic anaemia)

- B_{12} or folate deficiency
- Alcohol excess—or liver disease
- Reticulocytosis (eg with haemolysis)
- Cytotoxics, eg hydroxycarbamide
- Myelodysplastic syndromes
- Marrow infiltration
- Hypothyroidism
- Antifolate drugs (eg phenytoir

Haemolytic anaemias: (p322). These disorders do not fall elegantly into the ab classification as the anaemia may be normocytic, or, if there are many young (he larger) RBCs and reticulocytes, macrocytic. Suspect if there is a reticulocyt (>2% of RBCs; or reticulocyte count >100×10⁹/L), mild macrocytosis, haptoglob bilirubin↑ & urobilinogen↑. Often mild jaundice (but no bilirubin in urine haemolysis causes pre-hepatic jaundice).

Blood transfusion The decision on whether to transfuse depends on a numbe factors: the onset (acute or chronic), the severity of anaemia (one review sugg that transfusion is not essential for *most* patients unless Hb <7g/dL), if the co-morbidity (have a lower threshold to transfuse in ischaemic heart disease) whether the patient is symptomatic. If there is an acute cause (eg haemorrh with active peptic ulcer), transfuse up to 8g/dL. Chronic anaemia is be tolerated, and it is important to ascertain the cause eg in iron deficiency anae iron supplements will raise the haemoglobin in a safer and less costly way severe anaemia with heart failure, transfusion is vital to restore Hb to safe leve 6–8g/dL, but must be done with great care. Give packed cells *slowly* with 40mg furosemide IV/PO with alternate units (dose depends on previous exposu diuretics; do not mix with blood). Check for rising JVP and basal crackles. If CCF worse, stop and treat. If immediate transfusion is essential, a 2–3 unit excha transfusion can be tried, removing blood at same rate as it is transfused.

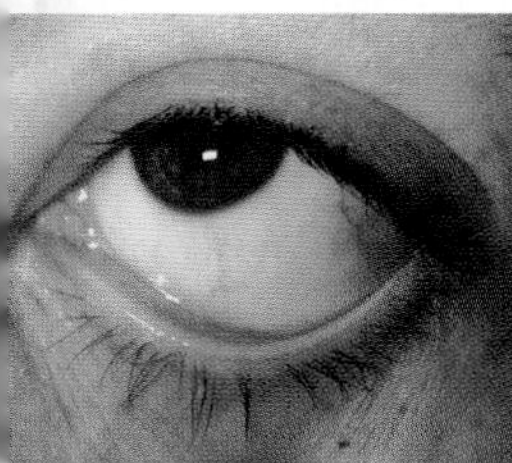

ȝ 1. 'Conjunctival pallor', *the* classic sign of anaemia, is confusing term as the conjunctiva is translucent, ansmitting the colour of the structures under it. The allor' in fact refers to the vasculature on the inner rface of the lid which lacks haemoglobin.

is this colour , whereas it should be more

e this: .

Iron-deficiency anaemia (IDA)

This is common (seen in up to 14% of menstruating women).

Causes: • Blood loss eg menorrhagia or GI bleeding (upper p244; lower p70).
• Poor diet may cause IDA in babies or children (but rarely in adults), those special diets, or wherever there is poverty.
• Malabsorption (eg coeliac disease) is a cause of refractory IDA.
• In the Tropics, hookworm (GI blood loss) is the most common cause.

Signs: Chronic IDA (signs now rare): koilonychia (fig 1 and p27), atrophic glossi angular cheilosis (fig 2), and rarely, post-cricoid webs (Plummer-Vinson syndron

Tests: Microcytic, hypochromic anaemia with anisocytosis and poikilocytosis (fi and 4). $\downarrow$MCV, $\downarrow$MCH & $\downarrow$MCHC. Confirmed by ferritin$\downarrow$ (also serum iron$\downarrow$ with $\uparrow$tc iron binding capacity—TIBC, but these are less reliable). $\uparrow$red cell protoporphy NB: Ferritin is an acute phase protein and $\uparrow$ with inflammation eg infecti malignancy. Serum transferrin receptors are also $\uparrow$ in IDA but are less affected inflammation. If MCV$\downarrow$, and good history of menorrhagia, oral iron may be start without further tests. Otherwise investigate for GI blood loss: gastrosco sigmoidoscopy, barium enema or colonoscopy, stool microscopy for ova if fore travel. Faecal occult blood is not recommended as sensitivity is poor. ►*I deficiency without an obvious source of bleeding mandates a careful GI work*

Treatment: Treat the cause. Oral iron eg ferrous sulfate 200mg/8h PO. SE: naus abdominal discomfort, diarrhoea or constipation, black stools. Hb should rise 1g/dL/week, with a modest reticulocytosis (ie young RBC, p314). Continue unti is normal and for at least 3 months, to replenish stores. Intravenous iron is alm never needed, but may be indicated if the oral route is impossible or ineffective functional iron deficiency in chronic renal failure, where there is inadequate mo ization of iron stores in response to the acute demands of erythropoietin thera

The usual reason that IDA fails to respond to iron replacement is that the pati has rejected the pills. Negotiate on concordance issues (p3). Is the reason for problem GI disturbance? Altering the dose of elemental iron with a differ preparation may help. There may be continued blood loss, malabsorption, anaer of chronic disease; or there is misdiagnosis, eg when thalassaemia is to blame

The anaemia of chronic disease

This is associated with many diseases, including chronic infection (eg osteomyelitis), vasculitis, rheumatoid arthritis, malignancy, renal failure. There cytokine driven inhibition of red cell production. ***Investigations:*** Mild normocy anaemia (eg Hb >8g/dL), ferritin normal or $\uparrow$. ***Treatment:*** Treat the underly disease. The anaemia of renal failure is partly due to erythropoietin deficiency a recombinant erythropoietin is effective in raising the haemoglobin level (SE: 'flu- symptoms, hypertension, mild rise in the platelet count). It is also effective raising Hb and improving quality of life in those with malignant disease.

Sideroblastic anaemia

Characterized by ineffective erythropoiesis, leading to $\uparrow$iron absorption, i loading (bone marrow) and occasionally haemosiderosis (endocrine, liver a cardiac damage due to iron deposition). It may be congenital (rare, X-linked) acquired—usually idiopathic as one of the myelodysplastic disorders, but can fol chemotherapy, irradiation, alcohol or lead excess, anti-TB drugs or myeloprc erative disease. Hypochromic RBCs are seen on the blood film with ring sideroble in the marrow (erythroid precursors with iron deposited in mitochondria in a r around the nucleus). ***Treatment:*** Remove the cause if possible. Pyridoxine may of benefit. Repeated blood transfusion may be needed in severe anaemia.

1 In one study, 11% presenting to their GP with IDA had GI carcinoma. Consider both upper and lc GI investigation as in another study, 29% (n=89) had abnormalities on both.

[I]nterpretation of plasma iron studies

	Iron	TIBC	Ferritin
[Ir]on deficiency	↓	↑	↓
[An]aemia of chronic disease	↓	↓	↑
[Ch]ronic haemolysis	↑	↓	↑
[H]aemochromatosis	↑	↓ (or ↔)	↑
[Pr]egnancy	↑	↑	↔
[Si]deroblastic anaemia	↑	↔	↑

TIBC: total iron binding capacity.

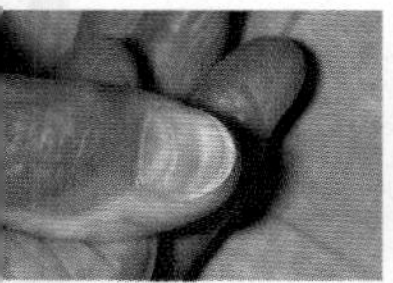

[Fig] 1. Koilonychia. Spoon-shaped nails, [fou]nd in iron deficiency anaemia.

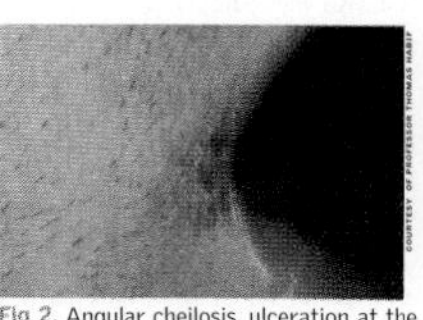

Fig 2. Angular cheilosis, ulceration at the side of the mouth, in iron deficiency anaemia. Also a feature of Vitamin B_{12} and B_2 (riboflavin) deficiency. 6

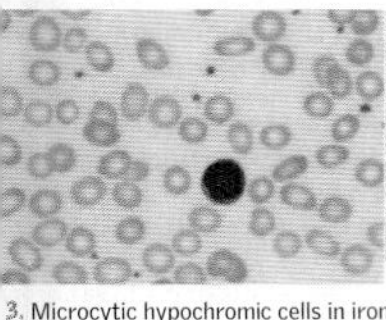

[Fig] 3. Microcytic hypochromic cells in iron [defi]ciency anaemia. 7

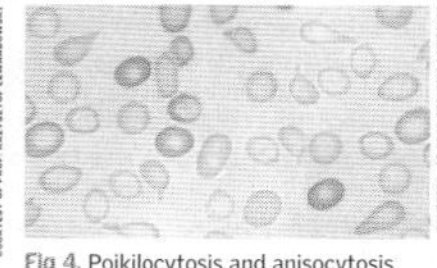

Fig 4. Poikilocytosis and anisocytosis seen in iron deficiency anaemia. 8

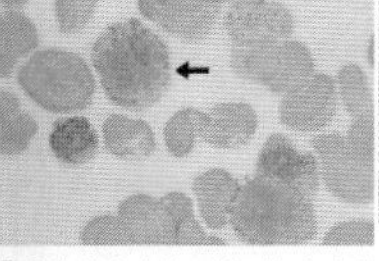

[Fig] 5. Pathological ring sideroblasts in the [bon]e marrow, with a perinuclear ring of iron [gra]nules, found in sideroblastic anaemia. 9

The peripheral blood film

►Many haematological (and other) diagnoses are made by careful examinatio the peripheral blood film. It is also necessary for interpretation of the FBC indi

Anisocytosis is variation in RBC size, eg megaloblastic anaemia, thalassaemia,

Acanthocytes: (fig 1) RBCs show many spicules due to an unstable red membrane lipid structure (eg in abetalipoproteinaemia).

Basophilic RBC stippling: (fig 2) Denatured RNA found in RBCs, indicating accelera erythropoiesis or defective Hb synthesis. Seen in lead poisoning, megalobla anaemia, myelodysplasia, liver disease, haemoglobinopathy eg thalassaemia.

Blasts: Nucleated precursor cells. They are not normally in peripheral blood, but seen in myelofibrosis, leukaemia or malignant infiltration by carcinoma.

Burr cells: Irregularly shaped cells occurring in uraemia.

Dimorphic picture: Two populations of red cells. Seen after treatment of Fe, B folate deficiency, in mixed deficiency (↓Fe with ↓B_{12} or folate), post-transfusio with primary sideroblastic anaemia, where a clone of abnormal erythrobl produce abnormal red cells, alongside normal red cell production.

Howell–Jolly bodies: DNA nuclear remnants in RBCs, which are normally remove the spleen (fig 8). Seen post-splenectomy and in hyposplenism (eg sickle disease, coeliac disease, congenital, UC/Crohn's, myeloproliferative disease, amyl Also in dyserythopoietic states: myelodysplasia, megaloblastic anaemia.

Hypochromia: (p312). Less dense staining of RBCs due to ↓Hb synthesis, see IDA, thalassaemia, and sideroblastic anaemia (iron stores unusable).

Left shift: Immature neutrophils are sent out of the marrow, eg in infection.

Leucoerythroblastic anaemia: Immature cells (myelocytes, promyelocy metamyelocytes, normoblasts) seen in film. Due to marrow infiltration (eg mal ancy) when these cells are displaced; also seen in anorexia, sepsis, severe haemol

Leukaemoid reaction: A marked leucocytosis (WCC>50×10⁹/L). Seen in se illness eg with infection or burns, and also in leukaemia.

Pappenheimer bodies: (fig 5) Granules of siderocytes containing iron. Seen in poisoning, carcinomatosis, and post-splenectomy.

Poikilocytosis is variation in RBC shape, eg in IDA, myelofibrosis, thalassaemia

Polychromasia: RBCs of different ages stain unevenly (young are bluer). This response to bleeding, haematinic replacement (ferrous sulfate, B_{12}, fola haemolysis, or marrow infiltration. Reticulocyte count is raised.

Reticulocytes: (normal range: 0.8–2%; or <85×10⁹/L) fig 6. Young, larger (contain RNA) signifying active erythropoiesis. Increased in haemol haemorrhage, and if B_{12}, iron or folate is given to marrow that lack these.

Right shift: Hypermature white cells: hypersegmented polymorphs (>5 lobe nucleus) seen in megaloblastic anaemia, uraemia, and liver disease. See p318, f

Rouleaux formation: (fig 7) Red cells stack on each other (it causes a raised p356). Seen with chronic inflammation, paraproteinaemia and myeloma.

Spherocytes: Spherical cells found in hereditary spherocytosis and autoimm haemolytic anaemia. See p324.

Schistocytes: Fragmented RBCs sliced by fibrin bands, in intravascular haemo (p324, fig 4) Look for microangiopathic anaemia, eg DIC (p336), haemolytic ura syndrome, thrombotic thrombocytopenic purpura (TTP: p300), or pre-eclampsi

Target cells: (also known as Mexican hat cells, fig 8). These are RBCs with cer staining, a ring of pallor, and an outer rim of staining seen in liver dise hyposplenism, thalassaemia—and, in small numbers, in iron-deficiency anaem

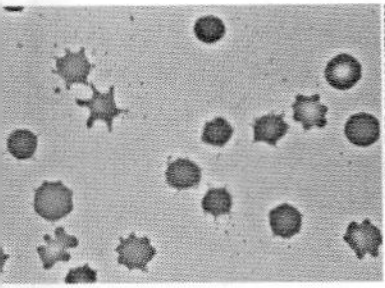

COURTESY OF DR. NIVALDO MEDEIROS

1. Acanthocytosis.[10]

COURTESY OF PROFESSOR BARBARA BAIN

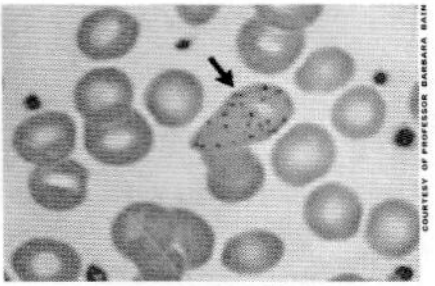

Fig 2. Basophilic stippling.[11]

COURTESY OF PROF. CHRISTINE LAWRENCE

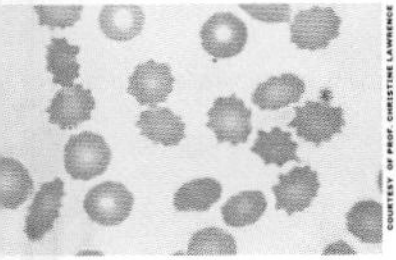

3. Burr cells.[12]

COURTESY OF DR. NIVALDO MEDEIROS

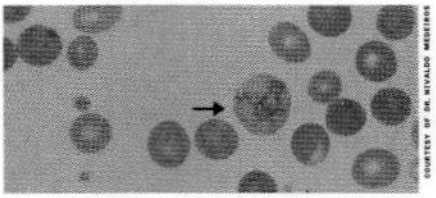

Fig 6. Reticulocytes. RNA in RBCs; supravital staining (azure B; cresyl blue) is needed.[13]

COURTESY OF PROF. CHRISTINE LAWRENCE & CROOKSTON COL.

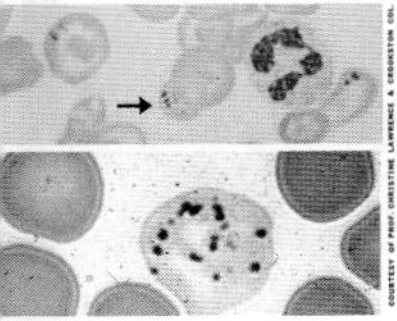

5. Pappenheimer bodies.[14] [15]

COURTESY OF PROF. KRZYSZTOF LEWANDOWSKI

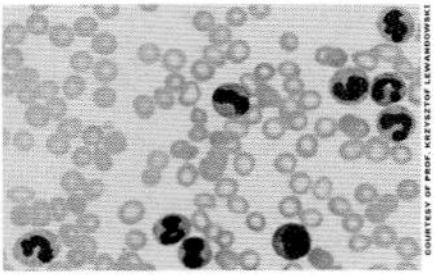

Fig 4. Left-shift: presence of immature neutrophils in the blood.[16]

COURTESY OF DR. NIVALDO MEDEIROS

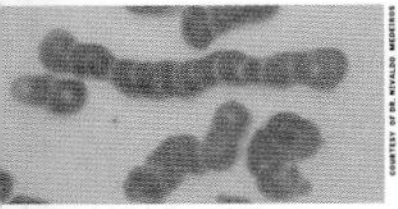

7. Rouleaux formation.[17]

COURTESY OF PROFESSOR BARBARA BAIN ©2005 MASSACHUSETTS MEDICAL SOCIETY

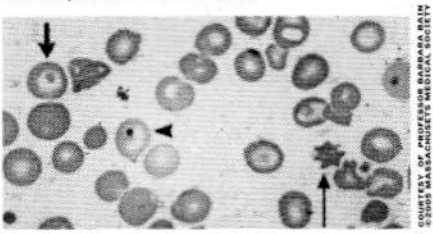

Fig 8. Film in hyposplenism: target cell (short arrow), acanthocyte (long arrow) and a Howell–Jolly body (arrow head).[18]

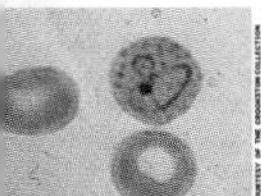

COURTESY OF THE CROOKSTON COLLECTION

Fig 9. A Cabot ring; these red/purple-staining filamentous figure-of-8 rings are often seen in RBCs with basophilic stippling.[19] They may be microtubules from mitotic spindles or nuclear remnants. They occur in severe or megaloblastic anaemia, leukaemia, and lead poisoning. It is easy to confuse them with malaria parasites, p385 (especially if stippling gives a 'chromatin dot' artefact, as here).[20]

The differential white cell count

Neutrophils 2–7.5 × 10^9/L (40–75% of white blood cells: but absolute values a
more meaningful than percentages).

Increased in neutrophilia:
- Bacterial infections.
- Inflammation eg myocardial infarction, polyarteritis nodosa.
- Myeloproliferative disorders.
- Drugs (steroids).
- Disseminated malignancy.
- Stress eg trauma, surgery, burns, haemorrhage, seizure.

Decreased in neutropenia: (see p336)
- Viral infections.
- Drugs eg post-chemotherapy, cytotoxic agents, carbimazole, sulfonamides.
- Severe sepsis.
- Neutrophil antibodies (SLE, haemolytic anaemia)—↑ destruction.
- Hypersplenism eg Felty's syndrome (p357).
- Bone marrow failure—↓ production (p348).

Lymphocytes 1.5–4.5 × 10^9/L (20–45%).

Increased in:
- Acute viral infections.
- Chronic infections eg TB, Brucella, hepatitis, syphilis.
- Leukaemias and lymphomas, especially chronic lymphocytic leukaemia.

Large numbers of abnormal ('atypical') lymphocytes are characteristically se with EBV infection: these are T-cells reacting against EBV-infected B-cells. They ha a large amount of clearish cytoplasm with a blue rim that flows arou neighbouring RBCs. Other causes of 'atypical' lymphocytes: see p389.

Decreased in:
- Steroid therapy; SLE; uraemia; Legionnaire's disease; HIV infection; marr infiltration; post chemotherapy or radiotherapy.

T-lymphocyte subset reference values: CD4 count: 537–1571/mm^3 (low in H infection). CD8 count: 235–753/mm^3; CD4/CD8 ratio: 1.2–3.8.

Eosinophils 0.04–0.4 × 10^9/L (1–6%).[21]

Increased in:
- Drug reactions eg with erythema multiforme, p546.
- Allergies: asthma, atopy.
- Parasitic infections (especially invasive helminths).
- Skin disease: especially pemphigus, eczema, psoriasis, dermatitis herpetiforn

Also seen in malignant disease (including lymphomas and eosinophilic leukaemi PAN, adrenal insufficiency,[22] irradiation, Löffler's syndrome (p696), and during t convalescent phase of any infection.

The hypereosinophilic syndrome[1] is a disease of unknown cause, with a sustain eosinophil count >1.5 × 10^9/L for more than 6wks, leading to end-organ dama (endomyocardial fibrosis causing restrictive cardiomyopathy, skin lesio thromboembolic disease, pulmonary disease, neuropathy, and hepatosplenomegal

Monocytes 0.2–0.8 × 10^9/L (2–10%). ***Increased in:*** Post chemo- or radiothera chronic infections (eg malaria, TB, brucellosis, protozoa), malignant disea (including M4 and M5 acute myeloid leukaemia—(p340), and Hodgkin's diseas myelodysplasia.

Basophils 0–0.1 × 10^9/L (0–1%). ***Increased in:*** Myeloproliferative disease, vi infections, IgE mediated hypersensitivity reactions (eg urticaria, hypothyroidisr and inflammatory disorders (eg UC, rheumatoid arthritis).

1 Many previously diagnosed with this have been recently found to have monoclonal gene abnormalities consistent with chronic eosinophilic leukaemia, with improved molecular techniques.

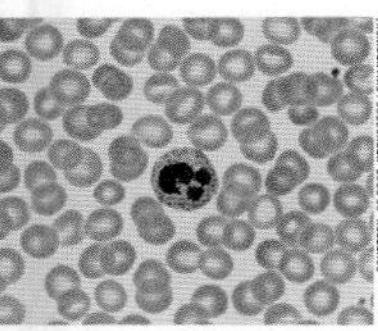

1. Neutrophil. These ingest and kill :teria, fungi and damaged cells.

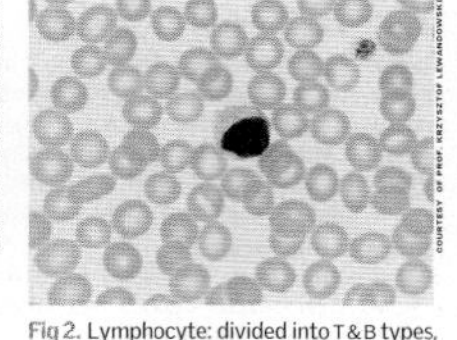

Fig 2. Lymphocyte: divided into T&B types, which have important roles in cell mediated immunity & antibody production.

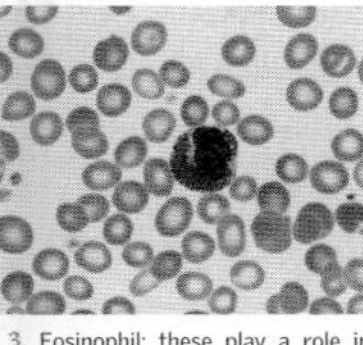

3. Eosinophil: these play a role in ergic reactions, and in defence against asitic infections.

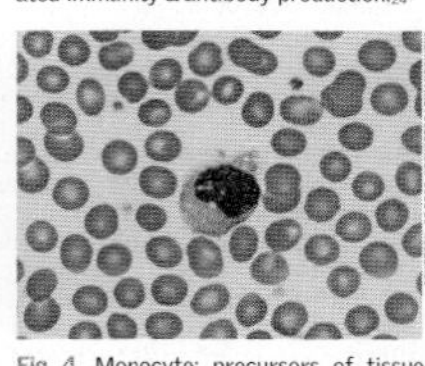

Fig 4. Monocyte: precursors of tissue macrophages.

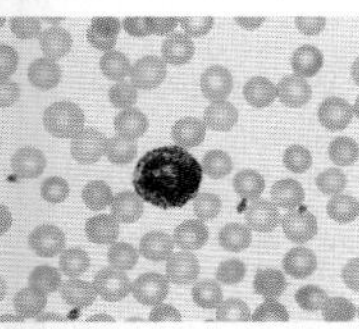

5. Basophil. The cytoplasm is filled :h dark staining granules, containing tamine, myeloperoxidase and other ymes. On binding IgE, histamine is eased from the basophil.

Macrocytic anaemia

Macrocytosis (MCV >96fL) is common, often due to alcohol excess without a accompanying anaemia. Although only ~5% are due to B_{12} deficiency, pernici anaemia is the most common cause of a macrocytic anaemia in Western countr B_{12} and folate deficiency are megaloblastic anaemias. A megaloblast is a cel which nuclear maturation is delayed compared to the cytoplasm. This occurs w B_{12} and folate deficiency, as they are both required for DNA synthesis.

Causes of macrocytosis

- ***Megaloblastic:*** B_{12} deficiency, folate deficiency, cytotoxic drugs.
- ***Non-megaloblastic:*** Alcohol, reticulocytosis (eg in haemolysis), liver disea hypothyroidism, pregnancy.
- ***Other haematological disease:*** Myelodysplasia, myeloma, myeloproliferat disorders, aplastic anaemia.

Tests: B_{12} and folate deficiency result in similar blood film and bone marrow bio appearances.
Blood film: Hypersegmented polymorphs in B_{12} and folate deficiency, (target c if liver disease).
Other tests: LFT (include γGT), TFT, serum B_{12} and serum folate (or red cell folate more reliable indicator of folate status, as serum folate only reflects *recent* intal
Bone marrow biopsy is indicated if the cause is not revealed by the above tests is likely to show one of the following four states:

1. Megaloblastic.
2. Normoblastic marrow (eg in liver disease, hypothyroidism).
3. Abnormal erythropoiesis (eg sideroblastic anaemia, leukaemia, aplasia).
4. Increased erythropoiesis (eg haemolysis).

Folate is found in green vegetables, nuts, yeast & liver; it is synthesized by gut ba eria. Body stores can last for 3–4 months. Maternal folate deficiency may ca neural tube defects in the fetus. It is absorbed by duodenum and proximal jejun

Causes of deficiency

- Poor diet: eg poverty, alcoholics, elderly.
- Increased demand: eg pregnancy or ↑cell turnover (seen in haemolysis, mal nancy, inflammatory disease and renal dialysis).
- Malabsorption: eg coeliac disease, tropical sprue.
- Drugs: eg alcohol, antiepileptics (phenytoin, sodium valproate), methotrexa trimethoprim.

Treatment: Assess for an underlying cause eg poor diet, malabsorption. Treat w folic acid 5mg/day PO for 4 months, ►never without B_{12} unless the patient known to have a normal B_{12} level, as in low B_{12} states, it may precipitate, or wors subacute combined degeneration of the spinal cord (p320). In pregnancy prop lactic doses of folate (400μg/day) are given from conception until at least 12 w this helps prevent spina bifida, as well as anaemia.

NB: In ill patients with megaloblastic anaemia (eg with CCF), it may be necessary treat before the results of serum B_{12} and folate are at hand. Do tests then tr with large doses, eg hydroxocobalamin 1mg/24h IM, with folic acid 5mg/24h Blood transfusions are very rarely needed, but see p310.

Folate and ischaemic heart disease Previous observational studies have indica that higher homocysteine concentrations are associated with a greater risk coronary heart disease. It has been suggested that folic acid supplementation m have a role in prevention of cardiac disease by lowering homocysteine lev However, trial results have so far been disappointing (further studies awaited One meta-analysis also showed no causal relationship between high homocyste concentrations and coronary heart disease risk in Western populations.[MET 29]

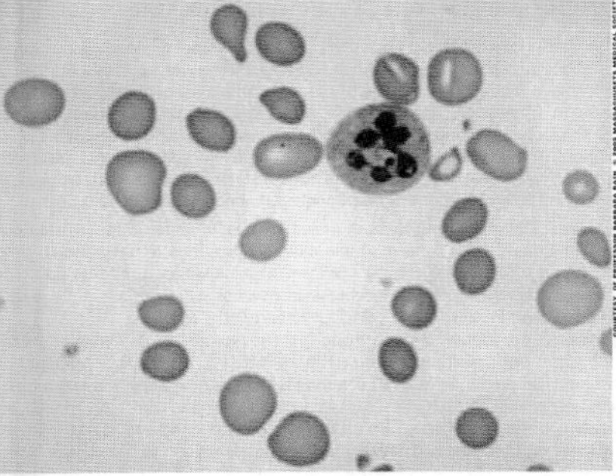

1. Megaloblastic anaemia: peripheral blood film showing many macrocytes and one ersegmented neutrophil (normally there should be ≤5 segments).

B_{12} deficiency and pernicious anaemia

Vitamin B_{12} is found in meat and dairy products, but not in plants. Body stores sufficient for 4yrs. It is protein bound and released during digestion. B_{12} then bi to intrinsic factor in the stomach, and this complex is absorbed in the term ileum. In B_{12} deficiency, synthesis of thymidine, and hence DNA, is impaired, so cell production is reduced. ***Causes of deficiency:*** • Dietary (eg vegans) • Mal orption: *Stomach* (lack of intrinsic factor): pernicious anaemia, post gastrecto *Terminal ileum:* ileal resection, Crohn's disease, bacterial overgrowth, tropical sp tapeworms (*Dyphyllobothrium*) • Congenital abnormalities in metabolism.

Features: ***General:*** Symptoms of anaemia (p310), 'lemon tinge' to skin due combination of pallor (anaemia) and mild jaundice (due to haemolysis), gloss (beefy-red sore tongue), angular cheilosis (also known as stomatitis, p312).
Neuropsychiatric: Irritability, depression, psychosis, dementia.
Neurological: Paraesthesiae, peripheral neuropathy. Also:
Subacute combined degeneration of the spinal cord: Onset is insidi (*subacute*) with peripheral neuropathy due to ↓B_{12}. There is a *combination* symmetrical posterior (dorsal) column loss, causing sensory and LMN signs, symmetrical corticospinal tract loss, causing motor and UMN signs (p438). Jo position and vibration sense are often affected first leading to ataxia, followed stiffness and weakness if untreated. The classical triad is: • Extensor plant (UMN) • Absent knee jerks (LMN) • Absent ankle jerks (LMN). It may present w falls at night-time, due to a combination of ataxia and reduced vision, which is seen with ↓B_{12}. Pain and temperature sensation may remain intact even in sev cases, as the spinothalamic tracts are preserved.
►Neurological signs with B_{12} deficiency can occur without anaemia.

Haematology

Pernicious anaemia (PA) This is caused by an autoimmune atrophic gastr leading to achlorhydria and lack of gastric intrinsic factor secretion.

Incidence 1 : 1000; ♀:♂≈1.6:1; usually >40yrs; higher incidence if blood grou

Associations Other autoimmune diseases (p539): thyroid disease (~25%), vitil Addison's disease, hypoparathyroidism. Carcinoma of stomach is ~3-fold m common in pernicious anaemia, so have a low threshold for upper GI endosco

Tests • Hb↓ (3–11g/dL) • MCV↑ • WCC & platelets ↓ in severe cases • Serum B_{12} • Reticulocytes ↓ or normal as production impaired • Hypersegmented polymor (p318) • Megaloblasts in the marrow • Specific tests for PA: 1 Parietal antibodies: found in 90% with PA, but also in 3–10% without. 2 Intrinsic factor antibodies: specific for pernicious anaemia, but lower sensitivity. These target binding sites (in 50%) or ileal binding sites (in 35%). 3 Schilling test (BOX).

Treatment Treat the cause if possible. Most cases are due to malabsorption injections are required. Replenish stores with hydroxocobalamin (B_{12}) 1mg alternate days eg for 2wks (or, if CNS signs, until improvement stops). Maintenar 1mg IM every 3 months for life (child's dose: as for adult). If the cause is diet then oral B_{12} can be given after the initial acute course. Initial improvemen heralded by a transient marked reticulocytosis and hence ↑MCV, after 4–5 day

Practical hints • Beware of diagnosing PA in those under 40 yrs old: look for malabsorption (small bowel biopsy, p272).
- Watch for hypokalaemia as treatment becomes established.
- Transfusion is best avoided, but PA with high output CCF may require exchar transfusion (p310), after doing tests for FBC, folate, B_{12}, and marrow sampli
- As haemopoiesis accelerates on treatment, additional iron may be needed.
- Hb rises ~1g/dL per week, WCC and platelet count should normalize in 1wk.

Prognosis Supplementation usually improves peripheral neuropathy within first 3–6 months, but has little effect on cord signs. Patients do best if treated soon as possible after the onset of symptoms: don't delay!

1 Plasma B_{12} levels are normal in many patients with subclinical B_{12} deficiency. Serum methylmal acid and homocystine levels are raised—and offer a more sensitive marker.

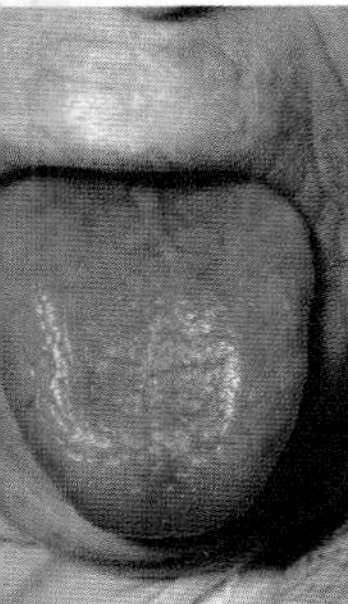

1. Glossitis in B_{12} deficiency.

chilling test

f there is B_{12} deficiency, and the parietal cell and intrinsic factor antibodies do ot give the answer, consider a Schilling test to help to identify the cause. This etermines whether a low B_{12} is due to malabsorption from the terminal ileum r due to a lack of intrinsic factor—by comparing the proportion of an oral dose Lμg) of radioactive B_{12} absorbed and hence excreted in urine, with and without e concurrent administration of intrinsic factor (the blood must be saturated by iving an IM dose of 1000μg of B_{12} first). If intrinsic factor enhances absorption ading to increased urine B_{12}, then lack of intrinsic factor, ie pernicious anaemia, likely to be the cause. Note that the Schilling test is rather cumbersome, and ome labs have stopped offering this test, hoping to rely on serology testing for arietal cell and intrinsic factor antibodies, and the plasma response to oral or M B_{12}.

An approach to haemolytic anaemia[1]

Haemolysis is the premature breakdown of RBCs, before their normal life span ~120d. It occurs in the circulation (*intravascular*) or in the reticuloendothe system ie macrophages of liver, spleen and bone marrow (*extravascular*). In sick cell anaemia, lifespan may be as short as 5d. Haemolysis may be asymptomatic, I if the bone marrow does not compensate sufficiently, a haemolytic anaemia resul

An approach is to first confirm haemolysis and then find the cause—try to answ these 4 questions:

1 ***Is there increased red cell breakdown?***
- Anaemia with normal or ↑MCV.
- ↑Bilirubin: unconjugated, from haem breakdown (prehepatic jaundice).
- ↑Urinary urobilinogen (no urinary conjugated bilirubin).
- ↑Serum lactic dehydrogenase (LDH), as released from the RBC.

2 ***Is there increased red cell production?***
- ↑Reticulocytes, causing ↑MCV (reticulocytes are large immature RBCs) a polychromasia.

3 ***Is the haemolysis mainly extra- or intravascular?***

Extravascular haemolysis may lead to splenic hypertrophy and splenomega Features of intravascular haemolysis are:
- ↑Free plasma haemoglobin: released from RBCs.
- Methaemalbuminaemia: some free Hb is broken down in the circulation to p duce haem and globin; haem combines with albumin to make methaemalbum
- ↓Plasma haptoglobin: mops up free plasma Hb, then removed by the liver.
- Haemoglobinuria: causes red-brown urine, in absence of red blood cells.
- Haemosiderinuria: occurs when haptoglobin binding capacity is exceed causing free Hb to be filtered by the renal glomeruli, absorption of free Hb the renal tubules and storage in the tubular cells as haemosiderin. This detected in the urine in sloughed tubular cells by Prussian blue staining week after onset (implying a *chronic* intravascular haemolysis)

4 ***Why is there haemolysis?*** Causes are on p324.

History Family history, race, jaundice, dark urine, drugs, previous anaemia, trav

Examination Jaundice, hepatosplenomegaly, gallstones (pigmented, due ↑bilirubin from haemolysis), leg ulcers (due to poor blood flow).

Investigation FBC, reticulocytes, bilirubin, LDH, haptoglobin, urinary urobilinog Thick and thin films for malaria screen if history of travel. The blood film may sh polychromasia and macrocytosis due to reticulocytes, or point to the diagnosi
- Hypochromic microcytic anaemia (thalassaemia).
- Sickle cells (sickle cell anaemia).
- Schistocytes (microangiopathic haemolytic anaemia).
- Abnormal cells in haematological malignancy.
- Spherocytes (hereditary spherocytosis or autoimmune haemolytic anaemia)
- Elliptocytes (hereditary elliptocytosis).
- Heinz bodies, "bite" cells[2], (glucose-6-phosphate dehydrogenase deficiency).

Further tests:
- *Direct antiglobulin (Coombs') test* (DAT) identifies red cells coated with antibo or complement. A positive result indicates an immune cause of the haemoly
- RBC lifespan may be determined by *chromium labelling* and the major site of R breakdown may also be identified. This test is rarely done now.

The cause may now be obvious, but further tests may be needed. Membra abnormalities are identified on the film and can be confirmed by *osmotic fragil* testing. *Hb electrophoresis* will detect haemoglobinopathies. *Enzyme assays* a reserved for situations when other causes have been excluded.

1 See *Oxford Handbook of Clinical and Laboratory Investigation*, OUP, p184.

2 On passing through the spleen, Heinz bodies may be removed, leaving an RBC with 'a bite taken ou it'. See p325 fig 2.

Causes of haemolytic anaemia

Acquired—these are divided into immune and non-immune causes.

- **Immune mediated** (=direct antiglobulin test +ve).
  - ***Drug-induced*** Causing formation of RBC autoantibodies from binding to the membrane (eg penicillin) or production of immune complexes (eg quinine).
  - ***Autoimmune haemolytic anaemia (AHA)*** Mediated by autoantibodies caus mainly extravascular haemolysis and spherocytosis. They are divided by th optimal binding temperature to RBCs. ***Warm AHA:*** IgG-mediated, bind at bo 37°C. ***Treatment:*** Steroids/immunosuppressants (± splenectomy). ***Cold A*** IgM-mediated, bind at lower temperature (<4°C), activating cell surf complement. Causes a chronic anaemia made worse by cold, often w Raynaud's or acrocyanosis. ***Treatment:*** Keep warm. Chlorambucil may h ***Causes:*** Most are idiopathic; secondary causes of warm AHA include lymp proliferative disease (eg CLL, lymphoma), drugs, autoimmune disease eg SLE. C AHA may follow infections eg *Mycoplasma pneumoniae*, EBV.
  - ***Paroxysmal cold haemoglobinuria*** is seen with viruses/syphilis. It is causec the Donath–Landsteiner antibodies, which stick to RBCs in cold, and ca complement-mediated haemolysis on rewarming. Haemolysis is self-limitin
- **Isoimmune** Acute transfusion reaction (p571); haemolytic disease of newbo
- **Microangiopathic haemolytic anaemia (MAHA)** A mechanical disruption of R in circulation, causing intravascular haemolysis and schistocytes. Causes inclu haemolytic–uraemic syndrome (HUS), TTP (p300), DIC, pre-eclampsia, eclamp Treat the underlying disease; transfusion or plasma exchange may be need Also caused by intravascular devices eg prosthetic heart valves.
- **Infection** eg malaria (p382): RBC lysis and 'blackwater fever' (haemoglobinur
- **Paroxysmal nocturnal haemoglobinuria** RBCs (also platelets, neutrophils) sensitive to complement-mediated lysis due to an inherited loss of surf glucosylphosphatidylinositol (GPI). There is chronic intravascular haemoly (especially at night→haemoglobinuria), pancytopenia, and ↑thrombosis (eg Buc Chiari syndrome, p688). ***Diagnosis:*** Urinary haemosiderin +ve. Cellular immu phenotype shows altered GPI. Ham's test +ve (*in vitro* acid-induced lysis, rarely done now). ***℞:*** Anticoagulation. Stem cell transplant may be curative.

Hereditary Is there a defect in RBC enzymes, membrane, or Hb? ***Enzyme defec***

- ***Glucose-6-phosphate dehydrogenase (G6PD) deficiency*** is the commonest enzyme defect. Inheritance is X-linked, affecting 100 million mainly ♂ in Afr Mediterranean and Middle/Far East. Most are asymptomatic, but are suscepti to oxidative crises due to ↓glutathione production, precipitated by many dru (eg primaquine, sulfonamides, aspirin), exposure to the broad bean *Vicia fa* (favism) or illness. During an attack, there is rapid anaemia and jaundice, w bite cells and blister cells on the film. ***Diagnosis:*** Enzyme assay. Don't do until 3 months after a crisis: young RBCs may have sufficient enzyme so results m appear normal. ***℞:*** Avoid precipitants; transfuse if severe.
- ***Pyruvate kinase deficiency*** Autosomal recessive, ↓ATP production caus shortened red cell survival. Homozygotes have neonatal jaundice; later, chro haemolysis with splenomegaly and jaundice. ***Diagnosis:*** Enzyme assay. ***℞:*** Of the condition is well tolerated. No specific therapy—splenectomy may help.

Membrane defect—Hereditary spherocytosis Autosomal dominant RBC membra defect. Less deformable spherical RBCs, so trapped in spleen → extravascu haemolysis. ***Signs:*** Splenomegaly, jaundice. ***Δ:*** Mild anaemia. Film (p314): ma spherocytes. Osmotic fragility tests: RBCs show ↑fragility in hypotonic solution

- ***Hereditary elliptocytosis*** Autosomal dominant, most are asymptoma ***Treatment:*** Folate, splenectomy is curative but reserved for severe cases.
- ***Haemoglobinopathy: Sickle-cell disease*** p326. • ***Thalassaemia*** p328.

Factors exacerbating haemolysis Infection leads to ↑haemolysis. The anaer may be exacerbated by parvoviruses (*OHCS* p142), producing a cessation of marr erythropoiesis, ie aplastic anaemia, with no reticulocyte formation (p348).

Haematology

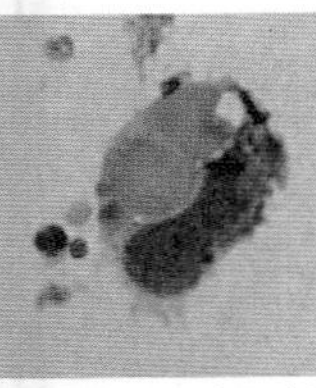

g 1. Autoimmune haemolytic ıaemia: antibody coated red cells ıdergoing phagocytosis by onocytes.

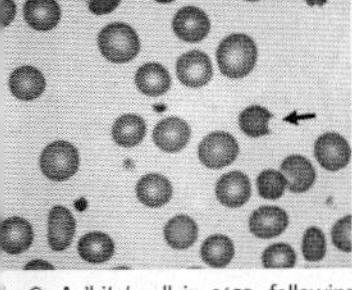

g 2. A 'bite' cell in G6PD, following emoval of Heinz bodies by the spleen. einz bodies are formed from oxidized, enatured Hb during oxidative crises.

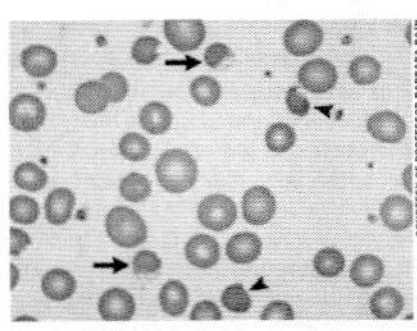

Fig 3. 'Blister' cells (arrows) in G6PD, following removal of Heinz bodies. Also contracted red cells (arrowheads).

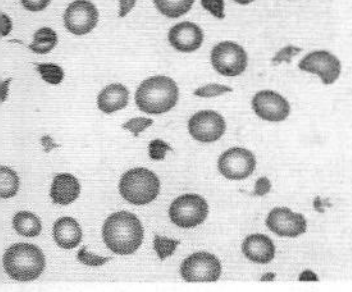

ig 4. Microangiopathic anaemia eg om DIC: numerous cell fragments schistocytes) are present.

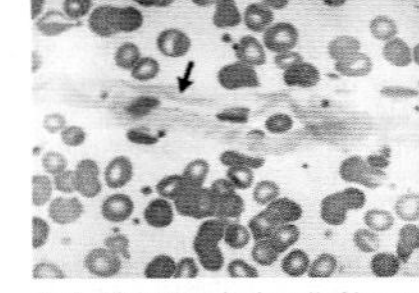

Fig 5. Fibrin strands, deposited in HUS & TTP (p300), slice up passing red cells (microangiopathic anaemia).

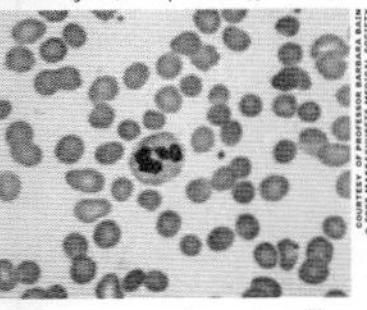

ig 6. Hereditary spherocytosis.

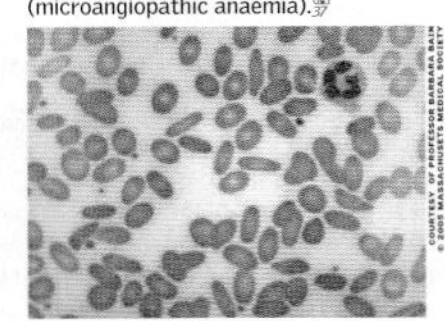

Fig 7. Hereditary elliptocytosis.

Sickle-cell anaemia

Sickle-cell anaemia is an autosomal recessive disorder causing production of abnormal β globin chains. An amino acid substitution in the gene coding for the chain (Glu → Val at position 6), results in the production of HbS rather than HbA. HbA_2 and HbF are still produced. It is common in people of African origin. The homozygote (SS) has sickle-cell *anaemia* (HbSS), and heterozygotes (HbAS) have sickle-cell *trait*, which causes no disability (and protects from *falciparum* malaria) except in hypoxia, eg in unpressurized aircraft or anaesthesia, when vaso-occlusive events may occur, so all those of African descent need a sickle cell test pre-op. Symptomatic sickling also occurs in heterozygotes with genes coding other Hb variants (eg HbC leading to HbSC, or β-thalassaemia trait leading to HbS/βthal).

Pathogenesis HbS polymerizes when deoxygenated, causing RBCs to deform. This produces sickle cells, which are fragile and haemolyse, and also block small vessels.

Tests Haemolysis is variable. Hb ≈ 6–9g/dL, ↑reticulocytes 10–20%, ↑bilirubin. *Film:* sickle cells and target cells. *Sickle solubility test:* +ve, but does not distinguish between HbSS and HbAS. *Hb electrophoresis:* Confirms the diagnosis and distinguishes SS, AS states, and other Hb variants. Aim for diagnosis *at birth* (cord blood) to aid prompt pneumococcal prophylaxis (vaccine, p152, or penicillin V).

Signs and symptoms are highly variable. There is a chronic haemolytic anaemia usually well tolerated unless there is a supervening crisis (below and see BOX). ***Vaso-occlusive 'painful' crises:*** Common, due to micro-vascular occlusion. Often affects the bone marrow, causing severe pain. Precipitated by cold, dehydration, infection or hypoxia. Hands and feet are affected in children <3yrs leading to dactylitis. Occlusion may also cause mesenteric ischaemia, mimicking an acute abdomen. Cerebral infarction occurs in ~10% of children, leading to stroke, seizures or cognitive defects. Transcranial Doppler ultrasonography indicates risk of impending stroke, and blood transfusions can be used to prevent this, by reducing HbS. Priapism may occur; if >12h, arrange prompt cavernosus-spongiosum shunting—prevents future erectile dysfunction (also occurs in CML, p342). ***Aplastic crises:*** This is due to Parvovirus B19, with sudden reduction in marrow production, especially RBCs. Usually self-limiting <2wks, transfusion may be needed. ***Sequestration crises:*** Mainly affects children as the spleen has not yet undergone atrophy. There is pooling of blood in the spleen ± liver, with organomegaly, severe anaemia and shock. Urgent transfusion is needed.

Complications • Splenic infarction occurs before 2yrs old, due to repeated microvascular occlusion, leading to ↑susceptibility to infection (p357) • Growth impairment • Bone necrosis due to ↓blood supply, especially the femoral head • Chronic renal failure • Chronic leg ulcers • Gallstones • Retinal disease and visual impairment • Multiple blood transfusions may lead to iron overload or blood-borne infection • Long-term lung damage—hypoxia, fibrosis and pulmonary hypertension, partly preventable by incentive spirometry—10 maximal inspirations/2h.

Management of chronic disease

- Consider hydroxycarbamide (hydroxyurea) if frequent crises.[1]
- Splenic infarction leads to hyposplenism. Prophylaxis, in terms of antibiotics and immunization should be given (p357).
- Febrile children risk septicaemia: repeated admission may be avoided by out-patient ceftriaxone (eg 2 doses, 50mg/kg IV on day 0 and 1). Admission may still be needed, eg if Hb <5g/dL, WCC <5 or >30 × 10^9/L, T° >40°C, severe pain, dehydration, lung infiltration. Seek expert advice.
- Bone marrow transplant can be curative, but remains controversial.

Prevention Genetic counselling; prenatal tests (*OHCS* p152–3). Parental education can help prevent 90% of deaths from sequestration crises.

1 Long-term hydroxycarbamide causes ↑production of fetal haemoglobin (HbF) and decreased HbS polymerization, causing reduction in painful crises, acute chest syndrome, admissions, blood transfusions and mortality. This may result from fewer episodes of bone marrow ischaemia and embolization.

Management of sickle-cell crisis[1]

▶Seek expert help early.

- Give *prompt*, generous analgesia, eg IV opiates (see p560).
- Crossmatch blood. FBC, reticulocytes, blood cultures, MSU ± CXR if fever or chest symptoms.
- Rehydrate with IVI and keep warm.
- Give O_2 by mask if $P_aO_2\downarrow$ or O_2 sats <95%.
- 'Blind' antibiotics (eg cephalosporin, p372) if fever T° >38°, unwell, or chest symptoms, after sending infection screen.
- Measure PCV, reticulocytes, liver, and spleen size twice daily.
- Give blood transfusion if Hb or reticulocytes fall sharply. Match blood for the blood group antigens Rh(C, D, E) and Kell, to prevent formation of antibodies. Red cell transfusion improves oxygenation, and is as good as exchange transfusion, which is reserved for those who are rapidly deteriorating.[43] ***Exchange transfusion*** is a process where blood is removed and donor blood is given in stages. Indications: severe chest crisis, suspected CNS event or multiorgan failure—when the proportion of HbS should be reduced to <30%.

The acute chest syndrome: Entails pulmonary infiltrates involving complete lung segments, causing pain, fever, tachypnoea, wheeze, and cough. It is a serious condition. Incidence: ~0.1 episodes/patient/yr. 13% in the landmark Vichinsky study needed ventilation, 11% had CNS symptoms, and 9% of those over 20 years old died. Prodromal painful crisis occur ~2.5 days before any abnormalities on CXR in 50% of patients. The chief causes of the infiltrates are fat embolism from bone marrow or infection with *Chlamydia*, *Mycoplasma*, or viruses.[44] **℞:** Oxygen, analgesia, empirical antibiotics (cephalosporin + macrolide) until culture results known. Bronchodilators (eg salbutamol, p167) have proved to be very effective in those with wheezing or obstructive pulmonary function at presentation. Blood transfusion (exchange if severe). *Take to ITU* if P_aO_2 cannot be kept above 9.2kPa (70mmHg) when breathing air.

Patient-controlled analgesia (PCA): An example with paediatric doses. First try warmth, hydration, and oral analgesia: ibuprofen 5mg/kg/6h PO (codeine phosphate 1mg/kg/4–8h PO up to 3mg/kg/d may also be tried, but is relatively ineffective). If this fails, see on the ward and offer prompt morphine by IVI—eg 0.1mg/kg. Start PCA with morphine 1mg/kg in 50mL 5% dextrose, and try a rate of 1mL/h, allowing the patient to deliver extra boluses of 1mL when needed. Do respiration and sedation score every ¼h + pulse oximetry if chest/abdominal pain.[45] For further advice, liaise with the local pain service.

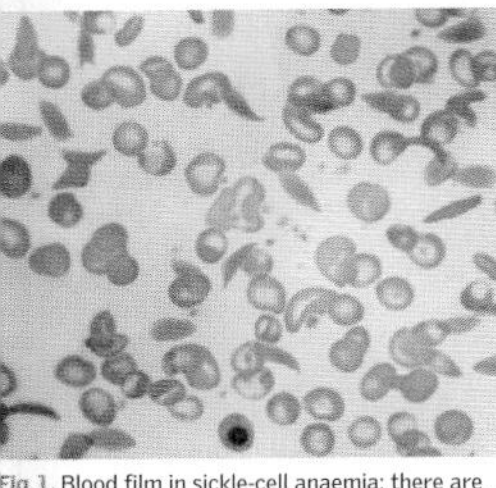

Fig 1. Blood film in sickle-cell anaemia: there are sickle cells, target cells, and a nucleated red cell.[46]

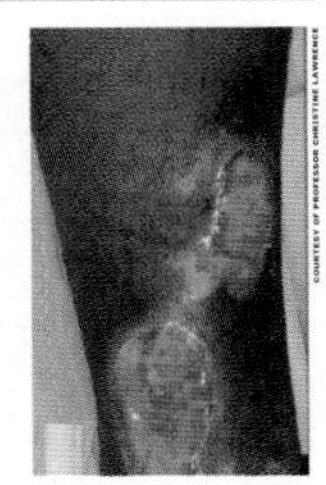

Fig 2. Leg ulcers in sickle cell disease.[47]

1 Brit. Committee for Standards in Haem. Management of the acute painful crisis in sickle cell disease.

Thalassaemia

The thalassaemias are genetic diseases of unbalanced Hb synthesis, as there underproduction (or no production) of one globin chain (BOX). Unmatched globi precipitate, damaging RBC membranes, causing their haemolysis while still in tl marrow. They are common in areas from the Mediterranean to the Far East.

The β thalassaemias are usually caused by point mutations in β-globin genes c chromosome 11, leading to ↓β chain production (β^+) or its absence (β^0). Variou combinations of mutations are possible (eg β^0/β^0, β^+/β^+, or β^+/β^0).

Tests FBC, MCV, film, iron, HbA_2, HbF, Hb electrophoresis.

β thalassaemia minor or trait (eg β/β⁺; heterozygous state): This is a carri state, and is usually asymptomatic. Mild, well-tolerated anaemia (Hb >9g/dL) whic may worsen in pregnancy. MCV <75fL, HbA_2 >3.5%, slight ↑HbF. Often confuse with iron deficiency anaemia.

β thalassaemia intermedia describes an intermediate state with moderat anaemia but not requiring transfusions. There may be splenomegaly. There are variety of causes including mild homozygous β thalassaemia mutations eg β^+/β^+, c co-inheritance of β thalassaemia trait with another haemoglobinopathy eg Hb thalassaemia (1 parent has the HbC trait, and the other has β^+). Sickle-cell β thalassaemia produces a picture similar to sickle-cell anaemia.

β thalassaemia major (Cooley's anaemia) describes abnormalities in bot β-globin genes, and presents within the 1st year, with severe anaemia and failure t thrive. Extramedullary haematopoiesis (production of RBCs outside the bor marrow) occurs in response to the anaemia, causing characteristic faci deformities eg skull bossing (fig 1) and hepatosplenomegaly (also due to hae molysis). Skull x-ray shows a 'hair on end' appearance due to increased marro activity. Life-long blood transfusions are needed, with resulting iron overload an deposition occurring after ~10yrs as endocrine failure (pituitary, thyroi pancreas→diabetes mellitus), liver disease, and cardiac toxicity. Long-term infusio of desferrioxamine helps to prevent iron loading. The film shows very hypochromi microcytic cells with target cells and nucleated RBCs. HbF↑↑, HbA_2 variable, Hb absent.

Treatment [48] • Folate supplements.

- Regular (~2–4 weekly) life-long transfusions to keep Hb >9g/dL, to suppress th ineffective extramedullary haematopoiesis and to allow normal growth.
- Iron-chelators to prevent iron deposition, eg desferrioxamine infusions given s for 8–12 hours per day. SE: pain, hearing loss, cataracts, retinal damage, ↑risk c *Yersinia* infection. Compliance can be a problem. The role of newer oral iror chelators, eg deferiprone, are under study (neutropenia may be a problem).
- Large doses of ascorbic acid also increase urinary excretion of iron.
- Splenectomy if hypersplenism persists with increasing transfusion requirement (p357)—this is best avoided until >5 yrs old due to risk of infections.
- Hormonal replacement or treatment for endocrine complications eg diabete mellitus, hypothyroidism. Growth hormone treatment has had variable success.
- A histocompatible marrow transplant can offer the chance of a cure.[50]

Prevention Approaches include genetic counselling or antenatal diagnosis usin fetal blood or DNA, then 'therapeutic' abortion.

The α thalassaemias There are two separate α-globin genes on each chromosom 16 ∴ there are four genes (termed αα/αα). The α thalassaemias are mainly cause by gene deletions. If all 4 α genes are deleted (--/--), death is *in utero (Bart hydrops)*. Here, HbBarts (γ_4) is present, which is physiologically useless. HbH diseas occurs if 3 genes are deleted (--/-α), there may be moderate anaemia and feature of haemolysis: hepatosplenomegaly, leg ulcers and jaundice. In the blood film, ther is formation of β_4 tetramers (=HbH) due to excess β chains, HbBarts, HbA an HbA_2. If 2 genes are deleted (--/αα or -α/-α), there is an asymptomatic carrie state, with ↓MCV. With one gene deleted, the clinical state is normal.

ructure of haemoglobin

e three main types of Hb in adult blood are:

pe	Peptide chains	% in adult blood	% in fetal blood
)A	$\alpha_2 \beta_2$	97	10–50
)A2	$\alpha_2 \delta_2$	2.5	Trace
)F	$\alpha_2 \gamma_2$	0.5	50–90

ult haemoglobin (HbA) is a tetramer of 2 α- and 2 β-globin chains each ıtaining a haem group. In the first year of life, adult haemoglobin replaces :al haemoglobin (HbF).

night be thought that because the molecular details of the thalassaemias are well worked out they represent a perfect example of the reductionist nciple at work: find out *exactly* what is happening *within* molecules, and you l be able to explain all the manifestations of a disease. But this is not so. We ve to recognize that two people with the identical mutation at their β loci may ve quite different diseases. Co-inheritance of other genes and conditions (eg α alassaemia) is part of the explanation, as is the efficiency of production of :al haemoglobin. The reasons lie beyond simple co-segregation of genes omoting the formation of fetal Hb. The rate of proteolysis of excess α-globin ains may also be important—as may mechanisms that have little to do with netic or molecular events. So the lesson the thalassaemias teach is more otle than the reductionist one: it is that if you want to understand the *whole* :ture, you must look at *every* level: genetic, molecular, physiological, social, and ltural. Each level influences the other, without necessarily determining them.

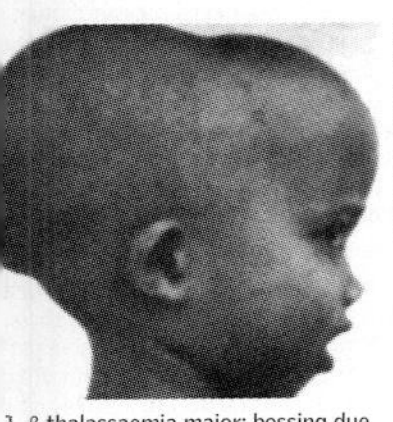

1. β thalassaemia major: bossing due xtra-medullary haematopoiesis.

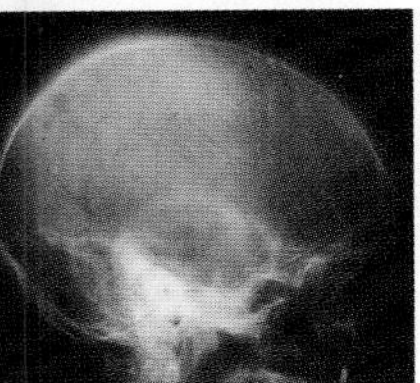

2. Thalassaemia major: skull X-ray.

her Reading: Drew Provan and John G Gribben 2004 *Molecular Hematology 2e*, Blackwell Publishing.

Bleeding disorders

After injury, 3 processes halt bleeding: vasoconstriction, gap-plugging by plate and the coagulation cascade. Disorders of haemostasis fall into these 3 groups pattern of bleeding is important—vascular and platelet disorders lead to prolo bleeding from cuts, bleeding into the skin (eg easy bruising and purpura), bleeding from mucous membranes (eg epistaxis, bleeding from gums, menorrha Coagulation disorders cause delayed bleeding into joints and muscle.

1 **Vascular defects** ***Congenital:*** Osler–Weber–Rendu syndrome (p700), conne tissue disease (eg Ehlers-Danlos syndrome OHCS p642, pseudoxanthoma elastic ***Acquired:*** Senile purpura, infection (eg meningococcal, measles, dengue fe steroids, scurvy (perifollicular haemorrhages), Henoch-Schönlein purpura (p6 painful bruising syndrome—women who develop tingling under the skin follo by bruising over limbs/trunk, resolving without treatment.

2 **Thrombocytopenia** ***↓marrow production:*** Aplastic anaemia (p348), meg blastic anaemia, marrow infiltration (eg leukaemia, myeloma), marrow suppres (cytotoxic drugs, radiotherapy). ***Excess destruction:*** *Immune:* Immune thron cytopenic purpura (ITP), other autoimmune causes eg SLE, CLL, drugs eg hep viruses; *Non-immune:* DIC p336, thrombotic thrombocytopenic purpura (TTP) or (p300), sequestration (in hypersplenism). **ITP** is caused by antiplatelet autoa bodies leading to phagocytic destruction. It is acute (usually in children, 2wks a infection with sudden self-limiting purpura: OHCS p197) or chronic (seen main adult women). Chronic ITP runs an indefinite fluctuating course of bleeding, pur (especially dependent pressure areas), epistaxis and menorrhagia. There is splenomegaly. ***Tests:*** ↑megakaryocytes in marrow, antiplatelet autoantibodies be present although not always. ***℞:*** Mild disease may not need treatmen symptomatic or platelets $<20 \times 10^9$/L, prednisolone 1mg/kg/d, and reduce a remission; aim to keep platelets $>30 \times 10^9$/L—takes a few days to work. If rela splenectomy cures ≤80%. If this fails: immunosuppression, eg azathioprine or cy phosphamide. Platelet transfusions are not used (except during splenectomy or threatening haemorrhage) as these are destroyed quickly by the autoantibodie immunoglobulin may temporarily raise the platelet count eg for surgery, pregna

Causes of ↓platelet function Myeloproliferative disease, NSAIDs, urea↑.

3 **Coagulation disorders** ***Congenital:*** Haemophilia, von Willebrand's dise (p704). ***Acquired:*** Anticoagulants, liver disease, DIC (p336), vitamin K deficier

- **Haemophilia A:** Factor VIII deficiency; inherited in an X-linked recessive pat in 1:10,000 male births—usually due to a 'flip tip' inversion in the Factor VIII g in the X chromosome. There is a high rate of new mutations (30% have no fa history). ***Presentation*** depends on severity and is often early in life or a surgery/trauma—with bleeds into joints leading to crippling arthropathy, into muscles causing haematomas, which may lead to nerve palsies compartment syndrome due to pressure. ***Diagnose*** by ↑APTT and ↓factor assay. ***Management:*** Seek expert advice. *Avoid NSAIDs and IM injections.* M bleeding: pressure and elevation of the part. Desmopressin (0.3µg/kg/12h over 20min) raises factor VIII levels, and may be sufficient. Major bleeds haemarthrosis) require factor VIII levels to be ↑ to 50% of normal and threatening bleeds (eg obstructing airway) need levels of 100%, eg v recombinant factor VIII. ***Genetic counselling:*** OHCS p154.
- **Haemophilia B (Christmas disease):** Factor IX deficiency (inherited, x-lin recessive); behaves clinically like haemophilia A.
- **Liver disease** produces a complicated bleeding disorder with ↓synthesis clotting factors, ↓absorption of vitamin K, and abnormalities of platelet funct
- **Malabsorption** leads to less uptake of vitamin K (needed for synthesis of fac II, VII, IX, and X). Treatment is IV vitamin K (10mg) or FFP for acute haemorrha

e intrinsic and extrinsic pathways of blood coagulation

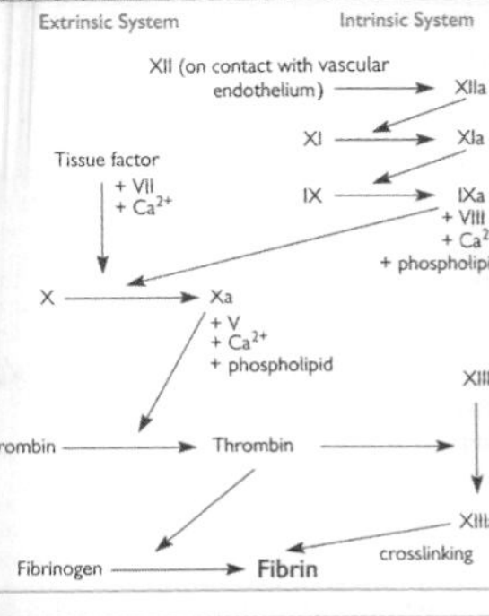

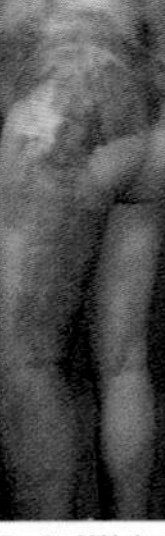

Fig 1. Mild haemophilia after an IM injection. Give vaccines etc SC.

brinolysis

ie fibrinolytic system causes fibrin dissolution and acts via the generation of asmin. The process starts with the release of tissue plasminogen activator -PA) from endothelial cells, a process stimulated by fibrin formation. t-PA nverts inactive plasminogen to plasmin which can then cleave fibrin, as well as veral other factors. t-PA and plasminogen both bind fibrin thus localizing brinolysis to the area of the clot.

echanism of fibrinolytic agents

iteplase (=rt-PA=Actilyse®; from recombinant DNA) is a fibrinolytic enzyme nitating t-PA, as above. Plasma $t_{½} \approx$ 5min.

treptokinase is a streptococcal exotoxin and forms a complex in plasma with asminogen to form an activator complex, which forms plasmin from unbound asminogen. Initially there is rapid plasmin formation which can cause uncon-olled fibrinolysis. However, plasminogen is rapidly consumed in the complex nd then plasmin is only produced as more plasminogen is synthesized. The ctivator complex binds to fibrin, so producing some localization of fibrinolysis.

An approach to bleeding

There are 3 sets of questions to be answered:

Is there an emergency?—needing immediate resuscitation or senior help?
- Is the patient about to exsanguinate (shock, coma, p774–9)?
- Is there hypovolaemia (postural hypotension, oliguria)?
- Is there CNS bleeding (meningism, CNS, and retinal signs)?

Why is the patient bleeding? Is bleeding normal, given the circumstances (surgery, trauma, parturition), or does the patient have a bleeding disorder?
- Is there a secondary cause eg drugs (warfarin), alcohol, liver disease, sepsi
- Is there unexplained bleeding, bruising, or purpura?
- Past or family history of excess bleeding eg during trauma, dentistry, surge
- Is the pattern of bleeding indicative of vascular, platelet, or coagulation proble (p330)? Are venepuncture or old cannula sites bleeding (DIC, p336)? Look associated conditions (eg with DIC).
- Is a clotting screen abnormal? Check FBC, platelets, PT, APTT and thrombin ti Consider D-dimers, bleeding time, and a factor VIII assay.

In the case of a bleeding disorder, what is the mechanism?

Coagulation tests (Sodium citrate tube; false results if under-filled)
- ***Prothrombin time (PT):*** Thromboplastin is added to test the *extrinsic system* is expressed as a ratio compared to control [International Normalized Ra (INR), normal range = 0.9–1.2]. It tests for abnormalities in factors I, II, V, VI Prolonged by: warfarin, vitamin K deficiency, liver disease, DIC.
- ***Activated partial thromboplastin time (APTT):*** Kaolin is added to test *intrinsic system*. Tests for abnormalities in Factor I, II, V, VIII, IX, X, XI, XII. Nor range 35–45s. Prolonged by: heparin treatment, haemophilia, DIC, liver disea
- ***Thrombin time:*** Thrombin is added to plasma to convert fibrinogen to fib Normal range: 10–15s. Prolonged by: heparin treatment, DIC, dysfibrinogenaer

D-dimers: These are a fibrin degradation product, released from cross-linked fib during fibrinolysis (p331). This occurs during DIC, or in the presence of ven thromboembolism—deep vein thrombosis (DVT) or pulmonary embolism (PE) dimers may also be raised in inflammatory states eg with infection or malignar

Bleeding time: This is a test of haemostasis, carried out by making two sm incisions into the skin of the forearm. Normal time <7 minutes. **NB:** This test seldom performed now, as results are very operator dependent.

Interpretation
- ***Platelets:*** If low, do FBC, film, clotting.
- ***PT:*** If long, look for liver disease or anticoagulant use.
- ***APTT:*** If long, consider liver disease, haemophilia (factor VIII or IX deficiency) heparin.
- ***Bleeding time:*** Raised in von Willebrand's disease (p704), or platelet disord Aspirin also prolongs the bleeding time.
- If both PT & APTT are very raised, with low platelets, and ↑D-dimers, consider D

Management depends on the degree of bleeding. If shocked, resuscitate (p778) bleeding continues, in the presence of a clotting disorder, or a massive transfusi discuss the need for FFP and platelets with a haematologist. In ITP (p330), stero ± IV immunoglobulin may be used. Especially in pregnancy (*OHCS* p88), consult expert. Is there overdose with anticoagulants (p826)? In haemophiliac blee *consult early* for coagulation factor replacement. *Never* give IM injections.

ɔrder[1]	INR	APTT	Thrombin time	Platelet count	Bleeding time	Notes
ɔarin	↑	↑↑	↑↑	↔	↔	
	↑↑	↑↑	↑↑	↓	↑	↑D-d, p336
ɜr disease	↑	↑	↔/↑	↔/↓	↔/↑	AST↑
telet defect	↔	↔	↔	↔	↑(↑)	
K deficiency	↑↑	↑	↔	↔	↔	
ɜmophilia	↔	↑↑	↔	↔	↔	see p330
ı Willebrand's	↔	↑↑	↔	↔	↑(↑)	see p704

Special tests may be available (factor assays: ►consult a haematologist).

ıfter *OTS*, p215. D-d = D-dimer.

Anticoagulants

Main indications

- ***Therapeutic:*** Venous thromboembolic disease: DVT and PE.
- ***Prophylactic:*** Prevention of DVT/PE in high-risk patients (p359), eg post-
Prevention of stroke, eg in chronic AF or prosthetic heart va

Heparin *1* ***Low molecular weight heparin (LMWH)*** Given SC. Molecular we ~5000 Daltons (Da), eg dalteparin, enoxaparin, tinzaparin. Inactivates facto (but not thrombin). T½ is 2–4-fold longer than standard heparin, and respons more predictable, and so only needs to be given once or twice daily, anc laboratory monitoring is usually required. It has replaced unfractionated hep (UFH) as the preferred option in the prevention and treatment of ver thromboembolism and in acute coronary syndrome. See *BNF* for doses. It accumul in renal failure: lower doses are used for prophylaxis, or UFH for therapeutic dose *2* ***Unfractionated heparin (UFH)*** IV or SC. ~13,000Da. A glycosaminoglycan, w binds antithrombin (an endogenous inhibitor of coagulation), increasing its ab to inhibit thrombin, factor Xa, and IXa. Rapid onset and has a short T½. Monitor adjust dose with APTT (p332).

SE for both: ↑Bleeding (eg at operative site, gastrointestinal, intracranial), hepa induced thrombocytopenia (HIT), osteoporosis with long-term use. HIT osteoporosis are less common with LMWH than UFH. Beware hyperkalaemia.

CI: Bleeding disorders, platelets <60×10⁹/l, previous HIT, peptic ulcer, cere haemorrhage, severe hypertension, neurosurgery.

Haematology

Warfarin is used orally once daily as long-term anticoagulation. The therape range is narrow, varying with the condition being treated (see BOX)—an measured as a ratio compared with the standard INR. Warfarin inhibits reductase enzyme responsible for regenerating the active form of vitami producing a state analogous to vit K deficiency. ***CI:*** Peptic ulcer, bleeding disord severe hypertension, pregnancy (teratogenic, see *OHCS* p640). Use with cautio the elderly and those with past GI bleeds. In the UK, warfarin tablets are 0.5 (white), 1mg (brown), 3mg (blue), or 5mg (pink). ►Interactions: p740.

Others: Fondaparinux is a pentasaccharide Xa inhibitor and may be used in p of LMWH for prophylaxis in certain situations. Ximelagatran, a direct thron inhibitor, may provide an alternative to warfarin that does not require monitor

Beginning therapeutic anticoagulation (follow local guidelines, and see *BNF* For treatment of venous thromboembolism, LMWH or UFH are used initially, warfarin is given in combination usually from day 1. Heparin should be contin until INR has reached target therapeutic range (see BOX) *and* until day 5, as warf has an initial prothrombotic effect.

LMWH Dose according to weight (see *BNF*).

UFH IV infusion: • Give heparin 5000iu IV bolus over 30min. (10000iu in severe
- Prepare syringe pump: Add 25,000iu to 50mL 0.9% saline (=500iu/mL).
- Start infusion at 1000–2000iu/h IVI (2.8mL/h=1400iu/h). Check APTT at 6h for APTT ratio 1.5–2.5 (see BOX). Measure APTT daily or 10h after dose chan

Warfarin is given daily; start with 10mg stat at 18.00. Do INR 16h later.
- If INR <1.8 (as is likely) the 2nd dose of warfarin is 5 or 10mg at 18.00 (24h a first dose). Give the lower dose if >60yrs, liver disease, or cardiac failure. B INR >1.8 (warfarin sensitivity; rare) give just 0.5mg.
- Do INR daily for 5d and adjust dose (see BOX—use 5mg, not 10mg dose 3 if c 60, or liver disease, or cardiac failure).
- Stop heparin after 5d and when INR >2 for 2d. Tell lab when stopped.
- Measure INR on alternate days until stable, then weekly or less often.

Antidotes If UFH overdose: stop infusion. If there is bleeding, protamine sulph counteracts UFH: discuss with a haematologist. Warfarin: see Box 2.

ırfarin guidelines and target levels for INR[1]

'ulmonary embolism and DVT. Aim for INR of 2–3; 3.5 if recurrent.
ıtrial fibrillation[2]: for stroke prevention (p116). Target INR 2–3. An alternative s aspirin (but less effective), if the risk of bleeding with warfarin is high (eg alls with risk of intracranial bleed, or difficulty with monitoring).
'rosthetic metallic heart valves: for stroke prevention. Target INR 3–4.

ration of anticoagulation in DVT/PE

f the cause will go away (eg post-op immobility):
 At least 6 weeks for below knee DVT.
 At least 3 months for above knee DVT or PE.
\t least 6 months if no cause found.
ndefinitely for identified, enduring causes, eg thrombophilia (p358).

ırfarin dosage and excessive anticoagulation

ow is a guide to warfarin dosing, for target INR of 2–3:

ː	<2	2	2.5	2.9	3.3	3.6	4.1
dose	10mg	5mg	4mg	3mg	2mg	0.5mg	0mg
ıintenance	≥6mg	5.5mg	4.5mg	4mg	3.5mg	3mg	*

*Miss a dose; give 1–2mg the next day (if INR >4.5, miss 2 doses). Lower doses are given in certain groups of patients (see TEXT).

cases of raised INR (see *BNF*):

R 4.5–6	Reduce warfarin dose or omit. Restart when INR <5.
-8	Stop warfarin. Restart when INR <5.
3, no bleed or inor bleed	If no bleeding: stop warfarin. 0.5–2.5mg vitamin K (oral) if risk factors for bleeding. Check INR daily.
ajor bleed, ıcluding tracranial ıemorrhage)	Stop warfarin. Give prothrombin complex concentrate (50units/kg; discuss with a haematologist). If unavailable, give FFP (15mL/kg ≈ 1L for a 70kg man). Also give 5–10mg vitamin K IV.

Minor bleeding includes epistaxis.

:amin K may take several hours to work, and can cause prolonged resistance ıen restarting warfarin, so should be avoided if possible when long-term ticoagulation is needed. Prothrombin complex concentrate contains a ncentrate of Factor IX, and provides a more complete and rapid reversal of ırfarin than FFP.

ıeparin dosing

TT ratio	>5	4–5	3–4	2.5–3	**1.5-2.5**	1.2–1.4	<1.2
ange rate (iu/h) by	Stop* -500	-300	-100	-50	**0**	+200	+400

* Stop for 1 hour then recheck APTT. Reduce dose by 500iu/h and restart if <5.

rit. Committee for Standards in Haematology. Guidelines on oral anticoagulation (warfarin): 3e 5.
or QALY-based decision analysis on who needs warfarin in AF, see R Thomson Lancet 355 956.

Leukaemia and the house officer

Leukaemic patients often fall ill suddenly and deteriorate quickly. Pro appropriate treatment is essential. Major concerns are infection, bleeding hyperviscosity (p356). Take non-specific confusion/drowsiness seriously: do b cultures, exclude hypoglycaemia, measure renal function, LFT, and Ca^{2+}. Cl clotting screen. Consider CNS bleeding—CT/MRI of brain if any doubt. Correct haemostatic defect urgently with platelets/FFP. (See p476 for delirium.)

Neutropenic regimen (for patients with a neutrophil count ≤1.0 × 10^9/L).
►Close liaison with a microbiologist and haematologist is essential.

- Full barrier nursing if possible, but simple hand-washing is probably n important. Use a side room.
- Avoid IM injections (danger of an infected haematoma).
- Look for infection (mouth, axilla, perineum, IVI site). Take swabs.
- Check: FBC, platelets, INR, U&E, LFT. Take cultures (blood×3—peripheral Hickman line; urine, sputum, stool if diarrhoea) and request a CXR.
- Wash perineum after defecation. Swab moist skin with chlorhexidine. A unnecessary rectal examinations. Oral hygiene (eg hydrogen peroxide mo washes/2h) and *Candida* prophylaxis are important (p230).
- TPR 4-hrly. High-calorie diet; avoid foods with high risk of micro contamination. Vases containing cut flowers pose a *Pseudomonas* risk.

Use of antibiotics in neutropenia ►Treat any known infection promptly.

- If T° >38°C or T° >37.5°C on separate occasions, 1–2h apart, or the patie toxic, assume septicaemia and start blind broad spectrum antibiotics, eg a pseudomonal penicillin/cephalosporin and aminoglycoside. Vancomycin (p3 may be added if suspected Hickman line sepsis. Check local preferences.
- Continue antibiotics until afebrile for 72 hours or 5d course, and until neu phils recover (>0.5×10^9/L). If fever persists despite antibiotics, consider CM fungal infection (eg *Candida* or *Aspergillus*, p428).
- May need to consider treatment for *Pneumocystis* (see p399 eg co-trimoxa =trimethoprim 20mg/kg with sulfamethoxazole 100mg/kg per day PO/IV in divided doses). Also remember TB.
- Genetically engineered recombinant human granulocyte-colony stimula factor (G-CSF) may be used to stimulate neutrophil production. Follow lo guidelines, and seek expert advice.

Other dangers • ***Tumour lysis syndrome:*** Caused by a massive destruction of leading to K^+↑, urate↑ and renal impairment. Prevent by giving a high fluid intal allopurinol pre-cytotoxics. For patients at high risk of cell lysis, eg children v high count ALL, recombinant uricase (rasburicase) may be given. Seek advice. • ***Hyperviscosity:*** (p356). If WCC is >100 × 10^9/L WBC thrombi may form in b lung, and heart (leucostasis). Avoid transfusing before lowering WCC, eg v hydroxycarbamide or leucopheresis, as viscosity rises (risk of leucostasis ↑). • ***Disseminated intravascular coagulation (DIC):*** This is pathological widespr activation of coagulation, due to release of procoagulant agents into the circulat Clotting factors and platelets are consumed, with ↑risk of bleeding. Fibrin stra fill small vessels, haemolysing passing RBCs, and fibrinolysis is also activa ***Causes:*** Malignancy, sepsis, trauma, obstetric: *OHCS* p88. ***Signs:*** Extensive bruis bleeding anywhere eg recent venepuncture sites, renal failure. ***Tests:*** Platele PT↑; APTT↑; fibrinogen↓ (correlates best with severity); fibrin degradation prod (D-dimers) ↑↑. Film: broken RBCs (schistocytes). ***℞:*** Treat the cause. (replacement therapy: platelets if <50×10^9/L, cryoprecipitate to replace fibrino FFP to replace coagulation factors. Heparin is controversial. Activated protei reduces mortality in DIC with severe sepsis or multi-organ failure. The use of transretinoic acid (ATRA) has significantly reduced the risk of DIC in ac promyelocytic leukaemia (the commonest leukaemia associated with DIC).

Leukaemias

These are divided into 4 main types depending on the cell line involved and the speed of disease progression:

	Lymphoid	Myeloid
Acute	Acute lymphoblastic leukaemia (ALL)	Acute myeloid leukaemia (AML)
Chronic	Chronic lymphocytic leukaemia (CLL)	Chronic myeloid leukaemia (CML)

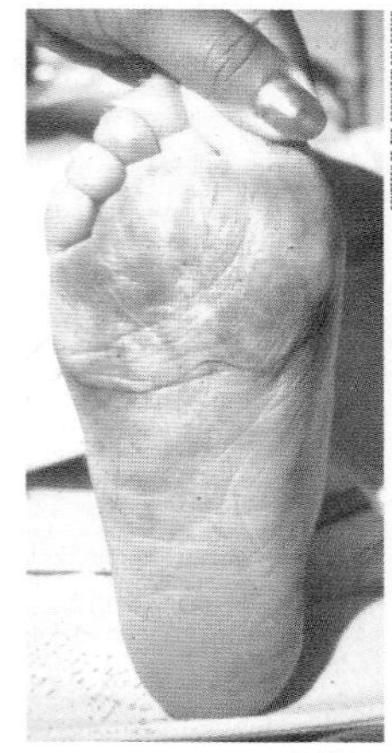

Fig 1. The appearance of DIC on the sole.

Acute lymphoblastic leukaemia (ALL)

This is a malignancy of lymphoid cells, affecting either B or T lymphocyte cell lin arresting maturation and promoting uncontrolled proliferation of immature bla cells, with bone marrow failure and tissue infiltration. It is thought to develop fro a combination of an environmental trigger in the presence of genetic susceptibili In most cases these are unknown, but predisposing factors include ionizi radiation (eg X-rays) during pregnancy, and syndromes including Down's. It is t commonest cancer of childhood, and is rare in adults. CNS involvement is commo

Classification is based on 3 systems:

1 ***Morphological*** The FAB[1] system divides ALL into 3 types (L1, L2, L3) by microscopic appearance. Provides limited information.

2 ***Immunological*** Surface markers are used to classify ALL into:
- Precursor B-cell ALL • T-cell ALL • B-cell ALL.

3 ***Cytogenetic*** Chromosomal analysis. Abnormalities are detected in up to 85 which are often translocations . Useful for predicting prognosis eg poor wi Philadelphia chromosome (see below), and for detecting disease recurrence.

Signs and symptoms are due to:
- Marrow failure: Anaemia (↓Hb), infection (↓WCC), and bleeding (↓platelets).
- Infiltration: Hepato- and splenomegaly, lymphadenopathy—superficial or med astinal, orchidomegaly, CNS involvement—eg cranial nerve palsies, meningism

Common infections: Especially chest, mouth, perianal and skin. Bacter septicaemia, Zoster, CMV, measles, candidiasis, *Pneumocystis* pneumonia (p398)

Tests • Characteristic blast cells on blood film and bone marrow. WCC usually hig
- CXR and CT scan to look for mediastinal and abdominal lymphadenopathy.
- Lumbar puncture should be performed to look for CNS involvement.

Treatment • ***Supportive care:*** Blood and platelet transfusions, IV fluids a allopurinol to prevent tumour lysis. Insert a Hickman line for venous access.
- ***Infections:*** These are dangerous, due to neutropenia caused by the disease ar treatment. Immediate IV antibiotics for infection. Start the neutropenic regim (p336): prophylactic antivirals, antifungals and antibiotics (eg co-trimoxazole prevent *Pneumocystis* pneumonia (p336), but beware: can worsen neutropeni
- ***Chemotherapy:*** Patients are entered into national trials. A typical programme i
  - ***Remission induction:*** This may be achieved with vincristine, prednisolon L-asparaginase, and daunorubicin.
  - ***Consolidation:*** High/medium-dose therapy in 'blocks' over several weeks.
  - ***CNS prophylaxis:*** Intrathecal (or high-dose IV) methotrexate ± CNS irradiatio
  - ***Maintenance:*** Prolonged chemotherapy, eg mercaptopurine (daily), methotre ate (weekly), and vincristine + prednisolone (monthly) for 2yrs. Relapse common in blood, CNS, or testis (so examine these sites at follow-up). Mo details: *OHCS* p194.
- ***Marrow transplant:*** (p340) Consider if poor prognosis or relapse. This is th only way to cure those with Philadelphia chromosome—see below.

Haematological remission means no evidence of leukaemia in the blood, a norm or recovering blood count, and < 5% blasts in a normal regenerating marrow.

Prognosis: Cure rates for children are 70–90%; for adults only 35% (<5% >65yrs old, where there is a 2nd peak in incidence). Poor prognosis if adult, ma Philadelphia chromosome (p342): BCR–ABL gene fusion due to translocation c chromosomes 9 & 22, presentation with CNS signs, WCC >100×10^9/L or B-cell AL PCR is used to detect minimal residual disease, undetectable by standard mean Prognosis is poor if seen in high amounts at presentation or during remission.

The future may lie in tailoring therapy to the exact gene defect, and according the individual's metabolism. Monoclonal antibodies, gene-targeted retinoid cytokines, vaccines, and T-cell infusions are all being studied.

1 FAB = French, American, British.

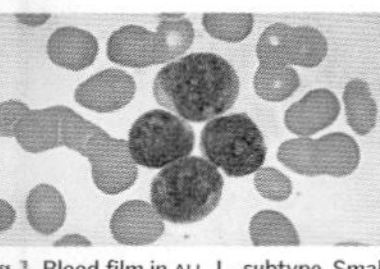

ig 1. Blood film in ALL, L_1 subtype. Small 'asts with scanty cytoplasm.

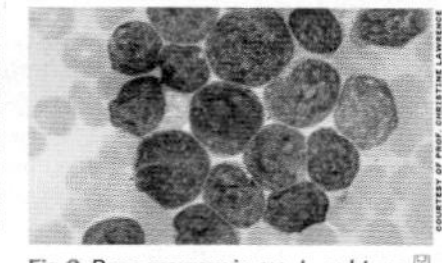

Fig 2. Bone marrow in ALL, L_1 subtype.

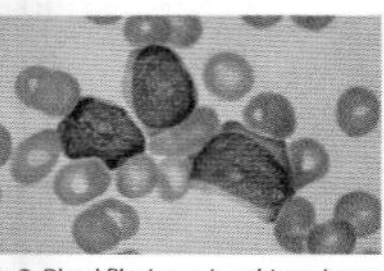

ig 3. Blood film in ALL, L_2 subtype. Larger last cells with greater morphological ariation, and more abundant cytoplasm.

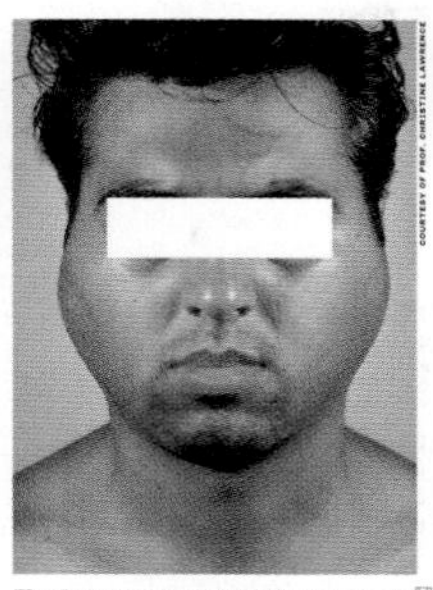

Fig 4. Bilateral parotid infiltration in ALL. (Enlarged parotid glands are also seen in mumps and sarcoidosis.)

Acute myeloid leukaemia (AML)

This neoplastic proliferation of blast cells is derived from marrow myelo elements. It is a very rapidly progressive malignancy (death in ~2 months untreated; ~20% 3-yr survival after chemotherapy).

Incidence 1/10,000/yr. Increases with age, and is the commonest acute leukaem of adults. Seen increasingly as a long-term complication of chemotherapy, eg f lymphoma. Also associated with myelodysplastic syndromes (see BOX), ionisir radiation and syndromes eg Down's.

Morphological classification now based on WHO histological classification, whic is complex and requires specialist interpretation. It recognizes the importa prognostic information from cytogenetics and molecular genetics. 5 main type:

- AML with recurrent genetic abnormalities.
- AML, other.
- AML multi-lineage dysplasia (usually 2° to preexisting myelodysplastic syndrom
- AML, therapy related.
- Acute leukaemias of ambiguous lineage (both myeloid and lymphoid phenotyp

Symptoms • ***Marrow failure:*** Patients usually present with symptoms of anaem infection or bleeding. DIC occurs in acute promyelocytic leukaemia, a subtype AML, where there is release of thromboplastin. Use of all-transretinoic acid wi chemotherapy reduces the risk of DIC (see p336).

- ***Infiltration:*** Hepato- and splenomegaly, gum hypertrophy, skin involvement. C involvement at presentation is rare in AML.

Diagnosis WCC is often ↑, but can be normal or even low. Blast cells may be few the peripheral blood, so diagnosis depends on bone marrow biopsy. Differentiati from ALL may be by microscopy (Auer rods are diagnostic of AML), but is now bas on immunophenotyping and molecular methods. Cytogenetic analysis (eg type mutation) affects treatment recommendations, and guides prognosis.

Complications • Infection is the major problem, related to both the disease ar during treatment. Be alert to septicaemia (p336). Infections may be bacteri fungal or viral, and prophylaxis is given for each during treatment. ***Pitfalls:*** AM itself causes fever, common organisms present oddly, few antibodies are made, ra organisms—particularly fungi (especially *Candida* or *Aspergillus*). • Chemothera causes ↑plasma urate levels (from tumour lysis)—so give allopurinol wi chemotherapy, and keep well hydrated with IV fluids. • Leucostasis (p336) m occur if WCC ↑↑.

Treatment • ***Supportive care*** As for ALL.

- ***Chemotherapy*** is very intensive, resulting in long periods of marrow suppressi with neutropenia + platelets↓. The main drugs used include daunorubicin, ar cytosine arabinoside, with ~5 cycles given in 1 week blocks to achieve remissi
- ***Bone marrow transplant (BMT)*** Pluripotent haematopoietic stem cells a collected from the bone marrow. *Allogeneic* transplants from HLA-match siblings or from matched unrelated donors (accessed via internation databases) is indicated during first remission in disease with poor prognosis. Th idea is to destroy leukaemic cells and the immune system by cyclophosphamide total body irradiation, and then repopulate the marrow by transplantation fron matched donor infused IV. BMT allows the most intensive chemotherapy regime because marrow suppression is not an issue. Ciclosporin ± methotrexate may b used to reduce the effect of the new marrow attacking the patient's body (gra vs host disease). ***Complications:*** Graft *vs* host disease (may help explain t curative effect of BMT); opportunistic infections; relapse of leukaemia; infertili ***Prognosis:*** Lower relapse rates ~60% long-term survivors, but significa mortality of ~10%. *Autologous BMT* where stem cells are taken from the patie themselves, is used in intermediate prognosis disease, although some studi suggest better survival rates with intensive chemotherapy regimes.
- Supportive care, or lower dose chemotherapy for disease control, may be mo appropriate in elderly patients, where intensive therapies have poorer outcom

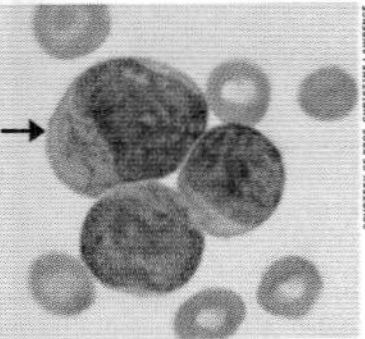

1. Auer rods found in AML myeloblast
s, representing crystals of coalesced
ıules.

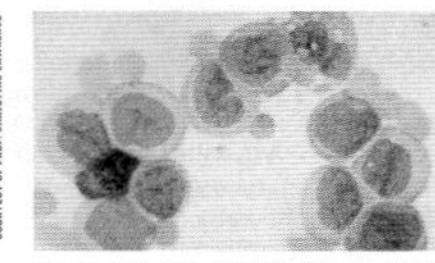

Fig 2. AML with monoblasts and myeloblasts on the peripheral blood film.

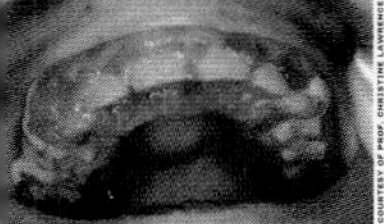

3. Gum hypertrophy, in AML.

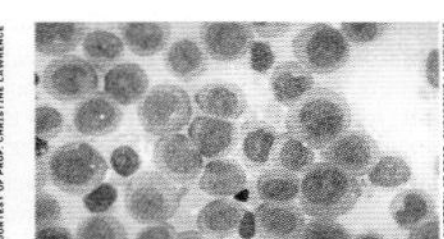

Fig 4. Bone marrow in AML: multiple monoblasts.

yelodysplastic syndromes (myelodysplasia)

ıese are a group of diseases where there is a neoplastic clonal disorder of ıltipotent haematopoietic stem cells, leading to progressive bone marrow ilure and ineffective haematopoiesis. This produces functional abnormalities of yeloid cells and peripheral cytopenias, with reduced numbers of red blood cells, utrophils, and platelets. A proportion of patients later undergo transformation AML. In most cases, these are primary disorders, but they may also develop condary to chemotherapy or radiotherapy, given for other malignancies.

inically, around half present >70 years old. There may be no symptoms with tection on blood tests, or they may present with anaemia, infections eutropenia), or easy bruising and bleeding (↓platelets). Tests show a ıncytopenia (p348), with a reduced reticulocyte count. Bone marrow llularity is usually increased due to the ineffective haematopoiesis. Ring leroblasts may also be seen in the marrow. There are different subtypes, ouped according to WHO classification.

eatment differs according to disease prognosis, and the individual. Allogeneic em cell transplantation offers a cure, but is associated with a risk of mortality, ıd is thus reserved for younger patients (<55yrs) with poor prognosis disease. ternatively, intensive combination chemotherapy may be used. In those where ere is a better prognosis, or in older patients where intensive treatment is sociated with poorer outcomes, single agent chemotherapy may be used to try obtain disease control. Multiple transfusions of red cells or platelets are often quired. Erythropoietin ± human granulocyte colony stimulating factor (G-CSF) ay be used to lower the transfusion requirement. Immunosuppressive agents ay also be used, eg ciclosporin or antithymocyte globulins.

ognosis Median survival: from 6 months to 6 years according to disease type.

Chronic myeloid leukaemia (CML)

CML is characterized by an uncontrolled clonal proliferation of myeloid cell accounts for 15% of leukaemias. It is a myeloproliferative disorder (p350) ha features in common with these diseases eg splenomegaly. It occurs most o between 40–60yrs, with a slight male predominance, and is rare in childhoo

Philadelphia chromosome (Ph) Present in >80% of those with CML. It is a hy chromosome comprising reciprocal translocation between the long arm chromosome 9 and the long arm of chromosome 22—t(9;22) forming a fusion g BCR/ABL on chromosome 22, which has tyrosine kinase activity. Those withou have a worse prognosis. Some patients have a masked translocation—cytogene do not show the Ph, but the rearrangement is detectable by molecular technic

Symptoms Mostly chronic and insidious: weight↓, tiredness, fever, sweats. T may be features of gout (due to purine breakdown), bleeding (platelet dysfunct and abdominal discomfort (splenic enlargement). ~30% are detected by char

Signs Splenomegaly (>75%)—often massive. Hepatomegaly, anaemia, bruisi

Tests WBC ↑↑ (often >100 × 10^9/L) with whole spectrum of myeloid cel ↑neutrophils, myelocytes, basophils, eosinophils. Hb↓ or normal, platelets vari Urate↑, B_{12}↑. Neutrophil alk phos score↓ (seldom performed now). Bone marro hypercellular. Ph found on cytogenetic analysis of blood or bone marrow.

Natural history Variable, median survival 5–6yrs. There are three phases: *chr* lasting months or years of few, if any, symptoms→ *accelerated phase*, v increasing symptoms, spleen size, and difficulty in controlling counts→ *b transformation*, with features of acute leukaemia ± death. **Treatment** See BC

Chronic lymphocytic leukaemia (CLL)

This is a monoclonal proliferation of non-functional mature B lymphocytes (T CLL occurs rarely). CLL constitutes 25% of all leukaemias. ♂:♀ 2:1. It is a diseas the elderly, median age at diagnosis is ~65 years. Staging correlates with surv

Stage 0	Lymphocytosis alone.	Median Survival >13yrs
I	Lymphocytosis + lymphadenopathy.	8yrs
II	Lymphocytosis + spleno- or hepatomegaly.	5yrs
III	Lymphocytosis + anaemia (Hb <11g/dL).	2yrs
IV	Lymphocytosis + platelets <100 × 10^9/L.	1yr

Symptoms (none in 25%) Infection, anaemia. If severe: weight↓, sweats, anore

Signs Enlarged, rubbery, non-tender nodes. Splenomegaly, hepatomegaly.

Tests ↑Lymphocytes—may be marked. Later: autoimmune haemolysis (p3 marrow infiltration: ↓Hb, ↓neutrophils, ↓platelets.

Complications 1 Autoimmune haemolysis. 2 ↑Infection due to hypogam globulinaemia (=↓IgG), bacterial, viral especially herpes zoster. 3 Marrow fail

Natural history Some remain in *status quo* for years, or even regr Usually nodes slowly enlarge (± lymphatic obstruction). Death is often du infection (commonly pneumococcus, haemophilus, meningococcus, *Candida* aspergillosis), or transformation to aggressive lymphoma (Richter's syndrom

Treatment If asymptomatic, the patient can be monitored. Chlorambucil is use ↓lymphocyte count, improve marrow function, and reduce node size. Dose: eg (0.2mg/kg daily PO. The purine analogue fludarabine is an alternative. Steroids used in autoimmune haemolysis. ***Radiotherapy:*** For relief of lymphadenopath splenomegaly. ***Supportive care:*** Transfusions, IV human immunoglobuli recurrent infections. Bone marrow transplant is currently experimental.

Prognosis Current treatments are mainly non-curative at present. Prognos often good: depends on stage and molecular/immunological factors.

Haematology

[Tre]atment of CML

[Ch]emotherapy

[I]matinib (Glivec®), a specific BCR/ABL tyrosine kinase inhibitor, has revolut[i]onized CML therapy. It is more effective than the previous gold standard of α-[i]nterferon—± cytarabine in chronic phase patients, in terms of preventing [d]isease progression. It is likely that this will be translated into a survival [a]dvantage; long term data are awaited. The drug may also be effective in acc[e]lerated phase and blast crises. Imatinib gives high haematological response [r]ates (>90%). Cytogenetic remissions are also common, but complete [e]radication of the Philadelphia clone, as detected by the most sensitive [m]olecular methods, is unusual (<5% patients). SE: usually mild: nausea, cramps, [o]edema, skin rash, headache, arthralgia. May cause myelosuppression.

[H]ydroxycarbamide may still be used in patients intolerant of imatinib, or [w]here imatinib has proved ineffective. Busulfan is very rarely used now.

[T]he use of α-interferon in CML has declined dramatically with the introduction [o]f imatinib, but α-interferon may still have a role in combination therapy.

[T]reatment of CML blast crisis is problematic. Patients not previously treated [w]ith imatinib may respond temporarily to this. Those with lymphoblastic trans[f]ormation may benefit from treatment as for ALL. Treatment of myeloblastic [t]ransformation with chemotherapy rarely achieves lasting remission and [a]llogeneic transplantation offers the only hope of long-term survival.

[Ste]m cell transplantation

[A]llogeneic transplantation from a HLA matched sibling or unrelated donor is [t]he only curative treatment but carries significant morbidity and mortality. [G]uidelines suggest that this approach should be used 1st line only in young [p]atients where mortality rates are lower. Other patients should be offered [i]matinib. Patients are then reviewed annually to decide whether to continue [i]matinib, or to offer combination therapy or stem cell transplantation.

The role of autologous transplantation, if any, in CML, remains to be defined.

Haematology

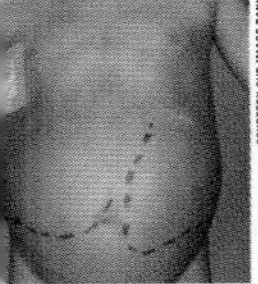

[Fig] 1. Hepatosplenomegaly in CML.

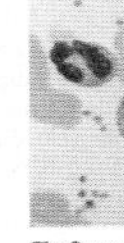

Fig 2. CML: Numerous granulocytic cells at different stages of differentiation.

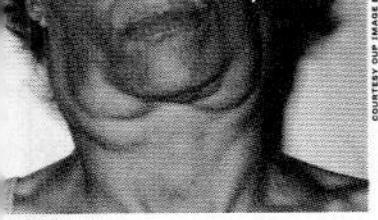

[Fig] 3. Bilateral cervical lymphadenopathy [in C]LL.

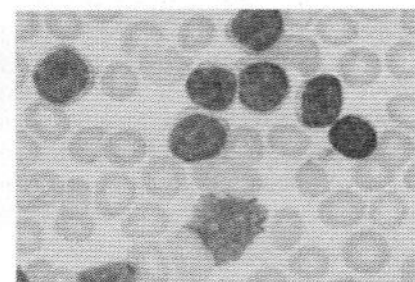

Fig 4. CLL: Numerous lymphocytes and a typical 'smear' cell: a fragile cell damaged in preparation.

Hodgkin's lymphoma

[Thomas Hodgkin, Guy's,UK 1798–18

Lymphomas are disorders caused by malignant proliferations of lymphocytes. T accumulate in the lymph nodes causing lymphadenopathy, but may also be four peripheral blood or infiltrate organs. Lymphomas are histologically divided Hodgkin's and non-Hodgkin's types. In Hodgkin's lymphoma, characteristic with mirror-image nuclei are found, called Reed–Sternberg cells.

Hodgkin's lymphoma: 2 peaks of incidence: young adults and elderly. ♂:♀≈2

Symptoms Often presents with enlarged, painless, non-tender, 'rubbery' superf lymph nodes, typically cervical (60–70%), also axillary or inguinal nodes. The siz the nodes may increase and decrease spontaneously, and nodes can bec matted. 25% have constitutional upset, eg fever, weight loss, night sweats, prur and lethargy. There may be alcohol-induced lymph node pain. Mediastinal lyr node involvement can cause features due to mass effect eg bronchial or obstruction (p514), or direct extension eg causing pleural effusions. *Pel-Ebs fever* implies a cyclical fever with long periods (15–28 days) of normal or temperature: it is, at best, rare—and some have called it mythical.[1]

Signs Lymph node enlargement. Also, cachexia, anaemia, spleno- or hepatomeg

Tests ***Tissue diagnosis*** Lymph node excision biopsy if possible. Image gui needle biopsy, laparotomy or mediastinoscopy may be needed to obtain a sam ***Bloods*** FBC, film, ESR, LFT, LDH, urate, Ca^{2+}. ↑ESR or ↓Hb indicate a worse progn LDH is raised as it is released during cell turnover.

Staging (Ann Arbor system) Influences treatment and prognosis. Done by CXR of thorax, abdo, pelvis ± bone marrow biopsy if B symptoms, or stage III–IV dise

I Confined to single lymph node region.
II Involvement of two or more nodal areas on the same side of the diaphra
III Involvement of nodes on both sides of the diaphragm.
IV Spread beyond the lymph nodes eg liver or bone marrow.

Each stage is subdivided into '**A**'—no systemic symptoms other than pruritus '**B**'—presence of B symptoms: weight loss >10% in the last 6 months, unexplai fever >38°C, or drenching night sweats (requiring change of clothes). '**B**' indica more extensive disease. Localized extra-nodal extension does not advance stage, but is indicated by subscripted '**E**', eg $I\text{-}A_E$.

Treatment This is with chemotherapy, radiotherapy or both. Radiotherapy ± sh courses of chemotherapy for stages I-A and II-A (eg with ≤3 areas involved). Lon courses of chemotherapy for II-A with >3 areas involved through to IV-B. standard regime is '**ABVD**': Adriamycin, Bleomycin, Vinblastine, and Dacarbaz More intensive regimens are used if poor prognosis or advanced disease relapsed disease, where disease recurs after treatment, high dose chemother with peripheral stem-cell transplantation may be used, involving autologous occasionally allogeneic) transplantation of peripheral blood progenitor cells restore marrow function after therapy.

Complications of treatment See p516–9: Radiotherapy may ↑ risk of sec malignancies—solid tumours (especially lung and breast, also melanoma, sarco stomach and thyroid cancers), ischaemic heart disease, hypothyroidism and l fibrosis due to the radiation field. Chemotherapy SE include myelosuppress nausea, alopecia, infection. AML (p340), non-Hodgkin's lymphoma and infertility r be due to both chemo- or radiotherapy—see page 519.

5-year survival Depends on stage and grade: >95% in I-A lymphocyte-predo nant disease; <40% with IV-B lymphocyte-depleted.

Emergency presentations Infection; SVC obstruction—JVP↑, sensation of fulln in the head, dyspnoea, blackouts, facial oedema (seek expert help; see p514).

1 Pel-Ebstein fever is dismissed by Richard Asher (*Talking Sense*), as existing only thanks to its having exotically named (the 1885 patients of Dr P Pel had no histology, and fevers in Hodgkin's are *usually* non-spec Another unfair reason for consigning it to myth is that the paper proving its existence and its relation to cy changes in node size doesn't come up in literature searches as Wilhelm *Ebstein* was spelled *Epstein* througho

Classification (In order of incidence)	Prognosis
Classical Hodgkin's lymphoma	
Nodular sclerosing	Good
Mixed cellularity*	Good
Lymphocyte rich	Good
Lymphocyte-depleted*	Poor

NB: nodular lymphocyte predominant Hodgkin's is recognized as a separate entity, behaving as an indolent B-cell lymphoma. **Higher incidence and worse prognosis if HIV +ve.*

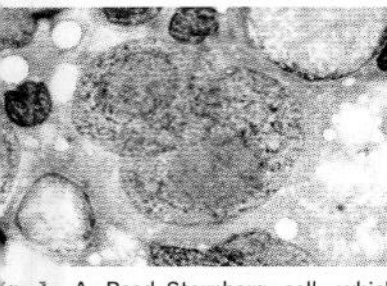

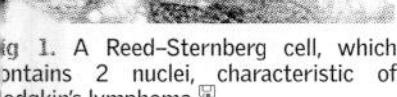

Fig 1. A Reed–Sternberg cell, which contains 2 nuclei, characteristic of Hodgkin's lymphoma.

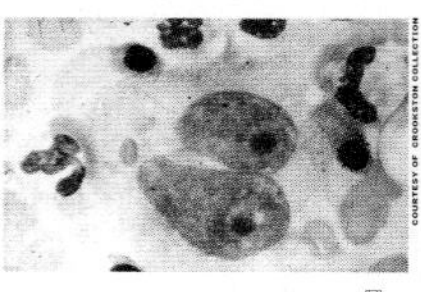

Fig 2. Another Reed–Sternberg cell.

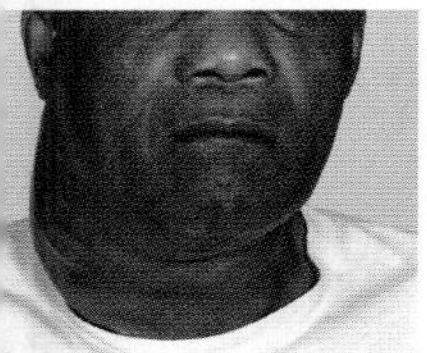

Fig 3. Cervical lymphadenopathy in Hodgkin's disease.

Non-Hodgkin's lymphoma

This includes all lymphomas without Reed–Sternberg cells, and is a ver diverse group of diseases. Most are derived from B-lymphocyte cell lines. Not all ar centred on lymph nodes (extranodal tissues generating lymphoma include mucosa associated lymphoid tissue—MALT. Gastric MALT is associated with *H. pylori*, an may regress when this is eradicated). The overall incidence of lymphoma ha doubled since 1970 (to 1 : 10,000). ***Causes:*** congenital immunodeficiency, acquire immunodeficiency eg drugs, HIV infection (usually high grade lymphoma), infectio (eg HTLV-1 p336, EBV, *H. pylori*) or environmental toxins.

Signs and symptoms • Nodal disease (75% at presentation): superficial lymph adenopathy • Extranodal disease (25%) involving the oropharynx, skin (especially cell lymphomas—p548), bone, gut, CNS, or lung. Disease of the oropharynge lymphoid tissue (Waldeyer's ring) causes sore throat and obstructed breathin • Systemic symptoms—fever, night sweats, weight loss (less common than i Hodgkin's lymphoma, and indicates disseminated disease) • Pancytopenia due t marrow involvement—anaemia, neutropenia (infection) and ↓platelets (bleeding

Tests As for Hodgkin's disease with the Ann Arbor system (p344). ***Diagnosi*** Lymph node biopsy. ***Bloods*** FBC, U&E, LFT, LDH. ↑LDH indicates worse prognosis as it released with cell turnover. ***Stage*** with CT or MRI of chest, abdomen, pelvis, an bone marrow aspiration. Send cytology of any effusion; lumbar puncture for cs cytology if any CNS signs.

Haematology

Histology This is something of a quagmire as classification systems are comple and changing. The current classification is based on the WHO classification c lymphoid neoplasms. Discuss diagnosis and management as a multidisciplinar team, bringing together information available from clinical evaluation, histolog immunology, molecular genetics, and imaging. *Generally:*

- Low-grade lymphomas are indolent, and are often incurable and wide disseminated at presentation. Include: follicular lymphoma, marginal zon lymphoma (includes MALT lymphomas), lymphocytic lymphoma (closely related t CLL and treated similarly), lymphoplasmacytoid lymphoma (associated wit production of IgM = Waldenström's macroglobulinaemia, p354).
- High-grade lymphomas are more aggressive, but long-term cure may b achievable. There is often a short history of rapidly enlarging lymphadenopath with systemic symptoms. Include: Burkitt's lymphoma (childhood disease wit characteristic jaw lymphadenopathy), lymphoblastic lymphomas (shares feature with ALL), diffuse large B-cell lymphoma.

Treatment Depends on disease subtype. ***Low grade:*** If symptomless, none may b needed. Radiotherapy may be curative in localized disease. Chlorambucil is used i diffuse disease. Remission may be maintained by using α-interferon or rituxima (see below). ***High grade:*** For diffuse large B-cell lymphoma (DLBCL), the 'CHO regime: **C**yclophosphamide, **H**ydroxydaunorubicin, vincristine (**O**ncovin®) ar **P**rednisolone plus rituximab may be used.[1] The addition of rituximab, an anti-CD2 monoclonal antibody, to this regimen has produced the first major advance in th treatment of this disorder for 30yrs.

Survival Histology is important. Prognosis is worse if at presentation: • Ag >60yrs • Systemic symptoms • Bulky disease (abdominal mass >10cm) • ↑LD • Disseminated disease. Typical 5-yr survival for treated patients: ~30% for high grade and >50% for low-grade lymphomas, but the picture is very variable.

1 NICE advice: rituximab is indicated in CD20+ve diffuse large-B-cell lymphoma (DLBCL) at stage II, III, IV. Do not use if CHOP is contraindicated. DLBCL denotes intermediate- to high-grade lymphomas that a rapidly fatal if untreated but often respond well to intensive chemotherapy. CD20 is a surface mark expressed on most B-cell lymphomas and testing for it is routine. CD20 occurs on normal and malignant cells, but not on precursor B cells, so obviating long-term B cell depletion. Rituximab kills CD20+ve cells antibody-directed cytotoxicity ± apoptosis induction. It also sensitizes cells to CHOP.

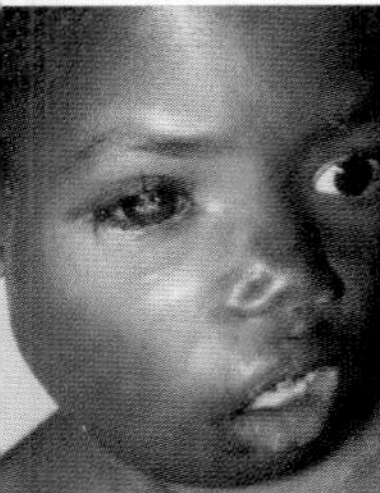

ig 1. Burkitt's lymphoma, with charact-
ristic jaw lymphadenopathy.

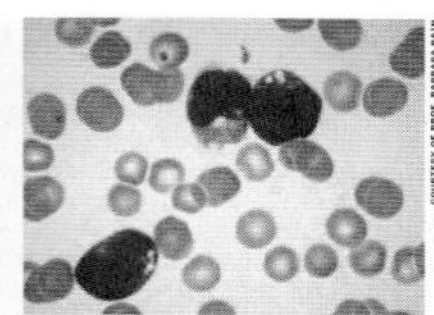

Fig 2. Burkitt's lymphoma, with 3 basophilic vacuolated lymphoma cells.

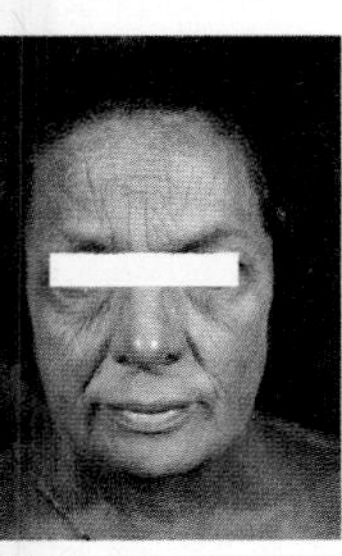

g 3. Cutaneous T cell lymphoma, hich has caused severe eryrroderma (Sézary syndrome) in a aucasian woman.

Pancytopenia, and bone marrow failure

The bone marrow is responsible for haemopoiesis. In adults, this normally take place in the central skeleton (vertebrae, sternum, ribs, skull) and proximal lon bones. In some anaemias (eg thalassaemia), increased demand produce haematopoiesis outside the bone marrow (extramedullary haematopoiesis), in th liver and spleen causing organomegaly. All blood cells arise from an ear pluripotent stem cell, which divides in an asymmetrical way to produce anothe stem cell and a progenitor cell committed to a specific cell line. Committe progenitors undergo further differentiation under myeloid or lymphocyte lineag before their release into the blood as mature cells.

Pancytopenia is reduction in all the major cell lines: red cells, white cells an platelets. Causes are due to 1 ↓***marrow production:*** aplastic anaemia, infiltratic (eg acute leukaemia, myelodysplasia, myeloma, lymphoma, solid tumours, TE megaloblastic anaemia, paroxysmal nocturnal haemoglobinuria (p324 myelofibrosis (p350), SLE. 2 ↑***peripheral destruction:*** hypersplenism.

Aplastic anaemia is a rare stem cell disorder leading to pancytopenia and hypoplastic bone marrow (the marrow stops making cells). Presents with featur of anaemia (↓Hb), infection (↓WCC) or bleeding (↓platelets). ***Incidence:*** ~5 cas per million/year. ***Causes:*** Most cases are autoimmune, triggered by drugs, (viruse eg Parvovirus, hepatitis) or irradiation. May also be inherited eg Fanconi anaemi (p690). ***Tests:*** A bone marrow examination is required for the diagnosi ***Treatment:*** Support the blood count (below). Asymptomatic patients do nc require specific treatment, but supportive treatment (eg neutropenic regimen) ma be required. The treatment of choice in young patients who are severely affected an allogeneic marrow transplantation from an HLA matched sibling, which can b curative. Otherwise, immunosuppression with ciclosporin and antithymocy globulin may be effective, although is not curative in most.

Marrow support Red cells survive for ~120d, platelets for ~8d, and neutrophils fo 1–2d, so early problems are mainly from neutropenia and thrombocytopenia.

Red cell transfusion: Transfusing 1U should raise Hb by ~1–1.5g/dL (p570). Tran fusion may drop the platelet count (you may need to give platelets before or afte

Platelets: Traumatic bleeds, purpura and easy bruising occur if platele $<50\times10^9$/L. Spontaneous bleeding may occur if platelets $<20\times10^9$/L, wi intracranial haemorrhage rarely. Platelets are stored at room temperature (22° not in the fridge). In marrow transplant or if severely immunosuppressed, platele may need irradiation before use, to prevent transfusion-associated graft-versu host disease (GVHD). Platelets should be ABO compatible. They are not used in IT (p330). Indications: • Platelets $<10\times10^9$/L • Haemorrhage, including DIC (p33 • Before invasive procedures (eg biopsy, lumbar puncture) to increase count to >5 $\times10^9$/L. 4U of fresh platelets should raise the count to $>40\times10^9$/L in adults; chec dose needed with lab.

Neutrophils: Use a 'neutropenic regimen' if the count $<0.5\times10^9$/L. See p336.

Bone marrow biopsy may provide diagnostic information where there a abnormalities in the peripheral blood, and is also an important staging test in th lymphoproliferative disorders. Ideally an aspirate *and* trephine should be take usually from the posterior iliac crest (aspirates can also be taken from the anteri iliac crest or sternum). The aspirate provides a film which is examined b microscope. The trephine is a core of bone which allows assessment of bor marrow cellularity, architecture and the presence of infiltrative diseas Coagulation disorders may need to be corrected pre-biopsy. Apply pressu afterwards (lie on that side for 1–2h if platelets are low).

The myeloproliferative disorders

These form a group of disorders caused by proliferation of a clone haematopoietic myeloid stem cells in the marrow. While the cells proliferate, th also retain the ability to differentiate into RBCs, WBCs or platelets.

Classification is by the cell type which is proliferating		
RBC	→	Polycythaemia rubra vera (PRV).
WBC	→	Chronic myeloid leukaemia (CML, p342).
Platelets	→	Essential thrombocythaemia.
Fibroblasts	→	Myelofibrosis.

Polycythaemia may be relative (↓plasma volume, normal RBC mass) or absolu (↑RBC mass). *Relative polycythaemia* may be acute and due to dehydration (e alcohol or diuretics). A more chronic form exists which is associated with obesi hypertension, and a high alcohol and tobacco intake. *Absolute polycythaemia* distinguished by red cell mass estimation, using radioactive chromium (^{51}C labelled RBCs. Causes are primary (***polycythaemia rubra vera***) or secondary due hypoxia (eg high altitudes, chronic lung disease, cyanotic congenital heart disea heavy smoking) or inappropriately ↑erythropoietin secretion (eg in renal carcinom hepatocellular carcinoma).

Haematology

Polycythaemia rubra vera This is a malignant proliferation of a clone deriv from one pluripotent marrow stem cell. The erythroid progenitor offspring a unusual in not needing erythropoietin to avoid apoptosis (p499). There is exce proliferation of RBCs, WBCs, and platelets, leading to thrombotic complications d to hyperviscosity. Usually affects older patients >60yrs.

Signs May be asymptomatic and detected on FBC, or present with vague signs d to hyperviscosity (p356): headaches, dizziness, tinnitus, visual disturbance. It after a hot bath, and erythromelalgia, a burning sensation in fingers and toes, a characteristic. Examination may show facial plethora and splenomegaly (in 60% Gout may occur due to ↑urate from RBC turnover. Features of arterial (cardi cerebral, peripheral) or venous (DVT, cerebral, hepatic) thrombosis may be prese

Investigations • FBC: ↑RCC, ↑Hb, ↑HCT, ↑PCV, often also ↑WBC and ↑platelets • B • Marrow shows hypercellularity with erythroid hyperplasia • Neutrophil alkali phosphatase (NAP) score is ↑ (↓ in CML) • ↓serum erythropoietin • Raised red c mass on ^{51}Cr studies and splenomegaly, in the setting of a normal P_aO_2, is diagnos

Treatment: Aim to keep HCT <0.45 to ↓risk of thrombosis. In younger patients low risk, this is done by venesection. If higher risk (age >60yrs, previc thrombosis), hydroxycarbamide (=hydroxyurea) is used. α-interferon is preferrec women of childbearing age. Low dose aspirin 75mg daily PO is also given.

Prognosis: Variable, many remain well for years. Thrombosis and haemorrha (due to defective platelets) are the main complications. Transition to myelofibro occurs in ~30% or acute leukaemia in ~5%. Monitor FBC every 3 months.

Essential thrombocythaemia A clonal proliferation of megakaryocytes leads persistently ↑platelets, often >1000 × 10⁹/L, with abnormal function, caus bleeding or arterial and venous thrombosis, and microvascular occlusior headache, atypical chest pain, light-headedness, erythromelalgia. Exclude otl causes of thrombocytosis (see BOX). ***Treatment:*** Low dose aspirin 75mg da Hydroxycarbamide is given to ↓platelets if >60yrs old or if previous thrombo

Myelofibrosis There is hyperplasia of megakaryocytes which produce plate derived growth factor, leading to intense marrow fibrosis and myeloid metapla (haemopoiesis in the spleen and liver)→massive hepatosplenomegaly. ***Presentati*** Hypermetabolic symptoms: night sweats, fever, weight loss; abdominal discomf due to splenomegaly; or bone marrow failure (↓Hb, infections, bleeding). ***Fi*** Leucoerythroblastic cells (nucleated red cells, p314); characteristic teardrop R (see fig 2). Hb↓. Bone marrow trephine for diagnosis. ***Treatment:*** Marrow supp (see p662). Allogeneic stem cell transplant may be curative in young people carries a high risk of mortality. ***Prognosis:*** Median survival 4–5 years.

Causes of thrombocytosis

↑Platelets >450 × 10^9/L may be a reactive phenomenon, seen with many conditions including:

- Bleeding
- Infection
- Chronic inflammation, eg collagen disorders
- Malignancy
- Trauma
- Post-surgery
- Iron deficiency

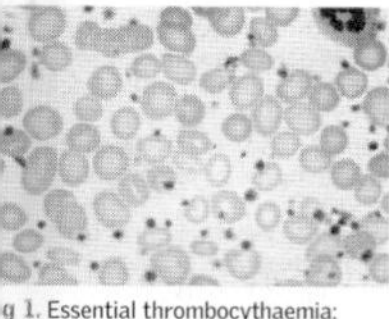

g 1. Essential thrombocythaemia: ımerous platelets seen.

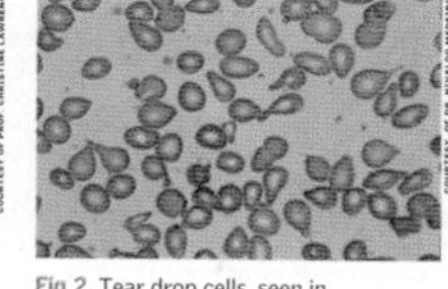

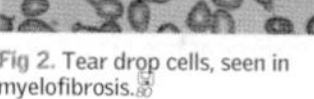

Fig 2. Tear drop cells, seen in myelofibrosis.

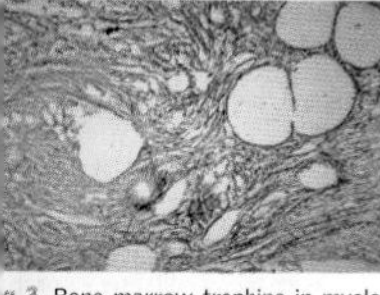

g 3. Bone marrow trephine in myelo- ɔrosis: the streaming effect is caused by tense fibrosis. Other causes of marrow ɔrosis include any myeloproliferative sorder, lymphoma, secondary carcinoma, , leukaemia, and irradiation.

Myeloma

Myeloma is a malignant clonal proliferation of B-lymphocyte derived plasma cel (fig 1). Normally many different plasma cells produce different immunoglobulir (Igs) which are polyclonal. In myeloma, a single clone of plasma cells produc identical Igs. This can be detected as a monoclonal band, or paraprotein, on serur and/or urine electrophoresis (see p678). ***Classification*** is based on the Ig produc which is IgG in ~⅔ and IgA in ~⅓. The small remainder are IgM or IgD. The other I levels are low. This is termed immunoparesis, causing increased susceptibility t infection. In ~⅔ of cases, the urine contains Bence-Jones protein, which are free I light chains of either kappa (κ) or lambda (λ) type, filtered by the kidney.

Incidence 5/100,000. Peak age: 70yrs. ♂:♀≈1. Afro-Caribbeans:Caucasians≈2:

Symptoms

- ***Osteolytic bone lesions*** causing unexplained backache, pathological fractur eg long bones or ribs, and vertebral collapse. ***Hypercalcaemia*** may result wi symptoms (p672). Lesions are due to ↑ osteoclast activation, from signalling b myeloma cells.
- ***Anaemia, neutropenia, or thrombocytopenia*** **may result from marro infiltration** by proliferating plasma cells, leading to symptoms of anaemi infection and bleeding.
- ***Recurrent bacterial infections*** due to immunoparesis, and also because neutropenia due to the disease and from chemotherapy.
- ***Renal impairment*** due to light chain deposition (p306 & p354).
- ***Systemic AL amyloidosis*** occurs in 15% (p354).

Haematology

Tests FBC—normocytic normochromic anaemia, film—rouleaux formation (p31 persistently ↑ESR or PV (p356), ↑urea and creatinine, ↑Ca^{2+} (in ~40%), alk ph usually normal (unless healing fracture). ***Screening test:*** Serum & urir electrophoresis. β_2-microglobulin (as a prognostic test). ***Imaging*** X-rays show lyt 'punched-out' lesions, eg pepper-pot skull, vertebral collapse, fractures osteoporosis. CT or MRI may be useful to detect lesions not seen on XR. ***Diagnos*** see BOX.

Treatment ***Supportive:*** • Bone pain should be treated with analgesia (avo NSAIDs due to risk of renal impairment). Give all patients a bisphosphona (clodronate, zolendronate or pamidronate), as they reduce fracture rates and bor pain. Local radiotherapy can help rapidly in focal disease. Orthopaedic procedur (vertebroplasty or kyphoplasty) may be helpful in vertebral collapse. • Anaem should be corrected with transfusion, and erythropoietin may be used. • Ren failure: Rehydrate, and ensure adequate fluid intake of 3L/day to prevent furth renal impairment by light chains. Dialysis may be needed in acute renal failu • Infections: Treat rapidly with broad spectrum antibiotics until culture results a known. Regular IV immunoglobulin infusions may be needed if recurrent.

Chemotherapy: In elderly patients, either melphalan or cyclophosphamide a used with prednisolone. This is usually effective in controlling disease for abo 1 year, reducing paraprotein levels and bone lesions. The disease may then becon uncontrollable and often resistant to treatment. One randomized trial (2006) fou the addition of thalidomide (a teratogenic immunomodulator) markedly improv event-free survival in the elderly.[RCT] Its use is non-standard. SE: birth defec drowsiness; neuropathy; neutropenia; sepsis; thromboembolism (anticoagulatio probably wise); orthostatic hypotension. In younger or fitter people, a mo aggressive approach is used (high-dose therapy and stem-cell rescue, HDT) with VAD type regime: Vincristine, Adriamycin and Dexamethasone. Autologous ste cell transplant may then be done, which improves survival but is not curati Allogeneic transplantation can be curative in younger patients, but carries ↑risk mortality (~30%). Thalidomide or bortezomib may be tried in relapsed disease

Prognosis Median survival is 3–4 years. A raised β_2-microglobulin is associat with a worse prognosis. Death is commonly due to infection or renal failure.

agnostic criteria

Monoclonal protein band in serum or urine electrophoresis
Increased plasma cells found on bone marrow biopsy
Evidence of end organ damage from myeloma
- Hypercalcaemia
- Renal insufficiency
- Anaemia
- Bone lesions: a skeletal survey is performed after diagnosis to detect bone disease, consisting of X-rays of chest; cervical, thoracic, and lumbar spine; skull and pelvis.

mplications of myeloma

Hypercalcaemia (p672). Occurs with active disease ie at presentation or relapse. Rehydrate vigorously with IV saline 0.9% 4–6L/d (careful fluid balance). IV bisphosphonates, eg zolendronate or pamidronate are useful for treating hypercalcaemia acutely.

Spinal cord compression (p458 & p515). Occurs in 5% of patients with myeloma. Urgent MRI if suspected. Treatment is with dexamethasone 8–16mg/24h PO and local radiotherapy.

Hyperviscosity (p356), causes reduced cognition, disturbed vision, and bleeding. It is treated with plasmapheresis, to remove light chains.

Acute renal failure is treated with rehydration. Patients may require urgent dialysis.

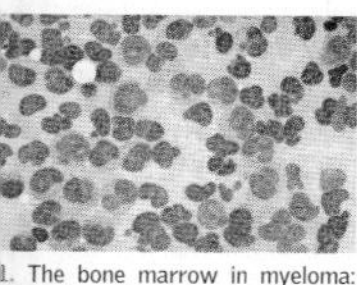

1. The bone marrow in myeloma: number of plasma cells with rmal forms.

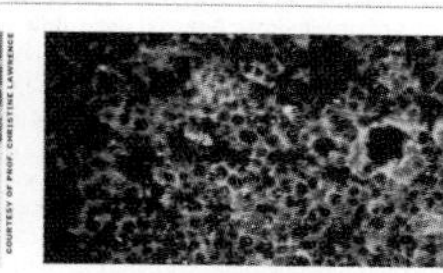

Fig 2. A bone marrow section in myeloma, stained with IgG kappa monoclonal antibody.

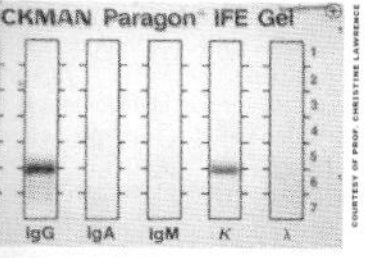

3. An IgG kappa paraprotein clonal band on electrophoresis (a ol sample has run on the left).

Paraproteinaemia

Paraproteinaemia denotes presence in the circulation of immunoglobulins prod by a single clone of plasma cells. The paraprotein is recognized as a monoc band (M band) on serum electrophoresis.[1] There are 6 major categories:

1. ***Multiple myeloma:*** See p352.
2. ***Waldenström's macroglobulinaemia:*** This is a lymphoplasmacytoid lymph producing a monoclonal IgM paraprotein. Hyperviscosity is common (p3 with CNS and ocular symptoms. Lymphadenopathy and splenomegaly are seen. ↑ESR, with IgM paraprotein on serum electrophoresis. **R:** Nor asymptomatic. Chlorambucil, fludarabine or combination chemotherapy ma used. Plasmapheresis[1] for hyperviscosity (p356).
3. ***Primary amyloidosis:*** See below.
4. ***Monoclonal gammopathy of uncertain significance*** (MGUS) is common >70yrs). There is a paraprotein in the serum but no myeloma, ma globulinaemia or lymphoma, with no bone lesions, no Bence-Jones protein a low concentration of paraprotein, with <10% plasma cells in the marro proportion of these patients develop myeloma or lymphoma in the future
5. ***Paraproteinaemia in lymphoma or leukaemia:*** Eg seen in 5% of CLL.
6. ***Heavy chain disease:*** This is where neoplastic cells produce free Ig h chains. α chain disease is the most important, causing malabsorption infiltration of small bowel wall. It may progress to lymphoma.

Haematology

Amyloidosis

This is a group of disorders characterized by extracellular deposits of a prote abnormal fibrillar form, resistant to degradation. The following are the syst forms of amyloidosis. Amyloid deposition is also a feature of Alzheimer's dis Type 2 diabetes mellitus and haemodialysis-related amyloidosis.

AL amyloid (primary amyloidosis): Due to clonal proliferation of plasma cells, production of amyloidogenic monoclonal immunoglobulins. In most cases, it o on its own as a primary amyloidosis, with occult plasma cell proliferation. It is seen in 15% of patients with myeloma, and smaller proportions Waldenströms, MGUS, or lymphoma. Deposition may occur in • Kidneys: Glome lesions—proteinuria and nephrotic syndrome • Heart: Restrictive cardiomyop ('sparkling' appearance on Echo), arrhythmias, angina • Nerves: Periphera autonomic neuropathy, carpal tunnel syndrome • Gut: Macroglossia (big ton malabsorption, perforation, haemorrhage, obstruction, and hepatome • Vascular: Purpura, especially periorbital—a characteristic feature.

AA amyloid (secondary amyloidosis): The amyloid here is derived from s amyloid A, an acute phase protein. It occurs with chronic inflammatic rheumatoid arthritis, inflammatory bowel disease, familial Mediterranean feve chronic infections—TB, bronchiectasis, osteomyelitis. It affects the kidneys, live spleen, and commonly presents with proteinuria, nephrotic syndrom hepatosplenomegaly. Macroglossia is not seen, and cardiac involvement is ra

Familial amyloidosis is a group of autosomal dominant disorder, most comm caused by mutations in transthyretin, a transport protein produced by the Usually causes a sensory or autonomic neuropathy ± renal or cardiac involve

Diagnosis is made with biopsy of affected tissue, and positive Congo Red sta with red–green birefringence under polarized light microscopy. The rectu subcutaneous fat are relatively non-invasive sites for biopsy and are +ve in 8

R: AA amyloidosis may improve if the primary disease is treated. AL may respo therapy as for myeloma. Liver transplant can be curative in familial amyloid

Prognosis Median survival is 1–2 years. Patients with myeloma and amylo have a shorter survival than those with myeloma alone.

1 Electro*phoresis* and plasma *pheresis* look as though they should share endings, but they do not *phoros=bearing* (*esis=process*), but *aphairesis* is Greek for *removal*.

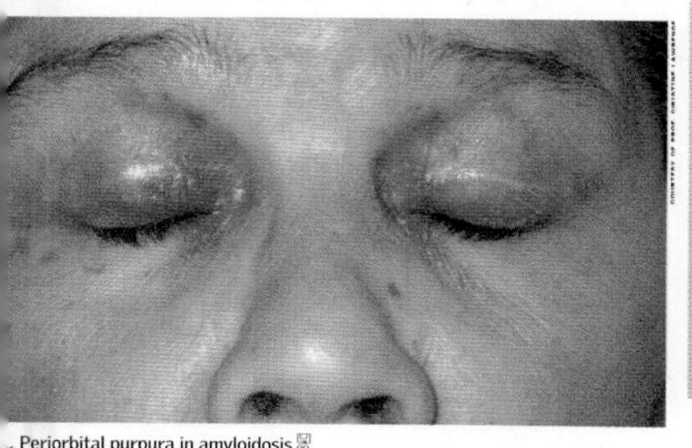

.. Periorbital purpura in amyloidosis.

COURTESY OF OTM

Isotope scan in
oidosis showing
of amyloid de-
on in the liver and
n.

Erythrocyte sedimentation rate (ESR)

Normal range: <20mm/h.

The ESR is a sensitive but non-specific indicator of the presence of diseas measures how fast RBCs fall through a column of anticoagulated blood over 1 certain proteins cover red cells, these cause RBCs to stick to each other in colu so they fall faster (the same phenomenon as rouleaux on the blood film, p314) main causes of a raised ESR are any inflammation eg infection, rheumatoid arth malignancy, myocardial infarction; or anaemia.

In those with a slightly raised ESR, the best plan is probably to wait a month repeat it. There is a group of patients whose vague symptoms would prompted nothing more than reassurance—were it not for a markedly raised E and in whom there are no pointers to specific disease. The same advice does hold true for those with a very high ESR (>100mm/h), where there is a predictive value for disease. In practice, most have signs pointing to the caus one survey, serious underlying disease later found in such patients incl myeloma, giant cell arteritis, abdominal aneurysm, metastatic prostatic carcin leukaemia, and lymphoma. Therefore, it would be wise (after history examination) to consider these tests: FBC, plasma electrophoresis, U&E, PSA, C and abdominal X-rays, ± biopsy of bone marrow or temporal artery.

ESR also rises with age. A simple, reliable way to allow for this is to calculat upper limit of normal, using the Westergren method, to be (for men) age in ye 2. For women, the formula is (years+10) ÷ 2.

Some conditions *lower* the ESR, eg polycythaemia (due to ↑red cell concentrat and sickle-cell anaemia. Even a slightly raised ESR in these patients should pr one to ask: *What else is the matter?*

Haematology

Plasma viscosity (PV)

Normal range: 1.50–1.72mPa/s.

In many laboratories, this has replaced the ESR, as it is less affected by ana and results can be produced in 15min. The PV is affected by the concentratio large plasma proteins and is raised in the same conditions as the ESR. The PV ESR are both raised in chronic inflammation and are less affected by acute cha under 24h in duration. The CRP is more sensitive in acute change (see p678).

Hyperviscosity syndrome

This occurs if the viscosity of blood rises enough to impair the microcirculati affects patients with a very high red cell count (haematocrit >50), white cell c (>100×10^9/L), or plasma components (usually immunoglobulins).

Causes: Polycythaemia rubra vera (↑red cells), acute or chronic leuka (↑peripheral blast cells), myeloma (p352), Waldenström's macroglobulina (p354, as IgM is larger and so ↑ viscosity more than the same amount of Ig

Presentation: Features include lethargy, confusion, spontaneous bleeding: GU CNS disturbance, visual disturbance, and retinopathy: engorged retinal v haemorrhages, exudates, and a blurred disc. The visual symptoms ('slow retinopathy') may be described as 'looking through a watery car windsc (Other causes of slow-flow retinopathy are carotid occlusive disease and Takay disease: p704).

Treatment: Urgent treatment is needed which depends on the cause. Venese is done in polycythaemia. Leucopheresis in leukaemias to remove white Plasmapheresis in myeloma and Waldenström's: blood is withdrawn via a pl exchange machine, the supernatant plasma from this is discarded, and the returned to the patient after being re-suspended in a suitable medium.

he spleen and splenectomy

ne spleen was a mysterious organ for many years; we now know that it plays a tal immunological role by acting as a reservoir for lymphocytes, and in dealing ith bacteraemias. Splenomegaly is a commonish problem and its causes are vided into *massive* (into the RIF) and *moderate*.

auses of massive splenomegaly CML, myelofibrosis, malaria (hyperreactive alarial splenomegaly), leishmaniasis, 'tropical splenomegaly' (idiopathic—Africa, E Asia), and Gaucher's syndrome.

loderate splenomegaly: See p624. • Infection (eg EBV, endocarditis, TB, alaria, leishmaniasis, schistosomiasis) • Portal hypertension (liver cirrhosis), Haematological (haemolytic anaemia, leukaemia especially CML, lymphoma) Connective tissue disease (RA, SLE) • Others: sarcoidosis, primary antibody eficiency (*OHCS* p198), idiopathic.

plenomegaly can be uncomfortable and may lead to *hypersplenism:* ancytopenia as cells become trapped in the spleen's reticuloendothelial system, ith symptoms of anaemia, infection, or bleeding. Splenectomy may be required severe.

'hen faced with a mass in the left upper quadrant, it is vital to recognize the pleen: • Dull to percussion • It enlarges towards the RIF • It moves down on spiration • You may feel a medial notch • 'You can't get above it' (ie the top argin disappears under the ribs). The last three features differentiate the pleen from an enlarged left kidney. Abdominal USS or CT are used to image the pleen. When hunting the cause for enlargement look for lymphadenopathy and ver disease, eg: FBC, ESR, LFT ± liver, marrow, or lymph node biopsy.

plenectomy Main indications: splenic trauma, hypersplenism, autoimmune aemolysis: in ITP (p330) or warm autoimmune haemolytic anaemia (p324), ongenital haemolytic anaemias. Splenectomy was historically performed for aging in Hodgkin's disease, but CT and MRI have replaced this role. Mobilise arly post-splenectomy as transient ↑platelets predisposes to thrombi. A naracteristic blood film is seen following splenectomy, with Howell–Jolly bodies, appenheimer bodies and target cells (see p314).

The main problem post-splenectomy is lifelong increased risk from infection. ne spleen contains macrophages which filter and phagocytose bacteria. Post-plenectomy infection is caused most commonly by encapsulated organisms: *treptococcus pneumoniae*, *Haemophilus influenzae*, and *Neisseria meningitidis*. educe this risk by giving:[1]

Immunizations:
- Pneumococcal vaccine (p152), at least 2 weeks pre-op to ensure good response, or as soon as possible after emergency splenectomy eg after trauma. Re-immunize every 5–10yrs. Avoid in pregnancy.
- *Haemophilus influenzae* type b vaccine (p381).
- Meningococcal C vaccine.
- Annual influenza vaccine (p390).

Lifelong prophylactic oral antibiotics (phenoxymethylpenicillin). Erythromycin if penicillin allergic.

Patient-held cards alerting health professionals to the infection risk.

Pendants or bracelets to alert medical staff.

Advice to seek medical attention if any signs of infection.

Urgent hospital admission if infection develops, for treatment with broad spectrum antibiotics.

If travelling abroad, warn of risk of severe malaria and advise meticulous prophylaxis, with nets, repellent, and medication.

ne above advice also applies to hyposplenic patients, eg in sickle-cell anaemia coeliac disease.

1 Newland A, Provan D, Myint S. Preventing severe infection after splenectomy. BMJ 2005; 331: 417.

Thrombophilia

Thrombophilia is an inherited or acquired coagulopathy predisposing to thrombo usually venous: DVT or PE (venous thromboembolism: VTE). Special precautions needed in *surgery, pregnancy,* and *enforced inactivity*. Risk is further increased obesity, immobility, trauma (accidents or surgery), pregnancy, and malignancy. Thrombocytosis and polycythaemia may also cause thrombosis (p350). Note o ~50% of patients with thrombosis and a +ve family history have an identifia thrombophilia: others may have abnormalities that are as yet unidentified.

Inherited • ***Activated Protein c (APC) resistance/Factor v Leiden:*** Common cause of inherited thrombophilia. Present in ~5% population, although most will develop thrombosis. Usually associated with a single point mutation in factc (Factor v Leiden), so that this clotting factor is not broken down by APC. Risk venous thromboembolism (DVT or PE) is increased 5-fold in patients who heterozygous for the mutation, and 50-fold in homozygotes. Thrombotic risk increased in pregnancy and those on oestrogens (*OHCS* p257 & p302).
• ***Prothrombin gene mutation:*** Leads to high prothrombin levels and increa thrombosis due to down-regulation of fibrinolysis, by thrombin-activa fibrinolysis inhibitor.
• ***Protein c and Protein s deficiency:*** These vitamin K-dependent factors together to cleave and thus neutralize Factors v and VIII. Heterozygotes defici for either protein risk thrombosis. Skin necrosis also occurs, especially if warfarin. Homozygous deficiency for either protein causes neonatal purp fulminans—fatal, if untreated.
• ***Antithrombin deficiency:*** Antithrombin is a co-factor of heparin, and inhi thrombin. Less common, affects 1 : 500. Heterozygotes' thrombotic risk is grea than Protein c or s deficiency by ~4-fold. Homozygosity is incompatible with l

Acquired Causes: newer '3rd generation' progesterones in the oral contraceptive and the *antiphospholipid syndrome* (APL: p540) when serum antiphospholi antibodies are found (lupus anticoagulant ± anticardiolipin antibody)—predispos to venous *and* arterial thrombosis, thrombocytopenia, and recurrent fetal los pregnant women. In most it is a primary disease, but it is also seen with SLE.

Who to investigate? *Consider special tests if:*

- Arterial thrombosis <50yrs (for APL)
- Venous thrombosis <40y with no risk factors
- Unexplained recurrent VTE
- Unusual site, eg mesenteric/portal vein thrombosis
- Familial VTE or with c contraceptives/pregna
- Recurrent fetal loss (≥
- Neonatal thrombosis

Liaise with a haematologist. Do FBC, film, clotting tests: PT, thrombin time, APTT, fibrinogen concentration. Further tests: APC resistance test, lupus anticoagulant anticardiolipin antibodies, and assays for antithrombin and proteins c an deficiency. Haematologists may advise DNA analysis by PCR for the Factor v Lei mutation if the APC resistance test is +ve, and for prothrombin gene mutat Ideally investigate while well, not pregnant, and not anticoagulated for 1 mo

Treatment Treat acute thrombosis as standard—heparin, then warfarin to tar INR of 2–3 (p335). If recurrence occurs with no other risk factors, lifelong warfa should be considered. Recurrence whilst on warfarin should be treated increasing target INR to 3–4. In antithrombin deficiency, high doses of heparin be needed so liaise with a haematologist. In protein c or s deficiency, mon treatment closely as skin necrosis may occur with warfarin.

Prevention Life-long anticoagulation is not needed in asymptomatic patie Patients should be advised of increased risk of VTE with the Pill or HRT, counselled as regards to the best form of contraception. Patients should also warned of other risk factors for VTE. Prophylaxis may be needed in pregnancy, e antiphospholipid syndrome. Get expert help: aspirin and prophylactic heparin used, as warfarin is teratogenic. Prophylactic SC heparin may also be indicate high risk situations, eg pre-surgery.

ther risk factors for thrombosis

rterial	*Venous*
• Smoking	• Surgery
• Hypertension	• Trauma
• Hyperlipidaemia	• Immobility
• Diabetes mellitus	• Pregnancy, oral contraceptive pill, HRT
	• Age
	• Obesity
	• Varicose veins
	• Other conditions: heart failure, malignancy, inflammatory bowel disease, nephrotic syndrome, paroxysmal nocturnal haemoglobinuria (p324).

r thrombophilia in pregnancy, see *OHCS* p33; for anticoagulant use in egnancy and thromboprophylaxis, see *OHCS* p16.

Immunosuppressive drugs

As well as being used in leukaemias and cancers, these are used in organ a marrow transplants, rheumatoid arthritis, psoriasis, chronic hepatitis, asthma, vasculitis (eg Wegener's, giant cell arteritis, polymyalgia, PAN), inflammatory bo and other diseases (so this page could figure in almost any chapter).

Prednisolone Steroids can be life-saving, but a number of points should be tal into consideration before initiating treatment.

- Certain conditions may be made worse by steroids, eg TB, hypertensi osteoporosis, diabetes: here careful monitoring is needed.
- Growth retardation may occur in young patients, and the elderly frequently more side effects from treatment.
- Interactions: [Prednisolone]↓ by antiepileptics (below) and rifampicin.
- Avoid pregnancy (may cause fetal growth retardation). If breast-feeding a prednisolone >40mg/day, see *BNF*.

Minimize side effects by using the lowest dose possible for the shortest perio time. Give doses in the morning, and alternate days if possible, to minimize adre suppression. Before starting long-term treatment (>3 weeks, or repeated cours observe these guidelines:

- Explain about not stopping steroids suddenly. Collapse may result, as endogen production takes time to restart. ►►See p818.
- Inform about the need to consult a doctor if unwell, and increase the dose steroid at times of illness/stress (eg flu or pre-op).
- Encourage to carry a steroid card saying dose taken, and the reason.
- You *must* warn patients about the listed side effects if they are receiving lo term treatment (over 6 weeks worth): see BOX.
- Avoid over-the-counter drugs, eg NSAIDs: aspirin and ibuprofen (↑risk of DU)
- Prevent osteoporosis if long-term use (p674): exercise, bisphosphonates, calci and vitamin D supplements, smoking cessation advice.

Do not stop long-term steroids abruptly as adrenal insufficiency may occur. Onc daily dose of 7.5mg of prednisolone is reached, withdrawal should be grad Patients on short-term treatment (<3 weeks) can be stopped immediately, unl they have had repeated courses of steroids, a history of adrenal suppressi greater than 40mg daily, or doses at night, where withdrawal should be grad

Azathioprine • SE: p533. • *Interactions:* mercaptopurine and azathioprine (whic metabolized to mercaptopurine) are metabolized by xanthine oxidase (XO). azathioprine toxicity results if XO inhibitors are co-administered (eg allopurin

Ciclosporin This is a calcineurin inhibitor, as is tacrolimus which works in a sim way. It has an important role in reducing rejection in organ and marrow transpl The main SE is dose-related nephrotoxicity. Doses are monitored by blood leve

- Other SE: Gum hyperplasia, tremor, BP↑ (stop if ↑↑), oedema, paraesthes confusion, seizures, hepatotoxicity, lymphoma, skin cancer—avoid sunbathir
- Monitor U&E and creatinine every 2 weeks for the first 3 months, then month dose >2.5mg/kg/d (every 2 months if less than this). ►Reduce the dose creatinine rises by >30% on 2 measurements *even if the creatinine is stil normal range*. Stop if the abnormality persists. Also monitor LFT.
- Interactions are legion: [Ciclosporin]↑ by: ketoconazole, diltiazem, verapamil, Pill, erythromycin, grapefruit juice. [Ciclosporin]↓ by: barbiturates, carbam epine, phenytoin, rifampicin. Avoid concurrent nephrotoxics: eg gentami Concurrent NSAIDs augment hepatotoxicity—monitor LFT.

Methotrexate An antimetabolite. Inhibits dihydrofolate reductase, whicl involved in the synthesis of purines and pyrimidines. See p533.

Cyclophosphamide An alkylating agent. • SE: marrow suppression (monitor F nausea, infertility, teratogenic, haemorrhagic cystitis due to an irritative urin metabolite. There is a slight ↑risk of later developing bladder cancer or leukaer

ide effects of steroid use

ystem:	Adverse reactions:
astrointestinal	Pancreatitis
	Candidiasis
	Oesophageal ulceration
	Peptic ulceration
1usculoskeletal	Myopathy
	Osteoporosis
	Fractures
	Growth suppression
ndocrine	Adrenal suppression
	Cushing's syndrome
NS	Aggravated epilepsy
	Depression; psychosis
ye	Cataracts; glaucoma
	Papilloedema
nmune	Increased susceptibility to, and severity of infections, especially chicken pox.

teroids can also cause fever and leucocytosis; steroids only rarely cause leucopenia.
xplain side effects in terms that patients understand: document this in the notes.

10 Infectious diseases (ID)

Alternative name: Climate chang poverty and pollution

Contents

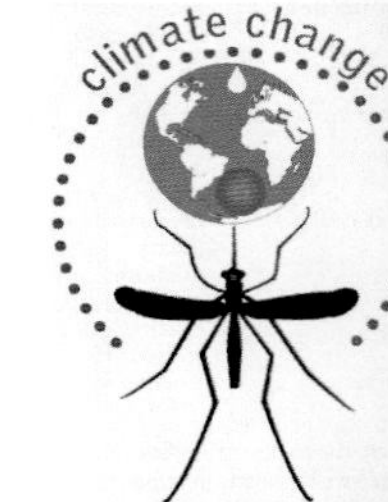

Fig 1. Interactions between polluti global warming, poverty, and infecti are often complex, and often fatal: W estimates that our warming clima partly caused by CO_2 pollution, co tributes to >150,000 deaths and million illnesses/yr. Global warmi compounds poverty, as poor areas a most vulnerable to the effects of cli ate change, which often worse access to clean water, and promot spread of mosquito-borne illness, malaria. Example: clima change→unstable housing→domes chaos→needle sharing ± random se HIV. ►France has a unique plan both issues: a tax on air travel (a cause of CO_2 emissions) to raise fur to fight HIV in developing nations.

We thank Dr Chris Conlon who is our Specialist Reader for this chapter.

K notifiable diseases[ND] ▸Inform the Consultant in Communicable Disease Control (CCDC).

nthrax	Malaria	Rubella
nolera	Measles	Scarlet fever
iphtheria	Meningitis (acute)	Smallpox; tetanus
ysentery (amoebiasis, typhoid, and paratyphoid)	Meningococcal sepsis	Tuberculosis
	Mumps	Typhus
	Ophthalmia neonatorum	Viral haemorrhagic fevers, eg yellow fever; Lassa fever
ncephalitis	Plague	
ood poisoning	Poliomyelitis	
eprosy	Rabies	Viral hepatitis
eptospirosis	Relapsing fever	Whooping cough

< Health Protection Agency www.hpa.org.uk. 020 7759 2700; webteam@hpa.org.uk

etting the balance right in studying infectious diseases

: is not possible for any ID chapter to be constructed so that it has the right alance throughout the world. Many of our readers come from communities here tetanus and malaria are daily problems—whereas, in UK consulting rooms, nest, GU, and ENT infections are likely to dominate.

In parts of Malawi, for example, 70% of adults are HIV+ve, and most atients cannot even begin to mount an immune response to approach the assic descriptions beloved of standard textbooks (eg there is meningititis ithout meningism, and pneumonia without fever etc etc)—and medicine *is* (so seems) no more than the pathology of immunosuppression.

In Western hospital specialist ID practice, the chief problems are:

- Respiratory tract infections (p152–60, and *Emergencies*, p800)
- Hospital acquired infections, eg p154, p408 (MRSA and *C. difficile*) & p238
- Infections in immunocompromised hosts, eg febrile neutropenia (p336)
- Infections associated with general surgery (p556 & p562)
- Infections in intensive care unit patients (examples on p548 & p613)
- Osteomyelitis (*OHCS* p696) and prosthetic joint infections (*OHCS* p706)
- HIV/AIDS (p396–402)
- Illness in a returning traveller (p378).

ll these, however, may be trumped by the arrival of pandemic flu which will nange everything (p155).

But in all areas and in all times, the pitfalls are the same: not taking time to nd out about your patient—where he has been, what his hobbies are (and his ork), and whom he or she has had contact with. Always have a high index of ıspicion for TB, and always remember that ID rarities are often very treatable.

Know your local emerging diseases (p378) and your local multi-resistant rganisms, and remember that it is common to have more than one infection. *Two heads are better than one: so when in doubt, get help.* The best help will ften be well-endowed microbiology and imaging departments. In many places nese are an impossible luxury—one chest x-ray can cost more than the entire early health budget allocated to each patient. If this is your predicament, try ot to give up the unequal struggle: bring your microscope to the bedside)373) and hope for, and campaign for, better times.

urces Many sources have contributed to this chapter—none more generously d at our disposal than the images belonging to Professor Steve Upton from the versity of Kansas. His web site provides very useful educational material, much it in the form of an quiz. See www.ksu.edu/parasitology/546tutorials.

The classification of pathogens

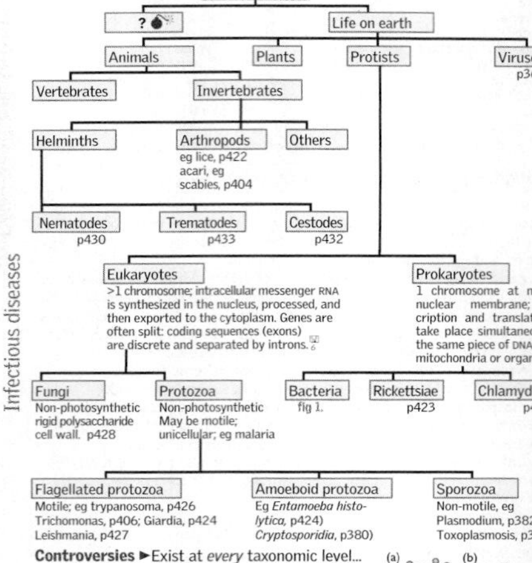

Controversies ►Exist at *every* taxonomic level...

- ***What is life?*** If a thing is organic and converts nutrients into progeny it is alive. If it does not do this, it is either non-living, dead, dying, or male. The average mind is always surprised to learn that long before birth, baby girls have their full complement of eggs for populating the next generation; but for biologists this fact is not so astounding: it is a proof of Aristotle's dictum that the defining essence of life is that it has a plan for its own survival and continuity.[8]
- ***Are viruses alive?***
- ***How many kingdoms?*** Seven, according to some: Archaebacteria, Eubacteria, Protozoa, Chromista (mainly photosynthetic; newly elevated to kingdomhood),[9] Plantae, Eumycota, Animalia. All Eumycota are fungi, and two of the phyla in Kingdom Chromista are also treated as fungi.[10]
- ***Are kingdoms the highest taxonomic category?*** No. There are 3 over-arching domains (or empires) according to some taxonomists: Archaea, Bacteria (also called Eubacteria), and Eucarya.[11]

(a) (b) (c)
(d) (e) (f)
(g) (h) (i)
(j) (k)

Fig 1. ***Bacteria:*** a coccus, b lococcus (gonococcus), c te of cocci, d streptococcus, e cina (cube of 8), f staphylo in random arrangement. ***Rods***: g bacterium, h bac ***Spiral:*** i vibrio (cholera), j illium, k spirochaete (syphil

xamples of pathogens from various types of bacteria

his table is not exhaustive; it is simply a guide for the forthcoming pages.

ram positive cocci
taphylococci (including MRSA, p408):
coagulase +ve, eg *Staph. aureus*
coagulase –ve, eg *Staph. epidermidis*
treptococci[1] (p408):
β-haemolytic streptococci, eg *Strep. pyogenes* Lancefield[1] group A
α-haemolytic streptococci
Strep. mitior
Strep. pneumoniae (pneumococcus)
Strep. sanguis
Enterococci (non-haemolytic)[2]:
Enterococcus mutans
E. faecalis
Anaerobic streptococci

ram positive bacilli (rods)
erobes
Bacillus anthracis (anthrax: p409)
Corynebacterium diphtheriae (p409)
isteria monocytogenes (p409)
Nocardia species
naerobes:
Clostridium
C. botulinum (botulism: p409)
C. perfringens (gas gangrene: p409)
C. tetani (tetanus: p412)
C. difficile (diarrhoea, p238)
ctinomyces: *Actinomyces sraelii* (p409), *A. naeslundii*
A. odontolyticus, A. viscosus

bligate intracellular bacteria:
hlamydia (p404, p154, OHCS p286)
C. trachomatis: Tropical eye disease
trachoma (OHCS p450)=serovars A–C
GU/cervicitis (p405)=serovars B–K
lymphogranuloma ven. (p404)=L_{1-3}
C. psittaci causes psittacosis (p154)
C. pneumoniae (atypical pneumonia)
oxiella burnetii (p422)
artonella (p422)
hrlichia (p422)
ickettsia (typhus, p423)
gionella pneumophilia (p154)
ycoplasma pneumoniae (p154)

Gram negative cocci
Neisseria: *Neisseria meningitidis* (meningitis, septicaemia)
N. gonorrhoea (gonorrhoea, p406)
Moraxella: *Moraxella catarrhalis* (pneumonia, p411)

Gram negative bacilli (rods)
Enterobacteriaceae (p380 & p410):
Escherichia coli
Shigella species (p414)
Salmonella species (p414)
Citrobacter freundii; C. koseri
Klebsiella pneumoniae; K. oxytoca
Enterobacter aerogenes; E. cloacae
Serratia marascens; Proteus mirabilis
Morganella morganii
Providencia species; Yersinia (*Y. pestis Y. enterocolitica, Y. paratuberculosis*)
Pseudomonas aeruginosa (p410)
Haemophilus influenzae (p410)
Brucella species (p410)
Bordetella pertussis (p410)
Pasteurella multocida (p411)
Vibrio cholerae (p414)
Campylobacter jejuni (p380)

Anaerobes:
Bacteroides (wound infections, p556)
Fusobacterium
Helicobacter pylori (p234)

Mycobacteria: *M. tuberculosis* TB, p386
M. bovis & M. leprae (leprosy, p416)
'Atypical' mycobacteria:
M. avium intracellulare (p398)
M. scrofulaceum, M. kansasii
M. marinum
M. malmoense
M. xenopi, M. gordonae
M. fortuitum, M. chelonae
M. flavescens
M. smegmatis-phlei

Spirochaetes (p418):
Treponema (syphilis; yaws; pinta)
Leptospira (Weil's dis.; canicola fever)
Borrelia (relapsing fever; Lyme dis.)

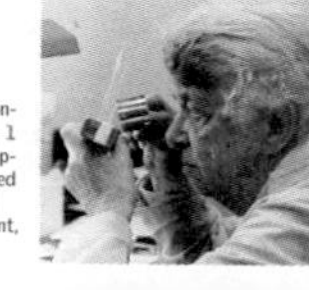

reptococci are grouped by haemolytic pattern (α, β-, or non-ιolytic) or by Lancefield antigen (A–G), or by species. Fig 1 s Rebecca Lancefield (1895–1981) with her hand lens, typ-treps with a variety of M protein-specific antibodies mixed a streptococcal extract by detecting the precipitin in a pipet.
inically, epidemiologically, and in terms of treatment, ococci behave unlike other streps.

DNA viruses—A) *Double-stranded* DNA	
• **Papovavirus**	Papilloma virus: human warts JC virus: Progressive multifocal leucoencephalopathy, PML
• **Adenovirus**	>30 serotypes; 10% of viral respiratory disease 7% of viral meningitis
• **Human herpes viruses**	Alphaherpesvirus$^{\alpha}$ (eg neurotropic) beta-$^{\beta}$ (eg epitheliotropic) and gammaherpesvirus$^{\gamma}$ (lymphotropic Herpes simplex virus$^{\alpha}$ (HSV) 1 & 2 (HHV-1 & HHV-2, p38 Herpes (varicella) zoster virus$^{\alpha}$ (HHV-3, p388) Cytomegalovirus$^{\beta}$—CMV, also called HHV-5, (p392) Herpes virus 6$^{\beta}$ & 7$^{\beta}$ (HHV-6 & 7): roseola infantum (mild, *OHCS* p143); also post-transplant, like CMV Epstein–Barr virus (EBV) (HHV-4, p389)$^{\gamma}$ –infectious mononucleosis (glandular fever) –Burkitt's lymphoma; nasopharyngeal carcinoma
Fig 1. Oral herpes (HSV1)	HHV-8: Kaposi's sarcoma (p694)
• **Pox viruses**	(1) Variola: smallpox (eradicated in 1979; some stocks l (2) Vaccinia, cowpox (3) Orf, cutaneous pustules, caught from sheep (4) Molluscum contagiosum, pearly umbilicated papules, typically seen in children or with HIV.
• **Hepatitis B virus**	See p394
***B) Single-stranded* DNA**	
• **Erythrovirus** (=parvovirus)	Erythema infectiosum (fifth disease, *OHCS* p142) 'slap cheek' appearance ± aplastic crises

RNA viruses—A) *Double-stranded* RNA	
• **Reovirus**	Eg rotavirus (p380), infantile gastroenteritis
***B) Positive single-stranded* RNA**	
• **Picornavirus** (fig 2.)	(1) Rhinovirus, common cold, >90 serotypes (2) Enterovirus (enteroviruses, esp echoviruses, are a important cause of meningoencephalitis and acut flaccid paralysis). See *J Med Virol* 2006 **78** 98 (i) Coxsackie A (meningitis, gastroenteritis) Coxsackie B (pericarditis, Bornholm disease) (ii) Hepatitis A virus (iii) Echovirus (30% viral meningitis) (iv) Poliovirus, p420 (fig 2 ©David Belnap; University of Ut; James Hogle; Harvard Med. Sch
• **Coronavirus**	Eg Urbani SARS-associated coronavirus (Dr Urbani des bed and died in an outbreak in Vietnam in 2003); ►p1
• **Togavirus**	(1) Rubella; (2) Alphavirus (3) Flavivirus (yellow fever, dengue, hepatitis C)
***C) Negative single-stranded* RNA**	
• **Orthomyxovirus**	Influenza A, B, C
• **Paramyxovirus**	Parainfluenza, mumps, measles, respiratory syncitial v
• **Arenavirus**	Lassa fever, some viral haemorrhagic fevers, lymphocytic-choriomeningitis virus (LCM)
• **Rhabdovirus**	Rabies
• **Bunyavirus**	Some viral haemorrhagic fevers

D) Retroviruses

• **Human immunodeficiency virus**—HIV-1, HIV-2. Types A & B predominate in UK (p3

• **Human T-lymphotropic virus**—HTLV-I, HTLV-II. *HTLV-I* causes adult T-cell leukaem lymphoma (ATLL); a definite role in mycosis fungoides & Sézary syndrome controversial. It is mostly asymptomatic, but 1–5% develop ATLL, a fatal expans of virus-infected CD4+ T cells. *HTLV-2* may be passed on by transfusions, inject drug users, or sexually. It may cause tropical spastic paraparesis (p508). I associated with ↑incidence of pneumonia and bronchitis, and arthritis.

Travel advice[1]

Most travel-related illness is not from infections, but due to accidents, violence, myocardial infarction etc. Most infections are due to ignorance or indiscretions. ►*Advice to travellers is more important than vaccination*: eg simple hygiene, malaria prophylaxis, and protective measures. Take time to advise travellers on the benefits of safer sex and the risks of HIV and other STDs. ***Malaria*** is a big killer; see p384 for prevention. ***Rabies:*** vaccinate if post-exposure vaccination is unlikely to be available (or their activities mean risk is ↑—or if they will be in a rabies area for >1month); seek immediate attention if bitten (wash the wound well); see p420. For ***cholera*** and ***traveller's diarrhoea***, see p414 & p380.

Vaccinations L = live vaccine	***Doses Needed***	***Gap between doses: 1st & 2nd***	***2nd & 3rd***	***Booster interval***
Yellow fever[L]	1			10yrs
Typhoid SC (Typhim VI®)*	1			3yrs
Tetanus	3	4 weeks	4 weeks	10yrs
Polio	3	>4 weeks	>4 weeks	10yrs
Rabies pre-exposure	3	7 days	21 days	3yrs
Meningococcal disease	1			3yrs
Japanese encephalitis	3	1–2 weeks	2–4 weeks	2yrs
Tick encephalitis	3	1–3 months	9–12 months	3yrs
Hepatitis A (Havrix monodose®)	1	6–12 months		not needed
if 1–15yrs use Havrix Junior®	1	6–12 months		
Hepatitis B	3	1 month	5 months	not needed if anti HBs >10miu/mL
if travelling soon:	3	1 week	3 weeks	1yr

*If live oral form used, give 3 doses (1 capsule on alternate days, 1h ac, with a cool drink).

If only one attendance is possible, all is not lost (make up *en route*): *malaria prophylaxis/advice:* p384. Suggested vaccines: ***Africa:*** Meningitis, typhoid, diphtheria, tetanus, polio, hepatitis A ± yellow fever. ***Asia:*** Typhoid, diphtheria, tetanus, polio, hepatitis A. Consider rabies and Japanese encephalitis. ***Meningitis and Hajj pilgrimage to Saudi Arabia:*** All >2yrs old *must* be vaccinated against meningococcal meningitis with quadrivalent vaccine (serogroups A,C, Y & W135); must be <3yrs ago but not within the last 10 days. If 3 months–2yrs of age, give 2 doses of the A vaccine separated by 3 months.

S. America: Typhoid, diphtheria, tetanus, polio, hepatitis A ± yellow fever ± rabies.

Travel if immunocompromised: Avoid live vaccines. Hepatitis B vaccine: p263.

Preventing traveller's diarrhoea

Water: If in doubt, boil all water. Chlorination is OK, but doesn't kill amoebic cysts (get tablets from pharmacies). Filter water before purifying. It is important to distinguish between simple gravity filters and water purifiers (which also attempt to sterilize chemically). Choose a unit which is verified by bodies such as the London School of Hygiene and Tropical Medicine (eg the MASTA *Travel Well Personal Water Purifier*). Make sure that all containers are disinfected. Try to avoid surface water and intermittent tap supplies. In Africa assume that all unbottled water is unsafe. With bottled water, ensure the rim is clean and dry. Avoid ice. Other water-borne diseases include schistosomiasis (p433).

Food: Hot, well-cooked food is best. Avoid salads and peel your own fruit. If you cannot wash your hands, discard the part of the food which you are holding (with bananas, careful unzipping obviates this precaution). In those in whom traveller's diarrhoea might be serious, consider a standby course of ciprofloxacin.

1 R Dawood *Traveller's Health*, OUP. Web: www.cdc.gov/travel (USA) or www.doh.gov.uk/traveladvice/index.htm.

Susceptibilities to antibiotics

Contact your local lab as there is much variation

Notes
S=usually sensitive
2=S, but may be 2nd choice
?=may be resistant (esp. if hospital-acquired)
R=resistance likely
0=not appropriate
sources: OTM & GAT (Sanford)

	Amoxicillin/ampicillin	Cefepime	Cefotaxime	Ciprofloxacin	Co-amoxiclav	Colistin	Erythromycin	Flucloxacillin	Gentamicin	Imipenem/meropenem	Metronidazole	Penicillin	Tetracyclines	Ticarcillin/piperacillin/azlocillin	Trimethoprim	Vancomycin/
STAPH AUREUS	R	S	S	?	R	0	?	S	R	2	R	R	?	R	?	S
STREP PNEUMONIAE	?	S	?	?	?	0	?	?	R	2	R	?	?	0	?	S
STREP PYOGENESE	S	S	S	S	S	0	?	S	R	2	R	S	?	0	?	S
ENTEROCOCCUS FAECALIS	?	S	R	S	S	0	R	R	R	2	R	?	R	2	?	S
N. GONORRHOEA	?	S	S	S	?	0	S	0	0	2	R	?	2	0	R	[illegible]
N. MENINGITIDIS	S	S	S	S	S	0	0	0	0	2	R	S	0	0	R	[illegible]
H. INFLUENZI	?	S	S	S	?	0	?	R	0	2	R	?	S	0	S	[illegible]
E. COLI	R	S	S	?	?	0	R	R	S	2	R	R	2	2R	?	[illegible]
KLEBSIELLA	R	S	S	S	R	2	R	R	S	2	R	R	?	2R	?	[illegible]
PROTEUS MIRABILIS	R	S	S	S	S	0	R	R	S	2	R	R	?	2R	?	[illegible]
SERRATIA SPECIES	R	S	S	S	R	0	R	R	S	2	R	R	R	R	?	[illegible]
PSEUDOMONAS AERUGINOSA	R	?	R	?	R	2	R	R	?	2	R	R	R	R	R	[illegible]
ACINETOBACTER BAUMANNII	R	R	R	R	R	2	R	R	R	?	R	R	R	R	R	[illegible]
BACTEROIDES FRAGILIS	R	R	R	R	R	0	?	R	R	2	S	R	?	R	R	[illegible]
CLOSTRIDIUM DIFFICILE	0	0	0	0	0	0	0	0	0	0	S	0	0	0	0	[illegible]

Penicillin-based antibiotics

Penicillin-based antibiotics	*Usual adult dose:*	*In renal failure*
Amoxicillin Uses as for ampicillin but better absorbed PO. For IV therapy, use ampicillin.	250–500mg/8h PO 3g/12h in recurrent or severe pneumonia	↓Dose if cc <1C (cc=creatinine c earance, mL/mi
Ampicillin Broader spectrum than penicillin; more active against Gram –ve rods, but β-lactamase sensitive. Amoxicillin is better absorbed PO.	500mg/4–6h IM/IV	↓If cc <10, give doses every 12-24h
Benzylpenicillin = penicillin G Most streps, meningococcus, gonococcus, syphilis, gas gangrene, anthrax, actinomycosis, and many anaerobes.	300–600mg/6h IV, 2.4g/4h in meningitis. If dose >1.2g, inject at rate <300mg/min	Anaphylaxis ris <1:100,000; hu doses cause Na^+ fits in renal failu
Co-amoxiclav Augmentin=amoxicillin 250 or 500mg + clavulanic acid 125mg confers β-lactamase resistance so broader spectrum, but LFT↑ may rise.	1 tab/8h PO IV form: p411.	If cc 10–50, giv 1 tab/12h; if cc <10, 1 tab/24h
Flucloxacillin For Gram +ve β-lactamase producers (staphylococci).	250–500mg/6h PO ½h before food. 0.5–2g/6h IV	Dose unaltered cc >10
Phenoxymethylpenicillin (=pen. v) Like penicillin G but less active; use as Prophylaxis or to complete IV course.	250–500mg/6h PO; take ½h before food	In severe renal failure, give dos every 12h
Piperacillin Very broad spectrum including anaerobes & *Pseudomonas*. Inactive against *Staphs*. Reserve only for those with severe infection. May be used with aminoglycosides (but not in the same IVI).	Tazocin®= tazobactam 500mg + piperacillin 4g: dose: 4.5g/8h IV over 3–5min	↓Dose if cc↓: cc 10–50: 2.25 6h cc <10: 2.25g/
Procaine penicillin (= procaine benzylpenicillin) Depot injection; good for syphilis; only available on a named patient basis in the UK.	Syphilis: 600mg/24h IM for 14d, gonorrhoea: start dose 3.6g if female, 2.5g if male	Dose unaltered renal failure
Ticarcillin Very broad spectrum, eg *Pseudomonas, Proteus*. Use with an aminoglycoside; more active than azlocillin or piperacillin.	Timentin®=3g ticarcillin +200mg clavulanic acid. Dose: 3.2g/8h IV (/4h in severe infections)	If cc 10–50 dos is 1–2g/8h If cc < 10, dose 1–2g/12h

ntibiotics: cephalosporins

ectrum Many cephalosporins are active against staphs (including β-lactamase ducers), streps (except group D, *Enterococcus faecalis & faecium*), pneumococci, *coli*, some *Proteus, Klebsiella, Haemophilus, Salmonella*, and *Shigella*. 2nd ıeration drugs (cefuroxime, cefamandole) are active against *Neisseria* and *emophilus*. 3rd generation drugs (cefotaxime, ceftazidime, ceftriaxone) have ter activity against Gram –ve organisms. Ceftazidime has less Gram +ve activity p. against *Staph aureus*) and is used in *Pseudomonas* infections.

es Oral cephalosporins (cefaclor, cefalexin, cefuroxime axetil) have a role in UTI, eumonia, and otitis media, but are not 1st-line (unless penicillin-allergic; but 10% l also be cephalosporin allergic). Their major use is parenteral, eg in surgical phylaxis or post-op infection. 3rd-generations drugs (eg ceftriaxone) may be ed in septicaemia. **SEs:** Hypersensitivity; warfarin potentiation.

ntibiotic	Adult dose	Notes For body surface area calculation, see *BNF*
faclor	250mg (max 1g)/8h PO	No dose change in RF
falexin	500mg/8h PO; Max: 4g/24h PO	↓Dose proportionately in RF if CC < 60 if CC <10: 750mg/24h
fepime[4]	1–3g/12h IVI	Good activity against *Pseudomonas*, enterobacter, other resistant Gram –ve organisms and *S. aureus*. If CC 10–50: 1–2g/12h; if CC ≤10: 1g/24h
fpirome[4]	1–2g/12h IV over 5min	Broad spectrum, used in polymicrobial infection; pyelonephritis; pneumonia. Not for MRSA (p408) or bacteroides. Good against enterobacter. In renal failure, load with 1–2g, then if: CC 20–50: 500mg–1g/12h; if CC 5–20: 500mg–1g/24h
fixime	Syrup: ½–1yr: 3.75mL/d 1–4yrs: 5mL/d 5–10yrs: 10mL/d Adults: 200mg/12–24h	Syrup = 100mg/5mL. Active against streps, coliforms, *Haemophilus*, *Proteus* and anaerobes, staphylococci, *E. faecalis*, and *Pseudomonas* are resistant. In RF: normal dose if CC >20mL/min
fotaxime[3]	1–2g/8h IV/IM; max 3g/6h (gonorrhoea: 500mg stat)	Broad spectrum for serious infections only (pneumonia, meningitis). Unreliable activity against *Pseudomonas*. If CC <10, give 2g/24h max. If CC <5 give 1g stat, then halve dose.
fradine	250–500mg/6h PO or 500mg–1g/12h PO or 500mg–2g/6h IM/IV	Less active than cefuroxime In RF load with 750mg, then give 500mg at frequency dictated by CC: if CC > 20: 500mg/6h CC 5–20: 250mg/6h CC < 5: 250mg/50–70h
tazidime[3]	UTI: 500mg–1g/12h Other: 1–2g/8h Max: 1g/8h if elderly Route: IV/IM but avoid IM if dose >1g	Broad spectrum, incl. most *Pseudomonas* but bad *vs* Gram +ves; for bad infections only; may help in blind ℞ of neutropenic sepsis (cefepime is better). In RF load with 1g, then if: CC 31–50: 1g/12h CC 16–30: 1g/24h CC 6–15: 500mg/24h CC ≤ 5: 500mg/48h
ftriaxone[3]	1–4g daily IM/IV; give ≤1g at each IM site. Use IVI, not IV, if dose >1g	Many Gram +ve and –ve infections. Used in meningitis (p370), pre-colonic surgery, and gonorrhoea. No activity against *Listeria*, enterococci, and *Pseudomonas*. Can use in RF if CC >10 (or limit dose to 2g/day and check levels)
uroxime	250–500mg/12h PO 750mg–1.5g/8h IV/IM; Max IV: 3g/8h. Give per 12h if CC 10–50.	Broad spectrum & good Gram –ve activity. Used in: surgical prophylaxis; cholecystitis; post-op infections; severe pneumonia.

breviations: RF = renal failure; CC = creatinine clearance; CC[M] = CC/1.73m² body area; [4] = 4th eration cephalosporin; not all are available in the UK; [3] = 3rd generation. Source: *GAT* 2006

Antibiotics: others

Antibiotic (and uses)	**Adult dose**	**Notes** CC=creatinine clearance, mL/r
Amikacin See gentamicin.	7.5mg/kg/12h IV; (~50% 12–18h if CC 10–50)	Resistance growing, but l common than for gentam
Azithromycin See clarithromycin, also good against *N. gonorrhoea*.	500mg PO for 3d.	SE: see erythromycin.
Chloramphenicol Rarely used 1st-line. May be used in typhoid fever and *Haemophilus* infection. Also in blind ℞ of meningitis if patient allergic to both penicillins and cephalosporins. Avoid late in lactation and pregnancy.	12.5mg/kg/6h PO or IV; 25mg/kg/6h may be used in septicaemia or meningitis	SE (rare): marrow aplas (check FBC often), neuri GI upset. Avoid long or repeated courses and in liver impairment or if CC <10mL/min. *Interaction* warfarin, rifampicin, phenytoin, sulfonylurea phenobarbital.
Ciprofloxacin Used in adult cystic fibrosis, typhoid, *Salmonella*, *Campylobacter*, prostatitis, and serious or resistant infections. Avoid overuse.	250–750mg/12h PO 200–400mg/12h IVI over ≥½h (over 1h, if 400mg used). If CC 10–50, give 50–75% of this dose.	A good oral anti-pseudomonal agent. β-lactamase-resistant. Halve dose if CC <10. SE: rashes, D&V, LFT ↑; potentiates theophylline
Clarithromycin A macrolide, like erythromycin, used for: *S. aureus*, streptococci, *Mycoplasma*, *H. pylori*, *Chlamydia*, MAI (p399).	250–500mg/12h PO for 7–14d. *H. pylori:* 500mg /12h PO for 1wk as triple therapy (p235). MAI may need 12wks (p399) If CC 10–50 give 75%.	Halve dose if CC <30. *Interactions:* ergot, warfarin, carbamazepin theophyllines, zidovudin never use with terfenad or pimozide.
Clindamycin Active against Gram +ve cocci including penicillin resistant staph, and anaerobes.	150–300mg/6h PO; max 450mg/6h PO. 0.2–0.9g/ 8h IV or IM (by IVI only, if >600mg used)	Stop if diarrhoea occurs (pseudomembranous col p239). Used in *Staph.* Bone/joint infection.
Co-trimoxazole Sulfameth-oxazole 400mg + trimetho-prim 80mg. 1st choice in *Pneumocystis jiroveci (=P. carinii*, p398), toxopl-asmosis and nocardia. **NB:** can act against *S. aureus*.	960mg–1.44g/12h PO/IVI; see *Pneumocystis* (p398)	SE (mostly ∵ sulfonamic elderly at ↑risk): jaundic Stevens–Johnson syndro marrow depression; folate↓. If CC 15–30, ha dose. Avoid if CC <15. C G6PD deficiency.
Doxycycline Used in travellers' diarrhoea, *Chlamydia*, leptospirosis, syphilis, and brucellosis.	200mg PO on 1st day then 100mg/24h; max 200mg/d in severe infections	As for tetracycline, but may be used in renal failure.
Erythromycin Macrolide, used in penicillin allergy. Used 1st line in atypical pneumonia, p154.	250–500mg/6h PO (≤4g/d in *Legionella*). 6.25–12.5mg/kg/6h IVI (adult and child)	SE: D&V; phlebitis in IV us Potentiates warfarin, the phylline, terfenadine, erg amine, carbamazepine.
Fusidic acid/sodium fusidate Anti-staph agent (incl. some MRSA, p408); used in osteomyelitis.	500mg/8h PO; 500mg/ 8h IVI over 6h; avoid intravenous route if possible.	Combine with another anti-staphylococcal dru SE: GI upset, reversible changes in LFTs.

Infectious diseases

ntibiotic (and uses):	Adult dose	Notes (eg use in renal failure)
entamicin Spectrum is de but poor against reps & anaerobes, so use th a penicillin ± metron-azole. Synergy with amp-llin against enterococci. r serious Gram –ve inf-tions or SBE prophylaxis.	►p738. *Once daily IV dose* over 15min: 5.1mg/kg[LBW] (7mg if very ill); aim for **peak** serum level of 16–24µg/mL 1h after dose 3; **trough:** <1µg/mL; levels *not* needed if only one stat dose used, eg in UTI.	►**Nomogram**, p738; ¾ dose if CC≈60mL/min. ½ dose or avoid if CC ≈30–40 mL/min (get help). **Avoid:** prolonged use, concurrent furosemide, use in pregnancy/myasthenia gravis.►Do U&E often. SE: oto- and nephrotoxicity.
nipenem (+cilastatin) ry broad spectrum: am +ve and –ve ganisms, anaerobes and robes. β-lactam stable.	250–500mg/6h IVI; if CC 50–90: ¼–½g/6–8h; if 10–50: ¼g/6–12h. CC <5: dialyse. High doses risk seizures.	Pregnancy/lactation: avoid. SE: fits; D&V; myoclonus, eo-sinophilia, WCC↓, Coombs' +ve; LFT abnormal. See package insert eg if <70kg.
nezolid An oxazolidinone tibiotic used against RSA, VISA, & VRE[1]	600mg/12h PO/IVI over 1h (even if renal failure); SE: D&V, gastritis, T°↑, tin-nitus, neuropathy, WCC↓	May cause pancytopenia if ≥2wks use; monitor FBC. CI: BP↑↑, phaeochromocytoma, carcinoid, thyrotoxicosis
eropenem e imipenem.	½–1g/8h IVI, max 2g/8h (if CC 10–50, 1g/12h)	Causes fewer fits than imipenem.
etronidazole 1st choice anaerobes, *Gardnerella, tamoeba histolytica, & ardia lamblia;* use PO in eudomembranous colitis.	400mg/8h PO. PR dose: 1g/8h for 3d then 1g/12h. IVI dose: 500mg/8h for ≤7d	Disulfiram reaction with alcohol, interacts warfarin, phenytoin, cimetidine; care if LFT↑. Pregnancy/breast-feeding: avoid high-doses.
inocycline pectrum > tetracycline.	100mg/12h PO	As tetracycline, but more SE (hepatitis, pneumonitis).
trofurantoin UTI.	50mg/6h PO with food	CI: CC <50.
xytetracycline	250–500mg/6h PO	See tetracycline.
fampicin[UK] = rifampin[US] ycobacteria, prophylaxis meningitis contacts.	Dose example: 450–600mg/24h PO before breakfast. See TB, p386	Caution in liver disease. Interferes with contra-ceptive Pill. SE: p386.
icoplanin See vanco-ycin, but not given PO.	IV/IM: 400mg/12h for 3 doses, then 200mg/24h	$t_{½}$ longer than vancomycin. (200mg/48h if CC 10–50)
tracycline Used in ronic bronchitis; 1st line in *hlamydia*, Lyme sease, mycoplasma, ucellosis, rickettsia.	250–500mg/6h PO ac 500–1000mg/12h IVI (not if liver disease). IV preparation not available in UK.	Avoid if <12yrs old, in pregnancy, and if CC <50. Absorption ↓by iron, milk, and antacids. SE: photosensitivity, D&V.
bramycin As ntamicin; better against *eudomonas.*	1mg/kg/8h IVI Dose↓ in renal failure	Monitor levels; reduce dose if CC ≤50
imethoprim Used in UTI, PD. Dose in prophylaxis: 0mg/24h PO.	200mg/12h PO	SE: depressed marrow, D&V. CC 10–50: 200mg/18h PO. CC <10: 200mg/24h PO.
ncomycin PO: pseudo-embranous colitis if etronidazole is contra-dicated; IV: MRSA or other am +ve organisms (not ysipelothrix species).	125mg/6h PO; ½g/6h IVI over 1h or 1g/12h IVI over 100min; do peak level 2h post-IVI, eg after dose 3; aim for <30mg/L & <10mg/L pre-dose 4	In renal failure, get help; nomograms are available, eg SE: renal and oto-toxicity. Do not overuse (↑risk of multiple resistance, p408).

1 MRSA, p408; VISA: vancomycin-intermediate resistance *S. Aureus*; VRE: vanco. resistant enterococci.

Blind ℞ for presumed septicaemia, pneumonia, et

History: A detailed history may reveal the source of infection: ask ab respiratory, GI and GU symptoms; any travel or possible immunocompromise?

Examination: Look at the temperature chart and examine for localizing signs

Tests: If time allows and the patient is not too ill, culture all possible sour before treating (blood, sputum, urine, faeces, skin/wound swabs, CSF, aspirat Also check FBC, ESR, CRP, U&E, LFT, clotting, serology, malaria film, acute phase ser save serum for virology, CXR, ABG (as clinically indicated). MSU/urine dipstick.

Prognosis: Poor if very old or young, BP↓, WCC↓, P_aO_2↓, DIC, hypothermia.

Treatment: Follow local guidelines. Change to the most appropriate drug o sensitivities are known. Treatment of most infections should not exceed Intravenous antibiotic therapy should preferably not exceed 48h; review the n and change to PO if possible. If in doubt, ask a microbiologist.

Infection	Treatment (*pen.=penicillin,* p36
Urinary tract infection	Trimethoprim 200mg/12h PO
Cellulitis	Co-amoxiclav (or flucloxacillin + pen., p368
Wound infection	Await swab result; if ill, flucloxacillin 1g/6h
Pneumonia	
Mild community-acquired	Amoxicillin 500mg/8h PO
Possible atypical pneumonia	Erythromycin 500mg/6h PO
Severe community-acquired	Cefuroxime 1.5g/8h IV + erythromycin 12.5mg/kg/6h IV
Hospital-acquired	Cefuroxime 1.5g/8h IV or Tazocin® 4.5g/8h
Meningitis (p806)	
Meningococcus *Pneumococcus*[2] *Haemophilus*	▸▸Ceftriaxone 2g/12h IV + benzylpenicillin 2.4g/4–6h slowly IV (1.2mg IM stat, pre-hospital)
Listeria	Add ampicillin 2g/4h IVI
If HSV encephalitis possible	Add aciclovir 10mg/kg/8h IVI
Endocarditis (p136)	
Empirical therapy	Flucloxacillin 2g/6h IV + gentamicin IV, p7
Strep. Viridans	Benzylpenicillin[2] + gentamicin IV
Enterococcus faecalis	Amoxicillin[2] + gentamicin IV
Staph. aureus or *epidermidis*	Flucloxacillin[2] + gentamicin IV
Prosthetic valve	Vancomycin + gentamicin + rifampicin
Osteomyelitis/Septic arthritis	Flucloxacillin 1g/6h IV then clindamycin PC
Septicaemia	
Urinary tract sepsis	Cefuroxime 1.5g/8h IV + gentamicin 5mg/kg *once daily* is typical max dose; rare 7mg/kg is needed, less if obese; p738
Intra-abdominal sepsis	Cefuroxime 1.5g/8h IV + metronidazole 500mg/8h IVI
Meningococcal sepsis	▸▸Ceftriaxone 2g/12h IV
Neutropenic sepsis	Tazocin® 4.5g/8h IV[1] over 3–5min + netilmicin eg 6mg/kg IV once daily
Skin or bone source	Flucloxacillin 1g/6h IV
Unknown cause	Cefuroxime 1.5g/8h IV + gentamicin 5.1–7mg/kg IV once daily, p7 + metronidazole 500mg/8h IVI

►All IV doses should be given slowly, eg over 5m

1 Tazocin = piperacillin 4g (p763) + tazobactam 500mg.
2 Use vancomycin if penicillin-allergic, or you suspect resistance to penicillins (eg MRSA)

sing a side-room laboratory (near-patient testing)

he main advantage of doing your own lab work is that it enables you to have itelligent chats with lab staff, and encourage their diligence (lab staff make rrors out of boredom; amateurs make errors out of ignorance). The great thing to understand the sources of error—and allow for them at the bedside.

rine Get used to microscoping your own urines. Dipstick analysis is OK but nisses casts etc (p278). If dipstick +ve for leucocytes, nitrites, blood, or protein, end for culture and testing for antibiotic sensitivities. If +ve for glucose, uspect diabetes. If heavily positive for protein, check 24h collection for protein.

lood Use universal precautions: all specimens could be HBV, HCV, or HIV +ve. To nake a ***thick blood film*** (malaria diagnosis), use fresh whole blood: a small blob nould be spread out somewhat untidily to cover ~1cm², thinly enough for watch ands to be seen through. The untidiness is helpful to the microscopist because it rovides areas of varying thickness, some of which will be ideal for what is often tricky task. Label and allow to dry. To make a ***thin blood film***, put 1 drop of ood near one end of the slide. Take another slide, place its end in the drop of lood, angled at 45°. Push the slide away from you to spread the blood into a nin film (practice makes perfect!). Allow the film to dry, fix in methanol for 5s, nen stain as follows.

eishman's stain: Cover with 10 drops of Leishman's stain. After 30s add 0 drops of water. Leave for 15min. Pick up the slide with forceps (to avoid urple fingers) and rinse in fast-flowing tap water—for 1s only. Allow to dry. ow examine under oil immersion. Note red cell morphology. Do a differential hite count. Polymorphs have lobed nuclei. Lymphocytes are small (just larger nan red cells) and round, having little cytoplasm. Monocytes are larger than mphocytes, but similar, with kidney-shaped nuclei. Eosinophils are like olymorphs, but have prominent pink-red cytoplasmic granules. Basophils are are, and have blue granules. See p309 & p317 for images. Learn to use a white ell counting chamber—don't expect this to be as accurate as electronic nethods.

eld's stain is easy to use and gives good (and quick) results for malaria, and lows detection of trypanosomes and filaria. Dip the slide in solution A for 5s nd solution B for 3s. Dip in tap water for 5s after each staining. Stand to y. Examine thick films for at least 5min before saying that it is negative. **NB:** ard ***serology tests***, eg *Para*Sight F® are available for *P. falciparum*, but cannot eplace microscopy as they are not 100% sensitive and parasites are not uantified (needed to plan treatment).

us (Gram stain) Make a smear; fix by gentle heat. Flood slide with cresyl violet or 30 seconds (s). Wash in running water. Flood with Lugol's iodine for 30s. Vash with running water. Decolourize with acetone for 1–3s until no blue colour ns out. Counterstain for 30s with neutral red or safranin. Wash and dry. Gram ve organisms appear blue-black; Gram –ve ones look red, but are easier to miss.

ear-patient chemistry In one sense this is less taxing than the above tests—e skill lies in the people who made the reagents easy to use. A problem is uality control and the black box effect: when we put a strip into a machine, eg measure cardiac enzymes, we cannot see the workings of the black box: it just ves a deceptively accurate-looking figure. Frequent calibration of equipment is nly a partial answer to this. It is only after you have spent a long time trying to et good results from near-patient analysers, and comparing paired samples ith the lab, that one appreciates the reproducibility, and reliability of the formal b. ►Speed of reporting is useless if you cannot trust the results.

Drug abuse and infectious diseases

►Always consider this when there are evasive answers or unexplained findi especially in younger patients. Ask direct questions: 'Do you use any drugs? H you ever injected drugs? Does your partner use any drugs? Do you share need Have you ever had an HIV test? How do you finance your drugs?' List drugs u and prescribed drugs, with names of prescriber. ***Behavioural clues:***

- Temporary resident seen by GP 'Just passing through your area'.
- Demands analgesia/antiemetics. Knows pharmacopoeia well: 'I just need s pethidine for my renal colic/sickle-cell crisis'.
- Erratic behaviour on the ward; unexplained absences; mood swings.
- Unrousable in the mornings; agitation from day 2.
- Heavy smoking; strange smoke smells (cannabis, cocaine, heroin).

Physical clues:

- Acetone or glue smell on breath (solvent abuse).
- Small pupils (opiates), reversed by naloxone.
- Needle tracks on arms, groin, legs, between toes; IV access hard.
- Abscesses and lymphadenopathy in nodes draining injection sites.
- Signs of drug-associated illnesses (endocarditis, p136; AIDS, p396, viral hepat

Common and possible presentations in drug abusers	
Unconscious	p774 Benzodiazepines (if in ITU consider flumazenil 0.2mg IV o 15s then 0.1mg/min as needed, to 1mg (2mg if on ITU).
Psychosis or agitation	Ecstasy (p827), LSD, amphetamine, anabolic steroids, benzodiazepines. Haloperidol may help (p13).
Asthma or dyspnoea	Is there opiate-induced pulmonary oedema? NB: Asthma may follow the smoking of heroin.
Lung abscess	Right-sided endocarditis (Staph) until proved otherwise
PUO	Is it endocarditis, eg with no cardinal signs (p136)?
Fever/PUO/shivering/headache	Do blood cultures; start eg gentamicin (p371 & p738).
Hyperpyrexia	p827
Abscesses	If over injection site, then often of mixed organisms. Eg on injecting suspended tablets into groin.
DVT	Any compression damage (compartment syndrome)? Do
Pneumonia	Pneumococcus, haemophilus, TB, pneumocystis (p398).
Tachyarrhythmia	(If young); cocaine, amphetamines, endocarditis.
Jaundice	Hepatitis A, B, or C; anabolic steroids (cholestasis).
'Glandular fever'	May be presentation of HIV seroconversion illness.
Osteomyelitis	Including spinal. *Staph. aureus*/Gram –ve organisms.
Constipation	If severe, opiate abuse may be the cause.
Blindness	Consider fungal ophthalmitis ± endocarditis.
Runny nose	Opiate withdrawal (+colic /diarrhoea, yawns, lacrimati dilated pupils, insomnia, piloerection, myalgia, mood↓; c occur in neonates if mother is an opiate abuser); cocain use.
Neuropathies	(And any odd CNS signs) Consider solvent abuse.
Infarctions	(eg of spinal cord, brain, heart): suspect cocaine use.

e vocabulary of drug abusers

e first step in helping a drug abuser is to communicate. To understand what he she is telling you, the following may be helpful.

nphetamines	Speed; whiz; Billy; pink champagne; crystal methamphetaime = 'meth' or 'chalk'
nyl-nitrate	Goldrush; poppers; snappers
biturates	Barbs; idiot pills
caine	Coke; Charlie; uncle; the white; the nice; snow; rock; crack; nuggets; wash; gravel
ydrocodeine	DFs
ug-induced sleep	Gauching; nodding; going on the nod
ug intoxication	Stoned; off it; bladdered; ripped; wiped out; off my box
roin	Smack; the nasty; gear; brown; scag; hit; Harry
stasy (MDMA)	E; X; echo; disco biscuit; love drug; XTC
roin with ecstasy	Party pack (2-for-1 deal when pusher's business is low)
brile reaction	Bad hit
ter	A bud (usually a cigarette tip, through which drugs are drawn before being injected)
ecting bcutaneous/IM/failed) bclavian)	Hitting up; jacking up; cranking; having a dig (skin popping/muscle popping/failed) (pocket shot)
tamine	Special K (Home Office class C drug, like cannabis); a 'K hole' is a dissociative state (hole in consciousness, p477)—may be a ketamine prelude to 'ego death'.
	Acid; trips; cardboard; tabs
arijuana	Weed; pot; draw; ganja; grass; resin; Mary; hash
thadone	Mud
edles	Spikes; nails
taining drugs	Score (selling drugs=deal)
	Angel dust; KJ; ozone; missile
yseptone ampoules	Amps
ostitution	Working the block/square; doing business; on the game; on the batter; flogging one's golly
ostitute's client	Mush; punter
ooting gallery	Supervised surroundings for injecting (conforming with some mythical British Standard of Hygiene)
oplifting	Grafting
oking heroin	Chasing the dragon (bonging=smoking cocaine)
ringes	Works; tools (barrel of a syringe=gun)
nazepam	Temazies
urniquet	Key
nted by police	'On me toes'; keeping head down
ite heroin	China white
thdrawing from opiates	Turkeying, clucking
piclone	Zim-zims

eral management of recreation drug users on the ward A non-judgemental roach will produce better cooperation and may avoid self-discharge. Establish n rules of acceptable ward behaviour. NSAIDs are useful for pain relief. Don't scribe benzodiazepines or clomethiazole. Methadone may be needed if opiate icts develop unacceptable withdrawal signs or symptoms in hospital. Get help. ommercial sex workers need an STD screen, speculum exam (*OHCS* p242), and vical cytology as carcinoma-*in-situ* is common (*OHCS* p273). Screen for syphilis 19), HIV (p396) and hepatitis B (vaccination, p263, use gloves); give safe sex safe injection advice. ►Liaise with community teams. See *OHCS* p362.

Pyrexia of unknown origin (PUO)

Contrary to Gustave Flaubert, most fevers are not caused by plums, melons, A
sunshine, etc.,[38] but by our immune responses to self-limiting viral infecti
resulting in production of interferons and cytokines. A PUO is defined as a fever
>3wks, eg resisting diagnosis after a week in hospital. Signs of bacteraemia incl
confusion, renal failure, neutrophilia, ↓plasma albumin,[39] and ↑CRP, p678.

Causes[40] Infection (23%); connective tissue diseases (22%); tumours (20%); d
fever (3%); miscellaneous (14%). PUOs resist diagnosis in 25% of patients.

- **Infections** *Abscesses* (lung, liver, subphrenic, perinephric, pelvic); empyer *bacteria* (*Salmonella, Brucella, Borrelia*, leptospira, p418); rheumatic fever; SBE (may be culture −ve, eg Q fever); TB (CXR may be normal, so culture sputur urine); other *granulomas* (actinomycosis, toxoplasmosis); *parasites* (eg amoe liver abscess, malaria, schistosomiasis, trypanosomiasis); fungi; HIV; typhus Asking ***'Where have you been'*** is vital: find an expert on that area, or else will miss diagnoses you may have never heard of, eg melioidosis (*Burkholde* p435, the chief cause of fatal bacteraemic pneumonia in parts of SE Asia).
- **Neoplasms** Especially *lymphomas* (any pattern: Pel–Ebstein fever, p344, is ra Occasionally *solid tumours* (GI; renal cell). Patients may be unaware of feve
- **Connective tissue disease** Rheumatoid arthritis, polymyalgia rheumatica, St disease, giant cell arteritis, SLE, PAN, Kawasaki disease.
- **Others** Drugs (T°↑ may occur months after starting but remits within days stopping; eosinophilia is a clue); pulmonary embolism; stroke; Crohn's; ulcerat colitis; sarcoid; amyloid; familial Mediterranean fever—recurrent polyseros (peritonitis, pleurisy) + fevers, abdominal pain, and arthritis; treat with colchic cause: gene defect, eg at 16p13.[42]

Examples of intermittent fevers Always think of malaria; septicaemia (eg fr
diverticular disease); UTI; pelvic inflammatory disease; IE/SBE; TB; filarial fever—
rarities, eg: amyloid; *Brucella*; occult thromboembolism;[43] Castleman's disease

- ***Daily spikes:*** Abscess; TB;[45] schistosomiasis. ***Twice-daily spikes:*** Leishmanias
- ***Saddleback fever*** (eg fever for 7d, then normal for 3d): Colorado tick fe Borrelia; Leptospira; dengue; Legionnaire's disease;[47] Ehrlichia[48] (p422).
- ***Longer periodicity:*** Pel–Ebstein (eg from lymphoma, p344).
- ***Remitting*** (diurnal variation, not dipping to normal): Amoebiasis; mala Salmonella; Kawasaki disease; CMV; TB.[49]

History Work; hobbies; sexual activities; eating raw animals; drug abuse; immunosuppression; distant travel (►p378); animal (or people) contacts; bites; cuts; surgery; rashes; diarrhoea; drugs (eg non-prescription); immunization; sweats; weight↓; lumps; and itching. ***Examine:*** Teeth; rectum; vagina; skin lesions; lymph nodes; hepatosplenomegaly (p624); nails; joints; temporal arteries; retina (Roth spots of SBE/IE, fig 1).

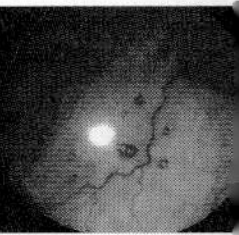

Fig 1. Roth spots: ΔΔ: mi
infarcts from hypertens
HIV,[50] connective tis
disease, anaemia, Behçe
viraemia, hypercoagulabi

Symptom-patterns Dialogue with experts ± decision support to diagnose fever with any other symptom. See www.emispdp.com.

ıges in the investigation of PUO

ıge 1 (the 1st days): FBC; ESR; U&E; LFT; CRP; FBC; blood cultures (several, from 'erent veins, at various times; prolonged culture for Brucella); baseline serum virology; HIV; sputum MC&S (specify TB); MSU; stools (ova; cysts; parasites); CXR. ' 'septicaemic' but blood culture –ve, exclude malaria, and typhus, p423.

ıge 2 Repeat history/exam daily for new symptoms and newly-remembered ıptoms or travel history. Protein electrophoresis; CT (chest; abdomen). eumatoid factor; ANA; antistreptolysin titre; Mantoux; ECG; marrow; lumbar ıcture. Consider withholding drugs, one at a time for 48h each. Consider ıporal artery biopsy (p542). HIV tests.

ıge 3 Follow leads uncovered, eg echocardiography; CT; IVU; liver biopsy; explor-ry laparotomy; bronchoscopy. Repeat serology (any change since 1st sample?).

ıge 4 ?Treat for TB, endocarditis, vasculitis, or trial of aspirin/steroids.

w and newly re-emerging infectious diseases

ny diseases preoccupying consultants in infectious diseases are new or vly re-emerging: food-borne *E. coli*, waterborne *Cryptosporidium*, airborne ȷionnaire's disease, blood-borne hepatitis C, and HIV have come to the fore y in the last 30 years. Why have these years been so tumultuous in the ID rld? The short answer is greed and exploitation. Examples: 1) Each year we ısume 4 centuries-worth of animal and plant life, so promoting ecological tability. 2) Economic drive builds dams (↑breeding grounds for vectors by ers of magnitude) and forces land development, putting people closer to tors, eg ticks, mosquitoes, and rodents. Intensive farming makes it easier infectious agents to jump the species barrier. Examples of viruses recently ssing species barriers to humans are hantavirus, haemorrhagic fever ıses, arboviruses, Nipah & Hendra viruses, avian influenza, monkeypox virus, s (p155), and CJD, p688). Consider also these 9 interacting causes:

amine and war (± threats of bioterrorism, eg with anthrax and smallpox).
Inprecedented movements of peoples, their animals and their parasites ıixing genes, cultures, customs, and behaviour, eg eating raw molluscs and rabs facilitates toxoplasma, trematode, cestode and nematode zoonoses.
licrobial adaptation and change making antibiotics less successful.
luman susceptibility to infection (increased immunocompromise).
limate change leading to shifting ecosystems and economic disaster (p362).
luman demographics (economic development and land use)—and related to n increasing world population (rising at ~86 million per year).
ourism and commerce. West Nile virus, for example, reached New York from s ancestral home in the Middle East on a bird carried by a ship or plane. Vith SARS, the precise tourists, businessmen, and doctors who took the virus rom Hong Kong to Hanoi, Singapore, and Toronto have been identified.
echnology and industry—easy to blame, but also part of the solution. Food ecurity for millions living on <$1/day depends on increasing rice yields thr-ugh high-tech genetic manipulation to produce insect- and saline resistant ice. Good crops from disease-free plants mean disease-free people.
Breakdown of public health measures with poverty and social inequality.

n we win against infectious diseases? No! All we can do is live with them. help us do this in ways which are not too destructive, we need robust public lth surveillance institutions, political will, quarantine laws, and above all, nness and cooperation. SARS and its spread emphasize this in a graphic y: as the Chinese and other less-than-open societies have found out, when it nes to reporting infectious diseases, lying means dying.

Winning or losing is the wrong image: infectious diseases have made us who are. The ability of genomes to produce and emit DNA/RNA sequences allows rizontal transmission of genes, and is one of the main motors of evolution.

GREED: GLOBAL WARMING: EMERGING DISEASES: POVERTY: WAR

Diagnosing the tropical traveller

Tropical medicine emergency advice^UK^ Liverpool 0151 708 9393, London 7388 9600, Birmingham 0121 766 6611. **In every ill traveller, consider:**

1 ***Malaria*** (p382 & p384): Fever, rigors, headaches, dizziness, 'flu sympt diarrhoea, thrombocytopenia. *Complications:* anaemia, renal failure, pulmo oedema, cerebral oedema. *Diagnosis:* serial thick and thin blood films. Mosquitoes may stowaway in luggage causing malaria in non-tropical area

2 ***Typhoid*** (p414): Presents with fever, relative bradycardia, abdominal pains cough, constipation, lymphadenopathy, headache, splenomegaly ± rose s (rare). *Complication:* GI perforation. *Diagnosis:* blood or marrow culture.

3 ***Dengue fever (DF)*** (p420): Presents with fever, headache, myalgia, rash (flus or petechial), thrombocytopenia, and leucopenia. *Diagnosis:* serology.

4 ***Amoebic liver abscess*** (p424): T°↑, jaundice, RUQ pain. Do ultrasound.

Examine all over: any bites/eschar, p423? Do serology, thick films & blood cultu

►***Know your locally re-emerging diseases!*** Examples: TB, Lyme disease, le spirosis, malaria, typhus, cholera, salmonella, hepatitis A, shigella, mumps, mea brucellosis. **NB:** A visit to the tropics doesn't preclude mundane fevers, eg '

Jaundice Think of viral hepatitis, cholangitis, liver abscess, leptospirosis, typh malaria, dengue fever, yellow fever, haemoglobinopathies.

Gross splenomegaly Malaria, visceral leishmaniasis (kala-azar).

Diarrhoea & vomiting (p380 & p238) *E. coli* (Travellers' diarrhoea) is commor Consider *Salmonella, Shigella, Campylobacter, Giardia lamblia, Vibrio cholerae,* (p380). See p238 for general management. If diarrhoea prolonged, cons protozoal infection of small bowel or tropical sprue (p272). In HIV: cryptospor microsporidia, and *Isospora belli* (need special stains—see fig 1, OPPOSITE).

Hepatosplenomegaly See p624; malaria; *Brucella*; typhoid; typhus; leishmani

Respiratory symptoms Common respiratory pathogens (p154), typhoid, *Legion* TB, Q fever, histoplasmosis, Löffler's (p696), HIV ± pneumocystosis. Do CXR &

Arthritis Gonococcus; septicaemia; viruses (Ross river, Chikungunya *et al* p421).

Erythema nodosum (p267) Causes: streps, TB, leprosy, fungi, Crohn's disease, u ative colitis, sarcoidosis, pregnancy, drugs (sulfonamides, contraceptive stero

Anaemia Hookworm, malaria, kala-azar, haemolysis, malabsorption.

Skin signs Scabies (itchy allergic rash + burrows, eg in finger web-spaces; p4 *OHCS* p608), orf (pustules), molluscum contagiosum (pearly, punctate, papu leprosy (p416, anaesthetic, hypopigmented areas), tropical ulcers, typhus ('esc =scab), leishmaniasis (ulcers/nodules), onchocerciasis (itchy nodules), my (nodules—larvae of various insects), drug reactions. Transitory migratory swell gnathostomiasis, Calabar swellings (loa loa, p431), urticaria, contact dermat

Acute abdomen Perforating typhoid ulcer, toxic megacolon in amoebic or baci dysentery, sickle-cell crisis, ruptured spleen.

Rarities to consider ►Use local emergency isolation policy.

- ***Rabies*** (p420) and other CNS viral infections, eg encephalitis (p388 & p80
- ***Yellow fever:*** (p420) Suspect in travellers from Africa.
- ***Lassa fever:*** Occurs in Nigeria, Sierra Leone, or Liberia. ***Signs:*** Fever; exuda sore throat; face oedema; collapse. **Δ:** *PCR/EM;* serology. **℞:** Isolate and refe
- ***Marburg and Ebola virus:*** Seen in Sudan, Zaire, Kenya. ***Signs:*** Fever, myalgia, pleuritic pain, hepatitis, shock, and bleeding tendency. A maculopapular rash app on day 5–7 and desquamates in <5d. Patients may bleed from all orifices gums. **Δ:** *PCR* or electron microscopy; serology. **℞:** Isolate and refer.
- ***Viruses causing haemorrhage:*** Dengue, Marburg, Lassa, Ebola, Crimea-Co fever, haemorrhagic fever with renal syndrome, yellow fever. ►See p420.

►Travel details (areas visited; immunization; prophylaxis; disease exposure) very important, even if you cannot interpret yourself, so seek expert opinion e

cubation times for fever in the tropical traveller

The incubation times below are typical, but considerable variation occurs.

14 days	14 days to 6wks	>6wks
ndifferentiated fever		
alaria	Malaria	Malaria
phoid	Typhoid	Hepatitis B or E
ptospirosis	Leptospirosis	Kala-azar
engue fever	Hepatitis A or E	Lymphatic filariasis
ckettsiae	Acute schistosomiasis	Schistosomiasis
cute HIV infection	Acute HIV infection	Amoebic liver abscess
ver with CNS signs		
ral and bacterial men-gitis and encephalitis	East African Trypanosomiasis	Rabies
ast African ypanosomiasis	Rabies	
oliomyelitis		
ver with chest signs		
fluenza	Tuberculosis	Tuberculosis
gionellosis	Q fever	
fever		
cute histoplasmosis		
RS		
ver with diarrhoea, p380		

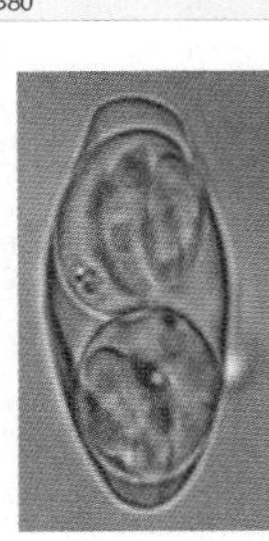

Fig 1. Sporulated (infective) oocyst of the protozoan *Isospora belli*; oocysts are passed unsporulated, but can sporulate in 1-3 days, depending on T°, and the presence of molecular oxygen.

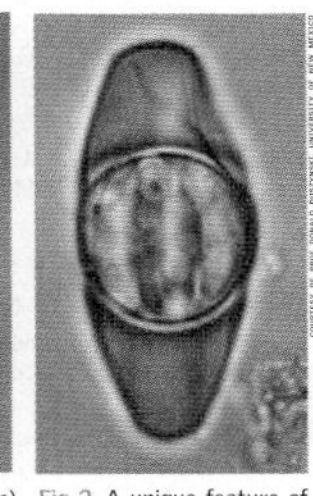

Fig 2. A unique feature of *I. belli* oocysts is that some develop irregularly, having 1 sporocyst with 8 sporozoites (Duszynski 1999). Isosporiasis is an AIDS-defining illnesses (diarrhoea ± haemorrhagic colitis).

Gastroenteritis

Ingesting certain bacteria, viruses, and toxins is a common cause of D&V (p' p238). Contaminated food and water are common sources, but often no spe cause is found. Ask about details of food and water taken, cooking method, tim onset of symptoms, and whether fellow-diners were affected. Ask a swimming, canoeing, etc. **NB:** *Food poisoning is a notifiable disease (p363) in th*

Organism/Source	Incubation	Clinical features	Notes/sources of infection
Staph. Aureus	1–6h	D&V, P, hypotension	Meat
Bacillus cereus	1–5h	D&V	Rice
Red beans	1–3h	D&V	
Heavy metals, eg zinc	5min–2h	V, P; with zinc, (delayed fever ± 'flu-like features after exposure at work)	
Scrombotoxin	10–60min	D, flushing, sweating erythema, hot mouth	Fish
Mushrooms	15min–24h	D&V, P, fits, coma, hepatic and renal failure	Image: p423
Salmonella	12–48h	D&V, P, fever, septicaemia	Meat, eggs, poultry
C. perfringens	8–24h	D, P afebrile	Meat
C. botulinum	12–36h	V, paralysis	Processed food
C. difficile	1–7d	Bloody D, P, GI perforation; toxic megacolon; hospital acquired (1000 deaths/yr[UK])	Antibiotic-associated; and getting more virulent (eg str BI/NAP1 with 20-fold ↑ in to A & B production)
Vibrio parahaemolyticus	12–24h	Profuse D; P, V	Seafood
Vibrio cholerae	2h–5d	See p414	Water*
Campylobacter	2–5d	Bloody D, P, T°↑	Milk, poultry, water*
Listeria		Meningoencephalitis; 'I've got flu'; miscarriages	Cheese, pâtés
E. coli type 0157	12–72h	Cholera/typhoid-like;*	Haemolytic-uraemic syn, p30(
Y. enterocolitica	24–36h	D, P, fever	Milk*
Cryptosporidium[1]	4–12d	D in HIV	Cow→water→man
Giardia lamblia	1–4wks	p424 (D, malabsorption)	*Nappies, cats, dogs, crows
Entamoeba histolytica	1–4wks	See p424	*
Noroviruses, eg Norwalk =SRVS (small round structured viruses)	36–72h	Fever, D & projectile V 'winter vomiting illness'	Fecal-oral (vomit is infectious very contagious, and commo
Rotavirus	1–7d	D&V, fever, malaise	* (RotaTeq vaccine ?available f infants aged from 6 weeks)
Shigella	2–3d	Bloody D, P, fever	Any food

V=vomiting; D=diarrhoea; P=abdominal pain. *May be food- or water-borne.

Tests ***Stool microscopy/culture*** if from abroad, an institution, or in day car an outbreak is suspected. In these circumstances culture of the food source help.

Prevention Hygiene; if abroad, avoid unboiled/unbottled water, ice cubes, sa and peel own fruit. Eat only freshly prepared hot food (or *thoroughly* rewarn

Management Usually symptomatic. Maintain *oral fluid intake* (±oral rehydra sachets). For severe symptoms (but not in dysentery), give *antiemetics* prochlorperazine 12.5mg/6h IM) + *antidiarrhoeals* (codeine 30mg PO/IM or lo amide 4mg stat, then 2mg after each loose stool). *Antibiotics are only indicat systemically unwell, immunosuppressed or elderly*; resistance is common.

- Cholera: tetracycline reduces transmission.
- *Salmonella*: ciprofloxacin 500mg/12h PO, 200–400mg/12h IVI over 60mi
- *Shigella* & *Campylobacter*: ciprofloxacin as above.

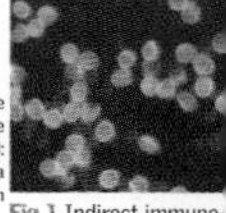

Fig 1 Indirect immuno-fluorescence (antibody to the inner oocyst wal

1 Cryptosporidium (fig 1) is a tiny fungus (5μm) causing diarrhoea/cramps—life threatening if HIV+ve; self-limiting if CD4 ≥100); if <100, 14L of diarrhoea can be lost/d (bad news). It's a UK crime to sell water with >1 oocyst/10L. Spread: unboiled water; cattle. If found in stool, quantify excretion. If ℞ needed, ask a microbiologist (℞ often fails); optimize anti-HIV ℞. Consider: nitazoxanide 0.5g/12h PO for 14d (if >12yrs old); azithromycin + paromomycin 1g/12h PO.

ve immunization stimulates the immune system (humoral+cellular immunity). *sive immunization* uses pre-formed antibody (nonspecific or antigen-specific).

ıe	Immunization (DoH[UK] 2006)
onths	**Pediacel®**, ie 5-in-1 diphtheria + tetanus + acellular pertussis + inactivated polio + haemophilus B (HIB); if prem, still give at 2 mths; can give if ≤10 yrs if missed vacs **+ Prevenar®** (7-valent pneumococcal).
onths	**Pediacel® + Neisvac C® or Meningitec®** (Meningitis C vaccine)
onths	**Pediacel® + Prevena® + Neisvav C or Meningitec®**
mths	**Menitorix®** (*H. influenzae* with meningitis C)
nths	**MMR II®L** or **Priorix®L** (Measles, Mumps & Rubella) **+ Prevenar®**
-5yrs	**Repevax®** or **Infanrix-IPV®** (Diphtheria, tetanus, pertussis & polio) **+ Priorix®L** or **MMR II®L**
18⁺yrs	**Revaxis®** (low-dose diphtheria, tetanus, inactivated polio; can also be used for primary vaccination if >10yrs).
' age	BCG[L]: (not for everyone, since 2004[uk]) If at ↑risk of TB, eg for all in high-risk areas (eg London), or in groups at ↑risk, eg TB contact, or (grand)-parents or from high-prevalence country, ie >40/100,000/yr—or a visitor to such a country for >1 month. May start at 3 days old. ***Hepatitis B:*** p263; universal (WHO advice) or if at ↑risk. ***MMR***[L] may be given at any age the above is missed. One-off ***pneumococcal vaccine*** with 23-valent Pneumovax II® (**Prevenar®**×2, as above, if <2yrs old); yearly ***'flu vaccine*** if caring for a vulnerable person or if chronic heart, chest, liver, or renal disease; DM; immunosuppression (eg HIV +ve, cirrhosis, on chemotherapy, or spleen function↓, eg ∵ coeliac or sickle cell disease). Consider 2nd pneumococcal vaccine if at ↑risk after >5yrs.
ılts	Tetanus and diphtheria booters (**Revaxis®**, as above). Travellers: p367.

' *acute febrile illness is a contraindication to any vaccine*. Give live vaccines ɜr together, or separated by ≥3wks. Caution with live vaccines in patients who mmune-deficient (transplants, cancer chemotherapy, steroids, HIV infection)— : expert advice. ►*Contraindications to vaccines*: see *OHCS* p151.

ıcille Calmette–Guérin (BCG) Live attenuated anti-TB vaccine (works in up to ɔ of subjects for ~10yrs, but there is much variation). Make a 7mm blanched weal veen the top and middle ⅓ of arm (deltoid's insertion) or, for cosmetic reasons, ıpper, outer thigh. Expect to feel marked resistance as the injection is given. If, ng injection, propagation of the weal stops, you are going too deep: re-insert ıeedle. A swelling appears after 2–6 weeks, developing into a papule or small r. Avoid air-occluding dressings. SE: pain, local abscess. CI: pyrexia, oral steroids, ıis, or eczema at vaccination site, immune pareses (eg AIDS and malignancy).

ıtoux test (p386) Offered to those at risk of TB (see BCG, above). It is now not ínely required for those <6yrs old being referred for BCG on the above criteria.

vel p367. Expert advice: *schools of tropical medicine*: London: 020 7636 8636; ·pool: 0151 708 9393); National Travel Health Network and Centre, www.nathnac.org. *lvice to travellers is more important than vaccination*: eg simple hygiene, ıria prophylaxis, and protective measures (mosquito nets, safe sex advice, etc).

ıunization in special situations If *splenectomized/hyposplenic (eg sickle cell):* polyvalent pneumococcal; Hib; annual 'flu vaccine. *Chronic lung, heart, liver or ey disease, diabetes:* pneumococcal; annual 'flu vaccine.

:her details Hepatitis B (p263); 'flu; pneumococcal (p152); meningococcal ngivac® = group A & C), for short-term use, eg travel abroad. Leave ≥2wks after ine MCC before giving Mengivac®. Ideally this gap should be >6 months, but lren <5yrs may not have responded well to their 1st dose of MCC.

MalariaND: clinical features and diagnosis

Malaria is one of the commonest causes of fever and illness in the tropics. ►Ch
for it in any sick patient from an endemic area. *Plasmodium falciparum* kills
million people each year. Summary of species differences:
P. vivax: incubation 10–17 days, '*benign tertian malaria*', symptoms 48hrly.
P. ovale: similar to *P. vivax*; except untreated infection lasts less long.
P. malariae: incubation 18–40 days, symptoms 72hrly, untreated infections ~2(
P. falciparum: incubation 7–10 days, symptoms 36–48hrly, fulminating disea

Plasmodium protozoa, injected by the female *Anopheles* mosquito (~
sporozoites/bite), multiply in RBCs (>10^8–10^{12} trophozoites per infection) caus
haemolysis, RBC sequestration, and cytokine release. Protective factors: sickle-
trait, Melanesian ovalocytosis, G6PD deficiency, certain HLA B53 allele (in many r
Europeans, enables killing of parasite-infected hepatocytes by cytotoxic T cel

P. falciparum* malaria *Incubation: ~7–10d. Most travellers present wit
2 months. ***Symptoms:*** Non-specific flu-like prodrome: headache, malaise, mya
and anorexia followed by fever and chills ± faints. Classic peric
fever (peaking every 3rd day, ie tertian) and rigors are unusual initially. ***Sig***
Anaemia, jaundice, and hepatosplenomegaly. No rash or lymphadenopa
Complications: *Cerebral malaria* (p385): confusion; coma ± fits. Focal si
unusual. May have variable tone, extensor posturing; upgoing plant
dysconjugate gaze; teeth-grinding. In children, seizures are common. Morta
~20%. *Metabolic (lactic) acidosis* giving laboured deep (Kussmaul's) breathir
also a major cause of death. *Anaemia* is common due to haemolysis of parasit
and unparasitized RBCs, and may be particularly severe in young child
Hyperparasitaemia (>5% of RBCs parasitized). *Hypoglycaemia* occurs in sev
malaria (25% of children, 8% of adults), pregnancy, or with quinine therapy. *A*
renal failure from acute tubular necrosis, sometimes with haemoglobin
(*'blackwater fever'*), and *pulmonary oedema* (ARDS, p170) are important cause
death in adults. Shock may develop in severe malaria (*algid malaria*) f
supervening bacterial septicaemia, dehydration or, rarely, splenic rupture
pregnancy, the risk of death (mother or fetus) is high (*OHCS* p27).
chemoprophylaxis in pregnant women in endemic areas of transmission.

Benign malaria has a very low mortality. The acute febrile illness is very simila
that of uncomplicated *falciparum* malaria. Incubation periods may be longer
10% of *P. malariae* malaria presents over 1yr after infection. Complicati
Relapse occurs as parasites lie dormant in the liver (*P. vivax* and *ovale*) or at
levels in the blood (*P. malariae*). Nephrotic syndrome (glomerulonephritis)
occur in chronic *P. malariae* infection.

Diagnosis Serial thin & thick blood films (needs much skill, don't always believe
reports, or reports based on thin film examination alone); if *P. falciparum*, wh
the level of parasitaemia? Rapid stick tests now available if microscopy canno
performed or previously treated seriously ill patient: see p373 for *Para*Sigh
Serology not useful. Other tests: FBC (anaemia, thrombocytopenia), clotting (
p336), glucose (hypoglycaemia), ABG/lactate (lactic acidosis) U&E and creati
(renal failure), urinalysis (haemoglobinuria, proteinuria, casts), blood culture.

Poor prognostic signs (Severe *falciparum* malaria) Age <3yrs, pregna
respiratory distress, fits, coma, absent corneal reflexes, papilloedema, pulmor
oedema, HCO_3^- <15mmol/L, plasma or CSF lactate >5mmol/L, glucose <2.2mm
hyperparasitaemia (>5% RBCs or 250,000/μL), Hb <5g/dL, DIC, creati
>265μmol/L. If ≥20% (or >10^4/μL) of parasites are mature trophozoite
schizonts, the prognosis is poor, even if few parasites seen (reflects critical mas
sequestered RBCs); malaria pigment in >5% of neutrophils.

alaria prophylaxis: a rough guide for adults and children

e	Weight (kg; a better guide than age)	Chloroquine (base) weekly (mg)	Proguanil daily (mg)	Mefloquine weekly (mg)	Doxy-cycline daily (mg)
2wks	<6	37.5	25	—	—
yr	6–9.9	75	50	62.5	—
3yrs	10–15.9	112.5	75	62.5	—
7yrs	16–24.9	150	100	125	—
12yrs	25–44.9	225	150	187.5	—
dult	>45	300	200	250	100

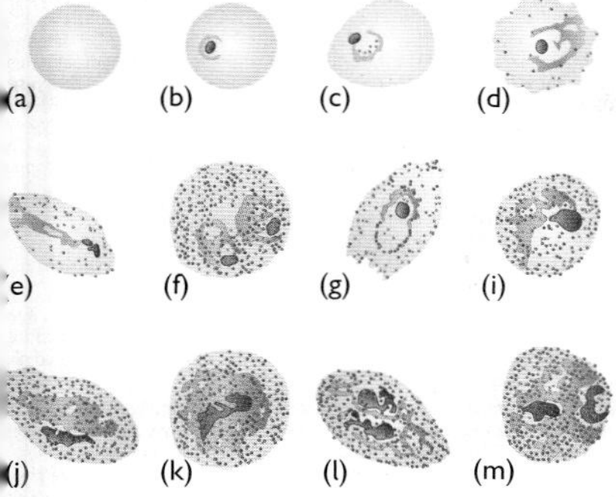

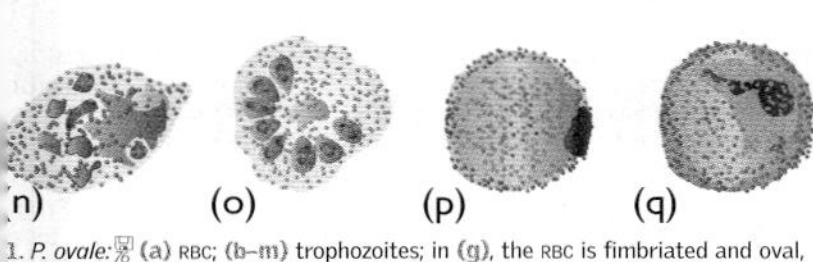

AFTER PAINTINGS BY GERTRUDE NICHOLSON, IN OATNEY GR. THE PRIMATE MALARIAS; U.S. DEPT. OF HEALTH, EDUCATION AND WELFARE

1. *P. ovale:* (a) RBC; (b–m) trophozoites; in (g), the RBC is fimbriated and oval, ng the species its name; (l–o) schizonts, ie segmentation; (p–q) ♀ & ♂ etocytes.

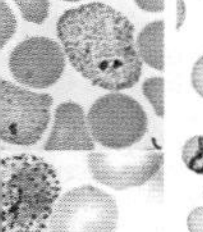

2. *P. vivax* forms partly en by uffner's dots

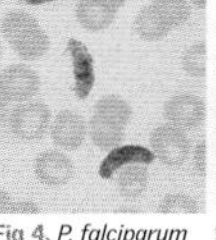

Fig 3. *P. malariae* ring & band forms from two specimens

Fig 4. *P. falciparum* sausage-shaped gametocytes within RBC ghosts

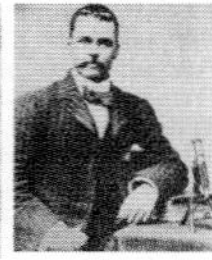

Fig 5. Ronald Ross who first described the malaria lifecycle

COURTESY OF PROF. S. UPTON, KANSAS UNIV.

Malaria: treatment and prophylaxis

Treatment If species unknown or mixed infection, treat as *P. falciparum*. Nea *P. falciparum* is now resistant to chloroquine and in many areas is also resista Fansidar® (pyrimethamine + sulfadoxine). If in doubt consider as resis Chloroquine is the drug of choice for benign malarias in most parts of the worl chloroquine-resistant *P. vivax* occurs in Papua New Guinea, Indonesia, some are Brazil, Colombia, and Guyana. Never rely on chloroquine if used alone as prophy

Falciparum malaria: As multi-drug resistance is common, artemisinins-comb ions are best (WHO). Artemisinins are 'OK' in children and in 2nd & 3rd trimeste pregnancy. If able to swallow and no severe signs:[1] **artesunate (AS)-amodiac (AQ)**; if a fixed combination pill is available (AS 100mg + AQ 270mg), the dose pills once daily for 3d. If aged ~7–13yrs, it is 1 pill/d for 3d. OR **arteme lumefantrine** (Riamet®) 4 tabs/12h for 6 doses. OR **dihydroartemis piperaquine** (2.1/16.8mg/kg daily for 3d, eg 3 Artekin® tabs/d) OR **artesu (4mg/kg/d for 3d) + mefloquine** (eg 5 Larium® tabs stat). These are better **quinine** regimens (eg 600mg quinine salt/8h PO for 7d, + **doxycycline** 100mg or **clindamycin** 450mg/8h for 5d). If seriously ill,[1] parenteral ℞ is needed (I artesunate, IM for artemether)—see BOX; take to ITU (fluid monitoring is vital may require a CVP line). NB: Resistance to artemisinins may have started.

Benign malarias: Give chloroquine PO as 600mg base, 300mg 6h later, 300mg/24h for 2d. If *P. ovale*, give primaquine 15mg/24h for 14d (30mg/2 *vivax*; CI pregnancy) after chloroquine to treat liver stage and prevent rel Screen for G6PD deficiency first.

Other treatments: Tepid sponging + paracetamol for fever. Transfuse if se anaemia. Consider exchange transfusion if patient severely ill. Treat 'algid' ma as malaria + bacterial shock (p778). Monitor TPR, BP, urine output, blood glu frequently. Daily parasite count, platelets, U&E, LFT.

Examples of prophylaxis ►*Prophylaxis does not give full protection*. Risk very variable; get local advice. Avoid mosquito bites between dusk and dawn: long-sleeved clothes, use repellents (DEET), insecticide-treated bed nets.

Except for Malarone® and mefloquine, take drugs from 1wk before trav reveal any SE) and continue for 4wks after return. None are required if just vis cities of East Asia. There is no good protection for parts of SE Asia.

Prophylaxis: Check up-to-date sources. *Caribbean, North Africa, Middle East:* cl quine ± proguanil. *S. America, sub-Saharan Africa, SE Asia, Oceania:* mefloc doxycycline, or Malarone®. South Asia: *chloroquine + proguanil.* Indonesia forests of Malaysia & Sarawak: *chloroquine + proguanil.* ►If area has poor me care and not pregnant, carry standby treatment course (eg Riamet®, Malarone

Adult prophylactic doses: **Chloroquine** (base[2]): 300mg/wk PO. **Progu** 200mg/24h PO. **Doxycycline**: 100mg/24h PO. **Mefloquine**: 250mg/wk PO for a if no risk of pregnancy; start 2½ weeks before travel. **Malarone®**: 1 tablet/2 starting 1d before travel, and continuing till 7d after return from malarious (other prophylactic drugs need to be continued for 4 weeks).

Antimalarial SE: *Chloroquine:* headache, psychosis, retinopathy (chronic use *Fansidar®:* Stevens–Johnson syndrome, erythema multiforme, LFT↑, blood dyscr *Primaquine:* Epigastric pain, haemolysis if G6PD-deficient, methaemoglobinaen *Mefloquine:* Nausea, dizziness, dysphoria, insomnia, neuropsychiatric signs, lon Ideally start prophylaxis 3wks prior to travel to reveal any SE. Avoid mefloqu • Low risk of chloroquine-resistant malaria, eg East African coastal resort • Pa family history of epilepsy, psychosis • Need for delicate work (pilots[etc]) • Ri pregnancy within 3 months of last dose. Interactions: quinidine, halofantrin *Malarone®*: Abdominal pain, nausea, headache, dizziness.

1 Prostration, consciousness↓, fits, respiratory distress, unable to drink, uncontrolled vomiting roscopic haemoglobinuria, jaundice, systolic BP ≤70mmHg, bleeding/DIC, inability to sit or stand.
2 150mg chloroquine base ≈ 250mg chloroquine phosphate (PO) ≈ 200mg chloroquine sulfate (

erebral malaria (*P. falciparum*)

alciparum malaria is one of the great killers, because it is swift and difficult to 'eat: so get expert help in anyone who could have travelled abroad particularly the last few months, who is feverish with ↓consciousness. But fever is not *'ways* a feature of malaria, and signs may be unusual if prophylaxis has been ven, and is partly effective. The central event in severe *Falciparum* malaria is equestration of parasitized erythrocytes in the microvasculature of vital organs. eath rate: ~1 million deaths/yr, worldwide.

ey questions What is the parasite count, the plasma bicarbonate and the 'eatinine? Are there complications: shock (algid malaria), metabolic acidosis, ypoglycaemia, renal failure, or acute respiratory distress syndrome (ARDS, p170).

reatment Take advice. Transfer to ITU. Give **artesunate** (if *immediately* available[1]) ' **quinine** (dihydrochloride) 20mg salt /kg IV (max 1.4g) over 4h, then after 8h ive 10mg/kg (max 700mg) over 4h every 8h (or give by constant IVI of 0mg/kg/d after loading dose).[2] Give IV until the patient can swallow; complete the ourse orally. Monitor for hypoglycaemia. **Artemether** (3.2mg/kg followed by 6mg/kg daily) is another alternative. In the UK, artemether is available on a amed patient basis: get local advice. Don't wait for an ideal drug if a good ternative is to hand: delay is fatal.

swallowing OK and no complications (shock; ARDS, renal failure) give either:

- **Artemether**-lumefantrine (80/480mg twice daily for 3d with food).
- **Malarone®** (atovaquone + proguanil; 4 tabs once daily for 3d with food).
- **Quinine** (600mg salt/8h PO for 7d), with either doxycyline 200mg daily or clindamycin 600mg/12h for 7d PO.

'U monitoring in cerebral malaria

- Fluid requirements vary widely; careful fluid management is critical. Haemofilter early if renal failure. Ventilate early if pulmonary oedema.
- Consider exchange transfusion in very seriously ill patients if feasible.
- Monitor blood lactate (or bicarbonate) and glucose: quinine may cause hypoglycaemia. Also do LFT and clotting studies and cross-match blood if haematocrit <20%.
- Repeated U&E (and arterial blood gases if ARDS).
- Arrange repeated skilled microscopy to monitor the parasite counts.

xpect a >75% decrease in the parasite count by 48h of treatment.

itfalls

- Failure to take a full travel history, including stop-overs in transit and failure to check if the patient has already received treatment which might make the blood smear negative.
- Delay in treatment while seeking lab confirmation.
- Failure to examine enough blood films before excluding the diagnosis.
- Belief that drugs will work, when the parasite is often one step ahead.
- Not having IV quinine available immediately. (Quinidine is an alternative.)
- Not observing *falciparum* patients closely for the first few days.
- Forgetting that malaria is an important cause of coma, deep jaundice, severe anaemia, and renal failure in the tropics.

Infectious diseases (ID)

Artesunate dose 2.4mg/kg as a bolus at 0, 12 & 24h, then daily. It is not universally available, but 'rks better than quinine (15% mortality *vs* 22%), and has fewer SEs, White N 2005 *Lancet* 366 717 RTC
Do not give **quinine** loading doses if the patient has already definitely had quinine, quinidine or floquine in last 24h. Warn about tinnitus. In some countries, IV quinine is not available; quinidine conate is an alternative, eg a loading dose of 10mg/kg over 1–4h then 0.02mg/kg/min IVI by pump 72h or until can swallow. ECG monitoring is essential when quinidine is given (not needed for quinine). p or ↓infusion if BP↓ or QTc prolonged by >25% (p84). Further details: A Omari 2004 *BMJ* **328** 154

Tuberculosis (TB)ND:

TB-with-HIV: p397; BCG: p3

TB kills 2 million people/yr; it is the cause of death of most people with HIV. T why the poor stay poor—and then die. If HIV+ve, risk↑ if CD4 cell count↓; ESR↑; m coinfections; poor nutrition; high viraemia. **UK incidence** 7000/yr; 350 deaths

Diagnosis Whenever TB is suspected, try hard to get the relevant clinical sam (sputum, pleural fluid, pleura, urine, pus, ascites, peritoneum, or CSF) for cultur establish the diagnosis and drug sensitivities. **Active case-finding:** ►Get advic testing contacts. In high-incidence areas, most transmission (≥80%) occurs out the household—so it may be necessary to spread your net wide.

Microbiology: Send multiple sputum for MC+S for AFB (acid-fast bacilli), ple aspiration and biopsy (p752) if there is an effusion. If sputum is nega bronchoscopy with biopsy and bronchoalveolar lavage may be helpful. Biopsy suspicious lesions in liver, lymph nodes or bone marrow. AFB are bacilli that re acid–alcohol decolourization under Ziehl–Neelsen (ZN) staining. Cultures unde prolonged incubation (up to 12 weeks) on Lowenstein–Jensen medium.

TB PCR: Allows rapid identification of rifampicin (and likely multi-drug) resista Occasionally useful for diagnosis in sterile specimens.

Histology: The hallmark is the presence of *caseating granulomata*.

CXR signs: Consolidation, cavitation, fibrosis, and calcification in pulmonary T

Immunological evidence of TB may be helpful:

- *Tuberculin skin test:* TB antigen is injected intradermally and the cell-medi response at 48–72h is recorded. A positive test indicates that the patient immunity. It may indicate previous exposure or BCG. A strong positive probably means active infection. *False negative tests* occur in imm suppression, including miliary TB, sarcoid, AIDS, lymphoma.
- *Mantoux test:* Serial dilutions of TB antigen provide 1, 10, and 100 tuber units (TU), respectively. The test is +ve if it produces ≥10mm induration, and if <5mm. This test is overrated in diagnosing TB and its use is controversia
- If active TB is strongly suspected, use 1 TU. If it is positive, infection is lik Otherwise, interpret in the clinical context.

Treatment of pulmonary TB ***Before treatment:*** Stress importance compliance/concordance (helps the patient and prevents spread of resistar Check FBC, liver, and renal function. Test colour vision (Ishihara chart) and ac before and during treatment as ethambutol may cause (reversible) ocular toxi ►Patients often forget to take pills, so consider *supervised* therapy as follow

- ***Initial phase*** (8wks on 4 drugs depending on susceptibilities):
  1 Rifampicin 600–900mg (child 15mg/kg) PO 3 times/wk.
  2 Isoniazid 15mg/kg PO 3 times/wk max 900mg + pyridoxine 10mg/24h.
  3 Pyrazinamide 2.5g PO (2g if <50kg) 3 times/wk (child 50mg/kg).
  4 Ethambutol 30mg/kg PO 3 times a week for 2 months, or streptom 0.75–1g/24h IM (see BNF; child 15mg/kg/24h).
- ***Continuation phase*** (16wks on 2 drugs) rifampicin and isoniazid at same dc Rifinah 300® = rifampicin 300mg + isoniazid 150mg; get advice about resista
- Give pyridoxine throughout treatment.
- Steroids are indicated in meningeal and pericardial disease.

Main side-effects ►Seek help in renal or hepatic failure, or pregnancy.

Rifampicin: Hepatitis (a small rise of AST is acceptable, stop if bilirubin ris orange discolouration of urine and tears (contact lens staining), inactivation of Pill, 'flu-like syndrome with intermittent use.

Isoniazid: Hepatitis, neuropathy, pyridoxine deficit, agranulocytosis.

Ethambutol: Optic neuritis (colour vision is the first to deteriorate).

Pyrazinamide: Hepatitis, arthralgia (CI: acute gout; porphyria).

WHO's/G8 '*Stop TB*' plan Sputum smear microscopy *et al* for all; directly obse therapy (**DOT**) in front of a health worker for 6 months; aiming to treat 50 mi people over 10yrs, and to reduce the required duration of therapy to 8 week

ıemoprophylaxis for asymptomatic tuberculous infection

ımigrant or contact screening may identify patients with TB without ·mptoms or radiographic changes. In such patients, chemoprophylaxis may be eful to kill the infective organisms and prevent possible disease progression at ater date. This involves administration of one or two anti-TB drugs for shorter riods than for symptomatic disease (eg rifampicin and isoniazid for 3 months, isoniazid alone for 6 months). Suitable patients for chemoprophylaxis include ults with documented recent tuberculin conversion, and some young ımigrants (16–34yrs) who are Mantoux +ve, without prior BCG vaccination.[99] Seek expert advice, or consult the latest British Thoracic Society guidelines ·ww.brit-thoracic.org.uk).

ɴ all cases, standard anti-TB therapy should be initiated once any evidence of tive disease (clinical or radiographic) is found.

·ophylaxis and dealing with latent TB

imary prophylaxis against TB is indicated in some HIV +ve patients. In Africa, 0% of those with HIV develop TB, and 80% with TB are HIV +ve. Isoniazid (eg)0mg/d PO; children 5mg/kg, max 300mg; give with pyridoxine) is the most ten used. Duration of prophylaxis is debated; 9 months is probably correct for ɔniazid,[100] lifelong prophylaxis is probably not helpful.[101] ►Seek expert advice rly. If prophylaxis is not used, monitor clinical state and CXR.

dications for primary prophylaxis:

If the patient has not had BCG and the Mantoux test is >5mm.
If BCG vaccinated (>10yrs ago), consider prophylaxis if Mantoux >10mm.
If there is recent exposure to someone with active TB.

3 meningitis (TBM)

►Ask about recent contact with TB.

odrome Fever, headache, vomiting, drowsiness, meningism, and delirium often ɔrsening over 1–3 weeks (rarely many months) ± seizures. ***CNS signs:*** Tremor, pilloedema; cranial nerve palsies. ***Diagnosis:*** LP (p806—the 1st few LPs may be rmal); TB PCR; Look for immunosuppression (HIV) and TB elsewhere (CXR etc). CT bstructive hydrocephalus and basal enhancement). There may also be CNS berculomas.[102] ***ΔΔ:*** Pyogenic meningitis, histoplasmosis, glioma, CNS lymphoma, scess, toxoplasmosis, neurocysticercosis, sarcoidosis, hydatid, and late ɔhilis.[103] ***R̸:*** **Isoniazid + rifampicin** for 12 months, with **pyrazinamide** and **reptomycin** during the 1st 2 months is often used (*OTM*). Ethambutol or hionamide are alternatives to streptomycin. Add pyridoxine 25–50mg/24h PO regimens using isoniazid to prevent neuropathies.[104] In adults, daily single ses of 300mg of isoniazid, 600mg of rifampicin, and 1500mg of pyrazinamide adequate. Higher doses are unnecessary and can cause hepatotoxicity. Always eck sensitivities of the causative organism, and discuss the chances of multi-ug resistant TB with a microbiologist. TBM with resistance to isoniazid and ampicin is likely to be fatal.[105] There is a role for **dexamethasone** (eg for month),[106] but tuberculomas may start to appear.[107] **Mannitol** for ICP↑ 813).[108] ***Complications:*** Hydrocephalus (may need surgery).[109] Cognition↓. Salt ısting states (hyponatraemia with high urinary Na^+ excretion and oddly high ine output even when dehydrated—it responds to fludrocortisone).[110]

ıti-TB drug use in liver and renal failure[111]

Monitor U&E +LFT before and after starting. In liver failure, get expert help.
creatine clearance=10–50mL/min: **Rifampicin**: ↓dose by 50%. **Ethambutol**: me dose every 36h (not /24h). No dose change for **ethionamide** or **isoniazid**.

Herpes virus infections

Herpes infections are like medical education: once you've had it, no one can ev take it away from you—and some people just can't help passing it on.

Herpes simplex virus (HSV) Manifestations of primary infection:

1 ***Genital herpes:*** HSV I or II (I is now overtaking II). Flu-like prodrome, th grouped vesicles/papules develop around genitals, anus, or throat. These bu forming shallow ulcers (heal in ~3wks). Also: urethral discharge ± dysuria (esp if urinary retention. *OHCS* p268. ***Tests:*** PCR. ***℞:*** Give analgesia + famciclo 250mg/8h (500mg if immunocompromise) PO for 5 days (recurrences: 1g/12h, 2 doses only, self-initiated[1]). If frequent (≥6/yr) or severe recurrenc continuous aciclovir ≤400mg/12h PO. *Prevention:* Condoms—even for oral s

2 ***Gingivostomatitis:*** Ulcers filled with yellow slough appear in the mouth.

3 ***Herpetic whitlow:*** Abrasions allow virus to enter the finger, causing a vesic

4 ***Herpes gladiatorum:*** Vesicles wherever HSV is ground into the skin by force

5 ***Eczema herpeticum:*** HSV infection of eczematous skin; usually children.

6 ***Herpes simplex meningitis:*** This is uncommon and usually self-limiting (typica HSV II in women during a primary attack).

7 ***HSV keratitis:*** Corneal dendritic ulcers. *Avoid steroids.* See *OHCS* p416.

8 ***Systemic infection*** eg fever, sore throat, and lymphadenopathy may pa unnoticed. If immunocompromised, it may be life-threatening with fev lymphadenopathy, pneumonitis, and hepatitis.

9 ***Herpes simplex encephalitis:*** Usually HSV I. Spreads centripetally, eg fro cranial nerve ganglia, to frontal and temporal lobes. ►*Suspect if* fever, f headaches, odd behaviour, dysphasia, hemiparesis, or coma or brainste encephalitis, meningitis, or myelitis. **Δ:** Urgent PCR on CSF (CT/MRI or EEG may sh temporal lobe changes but are non-specific and unreliable; brain biopsy rar required). Seek expert help: careful fluid balance to minimize cerebral oeder p812; ►►*prompt* aciclovir, eg 10mg/kg/8h IV for ≥10d, saves lives. Mortality: 19

Tests: Rising antibody titres in 1° infection; culture; PCR for fast diagnosis.

Recurrent HSV: Dormant HSV in ganglion cells may be reactivated by illne immunosuppression, menstruation, or sunlight. Cold sores (perioral vesicles) are c manifestation. Aciclovir cream may be disappointing.

Varicella zoster Varicella (=chickenpox) is a contagious febrile illness with crops of blisters of different ages starting on the back. Complications, eg purpura fulminans/DIC (get help; ►►may need heparin), pneumonitis, and ataxia are commoner in pregnancy and adults than in children. *Incubation:* 11–21d. *Infectivity:* 4d before the rash until all lesions are scabbed (~1 week). *OHCS* p144. After infection, virus is dormant in dorsal root ganglia. Reactivation causes **shingles** (affects 20% at some time; esp. if old or immunosuppressed). Pain in dermatomal distribution precedes malaise and fever by some days. See p446.

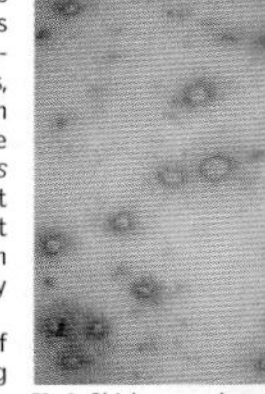

Fig 1. Chickenpox close-

Shingles ℞: Most will want antivirals (hoping to ↓risk of post-herpetic neuralgia); if seen early, give aciclovir eg 800mg 5 times a day PO for 5–7d. If immunocompromised, give 10mg/kg/8h slowly IVI for 10d. Alternatives: valaciclovir; famciclovir (more expensive; fewer SEs). Paracetamol ± amitriptyline (st with 10mg at night) for pain. If the conjunctiva is affected, apply 3% aciclovir ointm 5 times a day. Beware iritis. Measure acuity often. Say to report *any* visual loss at or SE of aciclovir: renal impairment (check U&E) vomiting, urticaria, encephalopathy. ***Po herpetic neuralgia*** in affected dermatomes can last years, and is hard to treat, a intolerable. Try amitriptyline or gabapentin (±carbamazepine, phenytoin, topical ca saicin counter-irritant); last resort: ablation of the ganglion; refer to a pain clinic.

1 F Aoki 2006 *Clin Infect Dis* 42 8 (RCT); if immunosuppressed try 500mg/12h for 7 days.

s is a common disease in the young which may be unnoticed or cause acute ess. Spread: saliva or droplet (presumed). Incubation 4–5wks.• Cause: Epstein–r virus (EBV, a DNA herpesvirus) infection of B-lymphocytes, causing proliferat- of T-cells ('atypical' mononuclear cells) which are cytotoxic to EBV-infected s. The latter are 'immortalized' by EBV infection and can, very rarely, proliferate a way indistinguishable from immunoblastic lymphoma in immunodeficient ividuals (whose suppressor T-cells fail to check multiplication of these B-cells).

Patient Sore throat, T°↑, anorexia, malaise, lymphadenopathy, palatal petechiae, enomegaly, hepatitis, haemolysis. ***Complications—CNS:*** • Meningitis • Encephalitis taxia[114] • Cranial nerve lesions (eg VII, bilateral in 40%[115]) ± Guillain–Barré drome • Neuropathy • Depression/fatigue• for a few for months, depending in t on features present at onset (eg less fit pre-morbidly, no delay in Monospot® coming +ve, and need for rest bed-rest—as determined by the patient).[116] igue is also part of 'severe chronic active EBV infection', eg with anaemia, platel-↓ and severe hepatosplenomegaly.[117] ***Others:*** Thrombocytopenia (±pancytopenia h a megaloblastic marrow),[118] ruptured spleen, splenic haemorrhage, upper ways obstruction (may need observation on ITU), hepatitis (± fulminant hepatic ure[119]), secondary infection, myo- or pericarditis, pneumonitis/fibrosis[120], renal ure, autoimmune haemolysis, and erythema multiforme. All are rare (or very rare).

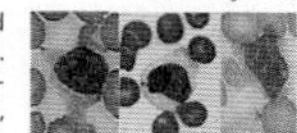
Fig 1. Atypical lymphocytes flowing around RBCs; dark cytoplasm at contact points.[121]

od film shows a lymphocytosis (eg 20% of WBC) and pical lymphocytes (large, irregular nuclei, fig 1). se may occur in many viral infections (CMV, HIV, par-irus, dengue), toxoplasmosis, typhus,[122] leukaemia, nphoma, drug hypersensitivity, and lead poisoning.

terophil antibody tests (Monospot®, Paul–Bunnell): erophil antibodies develop in 90% of patients by ek 3, disappearing after ~3 months (≤1yr).[123] They glutinate sheep RBCs and can be absorbed (and thus agglutination is prevented) ox RBCs, but not guinea-pig kidney cells. This pattern distinguishes them from er heterophil antibodies. These antibodies do not react with EBV or its antigens. ***se +ve*** Monospot® tests may occur in hepatitis, parvovirus infection, lymphoma, kaemia, rubella, malaria, carcinoma of pancreas, and SLE.[124] ***Other false trails:*** er patients may have little pharyngitis or adenopathy, but fever & LFT↑ are more longed, often with no telltale lymphocytosis or atypical lymphocytes.[125] So, if nospot –ve, they may be subjected to dangerous over-investigation unless you uest EBV-specific IgM—implies current infection (IgG reflects past infection). may reveal ↑↑serum EBV DNA levels and warn of fulminant infection.[126]

ferential diagnosis Streptococcal sore throat (may coexist), CMV, viral hepatitis, seroconversion illness, toxoplasmosis, leukaemia, diphtheria.

atment Avoiding alcohol 'to protect the liver' is traditional, but we can find no dence to support this ban. Prednisolone PO is recommended (rarely) for severe nptoms or complications such as severe thrombocytopenia[127] (eg 60mg on day 1, ering quickly); its use is non-standard. *Never give ampicillin or amoxicillin for e throats as they often cause a severe rash in those with acute EBV infection.*

oncogenicity Lymphoma[128] (eg post-transplant);[129] **nasopharyngeal cancer** (esp. sia), **leiomyosarcoma**[130] and **oral hairy leucoplakia** (p230; aciclovir-responsive).

ner EBV-associated diseases Crescentic glomerulonephritis;[131] **haemophago-ic syndrome** (EBV over-activates T-cells & macrophages, with overproduction of okines, eg causing fatal coagulopathy[132] ± central pontine myelinolysis).[133] The EBV **notti–Crosti rash** (self-limiting papular acrodermatitis of childhood) consists in e or red monomorphous 1–10mm papules and plaques placed symmetrically r extensor faces of limbs, buttocks, and face (also caused by streps, hepatitis B, echo, coxsackie, and respiratory syncitial viruses). forlag.fadl.dk/sample/derma/images/447.htm

Influenza

This is the most important viral respiratory infection because of its frequenc complication rate, particularly in the elderly. In pandemics (1918, 1957 & 1 millions die, particularly when new strains evolve (see BOX). WHO classific specifies: type/host origin/geographic origin/strain no./year of isolation/subty A/Swine/Taiwan/2/87/ (H3, N2)—see fig 1. **Spread** is by droplets. **Incub period** 1–4 days. **Infectivity** 1 day before to 7 days after symptoms start

Immunity Those attacked by one strain are immune to that strain only.

Symptoms Fever, headache, malaise, myalgia, prostration, nausea, vor conjunctivitis/eye pain (even photophobia). Also depression.

Tests ***Serology*** (paired sera; takes >2wks). ***Culture*** (1wk, from nasophary swabs). ***PCR:*** (eg 36h; sensitivity 94.2%; specificity ~100%).

Complications Bronchitis (20%, pneumonia (esp. *Staph. aureus*), sinusitis media, encephalitis, pericarditis, Reye's syndrome (coma, LFT↑).

℞ Bed rest ± aspirin. If severe pneumonia, take to ITU to prevent hypoxia and (cover *strep pneumoniae* and resistant staphs, eg **ciprofloxacin** & **co-amoxicl** ***Antivirals:*** **Zanamivir** (**Relenza®**, an inhaled neuraminidase inhibitor) sho attacks by ~36h; it is active against influenza types A and B. It is not a par consider if complications would be bad (cardiovascular or chronic respiratory disease; DM; immunosuppression; ≥65yrs old: see www.nice.org.uk). Dose: 2 bl (2×5mg)/12h for 5d (before any other inhalers); start only if within 4 symptom onset. NB: Inhalation is not an ideal route, eg if elderly. SE: bronchos oropharyngeal oedema. *Ensure your patient knows how to use the diskh*

Oseltamivir (***Tamiflu®***) eg 75mg/12h PO for 5d is an alternative (if >13yrs o. D&V, dyspepsia, headache, insomnia, dizziness, conjunctivitis, epistaxis, rash; hepatitis, Stevens–Johnson, p703 ± ?flawed reports of hallucinations in childr

M2 ion channel blockers (amantadine, rimantadine) are of low efficacy: don't seasonal flu in healthy people. ***SE:*** Hallucinations. Use in pandemics is unc

Prevention • Use whole ***trivalent vaccine*** (from inactivated viruses), rese split (fragmented virus) for those <13yrs old. It is prepared from current sero and takes <2wks to work. ***Indications:*** Diabetes; COPD; asthma* (not if mild), renal or liver failure; immunosuppression (eg splenectomy or on steroids); ha globinopathies, medical staff; those ≥65yrs old and their carers, especia institutions. The logistics of vaccinating all those in the at-risk groups p challenge in ageing populations. In addition, *routine* vaccination of children m worthwhile (might save ~100 deaths/yr). ***Dose:*** 0.5mL SC (once). In children r after 6wks (½ dose if <3yrs old). ***SE:*** Mild pain or swelling (17%). T°↑, heada and malaise are in ≤10%. Guillain–Barré and pericarditis are rare. *Vaccine ef* is 'modest' (eg relative risk of pneumonia falls from 1 to 0.88 after vaccinati the elderly living in the community; all cause mortality *is* slightly reduce • ***Oseltamivir*** Only use as **prophylaxis** after formal notice that influenza A c circulating ***and*** >1yrs old ***and*** <48h since exposure ***and*** in at-risk group, abov ***not*** needed if vaccinated >2wks ago with a well-matched vaccine ***unless*** livir rest- or nursing-home*et al* when it can be used ***whatever*** the vaccination stat Dose: 75mg/d (if 24–40kg, 60mg/d; 16–23kg, 45mg/d)—all for ≥10d. (If not at-risk group, UK guidelines allow us to give private prescriptions for prophyl

The common cold (coryza)

Rhinoviruses are the main culprits (>80 strains), and cause a self-limiting discharge (which becomes mucopurulent over a few days). ***Incubation:*** ***Complications:*** (6% in children) Otitis media, pneumonia, febrile convul ℞***:*** None is usually needed. If nasal obstruction in infants hampers feedin 0.9% saline nose drops. Zinc gluconate yields conflicting results in trials.

he ART of making and breaking new pandemics

Vhen an animal source of virus couples with human virus (reassortment[1]) to orm a novel hybrid with efficient replication and person-to-person transmis-ion—a pandemic is born. Millions of deaths occur if the human population is aive (no previous immunological exposure) and the new strain is highly athogenic. What can we do? The first clusters may be containable, but once ransmission is established, quarantine is probably futile and the pandemic will ecome global.[1] Nevertheless some strategic planning is possible:

- Buy time during spreading epidemics by moving free range chickens in-doors. (this was done in 2005–6, eg in Holland, to slow spread of H5N1 avian 'flu).
- Quarantine restrictions around clusters of animal infections, eg a 3km zone where entry and exit are banned, with movements restricted in a further 10km monitoring zone with checking of residents, and their birds destroyed. 145
- Stock-pile vaccine (if it can be made in time), antivirals, and vital supplies.
- Masks are recommended by WHO when health workers are within 1 metre of a probably-infected person (eg on entering a room with such patients). 146
- Seamless international co-operation with WHO and bodies such as the European Centre for Disease Prevention—eg to cancel mass events.
- Self-isolation at the 1st sign of human illness—and improved personal hygiene.
- Simulated exercises before the event to enhance preparedness.

revention, containment, health systems response, and communications This -part response to flu pandemics depends on how far we have progressed down he pandemic path. Preceding any pandemic there is an ***interpandemic period*** 10 new subtypes in humans but circulating animal virus may pose a risk) and hen a ***pandemic alert period***. 2006, for example, began with the *first phase* of he pandemic alert period, characterized by 'human infections with a new subtype, with] rare instances of spread to a close contact'. The next phase is 'small lusters of highly localized spread' (virus isn't well adapted to humans). The last hase before any ***pandemic phase*** of sustained transmission is one of large lusters of human-to-human spread, with full transmissibility less developed.

thomyxoviridae[RNA] divide into 2 genera: luenza A and B viruses—and influenza C, tinguishable by antigenic differences tween their nucleoproteins (NP) and matrix) proteins. Influenza B & C are almost clusively isolated from man (rarely pigs & als). Influenza A infects many birds and mmals; they are subtyped by surface coproteins (haemagglutinin, HA) and uraminidase (NA). So far, 15 different HAs to 15) and 9 NAs (N1 to 9) have been found ong all influenza viruses. 147

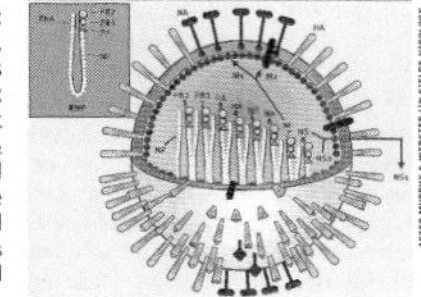

Fig 1. Influenza A.

1 In genetic reassortment, 2 viral sources shuffle genetic material in someone with a dual infection. Also, ple stepwise single mutations can accumulate to produce new strains. Coulombier D, *BMJ* 2005 414

Toxoplasmosis

The protozoan *Toxoplasma gondii* infects via gut (poorly-cooked meat), lung, broken skin. Life-cycle: fig 1. In humans, the oocysts release trophozoites, wh migrate widely, with a predeliction for eye, brain, and muscle. Toxoplasmosis occ worldwide, but is common in the tropics. Infection is lifelong. HIV may reactivate

The Patient ►*In any granulomatous uveitis or necrotizing retinitis, think toxoplasmosis, especially in the immunosuppressed.* Most infections are asymp matic: in the UK 50% have been infected by 70yrs. Symptomatic acqui toxoplasmosis resembles infectious mononucleosis, and is usually self-limiting. E infection, usually congenital, presents with posterior uveitis, often in the 2nd deca of life, and may cause cataract. In the immunocompromised (eg AIDS), myocard encephalitis, focal neurological signs, stroke or fits may occur.

Tests Acute infection is confirmed by a 4-fold rise in antibody titre over 4wks specific IgM (unreliable if HIV+ve). Reactivation of latent toxoplasmosis in presents problems (you may need to look for toxoplasma antigen and IgG).[148] may be rewarding.[149] Parasite isolation is difficult; lymph node or CNS biopsy may diagnostic. CT: characteristic multiple ring-shaped contrast-enhancing CNS lesio

Treatment• Often none is needed: seek expert advice.[150] If the eye is involved, in the immunocompromised, pyrimethamine 200mg PO on day one then 75mg/d for 4wks, + sulfadiazine ≤1g/6h PO *may* be needed. SE: renal stones. Folinic acid 1 20mg/d until 4wks after resolution. ►If pregnant, get expert help. Sampling of fe cord blood, eg at 21wks for IgM indicates severe infection. For HIV: p396.

Congenital toxoplasmosis (*OHCS* p34) May cause abortion, neonatal seizur choroidoretinitis, (fig 2), hydrocephalus, microcephaly, or cerebral calcificati Worse prognosis if early infection.

Cytomegalovirus (CMV)

CMV may be acquired by direct contact, blood transfusion, or organ transplantati After acute infection, CMV becomes latent but the infection may reactivate at tim of stress or immunocompromise. If immunocompetent, primary infection is usua asymptomatic, but acute hepatitis may occur. In transplant recipients or post marrow transplantation: fever > pneumonitis > colitis > hepatitis > retinitis. In AIDS: retinitis > colitis > CNS disease. (> = 'is commoner than')

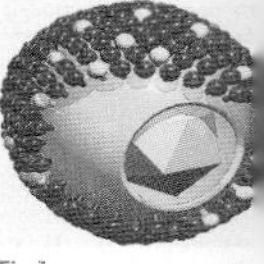
Fig 1. CMV.

Diagnosis of acute CMV infection is difficult; virus growth is slow and there may be prolonged CMV excretion from a distant source of infection. Serology is good; specific IgM indicates acute infection (unreliable if HIV +ve). CMV PCR (including quantitative tests) of blood/CSF/broncho-alveolar lavage is available.

Treat only if serious infection (eg immunocompromised), with ganciclo 5mg/kg/12h IVI over 1h via a central line. Alternatives: oral valganciclo foscarnet. Immunization is being explored. For CMV in HIV, see p398.

Prevention post-transplantation[151] If seropositive pre-op, ganciclovir, 2.5mg/kg/d IV for the first 2 post-op weeks. If sero–ve pre-op, valaciclovir 2g/6h for 90d reduces incidence and delays onset of CMV disease.[152] Use CMV–ve, irradiat blood when transfusing transplant recipients, leukaemics, or HIV patients.

Congenital CMV (*OHCS* p34) Look for: jaundice, hepatosplenomegaly, and purpu Chronic defects include mental retardation, cerebral palsy, epilepsy, deafness, a eye problems. Treatment: none is established.

Complications GU CMV reactivation in HIV +ve men leads to ↑ semen levels of HI

1 Semen transmission drives HIV spread, so this is important: Sheth P 2006 *Infect Dis* 193 45

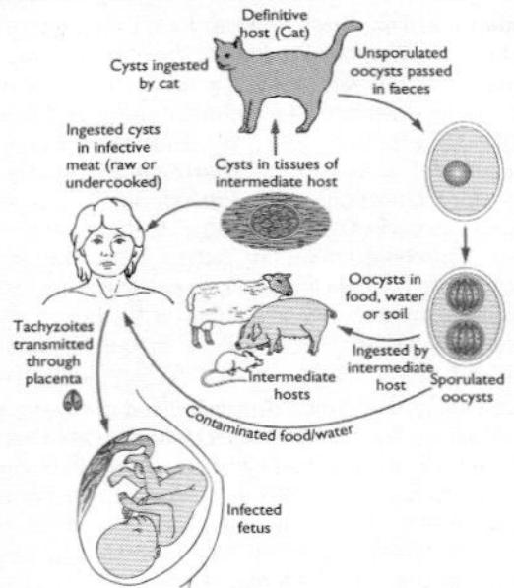

1. Oocysts in cat faeces can stay in the soil for months, where animals such as rats them. They get infected, and, under the direction of *Toxoplasma* in the amygdala, se rats lose their innate fear of cats, and so tend to get eaten. So parasites ensure r success by facilitating their jump from the intermediate to the definitive host.[155]

nans with toxoplasmosis may show these features

Confusion, seizures, and signs of brainstem or spinal cord injury.
latent phase of toxoplasmosis is recognized, as is subtle personality change. oss of fear of cats is *not* reported in us, but there are changes in willingness o accept group moral standards, in proportion to the latent period's length.[154]
Meningoencephalitis + localizing signs (fever + headache → drowsiness → coma → eath, eg over a days or weeks). CSF: mild lymphocytic pleocytosis & protein↑.
Multifocal myelin loss, and microglial nodules.
Pseudotumour cerebri syndrome: transient intracranial hypertension.
Space-occupying mass with ICP↑ mimicking a tumour or a brain abscess.
Multiple mass lesions that can be the cause of hemisensory abnormalities, emiparesis, cranial nerve palsy, aphasia, and tremors.
some areas, eg India, toxoplasmosis is the major HIV-associated CNS infection.[155]

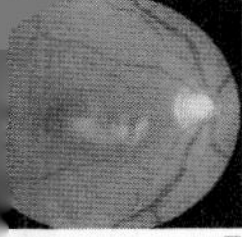

. Retinal toxoplasmosis.[158]

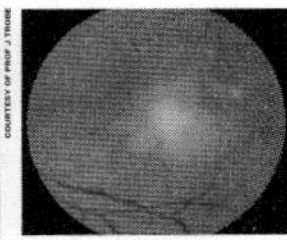

Fig 3. Ill-defined yellow infiltrates. ΔΔ: toxoplasmosis; herpes simplex/zoster; syphilis; sarcoidosis; leukaemia.[156]

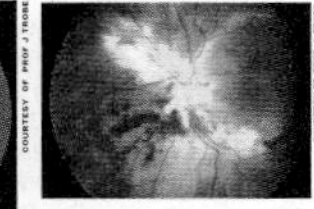

Fig 4. In HIV this 'pizza-pie' fundus means CMV retinitis. If CD4↓↓, re-examine in 2 days; ►is it progressing?[157]

Viral hepatitis

Hepatitis A virus (HAV) RNA virus. ***Spread:*** Faecal–oral, often in travelle institutions. Most infections occur in childhood. ***Incubation:*** 2–6wks. ***Sympt*** Prodromal symptoms include fever, malaise, anorexia, nausea, arthralgia. Jau develops ± hepatomegaly, splenomegaly, and adenopathy. ***Tests:*** Serum transa ases rise 22–40d after exposure. IgM rises from day 25 and signifies re infection. IgG remains detectable for life. ***Treatment:*** Supportive. Avoid alc Rarely, interferon-α for fulminant hepatitis. ***Prevention:*** Passive immunizatior normal human immunoglobulin (0.02mL/kg IM) gives <3 months' immunity to at risk (travellers, household contacts). Active immunization is with H Monodose®, an inactivated protein derived from HAV. ***Dose:*** if >16yrs old, 1 IM (1mL to deltoid) gives immunity for 1yr (10yrs if further booster is given months). Use Havrix Monodose Junior® if 1–15yrs old. ***Prognosis:*** Usually limiting. Fulminant hepatitis occurs rarely. Chronic liver disease does not oc

Hepatitis B virus (HBV, a DNA virus.) ***Spread:*** Blood products, IV drug ab (IVDU), sexual intercourse, direct contact. ***Risk groups:*** IVDU & their sexual par health workers; haemophiliacs and their carers (exposure to blood products– morticians/embalmers); haemodialysis (and chronic renal failure); the sex promiscuous; foster carers; close family members of a carrier or case; sta residents of day care or longterm institutions/prisons; babies of HBsAg +ve mot adopted child from endemic area. ***Endemic in:*** Far East, Africa & Mediterra ***Incubation:*** 1–6 months. ***Signs:*** Resemble hepatitis A but extrahepatic feature more common, eg arthralgia, urticaria. ***Tests:*** HBsAg (surface antigen) is pre from 1 to 6 months after exposure. HBeAg (e antigen) is present for 1½–3 mo after the acute illness and implies high infectivity. The persistence of HBsAg fo months defines carrier status and occurs in 5–10% of infections (ch infection). Antibodies to HBcAg (anti-HBc) imply past infection; antibodies to H (anti-HBs) alone implies vaccination. HBV PCR allows monitoring of respon therapy. ***Vaccination*** (►p263) may be universal in childhood or just for high groups. Passive immunization (specific anti-HBV immunoglobulin) may be giv non-immune contacts after high-risk exposure. ***Treatment:*** Supportive. A alcohol. Chronic HBV may respond to interferon-α or other antivirals, eg lamivu adefovir.[159] Immunize sexual contacts. ***Complications:*** Fulminant hepatic fa (rare); relapse; prolonged cholestasis; chronic hepatitis (5–10%); cirrh hepatocellular carcinoma (HCC: 10-fold ↑risk if HBsAg +ve, 60-fold ↑risk if HBsAg and HBeAg +ve);[160] glomerulonephritis; cryoglobulinaemia.

Hepatitis C virus (HCV) RNA flavivirus. ***Spread:*** Blood, IVDU, sexual, acupunct UK prevalence: 200,000–466,000.[161] Early infection is often mild/asympton ~85% develop chronic infection; 20–30% get cirrhosis within 20yrs; a few hepatocellular cancer (HCC). ***Tests:*** LFT (AST : ALT <1:1 until cirrhosis develops, p anti-HCV antibodies, recombinant immunoblot assay, HCV-PCR; liver biopsy if HC +ve to assess liver damage and need for ℞. Do HCV genotype (BOX). ***D*** Interferon-α + ribavirin in chronic infection; peginterferon-α is better than IFN IFN-α in acute infection may ↓ progression to chronic disease.[163]

Hepatitis D virus (HDV) Incomplete RNA virus, exists only with HBV. ***Spr*** Coinfection or superinfection with HBV. ***Clinical features:*** Increased risk of a hepatic failure and cirrhosis. ***Tests:*** Anti-HDV antibody. ***Treatment:*** Interferon- limited success in treatment of HDV infection.

Hepatitis E virus (HEV) RNA virus. Similar to HAV. Common in India. High mor in pregnancy. ***Diagnosis:*** Serology. No effective treatment/vaccine.

Hepatitis GB Parenterally transmitted. Causes asymptomatic post-transfu hepatitis. One type (HGB-C) can cause fulminant liver failure.

ΔΔ Alcohol; drugs; toxins; EBV/CMV; leptospirosis; malaria; Q fever; syphilis; yellow f chronic hepatitis (eg alcohol; drugs; autoimmune hepatitis, p260; Wilson's, p25

1 In elderly, HCV is a more important cause of hepatocellular cancer than HBV. Shin 2006 *Intervir*

rological markers of HBV infection

	Incubation	Acute	Carrier	Recovery	Vaccinated
Ts		↑↑↑	↑	Normal	Normal
bsAg	+	+	+		
beAg	+	+	+/−		
nti-HBS				+	+
nti-Hbe			+/−		
nti-HBc IgM		+	+/−		
nti-HBC IgG		+	+	+	

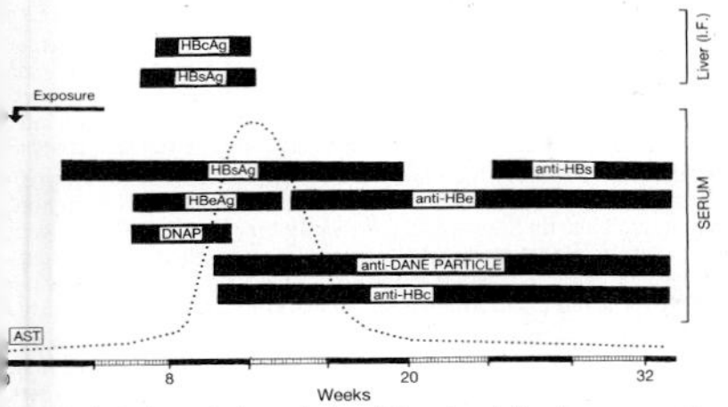

1. Virological events in acute hepatitis B in relation to serum amino-nsferase (AST) peak. IF=immunofluorescence; Ag=antigen; HBS=hepatitis urface; HBC=hepatitis B core; HBe=hepatitis B e antigen; DNAP=DNA polymerase.

ing ribavirin with peginterferon-α in HCV: *NICE* advice

is combination is indicated in moderate and severe chronic hepatitis C ection if liver biopsy shows necro-inflammation and fibrosis. Efficacy is less if: CV genotype G1, 4, 5, or 6 is involved[1] • ↑Viral load • Older patients • Excessive lay before ℞ starts • Blacks (*vs* Caucasians) • Males • HIV+ve.

: Pegylated interferon has an inert tail retarding its elimination (hence it may given SC once weekly). Giving these drugs is a specialist role, so the main ng is for non-specialists is to know the contraindications, to prevent appropriate referral. **CI:** • Allergy to or past use of interferon • Autoimmune patitis • Severe liver dysfunction or decompensated cirrhosis • Age <3yrs evere, unstable or uncontrolled heart disease in past 6 months • Past severe ychiatric conditions (esp. depression) • Pregnancy/lactation • Haemoglobin-athies (a contra-indication to ribavirin).

/ and hepatitis C HCV prevalence is ~7% for sexually transmitted HIV and 0% for IV drug abuse transmission. Untreated HIV seems to accelerate the ogression of HCV-induced liver fibrosis. Given the safety and efficacy of co-erapy with peginterferon + ribavirin and the bad effects of chronic hepatitis C, HIV/HCV co-infected patients should be evaluated for therapy. 164

terferon-α ℞ is either for 24wks (genotype 2 & 3) or 48wks for G1 (commonest in UK) & G4–6, if, 12 weeks, viral load is <1% of pre-treatment levels.

Human immunodeficiency virus (HIV)

Over 40 million people are HIV +ve (5 million/yr; 3 million deaths/yr); over ha in Africa and there is markedly increasing transmission in eastern Europe. HIV retrovirus) is responsible for most cases worldwide. HIV-2, a related virus, cau similar illness, perhaps with a longer latent period. >3 million have acq immunodeficiency syndrome (AIDS); most are women and children in Africa. N the news in Africa is bad: prevalence is falling in Kenya, for example (preval falling from 10% in the 1990s to 7% now).[165] UK *incidence:* >7250/yr—heterosexually acquired than homosexually since 1999.[166]

Transmission Sexual (75%, oral, in 3–7%[167][168]), infected blood, IV drug abu perinatally (vertical transmission causes ~600,000 child deaths/yr: see *OHCS* p

Immunology HIV binds, via its gp120 envelope glycoprotein, to CD4 recepto helper T-lymphocytes, monocytes, macrophages, and neural cells. CD4 +ve migrate to the lymphoid tissue where the virus replicates producing billions of virions. These are released, and in turn infect new CD4 +ve cells. As infe progresses depletion or impaired function of CD4 +ve cells ↓immune dysfunc

Virology (RNA retrovirus). After entry into the cell, the viral reverse *transcrip* enzyme makes a DNA copy of the RNA genome. The viral *integrase* enzyme integrates this into the host DNA. The core viral proteins are initially synthesiz large polypeptides that are cleaved by the viral *protease* enzyme into the enzy and building blocks of the virus. The completed virions are then release budding. The number of circulating viruses (viral load) predicts progression to A

Stages of HIV infection ***Acute infection*** is often asymptomatic. ***Seroconver*** may be accompanied by a transient illness 2–6wks after exposure: fever, mal myalgia, pharyngitis, maculopapular rash or meningoencephalitis (rare). A peri ***asymptomatic infection*** follows although 30% of patients will have ***persis generalized lymphadenopathy (PGL)***, defined as nodes >1cm diameter at ≥2 e inguinal sites, persisting for 3 months or longer. Later, constitutional sympt develop: T°↑, night sweats, diarrhoea, weight↓, ± minor opportunistic infection oral candida, oral hairy leucoplakia, herpes zoster, recurrent herpes sim, seborrhoeic dermatitis, tinea infections. This collection of symptoms and sig referred to as the ***AIDS-related complex (ARC)*** and is regarded as a prodrom AIDS. ***AIDS*** is a stage in HIV infection characterized by the presence of an indic disease (p398). CD4 count is usually <200 × 10⁶/L (prognosis ~2yrs if untreat

Diagnosis Look for anti-HIV antibodies in serum. Acute infection is detectab finding P24 antigen or HIV RNA by PCR and precedes the appearance of IgM and (within 3 months). During the asymptomatic period, there are high titres of Ig core and envelope proteins. As immunodeficiency develops, IgG titre to core pro falls, and P24 antigenaemia recurs. Rapid diagnostic kits for detecting anti antibodies are available.[169] The OraQuick® test uses oral fluid, and may be bo over the counter in some places; but false +ves are a problem.[170] ***HIV subtypes*** predominate in the UK; type D (commoner in Africa)[171] & hybrid/recombinant str carry a worse prognosis as they bind to immune cells more readily.

Prevention Blood screening; disposable equipment; perinatal antiretrovirals HIV+ve mothers ± **Caesarean birth ± bottle-feeding** (may ↑mortality if hygiene p ▶***A 'stop-HIV' sexual manifesto:*** Accurate *accessible* HIV **tests** and **informatio** TV, wind-up radios, eg in Africa; HIV issues in soap-operas are most influential).[172] V rehearsed **sexual negotiation** skills. **Condoms** for *all* sexual contact, or **abstine** (but..."I'd rather be dead than abstain"[173]). **Reframing of our bodies as a rout intimacy** rather than as instruments of gratification always entailing penetra **Fewer sexual partners.** NB: 3 *simultaneous* partners is more risky than 6 s partners. ↓**Alcohol use** (to avoid risky behaviour). NB: a randomized trial (unbl found that **circumcision** prevented 65% of HIV infections over 1½yrs. N=3128 hete sexuals <25 This didn't control for glans hygiene (washing/foreskin retraction if uncircumcis It is not a reliable preventive: uncircumcised men must not behave as if they are

/ and TB: a prime example of the complex interaction between /, diseases of poverty, and multi-drug resistance (MDR-TB)

is a common, serious, but treatable complication of HIV. 30–50% of those with s in the developing world also have TB. Morbidity due to HIV/AIDS/TB leads to astrous losses in productivity, and a poorly trained workforce due to senteeism from work & training. Health budgets become unbalanced in trying treat these preventable diseases—if only the context was not one of poverty d ignorance. Economies become uncompetitive, there is higher labour turnover, nce unstable national budgets and politics. Other interactions of HIV and TB:

- Mantoux tests may be negative and the presentation of TB may be atypical.
- Increased reactivation of latent TB.
- Previous BCG vaccination does not prevent development of TB.
- Smears may be –ve for AFB. Smears that are +ve often have few AFB. This makes culture very important (and vital to characterize drug resistance).
- Atypical CXR, eg lobar or bibasal pneumonia, hilar lymphadenopathy.
- Extrapulmonary and disseminated disease is much more common.
- TB R in poor countries entails a 4-drug initial phase (2 months of rifampicin, isoniazid, pyrazinamide & ethambutol) and a 2-drug continuation phase (4 months of rifampicin & isoniazid, or 6 months of isoniazid & ethambutol). HIV is known to increases case fatality and rates recurrent TB after this regimen.
- There is ↑toxicity (D&V, hepatitis, rash neuropathy) from combining anti-TB and anti-HIV drugs (eg stavudine, lamivudine & nevirapine as twice-daily generic tablet, often used in resource-poor/WHO HAART, p401). NB: it may be best to delay HAART until 1–2 months after TB R is started (unless CD4 <100×10⁶/L).
- As HAART reconstitutes CD4 counts, paradoxical worsening of TB symptoms may occur (the 'immune reconstitution inflammatory response', IRIS).
- HIV may or may not necessitate lifelong prophylaxis with isoniazid, but either way, regular clinical monitoring is vital.

Directly observed treatment strategy (DOTS) prevents MDR-TB. In areas where MDR-TB is common, DOTS-plus (use of 2nd-line drugs) may be a solution.

Respiratory isolation is vital if TB patients are near HIV +ve people. Nosocomial (hospital-acquired) and MDR-TB are major problems worldwide, affecting HIV +ve and HIV –ve people. Mortality is ~80% in patient-to-patient spread. Test TB cultures against 1st and 2nd line agents; 5+ drugs may be needed in MDR-TB :

First line antitubercular agents:		Second line antitubercular agents:	
Isoniazid	Streptomycin	Ofloxacin	Aminosalicylic acid
Rifampicin	Amikacin	Ciprofloxacin	Clarithromycin
Pyrazinamide	Kanamycin	Cycloserine	Azithromycin
Ethambutol	Capreomycin	Ethionamide	

Reducing MDR-TB Chief goals: early identification; full treatment; isolation.

- Early isolation of suspected patients. A suspicious CXR or a past history of MDR-TB is enough. Don't wait to prove the diagnosis.
- The ability to obtain Ziehl–Nielsen (ZN)/auramine stains 24h a day.
- Directly observing and confirming that patients take all prescribed drugs.
- Wearing of special masks by staff and the patient if s/he leaves the isolation room (avoid this if possible).
- Sputum induction/expectoration being confined to isolation rooms.
- Doors to isolation rooms having automatic closing devices.
- Providing negative air pressure in isolation rooms.
- Only stop isolation after ≥3 sputum samples are AFB –ve on culture for MDR-TB.
- Frequent tuberculin skin surveillance tests for workers and contacts.

Guidelines on MDR-TB are under review. Discuss treatment with a microbiologist, and refer early to a consultant in infectious diseases. Specific advice is available from the British Thoracic Society and the USA National Institutes of Health.

Complications of HIV infection

►All patients with a new diagnosis of HIV should have a tuberculin test an tested for toxoplasma, CMV, hepatitis B/C, and syphilis serology, to identify pa current infections that may develop as immunosuppression progresses.

- **Pulmonary *Pneumocystis jiroveci* (=*P. carinii*)** pneumonia: this fungus i commonest life-threatening opportunistic infection in AIDS (p154). ***R*:** high- co-trimoxazole IV (60mg/kg/12h for 14d PO or IV; special monitoring mu available) or pentamidine by slow IVI for 2–3wks. Steroids are benefic severe moderate to hypoxaemia. ***Primary prophylaxis:*** If CD4 c <200×10⁶/L: co-trimoxazole 960mg/24h PO—reducible to 480mg to imp tolerance or 960mg on alternate days (3 times a week), or 960mg/12 alternate days (3 times a week). Secondary prophylaxis is essential afte attack until CD4 count >200×10⁶/L.[186] Other pathogens include ***pyog bacteria*** (atypical presentation); ***M. tuberculosis*** (p386); ***M. av intracellulare*** (MAI); ***fungi*** (*Aspergillus*, cryptococcus, histoplasma); ***CMV***. ***Kaposi's sarcoma***, lymphoma, lymphoid interstitial pneumonitis, and non-spe pneumonitis.
- **Gut** Oral pain may be caused by ***candidiasis***, HSV or aphthous ulcers, or tum ***Oral Candida*** is treated with nystatin suspension or amphotericin lozen ***Oesophageal*** involvement causes dysphagia ± retrosternal discomfor fluconazole, ketoconazole, or itraconazole PO for 1–2 weeks. Relapse is com ***HSV*** and ***CMV*** also cause oesophageal ulceration which may be difficu differentiate from *Candida* by barium studies. ***Anorexia and weight los*** common in HIV infection. ***LFT* ↑ *and hepatomegaly*** are common; causes inc drugs, viral hepatitis, AIDS sclerosing cholangitis, or MAI. ***MAI*** causes fever, sweats, malaise, anorexia, weight↓, abdominal pain, diarrhoea, hepatome and anaemia. *Diagnosis:* blood cultures, biopsies (lymph node, liver, colon, marrow). *R*: ethambutol + clarithromycin + rifabutin/rifampicin (box). *Pri prophylaxis:*[187] eg azithromycin 1200mg weekly, while CD4<100×10⁶/L. ***Chr diarrhoea*** may be caused by bacteria (*Salmonella*, *Shigella*, *Campyloba atypical mycobacteria*, *C. difficile*), protozoa (*Cryptosporidium* p380, *M sporidium*, *Isospora belli* fig 1 p379, *cyclospora*), or viruses (*CMV*, *adenov* ***Perianal disease*** may be from recurrent HSV ulceration, perianal warts, squa cell Ca (rare). Kaposi's sarcoma (p694) and lymphomas can also affect the
- **Neurological *Acute HIV*** is associated with transient meningoencephalitis, opathy, and neuropathy. ***Chronic HIV*** is associated with several CNS syndro AIDS-related dementia, HIV-related meningitis, CMV encephalitis, PML, p366, vacuolar myelopathy. ***Toxoplasma gondii*** (p392) is the main CNS pathog AIDS, presenting with focal symptoms/signs. CT/MRI shows ring-shaped con enhancing lesions. Treat with pyrimethamine (and folinic acid) + sulfadiazi clindamycin for 6 months. Lifelong secondary prophylaxis is needed. Pneum tis prophylaxis also protects against toxoplasmosis.[187] ***Cryptococcus neof ans*** (p428) causes a chronic meningitis, eg with no neck stiffness. ***R*:** See
- ***Tumours*** affecting the CNS include primary cerebral lymphoma, B-cell non-Hod lymphoma. CSF JC virus PCR is useful in distinguishing lymphoma from PML.
- **Eye *CMV retinitis*** (acuity↓ ± blindness) may affect 45% of those with Fundoscopy shows characteristic 'mozzarella pizza' signs, fig 4 p393. ***Pri induction R*:** Valganciclovir 900mg/12h PO with food for 21d—or ganciclo or foscarnet, or cidofovir, or ganciclovir-containing intraocular implants (NB of post-op retinal detachment, one implant does not prevent disease in the eye). The need for maintenance therapy may be reviewed if CD4 ≥100×10 eg after immune restoration by HAART (p402), if retinitis is inactive.[189]
- **TB** p386.
- **Leishmaniasis** p427.
- **Kaposi's sarcoma** p694.

1 PML is caused by the JC virus (named after the initials of its first patient).

naging opportunistic infections in HIV

ction	Treatment/side-effects/prophylaxis
rculosis	The most lethal opportunistic infection; ►p386. If no active infection, prophylaxis may be needed if significant exposure, or tuberculin skin test >5mm induration (isoniazid 300mg/day + pyridoxine 50mg/day PO; get expert local help, eg on how long to continue prophylaxis for).[190]
umocystis jiroveci carinii) 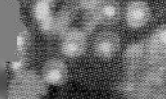 1. PCC (fluorescent 1 × 1000)[191] COURTESY OF SUBHASH K. MOHAN	***Co-trimoxazole*** (=trimethoprim 1 part + 5 parts sulfamethoxazole) 120mg/kg/d IVI in 3–4 divided doses for 14d. (SE: nausea, vomiting, fever, rash, myelosuppression) **or** ***Pentamidine isetionate*** 4mg/kg/d by slow IVI for 14–21d (SE: BP↓, hyper- or hypoglycaemia, renal failure, hepatitis, myelosuppression, arrhythmias). ***Prednisolone*** 40–60mg PO daily (reducing dose) if severe hypoxia. ***2nd line agents:*** primaquine + clindamycin, trimetrexate + calcium folinate, atovaquone. *Secondary prophylaxis,* eg co-trimoxazole 480mg/24h PO; same dose as 1° prophylaxis, essential after 1st attack.
idiasis e figures on p429)	*Local* ℞: ***Nystatin*** oral suspension or ***amphotericin*** lozenges/6h. *Systemic* ℞ ***if mucosal: Fluconazole*** 50–100mg/d PO for 7–30d; ***if invasive:*** 400mg/d for eg 8wks (SE: nausea, hepatitis, platelets↓) **or** ***ketoconazole*** **or** ***itraconazole*** (SE: CCF, nausea, hepatitis). ***Amphotericin B*** (p160) is for *severe* systemic infection. Relapse is common.
plasmosis 2, p392)	***Sulfadiazine*** 1g/6h (or ***clindamycin*** 600–1200mg/6h) + ***pyrimethamine*** eg 25mg/8h PO + folinic acid 15mg/d. *Secondary prophylaxis:* halve doses.
ptococcal meningitis COURTESY M. MCGINNIS 2. Cryptococcus	***Amphotericin B*** IV (p160) + flucytosine 25mg/kg/6h PO for 14d IV. 20% mortality. Normalizing ICP (repeated LPs ± shunts) may help. Give secondary prophylaxis (fluconazole) until CD4 >150×10⁶/L and cryptococcal antigen –ve.[193] Diagnosis: India ink stain (fig 2); CSF culture; cyptococcal antigen in blood & CSF. Note that the capsule is an essential virulence factor for this yeast.
/ retinitis 2 on p392)	Induction: ***ganciclovir*** 5mg/kg/12h IV for 14–21d (SE: myelosuppression) or ***foscarnet*** 60mg/kg/8h IV for 2wks, then reduce. SE: U&E↑↓, ulcers. Alternatives: ***valganciclovir*** 900mg/12h PO for 3wks, then 900mg/24h PO **or** ***cidofovir:*** start with 5mg/kg IV once weekly for 2wks (with probenecid & IV fluids), then reduce to alternate weekly doses. Oral ganciclovir (1g/8h with food) is less good. Maintenance ℞ may be discontinued in some patients with CD4 >150×10⁶/L.
Mycobacterium avintracellulare (=MAC, *vium* complex, p398).	***Clarithromycin*** 500mg/12h + ***ethambutol*** 15mg/kg/d + ***rifabutin*** 300mg/d ± ***ciprofloxacin*** 500mg/12h, all PO. Prophylaxis if CDC <50/mm³: ***azithromycin*** 1.2g/wk PO.
p. pneumoniae	Prophylaxis: 23-valent pneumococcal vaccine, p152.[194]

What every doctor should know about HIV

Preventing HIV spread ►Promote *lifelong* safer sex, barrier contraceptior reduction in partner numbers. Videos, followed by interactive discussions, i way to double condom use. Another way is the *100% condom programme* invc distribution of condoms to sex establishments, with enforcement. programmes are estimated to have prevented 2 million HIV infections in Tha

- Warn everyone about dangers of sexual tourism/promiscuity. Teach sk sexual negotiation. Explain how alcohol can undermine safe sex message
- Introduce drug users to needle exchange schemes ('don't share needles').
- Vigorous control of other STDs can reduce HIV incidence by 40%.
- Strengthen awareness of STD clinics (and support them in their work).
- Reduce unnecessary blood transfusions.
- Encourage HIV tests in pregnancy (±Caesarean sections if +ve, *OHCS* p34).

Post-exposure prophylaxis (eg needle-stick injury; split condom and HIV+v Seroconversion rate post-needle-stick: ~0.4% (HIV); 30% for hep B if HBeAg

- Wash well. If needle-stick, encourage bleeding; do not suck or immerse in bl
- Note name, address, and clinical details of 'donor'.
- Report incident to Occupational Health and fill in an accident form.
- Store blood from both parties (HIV, HBV & HCV tests). Immunize (active & pas against hepatitis B at once, if needed. Counsel (HIV risk <0.5% if 'donor' is HIV and test recipient at 3, 6, and 8 months (seroconversion may take this lon
- Weigh risks by questioning 'donor'; if HIV+ve, what is the CD4 and viral count? Before prophylaxis, do a pregnancy test. Get informed consent. Was a large inoculum? Was injury deep? (Mucous membrane exposure carries low risk.) Give 4wks of drugs, if possible within 1h of exposure: ***Low-risk*** antiviral medication. ***Higher-risk:*** Typically zidovudine 250mg/12h + lamiv 150mg/12h, and particularly for worst episodes (deep puncture from wide needle causing bleeding), indinavir 800mg/8h OR nelfinavir 750mg/8h, al

Infectious diseases

HIV test counselling If in doubt, get help from a genitourinary clinic.

- Determine level of risk (eg unprotected sex; sex overseas).
- Discuss test benefits: partner protection; avoiding vertical transmission; getti
- What are the difficulties? Will you tell family and friends? Explain possibl ects on: job, mortgage, insurance (we have no obligation to disclose HIV sta
- Do post-test counselling (eg to re-emphasize ways to ↓risk exposure).
- *Counselling throughout HIV illness:* A key issue when a person is dying from making a will. Legal help may be needed on housing, employment, guardianship of children. Making advance directives needs special skill. Dor iary genitourinary teams, GP, and hospices help with terminal care all have a

Acute seroconversion As HIV gets more treatable, recognizing this early p becomes more important. Signs are similar to infectious mononucleosis lymphadenopathy, myalgia, rash and headache); perform tests if there are un signs, eg oral candidiasis, recurrent shingles, leucopenia, or CNS signs (anti tests may be negative but viral p24 antigen and HIV RNA levels are ↑ in infection). As ever, the first best 'test' is to take a thorough history. If yo identify acute seroconversion illness, get expert help—and advise unambiguc on preventing transmission. It is not known if early therapy is worthwhile.

Questions for when you are seeing HIV+ve people •Have you been to ar clinic? (STDs promote spread of HIV). •Are you using condoms? •What is your cell count/HIV-1 RNA level? (viral load helps plan start of antiretrovirals; CD4 < <100, and <50/mm³ prompt prophylaxis for *Pneumocystis*, *Toxoplasma*, and *M bacterium avium* complex, respectively). •What is your CMV and toxoplasma t (if -ve, counsel to avoid infection, eg no uncooked meat; avoid cats etc). •Re CXR? (eg TB; pneumocystosis). •Recent cervical smear? (risk of neoplasia↑).

1 Without interventions, rate of vertical transmission is 15–20%; prolonged breastfeeding doub this, falling to <2% with antiretroviral prophylaxis, elective Caesars and bottle feeding. 2006 da

ims of highly active antiretroviral therapy (HAART) & other strategies

HAART aims to suppress plasma HIV RNA concentrations below the limit of detection and restore immune function. This is not a cure as latent replication-competent provirus in resting CD4+ T lymphocytes and persistent (but cryptic) viral replication remain intact.[198] Life-long suppression of plasma HIV RNA is problematic—hence the need for strategies to *eradicate* HIV.

Enfuvirtide (a 'fusion inhibitor' eg 90mg/12h SC) intensifies HAART by blocking the last step in the 3-part process by which virus enter cells (attachment→co-receptor binding→fusion). It modestly increases rate of decay of the number of cells containing replication-competent HIV.[199]

In theory, these effects can be helped by any therapy which blocks histone deacetylase 1 (HDAC1 mediates virion production). This is the rationale behind studies of HDAC1 blockers such as valproic acid—which has been shown ↓frequency of resting cell infection (mean reduction 75%).[200]

►HAART should be part of a holistic, integrated, individualized care plan proceeding with management of co-morbidities eg malnutrition, malaria etc.[1]

lonitoring HIV infection

ıere is more to monitoring HIV than periodic measurements of the CD4 count. asma ***HIV RNA levels*** strongly predict progression to AIDS and death, whatever e CD4 count. This test typically involves quantitative reverse transcriptase PCR amplify DNA copies of the target RNA. HIV patients in the lowest quartile of viral ad (HIV RNA ≤4530 copies/mL) have an 8% chance of progressing to AIDS in yrs compared with 62% in those in the highest quartile (>36,270 copies/mL). inical benefit from anti-HIV agents depends not only on improving the ***CD4 ount*** but also from decreasing HIV RNA to undetectable levels.

/hen to treat HIV infection

ong-term studies of various different populations with HIV and involving clinical ndpoints such as death are few or lacking. In general, start drugs if:

Any patient diagnosed with AIDS, or with severe/recurrent HIV-related illness.
Any patient with CD4 count ≤200×10⁶/L (≤275 *might* be a better threshold).[201]
Asymptomatic with CD4 count of 200–350 × 10⁶/L and a high viral load.
Asymptomatic with a CD4 count of 200–350 × 10⁶/L which is falling rapidly.

orbidity data suggest these levels may be too stringent in determining eligibility.[202]
Do CD4 counts and HIV RNA levels to monitor treatment, eg every 3 months. nere is an argument for changing treatment if HIV RNA level rebounds (>500 opies/mL on two consecutive tests), if there is a consistent fall in the CD4 count, if new symptoms occur. The new regimen should include at least two drugs ew to the patient. Request resistance tests, eg genotyping for HIV reverse anscriptase/protease mutations (if available). **NB:** Multi-drug therapy imposes fficulties both in terms of timing of doses and interactions with other drugs.

esource-limited settings Where HIV is most prevalent, CD4 counts are too xpensive. A reasonable alternative is the TLC—the total lymphocyte count: a TLC 1400/μL≈a CD4 count of 200/μL as far as risk of mortality from HIV goes.[203]

Useful web link: British HIV association: www.bhiv.org.

NICEF integrated management of childhood illness: Qasi S 2006 *Trans R Soc Trop Med Hyg* 100 10

Antiretroviral agents

This is an expensive luxury for most of the world's HIV patients. In many ways anti-HIV treatment is experimental so perhaps the best question to ask is not *w is the best treatment for HIV* but *which is the most appropriate trial to enter patient into?* ►Seek expert help early.

►HAART (highly active anti-retroviral therapy) involves combining two nucleos analogue reverse transcriptase inhibitors (NRTI) with *either* a protease inhibitor *or* a non-nucleoside reverse transcriptase inhibitor (NNRTI) *or* (in patients w relatively low viral loads) abacavir.[204] One example of comparative data: efavire tenofovir–emtricitabine is better than efavirenz–zidovudine–lamivudine.[205] [206]

Nucleoside analogue reverse transcriptase inhibitors (NRTI)

- ***Zidovudine (azidothymidine, AZT)*** was the first anti-HIV drug. Dose: 25 300mg/12h PO or 1–2mg/kg/4h IV. SE: anaemia, leucopenia, gastrointesti disturbance, fever, rash, myalgia. Stop treatment if ↑LFT, hepatomegaly, lac acidosis. CI: anaemia, neutropenia, breast-feeding.
- ***Didanosine (DDI; Videx EC®)*** 250mg/24h PO if wt <60kg; 400mg/24h if ≥60 SE: pancreatitis, peripheral neuropathy, hyperuricaemia, GI disturbance, reti and optic nerve changes, liver failure. Stop treatment if significant rise in LFT amylase. CI: breast-feeding.
- ***Lamivudine (3TC)***[207] is a well-tolerated antiretroviral. Dose: 150mg/12h PO, t without food. se: see zidovudine, but less common. Stop if ↑LFT, hepatomeg lactic acidosis, pancreatitis.
- ***Emtricitabine (FTC)*** It is like lamivudine, but is also active against hepatitis B
- ***Stavudine (D4T)*** 40mg/12h PO if weight ≥60kg; 30mg/12h PO if <60kg. Sto neuropathy or ↑LFT.
- ***Tenofovir*** 245mg/24h PO. SE: see lamivudine.
- ***Abacavir*** 300mg/12h PO. SE: hepatitis, lactic acidosis, hypersensitivity syndro (3–5%)—rash, fever, vomiting; may be fatal if rechallenged.

Protease inhibitors (PI) slow cell-to-cell spread, and lengthen the time to the fi clinical event. PIs are often given with low dose ritonavir (100mg/12hr PO), wh appears to enhance drug levels. All PIs are metabolized by the cytochrome p4 enzyme system. They may therefore increase the concentrations of certain drugs competitive inhibition of their metabolism, if administered concomitantly.[209] PIs cause metabolic syndrome (dyslipidaemia, hyperglycaemia, insulin resistance).

- ***Indinavir*** 800mg/8h PO, 1h before or 2h after a meal. SE: dry mouth, ta disturbance, rash, pruritus, hyperpigmentation, alopecia, nephrolithiasis, anaem neutropenia, myalgia, paraesthesiae, ↑LFT.
- ***Ritonavir*** Start with 300mg then ↑ to 600mg/12h PO. SE: see indinavir.
- ***Saquinavir*** 1g/12h PO within 2h of a meal. SE: oral ulcers, paraesthesiae, myal headache, dizziness, pruritus, rash, pancreatitis.
- ***Nelfinavir*** 750mg/8h PO. SE: hepatitis, neutropenia, flatulence, ↑CK.
- ***Lopinavir/Ritonavir (Kaletra®)*** is probably superior to nelfinavir.[210] Do 400mg (+100mg ritonavir)/12h PO. SE: see saquinavir.
- **Others:** ***amprenavir*** 1200mg/12h PO (it has a new pro-drug, ***fosamprenavi*** SE: see saquinavir; ***atazanavir***; ***tipranavir***.

Non-nucleoside reverse transcriptase inhibitors (NNRTI) These may interact w drugs metabolized by the cytochrome p450 enzyme system, which they eith induce or inhibit depending on the concomitantly administered drug.[211]

- ***Nevirapine*** 200mg/24h for 2wks, then 200mg/12h PO. Resistance emerg readily. SE: Stevens–Johnson syndrome, toxic epidermal necrolysis, hepatitis
- ***Efavirenz*** Dose: 600mg/24h PO. SE: rash, insomnia, dizziness. Avoid in pregnan

olden rules in HIV therapy

Start HAART early, ideally before CD4 count <200 x 10^6/L.
Explain to patients that regimens are complex and negotiate strict adherence.
Take time to harmonize pills with the patient's expectations and lifestyle.
Is the patient suitable to include in an on-going research trial?
Aim for no more than twice-daily dosing, if possible.
Use ≥3 drugs (minimizes replication and cross-resistance). No dual therapies.
Monitor plasma viral load & CD4 count; *what seems like elimination of HIV often turns into reactivation when treatment stops*. Aim for undetectable viral loads 4 months after starting HAART. Suspect poor adherence if viral load rebounds.
If viral loads remains high despite good adherence, if there is a consistent fall in CD4 count, or if new symptoms occur, change to a new combination of anti-HIV drugs and request resistance tests, eg genotyping for HIV reverse transcriptase/protease mutations (if available).
Stay informed about new drugs, and emerging classes of drugs.

tandard regimens and some practical problems

Other illnesses: no ddI if **pancreatitis**. If **polyneuropathy**, avoid d-drugs (ddI, ddC, d4T). **Non-insulin-dependent diabetes** may need insulin with PIs. Hepatotoxicity risk is ↑ for nevirapine or ritonavir if there are **liver problems**.
Common initial regimens consist of two nucleoside analogues, combined with either a protease inhibitor, an NNRTI or a third nucleoside analogue.[212]
Managing highly antiviral-experienced HIV-infected patients is complicated by drug resistance, patient intolerabilities, drug interactions and quality-of-life issues. So potent regimens need expert input to maximize activity against resistant virus, eg enfuvirtide and tipranavir/ritonavir, have shown promising results in HAART regimens in those with extensive treatment histories and resistance profiles, if used in combination with other active agents.[213]
A few studies on simplification have been completed: for example, switching from complex regimes to didanosine-tenofovir-efavirenz provides a virological suppression rate at 12 months similar to that seen in patients who do not change from more complex therapy (and may obviate dyslipidaemias).[214]
Combination tablet examples: Trizivir® is abacavir 300mg, lamivudine 150mg, and zidovudine 300mg. Combivir® is zidovudine with lamivudine.

3-by-5'→'10-by-10': free access to antiretroviral drugs?

Vhen WHO announces targets such as '***3-by-5***' (3 million extra to get HIV ℞ by 2005) or, when this failed, '***10-by-10***' (100% availability of free HIV drugs by 2010), some people look on with scepticism, confident of failure. This is very lever, but misses the point, which is to save lives *and* raise awareness by ushing the HIV pandemic (which judges us all) up political agendas and to spur overnments into action. Looked at it this way, WHO has had a major impact, vith 300,000 lives saved, and, in some places, prevalences falling (eg in Kenya rom 14% in 1997 to ~4% in 2006). In some places, wards full of people dying of AIDS have emptied as drugs enable people get off their knees and start *living* vith HIV.[215] From 2006, as a result of debt-cancellation and pressure from Médecins Sans Frontières, all people in Nigeria have access to free antiretroviral therapy. But sometimes drugs remain in warehouses beyond their xpiry date—owing to corruption, and lack of blood tests for monitoring.[216]

Can HIV ℞ save lives rather than just postpone death? Of course: if drugs eep a mother alive, her offspring stand a chance. In one chilling study from Gambia 100% of babies who lost their mother died within a year.[217]

WHO initiatives also make HIV less taboo. If people know that HIV is a ondition which can be managed, and not a death-warrant, a culture of passive dependency is replaced by one of interdependence, initiative, and practical optimism. This really is a better definition of health than being disease-free.

►Refer early to genitourinary medicine clinic (GUM) for full microbiologi investigation and contact tracing and notification. Most clinics see patie immediately during the working day; some offer an on-call service. Avoid giv antibiotics until seen in GUM clinic or at least discussed. For HIV, see p398.

UK incidence is rising alarmingly, by >10%/yr as 'safer sex' practices are be ignored. Prevalence of chlamydia is ~11%[UK] (>104,000 cases new cases of gen *Chlamydia*); 22,320 cases of gonorrhoea[UK], and >2250 cases of syphilis.[218]

History Ask about timing of last intercourse; contraceptive method; sex contacts; duration of relationship; sexual practices and orientation; past sex infections; menstrual and medical history; antimicrobial therapy.

Examination Detailed examination of genitalia including inguinal nodes and pu hair. Scrotum, subpreputial space, and male urethra. PR examination a proctoscopy (if indicated); PV and speculum examination.

Signs Vaginal/urethral discharge (p406), genital lesions: herpes (p388); syph (p419); *Chlamydia* (BOX). Genital warts (*OHCS* p268). Salpingitis (*OHCS* p286). L (*OHCS* p608).

Tests Refer to GUM clinic. Urine: dipstick and MSU for MC+S. Ulcers: take swabs for culture (viral transport medium) and dark ground microscopy for syphilis ***pallidum***). Urethral smear for Gram stain/culture for ***N. gonorrhoeae*** (send quickly lab in Stuart's medium); urethral swab for ***Chlamydia*** (free tests also available fr UK chemists, see BOX). High vaginal or swab in Stuart's medium for microscopy/cult (***Candida, Gardnerella vaginalis,*** anaerobes, ***Trichomonas vaginalis***); endocervi swab for ***Chlamydia trachomatis. Chlamydia*** (an obligate intracellular bacteria the trickiest STD to diagnose as it is asymptomatic, difficult to culture, and serolc may be unhelpful as it cross-reacts with *C. pneumoniae*. Nucleic acid amplificat assays (eg urine ligase chain reaction, PCR) are quite good screening tests, w sensitivity >90%. Other tests: include ***Chlamydia*** antigen and nucleic acid prc assays.[219] ***Blood tests:*** Syphilis, hepatitis, and HIV serology after counselling.

Follow-up At 1wk & 3 months, with repeat smears, cultures, and syphilis serolo

Scabies (*Sarcoptes scabei*, an arachnid) Spread is common in families. ***The patient:*** Papular rash (on abdomen or medial thigh; itchy at night) + burrows (in digital web spaces and flexor wrist surfaces). ***Incubation:*** ~6wks (during which time sensitization to the mite's faeces and/or saliva occurs). Penile lesions produce red nodules. ***Diagnosis:*** Tease a mite out of its burrow with a needle for microscopy. This may fail but if a drop of oil is placed on the lesion, a few scrapes with a scalpel may provide faeces or eggs. ***R̶:*** ►Treat all the household. Give written advice (*OHCS* p608). Apply 5% permethrin over wh body including scalp, face, neck and ears (BNF); wash off after 8–12h; repeat after Use 5% cream on hands if washed before the 8h elapses. Remember to paint parts, including soles (avoid eyes); wash off after 24h.

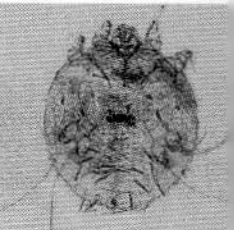
Fig 1. *Sarcoptes scabei.*

Lymphogranuloma ***Signs:*** Inguinal lymphadenopathy + ulceration ***Causes:*** *Lymph granuloma venereum* (*Chlamydia trachomatis;* serovar L_2 causes proctitis too, eg HIV +ve European men),[221] chancroid (*Haemophilus ducreyi*),[1] or granulor inguinale (*Klebsiella (Calymmatobacterium) granulomatis*, ie donovanosis). T latter causes extensive, painless, red genital ulcers and pseudobuboes (ingui nodes abscess), with possible elephantiasis ± malignant change. ***Diagnosis:*** 'clos safety-pin' inclusion bodies in cytoplasm of histiocytes. ***R̶:*** doxycycline 100mg/1 PO until all lesions epithelialized—or azithromycin, erythromycin, or tetracyclir

1 In the Tropics, chancroid is a common cause of sexually acquired genital ulcers, typically wit granular, yellow base, and ragged edges (± inguinal buboes, which may need draining via a wide-b needle); the cause is *Haemophilus ducreyi*. WHO recommends erythromycin 500mg/6h PO for ceftriaxone 250mg IM (1 dose), azithromycin 1g PO (1 dose). Chancroid facilitates spread of HIV.

hlamydia screening to prevent pelvic inflammatory disease NICE 2006

enital *Chlamydia trachomatis* is the commonest STI in the UK (>104,000 iagnoses in GUM clinics/yr). Highest rates are in men and women <24yrs old—nplying longterm morbidity, as salpingitis, infertility, or ectopic pregnancy will ccur in 2–4%.[222] These 2006 data (n=43,751) are at odds with older NICE data, asting doubt of some of NICE's strategies (below).

Shame, embarrassment about discussing STIs with partners, **lack of ppointments**, and having to go **out of one's way** to be sensible are the main bstacles. Dialogue is the key; you can help by talking frankly with your patients bout sex: see *OHCS* p328. As part of implementing the UK **National Chlamydia creening Programme**, UK high street pharmacies (Boots) offer **free chlamydia ests** (NHS funded) or those aged 16–24yrs (eg in London, and if +ve, to their artners, of *any* age). Uptake of this service is patchy and it may be hard to ıstain. Colleges, prisons, and armed forces are also targeted.[223] NB: Only 0.5% of oung adults respond to **mass media campaigns** inviting them in for screening.

Free home-based urine test kits may be distributed to garages, hairdressers, nd supermarkets with results texted to **mobile phones**—removing the need to rovide embarrassing samples at the doctor's surgery.

Walk-in STI clinics and **late-opening GP clinics** allow *prompt* treatment of ncomplicated genital chlamydial infection: **azithromycin** 1g PO as a single dose.

NICE advocates **opportunistic screening** of young adults (eg with nucleic acid mplification tests on urine) *wherever* they present to primary care, irrespective f presenting symptoms.[224] This might halve the incidence of pelvic inflam-ıatory disease. Issues about efficient contact tracing are unresolved. NB: There no good evidence to support using screening to halt transmission, of to reduce ates of orchitis,♂ ectopic pregnancy or infertility.

Vaginal discharge and urethritis

Non-offensive vaginal discharge may be physiological. Most which are smelly itchy are due to infection. Foul discharge may be due to a foreign body (eg forgot tampons, or beads in children). ►Discharges rarely resemble their class descriptions. ►Untreated GU inflammation ↑viral shedding of HIV-1 in semen 3-f

Thrush *(Candida albicans)* Thrush is the commonest cause of discharge an classically described as white curds. The vulva and vagina may be red, fissured, a sore. The partner may be asymptomatic. ***Risk factors:*** Pregnancy, immu deficiencies, diabetes, the Pill, antibiotics. ***Diagnosis:*** Microscopy: strings mycelium or oval spores. Culture on Sabouraud's medium. ***Treatment:*** A sin imidazole vaginal pessary, eg **clotrimazole** 500mg, + cream for the vulva (a partner) is convenient. Alternative: 1 dose of **fluconazole** 150mg PO. Reassure t thrush is not necessarily sexually transmitted. Recurrent thrush: see *OHCS* p28

Trichomonas vaginalis (TV) Produces vaginitis and a thin, bubbly, fishy smelling discharge. It is sexually transmitted. Exclude gonorrhoea (which may coexist). The motile flagellate may be seen on wet film microscopy, or cultured. ***℞:*** **Metronidazole** 400mg/12h PO for 5 days or 2g PO stat. Treat the partner. If pregnant, use the 5-day regimen.

Fig 1. *T. vaginalis.*

Bacterial vaginosis causes a fishy smelling discharge. The vagina is not inflamed. Itch is rare. Vaginal pH is >5.5, hence alteration of bacte flora ± overgrowth, eg of *Gardnerella vaginalis*, *Mycoplasma hominis*, peptostrep cocci, *Mobiluncus* and anaerobes, eg *Bacteroides* species with too few lactobacil There is ↑risk of pre-term labour and amniotic infection if pregnant. ***Diagno*** Stippled vaginal epithelial 'clue cells' on wet microscopy. Culture. ***℞:*** *OHCS* p284; **metronidazole** 400mg/12h PO for 5d, or **clindamycin** cream.

Gonorrhoea *Neisseria gonorrhoea* (gonococcus, GC) can infect any columnar epithelium, eg urethra, cervix, rectum, pharynx, conjunctiva. Incubation: 2–10d. ♂: Urethral pus ± dysuria; tenesmus; proctitis ± discharge PR if gay. ♀: Often asymptomatic, but may have vaginal discharge, dysuria, proctitis. Pharyngeal disease is often asymptomatic. ***Complications—Local:*** Prostatitis, cystitis, salpingitis, epididymitis, Bartholinitis. ***Systemic:*** Septicaemia, eg with petechiae, hand/foot pustules, arthritis; Reiter's syndrome; SBE (rare). ***Obstetric:*** Ophthalmia neonatorum[ND] (*OHCS* p36). ***Long-term:*** Urethral stricture, infertility. ***℞:*** **Cefixime**, eg 400mg PO stat (or **ciprofloxacin** 500mg stat PO, but resistance is a problem in eg in 36% in N England). Treat for chlamydia too (eg **doxycyline** 100mg/12h PO for 7d, or a stat dose of **azithromycin** 1g PO) as 50% of patients with urethritis or cervicitis also have *C. trachoma* Trace contacts (refer to special clinic). No intercourse or alcohol until cured.

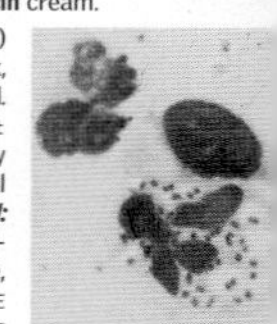

Fig 2. Gonococci in neut phils; pairs of diplococci (long axes parallel)—her stained at the bedside b Field's stain (p373).[226]

Non-gonococcal urethritis is commoner than GC. Discharge is thinner and sig less acute, but this may not help diagnosis. Women (typically asymptomatic) m have cervicitis, urethritis, or salpingitis (pain, fever, infertility). Rectum and phar are not infected. ***Organisms:*** *C. trachomatis* (►special swabs are needed, *O* p286); *Ureaplasma urealyticum*; *Mycoplasma genitalium*; *Trichomonas vagina* *Gardnerella*; Gram –ve and anaerobic bacteria; *Candida*. ***Complications:*** Simila local complications of GC. *Chlamydia* may cause Reiter's syndrome and neona conjunctivitis. ***Treatment:*** 1 week of **doxycycline** 100mg/12h PO. A single dos **azithromycin** 1g PO is an alternative where compliance is likely to be problema Trace contacts. Avoid intercourse during treatment and alcohol for 4 weeks.

Non-infective urethritis Traumatic; chemicals; cancer; foreign body.

/hen do antibiotic guidelines become outdated?

ıe emergence of antibiotic resistance amongst pathogens represents one of the ain obstacles in the fight against infectious diseases. Antibiotic guidelines, which cist on local, regional, and national levels help ensure optimal therapy, but must be ɔntinually updated in the vain task of trying to keep up with pathogens. To onitor resistance patterns, sample infective isolates from different UK regions ·e collected centrally and tested against a variety of antibiotics to determine ıeir sensitivities to the different drugs (as measured by the minimal inhibitory ɔncentration (MIC) of drug required to prevent organism growth in culture). ɹch results can highlight the need to revise antibiotic guidelines.

One example is the emergence of ciprofloxacin resistance in *Neisseria ɔnorrhoeae* isolates in England and Wales. Resistance was found in 36% of olates from N England in 2004–5—a big rise from 10% of isolates in 2002, ıd 3% in 2001, and 2% in 2000. National guidelines aim for chosen drugs to iminate gonococcal infection in >95% of patients. Ciprofloxacin, previously st-line, now has to be replaced by cephalosporins (eg cefixime) in new ɹidelines.

Miscellaneous Gram positive bacteria

Staphylococci When pathogenic, these are usually *Staph. aureus*. Typically, they inf skin, lids, or wounds. Severe *Staph. aureus* infections are: pneumonia, osteomyeli septic arthritis; endocarditis; septicaemia. Production of β-lactamase which destr many antibiotics (p368–70) is the main problem. *Staph. aureus* toxins cause fc poisoning (p380) and toxic shock syndrome toxin (TSST-1): shock, confusion, fever, a ra with desquamation, diarrhoea, myalgia, CPK↑, platelets↓ (associated with the use hyperabsorbent tampons). *Staph. epidermidis (albus)* is recognized as a pathogen in immunocompromized, particularly in connection with IV lines or any prosthesis. Wh isolated from a culture, *Staph. epidermidis* can usually be assumed to be a contamina It is often enough to remove infected lines. Deep *Staph.* infections need ≥4wks flucloxacillin 500mg/6h IV ± removal of foreign bodies, eg prostheses.

***Methicillin-resistant Staph. aureus* (MRSA)** is a high-profile hospital-acqui infection, causing pneumonia, septicaemia, wound infections, and death (risk ↑ fold),228 but MRSA only accounts for ~6% of total hospital acquired infect (~300,000/yr in England, with ~5000 deaths). ≥17 sub-types. NB: *C. difficile* a glycopeptide-resistant enterococci are just as bad. In the UK it is mandatory to recc all infections; despite stringent efforts rates are rising in 40% of UK hospitals— related to overcrowding, the inability to close affected wards, poor barrier-nursi facilities, and faulty hygiene (eg not washing hands between patients). Carria rates (nasal): 1–10%. Risk factors: HIV, dialysis, being on ITU. MRSA is communi acquired in up to 40%. ℞: Discuss with a microbiologist. Vancomycin or teicopla are used, but strains with reduced sensitivity (vancomycin-intermediate *Sta aureus* (VISA)—↓sensitivity to *both* drugs) have emerged.229 Here, linezolid quinupristin/dalfopristin (Synercid®) may be effective. Preventive measures:

- Isolate recently admitted patients with suspected MRSA. Group MRSA cases one ward (impractical if hospital has to run at 100% capacity).
- Wash your hands and your stethoscope! (also TV remote controls, etc).
- Ask about the need for eradication (with *mupirocin*).
- Be meticulous in looking after intravascular catheters when on ITU.
- Surveillance swabs of patients and staff during outbreaks.
- Use gowns/gloves when dealing with infected or colonized patients. Masks m be needed during contact with MRSA pneumonia.

Streptococci Group A streps (eg ***Strep pyogenes***) are common pathogens, causing wound and skin infections (eg impetigo, erysipelas, *OHCS* p598), tonsillitis, scarlet fever[ND], necrotizing fasciitis (p592), toxic shock, or septicaemia. Late complications are rheumatic fever and post-streptococcal glomerulonephritis. ***Strep. pneumoniae*** (pneumococcus, Gram +ve diplococcus) causes pneumonia, otitis media, meningitis, septicaemia, peritonitis (rare). Resistance to penicillin is a problem. ***Strep. sanguis, Strep. mutans,*** and ***Strep. mitior*** (of the 'viridans' group), ***Strep. bovis***, and ***Enterococcus faecalis*** all cause endocarditis. ***Enterococcus faecalis*** also causes UTI, wound infections, and septicaemia. ***Strep. mutans*** is a very common cause of dental caries. ***Strep. milleri*** forms abscesses, eg in CNS, lungs, and liver. Most streps are sensitive to the penicillins, but ***Enterococcus faecalis*** and ***Enterococcus faecium*** may present some difficulties. They usually respond to a combination of ampicillin and an aminoglycoside, eg gentamicin (p371 & p738). Vancomyc resistant enterococci (VRE) have been reported. Some strains of VRE are sensitive either teicoplanin or Synercid®; all appear to be sensitive to linezolid (p370).[1]

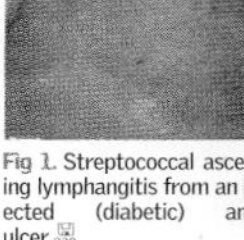

Fig 1. Streptococcal asce ing lymphangitis from an ected (diabetic) ar ulcer.230

1 See reports of vancomycin-resistant *S. aureus* (VRSA), containing a *vanA* resistance gene

Anthrax[ND] ***(Bacillus anthracis)*** Occurs in Africa, Asia, China, Eastern Europe, and Haiti. Spread is by handling infected carcasses; well-cooked meat poses *no* risk. Terrorists have used long-lasting anthrax spores (from the ear of a cow that died near Oxford in 1937)[231] as a biological weapon.[232] ***Signs:*** Common form: local cutaneous black pustule (anthrax=ανθηραξ=coal in Greek). Oedema may be a striking sign ± fever and hepatosplenomegaly. May cause lung or GI anthrax with dyspnoea ± big GI bleeds or meningoencephalitis. ***Tests:*** CXR (wide mediastinum). Gram stain is sometimes diagnostic (Gram +ve rod). ***℞:*** *Cutaneous disease:* ciprofloxacin 500mg/12h PO for up to 60d. *Pulmonary or GI anthrax:* Ciprofloxacin 400mg/12h IVI + clindamycin 900mg/8h IVI + rifampicin 300mg/12h IVI. Switch to oral drugs when able; treat for 60d. ***Prevention:*** Immunize animals at risk, and enforce sound food-handling and carcass-hygiene policies.[233]

Diphtheria[ND] is caused by *Corynebacterium diphtheriae* toxin. ***Signs:*** tonsillitis ± a pseudomembrane over the fauces and lymphadenopathy ('bull neck'). ENT details: *OHCS* p158. ***℞:*** Erythromycin 10–12mg/kg/6h IVI. ***Prevention:*** p381. Give non-immune contacts erythromycin 500mg/6h PO for 10d *before* swab results known.

Listeriosis is caused by *Listeria monocytogenes*, a Gram +ve bacillus with an odd ability to multiply at low temperatures. Possible sources of infection include pâtés, raw vegetables, unpasteurized milk, and soft cheeses (brie, camembert, and blue vein types). It may cause a non-specific 'flu-like illness, pneumonia, meningoencephalitis, ataxia, rash, or PUO, especially in the immunocompromised, in pregnancy, where it may cause miscarriage or stillbirth, and in neonates.[234] ***Diagnosis:*** Culture blood, placenta, amniotic fluid, CSF, and any expelled products of conception. ►*Take blood cultures in any pregnant patient with unexplained fever for ≥48h.* Serology, vaginal, and rectal swabs don't help (it may be a commensal here). ***Treatment:*** Ampicillin IV (erythromycin if allergic) + gentamicin; see p368 & p371 for doses. ***Prevention in pregnancy:*** • Avoid soft cheeses, pâtés, and under-cooked meat. • Observe 'use by' dates. • Ensure reheated food is piping hot; observe standing times when using microwaves; throw away any left-overs.

Nocardia* species** cause subcutaneous infection (eg Madura foot) in warm climes, and, if immunocompromised, abscesses (lung, liver, cerebral). Microscopy: branching chains of cocci. ***℞: Trimethoprim 5mg/kg/8h IVI + sulfamethoxazole 25mg/kg/8h IVI for 3wks (do serum levels) then reduce. 2nd-line: imipenem ½g/6h IVI + amikacin.

Clostridia Tetanus p412. ***C. perfringens*** causes wound infections and gas gangrene ± shock or renal failure after surgery or trauma (p592). ***℞:*** Debridement is vital; benzylpenicillin 1.2–2.4g/6h IV + clindamycin 900mg/8h IVI, antitoxin and hyperbaric O_2 may also be used. Amputation may be necessary. *Clostridia* food poisoning (p380). ***C. difficile:*** Diarrhoea (the cause of pseudomembranous colitis following antibiotic therapy, p239). ***C. botulinum:*** (Botulism) *C. botulinum* toxin blocks release of acetylcholine causing descending flaccid paralysis. Botulism is not spread from one person to another. There are 2 adult forms of botulism: food-borne and wound botulism. ►*Risk is high in IV drug abusers* if heroin is contaminated with *C. botulinum*. ***Signs:*** Afebrile, flaccid paralysis, dysarthria, dysphagia, diplopia, ptosis, weakness, respiratory failure. Autonomic signs: dry mouth, fixed or dilated pupils. ***Tests:*** Find toxin in blood samples or, in wound botulism, identify *C. botulinum* in wound specimens by prompt referral to a reference lab. Samples include: serum, wound pus, swabs in anaerobic transport media (in the UK, phone 020 8200 6868).[235] ***℞:*** Get help (on ITU). IM botulism antitoxin works if given early (eg 50,000U of types A & B + 5000U of type E). Also give to those who have ingested toxin but are as yet asymptomatic. *C. botulinum* is sensitive to benzylpenicillin and metronidazole. In the UK, if out of hours, antitoxin is sourced via CDSC doctors (tel. 020 7210 300).[236]

Actinomycosis is caused by ***Actinomyces israelii***. Usually causes subcutaneous infections, forming sinuses with pus which contains sulfur granules—eg on the jaw or IUCDs, *OHCS* p298). It may cause abdominal masses (may mimic appendix mass). ***℞:*** Benzylpenicillin (p368) for ≥2wks post-clinical cure. Liaise with surgeons.

Miscellaneous Gram negative bacteria

Enterobacteria Some are normal gut commensals, others environmenta organisms. They are the commonest cause of UTI and intra-abdominal sepsis especially post-operatively and in the acute abdomen. They are also a commor cause of septicaemia. Unusually, they may cause pneumonia (especially ***Klebsiella***) meningitis, or endocarditis. These organisms can be sensitive to ampicillin anc trimethoprim but resistance is growing. Resistance of *K. pneumoniae* to amikacin is seen in 50% (in some places), ceftazidime (90%) and tobramycin (90%)[237] sc imipenem may be needed. ***Salmonella*** & ***Shigella*** are discussed on p380 & p414

Pseudomonas aeruginosa is a serious pathogen (esp. if immunocompromised anc in cystic fibrosis). It causes pneumonia, septicaemia, UTI, wound infection, osteo myelitis, and cutaneous infections. The main problem is its increasing antibioti resistance. ***Treatment:*** Piperacillin (p368) or mezlocillin + an aminoglycoside Ciprofloxacin, ceftazidime, and imipenem (p371) are useful against *Pseudomonas*

Haemophilus influenzae typically affects unvaccinated children usually <4yrs olc It causes otitis media, acute epiglottitis, pneumonia, meningitis, osteomyelitis, anc septicaemia. In adults it may cause exacerbations of chronic bronchitis. ***R:*** Unrel iably sensitive to ampicillin; cefotaxime is more reliable. Capsulated types tend t be much more pathogenic than non-capsulated types. ***Prevention:*** Immunizatior with HIB vaccine (p381) has resulted in a dramatic fall in incidence.

Plague[ND] ***Cause: Yersinia pestis***. ***Incubation:*** 1–7d. ***Bubonic plague*** presents as suppurating lymphadenopathy (buboes). ***Pneumonic plague:*** 'Flu-symptoms, dyspnoea, cough, copious, bloody sputum, septicaemia, and a fatal haemorrhagic illness (± buboes). ***Diagnosis:*** Phage typing of bacterial culture, or a 4-fold rise in antibodies to F antigen.[239] ***R:*** Isolate suspects; streptomycin 15mg/kg/12h IM for 10d. If in 1st ⅓ of pregnancy, amoxicillin 250–500mg/8h PO; if later in pregnancy, co-trimoxazole 480mg/12h PO; children: co-trimoxazole.[240] Staying at home, quarantine (inspect daily for 1wk), insect sprays to legs and bedding, and avoiding dead animals helps stop spread. ***Post-exposure prophylaxis:*** Doxycycline 100mg/12h PO for 7d ***Prevention:*** Vaccines give no instant protection (multiple doses may be needed)

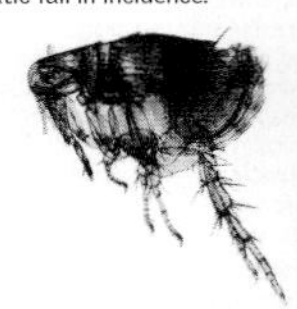

Fig 1. Rat fleas (*Xenopsylla cheopis*) spread plague; also cat fleas ± human-to-human droplet spread.[238]

Brucellosis This zoonosis (carried by domestic animals) is common in the Middl East. Typically affects vets or farmers. Cause: ***B. melitensis*** (the most virulent ***B. abortus***, ***B. suis***, or ***B. canis***. Symptoms may be indolent and last for years—e fever (PUO), sweats, malaise, anorexia, vomiting, weight loss, hepatosplenomegal constipation, diarrhoea, myalgia, backache, arthritis, sacroiliitis, rash, bursitis, orchitis depression. ***Complications:*** Osteomyelitis, SBE/IE (culture –ve), abscesses (liver spleen, lung), meningoencephalitis. ***Diagnosis:*** Blood culture (≥6wks but rapi culture systems available, contact lab); serology: if titres equivocal (eg >1 : 40 in non endemic zones) do ELISA ± immunoradiometric assays; pancytopenia. ***Treatment*** Doxycycline 100mg/12h PO for 6 weeks + streptomycin 1g/d IM for 2–3wk (↓relapse rate from 2–10% *vs* >20%).[241] If a child, get expert help.

Whooping cough[ND] is caused by ***Bordetella pertussis***. It begins with a prodroma catarrhal, fever, and cough. After a week or so, the child develops the characteristi paroxysms of coughing and inspiratory whoops. Most children recover wel although the illness may last months. Some, especially the very young, may develo pneumonia (±bronchiectasis) or convulsions and brain damage. ***R:*** Erythromycir given early, if only to limit spread. *Immunization* (p381) has not controlled th disease in Europe: incidence in adults doubled over a recent 5yr period.[242]

asteurella multocida is acquired via domestic animals, eg cat or dog bites. It can ause skin infections, septicaemia, pneumonia, UTI, or meningitis. ***R:*** Co-amoxiclav, 368 eg is 1g/6–8h IV over 3–4 min (expressed as amoxicillin).

ersinia enterocolitica In Scandinavia, this is a common cause of a reactive, symmetrical polyarthritis of the weight-bearing joints, and, in America, of nteritis. It also causes uveitis, appendicitis, mesenteric lymphadenitis, pyomyositis, lomerulonephritis, thyroiditis, colonic dilatation, terminal ileitis and perforation, nd septicaemia. ***Diagnosis:*** Serology is often more helpful than culture, as there ay be quite a time-lag between infection and the clinical manifestations. gglutination titres >1 : 160 indicate recent infection. ***Treatment:*** None may be eeded or ciprofloxacin 500mg/12h PO for 3–5d.

loraxella catarrhalis (Gram –ve diplococcus) is an increasingly recognized cause f pneumonia, exacerbations of COPD, otitis media, sinusitis, and septicaemia. ***reatment:*** Clarithromycin 500mg/12h PO.

ularaemia is caused by ***Francisella tularensis*** (Gram –ve bacillus), which may be cquired by handling infected animal carcasses. It causes rash, fever, malaise, onsillitis, headache, hepatosplenomegaly, and lymphadenopathy. There may e papules at sites of inoculation (eg fingers). ***Complications:*** Meningitis, steomyelitis, SBE/IE, pericarditis, septicaemia.

iagnosis: Contact local microbiologist for advice. Only use laboratories with afety cabinets suitable for dangerous pathogens. Swabs and aspirates must be ransported in approved containers. ***Treatment:*** Gentamicin or streptomycin .5–10mg/kg/12h IM for 2wks. Oral tetracycline may be suitable for hemoprophylaxis. ***Prevention:*** Find the animal vector; reduce human contact vith it as far as possible. Vaccination may be possible for high-risk groups.

at scratch disease Mostly due to ***Bartonella henselae*** (a small, curved, leomorphic, Gram negative rod) or ***Afepilis felis***. Think of this when any three of e following coexist: an inoculating cat scratch; regional lymphadenopathy (with egative lab tests for other causes of lymphadenopathy, p64); positive cat scratch kin test antigen response; or microabscesses in lymph nodes. In HIV-infected atients, the skin lesions may resemble Kaposi's sarcoma. ***Treatment:*** Usually esolves spontaneously within 1–2 months. One trial found that azithromycin speed of resolution of lymph nodes.[243] Other drugs that have been used include iprofloxacin, rifampicin and co-trimoxazole. Usually unresponsive *in vivo* despite usceptibility *in vitro*.

ee also **Spirochaetes** p418; ***Neisseria*** p368, and ***Legionella*** p154.

Tetanus[ND]

Essence Tetanospasmin, *Clostridium tetani's* exotoxin, causes muscle spasms an rigidity, cardinal features of tetanus (='to stretch').

Incidence ~50 people/yr in the UK. Mortality: 40% (80% in neonates).

Pathogenesis Spores of *C. tetani* live in faeces, soil, dust, and on instruments. A tin breach in skin or mucosa, eg cuts, burns, ear piercing, banding of piles, may adm the spores. Diabetics are ↑risk. Spores then germinate and make the exotoxin. Th travels up peripheral nerves and interferes with inhibitory synapses.

The Patient *15–25% will have no evidence of recent wounds.* Signs appear from 1 to several months from the (often forgotten) injury. There is a prodrome of feve malaise, and headache before classical features develop: *trismus* (=lockjaw; Gree trismos = grinding, hence difficulty in opening the mouth); *risus sardonicus* (a grir like posture of hypertonic facial muscles); *opisthotonus* (fig 1); *spasms* (which a first may be induced by movement, injections, noise, etc., but later are spontaneous they may cause dysphagia & respiratory arrest); autonomic dysfunction (arrhy thmias ± wide fluctuations in BP).

Differential diagnosis is dental abscess (both cause trismus), rabies, phenothiazin toxicity, and strychnine poisoning. Phenothiazine toxicity usually only affects faci and tongue muscles; if suspected, give benzatropine 1–2mg IV.

Poorer prognosis Short incubation; trismus leads to spasms in <48h; neonate elderly; postinfective; postpartum (a big cause of maternal mortality worldwide

Treatment ▸▸Get help on ITU. ABC (may need tracheostomy & ventilation). Monito ECG + BP + SpO_2 (keep >92%, eg with O_2 mask + reservoir); careful fluid balance.

- **Human tetanus immunoglobulin** (HTIG) 5000–10,000U IVI to neutralize toxin
- Aim to keep the patient asleep but rousable to obey simple command **Diazepam** 5–20mg/8h PO (mild disease) or, to control spasms, 0.05–0.2mg/kg/ IVI (≤140mg/d) ***or*** **phenobarbital** 1.0mg/kg/h IM or IV + **chlorpromazin** 0.5mg/kg/6h IM (IV bolus is dangerous) starting 3h after the phenobarbital. I this fails to control the spasms, paralyse and ventilate (get anaesthetist's help Dose example (*OTM*): **pancuronium** 2–4mg IV/½–2h (or by continuous IVI).

Prevention Active immunization with tetanus toxoid is part of the 3-stage vaccin during the 1st year of life (eg Pediacel®, p381). Boosters are given on startin school and in early adulthood. Once 5 injections have been given, revaccinate onl at the time of significant injury, and consider a final 1-off booster at ~65yrs.

Primary immunization of adults: 0.5mL tetanus toxoid IM repeated twice a monthly intervals. In the UK, the formulation is Revaxis®, p381.

Wounds: Any cut merits an extra dose of 0.5mL toxoid IM, unless already full immune (a full course of toxoid or a booster in last 10yrs). If non-immune: 2 further injections (0.5mL IM) at monthly intervals. If partially immune (ie has had a toxoid booster or a full course >10yrs previously), a single booster is enough.

Human tetanus immunoglobulin: Give if non-immune or partially immune, define above if wound is dirty, old (>6h), infected, devitalized, or soil-contaminated. Giv 250–500 units IM, using a separate syringe and site to the toxoid injection.

▸If immune status is unknown, assume that the patient is nonimmune. Routin infant immunization started in 1961, so many adults are at risk.

▸Hygiene education and wound debridement are of vital importance.

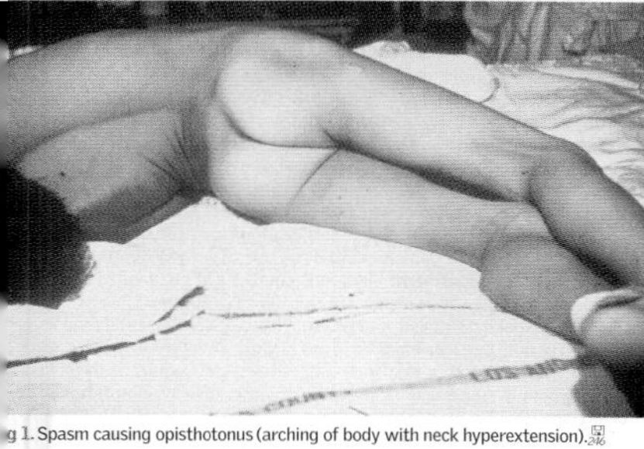

g 1. Spasm causing opisthotonus (arching of body with neck hyperextension).

Enteric fever[ND]

Typhoid and paratyphoid are caused by ***Salmonella typhi*** and ***S. paratyphi*** (types A, B, and C), respectively. (Other *Salmonella* cause D&V: p380 & p238.) ***Incubation:*** 3–21d. ***Spread:*** Faecal-oral. 1% become chronic carriers. ***Presentation:*** Usually malaise, headache, high fever with relative bradycardia, cough and constipation (or diarrhoea). CNS signs (coma, delirium, meningism) are serious. Diarrhoea is more common after the 1st week. Rose spots occur on the trunk of 40% but may be very difficult to see. Epistaxis, bruising, abdominal pain, and splenomegaly may occur. ***Tests:*** First 10d: blood culture; later: urine/stool culture. Bone marrow culture has highest yield (infiltration may cause ↓platelets & WCC, LFT↑. Widal test unreliable. DNA probes and PCR tests have been developed, but are not widely available. ***Treatment:*** Fluid replacement and good nutrition. There is good evidence that fluoroquinolones (eg ciprofloxacin 500mg/12h PO for 6d) are the best antimicrobial treatment for typhoid. Chloramphenicol is still used in many areas: 1g/8h PO until pyrexia diminishes, then 500mg/8h for a week and 250mg/6h to make up 14d (can be shorter). Other alternatives: cefotaxime, azithromycin, or amoxicillin (if fully susceptible). In severe disease, give IV ciprofloxacin or IV cefotaxime for 10–14d. In encephalopathy ± shock, give dexamethasone 3mg/kg IV stat, then 1mg/kg/6h for 48h. Drug resistance is an increasing problem, even with ciprofloxacin, eg due to mutations in the DNA gyrase enzyme of *S. typhi*.[247]

Complications: Osteomyelitis (eg in sickle-cell disease); DVT; GI bleed or perforation; cholecystitis; myocarditis; pyelonephritis; meningitis; abscess. Infection is said to have cleared when 6 consecutive cultures of urine and faeces are –ve. Chronic carriage is a problem; treat if at risk of spreading disease (eg food handlers). Ciprofloxacin 500mg/12h PO for 6 weeks; cholecystectomy may be needed. ***Prognosis:*** If untreated 10% die; if treated, 0.1% die. ***Vaccine:*** p381.

Bacillary dysentery[ND]

Shigella causes abdominal pain and bloody diarrhoea ± sudden fever, headache and occasionally neck stiffness. CSF is sterile. UK school epidemics are usually mild (often ***S. sonnei***), but imported dysentery may be severe (often ***S. flexneri*** or ***S. dysenteriae***). ***Incubation:*** 1–7d. ***Spread:*** Faecal–oral. ***Diagnosis:*** Stool culture. ***Treatment:*** Fluids PO. Avoid anti-diarrhoeal drugs. Drugs: ciprofloxacin 500mg/12h PO for 3–5d. Imported shigellosis is often resistant to several antimicrobials: sensitivity testing is important for all enteric fevers. There may be associated spondyloarthritis (p537).

Cholera[ND]

Caused by ***Vibrio cholerae*** (Gram negative comma-shaped rod, fig 1, on p364). Pandemics or epidemics may occur, eg outbreaks in Angola and the 1990s epidemic in S America and Bangladesh (Bengal *Vibrio cholerae 0139*). ***Incubation:*** From a few hours to 5d. ***Spread:*** Faecal–oral. ***Presentation:*** Profuse (eg 1L/h) watery ('rice water') stools, fever, vomiting, and rapid dehydration (the cause of death). ***Diagnosis:*** Stool microscopy and culture. ***Treatment:*** Strict barrier nursing. Replace fluid and salt losses meticulously (0.9% saline IVI if shocked), add 20mmol/L K^+ until U&E known (avoid plain Ringer's lactate: it may cause fatal K^+↓). Oral rehydration with WHO formula (20g glucose/L) is not so effective as cooked rice powder solution (50–80g/L) in reducing stool volume.[248] Its high osmolarity (310mmol/L vs 200mmol/L) is also unfavourable to water absorption. A dose of ciprofloxacin 1g PO may reduce fluid loss.[249] ***Prevention:*** Only drink boiled or treated water. Cook all food well; eat it hot. Avoid shellfish. Peel all vegetables. Heat-killed vaccine (serovar 01) gives limited protection, and is no longer needed for international travel; newer vaccines are non-standard.[250]

Whose deaths really matter? Enteric fevers suggest an answer

In 2006, DNA analysis of pulp in the teeth of Athenians dying in the great plague of 430BC revealed that the cause was typhoid fever. 30% of Athenians died, including Pericles, their leader. He gave us the Parthenon, juries, free theatre, and, in his own immortal oratory, the notion that it is better to die resisting than to live in submission. This is definitely *not* the right approach to infectious diseases: Pericles should have promulgated a third way: neither victory nor submission, but, more subtly, *accommodation*, or something even more symbiotic.

For the next 23 centuries, typhoid fever carried on killing, teaching us nothing much, until noon on 23 April 1851, when a little-known girl was quietly expiring in Malvern. Her name was Annie Darwin, her father's, Charles. Annie was his favourite fun-loving daughter, and with her lingering enteric death Darwin gave up all belief in a just and moral universe. Thus unimpeded, his mind was able to frame and compellingly justify the most devastating answer to the oldest question: that we are here by accident, thanks to natural selection, the survival of the fittest, and the 'wasteful, blundering, low & horridly cruel works of nature'.[1]

The next significant enteric death was 3 summers later at 40 Broad Street, in the Parish of St James, London, where a child became ill with diarrhoea in August, 1854, dying on September 2. Her mother rinsed the soiled nappies into the house drains. These led within feet of the supply to the Broad Street pump. Both the drain and the pump's well had faulty brickwork allowing the waters to mix. From this confluence sprung the discipline of Public Health, for many of the 500 or so ensuing late summer deaths from cholera clustered around this Broad Street pump, as diagrammed by the local doctor, Dr John Snow. He used his now famous diagrams locating each death to motivate the Board of Guardians of St James's parish at its meeting of Sept. 7th 'In consequence of what I said, the handle of the pump was removed the following day'[2]—so inaugurating the control of cholera. If Snow were alive today, he might be busy unplugging all our carbon-emitting power-stations (as killing as cholera), but note that Snow worked through committees to save his countless lives, not by direct action.

These events illustrate two counter-intuitive truths: knowledge of the microscopic cause of a disease is not required for public health measures to succeed (*Vibrio cholerae* was as yet undiscovered)—and even the most parochial Church Council is capable of prompt and decisive action affecting the lives of millions, when informed by an intelligent doctor in command of the facts.

There is one metaphysical truth revealed by these enteric deaths, which would not have escaped Pericles had he only taken the trouble to become a medical student for long enough to realise that his overvalued ideal of heroism is often pointless.[3] Pericles never gave his condolences to parents who lost their sons in battle, because, he said, a hero's death was the finest thing that could befall a man. We meet many heroic deaths on our wards, but they seem oddly pointless in retrospect. This is why we award the palm to Annie, whose unheroic death so transforms the inner landscapes of the mind. And with her in mind, we can confidently relieve our patients of the notion that they must die fighting.

1 A remark of Darwin's in 1856, before starting his *Origin of Species*, quoted in *Darwin* (Desmond & Moore, Penguin). This reminds us of Thomas Hobbes' (1588-1679) dictum: owing to scarcity of natural resources, there is constant war of all against all ('***bellum omnium contra omnes***'). Life in the state of nature is 'solitary, poor, nasty, brutish & short'. It was Thomas Hobbes who first brought Pericles to our attention through his great translations of Thucydides, the biographer of Pericles.

2 J Snow 1854 *Med Times Gaz* **9** 321. Snow (a teetotaller, a vegetarian, and a virgin) is unfairly portrayed as secular saviour; he was really just the man on the spot who took logical decisions.

3 If you doubt that heroism is often pointless, visit the Somme where lies buried the old lie '***dulce et decorum est pro patria mori***'. Wilfred Owen (1893–1918) wrote in a letter to his mother: 'The famous Latin tag [Horace] means *It is sweet and meet to die for one's country*. Sweet! and decorous!...'

Leprosy[ND]

►The diagnosis of leprosy (Hansen's disease) must be considered in all who hav visited endemic areas who present with painless disorders of skin and nerves. It i not just a tropical disease, and may occur in the USA, eg in Texas, Louisiana, an California, as well as Hawaii and Puerto Rico.

Mycobacterium leprae affects millions of people in the Tropics and subtropics Since the widespread use of dapsone, and WHO elimination campaigns, prevalenc has fallen (from 0.5% to 0.4/10,000 in Uganda; from 11% to 4/10,000 in parts c India). Incidence remains stable, however, at about 800,000 new cases/y worldwide, many of whom are children.

The Patient The incubation period is months to years, and the subsequent cours depends on the patient's immune response. If the immune response is ineffective ***'lepromatous'*** or ***'multibacillary'*** disease develops, dominated by foam histiocytes full of bacilli, but few lymphocytes. If there is a vigorous immun response, the disease is called ***'tuberculoid'*** or ***'paucibacillary'***, with granulomat containing epithelioid cells and lymphocytes, but few or no demonstrable bacill Between these poles lie those with 'borderline' disease.

Skin lesions: Hypopigmented anaesthetic macules, papules, or annular lesion (with raised erythematous rims). Erythema nodosum (fig 1 p267) occurs i 'lepromatous' disease, especially during the 1st year of treatment.

Nerve lesions: Major peripheral nerves may be involved, leading to much disabilit Sometimes a thickened sensory nerve may be felt running into the skin lesion (e ulnar nerve above the elbow, median nerve at the wrist, or the great auricula nerve running up behind the ear).

Eye lesions: ►*Refer promptly to an ophthalmologist.* The lower temperature of th anterior chamber favours corneal invasion (so secondary infection and cataract Inflammatory signs: chronic iritis, scleritis, episcleritis. There may be reduce corneal sensation (V nerve palsy), and reduced blinking (VII nerve palsy) an lagophthalmos (difficulty in closing the eyes; *lagos* is Greek for hare), ± ingrowin eyelashes (trichiasis).

Diagnosis Biopsy a skin lesion; *in vitro* culture is not possible. As an incidental curi armadillo (or mouse) foot-pad culture works, but don't taunt your lab by requestin this test! Split skin smears for AFB are +ve in borderline or lepromatous diseas Classification matters: it reflects biomass of bacilli, influencing treatment: the mor organisms, the greater the chance that some will be drug resistant. Other test neutrophilia, ESR↑, IgG↑, false +ve rheumatoid test.

Treatment Ask a local expert about: • Resistance patterns, eg to dapsone, whe ethionamide may (rarely) be needed • Using prednisolone for severe complicatior • Is surgery ± physiotherapy needed as well as drug therapy? In the UK, seek advic from the panel of Leprosy Opinion. In other areas, the administration of some drug should be supervised (S) whereas others need no supervision (NS). For multibacillar and borderline disease, WHO advises rifampicin 600mg PO monthly (S), dapson 100mg/24h PO (NS), and clofazimine 300mg monthly (S) + 50mg/24h (NS) for 2yr. In paucibacillary leprosy, rifampicin 600mg monthly (S) and dapsone 100mg/24 (NS) for 6 months. In single skin lesion paucibacillary disease, single-dose therap (rifampicin 600mg, ofloxacin 400mg, minocycline 100mg, all PO, together) is advise

►Beware sudden permanent *paralysis* from nerve inflammation caused by dyin bacilli (± *orchitis*, *prostration*, or *death*); this 'lepra reaction' may be mollified b thalidomide (*NOT* if pregnant). Liaise urgently with a leprologist. Supervised therap may be problematic as many patients find it hard to attend (nomads, jungle dwellers). WHO has proposed 'accompanied' multi-drug therapy, where someon close to the patient takes responsibility for ensuring treatment compliance. Th strategy is controversial.

/hat is more communicable than leprosy?

his page is dedicated to Joseph deVeuster of Kalawao, Molokai, in Hawaii, ·ho befriended sufferers of leprosy in a remote pacific colony. Here the prosy victims, arriving by ship, were sometimes told to jump overboard and vim for their lives, so frightened were the sailors of this island of contagion. ut when they arrived they found a friend who was both doctor and priest to em, whose self-imposed duty was to build their homes, their churches—and eir coffins. Without any distinction of race or religion, he gave a voice to the oiceless, building a unique community where the joy of being together gave eople new reasons for living.

It is said that after spilling hot water painlessly on his foot, he diagnosed s own leprosy. After that, his sermons beginning 'We lepers...' had added eracity.

He gave everything to leprosy—and leprosy took all it could from him, cluding, on April 15th 1889, his life.

We may look upon that water flowing over his foot not so much as a death entence, but as one of those initiation ceremonies devised by ancient amans who realized that it was by these close encounters with death that e augment our spirituality, and so are able to heal.

Joseph deVeuster also invalidates all our definitions of health, and, more nportantly, he demonstrates that optimism works and is more communicable an leprosy, proving that there is nothing that cannot be transcended.

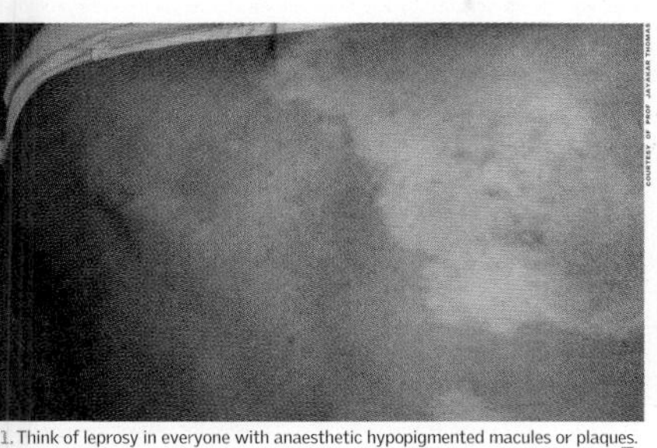

1. Think of leprosy in everyone with anaesthetic hypopigmented macules or plaques. ıld this be vitiligo? No: vitiligo is more demarcated and **de**pigmented (chalk white).[256] e fig 4 on p547.

Spirochaetes

Lyme disease is a tick-borne infection caused by *Borrelia burgdorferi*. Altho famously described in Lyme (Connecticut) it is now global, eg New Forest.[UK] ►≤7 remember the tick bite. ***Signs:*** Cognition↓; lymphadenopathy; arthralgia/arthr myocarditis; heart block; meningitis; ataxia; amnesia; cranial nerve palsies; neu pathy; lymphocytic meningoradiculitis (Bannwarth's syndrome). If the problem '?Lyme' skin condition, eg ACA (below) erythema migrans target lesions (p546) y need to ask about Bell's palsy[etc] *years* ago. **Δ:** Clinical ± serology; if –ve do, PCR. ***℞:*** Skin rash: doxycycline 100mg/12h PO (amoxicillin or penicillin V if <8yrs or pregnant) for 14–21d. Later complications: high-dose IV benzylpenicillin, ceftriaxone. ***Prevention:*** Keep limbs covered; use insect repellent; tick collars for pets; check skin often when in risky areas. Vaccination is available eg if living in high-risk areas. Advice differs on prophylaxis after a tick bites. A single dose of doxycycline 200mg PO given within 72h of a bite is effective prophylaxis; in highly endemic areas, this may be worthwhile (eg if risk is >1%). ***Removing tic*** Suffocate tick with, eg petroleum jelly, then remove by grasping close to mo parts and twisting off; then clean skin. Skin complications: **acrodermatitis chr ica atrophicans** (ACA; skin is as 'thin as cigarette paper'); **borellia lymphocyto** manifests eg as a blue/red discolouration of the earlobe; **erythema migrans**, p5

Lone star ti

Fig 1. *Amblyo americ*

Endemic treponematoses ***Yaws*** is caused by *T. pertenue* (serologically indistingu able from *T. pallidum*). It is a chronic granulomatous disease prevalent in childre the rural Tropics. Spread is by direct contact, via skin abrasions, and is promoted poor hygiene. The primary lesion (an ulcerating papule) appears ~4wks af exposure. Scattered secondary lesions then appear, eg in moist skin, but can anywhere. These may become exuberant. Tertiary lesions are subcutane gummatous ulcerating granulomata, affecting skin and bone. Cardiovascular a CNS complications do not occur. ***Pinta*** (*T. carateum*) affects only skin; seer Central and S America. ***Endemic non-venereal syphilis*** (*bejel; T. pallidum*) is s in Third World children, when it resembles yaws. In the developed world *pallidum* causes ***syphilis*** (p419). ***Diagnosis:*** Clinical. ***℞:*** Procaine penicillin (p36

Weil's disease[ND] is caused by ***Leptospira interrogans*** (eg serogroup *L. icte haemorrhagiae*). Spread is typically by contact with infected rat urine, eg in slu or while swimming, canoeing or cycling through puddles. After an incubation of 20d there is abrupt fever, myalgia/myositis, cough, chest pain ± haemoptysis—t recovery, or jaundice, meningitis, uveitis, and renal failure. **Δ:** Blood culture +ve c up to day 4 of illness; serology. ***℞:*** IV penicillin or amoxicillin. Prophyla doxycycline 200mg/wk *may* have a role—eg for water sports in dangerous plac

Canicola fever is an aseptic meningitis caused by *Leptospira canicola*.

Relapsing fever[ND] This is caused by ***Borrelia recurrentis*** (louse-borne) ***B. duttoni*** (tick-borne). It typically occurs in pandemics following war or disas and may kill millions. ***Incubation:*** 4–18d. ***Presentation:*** Abrupt onset fever, rig and headache. A petechial rash (which may be faint or absent), jaundice, and ten hepatosplenomegaly may develop. Serious complications include myocardi hepatic failure, and DIC. Crises of very high fever and tachycardia occur. When fever abates, hypotension due to vasodilatation may occur and be fatal. Relap occur, but are milder. ***Tests:*** Organisms are seen on Leishman-stained thin or th films. ***Treatment:*** Tetracycline 500mg PO or 250mg IV as a single dose (but for 1 for *B. duttoni*). Alternative: doxycyline 100mg/12h PO. The Jarisch–Herxheir reaction (p419) is fatal in 5%: meptazinol 100mg IV slowly is given as prophyla with the tetracycline, repeated 30min later (with the chill phase) and during flush phase (if systolic BP <75mmHg). Delouse the patient and their clothes Doxycycline (p370) is useful prophylaxis in high-risk groups.

yphilis: the archetypal spirochaetal disease

Any anogenital ulcer is syphilis until proven otherwise. UK incidence is rising, eg 2254 new infections/yr.[260] In a recent 5-yr period, rates rose by 213% in hetero- xual men, 1412% in men who have sex with men, and 22% in women, with rious outbreaks in London & Manchester[261] as safe-sex messages are forgotten, nored, or trounced.[262] *Treponema pallidum* (fig 1) enters via a graze, during sex. ll features are due to an endarteritis obliterans. *Incubation:* 9–90d. 4 stages:

Primary syphilis: Macule at site of sexual contact forms a painless hard ulcer (*primary chancre;* it is very infectious).

Secondary syphilis: Occurs 4–8wks after the chancre: rash (trunk, face, palms, soles), malaise, lymphadenopathy, T°↑, alopecia, condylomata lata (flattened, sometimes moist papules around or beyond the genitals),[263] palatal or buccal snail-track ulcers; rarely hepatitis, meningism, nephrosis, and uveitis.

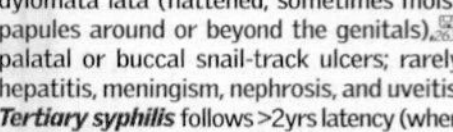

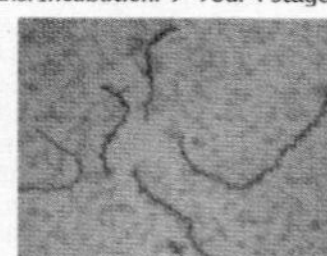

Fig 1. *T. pallidum.*[259]

Tertiary syphilis follows >2yrs latency (when patients are non-infectious): there are *gummas* (granulomas in skin, mucosa, bone, joints, viscera, eg lung, testis).

Quaternary syphilis *Cardiovascular:* Ascending aortic aneurysm/aortic regurgitation. *Neurosyphilis: (a) Meningovascular:* Cranial nerve palsies, stroke; *(b) General paresis of insane (GPI):* Dementia, psychoses (fatal untreated; treatment *may* reverse it); *(c) Tabes dorsalis:* Sensory ataxia, numb legs, chest, and bridge of nose, lightning pains ('like a bolt from the blue'), gastric crises, reflex loss, plantars ↑↑, Charcot's joints (p508). *Argyll Robertson pupil* (p70).

ardiolipin antibody: Not treponeme-specific. Detectable in primary disease but anes in late syphilis. Indicates active disease and becomes –ve after treatment. *alse +ves* (with –ve treponemal antibody): pregnancy, immunization, pneumonia, alaria, SLE, TB, leprosy. *Examples:* **venereal disease research laboratory slide est (VDRL), rapid plasma reagin (RPR), Wassermann reaction (WR).**

reponeme-specific antibody: Positive in 1° disease, remains so despite treatment. *xamples:* ***T. pallidum*** **haemagglutination assay (TPHA), fluorescent treponemal ntibody (FTA),** *T. pallidum* **immobilization test (TPI).** Non-specific, also +ve in on-venereal yaws, bejel, or pinta. ***ELISA:*** Syphilis ELISA IgG and ELISA IgM.

ther tests In 1° syphilis, treponemes may be seen by *dark ground microscopy* chancre fluid; serology at this stage is often –ve. In 2° syphilis, treponemes e seen in the lesions and both types of antibody tests are positive. In late philis, organisms may no longer be seen, but both types of antibody test sually remain +ve (cardiolipin antibody tests may wane). In neurosyphilis, CSF ntibody tests (particularly FTA and TPHA) are +ve. If HIV+ve, serology may be egative during syphilis reactivation. PCR may help.

eatment: Contact tracing; screening for other sexual infections (eg HIV) rocaine **penicillin** (=procaine benzylpenicillin) 600mg/24h IM for ~28d (14d in arly syphilis), or **doxycycline** 200mg/12h PO for 28d (100mg/12h PO for 14d in arly syphilis). Beware ***Jarisch–Herxheimer reaction:*** Fever, pulse↑, and asodilatation hours after the 1st dose of antibiotic. It is thought to be from udden release of endotoxin. Commonest in 2° disease; most dangerous in 3°. onsider steroids. If HIV+ve, penicillin may not stop neurosyphilis; consult icrobiologist. ***Congenital syphilis:*** *OHCS* p35.

Poliomyelitis[ND]

Polio is a highly contagious picornavirus (fig 1 BOX), though only a small proporti of patients develop any illness from the infection. ***Spread:*** Droplet or faeco–or ***The Patient:*** 7 days' incubation, then 2 days' 'flu-like prodrome, leading to a 'p paralytic' stage: fever, tachycardia, headache, vomiting, neck stiffness, a unilateral tremor. In <50% of patients this progresses to the paralytic stag myalgia, lower motor neurone signs, and respiratory failure—*with no sensory sig* ***Tests:*** CSF: WCC↑, polymorphs then lymphocytes, otherwise normal; paired sera (days apart); throat swab & stool culture identify virus. ***ΔΔ:*** *Non-viral causes flaccid paralysis: Borrelia*; mycoplasma; diphtheria; botulism; heavy meta transverse myelitis; polymyositis. ***Natural history:*** <10% of those with paraly die. There may be *delayed progression* of paralysis (post-polio syndrome, PPS). *R factors for severe paralysis:* Adulthood; pregnancy; post-tonsillectomy; mus fatigue/trauma during incubation period. ***PPS*** causes fatigue, weakness, joint a muscle pains, and worsening function (not necessarily in the sites origina affected). PPS management centres on just enough exercise to prevent wasting b no so much as to increase weakness in already damaged muscles. ***Vaccine:*** p38

Rabies[ND]

Rabies is a rhabdovirus spread by bites from any infected mammal, eg bats, do cats, foxes, or raccoons (bites may go unnoticed). ***The Patient:*** Usually 9–' days' incubation, so give prophylaxis even several months after exposu Prodromal symptoms: headache, malaise, abnormal behaviour, agitation, fever, a itching at the site of the bite. Progresses to 'furious rabies', eg with wate provoked muscle spasms often accompanied by profound terror (hydrophobia). 20%, 'dumb rabies' starts with flaccid paralysis in the bitten limb and spreads

Pre-exposure prophylaxis (eg vets, zoo-keepers, customs officials, bat handle travellers in rabies area for >1 month or at especial risk, or if access to pos exposure treatment is problematic): Give human diploid cell strain vaccine (1mL deltoid) on days 0, 7, & 28, and again at 2–3yrs if still at risk.

Treatment if bitten where rabies is endemic (if unvaccinated): Wash the wou well. ►Seek help (UK *virus reference lab, tel.:* 020 8200 4400). Observe the biti animal to see if it dies (but it is possible that it may not die of rabies before t patient does). Clean the wound. *If previously immunized:* give vaccine (1mL I on days 0 and 3. *If previously unimmunized:* give vaccine on days 0, 3, 7, 14, and and human rabies immunoglobulin (20U/kg on day 0; half given IM and half loca infiltrated around wound). Rabies is fatal once symptoms begin (but survival h occurred, with optimal CNS/cardiorespiratory support). Vaccinate attending sta

Viral haemorrhagic (and related) fevers[ND]

Yellow fever: An epidemic arbovirus disease spread by *Aedes* mosquitoes (Bra Bolivia, Peru, and Central and West Africa). *Immunization:* p367. *Incubati* 2–14d. *The Patient:* In mild forms, fever, headache, nausea, albuminuria, myalg and relative bradycardia. If severe: 3 days of headache, myalgia, anorexia ± naus followed by abrupt fever, a brief remission, then prostration, jaundice (± fat liver), haematemesis and other bleeding, oliguria. *Mortality:* <10% (day 5–1 *Diagnosis*: ELISA. *Treatment:* Symptomatic.

Lassa fever[ND], ***Ebola virus***[ND], ***Marburg virus***[ND], & ***dengue haemorrhagic fev*** (DHF—this 'unofficial' haemorrhagic fever is the commonest arbovirus disease). They start with sudden headache, pleuritic pain, backache, myalgia, conjunctivit prostration, dehydration, facial flushing (dengue), and T°↑. Bleeding soon superven There may be resolution, or renal failure, encephalitis, coma, and death. ***R:*** Primar symptomatic; ribavirin is useful in Lassa fever if given early in disease. ►*Use spec infection control measures (Lassa, Ebola, Marburg); get expert help at once.*

olio: a tantalizing exercise in prevention and (near) eradication

Pre-1950s, polio distribution was worldwide. In 1952, during an epidemic in Copenhagen, the cause of death was established as CO_2 retention. Mechanical ventilation began in special centres—the birth of intensive care units.[268]
12 April 1955: vaccination starts with Salk's inactivated vaccine.
1958: Sabin donated his 3 attenuated strains to Chumakov in Moscow, who produced the 3 vaccines, giving them to 15 million people in 1 year.
1960s: the 3 vaccines were mixed, to produce a single oral polio vaccine.
1988: Estimated 350,000 cases worldwide, occurring in 125 countries. The Global Polio Eradication Initiative, aiming to protect children worldwide through vaccination, is launched; the aim was eradication by the year 2000.
1991: Transmission interrupted in the West.
1993: China starts national immunization days; >80,000,000 vaccinated in 2 days; in 1994 only 5 cases of virus-confirmed wild polio.
1994: WHO declares the Americas polio-free.
1997: 1 case of wild polio in all of Europe.
1999: Only 7090 cases, worldwide.
2000: WHO declares Western Pacific polio-free.
2001: 483 cases in 10 endemic countries.
2002: WHO declares Europe polio-free.

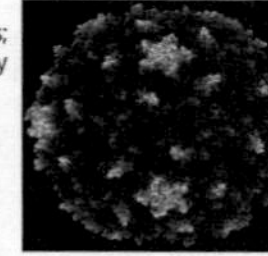
Fig 1. Poliovirus

2004: 6 polio-endemic countries: Afghanistan; India; Niger; Nigeria; Pakistan.[269]
2006: Transmission re-established in: Nigeria, Sudan, Egypt, Central African Republic, Mali, Côte D'Ivoire, Somalia, Burkina Faso, Uttar Pradesh.[270] [271]

efore 2005 most cases in the West were adult contacts of child vaccinees; these ases have stopped as live vaccine has been replaced by inactivated vaccine.
NB: Sabin viruses and their genetic revertants can cause chronic infection immunodeficient people, who may shed neurovirulent virus in faeces for years. programmes of oral vaccination should not continue one day longer than ecessary to eliminate disease caused by wild virus.[272]

engue fever (DF) and dengue haemorrhagic fever (DHF)

here is a global pandemic of this RNA flavivirus, related to poor vector control edes mosquitoes), urbanization,[1] poor waste disposal, and rapid migrations inging new strains (DEN-2) which become more virulent in those who have had ild dengue. Global warming is also important: a temperature rises of 1–3° creases transmission, leading to an extra 25,000 cases/yr. [WHO data] Incidence: 50–00×10⁶/yr; 250,000–500,000/yr get DHF.[2]

Infants typically have a simple febrile illness with a maculopapular rash. Older ildren/adults have flushing of face, neck, and chest or a centrifugal aculopapular rash from day 3—or a late confluent petechiae with round pale eas of normal skin—also headache, arthralgia, jaundice; hepatosplenomegaly; uria. ***Haemorrhagic signs:*** (Unlikely if AST normal).[273] Petechiae, GI, gum or se bleeds, haematuria; hypermenorrhoea.

onitor: BP; urine flow; WCC↓; platelets↓; PCV; +ve tourniquet test (>20 etechiae/inch²) + PCV↑ by 20% are telling signs (rapid endothelial plasma leak the key pathophysiology of DHF). **ΔΔ:** Chikungunya,[2] measles, leptospirosis, phoid, malaria. ***Exclusion:*** If symptoms start >2wks after leaving a dengue ea, or if fever lasts >2wks, dengue can be 'ruled out'. **℞:** Prompt IV resusc-ation, eg Ringer's lactate. ▸▸If shocked (mortality 40%), give a bolus of 5mL/kg; repeat every ½h until BP rises, and urine flow at >30mL/h.[274]

ities high in the Andes are free of Dengue—as the *Aedes* mosquito cannot survive high altitudes.
aemorrhagic features in Chikungunya virus infections are rare; arthralgia, fever, myalgia and a are more common, eg in Indian Ocean Islands.

Arthropod-borne bacteria

Q fever is caused by ***Coxiella burnetii*** (100 cases/yr in the UK). It is so nam because it was first labelled 'query' fever in workers in an Australian abattoir.

Epidemiology: Occurs worldwide, and is usually rural, with reservoirs in cattle a sheep. The organism is resistant to drying and is usually inhaled from infected du It can be contracted from unpasteurized milk, directly from carcasses in abatto sometimes by droplet spread, and rarely from tick bites.

Clinical features Suspect Q fever in anyone with a PUO or atypical pneumonia. may present with fever, myalgia, sweats, headache, cough, and hepatitis splenomegaly). If the disease becomes chronic, suspect endocarditis (typica 'culture-negative'). This usually affects the aortic valve, but clinical signs may absent. It also causes miscarriages and CNS infection.

Tests: CXR may show consolidation, eg multilobar or slowly resolving. Liver functi tests may be hepatitic and biopsy may show granulomata. Diagnosis is serologic phase I antigens suggest chronic infection; phase II antigens suggest acu infection. PCR may be used on tissue samples. CSF tests may be needed.

Treatment: Get expert microbiological help. ***Acute:*** Tetracycline or doxycycline 2wks. Minocycline, clarithromycin, ciprofloxacin (in pregnancy) and co-trimoxaz are used. ***Chronic:*** Ciprofloxacin + rifampicin for 2yrs ± valve replacement.

Prevention: Vaccination for those whose occupation places them at high risk.

Bartonellosis is caused by ***Bartonella bacilliformis***, a Gram –ve, motile, bacill like organism which parasitizes RBCs. Spread is by sandflies in the Andes, Pe Equador, Colombia, Thailand, and Niger. Transient immunosuppression leads other infections (eg *Salmonella*). ***Incubation:*** 10–210 days (mean=60d).

Signs: Fever, rashes, lymphadenopathy, hepatosplenomegaly, jaundice, cerebel syndromes, dermal nodules (verrugas), retinal haemorrhages, myocardi pericardial effusion, oedema, and rarely, meningo-encephalomyelitis.

Tests: Giemsa-stained blood films. Blood culture (prolonged). Coombs' – haemolytic anaemia, and hypochromic, macrocytic red cells with a megaloblas marrow. CSF pleocytosis. Serological tests are not widely available.

Treatment: Responds to penicillin, but chloramphenicol (p414) or ciprofloxa (500mg/12h PO for 10d) are often used because of frequent association with s monelloses. Steroids may be indicated if there is severe neurological involvement.

Cat scratch disease (p411) is caused by ***Bartonella henselae***.

Trench fever is caused by ***Bartonella quintana*** inoculated from infected lou faeces, not only in soldiers, but also in the homeless, and in alcoholics.

Clinical features: Fever, headache, myalgia, dizziness, back pain, macular rash, e pain, leg pain, splenomegaly, endocarditis (rare). In HIV-infected patients, the sk lesions may resemble Kaposi's sarcoma. It is not fatal; it may relapse.

Tests: Blood culture, serology, PCR. ***℞:*** Doxycycline 100mg/12h PO for 15 days

Ehrlichiosis is caused by ***Ehrlichia chaffeensis***, an obligate intracytoplasmic Gra –ve organism, related to Rickettsia. It is spread by ticks. It causes fever, headac anorexia, malaise, abdominal pain, epigastric pain, conjunctivitis, lymphadenopat jaundice, rash, confusion, and cervical lymphadenopathy.

Tests: Leucopenia, thrombocytopenia, AST↑. Serology/PCR are diagnostic.

Treatment: May respond to doxycycline 100mg/12h PO for 7–14d.

yphus: the archetypal rickettsial disease

ickettsiae are parasitic bacteria that are obligate intracellular parasites; they are igger than viruses but smaller than classical bacteria. They are carried by host rthropods and invade human mononuclear cells, neutrophils, or blood vessel ndothelium ('vasculotropic'). All the cataclysmic events of the last century war, revolution, flood, famine, genocide, and overcrowding) have favoured lice ıfestation. As a result, Rickettsia (especially typhus) have killed untold millions.

athology Widespread vasculitis and endothelial proliferation may affect any rgan and thrombotic occlusion may lead to gangrene.

linical features ►Think of typhus in all travellers or inhabitants of endemic reas who seem to have septicaemia, but have -ve blood cultures.[277] ıcubation: 2–23d. Infection may be mild/asymptomatic or severe/systemic, vith sudden onset of fever, frontal headache, confusion, and jaundice. With ome species, an *eschar* (dark crusty ulcer at the site of a bite) may be present. rickettsial rash may be macular, papular, petechial, or haemorrhagic. Test: aemolysis, neutrophilia, thrombocytopenia, clotting abnormalities, hepatitis, enal impairment. Patients die of shock, renal failure, DIC (p650), or stroke.

Epidemic typhus (*R. prowazeki*): *Spread*: human lice *Pediculus humanus* (fig 1) faeces are inhaled or pass through skin). It may recrudesce decades later (Brill–Zinsser disease). The rash is truncal, then peripheral (opposite to *R. rickettsii*).

Rocky Mountain spotted fever (*R. rickettsii*) is tick-borne (fig 2). Endemic in Rocky Mountains & south east USA. The rash (seen in 90%) begins as macules on hands/feet, spreading and becoming petechial or haemorrhagic in 50%.

Tick typhus (*R. conorii*; Mediterranean spotted fever) the chief imported rickettsial disease in the UK (endemic in Africa, the Mediterranean area, eg Croatia, and parts of Asia; sporadic in Laos, Korea etc). The rash starts in the axillae, becoming purpuric as it spreads. *Other signs*: Conjunctival suffusion; jaundice; deranged clotting; meningoencephalitis; cerebritis;[278] renal failure.

Scrub typhus (*Orienta tsutsugamushi*) Most common in SE Asia. Signs: Eschar from chigger bite (75%); hepatomegaly (65%); cough (60%); lymphadenopathy (46%);[279] tachypnoea (35%); constipation (25%); abdominal pain (20%); oedema (20%); splenomegaly (15%); vomiting (15%); rash (15%); petechiae (5%); sudden deafness.[280] CXR: bilateral infiltrations (85%).[281] Blood: LFT↑ (90%); platelets↓ (80%); neutrophilia (60%); lymphocytosis ± atypical lymphocytosis (5%). Complications: pneumonia ± pulmonary oedema, meningitis, and shock.

Murine (endemic) typhus (*R. typhi*) is spread by fleas from rats to humans. It is more prevalent in warm, coastal ports (eg Dalmatia, Laos).[282]

Rickettsialpox (*R. akari*) Variegate rash: macular, papular, or vesicular.

iagnosis This is difficult as often the picture is non-specific, the organisms are ifficult to grow, and traditional heterophil antibody Weil–Felix tests are insensive and nonspecific. A rise in antibody titre in paired sera is diagnostic. Latex gglutination, indirect immunofluorescence, ELISAs and PCR are available (may be one on the eschar).[283] An accurate, rapid dotblot immunoassay is available for crub typhus. Skin biopsy may be diagnostic in Rocky Mountain spotted fever.

reatment Doxycycline 100mg/12h PO/IV for 7d (or 48h after T° normal) **or** hloramphenicol 500mg/6h PO for 10–14d. Resistance has been reported in hailand. Azithromycin 500mg (1 dose) may work in tick and scrub typhus.[284]

oor prognostic factors Older age, male, Black, G6PD deficiency.

e human louse

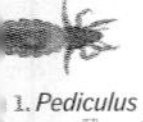

1. *Pediculus manus*,[285] vector epidemic typhus.

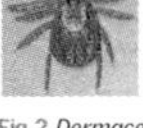

Fig 2 *Dermacentor variabilis* is one vector for Rocky Mountain spotted fever.

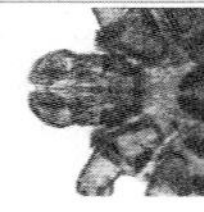

Fig 3 The 'dog tick'.

Some gastrointestinal protozoa

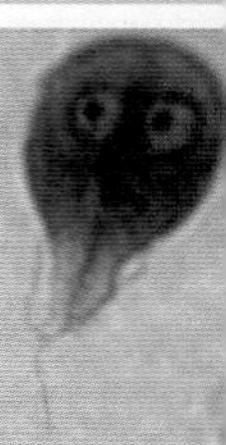

Fig 1. Giardia: the only dip monadid to trouble us.

Giardia lamblia is a flagellate protozoon, which lives in the duodenum and jejunum. Spread: faecal–oral (↑ risk if eg immunosuppression, travel, homosexuality, achlorhydria, playgroups, and swimming)—or from pets or birds. Drinking water may be contaminated.

The patient: Giardiasis is often asymptomatic. Lassitude, bloating, flatulence, abdominal pain, loose stools ± explosive diarrhoea are typical. Malabsorption, weight loss, and lactose intolerance may occur.

Diagnosis: Repeated stool microscopy for cysts/trophozoites may be –ve. Duodenal fluid analysis (aspiration or absorption on to a piece of swallowed string, Enterotest®) may be tried, or ELISA/PCR or therapeutic trial. **ΔΔ:** Any cause of diarrhoea (p378, p380, p580), tropical sprue (p272), coeliac (p272). **℞:** Scrupulous hygiene. Metronidazole 400mg/8h PO for 5d (avoid alcohol); if pregnant, paromomycin 500mg/6h PO. If treatment fails, check for compliance and consider treating *all* the famil diarrhoea persists, avoid milk as lactose intolerance may persist for 6wks.

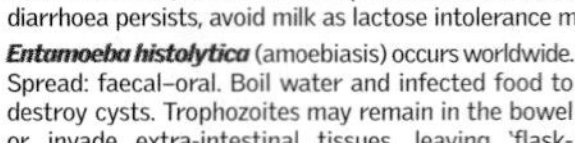

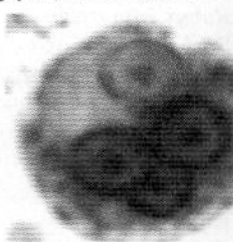

Fig 2. *E. histolytica* cyst with an endosome insid each of its 4 nuclei.

Entamoeba histolytica (amoebiasis) occurs worldwide. Spread: faecal–oral. Boil water and infected food to destroy cysts. Trophozoites may remain in the bowel or invade extra-intestinal tissues, leaving 'flask-shaped' GI ulcers. Presentation may be asymptomatic, with mild diarrhoea or with severe amoebic dysentery.

Amoebic dysentery[ND] may occur some time after initial infection. Diarrhoea begins slowly, becoming profuse & bloody. An acute febrile prostrating illness can occur but high fever, colic, and tenesmus are rare. May remit and relapse. *Diagnosis:* stool microscopy shows trophozoites, blood, and pus cells. Faecal antigen detection may also be useful. Serology indic previous or current infection and may be unhelpful in acute infection. **ΔΔ:** *N pathogenic amoebae* (eg *Entamoeba dispar*) are common in the tropics (cysts indistinguishable). *Bacillary dysentery* often starts suddenly; it may cause dehydra Stools are more watery. *Acute ulcerative colitis* has a more gradual onset and stools are very bloody. For other causes of bloody diarrhoea, see p414 & p23

Amoebic colonic abscess may perforate causing peritonitis.

Amoebomas are inflammatory masses, eg in the caecum (a cause of RIF mass

Amoebic liver abscess is usually a single mass in the right lobe, and cont 'anchovy-sauce' pus. There is usually a high swinging fever, sweats, RUQ pain, tenderness. WCC↑. LFT normal or ↑ (cholestatic). 50% have no history of amo dysentery. *Diagnosis:* ultrasound/CT ± aspiration; positive serology.

℞: Metronidazole 800mg/8h PO for 5d for acute amoebic dysentery (active aga vegetative amoebae), then diloxanide furoate 500mg/8h PO for 10d to destroy cysts (SEs rare). Diloxanide is also best for chronic disease when *Entamoeba* c not vegetative forms, are in stools. Amoebic liver abscess: metronida 400mg/8h IV for 10d; repeat at 2wks as needed; aspirate if no improvem within 72h of starting metronidazole; give diloxanide post-metronidazole. Ex intestinal amoebiasis (including liver abscess) and symptomless amoebic passers, metronidazole 400–800mg/8h for 5–10d (child 1–3 yrs: 100–200mg, 3–7yrs 100–200mg/6h; 7–10yrs 200–400mg/8h).

Other GI protozoa *Cryptosporidium* (p380), *Microsporidium* and *Isospora* (occ AIDS, p398), *Balantidium coli*, and *Sarcocyscocystis*.

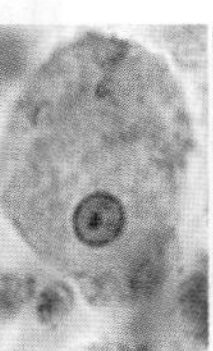

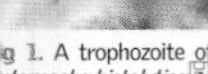

g 1. A trophozoite of ntamoeba histolytica.

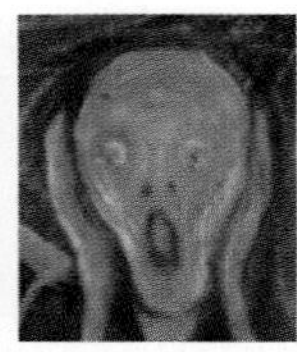

Fig 2. Edvard Munch, 1893 *The Scream*, crayon on paper

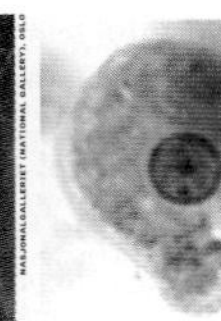

Fig 3. A 3rd trophozoite of *Entamoeba histolytica*.

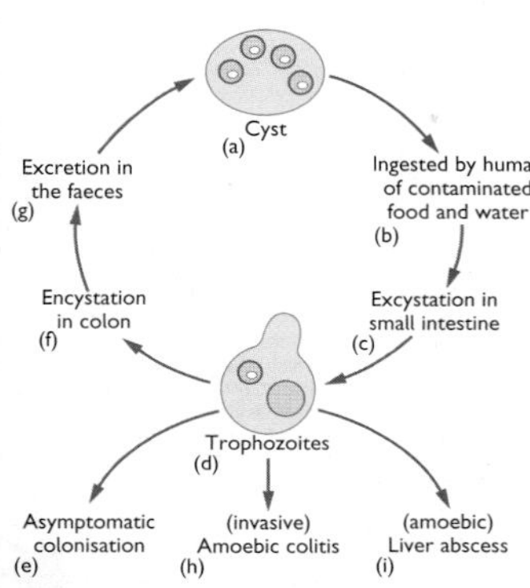

ig 4. The life cycle of *Entamoeba histolytica* is in 2 stages: cysts and trophozoites. ysts (10–15μm across) typically contain 4 nuclei; they are spread by ingesting faecally ontaminated food or water. During excystation in the gut lumen, nuclear division is ollowed by cytoplasmic division, giving rise to 8 trophozoites. Trophozoites (10–50μm cross) containing a single nucleus with a central karyosome, live in the caecum and olon. ~90% of individuals infected with *E. histolytica* are asymptomatic. Re-encystation f the trophozoites occurs in the colon, resulting in excretion of cysts in faeces and ontinuation of the life cycle.

Alternatively, trophozoites invade colonic epithelium, causing amoebic colitis (in 10%). *E. histolytica* can spread haematogenously after breaching colon epithelium and an establish persistent extra-intestinal infection (eg amoebic liver abscess).

Trypanosomiasis

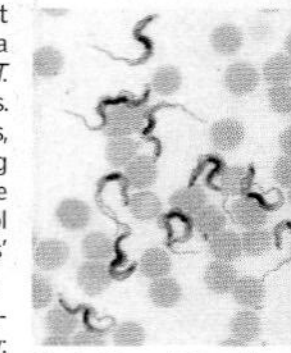

Fig 1. *T. gambiense* [293]

African trypanosomiasis (sleeping sickness) In West and Central Africa, *Trypanosoma gambiense* causes a slow, wasting illness with long latency. In East Africa, *T. rhodesiense* causes a more rapidly progressive illness. Trypanosome parasites, spread by tsetse flies, proliferate in blood, lymphatics, and CNS, causing progressive dysfunction, then death. Wars and famine caused an upsurge in the 1990s, now under control (prevalence ≤70,000) thanks to WHO, the Gates' foundation, Aventis, and Médecins Sans Frontières. [292]

Presentation: A tender, subcutaneous nodule (*chancre*) develops at the site of infection. 2 stages follow: ***Stage I (haemolymphatic):*** Non-specific symptoms including fever, rash, rigors, headaches, hepatosplenomegaly, lymphadenopathy, a joint pains. Winterbottom's sign (posterior cervical nodes↑) is a reliable sig particularly in *T. gambiense* infections. In *T. rhodesiense* infections, this sta may be particularly severe, with potentially fatal myocarditis. ***Stage (meningoencephalitic):*** Weeks (*T. rhodesiense*) or months (*T. gambiense*) aft initial infection, convulsions, agitation, and confusion—and then apathy, depressic ataxia, dyskinesias, dementia, hypersomnolence, and coma occur.

Diagnosis: Microscopy shows trypomastigotes in blood film, lymph node aspira or CSF. Serology is only reliable in *T. gambiense* infections.

Treatment: ►Seek expert help. Treat anaemia and other infections first; then:

- Early (pre-CNS) phase: pentamidine isethionate 4mg/kg/d IM for 10d. SE: WCC↓, ↓ ↓Ca^{2+}, ↑creatinine, platelets↓. Alternative: suramin (SE: proteinuria, ↑creatinin
- CNS disease: melarsoprol, eg '3 by 3' regimen IV: [294] 2–3.6mg/kg/d IV for thr doses. Repeat at 7d and once more after 10–21d. SE: pruritus, Jarisc Herxheimer-like reaction (p419), lethal encephalopathy in up to 10% (abnorm behaviour, fits, coma)—partly preventable with prednisolone (1mg/kg/24h, m 40mg/24h), starting the day before the first injection. Arseno-resista trypanosomiasis was always fatal until the introduction of eflornithine. Do example: 100mg/kg/6h IV over 1h for 14d. SE: anaemia, diarrhoea, seizur leucopenia, hair loss. Eflornithine has a role in more severe cases (a drug develop on a not-for-profit basis). Inhibitors of sterol biosynthesis, cysteine proteas other parasite biochemical pathways are being developed (with optimis promises of free availability). [295]

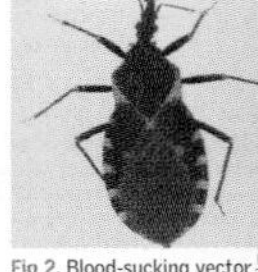

Fig 2. Blood-sucking vector

American trypanosomiasis (Chagas' disease) is caused by *T. cruzi*. Spread: blood-sucking reduviids (triatomine bugs, fig 2) in Latin America. Acute disease mostly affects children. An erythematous, indurated nodule (*chagoma*) forms at the site of infection which may then scar. ***Signs:*** T°↑, myalgia, rash, lymphadenopathy, hepatosplenomegaly ± unilateral conjunctivitis ± periorbital oedema (*Romaña's sign*) ± myocarditis/meningoencephalitis. In up to 30%, progression to chronic disease occurs after a latency of eg 20yrs. Multiorgan invasion causes megaoesophagus (dysphagia, aspiration), megacolon (abdominal distension, constipation) ± dilat cardiomyopathy (p138); CNS lesions, eg if immunosuppressed (HIV, lymphoma).

Diagnosis: Acute disease: trypomastigotes may be seen in or grown from blood, c or lymph node aspirate. Chronic disease: serology (Chagas' IgG ELISA).

Treatment: Unsatisfactory. Nifurtimox 2mg/kg/6h PO for 120d or benznidaz (3.7mg/kg/12h PO for 60d) in acute disease (toxic, and eliminate parasites in ≤50% Chronic disease can only be treated symptomatically. Surgery may be tried.

eishmaniasis

ishmania are protozoa (fig 1, inset, with 2 RBCs, from spleen aspirate) that cause granulomata. They are read by sandflies and occur in Africa, India, Latin nerica, the Middle East, and the Mediterranean. nical effects reflect: **1** The ability of each species to luce or suppress the immune response, to etastasize, and to invade cartilage, and **2** the speed d efficiency of our own immune response. *L. major*, example, is the most immunogenic and allergenic cutaneous Old World *Leishmania*, and causes most crosis. *L. tropica* is less immunogenic and causes s inflamed, slow-healing sores with relapsing sions and a tuberculoid histology.

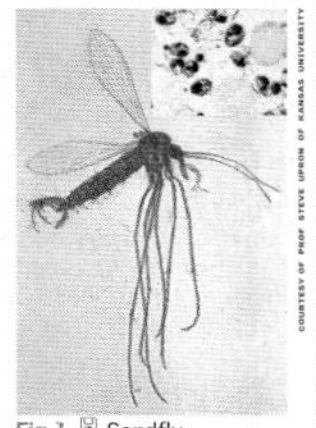

Fig 1. Sandfly.

taneous leishmaniasis (oriental sore) A major sease affecting >300,000 people eg in Africa, India, d S America caused by *L. mexicana, L. major, L. tropica* or *L. amazonensis*.[1] Lesions velop at the bite site, beginning as an itchy papule; crusts fall off to leave an ulcer *hiclero's ulcer*). Most heal in ~2 (old world disease) to 15 months, with scarring sfiguring if extensive). *L. mexicana* may cause pinna destruction (*Chiclero's ear*). ***agnosis:*** Microscopy and culture of aspiration from the base of the ulcer. ***℞:*** ay only be needed if unhealed by 6 months or lesion >4cm across (or multiple). t help. Fluconazole 200mg/d PO for 6wks can work against *L. major*; or ltefosine 2.5mg/kg/d PO for 4wks (teratogenic); sodium stibogluconate (Sb^V, ntavalent antimony) intralesional (no agreed dose) or IV (10mg/kg/12h IV; max 0mg/d) for 28d; paromomycin, eg 14mg/kg/d IM for 60d + 10mg Sb^V/kg/d IM.

ucocutaneous leishmaniasis (*L. brasiliensis*) occurs in S America. Primary skin sions may spread to the mucosa of the nose, pharynx, palate, larynx, and upper and cause severe scarring. Nasopharyngeal lesions are called *espundia*. ***Δ:*** As rasites may be scanty, a Leishmanin skin test may be needed to distinguish the ndition from leprosy, TB, syphilis, yaws, and cancer. Indirect fluorescent antibody sts and PCR tests are available. ***℞:*** Sodium stibogluconate (below). Treatment is satisfactory once mucosae are involved, so treat all cutaneous lesions early.

sceral leishmaniasis (kala-azar) Kala-azar means black sickness and is aracterized by dry, warty, hyperpigmented skin lesions. It occurs in Asia, Africa, America, and the Mediterranean. Cause: *L. donovani, L. chagasi*, or *L. infantum* (or rely, 'visceralizing' of *L. tropica*). Incubation: months to years. Protozoa spread a lymphatics from minor skin lesions and multiply in macrophages of the ticuloendothelial system (Leishman–Donovan bodies). There are 30 subclinical ses for every overt case. ♀:♂>3:1. It is HIV-associated. ***The patient:*** T°↑; sweats; rning feet; arthralgia; cough; epistaxis; abdo pain. *Signs:* Splenomegaly (96%); patomegaly (63%); lymphadenopathy; emaciation. ***Diagnosis:*** Leishman–Donovan dies in marrow (80%), node, or splenic aspirates (95%). Hypersplenism (Hb↓, atelets↓, WCC↓), albumin↓, IgG↑; –ve Leishmanin skin test. Solid-state serology for ld use (K39 antigen). Serology may be –ve if HIV+ve. ***℞:*** Get help. WHO regimen: dium stibogluconate (Sb^V) 20mg/kg/24h IV/IM, up to 850mg/d, for 30d. SE: alaise, cough, substernal pain, arrhythmias, Hb↓, urea↑, LFT↑. Regimens are anging as 25% fail to respond or relapse, eg 10mg/kg Sb^V/8h for 10d, without e 850mg limit. Alternative: pentamidine, eg 3–4mg/kg (deep IM) on alternate ys, up to 10 doses. SEs may be fatal (BP↓, arrhythmias, glucose↓, diabetes in %). Other agents: paromomycin, liposomal amphotericin B (AmBisome®). ltefosine (50mg/12h PO for 21d) is a promising oral alternative. ***Post kala-azar rmal leishmaniasis*** may occur months or years following successful treatment; sions resemble leprosy.

1 Visceralization may cause hepatitis & lymphadenopathy; *Trans R Soc Trop Med Hyg* 2006 100 79

Pathogenic fungi either produce toxins or allergic reactions, or infect directly. They are *superficial* (pityriasis versicolor), *cutaneous* (tinea/ringworm; intertrigo; restricted to keratinized skin, hair & nails), *subcutaneous* (mycetoma; madura foot or sporotrichosis; ℞ is complex and may need limb amputation)—or *systemic* (from the lung, spreading to many organs (eg histoplasmosis; blastomycosis; coccidioidomycosis; fungal meningitis).

Fig 1. Candida intertrigo.

Superficial and cutaneous mycoses *Candida* (fig 3). Dermatophytes (***Trichophyton*, *Microsporum*, *Dermatophyton***) cause tinea (ringworm). **Δ:** Skin scraping microscopy. **℞:** Topical clotrimazole 1%. Continue for 14d after healing. If intractable, try itraconazole (100–200mg/24h PO for 7d; SE: D&V; CCF), terbinafine (250mg/24h PO for 4wks) or griseofulvin 0.5–1g/24h (SE: agranulocytosis↓; SLE).

Malassezia furfur causes pityriasis versicolor: a macular rash which appears brown on pale skin and pale on tanned skin. ***Diagnosis:*** Microscopy of skin scrapings under Wood's light. **℞:** Ketoconazole 200mg/24h PO with food for 7d (also available as a cream); alternatively selenium sulfide lotio

Systemic mycoses *Aspergillus fumigatus* may precipitate asthma, allerg bronchopulmonary aspergillosis (ABPA), or cause aspergilloma (p160). Pneumon and invasive aspergillosis occur in the immunosuppressed. There is evidence th **voriconazole** is better than **amphotericin B** in invasive aspergillosis,[308] especially cerebral aspergillosis.[309] Systemic ***candidiasis*** also occurs in the immunocom romised: consider this *whenever* they get a PUO, eg *Candida* UTI in DM or as a ra cause of prosthetic valve endocarditis. Do repeated blood cultures. If infection do not resolve when the predisposing factor (eg IV line) is removed, the treatment **amphotericin B** IV (p180) or, if not neutropenic, **fluconazole** 400mg stat the 200mg/d PO. **Caspofungin** (70mg/d IVI if >80kg) is a new alternative.[310]

Cryptococcus neoformans causes meningitis or pneumonia. It is commonest the immunocompromised, eg AIDS, sarcoidosis, Hodgkin's, or on steroids. Th history may be long and there may be features suggesting ICP↑, eg confusio papilloedema, cranial nerve lesions. ***Diagnosis:*** Indian Ink CSF staining; bloc culture. Cryptococcal antigen is detected in CSF and blood by latex tests. **℞ amphotericin B** IV over 4h (Fungizone®) 0.5–0.8mg/kg/d + **flucytosine** 37.5m kg/6h PO until afebrile and culture –ve (≥2wks; 4 months if meningitis). Adju flucytosine to give a peak level of 70–80mg/L; trough 30–40mg/L. When culture ve, start fluconazole 200mg daily PO for 10wks. Monitor response clinically ar serologically. ***If HIV+ve:*** See p399 for **℞**. It may be necessary to lower CSF pressu by ~50% by removing CSF. Secondary prophylaxis with fluconazole 200mg/d PO needed until CD4 >150 × 10^6/L and cryptococcal antigen –ve (p398).

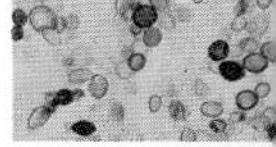
Fig 2. Histoplasma ×1000[311]

New World and Africa fungi causing deep infection: ***Histoplasma species, Coccidioides immitis, Paracoccidioides brasiliensis & Blastomyces dermatitidis*** may be asymptomatic or cause acute or chronic lung disease, or disseminated infection. Histoplasma pneumonitis features arthralgia, erythema nodosum (fig 1, p546), and multiforme (p546). Chronic disease causes upper-zone fibrosis ± CXR coin lesior Diagnosis: CXR, serology, culture, biopsy. **℞:** *Histoplasmosis:* **Amphotericin** 0.7mg/kg/d IV for ~3–10d, eg if HIV+ve & severe; liposomal form may be better (+le renal failure), then **itraconazole** 200mg/12h PO for 12wks. *Paracoccidioide* **Itraconazole** 200mg/d PO for 26wks. *Blastomycosis:* **Itraconazole**.

Candida on ITU: colonization→invasion→dissemination

Not everyone with +ve yeast cultures needs treatment: *Candida* is a common commensal (eg on skin, pharynx, or vagina, p230; p406) but if many sites (urine, sputum, or surgical drains) are colonized, risk of invasion rises, especially if:[312]

- Prolonged ventilation
- Urinary catheters
- Intravascular lines
- Broad-spectrum antibiotics
- Immunosuppression
- IV nutrition

Invasion implies fungus in normally sterile tissues. ***Dissemination*** involves infection of remote organs via the blood (eg endophthalmitis + fungi in lung or kidney). Consider IV amphotericin (OPPOSITE) or fluconazole (itraconazole if unresponsive) in these circumstances (esp. if your patient is deteriorating):[313]

- A single well-taken +ve blood culture—if risk factors present (above).
- Isolation of *Candida* from any sterile site except urine.
- Yeasts on microscopy on a sterile-site specimen, before cultures are known.
- Positive histology from normally sterile tissues in those at risk (above).
- Removal/change of IV lines is essential in patients with candidaemia.
- Consult an ID physician/microbiologist before starting systemic antifungals.

Preventing fungal infections if immunocompromized Fluconazole 50–400mg/24h after cytotoxics or radiotherapy, preferably started before onset of neutropenia, and continued for 1 week after WCC returns to normal.

Some facts about fungi They differ from bacteria in having chitin in their cell walls, being able to undergo mitosis—and being larger than bacteria (eg 8µm across). They mostly reproduce by budding or germ tubes (fig 6), not fission.

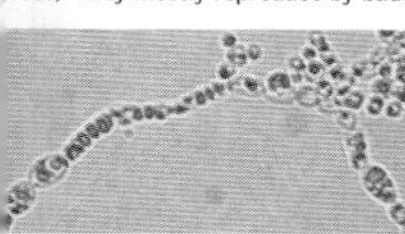

Fig 3. *Candida albicans*.[314] Yeasts usually occur as single cells or as clusters. Hyphae often occur in a mass of cells usually called moulds. A hyphal cell with cross-walls is called a mycelium. Some organisms grow as a yeast at 37°C but form mycelia at room temperature—ie they are dimorphic.

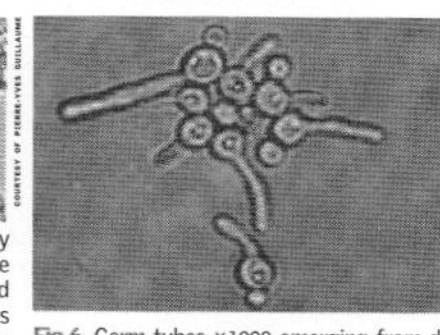

Fig 6. Germ tubes ×1000 emerging from dimorphic *Candida albicans* blastospores[315]

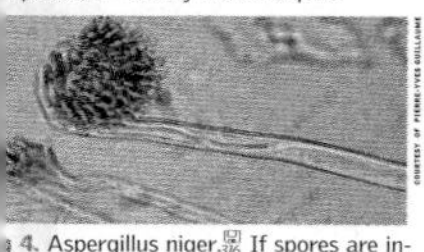

Fig 4. Aspergillus niger.[316] If spores are inhaled, aspergillosis can rarely occur, p161.[317]

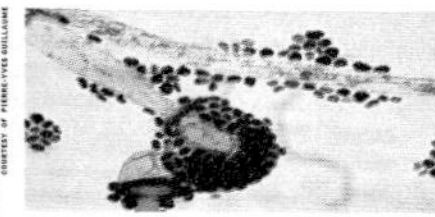

Fig 7. Mucor blastospores.[318] [319] Think of mucormycosis in diabetics with black pus in the nose ± proptosis/sinusitis or pneumonia. ℞: amphotericin B; posaconazole (if available).

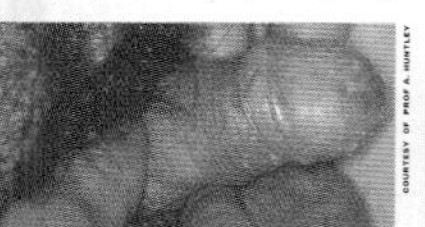

Fig 5. Candida of the glans.[320]

Fig 8. Web-space candida.[321]

COURTESY OF PIERRE-YVES GUILLAUME; COURTESY OF PROF A. HUNTLEY

Nematodes (roundworms)

1 billion people are hosts to nematodes (give or take a few hundred million). Many live with us quite peacefully (even helpfully); but ascariasis can cause obstruction, hookworms can stunt growth, necatoriasis can cause anaemia, a trichuriasis causes dysentery/rectal prolapse. Mass use of albendazole 400mg/2 PO for 3d to school children or immigrants from endemic areas may be benefic

Necator americanus & ***Ankylostoma duodenale* (hookworms)** occur in the Indian subcontinent, SE Asia, central/N Africa, and parts of Europe. Necator is also found in the Americas & sub-Saharan Africa. Many small worms attach to upper GI mucosa, causing bleeding (∴ Fe deficiency anaemia). Eggs are excreted in faeces and hatch in soil. Larvae penetrate feet, so starting new infections. Oral transmission of *Ankylostoma* occurs. Δ: Stool microscopy. ℞: Mebendazole 500mg PO stat (1 dose) ± iron.

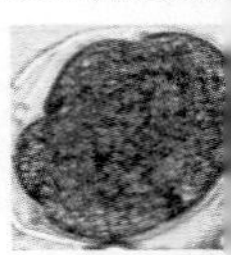

Fig 1. *Necator americanus* eggs ~70×38µm

Strongyloides stercoralis is endemic in the sub-tropics. Transmitted via skin, it causes migrating urticaria on thighs & trunk (*cutaneous larva migrans*) ± pneumonitis, enteritis/malabsorption (chronic diarrhoea; abdominal; pain). Worms may take bacteria into the blood, causing septicaemia; meningitis. Δ: Stool microscopy, serology, or duodenal aspiration. ℞: Ivermectin 0.2mg/kg/24h PO for 48h. Hyperinfestation occurs in immunocompromise; steroids; AIDS; consider albendazole 400mg/12h PO for 7–10d).

Ascaris lumbricoides looks like a garden worm (*Lumbricus*). It has 3 finely toothed lips. Transmission is faecal–oral. It migrates through liver & lungs, settling in small bowel. Often asymptomatic; GI obstruction/perforation is rare. If in bile ducts, cholangitis or pancreatitis can result. Worms may be >25cm long with a hooked end if ♂. Δ: Stool microscopy (ova stain orange in bile); worms on barium X-rays; eosinophilia (?not if immunosuppressed). ℞: Mebendazole 500mg PO stat (1 dose).

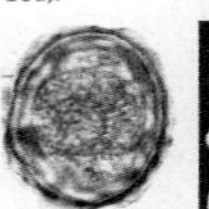

Fig 2. Ascaris eggs are 45×40µm. ♂

Enterobius vermicularis (threadworm; ~9mm long; fig 3) causes anal itch as it leaves the bowel to lay eggs on the perineum. Apply sticky tape there to identify eggs (~55 × 25µm) microscopically. ℞: Mebendazole 100mg PO stat. Repeat at 2wks if ≥2yrs. If aged <2yrs, try piperazine 0.3mL/kg/24h for 7d. Treat the whole family. *Hygiene is more important than drugs* as adult worms die after 6wks. Continued symptoms means *reinfection.*

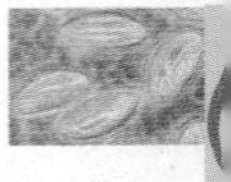

Fig 3. Enterobius: folded worm is s squirming in its egg.

Trichuris trichiura (whipworm) causes non-specific abdominal pain. Δ: Stool microscopy. ℞: Mebendazole 500mg stat. ***Trichinella spiralis*** (worldwide) Transmitted by uncooked pork migrates to muscle, causing myalgia, myocarditis, periorbital oedema ± fever. Albendazole 400mg/12h PO for 8–14d + prednisolone 40mg/d.

Toxocara canis is the main cause of *visceral larva migrans*. It presents with granulomas (squint, uveitis, blindness) or visceral signs (T°, myalgia, big liv asthma, cough). Δ: Fundoscopy, serology, histology. ℞: Mebendazole 1C 200mg/12h PO for 5d. Severe lung, heart, or CNS disease may warrant steroids eye disease, visible larvae can sometimes be lasered. *Toxocara* is often contrac by ingesting dirt, so de-worm pets often (exclude from play areas).

Dracunculus medinensis Guinea worm is the longest nematode (up to 70cm Ghana & Sudan); transmitted by water containing tiny crustaceans (copepods) ℞: Slow extraction of pre-emerging worms as they exit through the skin helped metronidazole 400mg/d PO (±steroids). WHO eradication date is set for 2009.

Filarial infection

This is common—prevalence of lymphatic filariasis: 120 million worldwide.

1 **Onchocerciasis** is caused by ***Onchocerca volvulus*** and is transmitted by the black fly. It causes river blindness in 72% of some communities in Africa and S America, affecting 17 million worldwide. A nodule forms at the site of the bite, shedding microfilariae to distant skin sites which develop altered pigmentation, lichenification, loss of elasticity, and poor healing. Disease manifestations are mainly due to the localized host response to dead/dying microfilariae. Eye manifestations include keratitis, uveitis, cataract, fixed pupil, fundal degeneration, or optic neuritis/atrophy. Lymphadenopathy and elephantiasis also occur. ***Diagnosis:*** Visualization of microfilaria in eye or skin snips. Remove a fine shaving of clean, unanaesthetized skin with a scalpel. Put on slide with a drop of 0.9% saline and look for swimming larvae after 30min. ***℞:*** Ivermectin 0.15mg/kg stat, repeated eg 6-montly to suppress dermal and ocular microfilariae. If the eye is involved start prednisolone 1mg/kg/24h PO a few days before starting ivermectin (it's probably OK in pregnancy). Worm survival requires symbiosis with Wolbachia bacteria (susceptible to doxycycline 100mg/d PO for 4–6 weeks).

2 **Lymphatic filaria** occur in Asia, Africa, and S America and is transmitted by mosquito vectors. Acute infections cause fever and lymphadenitis. ***Wuchereria bancrofti*** causes lower limb lymphoedema (elephantiasis) and hydrocoeles. ***Brugia malaya*** causes elephantiasis below the elbow/knee. *Wuchereria* life cycle: a mosquito bites an infected human→ingested microfilariae develop into larvae→larvae migrate to mosquito's mouth→Biting of another human→ Access to bloodstream →Adult filariae lodge in lymphatic system. ***Diagnosis:*** Blood film (fig 1), serology. A rapid immuno-chromatographic fingerprick test can be used in the field. ***Complications:*** Immune hyperreactivity may cause tropical pulmonary eosinophilia (cough, wheeze, lung fibrosis, high eosinophil counts, IgE↑ and IgG↑). It is a major public health problem and is a WHO target for elimination by the year 2020 (starting with Nigeria, Samoa, and Egypt). The current elimination strategy involves mass treatment with one yearly dose of 2 drugs for 5yrs: **albendazole** (400mg) + *either* **ivermectin** (200μg/kg) *or* **diethylcarbamazine** (6mg/kg).[328] Giving diethylcarbamazine-fortified salt to families for 1yr, has also been found to be effective.[329]

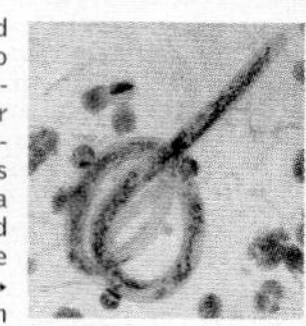

Fig 1. Blood smear of *Wuchereria bancrofti*; 290×8.5μm[327]

3 **Loiasis** is caused by ***Loa loa.*** Occurs in Africa; transmitted by the *Chrysops* fly. It causes painful 'Calabar' swellings of the limbs, eosinophilia, and may migrate across the conjunctiva. ***℞:*** Diethylcarbamazine 6mg/kg PO stat.

Cestodes (tapeworms)

Taenia solium (pork tapeworm) infection occurs by eating uncooked pork, or fro drinking contaminated water.[1] ***T. saginata*** is contracted from uncooked beef. Bot cause vague abdominal symptoms and malabsorption. Contaminated food ar water contain cysticerci which adhere to the gut and develop into adult worms. C swallowing the eggs of *T. solium* they may enter the circulation and dissemina throughout the body, becoming cysticerci within the human host (***cysticercosis*** This tapeworm encysts in muscle, skin, heart, eye, and CNS, causing focal sign ***Subcutaneous cysticercosis*** causes subcutaneous nodules (arms, legs, chest). ***Ocu lar cysticercosis*** causes conjunctivitis; uveitis; retinitis; choroidal atrophy; blindnes

Neurocysticercosis is the chief cause of seizures in some places, eg Mexico. Other features: focal CNS signs, eg hemiplegia, odd behavioural, dementia—or no symptoms. Cysticerci may cluster like bunches of grapes ('racemose' form) in the ventricles (causing hydrocephalus) and basal cisterns (causing basal meningitis, cranial nerve lesions, and raised ICP). Spinal cysticerci may cause radicular or compressive symptoms (p458). ***Diagnosis:*** •Stool microscopy and examination of perianal swabs. •Serology: indirect haemagglutination test. •CS may show eosinophils in neurocysticercosis, and a CSF antigen test is available. •C or MRI scan may locate cysts. •SXR and x-rays of soft tissues may show calcifie cysts. ***R:*** Get help (*tel:* 0151 708 9393[UK]). Niclosamide 2g PO in 2 doses, separated b 1h. Neurocysticercosis: albendazole 7.5mg/kg/12h PO with food, or praziquant 17mg/kg/8h PO for 30d. Allergic responses to dying larvae should be covered b dexamethasone 12mg/day PO for 21d. Cimetidine (800mg/d PO) can ↑concentratio of praziquantel. The role of steroids in the routine treatment of neurocysticercosis controversial. NB: If CSF ventricles are involved, you may need to shunt befor starting drugs. Drugs may worsen the acute phase of cysticercotic encephalitis.

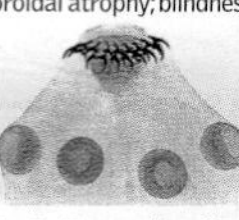

Fig 1. *Tinea solium* (not the two rows of hooks).

Hymenolepis nana; H. diminuta (dwarf tapeworm; rarely symptomatic). ***R:*** Pra iquantel 25mg/kg PO (1 dose; adults & children) or niclosamide 500mg/day for 3

Diphyllobothrium latum (fig 2) is a fish tapeworm (via uncooked fish) causing similar symptoms to *T. solium*. ***R:*** Niclosamide. It is a cause of vitamin B_{12}↓.

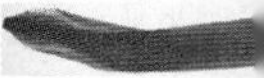

Fig 2.

Hydatid disease (fig 3) Cystic hydatid disease is a zoonosis caused by eating eggs of the dog parasite ***Echinococcus granulosus*** (fig 3) eg in rural sheep-farming regions. Hydatid is public health problem in parts of China, Russia, Alaska, Wales, and Japan. ***Sign*** Most cysts are asymptomatic, but liver cysts may present with hepatomegal obstructive jaundice, cholangitis, or PUO. Lung cysts present with dyspnoea, chest pain, haemoptysis, or anaphylaxis. Parasites migrate almost anywhere, eg CNS; or it turns up incidentally on CXR. ***Diagnosis:*** Plain X-ray, ultrasound, CT cysts. A good serological test has replaced the variably sensitive Casoni intradermal test. ***R:*** Get help. 1st-choice: albendazole before & after drainage (>60kg, 400mg/12h; if <60kg, 7.5mg/kg/12h with food). Excise/drain symptomat cysts. Beware spilling cyst contents (causes anaphylaxis; give praziquantel here The PAIR approach is often used: puncture→aspirate cyst→inject hypertonic salin → re-aspirate after 25min—and continue albendazole for 28 days to preve recurrence. (NB: Alveolar hydatid is caused by *E. multilocularis*.)

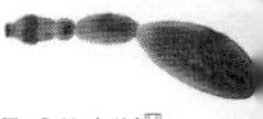

Fig 3. Hydatid

1 While eating undercooked pork is the only way to acquire intestinal *T. solium*, any food contaminat by faeces from hosts infected with cysticerci can carry the eggs that may lead to development cysticercosis. Even vegetarians are at risk. The lack of public awareness of this poses big problems.

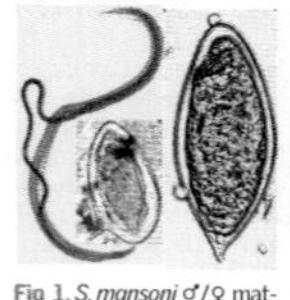

Fig 1. *S. mansoni* ♂/♀ mating; inset egg with sublateral spine (red arrow)
Fig 2. (enlarged) *S. haematobium*; terminal spine.

ıistosomiasis (bilharzia) is the most prevalent ɜase caused by flukes (~200 million people in Africa; v also introduced to S America/Caribbean). Snail tors release cercariae that penetrate skin, eg during ldling, causing itchy papular rashes ('swimmer's ı'). The cercariae shed their tails to become istosomules and migrate via lungs to liver where y grow. ~2wks later, there may be fever, urticaria, rhoea, cough, wheeze, and hepatosplenomegaly ('Katma fever'). In ~8wks, flukes are mature (14♂–mm long), mate (fig 1), and migrate to resting itats, ie bladder veins (*haematobium*) or mesenteric ıs (*mansoni* & *japonicum*). Eggs released from these s cause granulomata and scarring. Clinical signs ect our immune response to eggs (type IV hypersensitivity, eg for *S. mansoni*).

patient *S. mansoni:* abdominal pain; D&V; later, hepatic fibrosis, granulomatous ammation, anaemia,[1] and portal hypertension (transformation into true hosis has not been well-documented). *S. japonicum*, often the most serious, urs in SE Asia, tends to affect the bowel and liver, and may migrate to lung and ; ('travellers' myelitis'). Urinary schistosomiasis (*S. haematobium*) occurs in ica, the Middle East, and the Indian Ocean. Signs: frequency, dysuria, maturia (± haematospermia), incontinence. It may progress to hydronephrosis l renal failure. There is an ↑risk of squamous cell carcinoma of the bladder.

gnosis Eggs in urine (*S. haematobium;* fig 2, with 3 RBCs for scale) or faeces *mansoni* & *japonicum*) or rectal biopsy (all types). AXR may show bladder cification in chronic *S. haematobium* infection. Ultrasound (renal obstruction, ronephrosis ± thickened bladder wall). Schistosoma ELISA is most sensitive.

atment Praziquantel: 40mg/kg PO with food divided into 2 doses separated by 4–for *S. mansoni* & *S. haematobium*, or 20mg/kg/8h for 1d in *S. japonicum*. Sudden ısitory abdominal pain ± bloody diarrhoea may occur shortly after. Oxamniquine n alternative for *S. mansoni* infection. Artemether also shows promise, both for phylaxis in high-risk groups, and as a synergist to praziquantel.

sciola hepatica (liver fluke) is spread by sheep, water, and snails. It causes T°↑, lominal pain, diarrhoea, weight↓, jaundice, hepatomegaly, liver fibrosis and inophilia. ***Tests:*** Stool microscopy, serology. ***Ɍ:*** Get help. Triclabendazole 10mg PO, 1 dose, or bithionol 30mg/kg alternate days for 10–15 doses, max 2g/day IM.

isthorchis & ***Clonorchis*** are liver flukes common in Far East, where they cause cholangitis, cholecystitis, and cholangiocarcinoma. ***Tests:*** Stool micropy. ***Ɍ:*** Praziquantel 25mg/kg/8h PO for 1d.

sciolopsis buski is a big intestinal fluke ~7cm long sing ulcers or abscesses at the site of attachment. Praziquantel 25mg/kg/8h PO for 1d.

ragonimus westermani (lung fluke) is got by eating freshwater crabs and crayfish. Parasites migrate ough gut and diaphragm to invade lungs (hence gh, dyspnoea, haemoptysis, ± lung abscess/bronchıasis). It occurs in the Far East, S America, and ıgo; often mistaken for TB (similar signs & CXR). ***Tests:*** ıtun[egg] for CNS/lung lesions. ***Ɍ:*** Praziquantel (25mg/kg/8h PO for 2d).

Fig 3. *Clonorchis sinensis*

[1] erious in pregnancy (prevalence: 63% in Tanzania): Ajanga A 2006 *Trans R Soc Trop Med Hyg* 100 59

Exotic infections

Exotic infections may be ***community-acquired*** or ***nosocomial***, ie acqui in hospital. The increasing prevalence of immunosuppression, both drug indu and innate, and the widespread use of broad-spectrum antibiotics have resulte an increase in exotic infections. New techniques such as PCR have enabled identification of more putative infective agents. ***The history—and a good gos*** Don't expect to find the pertinent question in any textbook—eg "Are your c well at present?" (Mycobacterium marinum skin infection) or "Who has b licking your face recently?" (Pasteurella multocida); "Has your dog been holiday this year?" (monkeypox from prairie dogs); "Has your pet hedgehog l weight?" (Salmonella); "Did you have a stray pig living under your house when monsoon started?" (pigs + standing water + mosquitoes ≈ Japanese encephali

When you suspect infection (T°↑, sweats, inflammation, D&V, WCC↑, or unexplained symptom), ask about: • Foreign travel (recent and past) • Foreign boc (hip prosthesis, heart valve) • Work or hobby or family exposure to infectious age • Any bites/stings • Sexual exploits • Any necrotic tissue? • HIV risk or reason immunosuppression (eg pregnancy; steroids) • Any pets, exotic or otherwise?

Diagnosis Take appropriate cultures (blood, urine, stool, CSF) or swabs as clinic indicated. Liaise early with an infectious diseases physician or microbiolog Consider CXR, ultrasound, or CT as clinically indicated. If the infection appears t localized, consider surgical debridement ± drainage. Do not give up if you can culture an organism; tests may need to be repeated. Perhaps the organism 'fastidious' in its nutritional requirement or requires prolonged incubation? Eve culture *is* achieved, it may be that the organism is pathogenic, or it could b commensal (ie part of the normal flora for that patient). If culture is not possi look for antibodies or antigen in the serum or other body fluids. It is gener agreed that a 4-fold increase in antibody titres in convalescence (compared w the acute sera) is indicative of recent infection, although not diagnostic. PCR increasingly being used to make identifications; however, it is far from infalli and contamination with DNA from the lab or elsewhere is a frequent problem

Treatment Empirical therapy (p372) may be needed if the patient is ill. *The ta opposite is for reference purposes only:* no one can remember *all* the details ab even the common infectious diseases, let alone rare ones. Check with microbiologist for local patterns of disease and antibiotic sensitivity/resistar *Antibiotic doses:* Penicillins (p368); cephalosporins (p369); gentamicin;[1] ot agents (p370).

1 Prescribing by **surface area**, or **lean** body weight (LBW), eg for gentamicin, or **ideal** body weight (IB
Body surface area = 0.20247 × Height (metres)$^{0.725}$ × Weight(kg)$^{0.425}$
Lean body weight (♂) = (1.10 × Weight in kg) – 128 (Weight²/(100 × Height in metres)²)
Lean body weight (♀) = (1.07 × Weight in kg) – 148 (Weight²/(100 × Height in metres)²)
Ideal body weight (♂) = 50 + 2.3 for every inch over 5ft tall
Ideal body weight (♀) = 49 + 1.7 for every inch over 5ft tall. halls.md/ideal-weight/devine.htr

rganism	Site or type of infection IE=infective endocarditis	Treatment example
anthamoeba	Corneal ulcers	Propamidine + neomycin
netobacter calcoaceticus	UTI; CSF; lung; bone; conjunctiva	Gentamicin
tinobacillus	IE; CNS; UTI; bone; thyroid; lung	Penicillin ± gentamicin
:tinomycetemcomitans	Periodontitis; abscesses	
tinobacillus lignieresii	CSF; IE; wounds; bone; lymph nodes	Ampicillin ± gentamicin
tinobacillus ureae	Bronchus; CSF post-trauma; hepatitis	Ampicillin ± gentamicin
rococcus viridans	Empyema; UTI; CSF; bone; IE	Penicillin ± gentamicin
romonas hydrophila	IE; CSF; cornea; bone; D&V; liver abscess	Gentamicin
pia broomeae	Marrow; synovium	Imipenem or ceftriaxone
:aligenes species	Dialysis peritonitis; ear; lung	co-amoxiclav or cetazidime
achnia propionica	Actinomycosis; tear ducts; CNS	Penicillin
canobacterium	Throat; cellulitis; leg ulcer	Penicillin
besia microti (protozoa)	PUO ± haemolysis if old/splenectomy	Clindamycin + quinine
cillus cereus	Wounds; eye; ear; lung; UTI; IE	Gentamicin
idobacterium	Vagina; UTI; IE; peritonitis; lung	Penicillin
rdetella bronchiseptica	URTI; CSF (after animal contact)	Co-trimoxazole?
rkholderia cepacia, :c (formerly pseudomonas)	Wounds; feet; lungs; IE; CAPD; UTI ecthyma gangrenosa; peritonitis	Ceftazidime Clindamycin or gentamicin
rkholderia pickettii	CSF (formerly a pseudomonas)	Cefalosporin
rkholderia pseudomallei ormerly Pseudomonas seudomallei)	Melioidosis: self-reactivating septicaemia + multiorgan, protean signs eg in rice-farmers, via water/soil in Papua, Thailand, Vietnam, Torres Straits	Ceftazidime (14d) + Co-trimoxazole or co-amoxiclav for 3 months
pnocytophaga	Oral ulcer; stomatitis; arthritis	Penicillin or
chracea & C. sputagena	Blood; cervical abscess	ciprofloxacin
rdiobacterium hominis	IE (=infective endocarditis)	Penicillin + gentamicin
romobacterium violaceum	Nodes; eye; bone; liver; pustules	Erythromycin, chloramphenicol
robacter koseri/diversus	CSF; UTI; blood; cholecystitis	Cefuroxime + gentamicin
ynebacterium bovis/equi	IE; CSF; otitis; leg ulcer; lung	Erythromycin + rifampicin
rynebacterium ovis	Joints; liver; muscle; granulomata	Penicillin
ynebacterium ulcerans	Diphtheria-like ± CNS signs	Penicillin + Diphtheria antitoxin
clospora ayetanensis	Diarrhoea (via raspberries)	Co-trimoxazole
wardsiella tarda	Cellulitis; abscesses; BP↓; dysentery via penetrating fish injuries	Cefuroxime + gentamicin
enella corrodens	Sinus; ears; PE post-jugular vein phlebitis (postanginal sepsis) via bites	Penicillin + gentamicin
sipelothrix rhusiopathiae	Erysipelas-like (*OHCS* p598); IE	Penicillin
bacterium	Wounds; gynaecologic sepsis; IE	Penicillin
vobacterium neningosepticum	Lungs; epidemic neonatal meningitis; post-op bacteraemia	Penicillin
vobacterium multivorum	Peritonitis (spontaneous)	Cefuroxime
mella haemolysans	IE; meningitis after neurosurgery	Penicillin + gentamicin
licobacter cinaedia	Proctitis in homosexual men	Ampicillin or gentamicin
gella denitrificans kingae	Throat; larynx; eyelid; joint; skin	Penicillin ± gentamicin
rthia bibsonii/sibirica/zopfii	IE (infective endocarditis)	Penicillin
ctobacillus	Teeth; chorioamnionitis; pyelitis	Cephalosporins, Penicillin
gasphaera elsdenii	Anaerobic Gram-negative coccus; IE	Metronidazole
biluncus curtisii/mulieris	Vagina; uterus; septicaemia in cirrhosis	Cephalosporins or ampicillin
raxella osloensis and M. nonliquefaciens	Conjunctiva; wound; vagina; UTI; CSF CNS; bone; haemorrhagic stomatitis	Penicillin
isseria cani	Wounds from cat bites	Amoxicillin
isseria cinerea/mucosa + subflava; N. flavescens	IE; CNS; bone; post human bites or from peritoneal dialysis	Penicillin, cephalosporin
steurella multocida 340 (am-ve rod)	Skin; bone; lung; CSF; UTI; pericarditis epiglottitis. From cat or dog bite	β-lactam antibiotics or tetracyclines for >2weeks
steurella pneumotrophica	Wounds; joints; bone; CSF 341	Penicillin; cipro-/moxifloxacin
ptostreptococcus magnans	Bone/joint/discitis; wound; teeth; face	Penicillin or cephalosporins
siomonas shigelloides	D&V; eye; sepsis post fishbone injury	Ciprofloxacin
pionibacterium acnes	Face; wounds; CSF shunts; bone; IE; liver granuloma (botyromycosis)	Tetracycline or Penicillin
totheca wickerhamii 342 & ofii = achlorophyllous algae	Subcutaneous granuloma; plaques; bursitis; adenitis; nodules	Amphotericin or Ketoconazole
ovidencia stuartii	UTI; burn or lung infections	Gentamicin
eudomonas maltophilia	stenotrophomonas Wounds; ear; eye; lung; UTI; IE 343	Co-trimoxazole or cefepine
eudomonas putrefaciens	CSF post CNS surgery/head trauma	Cefotaxime
thia dentocariosa 344	Appendix abscess; infective emboli	Penicillin + gentamicin
rratia marcescens (may be non-pathogenic) 345	Wound; burns; lung; UTI; liver; CSF; bone; IE; red diaper/nappy syndrome	Imipenem, ceftazidime, ciprofloxacin
hingomonas paucimobilis	Superficial leg ulcer; CSF; UTI	Ceftazidime
reptococcus bovis	IE if colon cancer; do colonoscopy	Penicillin + gentamicin
brio vulnificus	Wounds; muscle; uterus; fasciitis	Tetracycline, penicillin

11 Neurology

Contents

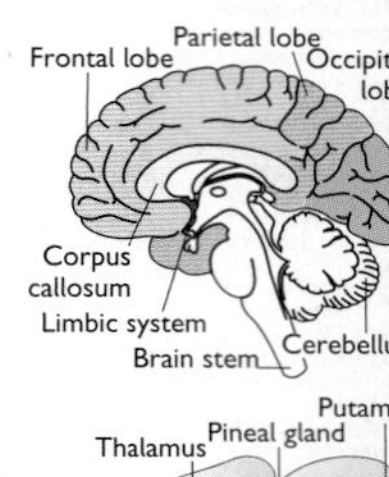

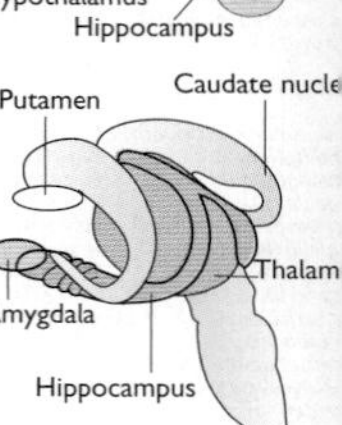

Fig 1. Cerebral hemispheres (top) a limbic system (middle & botto "We are very knowing. We know sorts of other things...about how the isn't a unitary ego—how we're made of conflicting, interacting system AS Byatt, *Possession*, p267.

Relevant pages elsewhere: CNS exam/cranial nerve lesions (p43–p45); mental s (p48); psychiatry (p13 & *OHCS* chapter 4); nystagmus (p44); facial pain (p60); Subac combined degeneration of the spinal cord (p320); LP (p756); headache emergen (p768); coma (p774); coma scale (p776); meningitis (p806); cerebral abscess (p8 status epilepticus (p808); head injury (p810); ↑ICP (p812).

We thank Dr Robert Clifford-Jones who is our Specialist Reader for this chapter.

We dedicate this page to those carers who find themselves responsible for a friend or relative who has a chronic neurological illness, eg stroke, rkinson's disease, Alzheimer's disease, or motor neurone disease. As a thought periment, try spending a morning imagining that you are such a carer— trying to expunge the smell of soiled sheets from your clothes, while awaiting visit from a neighbour, who said he would 'sit with him' so you can catch the s into town, and, like a guilty hedonist, play truant from your role as nurse for few sanity-giving hours of normal life. You wait. No one comes. You stop thering about the smell on your clothes, and turn towards your husband, out to say something, but when your eyes meet his, you realize he does not cognize you—and you keep your thoughts to yourself. Knuckles whiten as you asp his collar to lift him forward on the commode, and you seem to hear a ocking voice over your shoulder saying: '... so I see we're getting angry with n today, are we?' The ceaseless round from mouth to anus, from bed to chair, om twilight to twilight, continues, *ad infinitum*.

It is all we can do to spend *2 minutes* on this thought experiment, let alone a orning—or the rest of our lives. We need to be aware of the strategies we opt to avoid involvement with the naked truth of the shattered lives, which e a tragic subplot, stand behind the farce of morning surgery or out-patients which we hear ourselves for ever saying in plumy complacency: 'And how are u today Mrs Salt—your husband, I know... marvellous how you manage. You e a real support to each other. Let me know if I can do anything.' We pretend be busy, we ensure that we *are* busy, we surround ourselves with students, th white coats, and a miasma of technical expertise—we surround ourselves th *anything* to ensure that there is no chink through which Mrs Salt can shine r rays of darkness. Poor Mrs Salt. Poor us—to be frightened of the darkness, nicking at the thought that we might not have anything to offer, or that we ght be called to offer up our equanimity as a sacrifice to Mrs Salt. How dare e little grain upset our carefully contrived universe?

Respite care, medical charities, meals on wheels, laundry services, physio- erapy, occupational therapy (OT), transport, day care centres, clubs for carers, its from district nurses or from a nurse-matron specializing in chronic eases will go some way to mitigate Mrs Salt's problems. As ever, the way ward is by taking time to listen. Carers' needs evolve. First there is certainty, and the need for help in handling this. Next comes the moment of gnosis with the numbness, denial, and anger that may follow. Then there may an adjustment to reality, with frenzied searching for information and advice, a careful titration by the carer of how much information he or she can handle.

Issues of driving, mobility, finance, sex, and employment are likely to occur oughout the illness, and advice will need to be constantly tailored to suit ividual circumstances. But the best thing you can ever offer is the unwritten ntract that, come what may, you will be there, available, often ineffectual, but apable of being alienated by whatever the carer may disclose to you.

Revising for exams? You can skip this page, if you are *sure* your examiner is a narrow-minded bigot.

The chief questions of bedside neurology

Is there a **focal lesion** (illness of all cells in one part of the brain, eg a stroke)?-
- A **general insult**, eg trauma, encephalitis, anoxia, poisoning, or post-ictal sta
- **Widespread neurodegeneration** (may have specific local effects, eg amne
- Loss of **a specific type of nerve cell**, eg motor neurone disease; subacute c bined degeneration of the cord (B_{12}↓, p320); loss of pre-Bötzinger neurones in medulla causes central sleep apnoea (and death during sleep in the elderly
- **A disorder of function** (migraine; epilepsy) or **connectivity** (in autism, face p essing areas do not connect well to fronto-parietal areas directing attentior
- **Medically unexplained symptoms**, eg associated with psychological proble

A key feature in determining if a focal lesion is present is lack of symmet eg one pupil dilated, or an upgoing plantar response.

***Where* is the lesion?** Localizing the lesion depends on recognizing pattern cognitive, cranial nerve, motor, and sensory deficits occurring after lesion different sites in the nervous system. Analyse cognitive, cranial nerve, and m deficits first; the sensory examination is then used to confirm the site of the le

Patterns of motor deficits Weakness can arise from lesions of the cortex, cor radiata, internal capsule, brainstem, cord, peripheral nerves, neuromuscular junc or muscle. Is the pattern upper or lower motor neurone (UMN or LMN; see BOX ***Cortical lesions*** may show an unexpected pattern of weakness involving movements of a hand or foot, with normal or ↓tone—but ↑reflexes more proxin in the arm or leg will suggest an upper rather than lower motor neurone le ***Internal capsule*** and ***corticospinal pathway*** brainstem lesions cause contrala hemiplegia with a pyramidal distribution of weakness (1st BOX). If the hemipl occurs with epilepsy, ↓cognition, or homonymous hemianopia (p441), the lesion a cerebral hemisphere. A cranial nerve palsy (III–XII) contralateral to a hemipl implicates the brainstem on the side of the cranial nerve palsy. ***Cord lesions*** cau paraplegia (both legs) or quadriparesis/tetraplegia (all limbs) are suggeste finding a motor and reflex level (ie muscles are unaffected above the lesion, s LMN signs *at* the level of the lesion, and UMN signs *below* the lesion). ***Periph neuropathies:*** (p494) Most cause a distal weakness (foot-drop; weak hand), b Guillain–Barré syndrome weakness is often *proximal*. Involvement of a single n (mononeuropathy) occurs with trauma or entrapment (carpal tunnel, p495); ir vement of several nerves (mononeuritis multiplex) is seen eg in DM.

Sensory deficits Information about the site of a lesion is obtained chiefly from distribution of sensory loss; the range of sensory modalities involved (pain, te erature, touch, vibration, and joint position sense) can also add information, as and temperature sensations travel along small fibres in peripheral nerves tracts in the cord and brainstem. They are distinct from joint position and vibra sense, which travel in fibres in the large dorsal columns of the cord. Distal sen loss suggests a neuropathy and may involve all sensory modalities or be n selective, depending on the nerve fibre size involved in the peripheral ne Individual nerve lesions are identified by their anatomical territories which usually more sharply defined than those of root lesions (dermatomes, p446), w often show considerable overlap. The hallmark of a cord lesion is a sensory leve an area of decreased or absent sensation below the lesion (eg the legs) with no sensation above this level (eg in abdomen, trunk, and arms). Lateral cord lesions g Brown-Séquard syndrome (p688) with dorsal column loss on the side of the le and spinothalamic loss in the other leg. Cervical cord lesions (eg syringomy p508 or cord tumours) may cause selective loss of pain and temperature sens with sparing of joint position sense and vibration (ie 'dissociated' sensory l Lateral brainstem lesions show both dissociated and crossed sensory loss with and T° loss on the side of the face ipsilateral to the lesion, and contralateral and leg sensory loss. Lesions above the brainstem give a contralateral patte generalized sensory loss. In cortical lesions, sensory loss is confined to more su and discriminating sensory functions (2-point discrimination and stereognos

MN lesions (upper motor neurone)

ıese are caused by damage to motor pathways anywhere from motor nerve ells in the precental gyrus of the frontal cortex, through the internal capsule, ainstem, and cord, to the anterior horn cells in the cord. Typical characteristics e 'pyramidal'[1] in distribution, ie weakness involving physiological extensors of e arm (shoulder abduction; elbow, wrist, and finger extension; and the small uscles of the hand) and the flexors of the lower limb (hip flexion, knee flexion, ıd ankle dorsiflexion and everters). There is little muscle wasting and ***loss of illed fine finger movements*** may be greater than expected from the overall ade of weakness. ***Increased tone*** (spasticity) develops in stronger muscles (eg m flexors and leg extensors). It is manifest as resistance to passive movement at can suddenly be over-come (clasp-knife feel). There is ***hyperreflexia:*** flexes are brisk; ***plantars are upgoing*** (+ve Babinski sign) ± ***clonus*** (elicited by pidly dorsiflexing the foot; ≤3 rhythmic, downward beats of the foot are ›rmal; more suggest an UMN lesion) ± a positive ***Hoffman's reflex***: brief flexion thumb and index finger in a pincer movement following a flick to the pulp of e middle finger (it is a stretch reflex so the often-used way of flicking the ıger *towards* the palm isn't ideal). Neck extension is said to increase sensitivity this test. **NB:** UMN weakness affects ***muscle groups***, not individual muscles.

MN lesions (lower motor neurone)

ıese are caused by damage anywhere from anterior horn cells in the ›rd, nerve roots, plexi, or peripheral nerves. The distribution of weakness ›rresponds to those muscles supplied by the involved cord segment, nerve root, ırt of plexus, or peripheral nerve. See p444. A combination of anatomical ıowledge, good muscle testing technique, and experience is needed to stinguish, eg a radial nerve palsy from a C7 root lesion, or a common peroneal ›rve palsy from an L5 root lesion (p444).[2] The relevant muscles show ***wasting*** ± ›ontaneous involuntary twitching (***fasciculation***), and feel soft and floppy, oviding little resistance to passive stretch (***hypotonia/flaccidity***). ***Reflexes are duced*** or absent, the ***plantars remain flexor***. The chief differential is weak-ıss from primary muscle disease—here there is symmetrical loss, reflexes are st later than in neuropathies, and there is no sensory loss. Myasthenia gravis IG) causes weakness worsening with use of the affected muscles (↑fatigue); ere is little wasting, normal reflexes, and no sensory loss—see p504.
flexes and spinal cord level: p43. ***Spinal roots for each muscle:*** p444.
r mixed LMN and UMN signs, see p459 (B_{12}↓, syphilis etc).

uscle weakness grading (MRC classification)

ıde 0	No muscle contraction	**Grade 3**	Active movement against gravity
ıde 1	Flicker of contraction	**Grade 4**	Active movement against resistance
ıde 2	Some active movement	**Grade 5**	Normal power (allowing for age)

ade 4 Covers a big range: **4–**, **4**, and **4+** denote movement against slight, ›derate, and stronger resistance; avoid fudging descriptions—'strength 4/5 oughout' suggests a mild quadriparesis or myopathy. It is better to document or effort' and the maximum grade for each muscle tested.

yramidal neurones have basal dendrites and an apical dendrite pointing towards the dorsal cortical er. They are a distinctive cortical feature and are specialized in their dendritic morphology, projection erns, and localization within the 6 cortical layers. *'Extrapyramidal'* denotes CNS motor phenomena ing to the basal ganglia. Pyramidal lesions result in paresis and spasticity, but extrapyramidal lesions e abnormality in initiation and maintenance of movement—negative symptoms include ykinesia/akinesia (slow/absent movement) and loss of postural reflexes; positive symptoms are ıor, rigidity, and involuntary movements (p460, eg chorea, athetosis, ballismus, and dystonia).
'he booklet *Aids to the Examination of the Peripheral Nervous System* is invaluable here. ISBN 0-7020-2512-7

Cerebral artery territories

Knowledge of the anatomy of the blood supply of the brain helps in diagnosing a managing cerebrovascular disease (p462–470). Always try to identify the area brain that correlates with a patient's symptoms and identify the affected arte

Cerebral blood supply The brain is supplied by the two internal carotid arteries and the basilar artery (formed by the joining of the two vertebral arteries). These 3 vessels feed into an anastomotic ring at the base of the brain called the circle of Willis (below). This arrangement may lessen the effects of occlusion of a feeder vessel proximal to the anastomosis by allowing supply from unaffected vessels. The anatomy of the circle of Willis is, however, highly variable and in many people it cannot provide much protection from ischaemia due to carotid, vertebral, or basilar artery occlusion. Anastomotic supply from other vessels in the neck may mitigate occlusions of feeder vessels—occlusion of the internal carotid in the neck, eg may not cause infarction if flow from the external carotid artery enters the circle of Willis via its anastomosis with the ophthalmic artery.

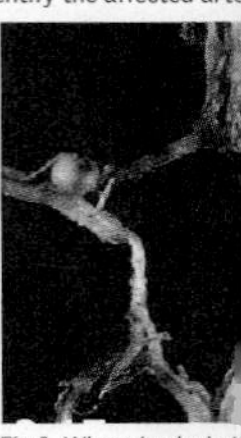

Fig 1. Where (and what) the lesion? Answer: p470

The circle of Willis at the base of the brain

see also CT on p47

Optic chiasm
Internal carotid artery
Posterior cerebral artery
Superior cerebellar artery
Basilar artery
Vertebral artery
Anterior spinal artery
Anterior cerebral artery
Anterior communicating artery
Middle cerebral artery
Posterior cerebral arter with posterior communicating artery connecting it to the middle cerebral artery
Internal auditory artery
Anterior inferior cerebellar artery
Posterior inferior cerebellar artery

Footnotes in history: Willis

Thomas Willis (1621–75) is one of those happy Oxford heroes belonging to Christ Chu College who hold a bogus DM degree—awarded in 1646 for his Royalist sympathies. had a busy life inventing terms such as 'neurology' and 'reflex'. Not only has his na been given to his famous circle, but he was the first to describe myasthenia gra whooping cough, and the sweet taste of diabetic urine. He was the first person (few h followed him) who knew the course of the spinal accessory nerve. He is unusual am Oxford neurologists in that, at various times, he developed the practice of giving lunch away to the poor. He also developed the practice of iatrochemistry: a theory medicine according to which all morbid conditions of the body can be explained disturbances in the fermentations and effervescences of its humours.

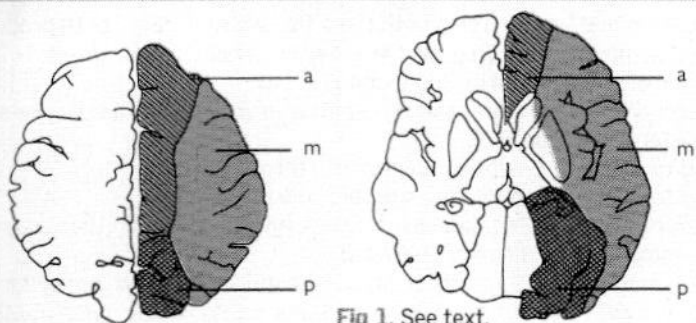

Fig 1. See text.

rotid artery Internal carotid artery occlusion may, at worst, cause total (and ıally fatal) infarction of the anterior two-thirds of the ipsilateral hemisphere ɗ basal ganglia (lenticulostriate arteries). More often, the picture is similar to niddle cerebral artery occlusion (below).

rebral arteries 3 pairs of arteries leave the circle of Willis to supply the ·ebral hemispheres; the anterior, middle, and posterior cerebral arteries. The terior and middle cerebrals are branches of the carotid arteries; the basilar :ery divides into the 2 posterior cerebral arteries. Ischaemia due to occlusion of y one of them may be reduced, if not prevented, by retrograde supply from eningeal vessels.

terior cerebral artery: (a in Fig 1) Supplies the frontal and medial part of ɛ cerebrum. Occlusion may cause a weak, numb contralateral leg ± similar, if lder, arm symptoms. The face is spared. Bilateral infarction can cause a kinetic ıtism from damage to the cingulate gyri (also a rare cause of paraplegia).

ddle cerebral artery: (m in Fig 1) Supplies the lateral (external) part of each misphere. Occlusion may cause: contralateral hemiplegia, hemisensory loss ıinly of face and arm; contralateral homonymous hemianopia due to ·olvement of the optic radiation, cognitive change including dysphasia if the minant hemisphere is affected, and visuo-spatial disturbance (eg cannot ɜss; gets lost) with non-dominant lesions.

sterior cerebral artery: (p in Fig 1) Supplies the :cipital lobe; occlusion gives contralateral homonıous hemianopia (often with macula sparing).

rtebrobasilar circulation Supplies the cerellum, brainstem, occipital lobes. *Occlusion cause:* mianopia; cortical blindness; diplopia; vertigo; stagmus; hemi- or quadriplegia; unilateral or ateral sensory symptoms; cerebellar symptoms; :cups; dysarthria; dysphasia; coma. Infarctions the brainstem can produce various syndromes, *Lateral medullary syndrome* (occlusion of one ·tebral artery or the posterior inferior cerebar artery). It is due to infarction of the lateral ɜdulla and the inferior cerebellar surface ısing vertigo with vomiting, dysphagia, stagmus, ipsilateral ataxia, soft palate paralysis, ipsilateral Horner's syndrome, d a crossed pattern sensory loss (analgesia to pin-prick on ipsilateral face and ntralateral trunk & limbs).

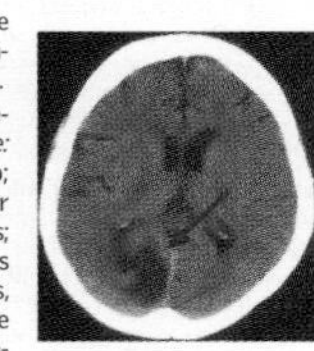

Fig 2. CT of stroke (arrow) in the distribution of the posterior cerebral artery.

bclavian steal syndrome: Subclavian artery stenosis proximal to the origin the vertebral artery may cause blood to be *stolen* by retrograde flow down s vertebral artery down into the arm, causing brainstem ischaemia typically :er use of the arm. Suspect if the BP in each arm differs by >20mmHg.

Drugs and the nervous system

The brain is a gland that secretes both thoughts and molecules: both products modulated by neurotransmitter systems. *Some target sites for drugs:*

1 Precursor of the transmitter (eg L-dopa).
2 Interference with the storage of transmitter in vesicles within the pre-syna neurone (eg tetrabenazine).
3 Binding to the post-synaptic receptor site (bromocriptine).
4 Binding to receptor-modulating site (benzodiazepines).
5 Interference with the breakdown of neurotransmitter within the synaptic c (monoamine oxidase inhibitors—MAOIs).
6 Reduce *reuptake* of transmitter from synaptic cleft into *pre-synaptic* (*selective serotonin reuptake inhibitors*, SSRIs, eg fluoxetine, *OHCS* p340). A SNRI (serotonin and nonadrenaline reuptake inhibitors). Nonadrenaline may more involved in the symptoms of anergia, fatigue and loss of drive in depress and 5-HT may be more involved in the alteration in subjective mood and anxiet
7 Binding to presynaptic autoreceptors. There are 3 kinds of autorecept neurotransmitter release modulators, synthesis modulators, and impulse mod ators. These offer sites for intervention. Augmenting antidepressant ther with 5-HT autoreceptor antagonists such as pindolol is possible.

The proven neurotransmitters include:

Neurology

Amino acids Glutamate & aspartate act as excitatory transmitters on NMDA & n NMDA receptors—relevant in epilepsy and ischaemic brain damage. γ-aminobut acid (GABA) is mostly inhibitory. ***Drugs enhancing GABA activity are used in:*** Epile (phenobarbital, benzodiazepines, vigabatrin); spasticity (baclofen, benzodiazepir

Peptides Opioids and substance P.

Histamine and **Purines** (such as ATP) Clinical relevance is not clear.

Dopamine (DA) ***Drugs enhancing DA activity:*** Used in Parkinson's; hyperprolac aemia; acromegaly. SE: vomiting; BP↓; chorea; dystonia; hallucinations and delusi ***Drugs which ↓ DA activity are used in:*** Schizophrenia (*OHCS* p360, D_2 antagonis delusions; chorea; tics; nausea; vertigo. SE: parkinsonism; dystonias; akathisia

Serotonin (5-hydroxytryptamine; 5HT) There are many types of receptors, $5HT_{1-4}$. $5HT_1$ has 5 subtypes ($5HT_{1A-E}$). ***Agonists:*** Lithium$_{1A}$; sumatriptan$_{1D}$. ***Par agonists:*** Buspirone$_{1A}$; LSD$_2$; ***Antagonists:*** Ondansetron$_3$, pizotifen$_{1\&2}$; me sergide$_{1\&2}$, clozapine$_{2C}$—known as low D_2–high $5HT_2$, while risperidone is high high $5HT_2$ (low D_2 means <60% D_2 occupancy at conventional doses; traditic antipsychotics are just high D_2, ie 60–80%). ***Reuptake inhibitors:*** Fluoxet sertraline, venlafaxine. Ecstasy increases nerve terminal 5HT release.

Adrenaline (epinephrine) and non-adrenaline (norepinephrine) 4 recep types: α1, α2, β1, β2. Norepinephrine is more specific for α-receptors but b transmitters affect all receptors. In the periphery: α-receptor stimulation lead arteriolar vasoconstriction and pupillary dilatation; β1 stimulation to increas pulse and myocardial contractility; β2 stimulation to bronchodilatation, ute relaxation, and arteriolar vasodilatation.

Drugs enhancing adrenergic activity are used in: Asthma (β2); anaphyla (adrenaline); heart failure (dobutamine); depression (MAOIs and tricyclics, the la may act by increasing synaptic norepinephrine in the CNS).

Drugs reducing adrenergic activity are used in: Angina, ↑BP, arrhythm thyrotoxicosis/anxiety (β1); ↑BP from phaeochromocytoma (α).

Acetylcholine (Muscarinic and nicotinic receptors) ***Centrally acting a cholinergic drugs are used in:*** Parkinsonism, dystonias, motion sickness. Cen toxic effects (especially in the elderly): confusion, delusions.

Peripheral antimuscarinic drugs are used in: Asthma (ipratropium); inco inence; to dry secretions pre-op; to dilate pupils; to ↑ heart rate (atropine).

Peripheral cholinergic agonists used in: Glaucoma (pilocarpine); myasthe (anticholinesterases). SE: sweating, hypersalivation, colic.

[N]eurotransmitters and CNS drugs

[He]re we list drugs used to modify CNS transmitters. When prescribing bear in [mi]nd that: • The drug (or a metabolite) must be able to pass through the blood–[br]ain barrier to have an effect. • The consequences of any sedative effects may [be] severe. • There will be short- and long-term side-effects (eg tardive dyskinesia [wi]th neuroleptic drugs). • Drugs may affect many neurotransmitters increasing [th]erapeutic scope (and uncertainty). • One neurotransmitter may have many [ef]fects—eg midbrain dopamine neurones go awry in Parkinson's disease, schizo[ph]renia, and in addiction to drugs and gambling, by affecting motor control, [mo]tivation, effort, reward, analgesia, stress, learning, attention, and cognition.

[Dr]ugs ↑ activity (≈agonists)	Drugs ↓ activity (≈antagonists)
[Do]pamine (L-dopa)	
[P]ergolide; apomorphine; amantadine	Major tranquillizers
[B]romocriptine (a D_2-agonist)	Benzisoxazoles (D_2) eg risperidone
[P]ramipexole (D_3) (to do with mood behaviour & rewards)	Some antiemetics
[S]elegiline (MAOI-B inhibitor)	
[No]n-adrenaline & adrenaline less (=norepinephrine & epinephrine)	
[S]albutamol (β_2); adrenaline	Propranolol (β) (atenolol is mostly β_1)
[T]ricyclic antidepressants	Clonidine (α_2-agonist)
[M]AOI	Phentolamine (α)
[5H]T	
[L]SD and other hallucinogens	Pizotifen
[S]umatriptan	Benzisoxazoles ($5HT_2$-antagonist) eg risperidone
[S]ome tricyclic antidepressants eg trazodone	Clozapine (*OHCS* p360 $5HT_{2A}$ antagonist)
[B]uspirone; lithium	
[F]luoxetine (*OHCS* p340)	Mianserin; ondansetron
[A]cetylcholine	
[C]arbachol	Atropine; Scopolamine
[P]ilocarpine	Ipratropium
[A]nticholinesterases	Benzhexol (=trihexyphenidyl)
eg pyridostigmine	Orphenadrine; Procyclidine
[G]ABA (inhibits other transmitters)	
[B]aclofen (GABA-B) (GABA=gamma aminobutyric acid)	Alcohol abuse[1]: *acute effects* block *N*-methyl-D-aspartate (NMDA) receptors; *with chronic use*, numbers of NMDA receptors rise, mediating alcohol
[B]enzodiazepines; valproate	
[B]arbiturates	
[A]camprosate (used in alcohol addiction; taurine & GABA analogue)	
[Gl]utamate[1]	
[A]n excitatory amino acid)	Lamotrigine (used in epilepsy)
	Topiramate (used in epilepsy *et al.*)[1]
	Acamprosate (↓craving in alcoholics)
	Memantine (Alzheimer's, p478)
	Zonisamide (+ carbonic anhydrase activity, and modulates T Ca^{2+} channels)

[N]ew drugs are often aimed at multiple neurotransmitters, eg *risperidone* [b]locks D_2, $5HT_2$, α_1 and α_2 adrenoceptors, *OHCS* p360). The smoking-cessation [dr]ug *bupropion* (=*amfebutamone*) is said to act by increasing dopamine in the [m]esolimbic system (mediates dependence) *and* via noradrenergic effects in the [lo]cus ceruleus (mediates symptoms of nicotine withdrawal).

1 Alcoholics have more glutamate binding sites, facilitating midbrain dopamine neurotransmission (path[wa]ys, which, in the ventral tegmental area, mediate alcohol's rewarding effects, eg craving). Topiramate [fac]ilitates GABA function, antagonizing glutamate at kainate receptors, and may ↓craving in alcoholism.

Testing peripheral nerves

Nerve root	Muscle	Test—by asking the patient to:
C3, 4	Trapezius	Shrug shoulder (via accessory nerve
C5, 6, 7	Serratus anterior	Push arm forward against resistan look for winging of the scapula, if we
C**5**, 6	Pectoralis major (p major) clavicular head	Adduct arm from above horizont and push it forward.
C6, **7**, 8	P major sternocostal head	Adduct arm below horizontal.
C**5**, 6	Supraspinatus	Abduct arm the first 15°.
C**5**, 6	Infraspinatus	Externally rotate semi-flexed ar elbow at side.
C6, **7**, 8	Latissimus dorsi	Adduct arm from horizontal position
C5, 6	Biceps	Flex supinated forearm.
C**5**, 6	Deltoid	Abduct arm between 15° and 90°.
Radial nerve		
C6, **7**, 8	Triceps	Extend elbow against resistance.
C5, **6**	Brachioradialis	Flex elbow with forearm half way between pronation and supination.
C5, **6**	Extensor carpi radialis longus	Extend wrist to radial side.
C6, 7	Supinator	Arm by side, resist hand pronation.
C**7**, 8	Extensor digitorum	Keep fingers extended at MCP joint.
C**7**, 8	Extensor carpi ulnaris	Extend wrist to ulnar side.
C**7**, 8	Abductor pollicis longus	Abduct thumb at 90° to palm.
C**7**, 8	Extensor pollicis brevis	Extend thumb at MCP joint.
C**7**, 8	Extensor pollicis longus	Resist thumb flexion at IP joint.
Median nerve		
C6, 7	Pronator teres	Keep arm pronated against resistanc
C6, 7	Flexor carpi radialis	Flex wrist towards radial side.
C7, **8**, T1	Flexor digitorum superficialis	Resist extension at PIP joint (with prc imal phalanx fixed by the examiner).
C7, **8**	Flexor digitorum profundus I & II	Resist extension at index DIP joint index finger.
C7, **8**, T1	Flexor pollicis longus	Resist thumb extension at interpl langeal joint (fix proximal phalanx).
C8, **T1**	Abductor pollicis brevis	Abduct thumb (nail at 90° to palm).
C8, **T1**	Opponens pollicis	Thumb touches base of 5th finger- (nail parallel to palm).
C8, **T1**	1st lumbrical/Interosseus (median & ulnar nerves)	Extend PIP joint against resistance w MCP joint held hyperextended.
Ulnar nerve		
C7, **8**, T1	Flexor carpi ulnaris	Flex wrist to ulnar side; observe tend
C7, C**8**	Flexor digitorum profundus III and IV	Resist extension of distal phalanx of 5 finger while you fix its middle phalar
C8, **T1**	Dorsal interossei	Finger abduction: cannot cross the middle over the index finger (tests index finger adduction too).
C8, **T1**	Palmar interossei	Finger adduction: pull apart a sheet c paper held between middle and rinc finger DIP joints of both hands; the paper moves on the weaker side.[1]
C8, **T1**	Adductor pollicis	Adduct thumb (nail at 90° to palm).
C8, **T1**	Abductor digiti minimi	Abduct little finger.
C8, **T1**	Flexor digiti minimi	Flex the little finger at MCP joint.

1 Also, metacarpophalangeal joint flexion may be more on the affected side as flexor tendons recruited—the basis of Froment's paper sign. Wartenberg's sign is persistent little finger abduction

wer limb Femoral nerve		
2, 3	Iliopsoas (also supplied via L1, 3, & 3 spinal nerves)	Flex hip against resistance with knee flexed and lower leg supported: patient lies on back.
3, 4	Quadriceps femoris	Extend at the knee against resistance. Start with the knee flexed.
turator nerve		
3, 4	Hip adductors	Adduct the leg against resistance.
ferior gluteal nerve		
S**1**, S2	Gluteus maximus	Hip extension ('bury heal into the couch')—with knee in extension.
perior gluteal nerve		
5, S1	Gluteus medius & minimus	Abduction and internal hip rotation with leg flexed at hip and knee.
iatic (and common peroneal*) and sciatic (and tibial) nerves**		
4, 5	Tibialis anterior	Dorsiflex ankle.
5, S1	Extensor digitorum longus	Dorsiflex toes against resistance.
5, S1	Extensor hallucis longus	Dorsiflex hallux against resistance.
5, S1	Peroneus longus & brevis	Evert foot against resistance.
5, S1	Extensor digitorum brevis	Dorsiflex proximal phalanges of toes.
.5, **S1**, 2	Hamstrings	Flex the knee against resistance.
.4, 5	Tibialis posterior	Invert the plantarflexed foot.
S1, 2	Gastrocnemius	Plantarflex ankle or stand on tiptoe.
.5, S**1**, **2**	Flexor digitorum longus	Flex terminal joints of the toes.
S1, 2	Small muscles of foot	Make the sole of the foot into a cup.

ick screening test for muscle power

oulder	Abduction	C5	**Hip**	Flexion	L1–L2
	Adduction	C5–C7		Adduction	L2–3
ow	Flexion	C5–C6		Extension	L5–S1
	Extension	C7	**Knee**	Flexion	L5–S1
ist	Flexion	C7–8		Extension	L3–L4
	Extension	C7	**Ankle**	Dorsiflexion	L4
gers	Flexion	C8		Eversion	L5–S1
	Extension	C7		Plantarflexion	S1–S2
	Abduction	T1	**Toe**	Big toe extension	L5

member to test proximal muscle power: ask the patient to sit from lying, to l you towards himself, and to rise from squatting (if reasonably fit).

bserve walking—easy to forget, even if the complaint is of walking difficulty!

oot numbers in bold indicate that that root is more important than its neighbour.
urces vary in ascribing particular nerve roots to muscles, and there is some biological variation in viduals. The above is a reasonable compromise, based on MRC/*Brain* 2001 guidelines: ISBN 0-7020-2512-7.
e don't react to nerve damage according to simple anatomy; eg ulnar neuropathy may initiate dystonic on or tremor of 4th & 5th digits by inducing a central motor disorder. [@8622720] [@2153273]

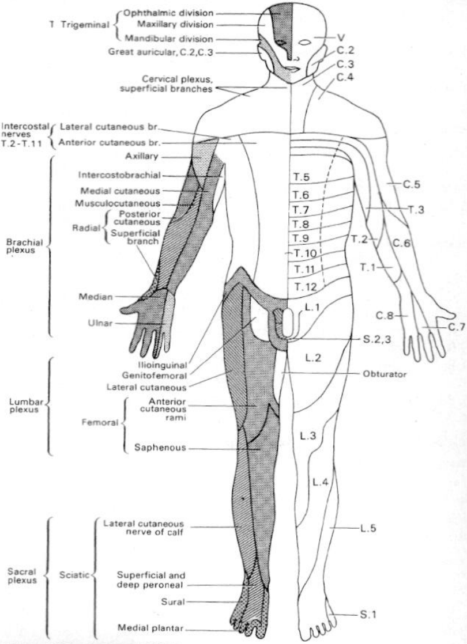

Dermatomes

V Trigeminal
Ophthalmic division
Maxillary division
Mandibular division
Great auricular, C.2, C.3
Cervical plexus, superficial branches
Intercostal nerves T.2–T.11
Lateral cutaneous br.
Anterior cutaneous br.
Brachial plexus
Axillary
Intercostobrachial
Medial cutaneous
Musculocutaneous
Radial
Posterior cutaneous
Superficial branch
Median
Ulnar
Lumbar plexus
Ilioinguinal
Genitofemoral
Lateral cutaneous
Femoral
Anterior cutaneous rami
Saphenous
Sacral plexus
Sciatic
Lateral cutaneous nerve of calf
Superficial and deep peroneal
Sural
Medial plantar

V
C.2
C.3
C.4
C.5
T.3
C.6
T.2
T.1
C.8
C.7
T.5
T.6
T.7
T.8
T.9
T.10
T.11
T.12
L.1
S.2,3
L.2
Obturator
L.3
L.4
L.5
S.1

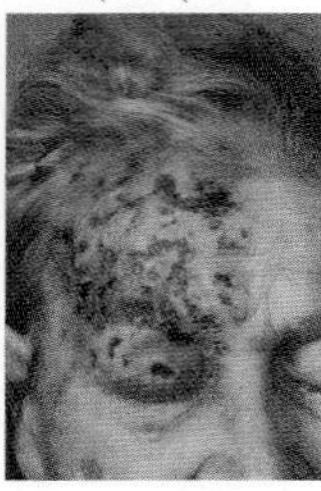

Pain in a dermatomal distribution suggests a probl with a cranial nerve or dorsal root ganglion (radic opathy)—where the cell bodies of sensory fibres live What is the dermatome? What is the lesion? S p388.

Dermatomes

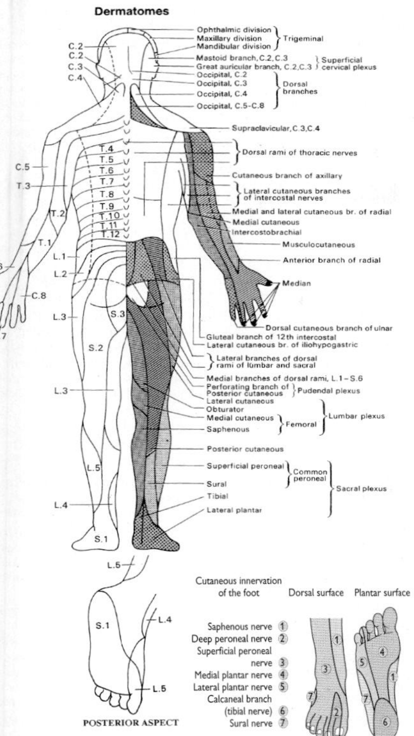
Ophthalmic division
Maxillary division
Mandibular division
Trigeminal
Mastoid branch, C.2, C.3
Great auricular branch, C.2, C.3
Superficial cervical plexus
Occipital, C.2
Occipital, C.3
Occipital, C.4
Occipital, C.5-C.8
Dorsal branches
Supraclavicular, C.3, C.4
Dorsal rami of thoracic nerves
Cutaneous branch of axillary
Lateral cutaneous branches of intercostal nerves
Medial and lateral cutaneous br. of radial
Medial cutaneous
Intercostobrachial
Musculocutaneous
Anterior branch of radial
Median
Dorsal cutaneous branch of ulnar
Gluteal branch of 12th intercostal
Lateral cutaneous br. of iliohypogastric
Lateral branches of dorsal rami of lumbar and sacral
Medial branches of dorsal rami, L.1–S.6
Perforating branch of Posterior cutaneous
Pudendal plexus
Lateral cutaneous
Obturator
Medial cutaneous
Saphenous
Femoral
Lumbar plexus
Posterior cutaneous
Superficial peroneal
Sural
Common peroneal
Tibial
Lateral plantar
Sacral plexus
C.2
C.2
C.3
C.4
C.5
T.3
T.2
T.1
.6
C.8
C.7
T.4
T.5
T.6
T.7
T.8
T.9
T.10
T.11
T.12
L.1
L.2
L.3
S.3
S.2
L.3
L.5
L.4
S.1
L.5
S.1
L.4
L.5
POSTERIOR ASPECT
Cutaneous innervation of the foot
Dorsal surface
Plantar surface
Saphenous nerve 1
Deep peroneal nerve 2
Superficial peroneal nerve 3
Medial plantar nerve 4
Lateral plantar nerve 5
Calcaneal branch (tibial nerve) 6
Sural nerve 7

Headache

Every day, *thousands* of patients visit doctors complaining of headache; t consultations are rewarding as the chief skill is in interpreting the history, n *taking* it, so much as in *allowing* it to unfold. Let patients tell you about al. headache's associations, or even *who* their headache is. Stress/tension headac the usual cause of bilateral, non-pulsatile headache (± scalp muscle tenderness without vomiting or sensitivity to head movement). Here, stress relief, eg mas or antidepressants, may have more to offer than a neurologist. But s headaches are disabling and treatable (migraine, cluster headache), while ot are sinister, eg space-occupying lesions, meningitis, subarachnoid haemorr (SAH), and giant cell arteritis. These are the headaches you must recognize:

Acute single episode	
Meningitis	p806, eg fever, photophobia, stiff neck, rash, coma
Encephalitis	p807, eg fever, odd behaviour, fits, or consciousness↓
Tropical illness	p378, eg malaria, +ve travel history, 'flu-like illness
Subarachnoid	p470, haemorrhage → *sudden* headache ± stiff neck
Sinusitis	p562 in *OHCS*, eg tender face + coryza + post-nasal drip
Head injury	p810, cuts/bruises, consciousness↓; lucid interval, amne
Acute recurrent attacks	
Migraine	p450, any pre-attack aura? Visual aura? Vomiti Sensitivity to light, noise, or movement
Cluster headache	p449, typically nightly pain in one eye for ~8wks then OK the next few months—then intermittently repeated
Glaucoma	p545, red eye; sees haloes, fixed big oval pupil; acuity↓
Recurrent (Mollaret's) meningitis	Suspect if T°↑ & fever; do LP + PCR for herpes simplex there access to the subarachnoid space via a skull fract or a recurring cause of aseptic meningitis (SLE, Behç sarcoid)?
Subacute onset	
Giant cell arteritis	p542; tender scalp; ≥50yrs old; threat to vision; ESR↑
Chronic headache (pain for >15d/month for >3 months)	
Tension headache	'a tight band round my head'; stress at work/home, mo
Chronically ↑ICP	Eg worse on waking, focal signs, BP↑, pulse↓
Medication misuse	p448; medication misuse headache eg from analgesic over

Acute single episode (eg meningitis, encephalitis, subarachnoid haemorrha If the headache is acute, severe, felt over most of the head and accompanie meningeal irritation (neck stiffness) ± drowsiness you must think of menin (p806), encephalitis (p807), or a subarachnoid (p470). Admit immediately urgent CT (and, if –ve, LP, looking for blood products in the CSF).

After head injury headache is common, eg at the site of trauma, or m generalized. It lasts ~2wks and is often resistant to analgesia. Bear in m subdural/extradural haemorrhage (p474). Sinister signs are drowsiness, focal si

Sinusitis causes dull, constant, aching pain over the frontal or maxillary sinus, tender overlying skin ± postnasal drip. Ethmoid or sphenoid sinus pain is felt de the midline at the root of the nose. Pain is worse on bending over. Often occurs coryza (p390). The pain lasts ~1–2 weeks. CT can confirm diagnosis (rarely need

Acute glaucoma: Mostly elderly, long-sighted people. Constant, aching develops rapidly around an eye, radiating to the forehead. ***Symptoms:*** Mark reduced vision, nausea, and vomiting. ***Signs:*** Red, congested eye; cloudy cor dilated, non-responsive pupil. Attacks may be precipitated by sitting in the dar the cinema, dilating eye-drops or emotional upset. Seek expert help at once. If d in treatment of >1h is likely, start IV acetazolamide, 500mg over several minu

ttacks of headache—*Cluster headache* (CH = *migrainous neuralgia*): One eory (among many) is that this is caused by superficial temporal artery smooth uscle hyperreactivity to 5HT. There are related hypothalamic grey matter ab- rmalities. An autosomal dominant gene also has a role. Onset: any age; ♂:♀ ≥ 5 : 1, mmoner in smokers. Pain occurs once or twice every 24h, each episode lasting 5–160min. Clusters typically last 4–12wks and are followed by pain-free periods of onths or even 1–2yrs before another cluster begins. Sometimes it is chronic rather an episodic. ***Symptoms:*** Rapid onset severe pain around 1 eye which may become atery and bloodshot with lid swelling, lacrimation, facial flushing, and rhinorrhoea. iosis ± ptosis (20% of attacks), being permanent in 5%. Pain is strictly unilateral d almost always affects the same side. ***The father in extremis:*** '...I am careful not wake the children as I make my way down the stairs. If they were to witness my ghtly cluster ritual, they would never see me the same way again. Their father, arless protector, diligent provider, crawling about in tears, beating his head on the rd wood floor. The pain is so intense I want to scream, but I never do. I go down 3 ghts of stairs where I can't be heard, and drop to my knees. I place my hands on e back of my neck, and lock my fingers together. I bind my head between my arms d squeeze as hard as I can in an attempt to crush my skull. I begin to roll around, nging my head on the floor, pressing my left eye with full force of my palm. I arch for the telephone that has always been my weapon of choice for creating a version, and I beat my left temple with the hand piece. I create a rhythm as I rike my skull, cursing the demon with each blow...' **℞: Acute attack:** 100% O_2 '–15L/min for ~15min; specify 'non-rebreathable mask and short-burst delivery to ve 100%'; CI: COPD)—or *sumatriptan* SC 6mg at the attack's onset. ***Preventives:*** erapamil; lithium; steroids; methysergide (SE: retroperitoneal fibrosis).

igeminal neuralgia: Paroxysms of intense, stabbing pain, lasting seconds, in the igeminal nerve distribution eg from anomalous intracranial vessels compressing e trigeminal root. It is unilateral, typically affecting mandibular or maxillary div- ions. The face screws up with pain (hence *tic doloureux*). ***Triggers:*** Washing fected area, shaving, eating, talking, dental prostheses. ***Typical patient:*** ♂ 50yrs old; in Asians ♀:♂≈2:1. ***Secondary causes:*** Aneurysm, tumour, chronic eningeal inflammation, MS, zoster, skull base malformation (eg Chiari). ***MRI*** is stifiable as secondary trigeminal neuralgia is not rare (~14%). ***Drugs:*** **Carba- azepine** (start at 100mg/12h PO; max 400mg/6h; **lamotrigine**; **phenytoin** 200– 00mg/24h PO; or **gabapentin** (p496). If drugs fail, surgery may be necessary. This ay be directed at the peripheral nerve, the trigeminal ganglion or the nerve root. ***licrovascular decompression:*** Anomalous vessels are separated from the trigem- al root. Stereotactic gamma knife surgery can work, but length of pain relief and e time to treatment response are limiting factors. ***Facial pain ΔΔ:*** p60.

eadaches of subacute onset ***Giant cell arteritis:*** p542. *Exclude in all >50yrs old ith a headache that has lasted a few weeks.* Look for tender, thickened, pulseless mporal arteries + ESR >40mm/h (↑CRP may be more sensitive). *Ask about:* Jaw audication during eating. Prompt diagnosis and steroids avoid blindness.

hronic headache ***Tension headache:*** See above.

aised intracranial pressure: Headache is a complaint of ~50% patients. lthough variable, headaches are typically present on waking or may awaken the atient. They may not be severe, and may be worse lying down. If accompanied by her signs of ↑ICP, such as vomiting, papilloedema, epilepsy, progressive focal eurology, or mental change, admit the patient urgently for diagnostic imaging. *LP contra-indicated*. Any space-occupying lesion (neoplasm, abscess, subdural aematoma) may present in this way, as may benign intracranial hypertension.

ledication misuse headache: Culprits are mixed analgesics containing codeine elf-medication), or prescribed opiates, ergotamine and triptans. It is a common eason for episodic headaches becoming daily headache. The culprit must be ithdrawn, and a preventive added (eg tricyclics, valproate, gabapentin, p496).

Migraine

Migraine causes much misery and costs the UK economy >£200 million a yea lost production. Its prevalence is 8%. ♀:♂≈2:1.

Symptoms *Classically:* • Visual (or other) aura lasting 15–30min followed wit 1h by unilateral, throbbing headache. *Or:* • Isolated aura with no headache • E sodic (often premenstrual) severe headaches, often unilateral, with naus vomiting ± photophobia/phonophobia but no aura; may have allodynia—all stir produce pain: 'I can't brush my hair, wear earrings or glasses, or shave, it's so pa ful'—(='*common migraine*'). Signs: none. Tests: none if typical presentation.

Aura Visual chaos (cascading, distortion, 'melting' and jumbling of print lines, d spots, zig-zag fortification spectra); hemianopia, hemiparesis, dysphasia, dysarth ataxia (basilar migraine). Mood or appetite ↑ or ↓, or ↑sensory awareness (eg sound) may occur hours before aura. Duration of aura is ≤1h, and typically bef headache. ***Sensory auras:*** eg paraesthesiae spreading from fingers to face, ***speech auras:*** (8% of auras; eg dysphasia; dysarthria; paraphasia, eg phone substitution). ***Diagnostic criteria if no aura:*** ≥5 headaches lasting 4–72h with eit nausea/vomiting or photophobia/phonophobia *and* ≥2 of: • Unilateral • Pulsat • Interferes with normal life • Worsened by routine activity, eg climbing stair

Pathogenesis Cerebral oligaemia leading to the aura followed by cerebral a extracranial hyperaemia leading to the headache. The underlying cause of vascular abnormalities may be dysfunction in the sensory modulation craniovascular afferents. Attacks are associated with changes in plasma 5HT.

Triggers—eg CHOCOLATE or: Cheese, oral contraceptives, caffeine (or withdrawal), alcohol, anxiety, travel, or exercise. In ~50%, no trigger is found, a in only a few does avoiding triggers prevent *all* attacks.

Associations: Obesity; patent foramen ovale (catheter closure may help).

Differential Cluster or tension headache, cervical spondylosis; ↑BP; intracrar pathology, sinusitis/otitis media, caries. TIAs may mimic migraine aura. Migrain rarely a sign of other pathology: don't look too hard for antiphospholipid syndror arteriovenous malformations, or microemboli (but in some they may be importa

Prophylaxis (eg if frequency > twice a month). If one drug does not work afte months, try another. Most (>65%) will achieve ↓in attack frequency of 50 Comparative trials are wanting—so select according to patient wish and SE prof

- **Pizotifen** 0.5–1mg/8h PO; or 1–3mg PO at night (5HT antagonist). SE: drow weight↑; ↑effects of alcohol; ↑glaucoma risk. Or **propranolol** 40–120mg/12h or **amitriptyline** 25–75mg nocte; SE: drowsiness, dry mouth, blurred vision.
- 2nd-line: **valproate** 400–600mg/12h; NSAIDs; **gabapentin** (p496); **topiramate**.

Treatment Low doses may fail as peristalsis is slow, so try *dispersible* high-dc **aspirin** 900mg/6h PO pc, or **paracetamol** 1g/6h PO 10min after metoclopram (5mg PO, ≤15mg/d; beware extrapyramidal SEs); ***or*** **ketoprofen** 100mg stat PO Studies comparing ergotamine, NSAIDs and triptans are few. In one QALY-bas study, **rizatriptan** was better/cheaper than **sumatriptan** which was better/chea than **Cafergot®** (below). Triptans are $5HT_{1B}/1D$ *agonists*, constricting crar arteries. Rare SEs: arrhythmias or angina ± MI, even if no pre-existing risk. CI: pa MI/IHD, coronary spasm, uncontrolled ↑BP, recent lithium, SSRIs, or ergot use.[1]

Ergotamine (a 5HT agonist, constricting cranial arteries) 1mg PO as headac starts, repeated at ½h, up to 3mg in a day, and 6mg in a week; or, better, as *Cafergot® suppository* (2mg ergotamine + 100mg caffeine up to 2 in 24h; then days without). Emphasize dangers of ergotamine (gangrene, vascular damage). the Pill (*OHCS* p301); peripheral vascular disease/ischaemic disease; pregnan breast-feeding; hemiplegic migraine; Raynaud's; liver or renal impairment; BP↑

1 Of the oral triptans, rizatriptan is said to have quick efficacy; rizatriptan & zolmitriptan are availabl rapid-dissolving wafers. Imigran Recover® may be had 'over the counter'. Almotriptan is similar to sumatriptan, but ?fewer SEs; 12.5mg is an effective, well-tolerated alternative if there is a p response to sumatriptan 50mg. A poor response to one triptan does not predict a poor response to a

igraine questions

hat is going on in migraine? The old theory was vascular: constriction during ıra, with dilatation causing pain. But MRIs during attacks show episodic rebral oedema, dilatation of intracerebral vessels, and ↓water diffusion not specting vascular territories, so the primary event may be neurological.[34]

s migraine due to a hyperexcitable brain? Magnetic studies have shown sting (interictum) hyperexcitability at least in the visual cortex, suggesting a ilure of inhibitory circuits.[35] Cortical hyperexcitability may relate to imbalance etween neuronal inhibition (mediated by GABA, p443) and excitation (via xcitatory amino acids). Putative causes: ↓cerebral Mg^{2+} levels, mitochondrial onormalities, dysfunctions related to ↑nitric oxide, and Ca^{2+} channelopathy.[36]

ow do triptans work? They block transmission from the trigeminal nerve to nd-order neurones in the trigeminal nucleus caudalis,[37] hence use in any process at activates trigeminal fibres, including migraine, cluster headache, SAH, p470.

f prophylaxis fails? Hyperexcitability *may* be reducible by anticonvulsants motrigine (*SE:* 'flu-like symptoms, drowsiness, diplopia, aggression), gabapentin 496), topiramate (*SE:* memory and language problems), tiagabine (*SE:* arrhoea, depression, concentration↓), levetiracetam (*SE:* somnolence; amnesia; ood swings). Patients will ask about these, and we must explain that there are de-effects, and the treatment is experimental. They are also expensive.

olistic care? Migraine often co-exists with other chronic conditions—and the ombined negative impact is immense. ►Don't treat each disease in isolation. ather, attempt to restore a good relationship with the self—and the recovery f the purpose of life. This is the hardest and the most rewarding task. Can ese structured holistic dialogues help? Yes, definitely,[38] so don't be daunted.

or those not wanting drugs, what other/alternative therapies help?

Some people find warm or cold packs to the head help abort attacks.

Spinal manipulation,[39] riboflavin[40] and magnesium may have a role.

Rebreathing into paper bag (raising P_aCO_2) may abort some attacks.[41]

If obese, weight loss makes sense (to ↓extra-ovarian production of oestrogen and estradiol in adipose tissue—but benefit is unproven).[42]

igraine, stroke, and the Pill *(combined oral contraception, coc)* Incidence f migraine + Pill-related ischaemic stroke is 8 : 100,000 if aged 20; and 80 : 00,000 in those aged 40yrs. Low-dose COCs only should be used. Those with igraine with aura are known to be at especial risk, precluding use of combined ills (but no problem with progesterone only or non-hormonal contraception). isk is further augmented by: • Smoking • Age >35yrs • BP↑ • Obesity (body ass index >30) • Diabetes mellitus • Hyperlipidaemia • Family history of rteriopathy when aged <45yrs. Warn women with migraine to stop Pills at nce if they develop aura or worsening migraine—see *OHCS* p301.

If the problem is migraine without aura in the pill-free interval consider: Alternative contraception method or a pill with a lower dose of the same rogestogen or lowest available dose of a different progestogen. • Tri-cycling: ake the pill continuously for 3 packets (9 weeks) followed by a 7 day pill-free terval, so that the number of menstrual bleeds is reduced. • Oestrogen upplements (below) from 3 days before menses, continuing for 7 days.

eri-menstrual migraine *Prophylaxis:* If no asthma, CCF, peptic ulcer etc, NSAID eg mefenamic acid) at onset of menses to last day of bleeding ± transdermal estradiol 50–100µg patches 3 days before menses, continue for 7 days. Prodigy guidance

regnancy Be optimistic: migraine often improves; if not, get help. *Prophylaxis:* top (or go on to amitriptyline). *1st choice anti-emetic:* **cyclizine** or **promethazine**. *nalgesia:* if **paracetamol** is insufficient, try partial agonist opioids eg if attacks ersist in the 2nd and 3rd trimesters (uncommon).[43] **Ibuprofen** (or **aspirin**) may be sed, up to 30 weeks' gestation. Don't use aspirin if breastfeeding. Prodigy guidance

Blackouts

History It is vital to establish exactly what patients mean by 'blackout'. Do th mean loss of consciousness (LOC)? a fall to the ground without loss consciousness? a clouding of vision, diplopia, or vertigo? Take a detailed histo from the patient *and* a witness (see BOX).

Vasovagal (neurocardiogenic) syncope Provoked by emotion, pain, fear standing too long and due to reflex bradycardia ± peripheral vasodilatation. Ons is over seconds (*not* instantaneous), and is often preceded by nausea, pall sweating. and closing in of visual fields (pre-syncope). It cannot occur if lyi down. The patient falls to the ground, being unconscious for ~2min. Incontinence urine is rare. Brief jerking of the limbs is uncommon, but there is no tonic → clor sequence. After an attack there is no prolonged confusion or amnesia.

Situation syncope ***Cough syncope:*** Weakness + LOC after a paroxysm of coughir

Effort syncope: Syncope on exercise; cardiac origin, eg aortic stenosis, HOCM.

Micturition syncope: Mostly men, at night.

Carotid sinus syncope: Carotid sinus hypersensitivity (on head-turning or shavin

Epilepsy presenting as blackout is most likely to be *grand mal* (LOC) or compl partial (impairment of consciousness). See p482. Attacks vary with the type seizure, but some features suggest epilepsy as a cause of blackout: attacks wh asleep or lying down; aura; identifiable precipitants, eg TV; altered breathir cyanosis; typical movements; urinary and faecal incontinence; tongue-bitir particularly the side of the tongue, is virtually diagnostic; post-attack drowsine or coma; amnesia; residual paralysis for <24h.

Stokes–Adams attacks Transient arrhythmias (eg bradycardia due to comple heart block) causing ↓cardiac output and LOC. The patient falls to the ground (oft with *no* warning except palpitation), pale, with a slow or absent pulse. Recovery in seconds, the patient flushes, the pulse speeds up, and consciousness is regaine Injury is typical of these intermittent arrhythmias. A few clonic jerks may occur an attack is prolonged. Attacks may happen several times a day and in any postu

Other causes ***Hypoglycaemia:*** Tremor, hunger, and perspiration herald ligh headedness or LOC; rare in non-diabetics but see p198. ***Orthostatic hypotensio*** Unsteadiness or LOC on standing from lying in those with inadequate vasomot reflexes: the elderly; autonomic neuropathy (p494); antihypertensive medicatio overdiuresis; multi-system atrophy (MSA). ►TIAs rarely cause blackouts.

Drop attacks Sudden weakness of the legs causes the patient, usually an old woman, to fall to the ground. There is no warning, no LOC and no confusi afterwards. The condition is benign, resolving spontaneously after a number attacks. Drop attacks also occur in hydrocephalus; these patients, however, m not be able to get up for hours.

Other causes ***Anxiety:*** Hyperventilation, tremor, sweating, tachycardi paraesthesiae, light-headedness, and no LOC suggest a panic attack. ***Factitio blackouts*** (Münchausen's, p698). ***Choking:*** If a large piece of food blocks t larynx, the patient may collapse, turn blue, and be unable to speak. Do the Heimli manoeuvre immediately to eject the food.

Examination Cardiovascular, neurological. BP lying and standing.

Tests Investigate unless obvious syncope. ECG;[1] 24h (or longer) ECG (arrhythmia, lo Q–T, eg Romano–Ward, p82), U&E, FBC, glucose. Perhaps tilt-table tests; EEG, slee EEG, echocardiogram, CT/MRI; HUT.[2] P_aCO_2↓ in attacks suggests hyperventilation the cause. ►*While the cause is being elucidated, advise against driving.*

1 Consider elevating V1–V3 leads from 4th to the 2nd intercostal space to reveal saddle-shaped ST elevatio telltale sign of **Brugada syndrome** (p687)—an autosomal SCN5A channelopathy predisposing to VT.
2 **Head-up tilt (HUT) tests** distinguish vasodepressor from cardio-inhibitory syncope. HUT is +ve symptoms are associated with a BP drop >30mmHg (vasodepressor; consider β-blockers to count ↑sympathetic activity)—or bradycardia (cardio-inhibitory; consider pacing).

Taking a history of blackouts

If a series of attacks, ask a witness: During a typical attack...

- Does the patient lose consciousness?
- Does the patient injure himself?
- Does the patient move? Floppy or stiff (suggests epilepsy)? NB: not everything that twitches is epilepsy. Ask for exact details of movements.
- Is there incontinence? (irrelevant if urine, but faeces suggests epilepsy).
- Is the complexion changed? (White or red suggests arrhythmia, but may occur in temporal lobe epilepsy).
- Does the patient bite the side of his tongue? (strongly suggests epilepsy).
- What is the patient's pulse like? (abnormalities suggest a CVS cause).
- Are there associated symptoms (palpitations, chest pain, dyspnoea)?
- How long does the attack last?
- Is the patient sleepy before an attack (narcolepsy, p692).

Before the attack:

- Is there any warning?—eg typical epileptic aura or pre-syncope (above).
- In what circumstances do attacks occur? (if watching TV, it is epilepsy).
- Can the patient prevent attacks?

After the attack:

- How much does the patient remember about the attack afterwards?
- Muscle pain afterwards suggests a tonic/clonic seizure.
- Is the patient confused or sleepy (post-ictal; narcolepsy)?

Background to attacks: Getting more frequent? Is anyone else in the family getting them? Sudden arrhythmic death[1] may leave no cardiac trace at *post mortem*, or there may be hereditary cardiomyopathy.

►Witnesses often give conflicting accounts: the most reliable may not be the one with the most medical knowledge. He or she may know what you expect to hear, and furnish you with extra (imagined) material.

Dizziness and vertigo

Complaints of 'dizzy spells' are very common and are used by patients to describ many different sensations. The key to diagnosis is to find out exactly what th patient means by 'dizzy' and then decide whether or not this represents vertigo.

Is this vertigo? ***Definition:*** An illusion of movement, often rotatory, of the patient or his surroundings. In practice, straightforward 'spinning' is rare—the floor may tilt, sink, or rise or 'I veer sideways on walking as if pulled to one side by a magnet'. Vertigo is always worsened by movement. ***Associated symptoms:*** Difficulty walking or standing; relief on lying or sitting still; nausea; vomiting; pallor; sweating. Attacks may even cause patients to fall suddenly to the ground. Associated hearing loss or tinnitus implies labyrinth or 8th nerve involvement. ***What is not vertigo:*** Faintness may be described as dizziness but is often due to anxiety with associated palpitations, tremor, and sweating. Anaemia can cause light-headedness as can orthostatic hypotension or effort in an emphysematous patient. But in all of these there is no illusion of movement or typical associated symptoms. Loss of consciousness during attacks should prompt thoughts of epilepsy or syncope rather than vertigo.

Causes of vertigo

Vestibular end-organ and vestibular nerve
- Ménière's disease
- Vestibular neuronitis (ie acute labyrinthitis)
- Benign positional vertigo (*OHCS* p554)
- Motion sickness
- Trauma
- Ototoxic aminoglycoside
- Zoster (ie Ramsay Hun syndrome, *OHCS* p652)

Brainstem, cerebellum, cerebello-pontine angle (Look for nystagmus and cranial nerve lesions)
- MS
- Infarction/TIA
- Haemorrhage
- Migraine (very rarely)
- Acoustic neuroma

Cerebral cortex
- Vertiginous epilepsy

Alcohol intoxication

Causes Disorders of the labyrinth, vestibular nerve, vestibular nuclei, or their central connections are responsible for practically all vertigo. Only rarely are other structures implicated (BOX

Labyrinthine vertigo ***Benign positional vertigo*** is due to canalolithiasis—mobil particles in the semicircular canal cause inappropriate endolymph flow on hea movement. It is curable by Epley manoeuvres (to reposition particles, *OHCS* p554

Vestibular nerve Damage in the petrous temporal bone or cerebello-pontine angl often involves the auditory nerve, causing deafness or tinnitus. Causes: trauma an vestibular schwannomas (acoustic neuromas).

Ménière's disease: Recurrent attacks of **vertigo** (eg lasting >20min ± nausea/vom iting), fluctuating sensorineural **hearing loss** (may become permanent), an **tinnitus** (or a sense of aural fullness) caused by endolymphatic hydrops. Dro attacks may rarely feature (no loss of consciousness or vertigo, but sudden fallin to one side). ℞: Acute attacks—bed rest and reassurance. An antihistamine (e cinnarizine) is useful if prolonged. Consider endolymphatic sac surgery or ablatio of the vestibular organ with gentamicin in very severe disease. Prophylaxis: low salt diets and diuretics may be tried—but there is no good evidence of efficac There is no evidence that tinnitus or deafness is alleviated or prevented b betahistine, diuretics, trimetazidine, or lithium. prodidgy +cochrane

Ototoxicity: (eg from aminoglycosides) may also cause vertigo and deafness.

Acoustic neuromas usually present with hearing loss, vertigo coming only late With progression, ipsilateral cranial nerves V, VI, IX, and X may be affected (als ipsilateral cerebellar signs). Paradoxically, there is rarely VII nerve involvement pre operatively. Signs of ↑ICP occur late, and indicate a large tumour.

They account for 80% of cerebello-pontine angle tumours (ΔΔ meningioma). Commoner in ♀; also in neurofibromatosis (esp. NF2, p506). Not all need removing

Acute labyrinthitis (vestibular neuronitis): Abrupt onset of severe vertig nausea/vomiting ± prostration. No deafness or tinnitus. Cause: virus; vascular lesio Severe vertigo subsides in days, complete recovery takes 3–4wks. Reassure. Sedat

Herpes zoster: Herpetic eruption of the external auditory meatus; facia palsy ± deafness, tinnitus, and vertigo (Ramsay Hunt syndrome).

Hearing loss

►See OHCS p550 for management

One reasonable bedside method to establish hearing loss is to whisper numbers increasingly loudly in one ear while blocking the other ear with a finger. Ask your patient to repeat the number. Make sure that failure is not from misunderstanding.

Tuning fork tests No single test is diagnostic but tuning fork tests do give useful information (also popular in exams). ***Rinne:*** Use a 512–256Hz tuning fork; strike it ⅓ from its free end on your patella and hold it so that the 2 prongs and the meatus lie on the same line (air conduction, AC). Then place the vibrating stem on the mastoid for bone conduction (BC). Ask: "which is louder?" ***Rinne negative:*** BC > AC. This occurs with conductive deafness >20dB (or with severe sensorineural hearing loss (SNHL)—ie a false –ve Rinne: the cochlea of the other ear picks up the sound by bone conduction—use of a Barany noise box to mask the other ear during the test prevents this). ***Rinne positive:*** AC > BC. Remember 'SNAC—rip': in sensorineural loss and normal ears, air conduction is better—and means Rinne positive.

Weber tuning fork test With the tuning fork on the vertex, forehead or upper incisors(!), ask the patient which ear the sound is heard in. Sound localizes to the affected ear with conductive loss (>10dB loss), to the contralateral ear in SNHL and to the midline if both ears are normal (or if bilateral sensorineural loss).

Conductive deafness Causes: wax (remove eg by syringing with warm water after softening with olive oil drops) or otosclerosis, otitis media, glue ear (*OHCS* p546).

Chronic sensorineural deafness Often due to accumulated environmental noise toxicity, ie presby(a)cusis or inherited disorders.

Sudden sensorineural deafness ►Refer promptly. Causes: noise exposure, gentamicin or other toxin; mumps; acoustic neuroma; MS; stroke; vasculitis; TB. Do ESR; FBC; LFT; viral titres; audiologist; evoked response audiometry ± CXR; Mantoux, MRI; pANCA; lymph node & nasopharyngeal biopsy for malignancy and TB culture.

Presbyacusis Loss of acuity for high-frequency sounds starts before 30yrs old. We do not usually notice it until hearing of speech is affected. Hearing is most affected in the presence of background noise. Hearing aids are the usual treatment.

Tinnitus

(See OHCS p552)

This is ringing/buzzing in the ears; it is common and may cause depression ± insomnia.

Causes Focal hyper-excitability in the auditory cortex (?the cause of common tinnitus);[45] hearing loss (20%); wax; viral; presbyacusis; noise (eg gunfire); head injury; septic otitis media; post-stapedectomy; Ménière's; head injury; anaemia; BP↑ (in up to 16%; it may not be causative).[46] ***Drugs:*** Aspirin; loop diuretics; aminoglycosides (eg gentamicin). ***Psychological associations:*** Redundancy, divorce, retirement. ♂:♀≈1:1. ►Investigate unilateral tinnitus fully to exclude a vestibular schwannoma (acoustic neuroma, p454). ***Mean age at onset:*** 40–50yrs.

Causes of pulsatile tinnitus: (eg audible with stethoscope; do MRI) Carotid artery stenosis/dissection;[47] AV fistulae; glomus jugulare tumours, *OHCS* p552.

Treatment Psychological support is very important (eg from a hearing therapist). Exclude serious causes; reassure that tinnitus does not mean madness or serious disease and that it often improves in time. **Cognitive therapy** helps, as does 'tinnitus coping training'. Patient support groups can help greatly.[48] **Drugs** are disappointing. Avoid tranquillizers, particularly if depressed (use tricyclic antidepressants here, eg amitriptyline[49] or nortriptyline).[50] Hypnotics at night may help. Carbamazepine is disappointing; if Ménière's disease is the cause, betahistine helps only a few. **Masking** may give relief. White noise (like an off-tuned radio) is given via a noise generator worn like a post-aural hearing aid. **Hearing aids** may help by amplifying desirable sounds. **Cochlear nerve section** can relieve disabling tinnitus in 25% (at the expense of deafness). Repetitive **focal transcranial magnetic stimulation** of the auditory cortex can help (a novel and non-standard therapy).[51]

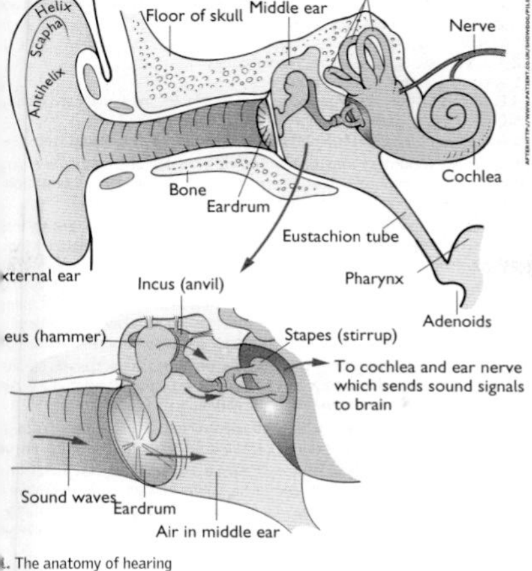

1. The anatomy of hearing

Weak legs and cord compression

Cord compression typically presents with weak legs. There are many cau weak legs (see BOX) but only 5 cardinal questions:

1 Was the onset gradual or sudden?
2 At what rate is the weakness progressing?
3 Are the legs spastic or flaccid?
4 Is there sensory loss?[1] A sensory level usually means spinal cord diseas
5 Is there loss of sphincter control (bowels, bladder)?
6 Any signs of infection (spine tenderness, WCC↑, eg in extradural absces

Progressive weakness *Rapidly progressing cord compression is an emer* Hours make a difference: untreated, irreversible loss of power and sensation the lesion's level, and a neurogenic bladder and bowel may ensue.

Symptoms: Spinal or root pain[1] may precede leg weakness and sensory los weakness is often less severe (suggests a cervical cord lesion). Bladder (anc sphincter involvement is late and manifests as hesitancy, frequency, and, la painless retention. ***Signs:*** Look for a motor, reflex, and sensory level, with r findings *above* the level of the lesion, LMN signs *at* the level (p439, especi cervical cord compression, see p500)—and UMN signs *below* the level; rem tone and reflexes are ↓ in acute cord compression (spinal shock, *OHCS* p76

Causes Secondary malignancy (breast, lung, prostate) in the spine is comm Rarer: Infection (epidural abscess), cervical disc prolapse, haematoma (war intrinsic cord tumour, atlanto–axial subluxation.

ΔΔ Transverse myelitis; MS; carcinomatous meningitis; Guillain–Barré (p694 vasculitis (PAN, syphilis); spinal artery thrombosis, trauma; dissecting aneu

Tests Do not delay imaging at any cost. Speed of imaging should parallel th of clinical progression. Spinal x-rays can be helpful, but MRI is the definitive i Biopsy or surgical exploration may be needed to identify the nature of any ***Screening blood tests:*** FBC, ESR, B_{12}, folate, syphilis serology, U&E, LFT, PSA CXR (primary lung malignancy, lung secondaries, TB).

Treatment If malignancy, give dexamethasone IV 4mg/6h while considering specific therapy, eg radiotherapy or chemotherapy ± decompressive laminec which is most appropriate depends on tumour type, quality of life, and prognosis. Epidural abscesses must be surgically decompressed and antibiotics

Cauda equina and conus medullaris lesions The big difference between lesions and those high up in the cord is that leg weakness is flaccid and are not spastic and hyperreflexic. ***Causes:*** As above plus congenital lumba disease; lumbosacral nerve lesions. ***Clinical features:*** Conus medullaris l show early urinary retention and constipation, back pain, sacral se disturbance, erectile dysfunction ± leg weakness. Cauda equina lesions fe back pain and radicular pain down the legs; asymmetrical, atrophic, are paralysis of the legs; sensory loss in a root distribution—and ↓sphincter pow

Paralysed patients need especial care Avoid pressure sores by turning. R weight-bearing areas often. Avoid thrombosis in paralysed limbs by fre passive movement and pressure stockings ± low molecular weight heparin (p Bladder care is vital; catheterization is only one option. Do not control inconti by decreasing fluid intake (*OHCS* p774). Bowel evacuation may be manual or by suppositories. Increasing dietary fibre intake may help. Exercise of unaffec partially paralysed limbs is important to avoid unnecessary loss of functior

1 *Nerve root sensations* may be sharp or dull (like angina if T3–T4 affected) or 'warm glow if icy bandages were wrapped round my leg' or rubbed with sandpaper, or sprayed with hot *Dorsal column damage* may cause hypersensitivity or vibratory feelings, as if on the deck c under full power, or the limbs may feel twice their normal size.
Spinothalamic symptoms may be 'as if my bones burned, and the flesh was torn away'.

er causes of leg weakness

hronic spastic paraparesis MS; intrinsic cord tumours (astrocytomas; pendymomas; haemangioblastomas; metastases, eg from melanoma, lung umours, etc.) syringomyelia; MND p498: subacute combined degeneration of ne cord (B_{12} deficiency, p320); syphilis; rare non-neoplastic lesions—eg istiocytosis X; schistosomiasis; other parasites (any eosinophilia?).

hronic flaccid paraparesis Tabes dorsalis; peripheral neuropathies (p496); nyopathies (rare; arms are usually involved too, see p502).

nilateral foot drop DM; stroke; prolapsed disc; MS; common peroneal nerve alsy.

Veak legs with no sensory loss MND; parasagittal meningioma (the rare xception to the 'rule' that weak legs mean cord or more distal problems).

bsent knee jerks and extensor plantars eg from combined cervical and umbar disc disease or a 'MAST': motor neurone disease, Friedreich's ataxia; ubacute combined degeneration of the cord (but knee jerks more often brisk); aboparesis (syphilis, p419).

ecific gait disorders

en the best professionals have to employ extraordinary tactics simply to *cribe* gaits accurately,[1] never mind *diagnose* them accurately.)

pastic: Stiff, circumduction of legs ± scuffing of the foot.

xtrapyramidal: Flexed posture, shuffling feet, slow to start, postural nstability. *Example*: Parkinson's disease.

praxic: Pathognomonic '**glueing-to-the-floor**' on attempting walking OTM3 3970 r a wide-based unsteady gait with a tendency to fall. Causes: normal ressure hydrocephalus; multi-infarct states.

taxic: Wide-based; falls; cannot walk heel-to-toe. May be caused by erebellar lesions (eg MS; posterior fossa tumours; alcohol; phenytoin toxicity) r by proprioceptive sensory loss (eg sensory neuropathies; subacute combined degeneration of the cord). Often worse in the dark, or with eyes closed.

Myopathic: Waddle (hip girdle weakness). Cannot climb steps.

sychogenic: Often a bizarre gait not conforming to any pattern of organic gait disturbance. Suspect if there is profound gait disturbance with inability even to stand, without any signs when examined on the couch ('astasia abasia')—but this may occur with midline cerebellar lesions, normal pressure hydrocephalus, and other rare tumours. Video analysis reveals 6 signs of psychogenicity, seen in 97% of patients in one study:

- Fluctuations in response to suggestion or distraction.
- Excessive hesitation of locomotion incompatible with CNS disease.
- 'Psychogenic' Romberg test with building-up of sway amplitudes.
- Uneconomic postures wasting muscular energy.
- 'Walking on ice' gait, ie small cautious steps, with ankle joints fixed.
- Sudden buckling of the knees, usually without falls.

sts Spinal X-rays. MRI; FBC, ESR, syphilis serology, serum B_{12}, U&E, LFT, PSA rostate cancer), serum electrophoresis (myeloma); CXR (TB, Ca bronchus); LP 756); EMG; muscle biopsy; sural nerve biopsy.

nda her brella mid piddle med puddle she ninnygoes nannygoes nancing by. James Joyce *Finnegans Wake*

Abnormal involuntary movements (dyskinesia

Movement disorders—ie ataxia, dystonic disorders, gait disorders (p Huntington disease (p694), myoclonus, parkinsonism, spasticity, tardive dyski tics and tremor—are clinically and pathologically heterogeneous and characterized by impairment of the planning, control or execution of movem

Tremor Note frequency, amplitude, and exacerbating factors (stress; fatigue). ***tremor*** is tremor abolished on voluntary movement. Cause: parkinsonism (p ***Intention tremor*** is irregular, large-amplitude, and worse at the end of purp acts, eg pressing a remote control. It suggests cerebellar disease, eg MS, st ***Postural tremor*** is absent at rest, present on maintained posture (arms outstret and may persist (but is not exaggerated) on movement. *Causes:* Benign ess tremor (autosomal dominant; helped by alcohol); thyrotoxicosis; anxiety; β agonis salbutamol). ***Re-emergent tremor*** is a postural tremor developing after a of ~10sec (eg in Parkinson's). Surgery/deep brain stimulation (DBS, below) some tremors.

Chorea, athetosis, and hemiballismus ***Chorea:***[1] Non-rhythmic, jerky, purpos movements flitting from one place to another—eg facial grimacing, raisin shoulders and flexing and extending the fingers. Causes: Huntington's or Sy ham's chorea (choreoathetoid movements; a rare complication of strep infect The anatomical basis of chorea is uncertain but it may be the pharmacolo mirror image of Parkinson's disease (L-dopa worsens chorea). ***Hemiballis*** Large-amplitude, flinging hemichorea (affects proximal muscles) contralatera vascular lesion of the subthalamic nucleus (often elderly diabetics). Rec spontaneously over months. ***Athetosis:*** Slow, sinuous, confluent, purpos movements (esp. digits, hands, face, tongue), often difficult to distinguish chorea. Commonest cause is cerebral palsy (*OHCS* p214). Most other patterns described as 'athetoid' may now be better characterized as one of the dysto

Tics Brief, repeated, stereotyped movements which patients may suppress while. Tics are common in children (and usually resolve). In *Tourette's synd* (p692), motor and vocal tics occur. Consider psychological support, clonazepa clonidine if tics are severe (haloperidol may help but risks tardive dyskinesia

Myoclonus Sudden involuntary focal or general jerks arising from cord, brainste cerebral cortex, seen in metabolic problems (eg renal failure), neurodegenerative di (eg lysosomal storage enzyme defects), CJD (p688), and myoclonic epilepsies (inf spasms). ***Benign essential myoclonus:*** General myoclonus begins in childho muscle twitches (eg autosomal dominant and has no other consequences). ***Aste ('metabolic flap'):*** Jerking (~1–2 jerks/sec) of outstretched hands, worse with w extended, from loss of extensor tone. ***Causes:*** liver or kidney failure; hyponatra thalamic stroke. ***Rx:*** Myoclonus may respond to valproate, clonazepam, or piracet

Tardive syndromes Tardive means after *chronic* exposure to dopamine rece blockers (eg antipsychotics, antiemetics). Tardive syndromes are a source of n distress and disability, and may be permanent, despite discontinuing all d ***Classification:*** • Tardive dyskinesia (orobuccolingual, truncal, or chorei movements, eg vacuous chewing and grimacing movements) • Tardive dyst (sustained, stereotyped muscle spasms of a twisting or turning character retrocollis and back arching/opisthotonic posturing • Tardive akathisia (unplea inner sense of restlessness or unease ± repetitive, purposeless movem (stereotypies; eg pacing) • Tardive myoclonus • Tardive tourettism (p692) • Ta tremor (may respond to donepezil). ***Treating tardive dyskinesia:*** Get Gradually withdraw neuroleptics and wait 3–6 months. If still a problem, cons tetrabenazine 12.5–50mg/8h PO. Quetiapine and olanzapine are exampl atypical antipsychotics that are less likely to cause tardive syndromes.

1 Paracelsus used the term chorea to describe the jerking movements of medieval pilgrims traveli the healing shrine of St. Vitus—reflecting the ancient Greek round dance accompanied by singing (chorus; choreography). He recognized 3 types: chorea arising from the imagination (chorea imagina or from sexual desire (chorea lasciva)—and chorea arising from corporeal causes (chorea natural

stonia

tonia entails prolonged muscle contraction causing abnormal posture or etitive movements due to many causes. Verbatim example of dystonic nptoms (writer's cramp, in this example): 'I cannot, for example, draw the rument [pen, pencil] toward me in a circular motion, eg the left arc of a le, or the letter O. If I force the move, the movements become jerky and I all smoothness in the character. The same thing will happen when eating trying to use a fork...I end up moving my mouth to the fork...instead of ving my hand to my mouth—awkward."[63]

ystonic disorders can be classified by **age of onset** (<12yrs old is childhood et, 13–20yrs is adolescent onset, and >20yrs is adult)—or by **part of body** ected, or by **cause**. Childhood onset suggests **idiopathic generalized tonia**, which often starts with dystonia in one leg, spreading to that side of body over 5–10yrs. Autosomal dominant inheritance is common (gene tests en show a deletion in DTY1). Treatment is challenging; exclude Wilson's disease dopa-responding dystonia (needs an L-dopa trial). High-dose trihexyphenidyl enzhexol, an anticholinergic) and deep-brain stimulation may help.[64]

ystonia may be confined to one part of the body—ie a **focal dystonia**, eg smodic torticollis (head pulled to one side), blepharospasm (*OHCS* p460; ie oluntary contraction of orbicularis oculi), **writers cramp** (see below). Focal tonias in adults are typically idiopathic, and they rarely generalize. They are rsened by stress; patients may develop a 'geste antagonistique' to try to st the dystonic posturing (eg a touch of the finger to the jaw in spasmodic ticollis).[65] Effective control of focal dystonia by botulinum toxin injections into overactive muscles (*OHCS* p460) is usually possible, but there may be SEs.[66]

Acute dystonia may occur in young men starting neuroleptics (head pulled k, eyes drawn upward, trismus). Use anticholinergics (benzatropine 1–2mg IV).

Writer's cramp (scrivener's palsy; graphospasm) When trying to write, the is driven into the paper and flow of movement is poor. "I would look at [my gers] and tell them to do one thing, and they would do jagged things instead, have full muscle control for everything—except putting a pen to a piece of er."[67] Look for hand and forearm spasm ± dystonic arm posture ± focal nor/myoclonus ± dominant hand muscle hypertrophy.[68] Association: obsessive npulsive disorder.[69] ***EMG:*** May correlate with the chief physiological events: ciprocal inhibition of wrist flexor motor neurones at rest, and ↑co-traction of antagonist muscles of the forearm during voluntary activity.[70] : Abnormal motor command (sensorimotor region β rhythm).[71] ***℞:*** β-blockers valproate often fail. Breath-holding or arm cooling may work, as may ulinum and EMG biofeedback.[72]

Stroke: clinical features and investigations

Strokes result from ischaemic infarction or bleeding into part of the brain, manif
rapid onset (over minutes) of focal CNS signs and symptoms. It is the major n
logical disease of our times (1.5/1000/yr, rising with age to 10/1000/yr at 7
Causes: • Thrombosis-*in-situ* or heart emboli (AF; endocarditis; MI—see BO
• Atherothromboembolism (eg from carotids)
• CNS bleeds (BP↑; trauma; aneurysm rupture)
• Failure of cerebral autoregulation of blood flow.[1]

Rare causes: Sudden BP drop by ≥40mmHg; vasculitis (p542); venous thrombosis (p472). ***In young patients suspect:*** Thrombophilia (p358); vasc subarachnoid haemorrhage; venous-sinus thrombosis (p472); carotid a dissection (spontaneous or from neck trauma or fibromuscular dysplasia).
►Do not hesitate to get a neurology, cardiology, or haematology opinion.

Risk factors BP↑, smoking, DM; heart disease (valvular, ischaemic, AF), perip vascular disease, past TIA, ↑PCV, carotid bruit, the Pill, lipids↑ (p682, statins by ~17%); alcoholism; clotting↑ (eg ↑plasma fibrinogen, ↓antithrombin III, p

Signs Sudden onset, or a step-wise progression over hours (rarely days) is ty In theory, focal signs relate to distribution of the affected artery (p440 collateral supplies cloud the issue. ***Cerebral hemisphere infarcts*** (50%) c contralateral hemiplegia—initially flaccid (floppy limb, falls like a dead w when lifted), then becomes spastic (UMN); contralateral sensory loss; homony hemianopia; dysphasia; visuo-spatial deficit (depending on site). ***Brain infarction*** (25%): wide range of effects which include quadriplegia, disturba of gaze and vision, locked-in syndrome (aware, but unable to respond). ***Lac infarcts*** (25%): small infarcts around basal ganglia, internal capsule, thalamus pons.[2] May cause pure motor, pure sensory, mixed motor and sensory sigr ataxia; intact cognition/consciousness.

Tests Prompt investigation to confirm diagnosis and avoid further stroke consider whether results will affect management. Look for:
- ***Hypertension:*** Look for retinopathy (p544) and a big heart on CXR. NB: ac raised BP is common in early stroke. In general, don't treat (p464).
- ***Cardiac source of emboli: Atrial fibrillation (AF):*** (p116) Emboli from th atrium may have caused the stroke. Look for a big left atrium (CXR; echo). ***MI:*** Mural thrombus is best seen by echocardiography. In stroke from AF or r thrombus do CT to exclude a haemorrhagic stroke, then start aspirin; wait be commencing full anticoagulation to avoid bleeds into infarcts. ***SBE/IE:*** (p 20% of those with endocarditis present with CNS signs due to septic emboli valves. Treat as endocarditis; ask a cardiologist's opinion.
- ***Carotid artery stenosis:*** In carotid territory (p441) TIA/small stroke, 2 trials show clear benefit of carotid surgery, so expert bodies say that ≥8 stenoses (on Doppler) merit referral for consideration of surgery in fit patier
- ***Hypoglycaemia, hyperglycaemia,*** and ***hyperlipidaemia***.
- ***Giant cell arteritis*** (p542) eg if ESR↑, or story of headache or tender scalp necessarily temporal). Give steroids promptly (p542).
- ***Syphilis:*** Look for active, untreated disease (p419).
- ***Thrombocytopenia*** and other bleeding disorders. • ***Polycythaemia*** (p35

Tests to exclude preventable causes of stroke		
Pulse and BP	FBC, platelets	Sickling tests, eg in Black
CXR + CT of head	ESR	Blood glucose
ECG	U&E	Syphilis serology if releva
Carotid Doppler	Lipids	Endocarditis tests (p136
Then consider echocardiography, carotid angiography & clotting		

1 This may explain stroke's association with morning arousal, stress, activity & winter (2006 da
2 Pontine stroke causes quadriplegia & small pupils ± coma; prognosis: poor.
3 '70%' or '80%' depends on perioperative stroke rate (2005 data); stenting may also be an optio

liac causes of stroke

ioembolic causes are the source of stroke in >30% of patients in population ies. These may recur, unless you prevent them.

examine the heart with as much attention as you examine the brain.

nvalvular atrial fibrillation is associated with an overall risk of stroke of 5% per year. Advancing age, prior stroke/TIA, diabetes and hypertension are ditive risks. Ischaemic strokes in AF are often worse than ischaemic stroke th sinus rhythm. Warfarin is effective for primary and secondary prevention ischaemic stroke, reducing ↓risk by 68%. Aspirin alone is adequate when ere are few or no additional risk factors. It is safer and needs no onitoring. Explain risks and benefits of warfarin, and let the patient decide, ving an evidence-based steer towards warfarin if there are additional risk ctors—provided there are no contra-indications (falls, poor compliance/ ncordance). If warfarin is chosen, aim for an INR of 2.5–3.5 (stroke risk is vice as much for those with an INR of 1.7 as opposed to 2). Adding aspirin to arfarin does not confer additional protection.

ternal cardioversion is complicated in 1–3% by peripheral emboli: armacological cardioversion may carry similar risks.

osthetic valves risk major emboli; anticoagulate (INR 3.5–4.5, p335).

cute myocardial infarct with large left ventricular wall motion abnormalities echocardiography predispose to left ventricular thrombus. Emboli arise in 0% of these patients in the next 6–12 months; risk being reduced by two- irds by warfarin anticoagulation.

aradoxical systemic emboli via the venous circulation in those with patent ramen ovale, atrial and ventricular septal defects can occur.

ardiac surgery, eg bypass graft, carries particular risk (0.9–5.2%).

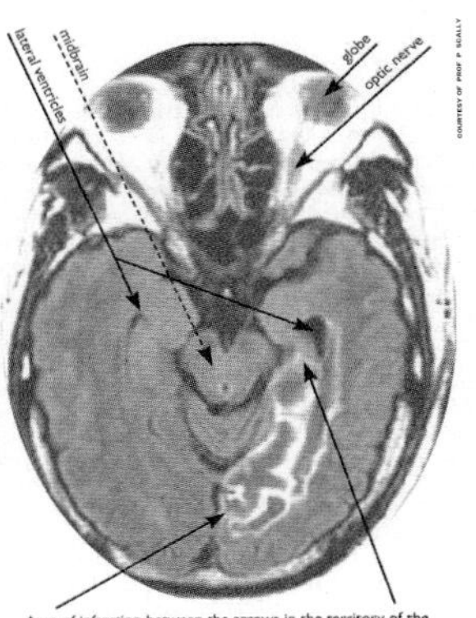

Area of infarction between the arrows in the territory of the posterior cerebral artery

Fig 1. MRI scan after a stroke (courtesy Prof P Scally)

Stroke: management and prevention

Imaging (p732) Prompt CT/MRI should now be the rule especially if:
- Unexpected deterioration after the first 24h.
- There are unusual features, or diagnosis remains unclear—eg onset slow known. Consider especially cerebral tumour and subdural haematoma.
- To distinguish between haemorrhage and ischaemic infarction (do scan w few days of stroke), eg if considering later anticoagulation.
- Cerebellar stroke—cerebellar haematomas may need urgent surgery.

ΔΔ CNS tumour; subdural bleed (p474); Todd's palsy (p704); migraine; hy caemia; overdose if comatose. Ischaemic and haemorrhagic stroke are *not* re distinguishable clinically but pointers to haemorrhage are: meningism, s headache, and coma within hours. Ischaemic pointers: carotid bruit, AF, pas

℞ (See p462 & p466.) Explain what has happened. ►*Communicate fully with patient, relatives and carers* over difficult decisions, eg deciding on the kindest level of intervention taking into account quality of life, coexisting conditions, and prognosis. Admission to stroke units for nursing/physio saves lives, and is a great motivator. 'Nil by mouth' if swallowing is a problem (try 1mL of water on a teaspoon first).

Emergency manage
⏩Ensure patent airw
⏩Ensure hydration
⏩Prevent hypoxia/asp
⏩Diagnose & treat fe
⏩Treat any hypergly mia or hypoglycaem
⏩Skilled nursing to pr ent pressure sores (

- Keep hydrated; don't overhydrate (cerebral oedema).
- Turn regularly and keep dry (consider catheter) to stop bed sores (fig 1).
- Monitor BP; but treating even very high levels may harm (unless th encephalopathy, or aortic dissection): even a 20% fall may impair ce perfusion, as autoregulation is impaired. NB: if on HRT—stop it.
- If cerebellar haemorrhage possible, immediate referral for evacuation m needed (familiarize yourself with local current management).

Acute antiplatelet measures: Unless you strongly suspect CNS bleeding, give aspirin 300mg/24h for 2wks, then 75mg/day. If CT confirms ischaemia, advice (2nd European stroke Prevention Study) is that dipyridamole be added (eg as Assantin Reta bd, aspirin 25mg + dipyridamole MR 200mg/tablet). If aspirin-intolerant, ad p198; if aspirin-hypersensitive, substitute clopidogrel (p468).

Mortality 60,000/yr;[uk] 20% at 1 month, then ≤10%/yr. **Full recovery** ≤40%; c siness≈poor prognosis. **Sequelae** Pneumonia; depression; contractures; cons ion; bed sores; 'I'm a prisoner in my body'; stress in spouse (eg alcoholism), p

Prevention ***Primary (ie before a stroke):*** Control risk factors (p462: BP,[1] smo DM, lipids, and, possibly folate[2]); exercise helps (HDL↑; glucose tolerance↑). *Hel smoking:* ►p79. In middle-aged men (esp. if ↑BP), quitting ↓risk of stroke, benefits seen in ≤5yrs. (Switching to pipes or cigars achieves little; former h smokers retain some excess risk.) ***Lifelong anticoagulants*** if rheumat prosthetic heart valves on left side. Consider warfarin in chronic non-rheuma especially if there are risk factors for vascular disease. Prevention post-TIA (p ***Secondary (ie preventing further strokes):*** Control risk factors. Several studies suggest considerable advantages from lowering BP and cholesterol (e not particularly raised). Aspirin (p468) or warfarin if an embolic stroke, chronic AF (p130). **NB:** Combining aspirin with twice-daily modified-releas pyridamole or use of clopidogrel in place of aspirin offers additional benefit p

The future for ischaemic stroke[3] Some trials suggest rapid assessment of ' attacks' (like 'heart attacks') and thrombolysis with alteplase (t-PA) *within onset of symptoms* ↓adverse outcomes by 12%.[4] CI: • Major infarct on CT • deficits • Recent surgery • Past CNS haemorrhage • Recent arterial puncture non-compressible site • Anticoagulants or PTT >15s • Platelets <100 × 10^9/L •

1 Reducing salt intake from 10g/d to 5g/day can lower systolic BP by 10mmHg, ↓stroke risk by ~
2 Folate ('good') and homocystein ('bad') have a complex link with risk of haemorrhagic stroke.

Neurology

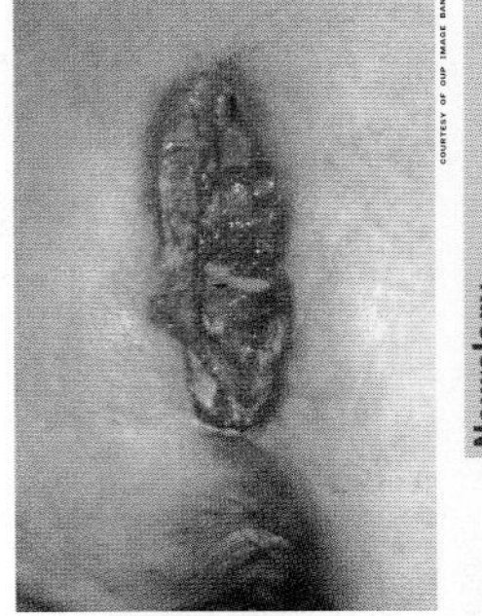

Fig 1. Sacral pressure sore after a stoke. Easy to prevent, given good nurses; so hard to treat, and so often a prelude to death.

3 *Thrombolysis cannot be recommended yet in the UK*, because the risk of harm has not been fully quantified for NHS patients outside the controlled environment of trials. The position may be different in hospitals which already have CNS thrombolysis teams with a dedicated imaging service on 24h call.

4 Although USA doctors may be sued for *not* giving thrombolysis in stroke, Cochrane meta-analyses are unconvinced: in the most favourable trial, the placebo group had worse strokes. Despite a favourable re-analysis of the data it remains true that unreasonable data assumptions may have been made.

Rehabilitation after stroke

(see p462 for acute stroke)

►*Good care requires attention to detail.* Principles are of those of *any* chronic disease (p467) and are best realized by specialist rehab or community teams (↓morbidity and institutionalization). *Special points in the early management:*

- Watch the patient swallows a small volume of water; if signs of aspiration (a cough or voice change) make *nil by mouth* for some days; use IV fluids, then semi-solids (eg jelly; avoid soups and crumbly food). Avoid early NG tube feeds (needed only in the few with established chronic swallowing problems). Speech therapists skilled in assessing swallowing difficulties are invaluable here.
- Avoid damaging patients' shoulders through careless lifting.
- Ensure good bladder and bowel care through frequent toileting. Avoid early catheterization which may prevent return to continence.
- Position the patient to minimize spasticity. Get prompt physiotherapy.
- In pseudo-emotionalism/emotional lability (sobbing unprovoked by sorrow, from failure of cortical inhibition of the limbic system), tricyclics or fluoxetine may help
- Measure time taken to sit up, and to transfer from lying to sitting in a chair; this is a good way to monitor progress with physio/occupational therapy.

Screen for depression[1] 33% are depressed, and, untreated (p13), this worsens motor function and ↑mortality (there's a known association with vascular disease).

Neurology

Tests Asking to point to a named part of the body tests *perceptual function*.
Copying matchstick patterns tests *spatial ability*.
Dressing or drawing a clock face tests for *apraxia* (p46).
Picking out and naming easy objects from a pile tests for agnosia (acuity OK, but cannot mime use; guesses are way-out, semantically, and phonetically).

Neurorehabilitation takes a functional approach building on what patients can do—with speech- and physiotherapy. Making it fun is an important route to motivation, eg swimming (a hemiplegic arm may be supported on a special float) and video games (which ↑recovery by aiding coordination). The aim is to promote cerebral reorganization. To this end, constraint of the good arm has been found to be helpful (*constraint-induced movement therapy*).

End-of-life decisions '...And thus the native hue of resolution is sicklied o'er with the pale cast of thought' *Hamlet* act iii:i—the more we think on these issues, the more we tie ourselves in knots. We intended these precepts to bisect these snares, not to reveal deep, hidden truths, but to provide a workable framework at the bedside.

- If the patient's views are known, comply with them, except perhaps where doing so entails an illegal act, or one that clearly harms others.
- No person has authority to impose his or her own views on end-of-life decisions. You cannot tell a nurse to stop feeding someone, and expect her to obey you. Consensus is the only practical way forward. Try to get the opinion of more than one relative, and more than one shift of nurses (eg at changeover time). Let everyone have their say. You may learn new and important facts about your patient, which make decisions easier—or harder.
- If consensus is impossible, recourse to the Courts is one option: but remember that judges have no special skill in this area.

Beware guidelines giving doctors special powers (such as the BMA guidelines). Doctors may be the worst decision-makers as closeness to life and death may make them tolerant of ending life—eg if the bed could be used for 'something better'. Even if *not* the case, if society thinks this, then doctors are in an untenable position. We *do* have a role, though, in facilitating consensus, and documenting it.

Success is often impossible (there are too many grey areas), but if you can stumble from one ambiguity to another without being disheartened, then that is good enough. Your patients will respect your honesty.

1 Have you been bothered by **little interest or pleasure** in doing things? Have you been **feeling down, depressed**, or **hopeless** in the last month? If 'yes' only 4 follow-up questions—on sleep disturbance, appetite change, low self-esteem, and anhedonia—are needed to confirm depression esp if 'yes' to: 'Have your feelings in the past month caused you significant distress, or impaired your ability to function?

Assessing handicap, disability, and independence in daily life

Handicap entails inability to carry out social functions. 'A disadvantage for a given individual, resulting from an impairment or disability, that limits or prevents the fulfilment of a role.' Two people with the same ***impairment*** (eg paralysed arm) may have different ***disabilities*** (one can dress, the other cannot). Disabilities are likely to determine quality of future life. Treatment is often best aimed at reducing disability, not curing disease. For example, Velcro® fasteners in place of buttons may enable a person to dress.

A person with a severe hearing impairment may seem to you to have no disability if they can lip-read. But ask yourself (and your patients, when you get to know them) about the price they pay for rising above their disabilities. Lip-reading, for example, is exhausting, requiring 100% vigilance to make sense of transitory and incomplete visual clues.

Barthel's index of activities of daily living

Bowels	0	Incontinent (or needs to be given enemas)
	1	Occasional accidents (once a week)
	2	Continent
Bladder	0	Incontinent, or catheter inserted but unable to manage it
	1	Occasional accidents (up to once per 24h)
	2	Continent (for more than seven days)
Grooming	0	Needs help with personal care: face, hair, teeth, shaving
	1	Independent (implements provided)
Toilet use	0	Dependent
	1	Needs some help but can do some things alone
	2	Independent (on and off, wiping, dressing)
Feeding	0	Unable
	1	Needs help in cutting, spreading butter, etc.
	2	Independent (food provided within reach)
Transfer	0	Unable to get from bed to commode: the vital transfer to prevent the need for 24-hour nursing care
	1	Major help needed (physical, 1–2 people), can sit
	2	Minor help needed (verbal or physical)
	3	Independent
Mobility	0	Immobile
	1	Wheelchair-independent, including corners, etc.
	2	Walks with help of one person (verbal or physical)
	3	Independent
Dressing	0	Dependent
	1	Needs help but can do about half unaided
	2	Independent (including buttons, zips, laces, etc.)
Stairs	0	Unable
	1	Needs help (verbal, physical, carrying aid)
	2	Independent up and down
Bath/shower	0	Dependent
	1	Independent (must get in and out unaided and wash self)

The aim is to establish the degree of independence from any help.

Barthel's paradox The more we contemplate Barthel's eulogy of independence, the more we see it as a mirage reflecting a greater truth about human affairs: ►there is no such thing as independence[1]—only **inter-dependence,** and in fostering this interdependence lies our true vocation.

Philosophy in action

Neurology

1 No man is an Island, intire of it selfe; every man is a peece of the Continent, a part of the maine; if a Clod bee washed away by the Sea, Europe is the lesse, as well as if a promontorie were, as well as if a Mannor of thy friends or of thine owne were. Any man's death diminishes me, because I am involved in mankinde; And therefore never send to know for whom the bell tolls: It tolls for thee. John Donne **1572–1631**; meditation XVII. What happens when we take up John Donne's offer of meditation? Some very interesting CNS events: brain activity slows, and blood is relocated to the anterior cingulate and dorsolateral prefrontal areas.

Transient ischaemic attack (TIA)

The sudden onset of focal CNS phenomena due to temporary occlusion, usually b emboli, of part of the cerebral circulation is termed a TIA if symptoms last <24 (often much shorter). Incidence: 0.4/1000/yr. 15% of 1st strokes are preceded b TIAs; they are also harbingers of MI, so... ➤*good management may avert disaste*

Attacks are single or many (the same or different for each TIA). ***Carotid territor*** (p441): Contralateral weakness/numbness; dysphasia; dysarthria; homonymou hemianopia; amaurosis fugax (one eye's vision is progressively blotted out 'like curtain descending over my field of view'). ***Vertebrobasilar territory:*** Hemiparesi hemisensory loss; bilateral weakness or sensory loss; diplopia; homonymous hemi anopia in cortical blindness; vertigo; deaf; tinnitus; vomiting; dysarthria; ataxia.

NB: *Global* events (syncope; dizziness) are **not** typical of TIAs.

Signs of causes Carotid bruit (p54); absence does not rule out a carotid source o emboli: tight stenoses often have *no* bruit.[97] BP↑. Heart murmur from valve disease ➤Identify and treat AF. Fundoscopy during TIAs may show retinal artery emboli.

Causes ***Atherothromboembolism*** from the carotid is the chief cause (may also b from heart (AF, mural thrombus post-MI, valve disease, prosthetic valve) ***Hyperviscosity*** (p356), eg polycythaemia, sickle-cell anaemia, WCC↑↑ (leukostasis may need urgent chemotherapy), myeloma[97] and ***vasculitis,*** eg cranial arteritis PAN, SLE, syphilis *et al* are rare causes, and perhaps shouldn't be classified as TIA.

Differential *Hypoglycaemia; migraine aura* (symptoms spread and intensify ove minutes, often with visual scintillations before headache); *focal epilepsy* (symptom spread over seconds and often include twitching and jerking); hyperventilation; MS retinal bleeds; peripheral neuropathy. Rare mimics of TIA: *Malignant hypertension hypoglycaemia; MS; intracranial lesions; phaeochromocytoma; somatization* (p635)

Tests Aim to find the cause and define vascular risk: FBC, ESR, U&E, glucose, lipids CXR, ECG, carotid Doppler ± angiography, MRI/CT (any existing infarcts?) ± cardia echo (rarely shows cardiac cause if no suggestive signs).

Treatment Begin after the 1st TIA: don't wait for the stroke! Control stroke risk factors (p462, eg smoking, BP, lipids, etc.) and MI (p79, risk equation, p642) *Reversible risk factors:* Hypertension (cautiously lower; aim for <140/85mmHg p142); hyperlipidaemia (p682); help to stop smoking (p79 & *OHCS* p512).

- *Antiplatelet drugs:* NICE recommends low-dose aspirin if no peptic ulcer (~75mg/ *day for life;*[1] probably ↓non-fatal strokes and MI by 25%, and vascular death by 15%) **and,** for the next 2yrs, dipyridamole (Assantin Retard® has dipyridamole MR 200mg + aspirin 25mg, so 1 tablet/12h is a good dose). Dipyridamole's effects: ↑cAMP & ↓thromboxane A2. *If aspirin-intolerant:* clopidogrel 75mg/day, a thienopyridine that ↓platelet aggregation by modifying platelet ADP receptors.
- *Warfarin indications:* heart emboli, eg AF, mitral stenosis, recent big septal MI.
- Carotid endarterectomy in carotid TIA if operative risk is good[2] and ≥75% stenosis at the origin of the internal carotid artery.[MET 93] [MET 94] For benefit to outweigh risk, the team's peri-operative stroke and mortality rate must be <3%.[95] Intraoperative transcranial Doppler can monitor middle cerebral artery flow. Using patches may reduce chances of restenosis. Do not stop aspirin beforehand. 50–70% stenosis may benefit from surgery only in the best hands; NNT=15.[MET 96]

Driving Avoid for ≥1 month; patients in the UK should inform the DVLA if multiple attacks in short period or residual deficit.

Prognosis The combined risk of stroke and MI is ~9%/yr; risk of stroke is 12% in year 1 and up to 10% subsequently if carotid stenosis is ≥70%. More frequent TIAs ↑risk further. Mortality is ~3-fold that of a TIA-free matched population. In one Dutch study in 2005, 60% of patients were dead within 10 years of a TIA.[97]

1 There is *no* dose–response relation for doses between 50 and 1500mg/d: E Johnson 2000 *E-BM* 5 9

2 *Who risks death/CVA from endarterectomy?* ♀ sex, >75yrs old, systolic BP↑, contralateral artery occluded; stenosis of ipsilateral carotid syphon/external carotid; wide-territory TIAs *vs* just amaurosis fugax.

Vhen should TIA lead to *prompt* or *emergency* referral?

patients with a suspected TIA should be referred to a specialist and seen nin 7 days (ideally!). A score of ≥6 (see TABLE) strongly predicts a stroke 5%) in the next week, so even this difficult target may be too lax.

Aged ≥60	1 point
BP ≥140/90	1 point
Unilateral weakness	2 points
Speech disturbance without weakness	2 points
Symptoms lasting >1h	2 points
Symptoms lasting 10–59 mins	1 point

scoring system is useful but should only be regarded as provisional: it has n formally validated only in 377 patients (from Oxfordshire; *Lancet* 2005).[98] n assessing urgency, bear in mind Warlow's 2005 data: in stroke patients who a preceding TIA, 17% occurred on the day of the stroke, 9% on the previous and 43% at some point during the 7 days before the stroke.[99] These figures uld remind us to rehearse routes for referral for emergency endarterectomy—resent this is typically performed >90 days post-TIA.[100]

Subarachnoid haemorrhage (SAH)

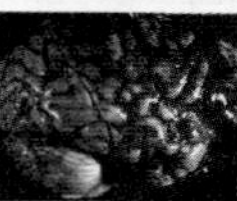

Fig 1. Middle cerebral ar SAH at the Sylvian fissur

Spontaneous bleeding into the subarachnoid space is often catastrophic. Incidence: 8/100,000/yr; typical age: 35–65. ***Causes:*** Rupture of saccular aneurysms (80%); arterio-venous (AV) malformations (15%). No cause is found in <15%. ***Risk↑ if:*** Smoking; alcohol misuse; BP↑;[1] bleeding disorders; mycotic aneurysm post-SBE; possibly lack of oestrogen (post-menopausal). ♀:♂ >1:1. Close relatives of those with SAH have a 3–5-fold ↑risk of SAH.[102]

Berry aneurysms Common sites: junction of posterior communicating wit internal carotid or of the anterior communicating with the anterior cerebral a or bifurcation of the middle cerebral artery (fig 1, p440). 15% are multiple. are hereditary. ***Associations:*** Polycystic kidneys, coarctation of the aorta, El Danlos syndrome (hypermobile joints + ↑skin elasticity, *OHCS* p642).

Symptoms Sudden (within seconds) devastating typically occipital headache ' *ught I'd been kicked in the head*'. Vomiting, collapse (± seizures), and coma follow. Coma/drowsiness may last for days. **Signs** Neck stiffness; Kernig's sign 6h to develop; retinal and subhyaloid haemorrhage. Focal neurology *at presen* may suggest site of aneurysm (eg pupil changes indicating a IIIrd nerve palsy a posterior communicating artery aneurysm) or intracerebral haematoma. deficits suggest ischaemia from vasospasm, or rebleeding, or hydrocephalu

Differential In primary care, only 25% of those with severe, sudden 'thunde headache have SAH. In 50–60%, no cause is found; the remainder have menir migraine, intracerebral bleeds, or cerebral venous thrombosis. See p472.

Sentinel headache SAH patients may earlier have experienced a sentinel heac perhaps due to a small warning leak from the offending aneurysm (~6% recall-bias clouds the picture.[104] As surgery is more successful in the least syr matic, be suspicious of any *sudden* headache especially with neck or back p

Tests In good hands, new CT scanners detect >90% of bleeds within the 1st 4 SAH;[106] older scanners miss small bleeds—so if the clinical suspicion is stron CT is –ve do an LP >12h after headache onset.[107] CSF in SAH is uniformly bloody on and xanthochromic (yellow) after a few hours. The supernatant from spun looked at photometrically to find breakdown products of Hb. Finding bili confirms SAH, showing that the LP was not a 'bloody tap' (don't rely on fi fewer CSF RBCs in each successive bottle).

Management ►Get neurosurgical help with all cases—immediately if ↓le consciousness, progressive focal deficit, or cerebellar haematoma is suspec

- Bed rest, and chart of BP, pupils, coma level (p776). ?Repeat CT if deterior
- Re-examine CNS often. Prevent the need for straining with stool softeners
- ***Surgery:*** Craniotomy and clipping aneurysms can stop rebleeds and is b those with few or no symptoms (≤grade II). SE: intra-operative rupture; pc epilepsy. If surgery is likely, do prompt angiography. ***Intraluminal platinum*** (Guglielmi[108]) are an alternative with less mortality (but rebleeding is a bit common after coils than after clipping).[109] [110] Intracranial stents and ba remodelling make possible the treatment of wide-necked aneurysms. Micrc eters can now traverse tortuous vessels to treat previously unreachable lesi AV malformations and fistulae may also benefit from this procedure.
- ***Medical:*** Cautiously control *severe* hypertension; analgesia for headache; bed sedation for ~4wks. Keep hydrated (running 'dry', out of respect for ICP↑, wc vasospasm). ***Vasospasm:*** Nimodipine (60mg/4h PO for 3wks, or 1mg/h IV Ca^{2+} antagonist that improves outcome (give to all if blood pressure allo

Rebleeding is a common mode of death. Rebleeding occurs in 30%, often in t few days. **Vascular spasm** follows a bleed, often causing ischaemia ± perm CNS deficit. If this happens, surgery is not helpful at the time but may be so

tality in subarachnoid haemorrhage

le	Signs	Mortality: %
	None	0
	Neck stiffness and cranial nerve palsies	11
	Drowsiness	37
	Drowsy with hemiplegia	71
	Prolonged coma	100

ost all the mortality occurs in the 1st month. Of those who survive the 1st th, 90% survive a year or more

uptured aneurysms: 'the time-bomb in my head'

ally, risks of preventive surgery outweigh any benefits, except perhaps in ng patients (more years at risk, and surgery is twice as hazardous if >45yrs [12] who have aneurysms >7mm in diameter, especially if located at the tion of the internal carotid and the posterior communicating cerebral artery, the rostral basilar artery bifurcation, and especially if there is uncontrolled ertension or a past history of bleeds.[113] Data from the 2003 International dy of Unruptured Intracranial Aneurysms (ISUIA) show that relative risks of ure for an aneurysm 7–12mm across is 3.3; if the diameter is >12mm, the tive risk is 17 times that for aneurysms <7mm across.[114]
ther patients, bear in mind the old adage: 'if it ain't broke; don't fix it'.
atients with a ***previous*** SAH have a high-ish risk for new aneurysm formation enlargement of untreated aneurysms. Screening these patients might be eficial, eg if multiple aneurysms, hypertension, or a history of smoking.[115]

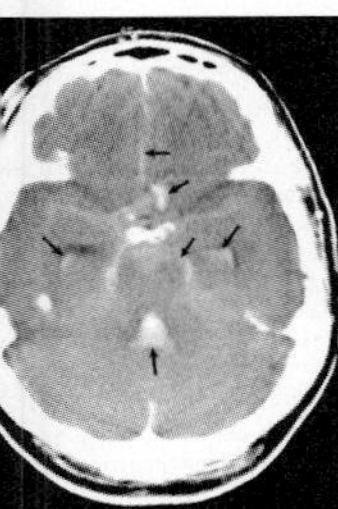

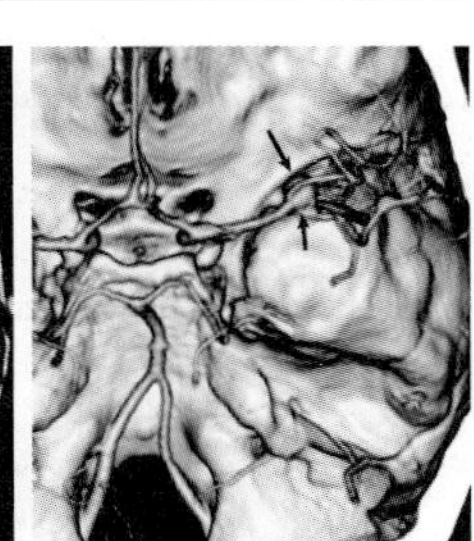

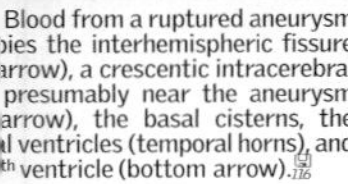
Blood from a ruptured aneurysm pies the interhemispheric fissure arrow), a crescentic intracerebral presumably near the aneurysm arrow), the basal cisterns, the al ventricles (temporal horns), and th ventricle (bottom arrow).[116]

Fig 2. CT images can be manipulated to show only high-density structures such as bones and arteries containing contrast. Here is a middle cerebral artery aneurysm.

We thank Professor Peter Scally for these CT images and the commentaries on them.

each 20mmHg rise in systolic BP, relative risks of ischaemic stroke, intracerebral haemorrhage, barachnoid hemorrhage are 1.8, 2.5, and 1.6 in ♂—and 1.6, 3.1, and 2.3 in ♀, respectively.

Intracranial venous thrombosis (IVT)

Isolated sagittal sinus thrombosis (47% of patients with IVT) ***Present*** Headache, vomiting, seizures, papilloedema (one cause of benign intrac hypertension). If venous infarction: focal signs occur, eg hemiplegia. Sagittal thrombosis is usually seen with thrombosis of other sinuses, eg ***lateral thrombosis*** (35%—eg headache, focal CNS signs, seizures, and papilloed ***cavernous sinus thrombosis*** (headache, oedematous eyelids/chemosis; prop and painful eye movements/ophthalmoplegia), ***sigmoid sinus throm*** (cerebellar signs, lower cranial nerve palsies), ***inferior petrosal sinus*** (v cranial nerve palsies, ie Gradenigo's syndrome).

Cortical (cerebral) vein thrombosis (CVT) may cause venous infarcts (± signs), encephalopathy, seizures, and headache (eg thunderclap headache sudden, severe headache). ***Signs:*** Evolving speech disorders, cognition↓, vis pareses.[118] It often coexists with sinus thromboses.[119] MRI may miss the diag unless T2-weighted conventional gradient echo sequences are used.[120]

Causes: Pregnancy/puerperium, oral contraceptives, head injury, dehydration, dyscrasias (eg mutations causing hypercoagulability), malignancies, recent LP. vein (vena magna Galani) thrombosis is a rare cause of CVT and is us associated with vascular malformation.[121] Rarer associations—see table:

Systemic diseases		Infections	Drugs
Hyperthyroidism	Hyperviscosity (p356)	Meningitis; TB	Androgens, eg
Nephrosis	Crohn's/UC (p264 & p266)	Cerebral abscess	(eg oxymetholo
Ketoacidosis[122]	Behçet's disease (p686)	Septicaemia	Antifibrinolytics
Heart failure	Protein C resistance (p358)	Fungal infections	Tranexamic acid
SLE	Antiphospholipid syndrome	Otitis media	Infliximab[123]
Homocystinuria	Klippel–Trénaunay syndrome	Cerebral malaria	IV steroids in MS
Paroxysmal nocturnal haemoglobinuria		HIV with nephrosis	(methylpredniso

Differential diagnosis (See subarachnoid differential diagnosis list on p Thunderclap headaches also occur in dissection of a carotid or vertebral arte well as in benign thunderclap headache.[126]

Emergency investigation of thunderclap headache[127] (ΔΔ: subarachnc pituitary bleed; CVT; idiopathic, triggered by Valsalva manoeuvre (cough, co

- Check that there are no signs of meningitis (p368).
- Do emergency MRI/CT scan. If normal, do LP; measure the opening CSF pressu high, and headache persists, and no subarachnoid bleed, suspect cerebra thrombosis if predisposing factors. Get neuroimaging help. MRI angiograp best.[128] **NB:** CT may be normal early; then at ~1wk develops the delta sign, w a transversely cut sinus shows a contrast filling defect. This may also be an sign. CSF may be normal, or show RBCs and bilirubin↑—with ↑opening pre

Management Seek expert help, eg in interpreting MRI ± MRI angiography small randomized study shows that heparin saves lives and improves outcor This may be important even in those with haemorrhagic venous infar Streptokinase & other fibrinolytics has been used via selective catheterizatio

Prognosis Variable. Causes of death are mainly transtentorial herniation unilateral focal mass effects or to diffuse oedema and multiple parench lesions. Independent predictors of death in one study were coma (odds rati 8.8), deep cortical vein thrombosis (OR≈8.5), posterior fossa lesion (OR≈6.5) intracerebral haemorrhage (OR≈3.4), and mental disturbance (OR≈2.5).[1]

1 Worsening of previous focal or new focal deficits also ↑risk of death; see *Stroke* 2005 (Jul 7

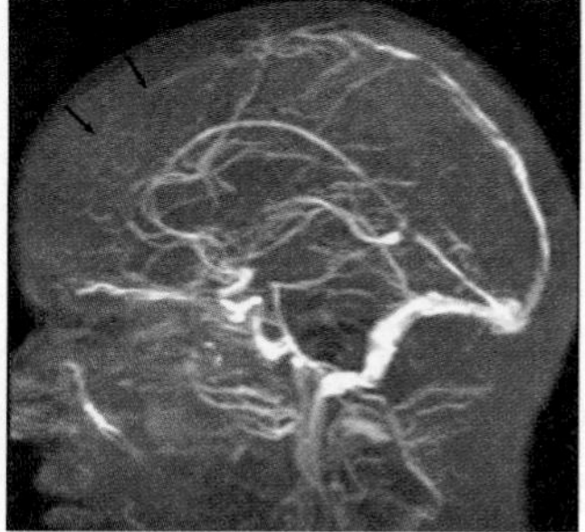

Fig 1. This magnetic resonance venogram (MRV) could look normal at first glance: the hardest thing to see in imaging is often that which is not there. Much of the superior sagittal sinus (SSS) is not demonstrated because it is filled with clot—a superior sagittal sinus thrombosis. The arrows point to where it should be seen. Posteriorly, the irregularity of the vessel indicates non-occlusive clot.

We thank Professor Peter Scally for the image and the commentary.

Subdural haemorrhage

►Consider this very treatable condition in all whose conscious level fluctuates, and also in those having an 'evolving stroke', especially if on anticoagulants. Bleeding is from bridging veins between cortex and venous sinuses (vulnerable to deceleration injury), resulting in accumulating haematoma between dura and arachnoid. This gradually raises ICP, shifting midline structures away from the side of the clot and, if untreated, eventual tentorial herniation and coning. Most subdurals are from trauma but they can occur without (eg intracranial hypotension;[1] dural metastases). *The trauma is often forgotten as it was so minor or so long ago (up to 9 months).* The elderly are most susceptible, as brain shrinkage makes bridging veins vulnerable. *Other risk factors:* falls (epileptics, alcoholics); anticoagulation.

Symptoms Fluctuating level of consciousness (seen in 35%) ± insidious physical or intellectual slowing, sleepiness, headache, personality change, and unsteadiness.

Signs ↑ICP (p812); seizures. Localizing neurological symptoms (eg unequal pupils, hemiparesis) occur late and often long after the injury (mean=63 days).

Imaging CT/MRI shows clot ± midline shift (but beware bilateral isodense clots). Look for crescent-shaped collection of blood over 1 hemisphere. The sickle-shape differentiates subdural blood from extradural haemorrhage.

ΔΔ Stroke, dementia, CNS masses (eg tumours, abscess, neurocysticercosis).

Treatment Irrigation/evacuation eg via burr twist drill and burr hole craniostomy can be considered 1st-line; craniotomy is 2nd-line, if the clot has organized. Address causes of the trauma (eg abuse; cataract *et al* causing falls, arrhythmia, etc)

Neurology

►►Extradural (epidural) haemorrhage

►*Suspect this if, after head injury, conscious level falls or is slow to improve, or there is a lucid interval.* Extradural bleeds are often due to a fractured temporal or parietal bone causing laceration of the middle meningeal artery and vein, typically after trauma to a temple just lateral to the eye. Any tear in a dural venous sinus will also result in an extradural bleed. Blood accumulates between bone and dura.

Symptoms and signs Look out for a deterioration of consciousness after any head injury that initially produced no loss of consciousness or after initial drowsiness post-injury seems to have resolved. This 'lucid interval' pattern is typical of extradural bleeds. It may last a few hours to a few days before a bleed declares itself by a deteriorating level of consciousness caused by a rising ICP. Increasingly severe headache, vomiting, confusion, and fits can follow, accompanied by a hemiparesis with brisk reflexes and an upgoing plantar. If bleeding continues, the ipsilateral pupil dilates, and coma deepens, bilateral limb weakness develops, and breathing becomes deep and irregular. Death follows a period of coma and is due to respiratory arrest. Bradycardia and raised blood pressure are late signs.

Tests CT shows a haematoma which is often lens-shaped (biconvex; the blood forms a more rounded shape because the tough dural attachments to the skull tend to keep it more localized). Skull x-ray may be normal or show fracture lines crossing the course of the middle meningeal vessels. Skull fracture after trauma greatly increases the risk of an extradural haemorrhage, and should lead to prompt CT. ►***Lumbar puncture is contraindicated.***

Management ►►Stabilize and transfer promptly (with skilled medical and nursing escorts) to a neurosurgical unit for clot evacuation (± ligation of the bleeding vessel). Care of the airway in an unconscious patient, and measures to ↓ICP often mandate intubation and ventilation (+ mannitol IVI, *p812*).

Prognosis Excellent if diagnosis and operation early. Poor if coma, pupil abnormalities, or decerebrate rigidity are present pre-op.

1 ***Intracranial hypotension*** (ICH) is due to CSF leaks, amenable to epidural blood patches over the leak. Suspect ICH if headaches are worse on standing. Causes: meningeal diverticula, after epidural anaesthesia; dehydration; hyperpnoea (↑tidal volume). *MRI:* engorged venous sinuses; meningeal enhancement; subdural fluid.

CT images

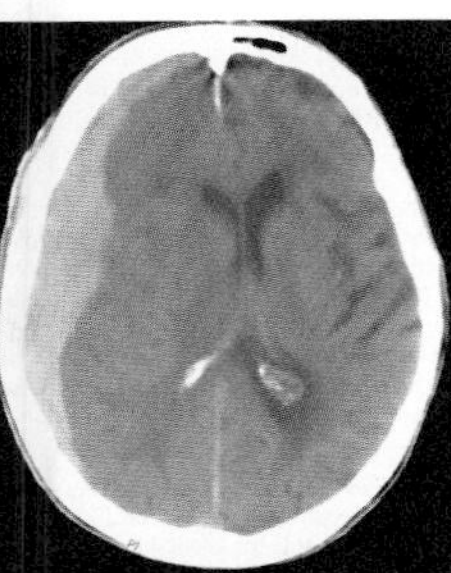

Fig 1. This image explains the cause as well as the pathology. On the patient's left, cerebral sulci are prominent and prior to this adverse event would have been even larger. The brain had shrunk within the skull as a result of atherosclerosis, and poor perfusion, leaving large subarachnoid spaces. A simple, quick rotation of the head is enough to tear a bridging veins, causing this ***acute subdural haematoma.***

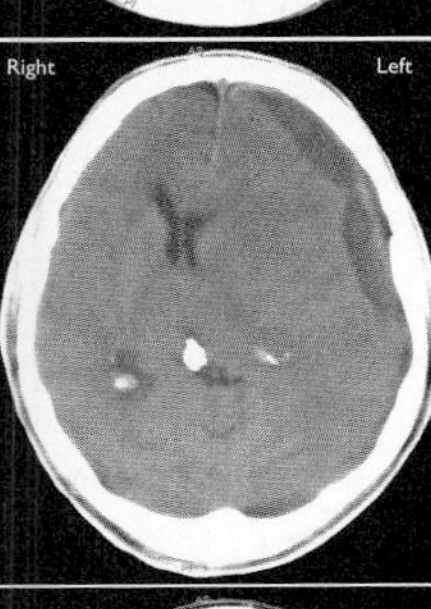

Fig 2. This fluid collection is of low attenuation compared to the brain, except for a small area of increased attenuation. It is an ***acute on chronic subdural haematoma***. But there is more! Look at the shift of midline structures across under the falx cerebri, subfalcine herniation. It is not just caused by the subdural. The left hemisphere is swollen as a result of the compression of the bridging veins in the subdural space, shifting the ventricles and calcified pineal across to the right.

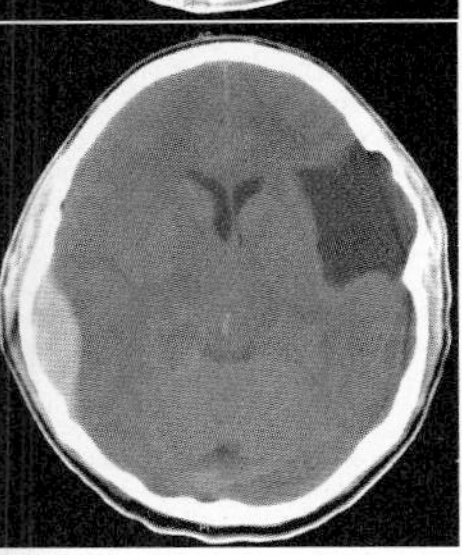

Fig 3. The blood (high attenuation, fusiform or biconvex collection) on the right side is limited anteriorly by the coronal suture and posteriorly by the lambdoid suture. This is therefore an ***extradural haematoma***. The low attenuation CSF density collection on the left is causing scalloping of the overlying bone. It is in the typical location of an arachnoid cyst; an incidental finding of a congenital abnormality.

Delirium (acute confusional state)

20% of elderly patients on medical and surgical wards have some form o delirium: consider ***any*** acute fluctuating baffling behaviour change as possible delirium. Look for organic causes (UTI, pneumonia, MI). The 8 signs of DELIRIUM are:

Disordered thinking: Slow, irrational, rambling, jumbled up, incoherent ideas.
Euphoria, fearful, depressed or angry: Labile mood, eg anxious then torpid.
Language impaired Speech is reduced or gabbling, repetitive and disruptive.
Illusions/delusions/hallucinations: Tactile or visual (unlike in schizophrenia)
Reversal of sleep–awake cycle: May appear drowsy or hypervigilant.
Inattention: Focusing, sustaining, or shifting attention is poor; no real dialogue
Unaware/disorientated: Doesn't know it's evening, or his own name, or location
Memory deficits: Often marked. (Later he may be amnesic for the episode.)

Summary: Globally impaired cognition and impaired awareness/consciousness.

Illustration from Conrad's *Heart of Darkness* 'The wastes of his weary brain were haunted by shadowy images now—images of wealth and fame...Sometimes he was contemptibly childish. He desired to have kings meet him at railway stations on his return from some ghastly Nowhere . . . "Close the shutter", said Kurtz suddenly "I can't bear to look at this." I did so. There was a silence. "Oh, but I will wring your heart yet!" he cried at the invisible wilderness.' Impaired consciousness is difficult to describe (which is why we have to resort to Conrad—the master of multi-layered descriptions). When you talk to the patient you have the sense that he is not with you, but away with the fairies—inaccessible and lost

Neurology

Causes (Pain and other psychological states are important co-factors.)

- Infection/contagion: pneumonia, UTI, malaria, wounds; IV lines.
- Drugs: opiates, anticonvulsants, L-dopa, sedatives, recreational, post-GA.
- Alcohol withdrawal (2–5d post-admission; raised LFTs with raised MCV; history of alcohol abuse), also drug withdrawal.
- Metabolic: hypoglycaemia, uraemia, liver failure, U&E↑↓, anaemia, malnutrition
- Hypoxia: respiratory or cardiac failure.
- Vascular: stroke, myocardial infarction.
- Intracranial infection: encephalitis, meningitis.
- Head injury—or ↑ICP (space occupying lesions, eg tumour, subdural haematoma)
- Epilepsy: status epilepticus (see BOX), post-ictal states.
- Nutritional: thiamine, nicotinic acid, or B_{12} deficiency.

Differential If agitated, is it **anxiety?** Check conscious level. If delusions or hallucinations, is it a **primary mental illness** (eg schizophrenia) but this is rare on the wards (esp if no past history) and delirium very is common in ill patients.

Tests Consider U&E, FBC, ABG, blood culture, malaria films; also LP, EEG, MRI.

Management After identifying and treating the underlying cause, aim to:

- Reduce distress and prevent accidents; encourage family to sit with the patient
- Use the **3M** non-drug cures for agitation: music, massage, and muscle relaxation
- Augment self-care. Discourage passive dependency and inappropriate napping
- Do not use physical restraints—and remove catheters and other impedimenta
- Hunt down hearing aids/glasses. If he's using ones from the patient next door.
- Nurse in a *moderately lit*, quiet room, ideally with the *same* staff in attendance (minimizes confusion) where the patient can be watched closely. Repeated reassurance and orientation to time and place can help.
- Minimize medication (esp. sedatives); but if disruptive, some sedation may be needed. Use a major tranquillizer—haloperidol 0.5–2mg IM/PO, p13—or chlorpromazine 50–100mg IM/PO (but not in the elderly, in whom it is liable to cause cardiac side-effects and hypotension). Wait 20min to judge effect—further doses can be given if needed. Benzodiazepines may be used for night-time sedation. NB in alcohol withdrawal do *not* use chlorpromazine, use diazepam instead (p274)

Tests of consciousness, and an explanation of dissociative states

Consciousness results wherever these four entities co-exist: perception, memory, emotion, and orientation in space and time. Remorse, for example, is a blend of these four constructs. If a black box exhibited remorse no further test would be needed to establish its consciousness. Patients are often like black boxes to us: we are never quite sure what is going on inside. How do we find out? Dialogue is the first method. Patients with clouding of consciousness often engage in dialogue, but we get the feeling that they are not quite with us. A conversation may suggest clouding of consciousness—until the moment when the patient makes an ironic remark, or we subconsciously detect a twinkle in their eye, banishing the need for formal tests of consciousness.

In general, if a patient knows where they are, the time of day, and passes tests of short and long term memory we tend to think there is not a problem of consciousness—and move on to more mundane issues. This is a pity because changes in consciousness are often subtle—and we need to ask others who know the patient well if there has been any change. Thus elucidating changes in consciousness depends on triangulation between three changing and interacting centres of consciousness—our own, the patient's, and a third party. These issues are exemplified in the next two boxes—where we illustrate the concept of derealization. Here, it is sufficient to say that ***depersonalization*** and ***derealization*** are part of the ***dissociative states*** (just one example of a disorder of consciousness). Dissociation is a mechanism of the mind that separates streams of memories or thoughts from normal consciousness. These mental fragments may then resurface and peruse a life of their own. Causes: migraine, epilepsy, head injury, stress, and, of course, prolonged sleeplessness (which is why all doctors instinctively understand this odd syndrome).

Non-convulsive status epilepticus (NCSE) as a cause of confusion

NCSE is under-diagnosed, and may manifest itself as confusion, impaired cognition/memory, odd behaviour, and dreamy derealization[139] (the external world appears unfamiliar and unreal—its objects, anchored neither in space nor time, float as in a more or less lucid dream). Other features of NCSE: aggression, psychosis ± abnormalities of eye movement, eyelid myoclonus, and odd postures. It may or may not occur in the context of classic seizures or ischaemic brain injury (eg subarachnoid haemorrhage).[140] Other causes and associations: drugs (eg antidepressants), infections (eg arboviruses; HIV; syphilis), neoplasia, dementias, sudden changes in calcium levels,[141] renal failure (eg with cephalosporin therapy or peritoneal dialysis). **Δ:** EEG evidence of rhythmical discharges (eg prolonged 3-per-second spike-wave complexes). Subsequent MRI may show focal oedema (eg in the hippocampus). **℞:** Valproate, ethosuximide, or IV benzodiazepines may be indicated (this requires specialist evaluation).[142]

Ganser syndrome—and example of dissociative symptoms

There are absurd or approximate answers to questions ('paralogias')—plainly wrong but suggesting that the answers are unconsciously known but have been passed by or half-ignored by the current (dissociated) stream of consciousness. There is also clouding of consciousness (or hypervigilance), somatic conversion symptoms (eg inexplicable paralysis—formerly known as hysterical symptoms), hallucinations, and amnesia regarding the episode.[143] Causes/associations: head injury, Munchausen's syndrome, solitary confinement, very stressful events.[144]

When asked to spell WORLD backwards, one Ganser patient replied "EBOLG". When asked to recall the words 'honesty', 'window', and 'lace', he replied "modesty, house, shoes".[145] NB: ►Ictal and post-ictal states may present with similarly impaired consciousness, perceptual abnormalities, and odd behaviour.

Dementia

Ameliorable causes
• T4↓; B_{12}/folate↓; thiamine↓ (eg alcohol); • Syphilis • Tumours (meningioma) • Subdural haematoma • Parkinson's (p486) • CNS cysticercosis (p432) • HIV (±cryptococcosis); • Normal pressure hydrocephalus[1] • Pellagra (p270) • Whipple's dis. (p708)

►Assume confusion is due to acute illness until proved otherwise (p476). Depression may mimic dementia (consider trial of therapy, p13). Dementia entails progressive deficits in several cognitive domains. The key is a good history: ask spouse, relatives, or friends about *progressively* impaired cognition/memory (autobiographical[2]; political etc.). Get *objective* evidence. Histories usually go back months or years. There is increasing forgetfulness, and normal tasks of daily living are done with increasing incompetence, eg going to buy sausages 6 times in a day, and then being baffled as to why there is a great mound of sausages in the kitchen. Sometimes the patient appears to have changed personality, e ↑apathy, uncharacteristically rude or depressed—or with slow, repetitious speech or literalness. For objective evidence, do tests of cognitive functioning (p47).

Epidemiology Rare below 55yrs of age. 5–10% prevalence above 65yrs. 20% prevalence above 80yrs, and 70% of those over 100yrs.

Commonest causes *Alzheimer's disease (AD)* *See* p480. ***Vascular dementia:*** ~25% of all dementias. It represents the cumulative effects of many small strokes. Look for evidence of vascular pathology (BP↑; past strokes; focal CNS signs): sudden onset and stepwise deterioration is characteristic (but often difficult to recognise).
Lewy body dementia: Characterized by Lewy bodies[3] in brainstem *and* neocortex; *fluctuating* cognitive loss, alertness; parkinsonism (p486); detailed visual hallucinations. It's the 3rd commonest dementia (15–25%) after AD and vascular causes. Older neuroleptics in these patients *often* cause neuropsychiatric SE. Rivastigmine *may* help.[MET 146]
Fronto-temporal dementia: (Frontal and temporal atrophy without Alzheimer histology, p480). *Signs:* Behavioural/personality change; early preservation of episodic memory and spatial orientation; disinhibition; hyperorality, stereotyped behaviour, and emotional unconcern. The disinhibition is not *always* bad.[4]
Rarer causes: Alcohol/drug abuse; pellagra (p270), Whipple's disease (p708); Huntington's (p694); CJD (p688); Parkinson's (p486); Pick's disease; HIV; cryptococcosis (p428); progressive leukencephalopathy.

Tests FBC, ESR; U&E; Ca^{2+}; LFT; TSH; autoantibodies; folate/B_{12} (treat low-normals); syphilis serology; CT/MRI (any structural pathology?). Consider EEG; CSF; functional imaging (PET; SPECT, ie single photon emission CT; cost ≈ $74,400 to $1.9 million per QALY).[148] Metabolic, genetic, and HIV tests after appropriate counselling, as indicated.

Management Neuropsychiatric referral: are specific drugs indicated? (p480)

- Nominate a key worker; make a *care management plan*; get support from social services ± Alzheimer's Society, p481. Ensure access to benefits (p481).
- Carer stress is inevitable (p437), causing ↑morbidity *and* mortality (↑ by 45%); ameliorate this by practical steps and unswerving loyalty (p437).
- GPs have a central role in 'couple focused planning', which acknowledges that needs combine in ways which are not simply additive.[149]

►Give any specific treatment (eg if TSH↑ or B_{12}/folate↓ or equivocal), and treat concurrent illnesses (these may contribute significantly to confusion).

1 Normal pressure hydrocephalus gives dilated ventricles *without* enlarged cerebral sulci (?from obstructed CSF outflow from the subarachnoid space). *Signs:* gait apraxia, incontinence; dementia. CSF shunts help.
2 Autobiographical and political memory is held in different areas: S Black 2004 *Neuropsychologia* **42** 25
3 Lewy bodies are eosinophilic intracytoplasmic neuronal inclusion bodies; there is overlap between Lewy body dementia and Alzheimer's and Parkinson's (PD), making treatment hard as L-dopa can precipitate delusions, and antipsychotic drugs worsen PD. Donepezil may help all 3. [@11981238]
4 An artist who had been constrained by over-adherence to one school of art had a fascinating blossoming of creativity and emotional insight with the arrival of fronto-temporal dementia. *Neurology* 2003 1707. This poses the question of what counts as a disease. If you can answer this question unequivocally perhaps you are over-endowed, fronto-temporally? Let some ambiguity in!

Neurology

The positive features of dementia (Auntie Kathleen's syndrome)

Positive features include wandering, aggression, flight of ideas, and logorrhoea:

> ***"Not for her a listless, dull-eyed wordless decline; with her it is all rush, gabble, celerity. She had always been a talker, but now her dementia unleashes torrents of speech...one train of thought switching to another without signal or pause, rattling across points and through junctions at a rate no listener can follow... Following the sense is like trying to track a particular ripple in a pelting torrent of talk."*** Alan Bennett *Untold Stories*, 87

Atypical antipsychotics may improve logorrhoea, wandering, agitation and aggression, without worsening cognition. SSRIs may help depressive symptoms, compulsions, food craving, and disinhibition in fronto-temporal dementia.[150]

Logorrhoea: when dialogue is *not* the answer

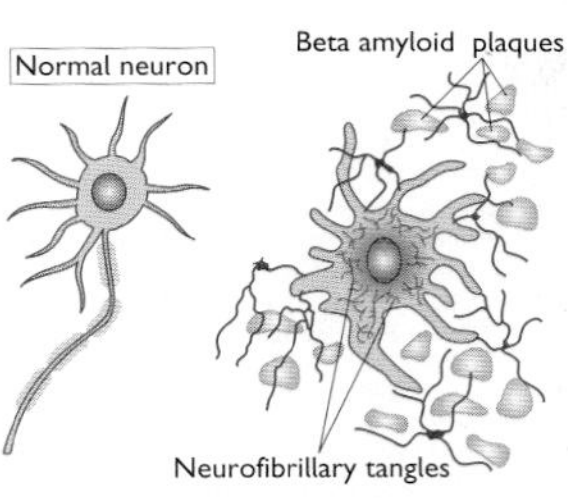

Fig 1. Amyloid plaques and neurofibrillary tangles in Alzheimer's disease. After micromedex.com.[151]

Alzheimer's disease (AD)

This leading cause of dementia is *the* big neuropsychiatric disorder of our times, dominating not just psychogeriatric wards, but the lives of countless children and spouses who have given up work, friends, and all accustomed ways of life to support relatives through the last long years. Their lives can be tormented—'*I am chained to a corpse*' (p437) or transformed, depending on how gently patients exit into their '*worlds of preoccupied emptiness*'. ***Mean survival:*** 7 years from onset.

Suspect Alzheimer's in adults with enduring,[1] acquired **deficits of visual-spatial skill** (gets lost easily), **memory**, and **cognition** (mental test scores + other neuropsychometric tests, p47). Early on there is **anosognosia**, ie lack of awareness—from the Greek *nosos* (disease) and *gnosis* (knowledge) of problems engendered by the disease, eg: missed appointments; misunderstood conversations or plots of films; mishandling of money and clerical work. Onset may be from 40yrs (earlier, in Down's syndrome). ***Cause:*** Accumulation β-amyloid peptide, a degradation product of amyloid precursor protein, resulting in progressive neuronal damage, neurofibrillary tangles, ↑numbers of senile plaques, and loss of the neurotransmitter acetylcholine. Neuronal loss is selective, and the hippocampus, amygdala, temporal neocortex and some subcortical nuclei, eg the nucleus basalis of Meynert are especially vulnerable (p436; 2006 data). Vascular effects are also important (see BOX).

Risk factors *Defective genes* on chromosomes 1, 14, 19, 21; the apoE4 variant brings forward age of onset. *Insulin resistance* (p191) *may* be important.

Diagnosis is often haphazard, as the exact form of dementia used not to matter (if B_{12} and TSH normal). This is hard to justify now that specifics are available for Alzheimer's. Brain imaging (CT; MRI; PET, p732) and neuropsychological tests help rule out fronto-temporal, Lewy body and vascular dementias. Another advantage of early diagnosis is that living will/advance directives may be made before the patient loses capacity to do this legally—the test is: can he **understand** and **retain** the information; **believe** it (no relevant delusions), and **weigh-up pros and cons**?

Presentation Memory/cognition↓; behavioural change (eg aggression, wandering, disinhibition); hallucinations; delusions; apathy; depression; irritability; euphoria. There is no standard natural history. Cognitive impairment is progressive, but behavioural/psychotic symptoms may go after a few months or years. Towards the end, often but not invariably, patients become sedentary, taking little interest in anything. Parkinsonism (p486), wasting, mutism, incontinence ± seizures may occur.

Treatment Evidence that **cholinesterase inhibitors** (see BOX) and **memantine** are modestly effective in treating AD is good. Cholinesterase inhibitors appear to be effective throughout the spectrum of AD, while memantine, alone or in combination with cholinesterase inhibitors, is effective in late stage disease. Memantine (see BOX) is an NMDA antagonist. (NMDA=N-methyl-D-aspartate, p443.) Manage arteriopathy (▶AD risk rises with increasing BP) so aim to normalize blood pressure.

We cannot recommend one cholinesterase over another, or suggest ginkgo biloba, oestrogen (neutral, at best, 2006 data), statins, or NSAIDs for prevention or treatment. Vitamin E gets support from one trial; data on other antioxidants is mixed.

Prevention Many ideas are being tested, eg cognitively stimulating hobbies, antihypertensives, statins, fish oils, ginkgo biloba, and other antioxidants—but good *replicated* randomized trials are lacking. (2006 data) Interventions are likely to be most effective if started early, and MRI/PET *can* predict decline/dementia in the cognitively normal,[2] but this science is most uncertain. Even if we could count neurofibrillary tangles with post-mortem accuracy we could not say 'this brain is becoming demented' as there is no simple relationship between structure and function.

1 'Enduring' doesn't mean unfluctuating: cognition comes and goes, allowing poetic insights, as in Iris Murdoch's poignant self-diagnosis: 'I am sailing into the dark'. 2 Jagust W 2006 *An Neurol*

ctical issues in managing Alzheimer's dementia

volve Social Services & family. UK Alzheimer's Disease Society: 0151 2982444.
clude *treatable dementias* (B_{12}, folate, syphilis serology, T4, ?HIV); *is this pression masquerading as dementia?* Antidepressant trials may be needed.
eticulous BP control; there is a complex interaction with AD: only 5% of AD tients have a pure form; 95% have mixed AD *and* vascular changes.[1] Optiise cerebral perfusion; it may be wrong to lower diastolic BP to ≤70mmHg.[1]
eat concurrent illnesses (many can make dementia worse). In most eople, the dementia remains and will progress.
oid drugs that may ↓cognition (neuroleptics, sedatives, tricyclics, p13).
range a well-lit, cognitively stimulating care setting. Try multisensory stimation, eg massage, music RCT 162 & aromatherapy etc. RCT 163 This can help mood, aggssion, anxiety, and speech. RCT 164 Structured conversation & exercise also lp. MET 165
See *Living with neurological disease*, p437. In late-stage AD, gastrostomy eding may be tried, but it is no better than oral feeding. 166 *Special help* is ailable for those caring for demented relatives at home, eg in the UK:

- Laundry services for soiled linen
- Car badge giving priority parking
- Carers' groups for mutual support
- Help from occupational therapist, district nurses, and community psychiatric nurses
- Attendance allowance
- Respite care in hospital
- Council tax rebate (forms from local council office)
- Day care/lunch clubs

cholinesterase inhibitors help embedding new memories more than essing old ones,[2] 167 and delay the need for institutional care, but not essarily its duration. 168 Liaise with a psychogeriatrician. NICE has found it ossible to develop acceptable guidelines for their use only partly because r effects are objectively modest. One cannot say 'stop these drugs as he has scored x on the mini-mental test score' (notoriously variable from day to if the wife says 'but he's brighter, more motivated'. 169 ►Be aware that g QALYs (p12) relentlessly can make us cruel; sentiment (the alternative to 's) may make us useless, but *it is better to be useless than cruel.* The ttish Intercollegiate Guidelines Network (SIGN) states that all AD patients d benefit from acetylcholinesterase inhibitors. Dose examples: **donepezil** at night (doubled after 4wks[2]); MET 170 **rivastigmine** 6mg/day;[3] **galantamine** ng/ day.[4] The SIGN meta-analysis did not take cost-effectiveness into ount.

iglutamatergic treatment: Randomized trials show that the NMDA antnist **memantine** helps eg moderate-to-severe Alzheimer's disease.[5] Its role ill undefined (SE: hallucinations, confusion, hypertonia, hypersexuality).

Neurology

eart failure there is a ~2-fold ↑risk of getting AD; excess risk ~halves if **hypotensives** are used.
)06 study of **transcranial doppler** middle cerebral artery monitoring for 1 hour, **small emboli** ed in 40% of those with Alzheimer's compared with ~15% for controls.
epezil cautions: heart conduction abnormalities; asthma/COPD; extrapyramidal signs; LFT↑. Chol- SE: D&V, cramps, incontinence; also headache, dizziness, heart block, psychiatric illness, LFT↑.
astigmine is a dual acetylcholinesterase/butyrylcholinesterase (ACHE/BUCHE) inhibitor (?better ACHE-selective inhibitors, eg donepezil & galantamine, vis-à-vis improving apathy, anxiety, sion, hallucinations & delusions (works in a wider range of dementias, eg in Parkinson's). Onceose is available. Pre-treatment orbitofrontal signs (agitation; disinhibition; odd motor activity) redict good response to donepezil; pre-℞ hallucinations predict response to rivastigmine.
antamine (Reminyl®) was originally isolated from daffodils. It is a specific, competitive, and ible acetylcholinesterase inhibitor. It is also an allosteric modulator at nicotinic cholinergic or sites potentiating cholinergic nicotinic neurotransmission. See Cochrane. CD001747.
mantine (a noncompetitive antagonist of NMDA receptors) is neuroprotective and cognitively es those with moderate-to-severe dementia. It can be combined with other drugs for AD.

Epilepsy: diagnosis

Epilepsy is a recurrent tendency to spontaneous, intermittent, abnormal ele activity in part of the brain, manifest as *seizures*.[1] These may take many forms given patient they tend to be stereotyped. *Convulsions* are the motor signs of rical discharges. Many of us would have seizures in abnormal metabolic ci stances—eg $Na^+\downarrow$, hypoxia (reflex anoxic seizures in faints): we would not no be said to have epilepsy. In deciding if an event is epileptic, don't pay *too* attention to associated incontinence and abnormal movement (not everythin twitches is epilepsy): but biting the side of the tongue and slow recovery of n mental functioning are very suggestive. Prevalence of active epilepsy is ~1%

The patient There may (rarely) be a *prodrome* lasting hours or days precedi seizure. It is not part of the seizure itself: the patient or others notice a cha mood or behaviour. An *aura*, which is part of the seizure, may precede its manifestations. The aura may be a strange feeling in the gut, or a sensation experience such as *déjà vu* (disturbing sense of familiarity), or strange sm flashing lights. It implies a partial seizure (a focal event), often, but not neces temporal lobe epilepsy (TLE). After a partial seizure involving the motor (Jacksonian convulsion) there may be temporary weakness of the affected li (Todd's palsy). After a generalized seizure, patients may feel awful with heac myalgia, confusion, and a sore tongue.

Diagnosis Decide first: is this epilepsy? (p452 for ΔΔ) A detailed descriptior a witness of 'the fit' is vital. Try hard not to diagnose epilepsy in error—thera significant side-effects, the diagnosis is stigmatizing and has implicatior employment, insurance, and driving. Decide next what type of seizure it is attack's *onset* is the key concern here: partial or generalized? If the seizure b with focal features, it is a partial seizure, however rapidly it is generalizec next: what if anything brings it on (eg flickering light (TV) or alcohol)? Can t avoided? TV-induced seizures—almost always generalized—rarely require d

Partial seizures Features are referable to a part of one hemisphere sugge structural disease.

- ***Elementary symptoms*** (consciousness unimpaired, eg focal motor seizu
- ***Complex symptoms*** (consciousness impaired, eg olfactory aura prec automatism). Usually TLE.
- ***Partial seizure with secondary generalization:*** Electrical disturbance st focally, then spreading widely, causing a secondary generalized seizure.

Primary generalized seizures No features referable to only one hemisphe

- ***Absences (petit mal):*** Brief (≤10s) pauses, eg suddenly stops talking ir sentence, then carries on where left off. Presents in childhood.
- ***Tonic–clonic*** (classical *grand mal*). Sudden onset, loss of consciousness, stiffen (tonic) then jerk (clonic); may have one without the other; drowsy
- ***Myoclonic jerk*** (eg thrown suddenly to ground, or a violently disobedient li patient described it as *my flying-saucer epilepsy*, as crockery which happer be in the hand would take off).
- ***Atonic*** (becomes flaccid) or ***Akinetic.*** Note also ***infantile spasms*** (*OHCS* p

Causes Often none is found. ***Structural:*** Trauma, space occupying lesions, s tuberous sclerosis, SLE, PAN, sarcoid, vascular malformations. ***Metabolic:*** Alco benzodiazepine withdrawal; glucose ↑ or ↓, $P_aO_2\downarrow$ (eg in bradyarrhythr uraemia, $Na^{2+}\uparrow$ or ↓, $Ca^{2+}\downarrow$, liver disease, drugs (eg phenothiazines, tric cocaine). ***Infection:*** Encephalitis, syphilis, cysticercosis, HIV.

1 ↑Membrane excitation (epileptogenicity) may be related to disorders of synaptic transmission, K nelopathies, or α-subunit mutations (eg SCN2A; SCN1A) of voltage-gated Na^+ channel. *Lancet* 2003 12

luation of an adult who has just had a first-ever seizure

status epilepticus, see p808; here structural lesions are especially likely.
, it really the first? Ask the family and patient about past funny turns/odd ehaviour. Déjà vu and odd episodic feelings of fear *et al* may well be relevant.
, it really a seizure? Convulsive syncope is problematic here; get help. Get as uch history as you can from the patient and witnesses; ask yourself: *are they eliable*? In the heat of the moment many witnesses may report twitching hen none in fact took place (perhaps they want to please you by seeming to e observant and they 'helpfully' fill in the gaps in reality—so, *beware*).
Vas the seizure provoked by a CNS insult, eg head injury, stroke, hypoglycae-nia, alcohol, drugs (clozapine, tramadol, theophylline, baclofen); T° ↑↑; U&E ↑↓? rovoked 1st seizures are less likely to recur (3–10%, unless there is an un-emovable condition, such as an infarct or glioma); if unprovoked, recurrence ates are 30–50%. Provoked seizures are also called 'symptomatic'.
Vas there a possible trigger to the attack (eg strobe lighting; TV)? Triggers re different to provocations: most people would have a seizure given ufficient provocation; but most people do not have seizures however many riggers they are exposed to—so triggered seizures mean an underlying pilepsy disorder. Triggered attacks tend to recur.
o U&E/LFT, glucose, • Ca^{2+}, PO_4^{3-} • FBC; INR/PTT.
erum & urine alcohol and toxin screens.
lood levels of medications. • Consider LP if CT shows no ↑ICP.
naging: don't assume that if one CT scan is OK, there is no structural lesion. f epilepsy worsens, do MRI to find small areas of cortical dysgenesis, tumours, ascular malformations, and cavernomas (surgically correctable sporadic or nultiple congenital malformations presenting with fits ± haemorrhage).
EG is problematic (often false +ve). Don't do if the likely diagnosis is simple yncope. EEG cannot *of itself* exclude or refute epilepsy; it forms part of the ontext for diagnosis. It helps classification and prognosis: in 1st unprovoked eizures, unequivocal epileptiform activity on EEG helps assess risk of recur-ence. Only do *emergency* EEGs if nonconvulsive status is the problem, p477.
dmission for ~24h is indicated (in <10%) for investigations and observation eg for intractable seizures or to substantiate ideas of pseudoseizures, p484).
Irgent treatment may be needed if seizures recur.
iet prompt neurological help for diagnosis, and *individualized* counselling on mployment, and possible dangers, eg swimming alone. This is a difficult rea—so get help. You must give advice against driving and (in the UK) advise he patient to contact DVLA (p145). Document your discussion carefully.
uggest treatment eg if the risk of recurrence is high or high-ish—eg if nprovoked, or structural brain lesion, or status, or epileptiform EEG or post-eizure Todd's paresis (p704). Start eg with carbamazepine if it is a focal eizure (or lamotrigine, gabapentin, topiramate) or, if generalized, valproate or lamotrigine or topiramate).

Anti-epilepsy drugs (AEDs)

►Status: p808; children: OHCS

►***Involve patients in all decisions.*** Compliance depends on communicatio doctor–patient concordance issues (p3). Living with *active* epilepsy creates problems (eg inability to drive, or operate machinery) and fears (eg of su death), and drug issues. A problem is that UK neurologists have little time to ex these issues as each could have 1500 people with epilepsy on their books. general practice will only have ~50 patients, but GPs may have no special inter epilepsy. One option is a yearly visit to a GP- or hospital-based **epilepsy nur** monitor drugs, address employment, leisure, and reproductive issues; and, a few seizure-free years, to see if drugs can be carefully withdrawn (see BOX). T nurses are skilful: respect their role! For **investigating first seizures,** see p4

Therapy Treat with *one* drug and with *one* doctor in charge only. Slowly bui doses (over 2–3 months) until seizures are controlled, or toxic effects are mar or maximum drug dosage reached. Beware drug interactions (consult formu Most specialists would not recommend treatment after 1 fit but would treatment after 2. ►Discuss options with the patient. If your patient has only every 2yrs, he or she may accept the risk (particularly if there is no need to or operate machinery) rather than have to take drugs every day.

Generalized: Try **sodium valproate** as 1st-line, then **lamotrigine** (which ma more effective as well as being preferred by patients—but is newer; see Also use **sodium valproate** or **ethosuximide** for absence seizures.

Partial with or without secondary generalization: **Carbamazepine** is 1st then **sodium valproate**. Levetiracetam and topiramate are new 2nd-line age

Commonly used drugs ***Carbamazepine:*** Start with 100mg/12h PO; maxi dose: 800–1000mg/12h. A slow-release form is available, which is use intermittent side-effects experienced when dose peaks. Toxic effects: rash, na diplopia, dizziness, fluid retention, hyponatraemia, blood dyscrasias.

Sodium valproate: Start with 300mg/12h PO after food; max 30mg/kg (or 2 daily. The *BNF* suggests LFT & INR during the first 6 months of therapy (but hepatic failure is in those <3yrs old on multi-drug regimens). Toxic eff sedation, tremor, weight↑, hair thinning, ankle swelling, hyperammona (causing encephalopathy), liver failure. Drug levels are not helpful.

Phenytoin: Although effective and well-tried, it is not 1st line for generaliz partial epilepsy owing to toxicity: nystagmus, diplopia, tremor, dysarthria, ataxia intellect↓, depression, poor drive, polyneuropathy, acne, coarse facial features, hypertrophy, blood dyscrasias. Dosage is difficult, and needs blood levels (p7

Other drugs: Phenobarbital; benzodiazepines; newer agents (see BOX).

Changing drugs ***Indications:*** On inappropriate drug; side-effects unaccept treatment failure; pregnancy/lactation desired. ***Method:*** Begin the new drug a starting dose. At the same time, withdraw the old drug, eg over 6wks (soor toxicity: get help). Slowly ↑ new drug to middle of its dose range.

Enzyme-inducing AEDs & contraception Non-enzyme inducing AEDs (valpro gabapentin, lamotrigine, levetiracetam) have no effect on the Pill. In other AE carbamazepine, phenytoin, phenobarbital, primidone) ≥50μg of oestrogen ma needed (Norinyl-1®; ↓pill-free days from 7 to 4; use condoms too) or Depo-Prove dose interval is unchanged (12 weeks). The coil is suitable for emerge contraception, or levonorgestrel (1.5mg) ►followed by 1.5mg 12h later.

Pre-conception counselling & AEP is vital ∵ teratogenicity—*OHCS* p2/p29. Use dose folic acid supplements (5mg/day) preconception and during all trimeste

When it all goes wrong **Sudden unexpected death in epilepsy (SUDEP)** is r common in uncontrolled epilepsy, and may be related to seizure-associated ap at night. Those with epilepsy have a mortality rate 3-fold that of controls. > epilepsy-related deaths are recorded/yr in the UK; up to 17% are SUDEPs. For with families of those with SUDEP, contact *'Epilepsy Bereaved'*, UK01235 7728

Neurology

ıcontrolled epilepsy and new antiepileptic drugs (AEDs)

k a neurologist to help. Is the diagnosis of epilepsy correct? (bear in mind n-epileptic attack disorder, below). If it *is* epilepsy, does the AED match the izure type? Has the top dose been prescribed and taken? Has an underlying ructural or metabolic abnormality been excluded? Low-grade gliomas, for ample, may not show on initial MRI. Aim to use 1 drug only. If seizures are not ntrolled, switch to the 2nd most appropriate drug. Only consider maintenance 2 drugs if all appropriate drugs have been tried singly at their top dose.

wer AEDs NICE asserts they are 2nd-line, ie if valproate and carbamazepine are ntraindicated or problematic, eg: poor seizure control; fertile women; or drug eractions. They are often cost-effective (but costly, eg £100/month *vs* £12.[179]

motrigine is used as monotherapy and as an add-on for secondary neralized epilepsy (also useful in primary generalized epilepsy.) Monotherapy se: 25mg/24h PO for 14d, ↑ to 50mg daily for a further 14d, then ↑ by up to –100mg every 7–14d; usual maintenance as monotherapy, 50–100mg/12h. 00mg daily may be needed.) ►Halve monotherapy doses if already on proate; double if on carbamazepine or phenytoin. *SE:* Rash (may be serious; ›ically occurs in 1st 8wks, esp if valproate co-prescribed; warn patients to see doctor at once if rash or 'flu symptoms associated with hypersensitivity velop; do FBC; U&E; LFT; INR). Other SEs: fever; malaise; 'flu symptoms; drowsi-ss; LFT↑; photosensitivity; diplopia; vision↓; vomiting; aggression; tremor; agit-on. Interactions (*BNF*): anticonvulsants (above); antimalarials; antidepressants.

vetiracetam & ***topiramate*** are powerful new AEDs for 2dary generalized fits. vetiracetam dose: if >50kg, initially 500mg/12h PO, adjust by ≤1g every 2–4 eeks; max 1.5g/12h. SE: D&V, dyspepsia, depression, drowsiness, diplopia, WCC↓.

bapentin is a weak anticonvulsant (a clearer indication is pain syndromes).

nisamide is a new-generation, broad-spectrum benzisoxazole-derived ıtamate inhibitor*et al* used in partial seizures (± secondary generalizations).[180]

gabatrin: Only use in infantile spasms (∵ high incidence of visual field defects).

her new AEPs Tiagabine and pregabalin (also used in neuropathic pain).

n-epileptic attack disorder *(pseudo or psychogenic seizures)* These are t infrequent: suspect this if there are uncontrollable symptoms, no learning sabilities, and CNS exam, CT, MRI, and EEG are normal.[181]

opping anticonvulsants

iscuss risks and benefits with patients. Informed choices are vital. Most tients are seizure-free within a few years of starting drugs. More than 50% main so when drugs are withdrawn. After assessing risks and benefits for the ividual patient (eg the need to drive), withdrawal may be tried, if the patient eets these criteria: normal CNS examination, normal IQ, normal EEG prior to thdrawal, seizure-free for >2yrs, and no juvenile myoclonic epilepsy. In one ıdy (*N*=459), over 5yrs 52% remained seizure-free, compared with 67% ntinuing their medication.[182] However in another study, resuming medication l not return the patient to his/her status quo, and not all seizures could be ntrolled (risk factors: cognitive deficits and partial epilepsy).[183]

One way to withdraw drugs in adults is to ↓the dose by 10% every 2–4wks r carbamazepine, lamotrigine, phenytoin, valproate, and vigabatrin) and by % every 4–8wks for phenobarbital, benzodiazepines, and ethosuximide.[184]

Alternative MRC regimen		Decrease every 4 weeks by:	
Phenobarbital	30mg	Valproate	200mg
Phenytoin	50mg	Primidone	125mg
Carbamazepine	100mg	Ethosuximide	250mg

ving and jobs (p145). ***Epilepsy in pregnancy*** (*OHCS* p29).

Parkinson's disease (PD) and parkinsonism NICE 20

Parkinsonism is a syndrome of *tremor, rigidity, bradykinesis (slowness)*, and loss postural reflexes. *Prevalence*: 1 : 200 if >65yrs old.

- ***Tremor:*** 4–6Hz (cycles per sec). It is most marked at rest and coarser th cerebellar tremor. It is typically a 'pill rolling' of thumb over fingers.
- ***Rigidity:*** ↑Resistance to passive stretch of muscles throughout range movement (lead-pipe); tone may be broken-up by tremor (cogwheel rigidit Unlike in spasticity, rigidity is present equally in flexors and extensors.
- ***Bradykinesis:*** Slowness of movement initiation with progressive reductior speed and amplitude of repetitive actions; also monotonous speech dysarthria). Expressionless face. Dribbling. Short shuffling steps with flexed tru as if forever a step behind one's centre of gravity (*festinant gait*). Feet behave if frozen to the ground'. Peristalsis↓. Blink rate↓. Fidgeting↓. Micrographia.

Parkinson's disease is one cause of parkinsonism (due to degeneration substantia nigra dopaminergic neurones; the pathological hallmark is Lewy boc in this area, p478). Degeneration may be related to mitochondrial c dysfunction. It usually starts after 50, and becomes ever more common with a

Management: ►***Get help***. Forge a humanizing ***therapeutic alliance*** betw neurologist, physiotherapist, specialist nurse, GP, patient, and carer: see p4 ***Respite care*** is much valued by carers. Episodes of multidisciplinary ***rehabilitat*** improve mobility and morale. Formal exercises regulating posture and har onizing this with mental strength can help mobility—eg Chinese qigong.[RCT 187]

- ***Assess disability*** and cognition regularly and objectively (eg time how long walk 10 metres; can he/she dress alone, and turn over in bed?).
- ***Start drugs*** when PD seriously interferes with life (not too soon, as L-dopa's e ects wear off with time; explain this to patients; let him choose); use lowest d giving symptom relief, without bad SEs. Dopaminergic drugs (BOX), eg **L-do** Start at 50mg/12h PO (with food, to avoid nausea/vomiting).[188] Increase dose 100mg/8h, then slowly ↑ to 800mg/24h in divided doses. Give enough periphe dopa-decarboxylase inhibitor (≥25mg/100mg L-dopa). Balance better mobi with L-dopa's SEs, eg nausea & unwanted movements (seen after ~2yrs) ± ort static hypotension, arrhythmias, psychosis, and compulsions (sex, gambling, foc
- Over years, drugs may get less effective with switching between times exaggerated involuntary movement and of immobility ('***on–off***'); **slow-rele L-dopa** (see BOX) aims to help this (evidence is poor); once it occurs, it may irreversible: there is evidence that early use of dopaminergic agonists **ropinirole**, see BOX) may reduce this, and allow lower doses of L-dopa.
- **Anticholinergics/antimuscarinics** (orphenadrine 50mg/8h PO; max 400mg help motor symptoms. CI: Urinary retention, porphyria, angle-closure glaucor GI obstruction, prostatism. SE: Dry mouth, dizziness, vision↓, urinary retenti pulse↑, anxiety, confusion, excitement, hallucinations, insomnia, memory↓.
- **Modafinil** (100–200mg bd before noon; CI: BP↑) helps daytime sleepiness.

Neuropsychiatric complications These are seen in ~50%, and often represent interplay of the illness and drug SEs. ***Depression*** tricyclics and SSRIs (p13) may of help. Psychosis and dementia often complicate PD; get help, p374. Older ar psychotics worsen PD, so consider atypical antipsychotics, eg quetiapine or olanzap Cholinesterase inhibitors (rivastigmine; donepezil, p481) may help memory proble

Treating drug-induced parkinsonism It may be unwise to reduce or stop culprit drug (eg in schizophrenia where relapse could spell catastrophe), so adding in an antimuscarinic (eg **procyclidine** 2.5mg/8h PO).

Rare causes Parkinsonism isn't *always* due to Parkinson's disease or neurolep (antiemetics; haloperidol *et al*), so look for **'VODKA' signs:** vascular events elsewh (stroke, MI) ≈ vascular causes; orthostatic hypotension + atonic bladder ≈ mu system atrophy (=MSA, p494 ≈ Shy–Drager syndrome); dementia + vertical ga paralysis ≈ supranuclear palsy (=Steele–Richardson–Olszewski syndrome); Kays Fleisher ring ≈ Wilson's disease; apraxic gait ≈ communicating hydrocephalus.

ugs combining L-dopa and dopa-decarboxylase inhibitors

ade name	L-dopa content (mg)	Benserazide (mg)	Carbidopa (mg)
adopar 62.5®	50	12.5	
adopar 125®	100	25	
adopar CR® controlled release	100	25	
adopar 250®	200	50	
nemet 62.5®*	50		12.5
nemet 110®*	100		10
nemet 275®*	250		25
nemet Plus®	100		25
lf Sinemet CR®	100		25
nemet CR®	200		50

*The proportion of carbidopa may be suboptimal.[190]

nerics: Madopar® is co-beneldopa (1 part benserazide to 4 parts L-dopa). Sine-t® is co-careldopa (carbidopa with L-dopa); doses are expressed as co-careldopa /, where *x* and *y* are strengths in mg of carbidopa and L-dopa, respectively; eg nemet 275® = co-careldopa 25/250 = 25mg carbidopa + 250mg L-dopa.

opaminergic drugs

romocriptine: *Week 1:* 1.25mg at night PO with food. *Week 2:* 2.5mg at night. *'eek 3:* 2.5mg/12h. *Week 4:* 2.5mg/8h. ↑ by 2.5mg/d at weekly intervals to ≤5 × 5mg/8h. SE: Hallucinations, BP↓, constipation, drowsiness, fibrosis.

ewer agents Ropinirole & **pramipexole** (dopamine D_3 agonist) are better lerated than L-dopa, and dosing is easier. They may be 1st-choice in younger atients to ↓risk of dyskinesias (and at any age as an adjunct to L-dopa). Claims at ropinirole ↓rate of loss of dopaminergic neurones compared with L-dopa ise from a one unreplicated PET study.[191] ***Ropinirole dose:*** eg 250µg/8h PO creased by small weekly increments to 3mg/8h if needed; tabs are 250µg, 1mg, ng, & 5mg. SE: drowsiness; nausea; hallucinations (17%).

ubcutaneous apomorphine (an injectable D_1 and D_2 dopamine agonist) may elp patients with severe on–off effects. Injections or continuous infusion may be quired. Liaise with a special PD centre.[192]

: the ergot-related agonists (pergolide, bromocriptine, and cabergoline) are eing used less owing to pleural and cardiac valve fibrosis.

ntacapone: This decreases peripheral L-dopa metabolism by catechol-O-ethyltransferase (COMT) inhibition. It may lessen the 'off' time in those with earing off effects. SE: red-brown urine, dyskinesia, nausea, vomiting, orthostatic ypotension, sleep disorders, hallucinations, dry mouth, Hb↓, LFT↑.[193]

urgery for PD • Destructive procedures interrupting overactive basal ganglia rcuits (eg subthalamic nuclei) by surgical lesions or deep-brain stimulation 460) are being tried in specialist centres in those inadequately controlled by ugs. • **Neural transplants**[1] with stem cells or dopaminergic neuroblasts from e brains aborted fetuses and **gene therapy** may be future (problematic) otions. MAOI-B inhibitors, eg **selegiline**, don't delay progression but may help otor fluctuations;[194] they have serious SEs (postural hypotension; AF).[195]

'wo placebo-controlled trials were disappointing: we have yet to resolve graft survival problems.
ther option is continuous infusion of glial cell line-derived neurotrophic factor into the putamen.

Multiple sclerosis (MS)

This relapsing/remitting disorder consists of plaques of demyelination (and a loss) at sites throughout the CNS (but not peripheral nerves). Pathogenesis invo focal disruption of the blood–brain barrier and associated immune response myelin damage—as well as axonal/neuronal neurodegenerative processes.[1]

Epidemiology Commoner in temperate areas (prevalence is very variable: Eng ≥42/100,000; SE Scotland 200/100,000; rarer in Black Africa and Asia). Life UK risk: ~1 : 1000. Adult travellers take their risk with them; children acquire risk of where they settle. ♀:♂≈2:1; mean age of onset is 30yrs.

Poor prognostic signs: Older males; motor signs at onset; many relapses early many MRI lesions.

Presentation is usually monosymptomatic: unilateral optic neuritis (pain on movement and rapid deterioration in central vision); numbness or tingling in limbs; leg weakness or brainstem or cerebellar symptoms such as diplopi ataxia. Less often there may be more than 1 symptom. Other signs: see Symptoms may worsen with heat (eg a hot bath) or exercise.

Progression/prognosis: Early on, relapses (which can be stress induced) ma followed by remission/full recovery. With time, remissions are incomplete disability accumulates. Steady progression of disability from the outset also occ while some patients experience no progressive disablement at all.

Examination Look carefully for deficits other than the presenting problem (E

Diagnosis This is clinical, requiring demonstration of lesions dissemin in time and space, unattributable to other causes. Isolated CNS deficits are n diagnostic, but may become so if a careful history reveals previous episodes unexplained blindness for a week. *The role of* MRI: See BOX.

Tests None is pathognomonic. ***CSF:*** up to 50 lymphocytes/mm³, protein ≤1g, oligoclonal bands of IgG on electrophoresis. Delayed visual, auditory, somatosensory ***evoked potentials. MRI*** is sensitive but not specific for pla detection and may exclude other causes, eg cord compression. Correlation of with clinical condition is poor. ***Antibodies to myelin oligodendro glycoprotein*** (MOG) and ***myelin basic protein*** (MBP) in those with a single MS clinical lesion can predict time to conversion to definite MS.

Treatment ***Methylprednisolone*** 1g/24h IV/PO for 3d shortens relapses; sparingly (≤ ×2/yr, ∵ steroid SEs, p361). It does not alter the overall prognos

Immuno-modulation with interferon (INF-1β; INF-1α) Trials show that these ↓relapses by ~30% in active relapsing-remitting MS (RRMS); they also ↓le accumulation on MRI. Their power to ↓disability is modest, as is their role in sec ary and primary progressive (SP & PP) MS. Licensed for use by neurologists, they expensive (eg ~£200/wk; €0.4–1.3×10⁶/QALY; 20×more expensive than **azathiopr** which may be just as good). SE: flu-like symptoms, depression, abortion depression, LFT↑, pregnancy, uncontrolled epilepsy. The UK DOH, the Assocⁿ of Br Neurologists, and the drug industry are making INF more available accordin agreed criteria and effectiveness monitoring. ***Glatiramer*** is a similar alterna There is no good, safe preventive treatment for those with primary progressive M

2nd-line drugs: **Alemtuzumab** (Campath-1H®; T-cell killing monoclonal antibo **Mitoxantrone** (doxorubicin analogue) ?helps in 2ᵈʳʸ progressive MS; safety is an is

Palliation: ►Help to live well with disability. ***Spasticity***: Start all drugs at a dose, and build up at weekly intervals. **Baclofen** 5–25mg/8h PO; **diazepam** 5 8–24h PO (addictive); **dantrolene** 25mg/24h (max 100mg/6h); **tizani** 2mg/24h PO; ↑at intervals of >3d in steps of 1mg/12h (max 9mg/6h). Intrath baclofen, phenol nerve block, botulinum toxin, and cannabis are less evidence-ba ***Urgency/frequency:*** If post-micturition residual urine >100mL teach intermit selfcatheterization; if <100mL, try **oxybutynin** 2.5mg/8h or **tolterodine**.

1 Simon JH *Radiol Clin North Am* 2006 44 79 (This paper discusses quantitative MRI technique

Clinical features of multiple sclerosis

Sensory:	dysaesthesia[1]	• GI: swallowing disorders; constipation.
	pins and needles	• Diplopia; hemianopia; optic neuritis;[2] nystagmus
	vibration sense↓	in the abducting eye on lateral gaze.[3] Pupil
	trigeminal neuralgia	defects[4] and visual defects (eg on exercise).[2]
Motor:	spastic weakness	• Cerebellum: truncal or limb ataxia; intention
	Hyperreflexia	tremor; scanning (ie monotonous) speech.
Cord:	transverse myelitis[5]	• Fatigue; cognition↓; memory↓; cognition↓.
	urgency; retention	• Depression (avoid ECT); mania; odd laughter p498
	erectile dysfunction	• Cranial nerve lesions; epilepsy; aphasia—all rare.

Proposed McDonald criteria for diagnosing MS

Warning: these criteria are provisional: it is likely that they err on the side of according too much weight to MRI: ►when in doubt, pay more attention to clinical signs.

Clinical presentation	Additional data needed
2 or more attacks (relapses) with 2 or more objective clinical lesions	None; clinical evidence will do; imaging evidence desirable; must conform to MS
2 or more attacks with 1 objective clinical lesion	Typical disseminated lesions on MRI • **or** +ve CSF **and** ≥2 MRI lesions consistent with MS • **or** 2nd attack at a new site
1 attack with 2 or more objective clinical lesions	Dissemination in time, shown by • MRI **or** 2nd clinical attack
1 attack with 1 objective clinical lesion (monosymptomatic presentation)	Dissemination in space: • MRI **or** +ve CSF if ≥2 MRI lesions consistent with MS • **and** dissemination in time shown by MRI **or** 2nd clinical attack[3]
Insidious neurological progression suggestive of MS (primary progressive MS)	+ve CSF **and** dissemination in space, ie: • MRI evidence of ≥9 T2 brain lesions • **or** 2 or more cord lesions • **or** 4–8 brain and 1 cord lesion • **or** +ve visual evoked potential (VEP) with 4–8 MRI lesions • **or** +ve VEP + <4 brain lesions + 1 cord lesion **and** dissemination in time seen on MRI • **or** continued progression for ≥1yr

Attacks: These must last >1h, eg motor weakness etc., see. BOX above.

Time between attacks: 30 days. ***MRI abnormality:*** 3 out of 4:
Gadolinium-enhancing **or** ≥9 T2 hyperintense lesions if no Gd-enhancing lesion
1 or more infratentorial lesions • **or** 1 or more juxtacortical lesions
≥3 periventricular lesions (1 spinal cord lesion = 1 brain lesion)

CSF: Oligoclonal IgG bands in CSF (and not serum) or ↑IgG index.

Evoked potentials: (EP) This counts if delayed but well-preserved waveform.

What provides MRI evidence of dissemination in time? A Gd-enhancing lesion demonstrated in a scan done at least 3 months following onset of clinical attack at a site different from attack, **or**
in absence of Gd-enhancing lesions at a 3-month scan, follow-up scan after an additional 3 months showing Gd-lesion or new T2 lesion.

1 In **Lhermitte's sign**, neck flexion causes 'electric shocks' in trunk/limbs also +ve in spondylosis & B_{12}↓
2 Optic neuritis symptoms: • Acuity↓ • Phosphenes (flashes) on eye movement • **Uhthoff's phenomenon** vision worsens on exercise, eating a hot meal, or in hot baths) • The **Pulfrich effect** (latencies between eyes are unequal, causing disorientation, eg in moving traffic as straight trajectories seem curved).
3 In internuclear ophthalmoplegia (a classic MS lesion) a lesion in the median longitudinal fasciculus causes weakness in adduction of the ipsilateral eye with nystagmus on abducting the contralateral eye.
4 Efferent or afferent defect (p68; ie poor response to light ∴ bigger); an **Argyle Robertson**-type pupil is rarer (p70; ΔΔ: syphilis, DM, MS or sarcoidosis—lesion in or near the **Edinger–Westphal** nucleus).
5 Loss of motor, sensory, autonomic, reflex, and sphincter function below the level of a lesion indicates transverse myelitis. **Devic's syndrome** is an MS variant of transverse myelitis with optic atrophy, p690.

Space-occupying lesions

Signs Features of ↑intracranial pressure, evolving focal neurology, seizures, fa localizing signs, cognitive or behavioural change, local effects (eg propto epistaxis). ***Raised ICP*** (p812): Headache (p448), vomiting, papilloedema (only 50% of tumours), altered consciousness. ***Seizures:*** Seen in ≤50% of tumou Suspect in all adult-onset seizures, especially if focal, or with a localizing aura post-ictal weakness (Todd's palsy, p704). ***Evolving focal neurology:*** Depends the site (see BOX for localizing signs). Ask first ***where*** the mass is then ***what it*** Frontal lobe, midline, and non-dominant temporal lobe masses present late. ***Fa localizing signs:*** These are caused by ↑ICP. VI nerve palsy is commonest (p44; c to its long intracranial course). ***Subtle personality change:*** Irritability, lack application to tasks, lack of initiative, socially inappropriate behaviour.

Causes Tumour (primary or secondary), aneurysm, abscess (25% multiple); chro subdural haematoma, granuloma p179 eg tuberculoma), cyst (eg cysticercos ***Histology:*** 30% secondaries (breast, lung, melanoma). Primaries: astrocytor glioblastoma multiforme (case–control studies now show probably *not* associa with mobile phone use 2006 data), oligodendroglioma, ependymoma (all <50% 5 survival), primary CNS lymphoma (eg as non-infectious manifestation of HI cerebellar haemangioblastoma (40% 20yr survival); meningioma (♀:♂≈2:1).

ΔΔ: Stroke, head injury, vasculitis (p542), eg SLE, syphilis, PAN, giant cell arteri MS, encephalitis, post-ictal (Todd's palsy, p704), metabolic, or U&E disturbance. A colloid cyst of the 3rd ventricle and benign intracranial hypertension (see belo

Tests CT; MRI (good for posterior fossa masses). Consider biopsy. Avoid LP (ri coning, ie cerebellar tonsils herniate through the foramen magnum).

Tumour management *Benign:* Removal if possible but some may be inaccessil *Malignant*: **Excision** of gliomas is hard as resection margins are rarely clear, b surgery does give a tissue diagnosis, it debulks pre-radiotherapy, and make cavity for inserting **carmustine wafers** RCT 208 (may cause serious cerebral oedema) If a tumour is inaccessible but causing hydrocephalus, a **ventriculo-periton shunt** can help. **Chemo-radiotherapy** is used post-op for gliomas or metastas and as sole therapy if surgery is impossible. Oligodendroglioma with 1p/1 deletions are especially sensitive. In glioblastoma, **temozolomide** (a new alkylat agent) ↑survival (benefit is mainly if tumours have methylated methylguan methyltransferase gene promoters and are thus unable to repair chemothera induced DNA damage). Prophylaxis for epilepsy is important, but often fails. Tre headache (eg **codeine** 60mg/4h PO). Cerebral oedema: **dexamethasone** 4mg/8h **mannitol** if ↑ICP acutely, p812. Plan meticulous palliative treatment (p520).

Prognosis Poor but improving in gliomas; benign tumours are curable by excisi

Third ventricle colloid cysts These congenital cysts declare themselves in ad life with amnesia, headache (often positional), obtundation (blunted consciousne incontinence, dim vision, bilateral paraesthesiae, weak legs, and drop attac ***Tests:*** CT scan/MRI. ***Treatment:*** Excision or ventriculo-peritoneal shunting.

Benign intracranial hypertension *(pseudotumor cerebri)* Think of this in the presenting as if with a mass (headache, ↑ICP and papilloedema)—*when none found.* Typical patients are obese women with blurred vision ± diplopia, VI ne palsy, and an enlarged blind spot, if papilloedema is present (it usually Consciousness and cognition are preserved. ***Cause:*** Often unknown, or secondary venous sinus thrombosis, or drugs, eg tetracycline, minocycline, nitrofurant vitamin A, isotretinoin, danazol, and somatropin.

R: Weight loss, acetazolamide, loop diuretics, and prednisolone (start at ~40mg/2 PO; more SE than diuretics) *may* reverse papilloedema. Consider optic nerve she fenestration or lumbar–peritoneal shunt if drugs fail and visual loss worsens.

Prognosis: Often self-limiting. Permanent significant visual loss in 10% (ie not benign). CSF shunting or optic nerve sheath fenestration can help vision.

Neurology

emporal lobe Remember the 'HAPPY-CLAPPY DJ' to remind you of excessive ligiosity, music-induced seizures, and states of surreal happiness and out-of-ody experiences which sometimes accompany temporal lobe lesions or auras temporal lobe epilepsy. The mnemonic stands for mostly less exotic features: emianopia (or upper quadrantanopia); automatisms (below); psychosis (delusns ± hallucinations of smell, taste, sound, eg repeating echoes, ie palinacousis); ecognition/persience (a sense of knowing what is about to happen); 'yells and lls to the floor' type of seizure or complex partial seizures; language disorders g dysphasia); amnesia; panic (or rage, or paroxysmal hypersexuality); pains—eg odominal pain (± ictal vomiting; or episodic fevers or D&V); you find ourself not believing your patient's bizarre story—examples are "canned music Tesco's always makes me cry and then pass out, unless I wear an earplug in e ear" or "I get orgasms when I brush my teeth" (right temporal lobe yper- and hypo-perfusion, respectively). Finally there are odd experiences ich as *déjà vu* (everything is familiar); *jamais vu* (everything is alien).

Automatisms are complex motor phenomena—eg oral (lip smacking; ewing; spitting; singing; kissing), or genital (repeated fondling, grabbing, or ratching)—or more complex and sometimes violent acts (homicide; arson). atients do not remember their automatisms after doing them.

ontal lobe Hemiparesis focal **motor seizures**, eg aversive seizures involving ead and eyes; **personality change** (indecent; indolent; indiscreet; facetious d a tendency to pun); **grasp reflex** (fingers drawn across palm are grasped) gnificant only if unilateral; **Broca's dysphasia**, p46, or more subtle difficulty ith initiating and planning speech with intact repetition and no anomia—but ss of coherence; also general lack of drive or initiative; loss of smell unilaterally. **oncrete thinking; perseveration** ± ↓verbal fluency—eg unable to switch from e line of thinking to another or to list words beginning with '*P*' (normal is ~15 in min). **Orbitofrontal syndrome:** Lack of empathy; disinhibition; ↓social skills; ver-eating; rash actions (mania); over-familiar; unconscious imitation of postures g when you put your feet on the desk, or sit on the floor); **'utilization behaviour'** whatever is provided is used, eg hand the patient spectacles, and he puts them , hand him another pair, and this goes on his nose too, ditto for a 3rd pair).

arietal lobe Hemisensory loss ↓2-point discrimination; **astereognosis** ability to recognize object in hand by touch alone); **sensory inattention**; **ysphasia** (p46); **Gerstmann's syndrome** (left–right disorientation etc, p692).

ccipital lobe Contralateral **visual field defects** (homonymous hemianopia); allucinations, eg **palinopsia** (persisting or recurring images, once the stimulus as left the field of view; Greek: *palin*=again). **Polyopia** is seeing multiple images.

erebellum ('DASHING') **dysdiadochokinesis**; **ataxia** (limb/truncal); **slurred speech**; **ypotonia**; **intention tremor**; **nystagmus**; **gait abnormality**. Dysdiadochokinesis impaired *rapidly alternating* movements, eg pronation–supination. NB: If uncal ataxia is worse on eye closure, blame the dorsal columns, not cerebellum.

erebellopontine angle (eg acoustic neuroma ie vestibular schwannoma) Ipsiteral **deafness**; **nystagmus**; **↓corneal reflex**, **facial weakness (rare)**; ipsilateral **erebellar signs** (above), **papilloedema**, **VI nerve palsy** (lateral rectus, p44).

orpus callosum (a rare site for lesions) Usually severe rapid **intellectual eterioration** with focal signs of adjacent lobes; signs of **loss of communication etween lobes** (eg left hand unable to carry out verbal commands).

idbrain (eg pineal tumours or midbrain infarction) **Failure of up or down gaze**; **ght/near dissociated pupil responses** (p68), with convergence globe-etracting **nystagmus** from co-contraction of opposing horizontal muscles, on ttempted up-gaze. Elicited by looking at a down-moving target. video link

Neurology

Bell's palsy (idiopathic facial nerve palsy)

Bell's palsy is partly a diagnosis of exclusion, but features distinguish it from facial palsy from other causes (BOX) are: abrupt onset (typically overnight or after a nap); complete unilateral facial weakness at 24 to 72h; ipsilateral numbness or pain around the ear; ↓taste (ageusia); hypersensitivity to sounds (ie hyperacusis from stapedius palsy).

Incidence 15–40/100,000/yr (~1 patient/2yrs/GP); risk ↑ in pregnancy (×3) & diabetes (×5). ♂:♀≈1:1

Other symptoms of VII palsy (from any cause)

- Unilateral sagging of the mouth (it is drawn towards the normal side on smiling, producing a grimace).
- Food trapped between gum & cheek; saliva leaks out.
- Speech difficulty because of adynamic lips.
- Failure of eye closure may cause a watery or dry eye, ectropion (sagging and turning-out of the lower lid), conjunctivitis, or injury from foreign bodies.

Ask the patient to wrinkle up the forehead and close the eyes forcefully; test buccinator by whistling/blowing out the cheeks (*buccina* is Latin for trumpet). Look for other cranial neuropathies (seen in 8%, eg V, XII).

Prognosis If **incomplete paralysis** and no axonal degeneration complete recovery in a few weeks is typical. If **complete paralysis** nearly all recover too (almost fully) but ~15% have axonal degeneration and recovery starts eg after 3 months, and may be complicated by aberrant reconne ions producing ***synkinesis***, eg eye blinking causes synchronous upturning the mouth. Misconnection of parasympathetic fibres (red in fig 1) can produ ***crocodile tears*** (gusto-lacrimal reflex) when eating stimulates unilate lacrimation, not salivation (intra-lacrimal gland botulinum toxin may help).

Causes of facial palsy
Bell's palsy (75% of cas
Ramsay Hunt syn: look for ear/ear-drum vesic les (herpes zoster otic
Lyme disease
Meningitis (eg fungal)
TB; viruses (HIV; polio)
Mycoplasma (rare)
Brainstem lesions
Stroke; tumour; MS
Cerebello-pontine an
Acoustic neuroma (p45
Meningioma
Systemic disease
Diabetes mellitus
Sarcoidosis
Guillain–Barré syn (ofte gives bilateral VII pals
ENT and other causes
Orofacial granulomatos
Parotid tumours
Cholesteatoma
Otitis media
Trauma to skull base
Diving (barotrauma+ten oral bone pneumocele)
Intracranial hypotension

Tests *Electroneurography* at 2 wks predicts delayed recovery by showing axo degeneration but doesn't influence treatment. ***Serology*** may show a 4-fold ↑ antibody to varicella zoster virus. ***MRI + LP*** to explore other diagnoses 'is only need in atypical presentations' experts say, but this misses some Lyme disease cases

Management If seen within 6d of onset, prednisolone (~50mg/24h PO for 5 10mg/day for 5 more days) may prevent weakness becoming paralysis ↓nerve oedema.[1] Evidence for prednisolone is not universally acknowledged. Many 'Bell's cases' are now thought to be due to herpes viruses, and some stud (with flaws) support antivirals (aciclovir or valaciclovir) + prednisolone. No has shown actively replicating virus, which may be why results are equivocal.

- Protect the eye with dark glasses and by instilling artificial tears (eg hyp mellose) if there is any evidence of drying.
- Encourage regular eyelid closure by pulling down the lid by hand.
- Use tape to close the eyes at night.
- If ectropion is severe, lateral tarsorrhaphy (partial lid-to-lid suturing) can help.

If no recovery in 1yr, plastic surgery to help lid closure and to straighten t drooping face can be tried. Botulinum toxin can augment facial symmetry, a hence self-esteem (beauty ***is*** symmetry according to Greek ideals—and *Vogue*)

In pregnancy, prognosis is worse if the palsy is complete (50% do badly 20% if non-pregnant). No advice on use of steroids is universally agreed.

1 Many neurologists give steroids 'to reduce oedema in the nerve', particularly if seen within 6d of on One helpful study—Shafshak T 1994 *J Laryng & Otol* **108** 940 showed that the extra benefit of sterc may be confined to those treated within 24h of onset. Spontaneous recovery is good in any case (85 NNT=3. Older randomized studies have been inconclusive, but did not look specifically at early treatm Older meta-analyses favour steroids (E-BM 1997 2 79) but not newer ones (Cochrane 2004).

Neurology

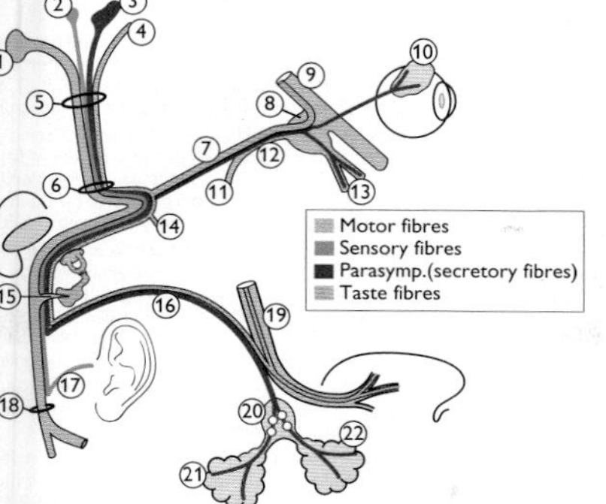

ɟ 1. Facial nerve branches. After Baylor College of Medicine www.bcm.edu/oto/studs/face.html

e motor part supplies moves the muscles of the face, scalp, and ears—also ccinator (puffs out the cheeks), and platysma, the stapedius, and the posterior ıly of the digastricus. It also contains the sympathetic motor fibres (vasodilator) the submaxillary and sublingual glands (via the chorda tympani nerve). The ısory part contains the fibres of taste for the anterior ⅔ of the tongue and a few natic sensory fibres from the middle ear region.

Facial nerve (VII) nucleus, deep in the reticular formation of lower pons
Spinal nucleus of V
Superior salivary nucleus
Solitary tract
Porus acusticus internus
Meatal foramen
Large petrosal nerve
8 Sphenopalatine ganglion
9 Superior maxillary nerve
10 Lacrimal gland
11 Large deep petrosal nerve
12 Vidian nerve
13 Nose & palate gland nerves
14 Small petrosal nerve at geniculate ganglion 249
15 Stapedial nerve
16 Chorda tympani
17 Auricular branch
18 Stylomastoid foramen
19 Lingual nerve—visceral motor[vii] & taste[vii] & general sensory to tongue (v^3) 250
20 Submandibular ganglion
21 Submandibular gland
22 Sublingual gland

Mononeuropathies

These are lesions of individual, including cranial, nerves. Trauma and entrapm are the main causes. *Others*: leprosy; DM. If ≥2 peripheral nerves are affected, term ***mononeuritis multiplex*** is used (causes: 'WARDS PLC': Wegener's (p706), AI amyloid, rheumatoid, diabetes mellitus, sarcoidosis, PAN, leprosy, carcinomatos

Median nerve C6–T1 ***At the wrist***: (eg lacerations; carpal tunnel syndrome— BOX) Weakness of abductor pollicis brevis and sensory loss over the radial fingers and palm. Lesions confined to the anterior interosseous nerve (neura amyotrophy;[1] trauma): weakness of flexion of the distal phalanx of the thumb index finger. ***Proximal lesions*** (eg at the elbow) may show combined defects.

Ulnar nerve C7–T1 Vulnerable to elbow trauma; ***Signs:*** Weakness/wasting of me (ulnar side) wrist flexors; weakness/wasting of the interossei (cannot cross the fi ers in the good luck sign) and medial 2 lumbricals (claw hand); hypothenar emine wasting (∴ weak little finger abduction) and sensory loss over medial 1½ fingers ulnar side of the hand. Flexion of 4th & 5th DIP joints is weak. Treatment: see With lesions at the wrist (digitorum profundus intact), claw hand is more mar

Radial nerve C5–T1 This nerve opens the fist. Damaged by compression agai the humerus. Test for wrist and finger drop with elbow flexed and arm pronat Sensory loss: variable; test dorsal aspect of root of thumb.

Sciatic nerve L4–S2 Damaged by pelvic tumours or fractures to pelvis or fe Lesions affect the hamstrings and all muscles below the knee (foot drop), with l of sensation below the knee laterally. **Common peroneal nerve L4–S2** Of damaged as it winds round the fibular head (trauma; sitting cross-legged). *Sig* foot drop + weak ankle dorsiflexion/eversion, and sensory loss over dorsum of f

Tibial nerve S1–3 Lesions lead to an inability to stand on tiptoe (plantarflexi invert the foot, or flex the toes. Sensory loss over the sole.

Autonomic neuropathy (sympathetic[S] & parasympathetic[P]

This may be isolated or part of a generalized sensory motor peripheral neuropa

Causes DM; amyloid; Guillian–Barré; HIV; leprosy; SLE; paraneoplastic; to genetic.

Signs Postural hypotension[S] (faints on standing, eating, or hot bath); erectile d function[P]/ejaculatory failure[S] (remember 'point & shoot'); sweating↓[S]; constipati nocturnal diarrhoea; urine retention[P]; Horner's[S] (p694); Holmes–Adie pupil[P] (p70

Autonomic function tests Postural drop of ≥20/10mmHg is abnormal (p68
- A variation of <10bpm with respiration is abnormal (do resting ECG).
- Bladder pressure studies (*cystometry*). • *Pupils*: Instil 0.1% epinephrine (dilat post-ganglionic sympathetic denervation, not if normal); 2.5% cocaine (dilat normal; not if sympathetic denervation); 2.5% methacholine (constrict parasympathetic lesion). These are rarely used.
- Antibodies: anti-HU & anti-nicotinic acetylcholine receptor antibodies may be

Primary autonomic failure Occurs alone, as part of MSA[2] or with parkinsoni Typical patient: middle-aged/elderly man. Onset: insidious (symptoms as abo

Treating postural hypotension Compression stockings; "stand slowly". Head-up of the bed at night ↑renin release, so ↓fluid loss and ↑standing BP. If post-pran dizziness, advise eating little and often, and to ↓carbohydrate & alcohol intake. Fl retaining drugs (fludrocortisone 0.1mg/24h PO, ↑ as needed) for severe disea

1 Brachial plexus neuropathy (eg after an infection or an immunization into deltoid) causes pain weakness (may involve the diaphragm). It resolves over months.

2 **Multisystem atrophy** is parkinsonism (p486) + autonomic dysfunction + cerebellar ataxia (refle olivopontocerebellar atrophy) ± dystonia, rhythmic myoclonus, emotional incontinence, sleep disturb sleep-related movement problems, and vasomotor signs. Extra-pyramidal symptoms may pre autonomic failure. MSA may be unmasked by a sudden worsening of mild postural hypotension w presumed classical Parkinson's is treated with L-dopa. Survival: rarely >10yrs after diagnosis of M

:arpal tunnel syndrome: the commonest mononeuropathy

tendons and the median nerve compete for space within the wrist. Compres-ion is common, especially in women who have narrower wrists but similar-sized endons to men; for similar reasons, the tibial nerve may be compressed: the tarsal unnel syndrome, causing unilateral burning sole pain, eg on walking or standing.

'he patient: Aching pain in the hand and arm (especially at night), and araesthesiae in thumb, index, and middle fingers, all relieved by dangling the and over the edge of the bed and shaking it. There may be sensory loss and veakness of abductor pollicis brevis ± wasting of the thenar eminence. Light ouch, 2-point discrimination, and sweating may be impaired. ***Associations:*** 'regnancy, rheumatoid, DM, hypothyroidism, acromegaly, dialysis, trauma.

'ests: Neurophysiology helps by confirming the lesion's site and severity (and kelihood of improvement after surgery). Maximal wrist flexion for 1min Phalen's test) may elicit symptoms (unreliable!). Tapping over the nerve at the vrist induces tingling (Tinel's test; also rather non-specific).

'reatment: Splinting, local steroid injection (*OHCS* p710) ± decompression urgery; many alternative therapies are tried: meta-analyses are doubtful.[1]

1anaging ulnar mononeuropathies from entrapments

he ulnar nerve 'asks for trouble' in at least 5 places around the elbow, eginning proximally at the arcade of Struthers (a musculofascial band ~8cm roximal to the medial epicondyle) and ending distally where it exits the flexor arpi ulnaris muscle in the forearm. Most commonly compression occurs at the picondylar groove or at the point where the nerve passes between the 2 heads f the flexor carpi ulnaris muscle (true ***cubital tunnel syndrome***). Trauma can asily damage the nerve against its bony confines (the medial condyle of the umerus—the 'funny bone'). Normally, the ulnar nerve suffers stretch and ompression forces at the elbow that are moderated by its ability to glide in its roove. When normal excursion is restricted, irritation ensues. This may cause a icious cycle of perineural scarring, consequent loss of excursion, and rogressive symptoms—without there being any antecedent trauma.

Rest and avoiding pressure on the nerve helps but if symptoms continue, ight-time soft elbow splinting (to prevent flexion to >60°) is warranted, eg or 6 months. For chronic neuropathy associated with weakness, or if splinting ails, a variety of surgical procedures have been tried. For moderately severe europathies, decompressions *in situ* may help, but often fail. Medial picondylectomies are effective in ≤50% (but many will recur). Subcutaneous erve re-routing (transposition) may be tried. Intramuscular and submuscular ransposition are more complicated, but the latter may be preferable.

Compressive ulnar neuropathies at the wrist (***Guyon's canal***—between the isiform and hamate bones) are less common, but they can also result in isability. ***Thoracic outlet compression*** is another cause of a weak numb hand. lectromyography (EMG) helps define the anatomic site of lesions.

Cochrane meta-analysis of 21 carpal tunnel trials: 7 (but not 2) weeks' ultrasound can help. Compared to cebo, diuretics & NSAIDs gave no benefit. Vit. B6 did not help (N = 50). Those adopting the namaste ayer) posture in yoga may obviate need for surgery: the forced wrist extension helps (N = 53). Trials of onomic keyboards give equivocal results for pain and function. Trials of magnet therapy, laser ıpuncture, and exercise showed no benefit. Chiropractic care can increase distress.

Polyneuropathies

Polyneuropathies are generalized disorders of peripheral nerves or cranial nerves whose distribution is usually bilaterally symmetrical and widespread often with distal muscle weakness and sensory loss ('glove & stocking anaesthesia'). They may be classified by time course (acute or chronic); by the functions disturbed (motor, sensory, autonomic, mixed); or by the underlying pathology (demyelination, axonal degeneration, or both). Guillain–Barré syndrome (p694), eg, is an acute, predominantly motor, demyelinating neuropathy, whereas chronic alcohol abuse leads to a chronic, initially sensory then mixed, axonal neuropathy.

Mostly motor	**Mostly sensory**
Guillain–Barré syndrome, p694	Diabetes mellitus
Lead poisoning	Uraemia
Charcot–Marie–Tooth syndrome	Leprosy

Symptoms ***Sensory neuropathy:*** Numbness; 'feels funny'; tingling or burning sensations eg affecting the extremities first ('glove & stocking' distribution). There may be difficulty handling small objects such as needles. ***Motor neuropathy:*** Often progressive (may be rapid) weakness or clumsiness of the hands; difficulty walking (falls; stumbling); respiratory difficulty. Signs are of LMN lesion: wasting and weakness most marked in the distal muscles of hands and feet (foot or wrist drop). Reflexes are reduced or absent. Involvement of the respiratory muscles may be shown by a falling vital capacity. ***Cranial nerves:*** Swallowing/speaking difficulty; diplopia. ***Autonomic neuropathy:*** See p494.

Diagnosis The history is vital; be clear about the illness's time course; the precise nature of the symptoms; any preceding or associated events (eg *Campylobacter* D&V before Guillain–Barré syndrome; weight↓ in cancer; arthralgia from a connective tissue disease); travel; sexual infections; alcohol and drug use; family history. Pain is typical eg neuropathy from DM or alcohol. ***Examination:*** Do a careful neurologic examination looking for lower motor signs (weakness, wasting, reduced/abse reflexes) and sensory loss (map out for each modality). Test the autonomic syste (p494) and cranial nerves (p44). Look for signs of trauma (eg finger burr indicating ↓sensation. Scuff marks on shoes suggest foot drop. If there is ner thickening think of leprosy or Charcot–Marie–Tooth. Examine other systems f clues to the cause, eg alcoholic liver disease.

Tests FBC, ESR, glucose, U&E, LFT, TSH, B_{12}, electrophoresis, ANCA (p539), ANA, C› urinalysis, and consider an LP ± specific genetic tests for inherited neuropathies (‹ Charcot–Marie–Tooth, p688), lead levels, and antiganglioside antibodies. Ner conduction studies help distinguish demyelinating from axonal neuropathies.

Treatment Treat causes. Involve **physio** & OT (p437). **Foot care** and **shoe choice** important in sensory neuropathies to minimize trauma. In Guillain–Barré (p694) CIDP,[1] IV **immunoglobulin** helps. **Steroids**/immunosuppressants may help vasculi causes. **Amitriptyline** ≥10mg PO at night may help neuropathic pain (NNT≈2; may n work in HIV neuropathy). If this fails, try **gabapentin**[2] (NNT≈3) or **pregabalin.**

Typical causes

Metabolic
Diabetes mellitus,
Renal failure,
Hypothyroidism,
Hypoglycaemia,
Mitochondrial disorders

Vasculitides (p542)
Polyarteritis nodosa,
Rheumatoid arthritis,
Wegener's granulomatos

Malignancy
Paraneoplastic syndrom
Polycythaemia rubra vera p3

Inflammatory
Guillain–Barré synd. CID
Sarcoidosis

Infections HIV
Leprosy Syphilis
Lyme disease (p418),

Vitamin pathologies
Lack of B_1, B_6, B_{12} (eg alcoholic), folate
Excess vit B_6 (>100mg/

Inherited syndromes
Refsum's (p702)
Charcot–Marie–Tooth, p6
Porphyria (p684)
Leukodystrophy *et al*

Toxins Lead; arsenic

Drugs Vincristine
Alcohol Cisplatin
Isoniazid Nitrofurantoi
Phenytoin Metronidazol

Others
Paraproteinaemias
Amyloidosis (p354)

1 Chronic inflammatory demyelinating polyradiculoneuropathy is an autoimmune demyelinating disea of peripheral nerves. Signs: weakness & sensory loss in limbs; peripheral nerve enlargement. CSF protein
2 300 mg on day 1, 300mg/12h on day 2, 300mg/8h on day 3, then ↑ according to response in steps 100mg/8h; max. 600mg/8h. SE: diarrhoea, dry mouth, dyspepsia, vomiting; peripheral oedema; dizzine

Bulbar palsy

This is palsy of the tongue, muscles of chewing/swallowing, and facial muscles c to loss of function of motor nuclei in the medulla. Signs are of a *LMN lesion*; flaccid, fasciculating tongue (p44, like a sack of worms); jaw jerk is normal absent, speech is quiet, hoarse, or nasal. ***Causes:*** MND (below); Guillain–Barré; po syringobulbia (p508); brainstem tumours; also as part of *central pont myelinolysis* (CPM, in malnourished alcoholics or in rapid correction of hy natraemia). CPM causes progressive and fatal quadriparesis, mutism, dysarth and bulbar palsy (but recovery can occur—demonstrable by serial MRI scans)

Pseudobulbar palsy *UMN lesion* of muscles of eating, swallowing, and talking c to bilateral lesions above the midpons eg corticobulbar tracts (MS, MND, stroke). I commoner than bulbar palsy. ***Signs:*** Spastic tongue; ↑jaw jerk; Donald Duck spee weeping unprovoked by sorrow or mood-incongruent giggling (emotional incontine *without* mood change, ie 'hollow laugher', is also seen in dementia & head injury)

Motor neurone disease (MND)

MND is caused by degeneration of neurones in motor cortex, cranial nerve nuc and anterior horn cells. Upper and lower motor neurones are affected but ther *no* sensory loss or sphincter disturbance, so distinguishing MND from MS and pc neuropathies. MND never affects external eye movements (III, IV, VI) distinguish it from myasthenia (p504). Fronto-temporal dementia is seen in 10–35%. ***Cause:*** Unknown, but as MND, like polio, affects anterior horn cells, viruses suggested. There is no diagnostic test. 3 clinical patterns:

- ***Bulbar palsy*** See above. This accounts for about 25% of patients.
- ***Amyotrophic lateral sclerosis (ALS)*** (50%) Combined LMN wasting and U signs (p439) contribute to weakness. Risk↑ ~2-fold in Gulf war veterans. familial, suspect copper/zinc superoxide dismutase mutations (SOD1).
- ***Progressive muscular atrophy*** (25%) Anterior horn cell lesion, affecting dis muscles before proximal. Better prognosis than ALS.

►Think of MND in those >40yrd old with stumbling (spastic gait, foot-drop), we grip (door-handles are difficult), or aspiration pneumonia. Look for UMN sig weakness; spasticity; brisk reflexes; plantars↑; and LMN signs: weakness; wasti fasciculation of tongue, abdomen, back, thigh. Is speech or swallowing affecte Diagnosis is strongly supported by combinations of progressive UMN and LMN sig with involvement of ≥2 limbs, or a limb and bulbar muscles. Fasciculations are r enough to diagnose an LMN lesion: look for weakness too. MRI of brain and cc helps exclude structural causes; LP helps to exclude inflammatory ones, a neurophysiology can detect subclinical denervation and help exclude mo neuropathies. *Prevalence:* 7/10,000. ♂:♀≈3:2. ≤10% are familial.

Prognosis MND is incurable (often fatal within 5yrs; median UK age at death 60yrs). Prognosis is worse with bulbar-onset disease (≤1.5yrs from diagnosis

Treatment Due to MND's rapid course, its rarity, and its frightening nature, a mu disciplinary approach is best: neurologist; palliative nurse; hospice; physio; speech therapist; dietician; social services—all orchestrated by the GP. Death choking is rare, so warmly reassure that a dignified end is the rule. mndassociation tel.UK 08457 626

- ***Antiglutamate drugs:*** Riluzole (see BOX) prolongs life by ~3 months; it is cos It is licensed for use in MND. **Cautions:** LFT↑. Do regular LFT every month 3 months, then every 3 months for a 9 months and annually thereafter. vomiting, weakness, pulse↑, somnolence, headache, dizziness, vertigo, pain, LF
- ***Drooling:*** Propantheline 15–30mg/8h PO; amitriptyline 25–50mg/8h PO.
- ***Dysphagia:*** Blend food; would he or she like a nasogastric tube, or percutanec catheter gastrostomy?—or would this prolong death? ***Spasticity:*** See MS (p48
- ***Joint pains and distress:*** Analgesic ladder (p521) NSAIDs etc; then opioids.
- ***Respiratory failure (± aspiration pneumonia and sleep apnoea):*** Non-invas ventilation at home in selected patients may give valuable palliation.

ɔllowing in the footprints of free radicals

ostmortem studies show that changes to proteins and DNA which are signs or ootprints' of free radical damage are more pronounced in MND brains than in ɔntrols.[271] Also, cultured fibroblasts from MND brains show high sensitivity to xidative insults. But these findings don't explain two key MND phenomena:

/hy is there predilection for motor neurones? One answer may be the sheer ɛngth and complex cytoarchitecture of motor cells, with their 1 metre axons nd high levels of neurofilament proteins, and low levels of Ca^{2+}-buffering roteins (thought to be protective). We note that motor cells with the shortest xons (to the eye's external muscles) are unaffected in MND; this is not true of ıe tongue which only requires slightly longer axons. Another answer is that it is *ot* only motor neurones which are affected: changes are seen in other areas, nd we note that specific aphasia-dementia syndromes occur in MND.[272]

/hy do some MND brains have excess levels of glutamate? (Glutamate is the hief excitatory neurotransmitter.) This is thought to be from ↓ activity of ıe excitatory amino acid transporter (EAAT2), which mops up glutamate—hence ıe notion that MND is an 'excitotoxic' phenomenon. Motor cells have high levels f Cu/Zn superoxide dismutase (thought to protect normal motor cells from lutamate toxicity/oxidative stress). But a high level may itself be damaging, iven certain genetic or acquired vulnerabilities.[273] Transgenic mice exhibiting igh levels of superoxide dismutase do indeed develop an MND phenotype.

These ideas are speculative,[274] but important, perhaps, in understanding and riticizing future therapeutic options. ***Riluzole*** is an Na-channel blocker inhibiting lutamate's release. Neurotrophic factors can protect motor neurones in animal tudies, but clinical trials have proved disappointing. CI: hepatic and renal npairment. Effects of free radical manipulation can be unpredictable.[275] The ntioxidant **vitamin E** protects transgenic mice from developing an MND-like icture, and in at least one human trial high intake of polyunsaturated fatty cids and vitamin E was associated with a 50% decreased risk of developing ALS these nutrients appear to act synergistically).[276]

Apoptosis is a hallmark of MND,[277] and genetically induced overexpression of roteins inhibiting cell death via apoptosis (Bcl-2) in transgenic mice can slow ıotor neurone degeneration.[278]

thical problems: beyond autonomy

'atients with MND may be ventilated, for example—and then decide that they vant this intervention withdrawn.[279] In some patients, this is likely to be fatal—ıaking these decisions difficult for everyone. Ethicists tend to speak in black-nd-white prose—'do whatever promotes autonomy' and this is the *raison d'être* f assisted suicide organizations such as Dignitas[280] (increasingly popular, vorldwide, even where illegal). But sometimes nature contrives something more mbiguous and poetic, in which rationality and rage,[281] and uncertainty and the orked emotions of hope and despair produce a heady internal world which the thicist can never quite catch or tame. If this internal world is one of perpetual hange and oscillating will, ideas of autonomy become incoherent. Rather than iming to apply Kantian universal rules (p17), our role may be more to offer a vell-placed hug to signal metaphysical complicity, and to stand beside our atients, come what may.

Cervical spondylosis

Cervical spondylosis with compression of the cord (myelopathy) and nerve roo the leading cause of progressive spastic quadriparesis with sensory loss below neck:[282] but most people with cervical spondylosis have no impairment— degeneration of the annulus fibrosus of cervical intervertebral discs ± bony sp which narrow the spinal canal and intervertebral foramina. As the neck flexes extends, the cord is damaged as it is dragged over these protruding osteophy anteriorly and indented by a thickened ligamentum flavum posteriorly.

Signs: Limited, painful neck movement ± crepitus—be careful! Neck flexion may produce tingling down the spine—a positive Lhermitte's symptom. This does not help decide if cord or roots or both are involved.

Arm: LMN signs at the level of the compressed cord or roots and UMN signs below. Visible atrophy of hand and forearm muscles. Sensory loss (esp. pain & T°).

Leg: Spasticity; weakness; brisk reflexes; plantars↑↑. Position & vibration sense↓. Examine skin sensation from below upwards to show any sensory level (eg several segments below level of cord compression).

Root compression (radiculopathy) Pain in arms & fingers and ↓reflexes, dermatomal sensory disturbance (numbness, tingling), LMN weakness and eventual wasting of muscles innervated by the affected root.

Complaints may be of:
- Neck stiffness (unhel as common in anyone over 50 years old)
- Crepitus on moving ne
- Stabbing or dull arm p (brachialgia)
- Forearm/wrist pain

Signs of cord compressi
- Spastic leg weakness
- Weak, clumsy hands
- Numbness in hands
- Weakness (often more marked in 1 leg)
- 'Heavy' weak legs
- Foot-drop/poor walkinc
- Incontinence/hesitanc urgency are often late

Typical motor and sensory deficits from individual root involvement	
C5/C6	Weak biceps and deltoid; ↓supinator and biceps jerks, Numb thumb
C7	Weak triceps and finger extension; ↓triceps jerks; numb middle fing
C8/T1	Weak finger flexors and small muscles of the hand; numb 5th & ring fin
C4/C5	Elbow sensation, supraspinatus.

Tests MRI is the best localizing image. AP compression ratio is ≥30% typically induces histopathological changes in the cord (cadaver studies). Time to walk 30m helps monitor progress (valid & cheap).[284]

Differential diagnosis MS, nerve root neurofibroma, subacute combined degeneration of the cord (B_{12}↓).

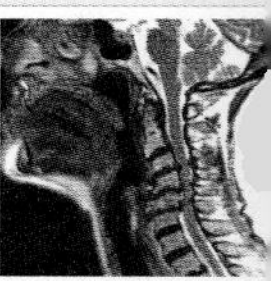

Fig 1. A T2 weighted MR imag (so CSF looks bright). The spir cord is compressed between t osteophytes anteriorly and t ligamentum flavum posteriorly

Treatment A firm neck collar restricts anterior-posterior movement of the neck so may relieve pain, but patients dislike them. Don't dismiss those with chronic root pain in the arm as suffering simply from 'wear and tear' spondylosis. Be optimistic: they may improve over months; if not, they *may* benefit greatly from surgical root decompression (**laminectomy,** fig 2 or **laminoplasty,** fig 3) if there is significant abnormality.[285] Consider if objective evidence of a root lesion or myelopathy, especially if the history is short, and the neurological deficit is progressing. A rule of thumb, opt for conservative treatment if the spinal transverse are >70mm², the patient is elderly, and motor conduction time is normal.[RCT 286] If surg *is* done, progression is usually halted and leg weakness may improve. Operative is less than with **anterior spinal fusion** (requires bone grafts with additic complications with no extra benefit).[287] **Transforaminal steroid injectio** gaining popularity on the rationale that nerve root inflammation causes radic pain. Pain reduction can be demonstrated, but we await randomized trials.

Rare complications Diaphragm paralysis;[288] spinal artery syndrome mimick angina (∵ spinal artery compression; pain & T° are lost before vibration sense)

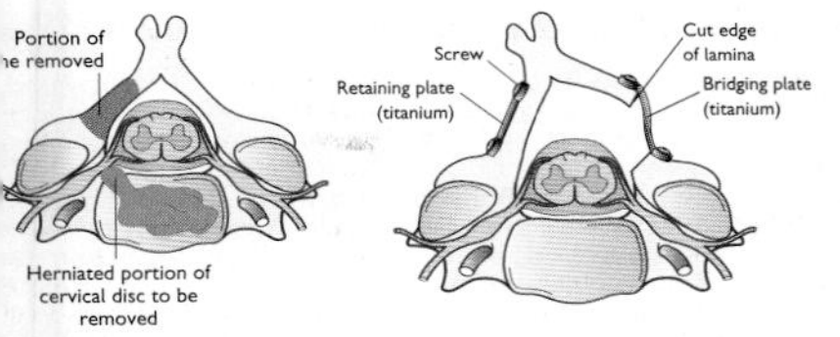

ɡ 2. Laminectomy

Fig 3. Laminoplasty (screws & plates)

minectomy or laminoplasty? Laminectomy and laminoplasty improve gait, ength, sensation, pain, and degree of myelopathy. To a roughly equal extent, but one study of 44 consecutive patients, laminoplasty was associated with more in reduction and fewer late complications (but there was more neck stiffness). appropriate level, the ligamentum flavum (overlies the dura) is incised and cut ay with part of adjacent laminae, as necessary to expose the extradural space.

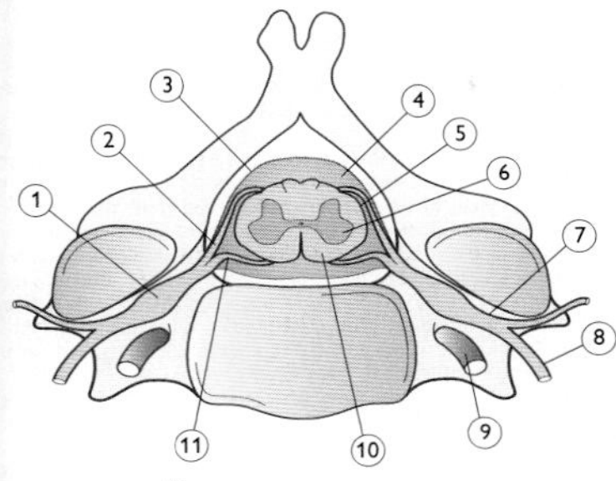

Fig 4. Cervical vertebra. (After Dr Carey Carpenter)

1 Dorsal root ganglion
2 Dorsal root
3 Dura mater
4 Subarachnoid space
5 Pia mater
6 Grey matter
7 Spinal nerve
8 Ventral ramus
9 Vertebral artery in the transverse foramen
10 White matter
11 Ventral spinal nerve

Primary disorders of muscle (myopathies)

Myopathy or neuropathy? In favour of myopathy: • Gradual onset of symmet *proximal* weakness—difficulty combing hair & climbing stairs (but note: weaknes *distal* in myotonic dystrophy). • Neck flexion weaker than neck extension • Tend reflexes preserved. A neuropathy is more likely if there are paraesthesiae, bladc problems or distal weakness (unless it's Guillain–Barré). Rapid onset suggest neuropathy or a toxic, drug, or metabolic myopathy. ***Excess fatigability*** (weakn increases with exercise) suggests myasthenia (p504). Spontaneous ***pain*** at r occurs in inflammatory disease as does local tenderness. Pain on exercise sugge ischaemia or metabolic myopathy (eg McArdle's disease). ***Oddly firm*** muscles (d to infiltrations with fat or connective tissue) suggest pseudohypertrophic muscu dystrophies. Muscle ***tumours*** are rare; common causes of ***lumps*** are herniation muscle through fascia, haematoma, and tendon rupture. ***Fasciculation*** (spontaneo irregular, brief contractions of part of a muscle) suggests anterior horn cell or rc disease. Look for evidence of systemic disease. ***Tests:*** ESR, CK, AST & LDH may be Do EMG and tests relevant to systemic causes (eg TSH ↑ or ↓ p200). Many gene disorders of muscle are detectable by DNA analysis: reserve muscle biopsy for wh genetic tests are non-diagnostic. ***6 types:***

1 ***Muscular dystrophies*** are a group of genetic diseases with progressi degeneration and weakness of specific muscle groups. The primary abnormal may be in the muscle membrane. Secondary effects are marked variation in si of individual fibres and deposition of fat and connective tissue. The commone is **Duchenne's muscular dystrophy** (pseudohypertrophic; sex-linked recessive 30% from spontaneous mutation) and is (almost always) confined to boys. T Duchenne gene is on the short arm of the X chromosome (Xp23), and product, dystrophin, is absent (or present in very low levels). Serum creati kinase is raised >40-fold. It presents at ~4yrs old with increasingly clum walking, progressing to difficulty in standing and respiratory failure. Sor survive beyond 20yrs. There is no specific treatment. Home ventilation is use Genetic counselling is vital. **Fascioscapulohumeral muscular dystrophy (Lan ouzy–Dejerine)** is almost as common. *Inheritance:* Autosomal dominant (4q3 *Typical age of onset:* 12–14yrs. *Early symptoms:* Inability to puff out t cheeks, difficulty raising the arms above the head (eg changing light-bulb *Signs:* Weakness of face ('ironed out' expression), shoulders, and upper arr (often asymmetric with deltoids spared) ± foot-drop ± winging of the scapul (due to weakness of thoracoscapular muscles) ± scoliosis ± anterior axilla folds ± horizontal clavicles. ≤20% need a wheelchair by 40yrs old.

2 ***Myotonic disorders*** cause tonic muscle spasm (myotonia); muscle histoloc shows long chains of central nuclei within fibres. The chief one is **dystroph myotonica** (=DM1) a **Cl⁻ channelopathy.** Typical onset: 25yrs with weakne (hands, legs, sternomastoids) and myotonia. Muscle wasting and weakness the face gives a long, haggard appearance. Also: cataract; frontal baldness testis/ovary atrophy; cardiomyopathy; mild endocrine abnormalities (eg DM and mental impairment. Most patients die in middle age of intercurrent illnes Mexiletine, phenytoin and acetazolamide may help. Genetic counselling important. **Na⁺ channelopathy** causing myotonia: paramyotonia congenit adynamia episodica hereditaria.

5 ***Acquired myopathies of late onset*** are often part of systemic disease—(hyperthyroidism); cancer; Cushing's; hypo- and hypercalcaemia.

6 ***Inflammatory myopathies:*** **Inclusion body myositis** is the chief example if age >50yrs. Aggregates of Alzheimer tau proteins suggest a 'peripheral tauopathy'. Signs: weakness starts with quads, finger flexors or pharyngeal muscles. Ventr extremity muscle groups are more affected than dorsal or girdle group Wheelchair dependency: <3%. Histology: ringed vacuoles + intranuclear inclusior ℞: nothing is consistently effective. For **polymyositis**[et al], see p538.

7 ***Neuromuscular junction disorders:*** **Myasthenia gravis** (p504).

8 ***Toxicity:*** Alcohol; statins; steroids; chloroquine; zidovudine; vincristine; cocain

Myasthenia gravis (MG)

MG is an autoimmune disease mediated by antibodies to nicotinic acetylcho receptors (AChR), interfering with the neuromuscular transmission via depletion working postsynaptic receptor sites. Cause: B- and T-cells are implicated.

Presentation Increasing muscular fatigue. If <50yrs old, MG is commoner women, associated with other autoimmune diseases and thymic hyperplasia. O 50, it is commoner in men, and associated with thymic atrophy or thymic tum Muscle groups affected, in order: extraocular; bulbar (swallowing; chewing); fa neck; limb girdle; trunk. Look for: ptosis; diplopia; myasthenic snarl on smiling; 'pe sign'.[1] On counting to 50, the voice deteriorates. **Reflexes:** normal. Weakness worsened by: pregnancy, K^+↓, infection, overtreatment, change of climate, emoti exercise, gentamicin, opiates, tetracycline, quinine, procainamide, β-blockers.

Associations: Thymic tumour; hyperthyroidism; rheumatoid arthritis; SLE.

Tests Tensilon® test: If resuscitation facilities and atropine are to hand, prepar syringes, 1 with 10mg edrophonium and 1 with 0.9% saline. Give 1st 20% of e separately IV as test dose. Ask an independent observer to comment on the eff of each; wait 30s before giving rest of each syringe. The test is +ve if edrophoni improves power in ~1min. The test may not be as dramatic as is stated. Othe ***Antiacetylcholine receptor antibody:*** ↑ in 90% (70% in ocular-confined MG sero–ve look for musk antibodies (muscle specific tyrosine kinase; ♀/♂≈15:2) ***Neurophysiology:*** Decremental muscle response to repetitive nerve stimulation single-fibre jitter. CT **of thymus** (5mm slices). NB: ptosis improves by >2mm af **ice application** to the (shut) affected lid for >2min: a nice, non-invasive test.

Treatment *Symptom control* Anticholinesterase eg **pyridostigmine** 60–120mg up to 6×daily; SE: diarrhoea; colic (controllable by propantheline 15mg/8h cholinergic SE: salivation↑; lacrimation; sweats; vomiting; miosis).
Immunosuppression **Prednisolone** (single-dose alternate day regimen + osteop osis prophylaxis); start at 5mg; ↑by 5mg/wk up to 1mg/kg on each treatment d ↓dose on remission (may take months). SE: weakness (hence low starting dos may be combined with azathioprine 2.5mg/kg/day (do FBC & LFT weekly for 8w then 12-weekly) or weekly methotrexate. IV methylprednisolone has a rc
Thymectomy: Consider if onset before 50yrs old and disease is not eas controlled by anticholinesterases. Expect remission in 25% and worthwhile bene in a further 50%. Thymectomy is also necessary for thymomas to prevent lo invasion (but MG symptoms are often unaffected).
Plasmapheresis or IV immunoglobulin (IVIg) gives ~2–4wks' benefit (useful crises or pre-thymectomy, eg IVIg 0.4g/kg daily for 5 days pre-op). Ventilato ***support*** This is unlikely to be needed if vital capacity >20mL/kg.

Prognosis Relapsing or slow progression. If thymoma, 5yr survival is 68%.

Other causes of muscle fatigability Polymyositis; SLE; botulism; Takayas arteritis (fatigability of the extremities). For other myopathies, see p502.

Lambert–Eaton myasthenic syndrome (LEMS=ELM

This para-neoplastic (small-cell lung cancer) or autoimmune disease[2] is unlike tr MG as there is: • Gait difficulty before eye signs • *Autonomic involvement* (c mouth; constipation; impotence) • *Hyporeflexia* • *Increased* strength post-exerci • Less response to edrophonium • Antibody to the *presynaptic* membrane's voltag gated Ca^{2+} channels (VGCC). • Electrical post-tetanic *potentiation* + >60% *increm* in post-exercise facilitation of abductor digiti quinti. • Anti-P/Q VGCC antibod are +ve in 85%. ***R̸:*** (by experts) 3,4-diaminopyridine or IV immunoglobulin.
►Do regular CXRs as symptoms may predate the cancer by more than 4 years.

1 After brief opposition to gentle sustained lid closure, the lids separate ('peek') to show white sclerae
2 64% of those with non-tumour LEMS have a family member with autoimmune thyroid disease or DM.

Neurology

Neurofibromatosis[1]

Type 1 neurofibromatosis (NF1, von Recklinghausen's disease) Prevalence: 2500, ♀:♂≈1:1; no racial predilection. Inheritance: autosomal dominant (g chromosome 17). Expression NF1 is variable, even within a family.

Signs ***Café-au-lait spots*** are flat, coffee-coloured patches of skin seen in the year of life (clearest in UV light), increasing in size and number with age. Ad have ≥6, >15mm across. They do *not* predispose to skin cancer.

Freckling typically occurs in skin-folds (axillae, groin, neck base, and submamm area♀) and is usually present by age 10.

Dermal neurofibromas appear at puberty and are small, violaceous nodu gelatinous in texture. They may become papillomatous. They are not painful may itch. Numbers increase over time.

Nodular neurofibromas arise from nerve trunks. Firm and clearly demarcat they can give rise to paraesthesiae if pressed.

Lisch nodules are tiny harmless regular brown/translucent mounds (hamartomas) on the iris (use a slit lamp) ≤2mm in diameter. They develop by 6yrs old in 90%. Also look for short stature and macrocephaly.

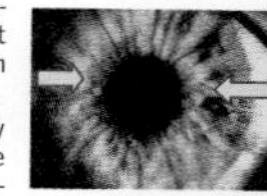

Fig 1. Many Lisch nodules (arrows) on the iris.

Complications (seen in 30%). Mild learning disability is common. ***Local effects of neurofibromas:*** Nerve roots—compression; gut—bleeds, obstruction; bone—cystic lesions; scoliosis pseudarthrosis. Hypertension (6%) from renal artery stenosis or phaeochromocytoma. Plexiform neurofibromas (large, subcutaneous swellings). Malignancy (5% patients with NF1): optic glion sarcomatous change in a neurofibroma. Epilepsy risk ↑ (slight). There is a ra association with carcinoid syndrome (p270).

Management Multidisciplinary team with geneticist, neurologist, and surge orchestrated by a GP. Yearly measurement of BP and cutaneous survey is advis Dermal neurofibromas are unsightly, and catch on clothing; if troublesome, exci but removing all lesions is unrealistic. Genetic counselling is vital (*OHCS* p154).

Type 2 neurofibromatosis (NF2)

Autosomal dominant inheritance. Much rarer than NF1 with a prevalence of only in 35,000. The gene responsible is on chromosome 22.

Signs ***Café-au-lait spots*** are fewer than in NF1. ***Bilateral vestibular schwannomas*** (acoustic neuromas) become symptomatic in the teens or twenties wh sensorineural hearing loss is the 1st sign. There may be tinnitus and vertigo. T rate of tumour growth is unpredictable and variable. The tumours are benign b cause problems by pressing on local structures and by ↑ICP. ***Juvenile posterior subcapsular lenticular opacity*** (a form of cataract) occurs before other manifestations and can be useful in screening those at risk.

Complications: Schwannomas of other cranial nerves, spinal nerve roots, or nerv Meningiomas (45% NF2; may be multiple). Glial tumours are less common. Consid NF2 in any young person presenting with one of these tumours in isolation.

Management Hearing tests yearly from puberty with CNS MRI if abnormality detected. A normal MRI in the late teens is helpful in assessing risk to any offsprin A clear scan at 30yrs (unless a family history of late onset) indicates that the ge has not been inherited. Treatment of vestibular schwannomas is neurosurgical a complicated by hearing loss/deterioration and facial palsy. Mean survival fro diagnosis has been reported at 15yrs, but with best practice this will be bett

1 Do not be put off by the excessive amount of detail on this page: you an always leave this topic unt later, when vague memories are stirred by coffee stains on the skin, or a lump in an unusual place.

agnostic criteria for neurofibromatosis

1 (von Recklinghausen's disease)

agnosis is made if 2 of the following are found:

. ≥6 *café-au-lait* macules >5mm (prepubertal) or >15mm (post-pubertal)
 ≥2 neurofibromas of any type or 1 plexiform
 Freckling in the axillary or inguinal regions
 Optic glioma
 ≥2 Lisch nodules
 Distinctive osseous lesion typical of NF1, eg sphenoid dysplasia
 First degree relative with NF1 according to the above criteria

fferential: McCune–Albright syndrome (*OHCS* p650), multiple lentigenes,[1] ticaria pigmentosa (*OHCS* p610).

2

agnosis is made if either of the following are found:

 Bilateral vestibular schwannomas seen on MRI or CT
 First degree relative with NF2 and either:
  (a) Unilateral vestibular schwannoma
  (b) One of the following:
   Neurofibroma
   Meningioma
   Glioma
   Schwannoma
   Juvenile cataract (NF2 type).

ifferential: NF1.

 May be part LEOPARD syndrome: autosomal dominant Lentigines, ECG anomalies, Ocular pertelorism (eyes wide-spaced), Pulmonary stenosis, Anomalies of genital organs, Retarded growth, eafness.

Syringomyelia

Syrinx was one of those versatile virgins of Arcadia who, on being pursued by
beside the river Ladon, turned herself into a reed, from which Pan made his pi
so giving her name to various tubular structures, eg syringes, and syrinxes, wh
are tubular or slit-like cavities in or close to the central canal of the cervical co
They may extend up or down. Incidence: 8/100,000/yr. See fig 1 p689.

Cause Typical cause: blocked csf circulation without 4th ventricular commun
ation), with ↓flow from the basal posterior fossa to the caudal space. The ch
example is Arnold–Chiari malformation (cerebellum extends through the foram
magnum; can cause communicating syringomyelia)—also basal arachnoiditis (af
infection, irradiation, subarachnoid haemorrhage); basilar impression/invaginatio
meningeal cancer; masses (cysts, rheumatoid pannus, encephalocele, tumours
Less commonly, syrinxes develop after myelitis, cord trauma or damage fr
rupture of an A–V malformation,[316] or within spinal tumours ∵ fluid secreted fr
neoplastic cells or haemorrhage typically in an ependymoma or hemangioblastor

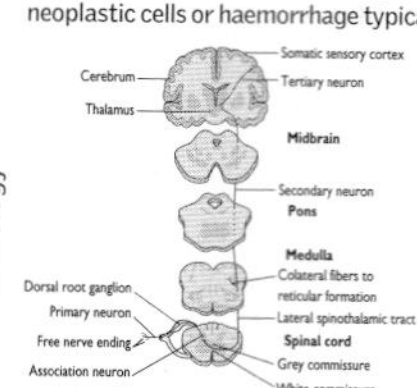

Fig 1. Spinothalamic decussations.[317]

Signs—*cardinal:* **Wasting/weakness**
hands (± **claw-hand**—then arms, then sh
ulders, then respiratory muscles) + **loss**
pain & **T° sensation** (eg with **painle**
burns with preserved light touch, vibrati
and joint-position sense, ie **dissociat**
sensory loss, p438, typically over trunk
arms, eg in a cape distribution (suspend
sensory loss). Fibres for pain and T° are lo
early as they decussate anteriorly in t
cord. Anterior horn cells are simila
vulnerable. ***Others:*** **Horner's syndro**
(cervical sympathetics) & **UMN leg signs**
body asymmetry, limb hemihypertroph
or odomegaly/ chiromegaly (unilateral enlarged hand or foot, perhaps from relea
of trophic factors via anterior horn cells). **Eye movement abnormalities** (eg dow
beat nystagmus, diplopia, oscillopsia,[2] and tunnel vision) are from base of bra
(foramen magnum) abnormality.[318] **Charcot's (neuropathic) joints:** On losi
sensation, joints are destroyed by ↑ range of movement, becoming swollen ar
mobile.[319] Causes: tabes dorsalis (eg knee), paraplegia (eg hips),[320] syringomye
(shoulder; wrist),[321] leprosy, spinal osteolysis/cord atrophy (systemic sclerosis).

MRI imaging How big is the syrinx? Any base-of-brain (Chiari) malformation?

Natural history Mean age of onset: 30yrs. Symptoms may be static for years, b
then worsen fast—eg on coughing or sneezing, as rises in venous pressure caus
extension eg into the brainstem (*syringobulbia*)[323] this causes nystagmus, tongu
atrophy, dysphagia, pharyngeal/palatal weakness and Vth nerve sensory signs.

Surgery Don't wait for gross deterioration to occur. Decompression at the forame
magnum may be tried in Chiari malformations, to promote free flow of cs
preventing syrinx dilatation. Surgery may relieve pain, and slow progression.[324]

Retroviruses and neurology

HIV/AIDS is part of the differential diagnosis of meningitis (eg fungal/TB), intr
cranial mass lesions (toxoplasmosis), dementia, encephalomyelitis, cord problems,
and peripheral nerve problems, eg mononeuritis multiplex; Guillain–Barré syndrom

Tropical spastic paraplegia/HTLV-1 myelopathy is a progressive spast
paraplegia, with paraesthesiae, sensory loss, and disorders of micturition.

1 The top of the odontoid process (part of C2) migrates upwards (congenitally or in rheumatoid arthrit
or osteogenesis imperfecta) causing foramen magnum stenosis ± medulla oblongata compressio
Consider basilar invagination if the odontoid tip is ≥4mm above McGregor's line (drawn from the upp
surface of the posterior edge of the hard palate to the most caudal point of the occipital curve).
2 Oscillopsia (sensation of oscillation of objects viewed) in brainstem disorders not causin
nystagmus is attributed to failure of vestibular-ocular reflex to compensate for head movement.

lodels of brain functioning

uperficial reading of the foregoing pages might lead one to the conclusion that structure of the adult brain is fixed, and that a circumscribed lesion will duce reproducible, predictable results (if we remember our neuroanatomy rectly). Furthermore, if a certain phenomenon appears when part of the brain y area a) is stimulated, and is lost when the same part of the brain is injured, we pily conclude that area a is the centre for laughter, fear, or whatever the nomenon is. A lesion here, and you will stop laughing for ever, we might think. area on the hard disk of our mind has been scratched. The grey cells do not enerate themselves, so the brain carries on as before with this one defect. The re we look at the brain, the more wrong this model becomes.

f our brains were like a computer, the more tasks we did at the same time, the wer we would do any one task. In fact, our performance can improve, the more ultaneous tasks we take on. This is why music helps some of us concentrate. eriments using functional MRI show that listening to polyphonic music recruits mory circuits, promoting attention, and aids semantic processing, target ection, and some forms of imagery.[1]

Another way in which our brains are not like a computer is that we are born h certain predispositions and expectations. Our hard disk was never blank. Just the skin on the feet of new-born babies is thicker than other areas (as if feet e made with a pre-knowledge of walking, or somehow expecting walking), so brains are made expecting a world of stimuli, which need making sense of by aming sequential events in terms of cause and effect. We cannot help onsciously imposing cause and effect relationships on events which are purely uential. This unconscious reframing no doubt has survival value.

The model we have of brain function is important because it influences our tude to our patients. If we are stuck with a neuroanatomical model, we will be her pessimistic and guarded in our assessment of how patients may recover er neurological events. If we use a model which is more holistic and reality ed, such as the Piaget-type model in which the brain is seen as intrinsically table and continually re-creating itself, we will grant our patients more sibilities. Our model of the brain must encompass its ability to set goals for lf, and to be self-actuating. Unstructured optimism is unwarranted, but ictured optimism is to some extent a self-fulfilling prognosis. For many medical ditions, the more optimistic we are, and the more we involve our patients in ir own care and its planning, the faster and better they will recover. If we nbine this with the observed fact that those with an optimistic turn of mind are s likely to suffer stroke,[2] we can reach the conclusion that emotional well-being dicts subsequent functional independence and survival. When this hypothesis is ted directly in a prospective way, the effect of emotional well-being is found to direct and strong and independent of other factors such as functional status, iodemographic variables, chronic conditions, body mass index, etc.

So the conclusion is that the brain has an unknown amount of inherent plasticity, l an unknown potential for healing after injury—uninjured areas may take on v functions, and injured parts may function in new ways.[3] The great challenge of rology is to work to maximize this potential for recovery and re-creation. This nands knowledge of your patient, as well as knowledge of neuroanatomy and rophysiology. The point is that there is no predefined limit to what is possible.

Neurology

1 Janata 2003 *Cogn Affect Behav Neurosci* **2** 121
2 Ostir 2001 *Psychosom Med* **63** 210. N = 2478 (6yr prospective population-based cohort study).
3 n early frontotemporal dementia, artistic creativity may blossom—suggesting that language is not ired for, and may even inhibit, certain types of visual creativity. B Miller 2003 *Neurology* **60** 1707

12 Oncology and palliative care

Contents

Relevant pages in other chapters: Leukaemias/lymphomas (pp336–346); myel (p352); immunosuppressive drugs (p360); pain (p560); dying at home (*OHCS* p4 facing death (p7). For specific cancers, see relevant chapters, eg *Surgery*, p5

Communication

This forms the first step in understanding, treating, or coming to terms w cancer. A range of overwhelming feelings can surface on receiving this diagno including shock, numbness, denial, panic, anger and resignation ('I knew along...'). Some doctors instinctively turn away from 'undisciplined squads emotions' and try to stop them taking over consultations. A more posit approach is to try to use these to benefit and motivate your patient—throu listening to, and addressing, their worst fears. ►*Include your patient in decision-making processes.* Many patients (not just the young and w informed) will appreciate this—and the giving of information and the sharinc decisions is known to reduce treatment morbidity. So, even when this physically exhausting (the same ground may need covering many times) i definitely worth spending this time. A huge amount is forgotten or fails register initially, so videos and written information are important. Be sure question, in an open way, about use of alternative therapies which can indic psychosocial distress and is frequently a sign of undisclosed worry recurrence.[1][2] Ask about this and through good communication and promotion of autonomy, your patient's fear-driven wish to try dangerous untried therapies may be trumped by a spirit of rational optimism.

This chapter's updating and reworking is the work of Dr Emma Smith whose contribution we acknowledge. We thank Dr Ian Cairns, who is our Specialist Reader for this chapter.

oking after people with cancer

rules guarantee success, but getting to know your patient, making an agreed anagement plan, and seeking out the right expert for each stage of treatment need to be central activities in oncology. The patient will bring worries from aspects of their family, working and social life. Communication is central to solving these issues and the personal attributes of the doctor as a physician e key. Remember, it is never too early to start palliative care (*with* other eatments) and that *quality of life* is of the utmost importance.

ychological support Examples include:

- Allowing the patient to express anger, fear—or any negative feeling (anger can anaesthetize pain).
- Counselling, eg with a breast cancer nurse (mastectomy preparation).
- Biofeedback and relaxation therapy can ↓side-effects of chemotherapy.[3]
- Cognitive and behavioural therapy reduces psychological morbidity associated with cancer treatments. See OHCS p370.
- Group therapy (OHCS p376) reduces pain, mood disturbance, and the frequency of maladaptive coping strategies.
- Meta-analyses have suggested that psychological support can have some effect on improving outcome measures such as survival.[4]

reamlining care pathways Care pathways map patient journeys in a health stem: symptoms felt→GP appointment→referral→hospital appointment→consultant clinic→imaging→1st treatment (surgery, etc). Each arrow represents a ssibly fatal delay. 48h access to GPs, GP referral under a '2-week rule' (hospital ist see within 2wks, inevitably making other equally or more deserving patients it longer) and *e*-booking (like on-line airline seat reservations) are unreliable ys of speeding up the crucial arrow pointing to 1st treatment.[5] The only way do this is to increase capacity (beds, nurses, doctors, equipment, and theatres).

ts on breaking bad news [6]

- Set the environment up carefully. Choose a quiet place where you will not be disturbed. Make sure family are present if wanted. Be sure of your facts.
- Find out what the patient already knows or surmises (often a great deal). This may change rapidly, and different perceptions may all be relevant.
- Ascertain how much the person wants to know. You can be surprisingly direct. 'If anything were amiss, would want to know all the details?'
- Give some warning — 'there is some bad news for us to address'. Offer small amounts of information at a time, as this can soften the impact.
- Share information about diagnosis and treatments, Specifically list supporting people (eg nurses) and institutions (eg hospices). Ask 'Is there anything else you want me to explain?' Don't hesitate to go over the same ground repeatedly. Allow denial: don't force the pace, give them time.
- 'Cancer' has negative connotations for many people. Address this, and explain that ~50% of cancers are cured in the developed world.[7]
- Listen to any concerns raised; encourage the airing of feelings and empathise.
- Prognosis questions are often hardest to answer, doctors are usually too optimistic.[8] Encourage an appropriate level of hope, refer to an expert.
- Summarize and make a plan. Offer availability.
- Follow through. The most important thing is to leave the patient with the strong impression that come what may, you are with them, and that this unwritten contract will not be broken.

n't imagine that a single blueprint will do for everyone. ►Be prepared to use *atever* the patient gives you.[9] Closely observe both verbal and non-verbal es. Practise in low-key interactions with patients—so when great difficulties se, you have a better chance of helping. As humans are very complex, we all quently fail. Don't be put off: keep trying, and recap with colleagues erwards, so you keep learning.

Some commoner cancer-predisposing gene mutations are given in the BOX.

Familial breast/ovarian cancer Most breast and ovarian cancer is sporadic, ~5% are due to germline mutation in BRCA1 (17q) or BRCA2 (13q). Both ge function as tumour suppressors. Carrying a BRCA1 mutation confers a lifetime of developing breast cancer of 70–80%, and ovarian cancer of 30–40%. Mutati in BRCA2 are much less likely to cause ovarian cancer, but may cause male bre cancer. Incidence of mutations varies among populations. In families with ≥4 ca of breast cancer collected by the Breast Cancer Linkage Consortium, the dise was linked to BRCA1 in 52% of families and BRCA2 in 32%. Individuals from fam in which a mutation has not been detected can be given risk estimation basec number of individuals affected and age of onset of cancer. There is no consensus efficacy of mammographic and ovarian ultrasound screening or analysis of ca1 and CEA (carcionembryonic antigen) serum markers in individuals at moderate

There is debate about cost–benefits of screening and risks of radiation expos from regular mammography. MRI assists early detection. Those at high risk breast or ovarian cancer may opt for prophylactic mastectomy and oophorectc both of which lower, but do not remove, the risk of developing cancer derived f those sites. Drugs have an uncertain role in prevention in high-risk patie tamoxifen is associated with unacceptable adverse side effects, anastrozol more promising but still under trial (IBIS-II and MAP III).

Familial colorectal cancer ~20% of those with colorectal cancer have a far history of the disease. Personal risk of colorectal cancer is proportionate to the deg of family history: the relative risk (RR) is about: ×2 for people with any family hist ×5 if 2 affected 1st degree relatives; and ×3 for an affected 1st degree relative a <45yrs at diagnosis. On the basis of empirical risk estimation, some people may recommended colonoscopic surveillance, but weigh against the dangers of lc term, invasive screening for at-risk individuals.

Hereditary non-polyposis colorectal cancer (HNPCC) is a syndrome of fam aggregation of colorectal (mainly), endometrial, ovarian, gastric, upper urir tract, small intestinal, pancreatic, and other cancers. Many HNPCC families h mutations in 1 of 5 DNA mismatch repair genes. Lifetime risk of colorectal car for relatives who carry a mutation is 60%, and women with a mutation hav 40% lifetime risk of endometrial cancer. Surveillance for HNPCC families is 2-ye with colonoscopy ± gynaecological surveillance, or even prophylactic surg These mutations cause ~2% of all UK colorectal cancers. Suspect if: ≥3 1st-deg relatives from ≥2 generations have colorectal cancer with one <50yrs ol provided familial adenomatous polyposis has been excluded.

Familial adenomatous polyposis is due to germline mutations in the APC ge Offspring are at 50% of risk of being a gene carrier, and gene penetra approaches 100% for colorectal cancer by 50yrs old. ***Peutz–Jeghers' syndro*** has a 10–20% lifetime risk of colorectal cancer, and has been shown to be du germline mutations in STK11, a serine threonine kinase (locus: 19p14).

Familial prostate cancer ~5% of those with prostate cancer have a family hist the genetic basis is multifactorial. There is a modestly elevated life time risk prostate cancer for male carriers of BRCA1 and BRCA2 mutations, although molecular basis of this remains to be elucidated. Mutations in BRCA1/BRCA2 c the genes on chromosomes 1 and X do not account for all family clusters prostate cancer and so it is clear that other genes must be involved. In one t study, 42% of the risk was found to be genetic.

Genetic tests can also tell if chemotherapy is likely to work: chemotherapy fai 17% of colon cancer patients—ie those with certain mutations.[1]

1 Shown by the microsatellite instability status being 'high-frequency'. Microsatellites are stretches of in which a short section is repeated several times. 5-fluorouracil only improves survival in microsat stable or low-frequency microsatellite unstable tumours. S Gallinger 2003 *NEJM* **249** 209

Oncology and palliative care

amples of cancers with a familial predisposition

ncer/syndrome	Gene	Chromosome	
east and ovarian cancers	BRCA1	17q	(OPPOSITE)
	BRCA2	13q	
reditary non-polyposis colorectal cancer (HNPCC)	MSH2	2p	(OPPOSITE)
	MLH1	3p	
	PMS2	7p	
milial polyposis (colorectum)	APC	5q	
n Hippel–Lindau (kidney, CNS)	VHL	3p	(p207)
rney complex	PRKAR1A	17q	(p207)
ltiple endocrine neoplasia Type I (pituitary, pancreas, thyroid)	MEN1	11q	(p207)
ltiple endocrine neoplasia Type 2	RET	10q	(p207)
sal cell naevus syndrome (CNS, skin)	PTCH	9q	
tinoblastoma (eye, bone)	Rb	13q	(*OHCS* p421)
-Fraumeni syndrome (multiple)	TP53	17p	(*OHCS* p648)
urofibromatosis Type I (CNS; rare)	NF1	17q	(p506)
urofibromatosis Type 2 (common) (meningiomas, auditory neuromas)	NF2	22	(p506)
milial melanoma	INK4a	9p	

Oncological emergencies

►A patient who becomes acutely unwell can often be made more comfortable simple measures, but some problems require specific treatment.

Febrile neutropenic patients See p336.

Spinal cord compression Requires urgent and efficient treatment to pres neurological function. A high index of suspicion is essential. ***Causes:*** Typi extradural metastases. Others: extension of tumour from a vertebral body, d extension of the tumour, or crush fracture. ***Signs & symptoms:*** Back pain w root distribution, weakness and sensory loss (a level may be found), bowel bladder dysfunction. ***Tests:*** Urgent MRI of the whole spine. ***Managem*** **Dexamethasone** 8–16mg IV then 4mg/6h PO. Discuss with neurosurgeon clinical oncologist immediately.

Superior vena cava (SVC) obstruction with airway compromise SVC obstruc is not an emergency unless there is tracheal compression with *airway compro* usually there is time to plan optimal treatment, which is to be preferred, ra than rushing into therapy which may not be beneficial.[15] ***Causes:*** Typically cancer; rarely from causes of mediastinal enlargement (eg germ cell tum lymphadenopathy (lymphoma); thymus malignancy; thrombotic disorders Behçet's or nephrotic syndromes); thrombus around an IV central line; hamart ovarian hyperstimulation (*OHCS* p311); fibrotic bands (lung fibrosis after che therapy). ***Signs & symptoms:*** Dyspnoea; orthopnoea; swollen face & arm; co plethora/cyanosis; headache; engorged veins. ***Pemberton's test:*** On lifting arms over the head for >1min, there is ↑facial plethora/cyanosis, JVP↑ (pulsatile), and inspiratory stridor. ***Tests:*** Sputum cytology, CXR, CT, venogra ***Management:*** Get a tissue diagnosis if possible, but bronchoscopy may hazardous. Give **dexamethasone** 4mg/6h PO. Consider balloon **venoplasty** and stenting,[16] eg prior to radical or palliative **chemo-** or **radiotherapy** (dependin tumour type).

Hypercalcaemia Affects 10–20% of patients with cancer, and 40% of those w myeloma. ***Causes:*** Lytic bone metastases, production of osteoclast activa factor or PTH-like hormones by the tumour. ***Symptoms:*** Lethargy, anorexia, nau polydipsia, polyuria, constipation, dehydration, confusion, weakness. Most obv with serum Ca^{2+} >3mmol/L. ***Management:*** **Rehydrate** with 3–4L of 0.9% salir over 24h. Avoid diuretics. Give **bisphosphonate** IV; consider maintenance ther IV or PO, p672). The best treatment is control of underlying malignancy resistant hypercalcaemia, consider **calcitonin**.

Raised intracranial pressure Due to either a primary CNS tumour or metast disease. ***Signs & symptoms:*** Headache (often worse in the morning), nau vomiting, papilloedema, fits, focal neurological signs. ***Tests:*** Urgent CT is impor to diagnose an expanding mass, cystic degeneration, haemorrhage with tumour, cerebral oedema, or hydrocephalus due to tumour or blocked shunt si the management of these scenarios can be very different. ***℞:*** **Dexamethas** 4mg/6h PO, radiotherapy, and surgery as appropriate depending on cause. **M nitol** may be tried for symptom relief for cerebral oedema (not evidence-basec

Tumour lysis syndrome Rapid cell death on starting chemotherapy for rap proliferating leukaemia, lymphoma, myeloma, and some germ cell tumours result in a rise in serum urate, K^+, and phosphate, precipitating renal fail Prevention is with good **hydration** and **allopurinol** 24h *before* chemotherapy; d example if renal function OK: 300mg/12h PO. If creatinine >100µmol/L: 10C alternate days.[18] Haemodialysis may be needed in renal failure. More pot uricolytic agents: recombinant urate oxidase (**rasburicase**) 200µg/kg/d IVI 5–7d; SE: fever; D&V; headache; rash; bronchospasm; haemolysis.[19] It may inter with uric acid tests; see *datasheet*.

Inappropriate ADH secretion p666; **febrile neutropenic regimen** p336.

reating hypercalcaemia with bisphosphonates

nsure adequate hydration (eg with 0.9% saline IVI). Zoledronic acid and amidronate are 2 options.

Disodium pamidronate doses

Calcium (mmol/L; corrected)[20]	Single-dose pamidronate (mg)
<3	15–30
3–3.5	30–60
3.5–4	60–90
>4	90

nfuse slowly, eg 30mg in 300mL 0.9% saline over 3h via a largish vein. lax dose: 90mg. Response starts at ~3–5d, peaking at 1wk.

E: 'Flu symptoms, bone pain, PO_4^{3-}↓, bone pain, myalgia, nausea, vomiting, eadache, lymphocytopenia, Mg^{2+}↓, Ca^{2+}↓, seizures (rare).

oledronic acid is significantly more effective in reducing serum Ca^{2+} han previously used bisphosphonates.[21] Usually, a single dose of 4mg IVI over h will normalize plasma Ca^{2+} within a week. A higher dose should be used if orrected Ca^{2+} is >3mmol/L. ***SE:*** 'Flu symptoms, bone pain, PO_4^{3-}↓, confusion, hirst, taste disturbance, nausea, pulse↓, WCC↓, creatinine↑.

odium clodronate and ***ibandronic acid*** are other bisphosphonates.

orrected calcium in mmol/L = serum Ca^{2+} – [0.02 × serum albumin in g/L] + 0.8.

Cancer therapy

Cancer affects 30% of the population; 20% die from it. Management require multidisciplinary team; communication is vital (p510). Most patients wish to ha some part in decision making at the various stages of their treatment, and to informed of their options. Patients are becoming better informed through self-h groups and access to the internet. Most patients undergo a variety of treatme during the treatment of their cancer and your job may be to orchestrate thes

Surgery In many cases a tissue diagnosis of cancer is made with either a biopsy formal operation to remove the primary tumour. Although it is sometimes the o treatment required in early tumours of the GI tract, soft tissue sarcomas, a gynaecological tumours, it is often the case that best results follow combination of surgery and chemotherapy. Surgery also has a role in palliat advanced disease.

Radiotherapy Uses ionizing radiation to kill tumour cells. See p518.

Chemotherapy Cytotoxics should be given under expert guidance by peo trained in their administration. Drugs are often given in combination with a vari of intents: *Neoadjuvant*—to shrink tumours to reduce the need for major surg (eg mastectomy). There is also a rationale which considers early control of mic metastasis. *Primary therapy*—as the sole treatment for haematologi malignancies. *Adjuvant*—to reduce the chance of relapse, eg breast and bo cancers. *Palliative*—to provide relief from symptomatic metastatic disease a possibly to prolong survival.

Important classes of drugs include:

- Alkylating agents, eg cyclophosphamide, chlorambucil, busulfan.
- Antimetabolites, eg methotrexate, 5-fluorouracil.
- Vinca alkaloids, eg vincristine, vinblastine.
- Antitumour antibiotics, eg actinomycin D, doxorubicin.
- Others, eg etoposide, taxanes, platinum compounds. Examples of new class monoclonal antibodies/epidermal growth factor receptor inhibitors (gefiti erlotinit), EFGR. Over expression of EFGR correlates with poor prognosis in ma cancers.

Side-effects depend on the types of drugs used. Nausea/vomiting are most fea by patients and are preventable or controllable in most. Alopecia can also hav profound impact on quality of life. Neutropenia is most commonly seen 10–1 after chemotherapy (but can occur within 7d for taxanes) and sepsis requi immediate attention. ⏩See p336.

Extravasation of a chemotherapeutic agent: Suspect if there is pain, burning swelling at infusion site. ***Management:*** Stop the infusion, attempt to aspir blood from the cannula, and then remove. Take advice. Administer steroids consider antidotes.[1] Elevate the arm and mark site affected. Review regula and apply steroid cream. Apply cold pack (unless a vinca alkaloid, in which cas heat compress should be applied). Consider report to National Extravasat Scheme. Early liaison with plastic surgeon may be needed.

Communication ►*Include the patient in the decision-making process,* p510.

1 Some recommend (on scant evidence) topical dimethylsulfoxide (DMSO) and cooling after ext asation of anthracyclines or mitomycin, locally injected hyaluronidase if vinca alkaloids involved, locally injected sodium thiosulfate (sodium hyposulfite) if chlormethine (mechlorethamine; must

voiding pointless procedures in patients with cancer

urgery is often curative (eg for colorectal cancers), while other operations estore function, or deal with local recurrence, or reduce tumour bulk. But mbitious surgery is often pointless if the cancer has already spread beyond the rgan in question. A key process in planning the right procedure is to interest a adiologist in your problem. This may require more than scrawling a request on n x-ray form. The range of imaging available is constantly changing, and the adiologist may need detailed information to allow best use of the scans vailable—eg:

omputer tomography (CT): Extensive application in many cancers.

MRI: Allows precise staging in areas occult to CT (eg marrow); see p720.

one scan: Helps staging/follow-up of prostate, breast, and lung ca.

estamibi scan: Localizing active disease in breast cancer and thyroid eg if not iodine-avid). Like bone scans, it uses technetium (^{99m}Tc).

hallium scan: Helps localize viable tissue, eg in brain tumours.

allium scan: Helps staging and follow-up in lymphoma.

ctreotide scan: Localizes cancers with somatostatin receptors (eg pancreas, nedullary thyroid, neuroblastoma, and carcinoid tumours).

Monoclonal antibodies: (^{99m}Tc-labelled tumour antibodies). Helps staging y detecting tumour antigen, eg in lung, colon, and prostate cancer.

DG PET: Positron emission tomography (PET) detects high rates of aerobic netabolism, eg in lung, colon, breast, and testis. FDG = 2-[18F] fluoro--deoxy-D-glucose.

MIBG scan (^{131}I): Localizing noradrenaline production, eg phaeochromo-ytoma. MIBG = meta-iodobenzylguanidine.

Radiotherapy

Radiotherapy uses ionizing radiation to produce free radicals which damage DN Normal cells are better at repairing this damage than cancer cells, so are able recover before the next dose (or fraction) of treatment.

Radical treatment is given with curative intent. The total doses given range fro 40–70Gy (1Gy = 100cGy = 100rads) in 15–35 daily fractions. Some regime involve giving several smaller fractions a day with a gap of 6–8h. Combin chemoradiation is used in some sites, eg anus and oesophagus, to increase respon rates.

Palliation aims to relieve symptoms. Doses: 8–30Gy, given in 1, 2, 5, or 1 fractions. Bone pain, haemoptysis, cough, dyspnoea, and bleeding are helped >50% of patients. ***'Will this patient benefit from radiotherapy?'*** is a frequent asked question. When in doubt, ask an expert (or 2).

Early reactions Occur during, or soon after treatment.

- Tiredness: common after radical treatments; can last weeks to months.
- Skin reactions: These vary from erythema to dry desquamation to moi desquamation to ulceration; on completing treatment, use moisturizers.
- Mucositis: all patients receiving head and neck treatment should have a dent check-up before commencing therapy. Avoid smoking, alcohol, and spicy fooc Antiseptic mouthwashes may help. Aspirin gargle and other soluble analgesi are helpful. Treat oral thrush eg with Nystatin pastilles® chewed every 6 hou
- Nausea and vomiting: occur when stomach, liver, or brain treated. Try a dopami serotonin antagonist 1st. If unsuccessful, try $5HT_3$ serotonin antagonist, p438.
- Diarrhoea: usually after abdominal or pelvic treatments. Maintain goc hydration. Avoid high-fibre bulking agents; try loperamide.
- Dysphagia. Thoracic treatments.
- Cystitis. Pelvic treatments. Drink plenty of fluids. NSAIDs, eg diclofenac.
- Bone marrow suppression. More likely after chemotherapy or when large are are being treated. Usually reversible.

Late reactions Occur months, or years after the treatment.

- CNS: somnolence, 6–12wks after brain radiotherapy. Treat with steroids. Spin cord myelopathy—progressive weakness. MRI is needed to exclude cord com ression. Brachial plexopathy—numb, weak, and painful arm after axillary radi therapy. Reduced IQ can occur in children receiving brain irradiation if <6yrs o
- Lung: pneumonitis may occur 6–12wks after thoracic treatment, eg with d cough ± dyspnoea. Treatment: prednisolone 40mg reducing over 6wks.
- GI: xerostomia—reduced saliva. Treat with pilocarpine 5mg/8h or artificial saliv with meals. Care must be taken with all future dental care as healing is reduce Benign strictures—of oesophagus or bowel. Treat with dilatation. Fistulae—nee surgical intervention.
- GU: urinary frequency—small fibrosed bladder after pelvic treatment Fertility—pelvic radiotherapy (and cytotoxics) may affect fertility, so ova c sperm storage should be considered. This is a complex area: get expert hel See BOX. In premature female menopause or reduced testosterone—repla hormones. Vaginal stenosis and dyspareunia. Impotence—can occur sever years after pelvic radiotherapy.
- Others: panhypopituitarism, following radical treatment involving pituitary foss Children need hormones checking regularly as growth hormone may be require Hypothyroidism—neck treatments, eg for Hodgkin's lymphoma. Cataract Secondary cancers, eg sarcomas usually 10 or more years later.

Fertility issues in cancer patients

Plan with patients *before* treatment.

Chemotherapy and radiotherapy often damage germ-cell spermatogonia (∴ impaired spermatogenesis ± sterility in the male), and may hasten oocyte depletion (premature menopause in women). GNRH agonists may offer some benefit to females if taken during chemotherapy.[26] As treatments become more effective and survival improves, there are more survivors in the reproductive years for whom parenting is a top priority.[27] There is nothing like the hope of creating new life to sustain patients through the difficult times of radio- and chemotherapy, so make sure this hope is well founded.[28]

Semen cryopreservation from men and older boys with cancer must be offered before therapy. With modern fertility treatment (*OHCS* p293), even poor quality samples can yield successful pregnancies.[29] Another option is use of sperm from cryopreserved testicular tissue followed up with intracytoplasmic sperm injection (ICSI). If your patient is a man some years after cancer therapy who is unable to have children, refer him to a specialist. ►*Do not write him off as infertile:* testicular sperm extraction (TESE) with ICSI can yield normal pregnancies.[30]

Cryopreservation of embryos and ***ovarian tissue banking*** are harder options in women.[31] Harvesting and storing ovarian cortical tissue from girls and young women before potentially gonadotoxic therapy is only available in some centres.[32] Success depends on the integrity of the uterus, and in some cancers this may have been badly affected by radiotherapy.

For ethical issues and the UK Human Embryology Authority, see *OHCS* p293.

Survival—European figures

On average, 40.5% of men and 53.6% of women survive >5yrs after a cancer diagnosis (respectively, in England, 37.1% of men and 50.8% of women).[33] These statistics are based on 1.8 million adults and 24,000 children diagnosed between 1990 and 1994 and followed to 1999. (England has probably caught up since then—see the Cancer Plan/Care Pathways, p511.) Early diagnosis, a full range of treatment options, and the money spent by nations on health care all have an impact on survival.[34]

Palliative care

This does not just apply to those with cancer but anyone in the last stages of illness. Take time to find out exactly what is troubling a patient and approa problems holistically. Attention to detail is the key. Remember each person com with a set of emotions, preconceptions and a family already attached. Mc hospitals now have a dedicated palliative care team for help and advice.

Pain One of the most feared sequelae of a terminal diagnosis yet larg preventable. Studies show that cancer pain especially is poorly managed in mc settings particularly in the elderly. No patient should live or die with unreliev pain, aim to prevent or eliminate it.

Types: Don't assume a cause, take a detailed history and examine to understa the aetiology. If there is nerve infiltration or local pressure damage amitryptili may be more appropriate than opioids. Evaluate severity, nature, functional defi and psychological state – depression occurs in up to 25% of cancer patients.

Management: Explain and plan rehabilitation goals, aim to modify the pathologic process when possible, eg radiotherapy; hormones; chemotherapy; surgery. Effecti analgesia is possible in 70–90% of patients by adhering to 5 simple guidelin

1 *By the mouth* – give orally wherever possible.
2 *By the clock* – at fixed intervals to give continuous relief.
3 *By the ladder* – following the WHO stepwise approach opposite.
4 *For the individual* – there are no standard doses for opiates, needs vary.
5 *With attention to detail* – inform, set times carefully, warn of side effects.

Use the WHO ladder shown opposite until pain is relieved. Monitor the respon carefully, review of results and side effects is crucial to good care. Start regul laxatives and anti-emetics with strong opiates. Paracetamol PO/PR/IV at step 1 m have an opiate-sparing effect, and should be continued at steps 2 and 3. *Adjuvants* – NSAIDs, steroids, muscle relaxants, anxiolytics, anti-depressants

Morphine – Start with oral solution 5-10mg/4h PO with an equal breakthrou dose as often as required. A double dose at bedtime can enable a good night sleep. Patient needs will vary greatly and there is no maximum dose, aim to contr symptoms with minimum side effects. Change to modified release preparatio (MST 12h) once daily needs are known by totalling 24h use and dividing by 2. Gi 1/6 of the total daily dose as breakthrough. Side effects (common) – drowsine nausea and vomiting, constipation, dry mouth. Hallucinations and myoclonic jer are signs of toxicity and should prompt dose review. ►*If the oral route unavailable* try diamorphine IV/SC (see BOX for conversions), oxycodone IV/SC is newer more potent opioid as effective as morphine, which may have fewer sic effects. Oxynorm is the liquid form. There are also ***Fentanyl transderm patches:*** which should usually be started under specialist supervision in tho already opiate-exposed for easy titration. Remove after 72h, and place a new pat at a different site. 25, 50, 75, and 100µg/h patches are made. $t_{½}$ ≈ 17h. See BN ***Suppositories*** for pain: try oxycodone 30mg PR (eg 30mg/8h ≈ 30mg morphine Agitation: try diazepam 10mg/8h suppositories. ***Syringe drivers*** See BOX

Unfounded fears Patients often shrink from using morphine analgesia, usually as result of common misconceptions—that it is addictive, for the dying, signifyir 'The End'. It is important to address and allay these fears. Addiction is not problem in the palliative care setting, neither is respiratory depression with corre titration—pain stimulates the respiratory centre. Reassure that it is simply a goo painkiller, used in many situations. There is evidence it has no effect on li expectancy. ►*Prescribing for morphine and other controlled drugs:* include th total quantity in both words and figures, and include the formulation (tablet capsules, oral liquid etc). On charts rewrite medications in full if doses change an always give the amount in milligrams, especially when using liquid preparation

In morphine-resistant pain consider adjuvants, methadone or ketamine.

analgesic ladder

(See p560 for NNT)

ng 1	*Non-opioid*	Aspirin; paracetamol; NSAID
ng 2	*Weak opioid*	Codeine; dihydrocodeine; tramadol
ng 3	*Strong opioid*	Morphine; diamorphine; hydromorphine; oxycodone; fentanyl ± adjuvant analgesics.

ne drug fails to relieve pain, move up the ladder; do not try other drugs at same level. In new, severe pain, rung 2 may be omitted.

nge drivers deliver opioids, haloperidol, cyclizine and metoclopramide, levo-romazine, hyoscine, and glycopyronium amongst others, giving 24h cover g the subcutaneous route. They enable continuous administration whilst ding cannulation.

ate dose equivalents

	Daily dose, mg	4h dose, mg	Relative potency to morphine PO
phine PO	30	5	1×
phine IV	15	2.5	2×
norphine IV	10	2	3×
codone PO	15	2.5	2×
codone IV	10	2	3×
anyl patch	0.2	—	150×

se conversions are not exact, the table is intended only as a rough guide. The ency figures particularly can vary widely. If in doubt, use a dose below your nate when converting between opioids and titrate up according to response.

Nausea and vomiting: There are many causes to consider including chemot constipation, obstruction, drugs, severe pain, cough, squashed stomach syn oral thrush, infection and uraemia. ***Management:*** Full history and exami first aim to prevent, then treat the reversible with laxatives, fluconazole, an and antibiotics as appropriate. Consider stopping, reducing or changing d route. Anti-emetic choice should be based on mechanism and site of drug oral if possible, but remember alternative routes (IV/SC/IM/PR) and give reg monitoring response. A third will need more than one medication.

►***In chemotherapy*** vomiting is a source of much anxiety and should be pre before the 1st dose, thus avoiding anticipatory vomiting later, dexamet 4mg/12h, **metoclopramide** 10mg 8h and **ondansetron** 4–8mg 8h can be eff

Oral agents: *First line:* **Cyclizine** 50mg/8h—antihistamine, central action, most causes; **metoclopramide** 10–20mg/8h—prokinetic, good in gastric **haloperidol** 0.5-1.5mg/12h—antipsychotic, effective in drug or metabolic i nausea. *Others:* **Ondansetron** 4–8mg/8h—serotonin antagonist; if morphin ced: **levomepromazine** 3–12.5mg/12h is broad spectrum but can sedate.

Constipation: Very common with opiates, better prevented than treate **bisacodyl** 5mg at night or combine a stimulant with a softener (**co-danth** suspension 5–10mL nocte). **Movicol** sachets 2–4/12h are useful in resistan if oral therapy fails, try **glycerol** suppositories, or an arachis oil enema.

Breathlessness: Consider fans, air supply, and **supplementary O_2** or mor Use of relaxation techniques and benzodiazepines can be useful. Assess for or pericardial effusion. If there is significant pleural effusion, consider th centesis ± pleurodesis. If there is a malignant pericardial effusion, co pericardiocentesis (p761), pericardiectomy, pleuropericardial windows, ex beam radiotherapy, percutaneous balloon pericardiotomy, or pericardial lation of immunomodulators or sclerosing bleomycin.

Coated/dry mouth: Treat any candida, infection or other underlying cause. measures such as chewing ice chips, pineapple chunks (release prot enzymes) or gum should be tried, good oral hygiene with mouth w chorhexidine and saliva substitutes, such as Oralbalance® gel can help.

Pruritus (itching): See p64.

Venepuncture problems: Repeated venepuncture with the attendant painful extravasation and phlebitis may be avoided by insertion of skin tun catheter (eg a Hickman line)—a single or multilumen line—into a major centr (eg subclavian or internal jugular) using a strict aseptic technique. Patien look after their own lines at home, and give their own drugs. Problems in infection, blockage (flush with 0.9% saline or dilute heparin, eg every axillary, subclavian, or superior vena cava thrombosis/obstruction, an slippage. Even more convenient portable delivery devices are available, all drugs to be given at a preset time, without the patient's intervention.

The last days and weeks of life: Once a decision has been made that a pat entering the very final weeks of their illness, comfort should be the main co Think about stopping observations, unnecessary blood tests and medications as those for long term prophylaxis). Ensure that a decision regarding resusci status has been made and clearly documented; this should usually be don senior doctor. Syringe drivers and fluids subcutaneously are often helpful, av repeated cannulation attempts. *Terminal secretions* can be eased with antic ergics such as **glycopyrronium** 200µg SC. Relieve pain, *agitation* can be distressing for relatives, **midazolam** 0.5–2.5mg SC can help.

Consider with the family and patient whether transfer to an alternative loca hospice may be appropriate and if going home is a priority—this can be arr at very short notice to enable comfort during final hours.

er agents

er agents and procedures to know about (alphabetically listed)

h)olestyramine 4g/6h PO (1h after other drugs) helps itch in jaundice.

uconazole 50md/24h PO for candida

-antagonists (eg **cimetidine** 400mg/12h PO) help gastric irritation—associated with gastric carcinoma.

aloperidol 0.5–5mg/24h PO helps agitation, nightmares, hallucinations, and miting.

yoscine hydrobromide 0.4–0.6mg/8h SC or 0.3mg sublingual: vomiting from per GI obstruction or noisy bronchial rattles.

erve blocks may lastingly relieve pleural or other resistant pains.

ow-residue diets may be needed for post-radiotherapy diarrhoea.

etronidazole 400mg/8h PO mitigates anaerobic odours from tumours; so do **arcoal dressings** (Actisorb®).

aproxen 250mg/8h with food: fevers caused by malignancy or bone pain om metastases (consider splinting joints if this fails).

odium chloride nebulisers 5mL as needed, can aid persistent cough

pironolactone 100mg/12h PO + **bumetanide** 1mg/24h PO for ascites.

teroids: **dexamethasone**: give 8mg IV stat to relieve symptoms of superior ena cava or bronchial obstruction—or lymphangitis carcinomatosa. Tablets are mg (≈15mg prednisolone). 4mg/12–24h PO may stimulate appetite, or reduce P headache, or induce (in some patients) satisfactory sense of euphoria.

Urgent referral in possible malignancy

A variety of clinical scenarios and symptoms should alert you to the pos presence of malignancy and prompt urgent referral to the appropriate specialist list below is by no means exhaustive but covers the commonest presentation

Lung • Immediate referral if there are signs of superior vena caval obstructic stridor • Urgently with persistent haemoptysis (smokers or non-smokers over • Suggestive CXR (pleural effusion, slowly resolving consolidation) • Normal CX high suspicion • History of asbestos exposure and recent chest pain or dysp • Unexplained systemic symptoms with suspicious CXR. ►*High risk groups:* ex current smokers, COPD, asbestos exposure, history of cancer.

Upper gastrointestinal • Urgent referral should be regardless of *H. Pylori* sta there is *dyspepsia* and one of the following; chronic GI bleeding, dysph progressive unintentional weight loss, persistent vomiting, iron deficiency anae an epigastric mass, suspicious barium meal result. Also if: • Isolated dysph • Unexplained upper abdominal pain and weight loss, with or without back • Upper abdominal mass without dyspepsia • Obstructive jaundice • Consid vomiting or iron deficiency anaemia with weight loss, or dyspepsia with; Barr oesophagus, dysplasia, atrophic gastritis or old (>20yrs ago) peptic ulcer surg ►*For endoscopy:* those over 55 with persistent unexplained recent onset dyspe

Lower gastrointestinal if there are equivocal symptoms and you are not anx it is reasonable to watch and wait. Do PR examination and FBC in • Over 40 with PR bleeding and bowel habit change (more loose/frequent weeks) • Over 60 with PR bleed or change of bowel habit >6 weeks • Any age a right lower abdominal mass likely to be bowel • Palpable rectal mass • Me non-menstruating women with unexplained iron deficiency anaemia and Hb than 11 or 10 respectively. ►*High risk groups:* Ulcerative colitis; it is unprc whether a family history of colon cancer assists decisions in symptomatic patie

Breast • Discrete, hard lump with fixation • Over 30 with a discrete lump pers ing after a period or presenting post-menopause • Under 30 with an enlarg lump, fixed and hard lump, or family history • Previous breast cancer with a lump or suspicious symptoms • Unilateral eczematous skin or nipple cha unresponsive to topical treatment • Recent nipple distortion • Spontaneous blo unilateral nipple discharge • Men over 50 with a unilateral firm subareolar m ►consider referral if under 30 with a lump or persistent breast pain.

Gynaecology • Examination suggestive of cervical cancer (don't wait for a sm test) • Postmenopausal bleeding in non-HRT patients or those on HRT after 6 we cessation • Vulval lump or bleeding • consider in persistent intermenstrual bleed ►*Ultrasound:* any abdominal or pelvic mass not GI or urological in origin. Do pe and abdominal examinations, with speculum as appropriate.

Urology • Hard irregular prostate (refer with PSA result) • Normal prostate raised PSA (p681) ± urinary tract symptoms • Urinary symptoms and a high • Painless macroscopic haematuria at any age • Over 40 with persistent recurrent UTI and haematuria • Over 50 with unexplained microscopic haemat • Any abdominal mass arising from the urological tract • A swelling or mass in body of the testis • Ulceration or mass in the penis suggestive of cancer.

Central nervous system • Symptoms including progressive neurological def new-onset seizures, headaches, mental changes, cranial nerve palsy, unilat sensorineural deafness or a suspicion of brain tumour • Recent-onset headac with suggestion of raised intracranial pressure eg. vomiting, drowsiness, postu related headache, pulse-synchronous tinnitus, or other CNS symptoms • A new different unexplained headache of progressive severity • Suspected recent-on seizures ►consider in rapid progression of subacute focal deficit, unexplai cognitive impairment, or personality change with features indicative of a tumc

Haematological p336; ***Thyroid*** p622.

:he energy we expend in speeding up referrals paying off?

sibly not. There is evidence that reducing breast cancer waits from a few ıths to a few weeks is helpful—but there is little evidence that a few weeks e or there make any difference in colon and other cancers.[48] There are blems with the guidelines in that patients can meet national criteria and still deemed 'inappropriate' by the consultant, while patients not meeting the eria can present with suspicious signs—but they will not be seen soon ause these possibly less serious cases are forced to jump the queue. This is one example of the aphorism that ***all targets distort clinical priorities***.

n one NHS trust ~66% of referrals for suspected cancer of breast, skin, and on problems were deemed 'appropriate', and 80–100% of gynaecological, er GI, lung, and urological cancer referrals were judged appropriate.[49]

tudies of how well dermatology cancer guidelines work conclude that the t way forward is by education regarding recognition of benign conditions.[50] lso seems likely that dialogue between local consultants and referring GPs is ey factor—and that this dialogue will become harder and less coherent as rent moves for 'choose and book' and patient-choice agendas lead to errals over ever wider geographical areas.

On the good side, establishing clear referral responsibilities forces everyone to k at what they are doing—and this has facilitated many care pathways.

13 Rheumatological and related illnes

Contents

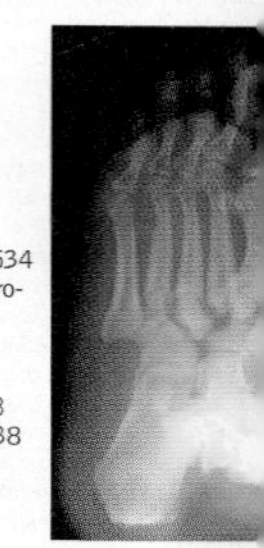

Fig 1. Oblique view of cot's joints in the foo

Relevant pages elsewhere: Charcot's joints (fig 1 & p508); Behçet's d (p686); Sjögren's syndrome (p702); Wegener's granulomatosis (p706).

Points to note in the rheumatological history

Age, occupation, origin (eg SLE is commoner in Afro-Caribbeans and Asian

- ***Presenting symptoms***

Joints: Pain, morning stiffness (eg RA)
Pattern of distribution
Swelling, loss of function

Extra-articular: Rashes, photosensitivity (eg SLE)
Raynaud's (SLE; CREST, p538; poly- and dermatomyositis)
Dry eyes or mouth (Sjögren's)
Red eyes (eg ank. spond., p536)
Diarrhoea/urethritis (Reiter's)
Nodules or nodes (RA; TB)
Mouth/genital ulcers (Behçet's)
Weight loss (eg TB; arthritis)

- ***Related diseases:*** eg Crohr in ankylosing spondylitis; psoriasis; gonorrhoea; Reite associated arthritis.
- ***Current & past drugs:*** Dise modifying drugs (p533), NS
- ***Family history:*** Arthritis, psoriasis, autoimmune dise
- ***Social history:*** Functioning eg dressing, writing, walkin domestic situation, social support, home adaptations. Smoking (may worsen RA).

Existential approaches to rheumatology patients We like to see rheumat patients early *before* destructive changes take place—but all too often, like ois Verret productions, our encounters are multimedia affairs, with confl lines of story and mime, ever-changing charts of painful, disjointed images, pu manifestations, disorganized articulations, and oblique views (fig 1). The diag you arrive at will depend on which layer of this multimedia event you attend single interpretation is universally valid, and in your attempts to lead an auth life on the wards and in clinics you may frequently need to change your an approach. When in doubt (the only valid state of the thinking doctor), ask patient what is most important. Their answers often focus on other peopl their relationships—so find out how these interact with their joint sympton

We thank Dr Andrew Brown who is our Specialist Reader for this chapter.

ts to note when assessing the locomotor system

aims to screen for most rheumatological conditions, and to assess motor ility. It is based on the GALS locomotor screen (below).

nce Ask questions; "look, 'feel' and move" (active and passive). If a joint *normal* to the patient, *looks normal* to you, and has *full range of movement,* ally *is* normal. Make sure the patient is comfortable, and obtain their ent before examination: expose the limb, including the joint above the one examined.

eening questions
Are you free of any pain or stiffness?
Can you dress all right?
Can you manage stairs?
s' to all 3, muscle/joint problems are unlikely. If 'No' to any, go into detail.

screening examination To be done in light underwear.

e: *Observe from behind:* Is muscle bulk OK (buttocks, shoulders)? Is the straight? Symmetrical paraspinal muscles? Swellings/deformities? *Observe the side*: Normal cervical and lumbar lordosis? Kyphosis? *'Touch your toes, se'*: Is lumbar spine flexion normal? *Observe from in front* for the rest of the nination. Ask him to: *'Tilt head towards shoulders'* (without moving the lders): is lateral neck flexion normal? Palpate for typical fibromyalgia tender s.[1]

s: *'Try putting your hands behind head'*—tests functional shoulder ement. *'Arms straight'*: Tests elbow extension. Also tests forearm nation/ pronation. *Examine the hands*: See p27. Any deformity, wasting, or lings? *Squeeze across 2nd–5th metacarpophalangeal joints.* Pain may denote or tendon synovitis. Repeat for metatarsophalangeal joints. *'Put index r on thumb'*—tests pincer grip. Assess dexterity.

: *Observe legs*: Normal quadriceps bulk? Any swelling or deformity ngth discrepancy? *Internally/externally rotate each hip in flexion.* Passively knee and hip to the full extent. Is movement limited? Any crepitus? *Find any effusion*: With patient supine, do the patella tap test. If there is fluid, ider aspirating and testing it for crystals or infection. *Observe feet*: Any rmity? Are arches high or flat? Any callosities? These may indicate an ormal gait of some chronicity.

: *'Walk over there please'*: Is the gait smooth? Good arm swing? Stride th OK? Normal heel strike and toe off? Can he turn quickly?

GALS system for quickly recording your findings

G (Gait) ✓

	Appearance:	Movement:
A (Arms)	✓	✓
L (Legs)	✓	✓
S (Spine)	✓	✓

✓ means normal. If not normal, then put a cross with a note to explain what the exact problem is.

ge of joint movement is noted in degrees, with anatomical position being neutral position eg elbow flexion 0°–150° normally, with fixed flexion and ed movement, range may be 30°–90°. A valgus deformity points (deviates) y from mid-line (laterally); a varus deformity points towards.

omyalgia (fibrositis) denotes an ill-understood set of symptoms, eg in menopausal women who ain of multiple musculoskeletal aches, sometimes with trigger points, eg to palpation over trapezius, knee, and the lateral epicondyle of the elbow.

Back pain

This is very common, and often self-limiting; but *be alert to sinister cau* malignancy, infection or inflammatory causes. Key points: **1** Onset: sudden (r to trauma?) or gradual? **2** Motor or sensory symptoms? **3** Is the bladder or affected? **4** Is there sciatica? True sciatica radiates into the buttock, back thigh, and *below* the knee into the calf and ankle. This is caused by sciatic irritation, and is usually due to a prolapsed disc.

Examination: 1 With the patient standing, gauge the extent and smoothn lumbar forward/lateral flexion and extension.[1] **2** Neurological deficits: test limb sensation, power and reflexes (BOX)—if there is any abnormality, do a perianal tone and sensation. **3** Examine for nerve root pain: this is distribu relevant dermatomes, and is worsened by coughing or bending forward. Str leg test is +ve if raising the leg with the knee extended causes pain below the which ↑ on foot dorsiflexion. It suggests irritation to the sciatic nerve (L4, L5 The main cause is lumbar disc prolapse. **4** Signs of generalized dise malignancy? Also examine other systems (eg abdomen) as pain may be ref

Causes Age determines the most likely causes:

- 15–30yrs: Prolapsed disc, trauma, fractures, ankylosing spondylitis p536), spondylolisthesis (a forward shift of one vertebra another, which is congenital or due to trauma), pregnancy.
- 30–50yrs: Degenerative spinal disease, prolapsed disc, malignancy (pri or secondary from lung, breast, prostate, thyroid or kidney
- >50yrs: Degenerative, osteoporotic vertebral collapse, Paget's, maligr myeloma, spinal stenosis.

Rarer: Cauda equina tumours, spinal infection (eg discitis, usually staphyloc also *Proteus*; *Escherichia coli*; *S. typhi*; TB): there are often no systemic signs

Red flags signalling to you that "*this back pain is sinister!*"

• Aged <20yrs or >55yrs old	• Thoracic back pain
• Acute onset in elderly people	• Bilateral or alternating symptoms
• Constant or progressive pain	• Neurological disturbance
• Nocturnal pain	• Sphincter disturbance
• ↑Pain on being supine	• Leg claudication (spinal stenosis)
• Morning stiffness	• Current or recent infection
• Fever, night sweats, weight loss	• Immunosuppression eg, steroids/H
• History of malignancy	• Abdominal mass

►**Neurosurgical emergencies** •***Acute cauda equina compression:*** Alternati bilateral root pain in legs, saddle anaesthesia (around anus), loss of anal tone bladder ± bowel incontinence •***Acute cord compression:*** Bilateral pain, LMN at level of compression, UMN and sensory loss below, sphincter disturbance. ***Causes*** (same for both): bony metastasis (look for missing pedicle on X-ray), disc protrusion, myeloma, cord or paraspinal tumour, TB (p386), abscess. ►►Urgent treatment prevents irreversible loss, eg laminectomy for disc protrus radiotherapy for tumours, decompression for abscesses.

Tests are usually only needed if red flags are present: FBC, ESR & CRP (myel infection, tumour), U&E, ALP (Paget's), serum/urine electrophoresis (myeloma) X-ray may show Paget's, vertebral collapse or spondylolisthesis. MRI is best fo prolapse, cord compression, cancer, infection or inflammation (eg sacroiliitis

R: If there is no serious pathology, focus on education and encouragement, as cases are self-limiting. Analgesia (regular paracetamol ± NSAIDs ± codeine) returning to normal activities as soon as possible is better than bed rest (w should not be advised). Avoid precipitants and refer to physiotherapy i improving. Address psycho-social issues (see BOX). Local injections, eg facet jo may have a role. Surgical options may be considered in a small group of sele patients with intractable symptoms who fail to respond to other measures.

'ellow flags

'sycho-social risk factors for developing persisting chronic pain and long-term ısability have been termed 'yellow flags'. These include:

- Belief that pain and activity are harmful.
- Sickness behaviours such as extended rest.
- Social withdrawal.
- Emotional problems such as low or negative mood, depression, anxiety, stress.
- Problems and/or dissatisfaction at work.
- Problems with claims or compensation or time off work.
- Overprotective family or lack of support.
- Inappropriate expectations of treatment eg low active participation in treatment.

ıerve root lesions

ıerve root	Pain	Weakness	Reflex change
.2	Across upper thigh	Hip flexion, adduction	Nil
.3	Across lower thigh	Hip adduction, knee extension	Knee
.4	Across knee to medial malleolus	Knee extension, foot inversion and dorsiflexion	Knee
.5	Lateral shin to dorsum of foot and big toe	Hip extension and abduction Knee flexion Foot and great toe dorsiflexion	Nil
51	Posterior calf to lateral foot and little toe	Knee flexion Foot and toe plantar flexion Foot eversion	Ankle

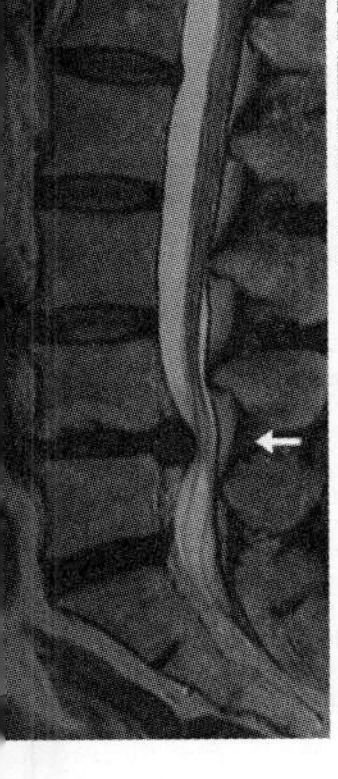

Fig 1. Sagittal T2 weighted MRI of the lumbar spine showing a herniated disc at the L4–L5 space.

Schober's test: this is a test of lumbar spine flexion. A mark is made on the lumbar spine at the vel of the posterior iliac spine. A line is measured 5cm below and 10cm above this. The patient is ked to bend forwards as far as they can. If the line does not increase by at least 5cm, this dicates a limitation of lumbar flexion eg in ankylosing spondylitis.

Arthritis—general points

Features of inflammatory arthritis Pain, stiffness (especially early morning >3 minutes), joint inflammation (swelling, redness, warmth) and loss of function.

Causes of inflammatory arthritis and their common presentations

Monoarthritis (1 joint)	Oligoarthritis (≤5 joints)	Polyarthritis (>5 joints)
Septic arthritis	Crystal arthritis	Rheumatoid arthritis
Crystal arthritis (gout, CPPD)	Psoriatic arthritis	Psoriatic arthritis
Osteoarthritis	Reactive arthritis	Reactive arthritis
Trauma (haemarthrosis)	Ankylosing spondylitis	Osteoarthritis
	Osteoarthritis	Systemic conditions[1]

Diagnosis ►Consider septic arthritis in any acutely inflamed joint, as this ma destroy a joint within 24h. All such joints should be aspirated, and if in doubt trea with antibiotics until results are known. NB: inflammation may be less overt immunocompromised or if there is underlying joint disease.

Assess Distribution of joint involvement (including spine), symmetry, disruption c joint anatomy, limitation of movement (by pain or contracture), joint effusions an peri-articular involvement (see p527 for full assessment). Look for extra-articula features: skin, nail or eye involvement; dysuria or genital ulcers; lungs, kidneys heart, GI (eg mouth ulcers, bloody diarrhoea in Crohn's/UC) and CNS systems.

Blood tests: Culture if septic arthritis. Do FBC, ESR, urate, U&E, CRP. Conside rheumatoid factor, antinuclear antibody, other autoantibodies (p539), and HLA B2 (p536) guided by presentation. Consider causes of reactive arthritis (p536) eg vira serology, urine chlamydia PCR, hepatitis and HIV serology if risk factors are presen

Radiology: Look for erosions, calcification, widening or loss of joint space, change in underlying bone of affected joints (eg periarticular osteopenia, sclerotic areas osteophytes). Image sacroiliac joints if considering a spondyloarthritis (there i irregularity of the lower half on XR or on MRI, which is more sensitive). Do a CXR fo RA, SLE, vasculitis, TB and sarcoid. In septic arthritis, X-rays may be normal, as ma ESR and CRP (if CRP ↑, expect it to fall with treatment). Other imaging (ultrasoun or MRI) may be more sensitive in identifying joint inflammation or damage than XR

Joint aspiration: See *OHCS* p708. Attempt to aspirate any joint suspected of being infected. Send synovial fluid for white cell count, polarized light microscopy (fo crystals, p531) and microbiology for urgent Gram stain and culture. The risk o inducing septic arthritis, using sterile precautions, is <1:10000.[8]

Treatment is determined by the cause. If **septic arthritis** is suspected,[2] give goo analgesia and ensure blood cultures and synovial fluid have been taken. Then star empirical IV antibiotics until sensitivities are known: flucloxacillin (in adults: ½- 1g/6h slowly IV) + benzylpenicillin 1.2g/4h IV ± gentamicin (p738).[9] In infants *Haemophilus* is common, so give cefotaxime too (50mg/kg/12h IV slowly). If HI +ve, look for atypical mycobacteria and fungi. Ask a microbiologist how long t continue treatment (eg ≥2wks IV, then 4wks PO).[10] Ask for orthopaedic advice fo consideration of aspiration (arthrocentesis), lavage, and debridement, especially i there is a prosthetic joint involved.[11] This may be done by arthroscopic means (eg for knee) or open (eg for hip or shoulder, with GA; this allows biopsy—helpful for TB) Splint for ≤48h; then give physiotherapy. ►*Ask yourself* 'how did the organism ge there?' Is there immunosuppression, or a focus of infection (eg pneumonia is presen in up to 50% of those with pneumococcal arthritis)?[12]

1 Eg: connective tissue disease (eg SLE), malignancy (eg leukaemia), endocarditis, haemochromatosis sarcoidosis, sickle cell anaemia, familial Mediterranean fever, Behçet's, relapsing polychondritis.

2 Common organisms are *Staph aureus*, *Streptococcus*, *Neisseria gonococcus*, Gram –ve bacilli. More common in those with RA and in those with joint prostheses—where infection is particularly difficult to treat. See *Rheum Dis Clin North Am* 2003 **29** 61 *Advances in managing septic arthritis*.

Synovial fluid in health and disease

Aspiration of synovial fluid is used primarily to look for infection or crystal (gout or CPPD crystal arthropathy, p534).

	Appearance	Viscosity	wbc/mm³	Neutrophils
Normal	Clear, colourless	↑	≤200	None
Osteoarthritis	Clear, straw	↑	≤1000	≤50%
Haemorrhagic[1]	Bloody, xanthochromic	Varies	≤10,000	≤50%
Acutely inflamed	Turbid, yellow	↓		
• RA			1–50000	Varies
• Crystal			5–50000	~80%
Septic	Turbid, yellow	↓	10–100000	>90%

Early treatment of rheumatoid arthritis

Therapeutic strategies for the treatment of rheumatoid arthritis have changed considerably over the past decade, with emphasis shifting towards early assessment, diagnosis and therapy. This has arisen from the concept that there is a 'window of opportunity' in early disease, where using combinations of disease modifying agents ± biological agents (see p533) may alter the disease course, reduce joint damage and provide life-long benefit. Imaging techniques, such as ultrasound and MRI, can help to identify synovitis more accurately, even in joints with normal clinical examination, and have greater sensitivity in detecting bone erosions than conventional XR.

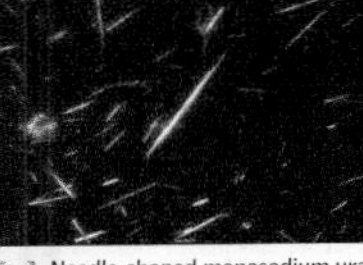

Fig 1. Needle-shaped monosodium urate crystals found in gout, displaying negative birefringence under polarised light.

Fig 2. Calcium pyrophosphate dihydrate crystals found in pseudogout, displaying positive birefringence under polarised light.

1 Eg seen with trauma, haemophilia or tumours.

Rheumatoid arthritis (RA)

RA is a chronic systemic inflammatory disease, characterised by a symmetri deforming, peripheral polyarthritis. Peak onset: 4th–5th decade. ♀:♂ >: Prevalence: ~1% (↑ in smokers). HLA DR4/DR1 linked (associated with ↑severit

Presentation Typically with symmetrical swollen, painful, and stiff small joint hands and feet, worse in the morning. This can fluctuate and larger joints becc involved. Less commonly presents as a sudden onset of widespread arthritis,

1. Recurring mono/polyarthritis of various joints (*palindromic—'was I saw!'*)
2. Persistent monoarthritis (often of 1 knee, shoulder or hip).
3. Systemic illness with extra-articular symptoms eg fever, fatigue, weight lc pericarditis, pleurisy. Minimal joint problems at first (commoner in men).
4. Polymyalgic onset—vague limb girdle aches.

Signs Early (inflammation, no joint damage): joint swelling, esp. symmetrical M PIP, wrist, metatarsal joints. Look for tenosynovitis or bursitis. Later (joint dama deformity): ulnar deviation of the fingers and dorsal wrist subluxation. Boutonni and swan-neck deformities of fingers or Z-deformity of thumbs occur. Ha extensor tendons may rupture. Foot changes are similar. Larger joints can involved. Atlanto-axial joint subluxation may threaten the spinal cord.

Extra-articular Nodules—elbows & lungs; lymphadenopathy; vasculitis; fibros alveolitis, obliterative bronchiolitis; pleural & pericardial effusion; Raynaud's; car tunnel syndrome, peripheral neuropathy; splenomegaly (in 5%; but only 1% h Felty's syndrome: RA + splenomegaly + neutropenia, p690); episcleritis, scleri scleromalacia, keratoconjunctivitis sicca; osteoporosis; amyloidosis (p354).

Tests *Rheumatoid factor* (RhF) is +ve in ~70% (p539). A high titre is associa with severe disease, erosions and extra-articular disease. Citrullinated pept antibodies (anti-CCP) are highly specific, but not widely available. There is of anaemia of chronic disease. Inflammation causes ↑platelets, ↑ESR, ↑CRP. ***X-ra*** show soft tissue swelling, juxta-articular osteopenia and ↓joint space. Later th may be bony erosions ± subluxation ± complete carpal destruction.

Diagnostic criteria (for research) include 4 out of 7 of: Morning stiffness (>1 hc lasting >6 weeks), arthritis of ≥3 joints, arthritis of hand joints, symmetri arthritis, rheumatoid nodules, +ve rheumatoid factor and radiographic changes

Management ►Refer early to a rheumatologist for specialist assessment.

- Early use of DMARDs improves symptoms and long term outcomes (see BOX).
- *Steroids*: Rapidly reduce inflammation and control symptoms in the short-te They are useful for treating acute exacerbations ("flares") of disease eg with depot injections of methylprednisolone 80–120mg. Intra-articular steroids a have a rapid but short-term effect (technique see *OHCS* p708–711). Oral stero may control difficult symptoms—eg prednisolone 7.5mg/d PO, but long te treatment is not routinely recommended, due to their significant side effect
- Most will need an *NSAID* to control symptoms, as paracetamol ± weak opiates a rarely effective. NSAIDs are CI in asthma or with an active peptic ulcer. O cannot predict which NSAID a patient will respond to, so different ones can tried eg ibuprofen, diclofenac, etodolac (see p535). Patients who are >65 or w have a previous history of peptic ulcer need gastric protection eg lansopraz 30mg/d PO. NSAIDs have little effect on disease progression.
- Encourage regular exercise; physio- and occupational therapy eg for aids, splir
- Surgery may be considered in the long-term to relieve pain, improve functi and to prevent disease complications (eg ulna stylectomy, joint replacement
- Risk of cardiovascular and cerebrovascular disease is ↑, as atherosclerosis accelerated in RA. Manage risk factors (p79). Smoking also ↑symptoms of R

1 *Palin dromo* is Greek for 'to run to and fro' or 'to recur'. Verbal palindromes read equally w forwards or back, to and fro, as in *Lager, Sir, is regal*. In rheumatological palindromes, arthritis last hours or days runs to and fro, visiting and revisiting 3 or more sites, typically knees, wrists, & MCP joir It may presage RA, SLE, Whipple's, or Behçet's disease. Remissions are (initially) complete, leaving radiological mark. Patient diaries *might* reflect **w**rist, ankle, shoulder, and interphalangeal arthritis, ten ting obsessive diagnosticians to hope (unreasonably) for a perfectly palindromic week, eg *Was I sa*

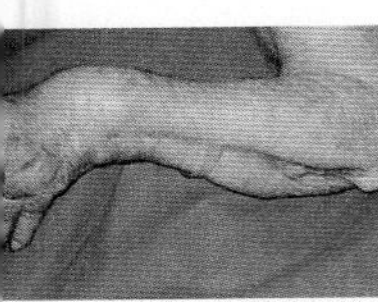

Fig 1. Rheumatoid Arthritis. Note ulna deviation of the fingers.

fluencing biological events in RA

e chief biological event is inflammation. Monocytes traffic into joints, tokines are produced, fibroblasts and endothelial cells are activated, and tissue oliferates. Fluid is generated (effusion) and cytokines and cellular processes ode cartilage and bone. Cytokines also produce systemic effects: fatigue, celerated atherosclerosis, and accelerated bone turnover.

sease-modifying drugs (DMARDs)[1] modulate the above reaction and slow or op disease progression. Early DMARD therapy is associated with better long m prognosis. They can take up to 6–12 weeks for symptomatic benefit. ethotrexate and sulfasalazine are typical 1st line choices and may be used gether. Regular blood test monitoring is required.

ethotrexate Given weekly. Avoid in liver disease, pregnancy and if alcohol nsumption↑; caution if pre-existing lung disease. SE: oral ulcers, nausea, hargy, myelosuppression, hepatotoxicity, pneumonitis (rare, but can be life-reatening). Give concurrent folic acid to ↓SE, eg 5mg/2–3 times per wk, PO.

lfasalazine SE: Myelosuppression, nausea, rash, oral ulcers, ↓sperm count.

flunomide may be an alternative to sulfasalazine. SE: Rash, oral ulcers, arrhoea, ↑BP, myelosuppression, hepatotoxicity. CI: Pregnancy.

old Usually by IM injection. More toxicity than methotrexate or sulfasalazine. : Myelosuppression, renal toxicity, rash, mouth ulcers, photosensitivity.

nicillamine SE: Myelosuppression, renal toxicity, loss of taste, oral ulcers, yasthenia gravis-like syndrome.

droxychloroquine Least toxic, but probably least effective. SE: Rash, tinopathy (check vision with an Amsler chart every 12 months, see p540).

athioprine SE: Myelosuppression, nausea, LFT↑. See p360.

closporin SE: Nausea, tremor, gum hypertrophy, ↑BP, renal impairment (p360).

Myelosuppression (bone marrow suppression) is a potentially serious SE of ARDS which can result in pancytopenia, with ↑susceptibility to infection and erwhelming sepsis due to neutropenia.

ti-cytokine therapy Tumour necrosis factor α (TNFα) and interleukin-1 (IL- are cytokines over-produced in RA synovium. TNFα blockers include ***infliximab*** himeric murine/human anti-TNF antibody, IV every 8wks p267), ***etanercept*** NFα receptor/IgFc fusion protein, SC twice weekly), and ***adalimumab*** (fully man anti-TNF monoclonal antibody, SC every 2wks). These biological agents e approved by NICE for severe active RA after failure to respond to 2 DMARDs. inical response can be striking, and improved outcomes have been shown. CI: egnancy, breast feeding, active infection, severe heart failure, demyelinating sease, previous Ca. *SE:* (Usually well tolerated): injection reaction, infections, activation of TB (∴ screen & consider prophylaxis), worsening of heart failure. ng-term safety is unknown (no clear evidence for ↑cancer). Neutralizing tibodies may ↓efficacy with infliximab; ANA and reversible SLE-type illness may olve. ***Anakinra***, an IL-1 inhibitor, and many more agents are being evaluated.

[1] See *BNF* for dosages and further details.

Osteoarthritis (OA)

OA is the commonest joint condition. ♀:♂≈3:1, usually >50yrs. It is usually prim
but may be secondary to joint disease or other conditions (eg haemochromato

Signs & symptoms In localised disease (usually knee or hip): pain on mover
and crepitus, worse at end of day; background pain at rest; joint gelling—stiff
after rest up to ~30mins; joint instability. In generalised disease—with Heberc
nodes ('nodal OA'; seen mainly in post-menopausal ♀), commonly affected joints
the DIP joints, thumb carpo-metacarpal joints and the knee. There may be
tenderness, derangement ± bony swelling (Heberden's nodes: bony lumps at
Bouchard's nodes: PIP; "squared" thumb), ↓range of movement and mild synov

Tests XR shows loss of joint space, subchondral sclerosis and cysts, and marg
osteophytes (see Figure). CRP can be elevated slightly.

Treatment Do **exercises** (quadriceps exercises to ↑muscle strength and
stability in knee OA) and keep active. Regular **paracetamol** ± **codeine** for
Consider NSAIDs (see BOX). **Reduce weight** if BMI >28, **walking aids**, suppo
footwear, **physio**; **topical NSAIDs** and **capsaicin** (derived from chillies) may
The role of hyaluronic acid injections is unclear; glucosamine & chondroitin su
'failed' a 2006 *NEJM* trial. **Intra-articular steroid injections** help severe s
ptoms temporarily. **Joint replacement** is the best way to deal with severe OA

Rheumatology

Crystal arthropathies

Gout When acute, there is severe joint redness, pain, and swelling. It often aff
one joint, eg the metatarsophalangeal joint of the big toe (podagra), but ca
polyarticular. Gout is associated with ↑plasma urate, and attacks are due to
deposition of monosodium urate crystals in and near joints (may be precipitate
trauma, surgery, starvation, infection or diuretics). With long-term hyperuricae
urate deposits (tophi) in the peripheries (pinna, tendons, joints), and renal dis
(stones, interstitial nephritis) may occur. ***Prevalence:*** ~1%. ♂:♀≈5:1.
Causes of ↑urate: Hereditary, dietary purines, alcohol excess (esp beer), diure
leukaemia, cytotoxics (tumour lysis), renal impairment. ***Diagnosis*** depends
finding urate crystals in tissues and synovial fluid (serum urate may be norma
Polarized light microscopy of synovial fluid shows *negatively birefringent* crys
X-rays show only soft-tissue swelling in the early stages. Later, well-def
'punched out' erosions are seen in juxta-articular bone. There is no scler
reaction, and joint spaces are preserved until late. ***Treating acute gout:*** U
strong NSAID (eg indomethacin). If CI (eg peptic ulcer), use **colchicine** 0.5
8–12h, or 0.5mg/2–3h PO until pain goes or D&V occurs or 6mg given. N
renal impairment, NSAIDs and colchicine are problematic. **Steroids** (oral, IM or ir
articular) may be effective. ***Preventing attacks:*** Avoid prolonged fasts, alc
excess, and purine rich food.[1] Lose weight. Avoid low-dose aspirin (it ↑ se
urate). Consider reducing serum urate with long-term **allopurinol** if there
recurrent attacks, tophi or renal stones. Introduction of allopurinol may caus
attack so wait until 3wks after an acute episode, and start with regular NSAI
colchicine cover. ***Allopurinol dose:*** Typically 200mg/24h; max 300mg/8h. Ac
according to serum urate levels. SE: rash, fever, WCC↓. Caution in renal impairm

Calcium pyrophosphate dihydrate (CPPD) arthropathy ***Risk factors:*** Old age
hyperparathyroidism, haemochromatosis, hypothyroidism, ↓PO_4^{3-}, ↓Mg^{2+}. ***Ac
CPPD (pseudogout):*** Similar to gout, presenting as a monoarthritis. It aff
different joints: knee, wrist or hip. Usually spontaneous, self-limiting, and ca
provoked by illness, surgery or trauma. ***Chronic CPPD:*** Destructive changes like
but more severe. Can present as a polyarthritis (pseudo-rheumatoid). Te
Polarized light microscopy of joint fluid: crystals are *weakly positively birefring*
It is associated with chondrocalcinosis—soft-tissue calcium deposition on X-ray
triangular ligament in wrist, or in knee cartilage. ***℞:*** Analgesia, NSAIDs. If
working, try steroids (intra-articular, IM or PO) or hydroxychloroquine 200mg

›scribing NSAIDs: dialogue with patients

y prescribe NSAIDs after careful risk-benefit analysis individualized for each :ient, including indication, dosage, proposed duration of therapy, and medical morbidity. The main serious SE are GI bleeding and renal impairment.

ny patients prescribed NSAIDs do not need them all the time, so say "Take the ⁄est possible dose for the shortest possible time." *Bleeding is more common in* ›*se who know less about their drugs.*[24] Explain:

›rugs are for relief of symptoms: *on good days none may be needed.*

›bdominal pain may be a sign of impending gut problems: stop the tablets, nd come back for more advice if symptoms continue.

Jlcers may occur with no warning: report black motions (± faints) at once.

›on't supplement prescribed NSAIDs with ones bought over the counter ›eg ibuprofen): mixing NSAIDs can increase risks 20-fold.

›moking and alcohol ↑NSAID risk.

›en should COX-2 selective NSAIDs be considered? Not often: perhaps **only** en an NSAID is essential **and** there is past peptic ulceration (but risk is not ıinated, and bleeds that do occur may be very serious) **if** an ordinary NSAID with (proton pump inhibitors, eg omeprazole, the preferred regimen) is problem- :—**or** >65yrs old (not on aspirin)—**or** needing high-dose NSAID over a long e. PPIs may also be given with COX-2 inhibitors;[25] it is not known if this works. X-2 (cyclo-oxygenase-2) selective NSAIDs are not as safe as we had hoped. ›ere is ↑risk of heart failure, MI & stroke.[MET 26] This ↑risk may also apply to ıventional NSAIDs.[27] So avoid if known renal failure or vascular disease (past ⁄stroke). There is insufficient experience with new COX-2 selective inhibitors oricoxib, parecoxib, and lumiracoxib) to recommend their use as 1st-line COX-2 ›ents.[28]

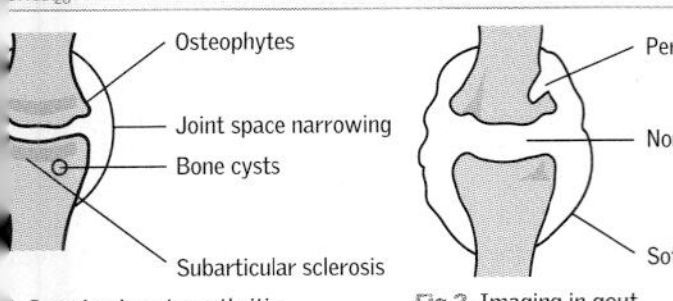

‹. Imaging in osteoarthritis

Fig 2. Imaging in gout

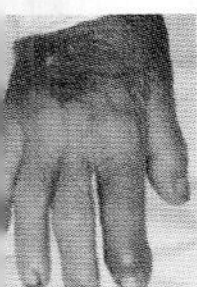

›. Acute mono- ›ritis in gout.

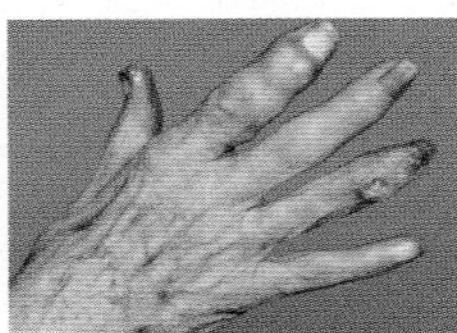

Fig 4. Ulcerated tophi in gout.

large prospective study (n=47150) showed an increased risk of gout with high meat ›cially beef, pork or lamb) and seafood consumption, but not with consumption of purine rich ›tables or protein. A lower risk was seen with high consumption of low fat dairy products.

Spondyloarthritides

1 Ankylosing spondylitis (AS) is a chronic inflammatory disease of the spine sacroiliac joints, of unknown cause. ***Prevalence:*** 0.25–1%. *Men present ear* ♂:♀≈6:1 at 16yrs old, and ≈ 2:1 at 30yrs old. >95% are HLA B27+ve.

Symptoms: The typical patient is a man <30yrs old with gradual onset of low b pain, worse at night, with spinal morning stiffness relieved by exercise. Pain ra ates to the sacro-iliac joints and the hips, and usually improves towards the en the day. There is progressive loss of spinal movement (all directions)—he ↓thoracic expansion. The disease course is variable. In a few, there is progress to kyphosis, neck hyperextension (question mark posture), and spino-cra ankylosis (fig 1). Other features include enthesitis (see BOX), especially at the h (Achilles tendon at the calcaneum and the plantar fascia), tibial and isc tuberosity, and iliac crests; anterior mechanical chest pain due to costochon inflammation and fatigue may feature. Acute anterior uveitis (iritis) occurs in ~ patients, which may lead to blindness if untreated. AS is also associated w aortitis and aortic regurgitation, pulmonary apical fibrosis, amyloidosis, and ot spondyloarthritides.

Tests: Diagnosis is clinical. Sacroiliitis is the earliest feature (XR may be norma early disease, MRI is more sensitive): look for irregularities, erosions, or scler affecting the lower half of the sacroiliac joints, especially the iliac side. The spir affected with characteristic *syndesmophytes*: bony proliferations due to enthes between ligaments and the vertebrae. These fuse with the above vertebral bo causing ankylosis. In later stages, calcification of ligaments with ankylosis lead 'bamboo spine' appearance. Also: FBC (normochromic anaemia), ↑ESR, ↑CRP, HLA-B

R̸: Exercise, not rest, for backache; there are intense exercise regimens to maint posture and mobility if able to manage. If no contraindications, use NSAIDs ibuprofen, diclofenac or naproxen) as symptoms are usually relieved within 4 and they may slow radiographic progression. The TNFα blockers etanerce infliximab and adalimumab are licensed in AS but await NICE approval (p533; Local steroid injections provide temporary relief. Surgery includes hip replacem to improve pain and mobility if the hips are involved, and rarely spinal osteoto There is ↑risk of osteoporotic spinal fractures (bisphosphonates may prevent th

Mortality: Higher than expected ×1.5–4 (eg secondary amyloidosis, heart disea

2 Enteropathic spondyloarthropathies Associated with Crohn's/UC. Also bypass surgery, and possibly coeliac and Whipple's disease (p709).

3 Psoriatic arthritis (*OHCS* p594) Occurs in 10–40% with psoriasis and present before skin changes. Patterns are (1) Polyarthritis (RA like) (2) DIP joi (3) Asymmetrical oligoarthritis (4) Spinal (AS like) (5) Psoriatic mutilans (ra severe deformity). XR: erosive changes, with 'pencil-in-cup' deformity in sev cases. Associated with nail changes in 80% (fig 2), synovitis (dactylitis—see B acneiform rashes and palmo-plantar pustulosis. Treatments used include NSA sulfasalazine, methotrexate and ciclosporin. Anti-TNF agents are also effective

4 Reactive arthritis A *sterile* arthritis, typically affecting the lower limb ~ weeks following urethritis (p404; *Chlamydia* or *Ureaplasma* species), or dysent (*Campylobacter, Salmonella, Shigella,* or *Yersinia* species). It may be chronic relapsing. Also there may be iritis, keratoderma blenorrhagica (brown, rais plaques on soles and palms), circinate balanitis (a painless serpiginous per ulceration secondary to *Chlamydia trachomatis*), mouth ulcers, enthesitis (plan fasciitis, Achilles tendonitis) and aortic incompetence (rare). ***Reiter's syndrom*** a triad of urethritis, arthritis and conjunctivitis. ***Tests:*** ESR & CRP↑. Culture sto diarrhoea, serum for serology. Consider a sexual health review. XR (or ultrasou may show enthesitis with periosteal reaction. ***R̸:*** Rest; splint affected joints; tr with NSAIDs or local steroid injections. Consider sulfasalazine or methotrex Treating the original infection may make little difference to the arthritis.

Spondyloarthritides typically hold these features in common

1. Seronegativity (rheumatoid factor –ve).
2. HLA B27 association (also in ~5% UK population, most do not have disease)
3. 'Axial arthritis': Pathology in spine (spondylo-) and sacroiliac (SI) joints.
4. Asymmetrical large-joint oligoarthritis (ie <5 joints) or monoarthritis.
5. Enthesitis: Inflammation of the site of insertion of tendon or ligament into bone, eg plantar fasciitis, Achilles tendonitis, costochondritis.
6. Dactylitis: Inflammation of an entire digit ("sausage digit"), due to soft tissue oedema, and tenosynovial and joint inflammation.
7. Extra-articular manifestations eg anterior uveitis, psoriaform rashes, oral ulcers, aortitis and aortic regurgitation, Crohn's or UC.

Spondyloarthritides show much overlap, with shared clinical features.

Juvenile idiopathic arthritis (JIA)

This is the commonest rheumatic disease of childhood, defined as a persistent arthritis lasting more than 6 weeks with an onset <16 yrs old. Recent studies have shown that most children never achieve complete remission. It is therefore important to recognise the disease and treat early, before irreversible deformity and joint damage occurs.

JIA is classified into the following forms:

- Systemic arthritis (formerly Still's disease): swinging pyrexia, rash, arthritis.
- Oligoarthritis: 1–4 joints affected in first 6 months.
  - Persistent: prognosis is generally good, most are self-limiting.
  - Extended: affects other joints after 6 months, with worse prognosis.
- Polyarthritis (RhF +ve: aggressive destructive symmetrical polyarthritis)
- Polyarthritis (RhF –ve: asymmetrical, less severe than RhF +ve disease)
- Psoriatic arthritis: similar to the adult form
- Enthesitis-related arthritis: HLA-B27 linked, asymmetrical lower limb arthritis and enthesitis. There is a risk of developing acute anterior uveitis.

Patients should be referred to a specialist. Treatment is based on NSAIDs, corticosteroids and early use of disease modifying drugs (p533) such as methotrexate, sulfasalazine, leflunomide or anti-TNF agents in severe forms. Corticosteroids have the SE of growth suppression; intra-articular injections may be used to minimise this.

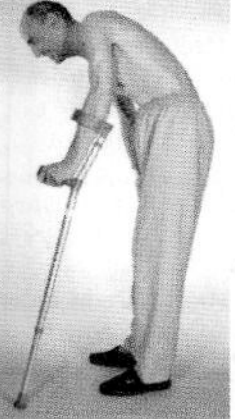

Fig 1. Question mark posture in ankylosing spondylitis.

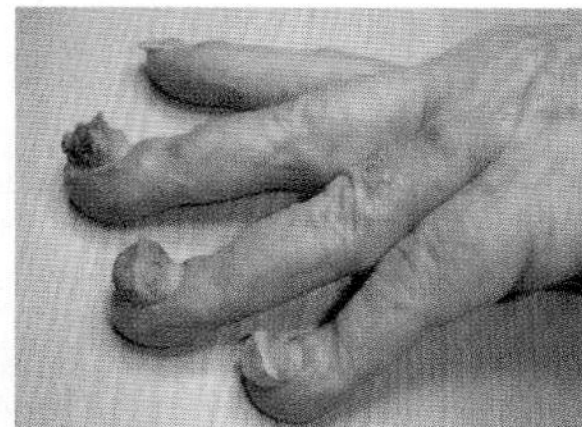

Fig 2. Nail changes in psoriasis: gross onycholysis is seen.

Autoimmune connective tissue diseases

Essence Included under this heading are: SLE (p540), diffuse and limited systemic sclerosis, primary Sjögren's syndrome (p702), idiopathic inflammatory myopathies, mixed connective tissue disease, relapsing polychondritis, and Behçet's disease (p686). They overlap with each other, affect many organ systems, and often require immunosuppressive therapies (p360). Consider connective tissue disease in ill patients with multi-organ involvement, especially if there is no infection.

Systemic sclerosis features scleroderma (skin fibrosis) and vascular disease:

- ***Limited systemic sclerosis:*** (of which CREST syndrome is part) Calcinosis (subcutaneous tissues), Raynaud's, oesophageal and gut dysmotility, Sclerodactyly, and Telangiectasia. Skin involvement is limited to the face, hands and feet. It is associated with anticentromere antibodies in 70–80%, and pulmonary hypertension (may be subclinical initially).
- ***Diffuse systemic sclerosis:*** 'Diffuse' skin involvement, whole body in severe cases. More profound organ fibrosis: lung, cardiac, and renal disease (p306). Anti-topoisomerase-1 [scl70] antibodies are found in 40% and anti-RNA polymerase in 20%. *Prognosis:* Often poor; monitor with annual echocardiogram & spirometry.
- ***Therapy:*** Currently no cure. Immunosuppressive regimes, including IV cyclophosphamide, are used for organ involvement or progressive skin disease. Raynaud's: Hand warmers, calcium antagonists, ACE-i, A2R blockers or intermittent IV prostacyclin are used. Regular ACE-i ↓risk of renal crisis (p306).

Mixed connective tissue disease (MCTD) combines features of systemic sclerosis, SLE and polymyositis. There is debate as to whether this is a distinct disease.

Relapsing polychondritis attacks cartilage, affecting the pinna (floppy ears), nasal septum ± larynx (hence stridor). Associations: aortic valve disease, polyarthritis and vasculitis. ***R̶:*** Steroids and immunosuppressives.

Polymyositis and dermatomyositis

Both feature progressive symmetrical proximal muscle weakness from *striated* muscle inflammation. Muscle weakness may also cause dysphagia, dysphonia (problems with the mechanics, not the idea, of speech production, ie phonation), or respiratory weakness. There is ↑ risk of malignancy, especially in dermatomyositis.

Dermatomyositis also features skin signs: • Macular rash (***shawl sign*** is +ve if over back & shoulders) • lilac-purple ***(heliotrope)*** rash on eyelids often with oedema • nail-fold erythema ***(dilated capillary loops)*** • roughened red papules over the knuckles, also seen on elbows, knees ***(Gottron's papules***—pathognomonic if CK↑ + muscle weakness) • subcutaneous calcifications • ***Mechanic's hands:*** a painful rough skin cracking, affecting the tips and lateral aspects of the fingers.

Extra-muscular signs in both conditions include fever, arthralgia, Raynaud's, lung (interstitial fibrosis) and myocardial involvement (myocarditis, arrhythmias).

Diagnosis Muscle enzymes (ALT & CK) ↑ in plasma; electromyography (EMG: shows fibrillation potentials); muscle biopsy confirms the diagnosis. ***Autoantibody associations:*** anti-Mi-2, anti-Jo1—associated with a syndrome of acute onset, fever, interstitial lung fibrosis, Raynaud's, arthritis and Mechanic's hands.

Differentials Carcinomatous myopathy, inclusion-body myositis, muscular dystrophy, endocrine/metabolic myopathy (including steroids), rhabdomyolysis, infection (eg HIV), drugs (penicillamine, colchicine, statins or chloroquine).

Management Screen for malignancy.[1] Start prednisolone (eg 1mg/kg/24h PO). Immunosuppressives (p360) and cytotoxics are used early in resistant cases, eg azathioprine, methotrexate, cyclophosphamide or ciclosporin. Hydroxychloroquine, dapsone, thalidomide or topical tacrolimus may help with skin disease. A more aggressive form with prominent vasculitis and calcinosis occurs in children.

1 This is usually limited to annual examination, CXR, abdominal & pelvic ultrasound ± CT, breast mammography ± flexible sigmoidoscopy (depending on age and family history). Lancet 2003 **362**: 971.

Plasma autoantibodies (Abs): disease associations

Always interpret in the context of clinical findings:

Rheumatological

Rheumatoid Factor (RhF): +ve in (%)

Sjögren's syndrome	≤100	Mixed connective tissue disease	50
Felty's syndrome	≤100	SLE	≤40
RA	70	Systemic sclerosis	30
Infection (endocarditis, Hepatitis)	≤50	Normal	2–10

Anti-nuclear antibody (ANA) Detected by immunofluorescence methods:

SLE	>95	RA	30
Autoimmune hepatitis	75	JIA (p299)	16
Sjögren's syndrome	68	Normal	0–2
Systemic sclerosis	64		

ANA titres are expressed according to dilutions at which antibodies can be detected ie 1:160 means antibodies can still be detected after the serum has been diluted 160 times. Titres of 1:40 or 1:80 may not be significant.

The pattern of staining may indicate the disease (although these are not specific):

- *Homogeneous* SLE
- *Speckled* Mixed connective tissue disease
- *Nucleolar* Systemic sclerosis
- *Centromere* Limited systemic sclerosis

Anti-histone Ab: Drug-induced SLE (~100%).

Anti-double stranded DNA (dsDNA): SLE (60%, more specific than ANA).

Anti-phospholipid Ab (eg anti-cardiolipin Ab): antiphospholipid syndrome, SLE.

Anti-centromere Ab: limited systemic sclerosis.

Anti-extractable nuclear antigen (ENA) antibodies (usually with +ve ANA)

- **Anti-Ro (SSA)** SLE, Sjögren's syndrome, systemic sclerosis. Associated with congenital heart block.
- **Anti-La (SSB)** Sjögren's syndrome, SLE (15%).
- **Anti-Sm** SLE (20–30%)
- **Anti-RNP** SLE, mixed connective tissue disease.
- **Anti Jo-1; Anti-Mi-2** Polymyositis, dermatomyositis.
- **Anti-Scl70** Diffuse systemic sclerosis.

Gastrointestinal

Anti-mitochondrial Ab (AMA): Primary biliary cirrhosis (PBC: >95%).
Also: autoimmune hepatitis (30%), idiopathic cirrhosis (25–30%).
Anti-smooth muscle Ab (SMA): Autoimmune hepatitis (70%), PBC (50%), idiopathic cirrhosis (25–30%).

Gastric parietal cell Ab: Pernicious anaemia (>90%), atrophic gastritis (40%). Also: autoimmune thyroid disease (40%), 'normal' controls (10–15%).

Intrinsic factor Ab: Pernicious anaemia (50%).

α-gliadin Ab, anti-tissue transglutaminase, anti-endomysial Ab: Coeliac disease.

Endocrine **Thyroid peroxidase Ab (TPO):** Hashimoto's thyroiditis (80–95%), Graves' (50–80%).

Islet cell Ab (ICA), glutamic acid decarboxylase (GAD) Ab: Type 1 DM (75%).

Renal **Glomerular basement membrane Ab (GBM)**: Goodpasture's syndrome.

Anti-neutrophil cytoplasmic Ab (ANCA):

- **Classical cytoplasmic (c-ANCA)**, with specificity for serine proteinase-3 (PR3 +ve). Wegener's granulomatosis (90%). Also microscopic polyangiitis (30%), PAN (11%).
- **Perinuclear (p-ANCA)**, with specificity for myeloperoxidase (MPO +ve). Microscopic polyangiitis (45%), Churg–Strauss, Goodpasture's.

ANCA may also be +ve in UC/Crohn's, primary sclerosing cholangitis, autoimmune hepatitis, Felty's, RA, SLE, or drugs (antithyroid, allopurinol, sulfasalazine, ciprofloxacin).

Neuromuscular **Acetylcholine receptor (ACR) Ab**: Myasthenia gravis (90%).

Systemic lupus erythematosus (SLE)

SLE is a multi-systemic autoimmune disease in which autoantibodies are produce against a variety of autoantigens (eg ANA). Immunopathology results in polyclonal B-cell secretion of pathogenic autoantibodies and subsequent formation of immun complexes which deposit in sites such as the kidneys. ♀:♂ ≈ 9:1, typicall women of child-bearing age. ***Prevalence:*** ~0.2%. ***Common in:*** Afro-Caribbean Asians, and if HLA B8, DR2 or DR3 +ve. ~10% of relatives may be affected.

Clinical features It is a remitting and relapsing illness. See BOX. Also: fatigue (ca be disabling), pyrexia during flares, weight loss, myalgia, lymphadenopathy, alopecia nail-fold infarcts, non-infective endocarditis (Libman–Sacks syndrome), serositis Raynaud's (in ⅓; image p701), CNS disturbance (partly due to antiphospholipi syndrome—see below): psychosis, seizures, migraines (40%), and retinal exudates There is an increased long-term risk of CVS disease and osteoporosis.

Immunology >95% are ANA +ve. A high titre of antibodies directed against double stranded DNA (dsDNA) is almost exclusive to SLE, but only ~60% of cases are +ve 40% are Rh factor +ve. There may be false +ve syphilis serology due t anticardiolipin antibodies (see below). SLE is associated with other autoimmun conditions: Sjögren's (15–20%), autoimmune thyroid disease (5–10%).

Rheumatology

Monitoring activity ***3 best tests:*** (1) Double-stranded (anti-ds) DNA antibod titres. (2) Complement: c3↓, c4↓ (denotes consumption of complement, hence c and c4↓, and c3d and c4d↑, their degradation products). (3) ESR. Also: BP, urinalysi for blood or protein, FBC, U&E, LFT, CRP. CRP is often normal: *think of SLE wheneve someone has a multisystem disorder and ESR↑ but CRP normal.* If CRP is raised, think instead of infection, serositis or arthritis. Skin or renal biopsies may be diagnostic

Drug induced lupus Causes (>50 drugs) include isoniazid, hydralazine (i >50mg/24h in slow acetylators), procainamide, chlorpromazine, minocycline phenytoin. It is associated with antihistone antibodies in up to 100%. Skin and lun signs prevail (renal and CNS are rarely affected). The disease remits if the drug is stopped. Sulfonamides or the oral contraceptive pill may worsen idiopathic SLE.

Antiphospholipid syndrome Occurs 'secondary' to SLE (in 20–30%) or as a primary disease (the majority). Antiphospholipid antibodies are present: anti cardiolipin antibody and lupus anticoagulants. These produce features of **CLOT** Coagulation defect, Livedo reticularis (p542), Obstetric: recurrent miscarriage Thrombocytopenia (↓platelets). There is a prothrombotic tendency, affecting the cerebral (stroke), renal and cardiovascular circulation. ***℞:*** Low dose aspirin, o warfarin if recurrent thromboses (aim INR of 2–3). Seek advice in pregnancy.

Treatment • High factor ***sun-block creams*** (*OHCS* p602).

- ***Hydroxychloroquine*** if joint or skin symptoms uncontrolled by NSAIDs, 200-400mg/day PO. SE: irreversible retinopathy—do baseline and annual assessment.[1]
- ***Low-dose steroids*** may be of value in chronic disease.
- ***High-dose prednisolone*** (PO/IV) is used, often with IV cyclophosphamide, fo severe flares of SLE (eg haemolytic anaemia, nephritis, severe pericarditis or CNS disease). Azathioprine may be used as maintenance treatment. **NB:** immuno-suppressed patients are prone to infection, which can present atypically.

Lupus nephritis: (p306) Requires intensive immunosuppression, usually steroids + cyclophosphamide (monthly IV or daily oral doses). SE (p360): myelosuppression nausea, alopecia, haemorrhagic cystitis, infertility (important in this patient group) Azathioprine or mycophenolate are alternatives. BP control is vital: ACE-i, α-blockers (eg doxazosin) or calcium channel blockers (eg nifedipine) are used. Rena replacement (dialysis or transplant) may be needed if disease progresses; nephritis recurs in ~50% post-transplant, but is a rare cause of graft failure.

The future A more targeted approach, such as using the B-cell depleting anti-CD20 monoclonal antibody rituximab (p346), has shown promise.

1 Refer to ophthalmology for assessment if there is visual impairment, changes in acuity or >5 years treatment. Royal College of Ophthalmologists Guidelines 2004.

Revised criteria (serial or simultaneous) for diagnosing SLE [37]

Diagnose SLE in an appropriate clinical setting if ≥4 out of 11 criteria are present.

1 ***Malar rash (butterfly rash):*** Fixed erythema, flat or raised, over the malar eminences, tending to spare the nasolabial folds. Occurs in up to ⅓.
2 ***Discoid rash:*** Erythematous raised patches with adherent keratotic scales & follicular plugging ± atrophic scarring. Think of it as a 3-stage rash affecting ears, cheeks, scalp, forehead, and chest: erythema→pigmented hyperkeratotic oedematous papules→atrophic depressed lesions.
3 ***Photosensitivity:*** on exposed skin representing unusual reaction to light. Exposure to sun may also cause disease to flare, so sunblocks are advised.
4 ***Oral ulcers:*** Oral or nasopharyngeal ulceration, usually painless.
5 ***Non-erosive arthritis:*** involving ≥2 peripheral joints (tenderness, swelling, or effusion). Joint involvement is seen in 90% of patients, and may present similar to RA. A reversible deforming arthropathy may occur due to capsular laxity (Jaccoud's arthropathy). Aseptic bone necrosis may also occur.
6 ***Serositis:*** (a) **Pleuritis** (presents as pleuritic pain or dyspnoea due to pleural effusion—80% have lung function abnormalities) OR (b) **Pericarditis** (chest pain, ECG, pericardial rub or signs of pericardial effusion).
7 ***Renal disorder:*** (a) **Persistent proteinuria** >0.5g/d (or >3+ on dipstix) OR (b) **Cellular casts**—may be red cell, granular, or mixed. See p306.
8 ***CNS disorder:*** (a) **Seizures**, in the absence of causative drugs or metabolic imbalance, eg uraemia or ketoacidosis, OR (b) **Psychosis** in the absence of causative drugs/metabolic derangements, as above.
9 ***Haematological disorder:*** (a) **Haemolytic anaemia** (p322) OR (b) **Leukopenia**, ie WCC $<4\times10^9$/L on ≥2 occasions OR (c) **Lymphopenia**, ie $<1.5\times10^9$/L on ≥2 occasions OR (d) **Platelets** $<100\times10^9$/L in the absence of a drug effect.
10 ***Immunological disorder:*** (a) **Anti-dsDNA** antibody (b) **Anti-Sm** antibody OR (c) Antiphospholipid antibody +ve based on:
- An abnormal serum level of IgG or IgM anticardiolipin antibodies,
- Positive result for lupus anticoagulant using a standard method, or
- False +ve syphilis serology, +ve for >6 months and confirmed by –ve *Treponema pallidum* immobilization & fluorescent treponemal antibody absorption tests.[39]

11 ***Antinuclear antibody (ANA):*** +ve in >95%.

A useful mnemonic is '**A RASH POINTS** an **MD**'....to a possible diagnosis.[40] Arthritis, Renal disorder, ANA, Serositis, Haematological, Photosensitivity, Oral ulcers, Immunological disorder, Neurological disorder, Malar and Discoid rash.

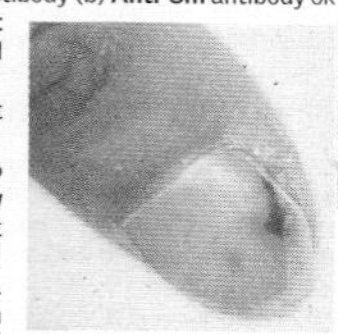

Fig 1. Nail-fold infarct. Sometimes immunological events are seen directly, as here—under the nail.[38]

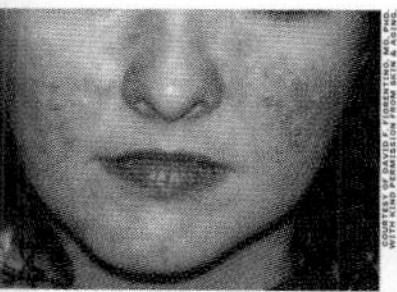

Fig 1. Malar rash; nasolabial folds spared.[41]

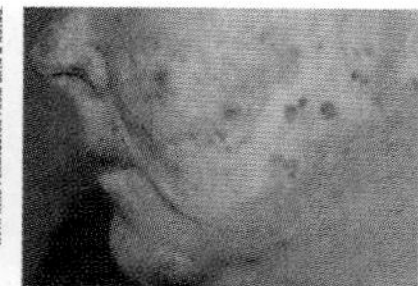

Fig 2. Discoid rash.[42]

Vasculitis

Vasculitis is defined as an inflammatory disorder of blood vessel walls and can affect vessels of any organ. They are divided according to the main size of blood vessel affected: ***Large***: Giant cell arteritis, Takayasu's arteritis (p704); ***Medium***: Polyarteritis nodosa (BOX), Kawasaki disease; ***Small***: Subdivided into **ANCA+ve**—these are associated with glomerulonephritis: Wegener's granulomatosis (p706), microscopic polyangiitis[1], Churg–Strauss syndrome (p688); **ANCA–ve**: Henoch Schönlein purpura (p694), cryoglobulinaemia, Goodpasture's disease (p692). Vasculitis may also be secondary to other diseases eg SLE, RA, hepatitis B and C, HIV. ►*Consider vasculitis as a diagnosis in any unidentified multisystem disorder*. Organ damage may result from acute vasculitis, recurrent attacks, or treatment.

Features seen in many vasculitides (see also individual disease): Systemic: fever, malaise, weight↓, arthralgia, myalgia. By organ:

- Skin: Purpura, ulcers, livedo reticularis, nailbed infarcts, digital gangrene.
- Eyes: Episcleritis, ulcers, visual loss.
- ENT: Epistaxis, nasal crusting, stridor, deafness.
- Pulmonary: Haemoptysis, dyspnoea.
- Cardiac: Heart failure, angina/MI.
- GI: Pain, malabsorption, due to chronic ischaemia.
- Renal: BP↑, haematuria, proteinuria, casts, acute or chronic renal failure.
- Neurological: Mononeuritis multiplex, sensorimotor neuropathy, stroke, fits, chorea, psychoses, confusion, cognition↓, mood↑↓.

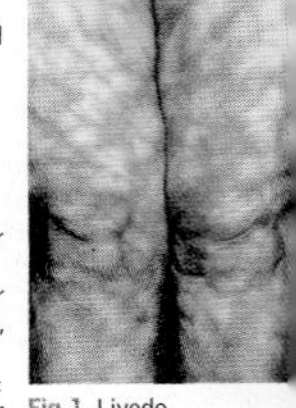

Fig 1. Livedo reticularis.[2]

Diagnosis: Clinical findings, supported by histology (± angiographic findings). ESR/CRP↑. ANCA may be +ve. ***℞:*** Large vessel vasculitis: steroids in most cases. Medium/Small: standard therapy is steroids (10mg/kg IV) + cyclophosphamide (15mg/kg IV). Azathioprine may be used as maintenance treatment.

Giant cell (or cranial or temporal) arteritis (GCA)

GCA is associated with polymyalgia in 25% of patients. Common in the elderly, it is rare <55yrs. ***Symptoms:*** Headache, temporal artery and scalp tenderness (eg on combing hair), jaw claudication, amaurosis fugax or sudden blindness in one eye. The risk is irreversible visual loss, which occurs in the 2nd eye if not treated. ***Tests:*** ESR and CRP↑, platelets↑, alk phos↑, Hb↓. ►If you suspect GCA, do an ESR and start prednisolone 40–60mg/24h PO *immediately*. Some advocate higher doses (?IV) if visual symptoms (ask an ophthalmologist). Get a temporal artery biopsy within 3–4 days. Skip lesions occur, so don't be put off by a negative biopsy. **NB:** in the longer term, the main cause of death and morbidity in GCA is steroid treatment! Reduce prednisolone after 5–7d in the light of symptoms and ESR; ↑dose if symptoms recur. Give osteoporosis prophylaxis. Typical course: 2yrs, then complete remission.

Polymyalgia rheumatica (PMR)

Common in those >70yrs (rare <60yrs) with gradual onset symmetrical aching, tenderness and morning stiffness in shoulders and proximal limb muscles ± systemic features: fatigue, fever, weight↓, anorexia and depression ± mild polyarthritis, tenosynovitis, and carpal tunnel syndrome (in 10%). It overlaps with GCA. ♀:♂≈2:1 ***Tests:*** CRP, plasma viscosity & ESR usually ↑; CK ↔; alk phos may be ↑. ***Differentials:*** Recent onset RA, polymyositis, hypothyroidism, primary muscle disease, occult malignancy or infection, osteoarthritis (esp. cervical spondylosis, shoulder OA), neck lesions, bilateral subacromial impingement (*OHCS* p664), spinal stenosis (*OHCS* p674). ***℞:*** Prednisolone 15mg/24h PO—expect a dramatic response within 4 days. ↓dose slowly, eg by 1mg/month (according to symptoms & ESR). Most need steroids for ≥2yrs, so prevent osteoporosis (p674).

Polyarteritis nodosa (PAN)

PAN is a necrotizing vasculitis that causes aneurysms and thrombosis in medium-sized arteries, leading to infarction in affected organs, with severe systemic symptoms. ♂:♀≈2:1. It may be associated with Hepatitis B, and is rare in the UK.

Signs and symptoms:

- General features: Fevers, malaise, weight↓, arthralgia.
- Skin: Urticaria, palpable purpura, infarcts, livedo reticularis,[2] nodules.
- Renal: (75%) Main cause of death. Renal cortical infarcts lead to hypertension, haematuria, proteinuria and renal failure (glomerulonephritis is not seen).
- Cardiac: (80%) Second commonest cause of death in PAN. Coronary arteritis causes consequent angina or myocardial infarction. Heart failure and pericarditis are also seen. In Kawasaki disease (childhood PAN variant, *OHCS* p646) coronary aneurysms occur.
- CNS: (70%) Arteritis of the vasa nervorum leads to mononeuritis multiplex or polyneuropathy. Stroke, seizures or psychoses are also seen.
- GI: (70%) Abdominal pain (any viscus may infarct), bleeding, perforation, malabsorption because of chronic ischaemia.
- GU: Orchitis—testicular pain or tenderness.

Tests: Often WCC↑, mild eosinophilia (in 30%), anaemia, ESR↑, CRP↑. ANCA is –ve.

Diagnosis: This is often made from clinical features with renal or mesenteric angiography. Biopsy can also be diagnostic.

Treatment: Treat hypertension meticulously. Refer to experts. Most respond to corticosteroids and cyclophosphamide. Hepatitis B should be treated with an antiviral (lamivudine or interferon-α) after initial treatment with steroids.

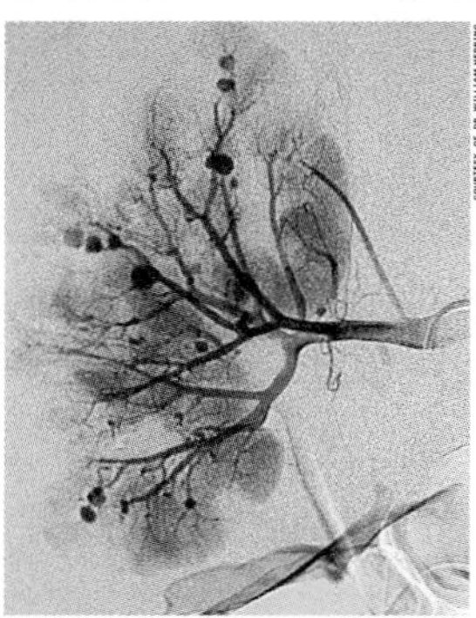

Fig 1. Angiographic appearances of the right kidney in PAN. Multiple aneurysms are present.

1 Microscopic polyangiitis (MPA) is a necrotizing vasculitis affecting small and medium sized vessels. A rapidly progressive glomerulonephritis usually features, pulmonary haemorrhage occurs in up to 30%, other features are rare. Blood tests: pANCA +ve, with positive MPO titre (see p539).

2 Livedo reticularis is pink-blue mottling of the skin caused by capillary dilatation and stasis in skin venules which may be physiological eg in cold weather (cutis marmorata), or due to a vasculitic process.

Systemic conditions causing eye signs

The eye is host to many diseases: the more you look, the more you'll see, and the more you'll enjoy, not least because the eye is as beautiful as its signs are legion.

Granulomatous disorders Syphilis, TB, sarcoidosis, leprosy, brucellosis, and toxoplasmosis may all inflame the eye; either front chamber (anterior uveitis/iritis) or back chamber (posterior uveitis/choroiditis). Refer to an ophthalmologist.

Connective tissue diseases cause inflammation of the eye coat (episcleritis/scleritis). Conjunctivitis is found in Reiter's; episcleritis in PAN and SLE; uveitis in ankylosing spondylitis and Reiter's (p536). Scleritis in RA and Wegener's may damage the eye. Refer immediately if eye pain. In dermatomyositis, there is orbital oedema with retinopathy showing cotton-wool spots (micro-infarcts).

Keratoconjunctivitis sicca is a reduction in tear formation, tested by the Schirmer filter paper test (<5mm in 5min). It causes a gritty feeling in the eyes, and a dry mouth (xerostomia from ↓saliva production). It is found on its own (Sjögren's syndrome, p702), or with other diseases eg SLE, RA, sarcoidosis. Treatment: artificial tears/saliva (eg tears naturale, hypromellose drops, Salivaese Oral Spray®).

Vascular retinopathy (p124) may be *arteriopathic* (arteriovenous nipping: hardened arteries nip veins where they cross) or *hypertensive*, with arteriolar vasoconstriction and leakage (hard exudates, macular oedema, haemorrhages, and papilloedema if severe). Thickened arterial walls are shiny ('silver wiring'). Narrowed arterioles lead to localized infarction of the superficial retina, seen as cotton-wool spots. Leaks from these appear as hard exudates ± macular oedema or papilloedema. The grading of hypertensive retinopathy from I to IV is considered obsolescent by some, partly because changes due to arteriopathy and those due to hypertension are confused, and also because some grades exist in normotensive, non-diabetic people.

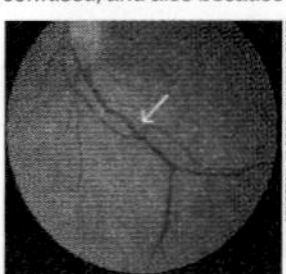

Fig 1. AV nipping.

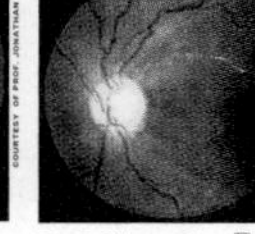

Fig 2. Silver wiring.

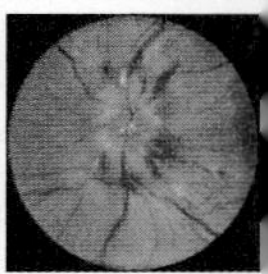

Fig 3. Papilloedema.

Emboli passing through the retina produce *amaurosis fugax* (p468). *Retinal haemorrhages* occur in leukaemia; comma-shaped *conjunctival haemorrhages* and retinal *new vessel formation* may occur in sickle-cell disease; *optic atrophy* in pernicious anaemia and *Roth spots* (small retinal infarcts) in SBE/IE.

Retinal vein occlusion is caused by BP↑, age, or hyperviscosity (p356). Suspect in any acute fall in acuity. If it is the central vein, the fundus is like a stormy sunset (those angry red clouds are haemorrhages). In branch vein occlusion, changes are confined to a wedge of retina. Get expert help.

Metabolic disease Diabetes: p190. Hyperthyroid exophthalmos: p203. Lens opacities are seen in hypoparathyroidism. Conjunctival and corneal calcification can occur in hypercalcaemia. In gout, conjunctival urate deposits may give sore eyes.

Systemic infections Septicaemia may seed to the vitreous causing endophthalmitis. Syphilis (above) can cause iritis (+ pigmented retinopathy if congenital).

AIDS & HIV (p396) CMV retinitis (pizza-pie fundus, p393): This may be asymptomatic but can cause sudden visual loss. If present, it implies full-blown AIDS (CD4 count <100 × 10^6/L). Cotton-wool spots on their own indicate HIV retinopathy and may occur before the full HIV picture. Candidiasis of the vitreous is found in IV drug abusers and is hard to treat. Kaposi's sarcoma may affect the lids or conjunctiva.

Differential diagnosis of 'red eye'

	Conjunctiva	Iris	Pupil	Cornea	Anterior chamber	Intraocular pressure	Appearance
Acute glaucoma	Both ciliary and conjunctival vessels injected Entire eye is red See *OHCS* p430	Injected	Dilated, fixed, oval	Steamy, hazy	Very shallow	Very high	
Anterior uveitis (Iritis)	Redness most marked around cornea Colour does not blanch on pressure (See *index* for list of causes.)	Injected	Small, irregular due to adhesions between the anterior lens and the pupil margin	Normal	Turgid	Normal	
Conjunctivitis	Conjunctival vessels injected, greatest toward fornices Blanch on pressure Mobile over sclera Purulent discharge	Normal	Normal	Normal	Normal	Normal	
Subconjunctival haemorrhage	Bright red sclera with white rim around limbus (*Causes:* BP↑; leptospirosis; bleeding disorders; trauma: snake venom; haemorrhagic fevers.)	Normal	Normal	Normal	Normal	Normal	

After RD Judge, GD Zuidema, FT Fitzgerald *Clinical diagnosis* 5 ed, Little Brown, Boston. Images courtesy of Prof. Jonathan Trobe.

Skin manifestations of systemic diseases

Erythema nodosum Painful, blue-red, raised lesions on shin fronts (± thighs/a *Causes*: sarcoidosis, drugs (sulfonamides, the Pill, dapsone), streptococcal infe *Less common*: Crohn's/UC, BCG vaccination, leptospirosis, *Mycobacterium* leprosy), *Yersinia* or various viruses and fungi. See p267.

Erythema multiforme 'Target' lesions: symmetrical ± central blister palms/soles, limbs, and elsewhere. Occasionally severe with fever and mu involvement—mouth, genital, and eye ulcers (this is the Stevens–Joh syndrome). It is associated with a hypersensitivity reaction to drugs (barbitur sulfonamides) or infections (herpes, *Mycoplasma*, orf—p366). Also seen in coll disorders. 50% of cases are idiopathic. Get expert help in severe disease.

Erythema chronicum migrans Presents as a small papule which develops i spreading large erythematous ring, with central fading. It lasts from 48 3 months. May be multiple. *Cause*: Lyme disease (p418).

Erythema marginatum Pink coalescent rings on trunk which come and go. seen in rheumatic fever (or rarely other causes, eg drugs).

Pyoderma gangrenosum Recurring nodulo-pustular ulcers, ~10cm wide, tender red/blue overhanging necrotic edge, purulent surface, and healing cribriform scars on leg, abdomen, or face. *Associations*: UC/Crohn's, autoimr hepatitis, Wegener's, myeloma, neoplasia. ♀:♂ >1:1. *Treatment*: Get help. S toilet, high-dose oral or topical steroids ± ciclosporin ± topical antibiotic.

Vitiligo (Fig.4) *Vitellus* is Latin for *spotted calf*: typically white patches ± hy pigmented borders. Sunlight makes them itch. *Associations*: Autoimmu including Graves', Addison's, Hashimoto's, DM, alopecia areata, hypoparathyroi premature ovarian failure. Treat by camouflage cosmetics and sunscr (± steroid creams ± dermabrasion). UK vitiligo society: 0800 018 2631.

Rheumatology

Specific diseases and their skin manifestations

Diabetes mellitus Ulcers, *necrobiosis lipoidica* (shiny area on shin with yello skin ± telangiectasia), *granuloma annulare* (OHCS p586), *acanthosis nigrican*

Gluten-sensitive enteropathy (coeliac disease) *Dermatitis herpetiformis*— blisters, in groups on knees, elbows, and scalp. The itch (which can drive patier suicide) responds to dapsone 25–200mg/24h PO within 48h—and this may be as a diagnostic test. The maintenance dose may be as little as 50mg/wk. A gl free diet should be adhered to, but in 30% dapsone will need to be continue (dose related): haemolysis (CI: anaemia; G6PD-deficiency), hepatitis, agranulocy (monitor FBC and LFT). There is an ↑risk of small bowel lymphoma with cc disease *and* dermatitis herpetiformis—so surveillance is needed.

Malabsorption Dry pigmented skin, easy bruising, hair loss, leuconychia.

Hyperthyroidism *Pretibial myxoedema*—red oedematous swellings above la malleoli, progressing to thickened oedema of legs and feet, *thyroid acropac* clubbing + subperiosteal new bone in phalanges.

Other endocrine diseases See p188.

Neoplasia *Acanthosis nigricans:* Pigmented, rough thickening of axillary, ne groin skin with warty lesions, associated with stomach cancer. *Dermatomy* (p538). *Skin metastases*. *Acquired ichthyosis*: Dry scaly skin associated lymphoma. *Thrombophlebitis migrans*: Successive crops of tender nodules affe blood vessels throughout the body, associated with pancreatic cancer (espe body and tail tumours).

Crohn's Perianal/vulval ulcers; erythema nodosum; pyoderma gangrenosum

Liver disease Palmar erythema; spider naevi; gynaecomastia; decrease in p hair; jaundice; bruising; scratch marks.

Dermatomyositis Gottron's papules; shawl sign; heliotrope rash on eyelids (p

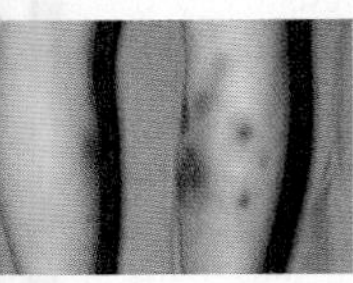

… Erythema nodosum.

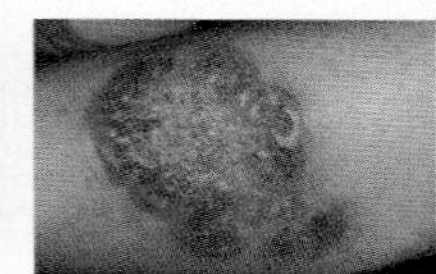

Fig 2. Pyoderma gangrenosum.

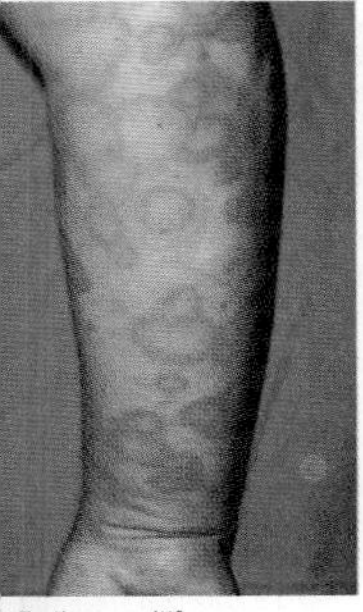

… Erythema multiforme.

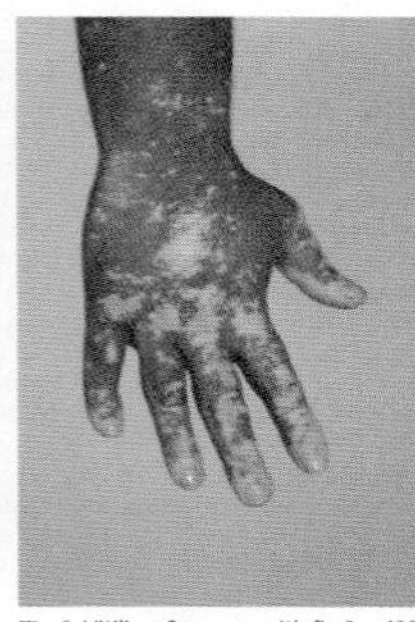

Fig 4. Vitiligo. Compare with fig 1, p417.

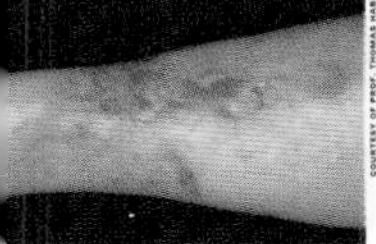

… Necrobiosis lipoidica.

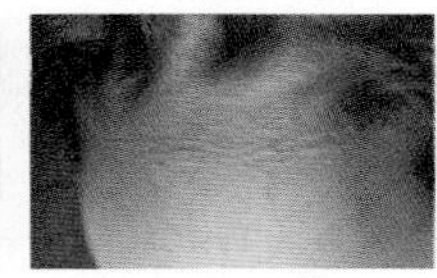

Fig 6. Acanthosis nigricans.

Skin diagnoses not to be missed

Malignant tumours

1 Malignant melanoma ♀:♂ ≈ 1.5 : 1. UK incidence: 3500/yr, with 800 deaths, (up ≥80% in last 20yrs), these metastasise early. Sunlight is a major cau particularly in the early years. They may occur in pre-existing moles. Diagnosis be tricky, so ►if in doubt, refer. Refer if there are ≥3 points on the Glasgow scale for major feature, 1 for minor feature), or with 1 point if suspicious.

Major	Minor	Less helpful signs
• Change in size	• Inflammation, crusting, or bleeding	• Asymmetry
• Change in shape	• Sensory change	• Irregular colour
• Change in colour	• Diameter >7mm (unless growth is in the vertical plane: beware)	• Elevation • Irregular border

Neighbouring 'satellite' lesions may occur in melanoma. If smooth, well-demarca and regular, it is unlikely to be a melanoma. Treatment: urgent excision. *OHCS* p5

2 Squamous cell cancer This usually presents as an ulcerated lesion, with ha raised edges, in sun-exposed sites. They may begin in solar keratoses (below), or found on the lips of smokers or in long-standing gravitational leg ulc (=Marjolin's ulcer). Metastases are rare, but local destruction may be extensi ***Treatment:*** Excision. NB: the condition may be confused with a keratoacanthom a fast-growing, benign, self-limiting papule plugged with keratin.

3 Basal cell carcinoma (rodent ulcer) Typically, a pearly nodule with ro telangiectatic edge, usually on the face on a sun-exposed site. Metastases are v rare. It slowly causes local destruction if left untreated. Lesions on the trunk appear as red scaly plaques with a raised smooth edge. *Cause*: UV exposu ***Treatment:*** Excision is best; radiotherapy may be used for larger lesions in elderly, if surgery is to be avoided.

Pre-malignant tumours

1 Solar (actinic) keratoses appear on sun-exposed skin as crumbly, yellow-wh crusts. Malignant change to squamous cell carcinoma may occur after seve years. ***Treatment:*** cautery, cryotherapy or twice-daily 5% 5-fluorouracil (5- cream—this works by causing: erythema → vesiculation → erosion → ulceratio necrosis → healing epithelialization, leaving healthy skin unharmed. Treatment w 5-FU cream is usually for 4wks, but may be prolonged. There is no signific systemic absorption if the area treated is <500cm^2. Avoid in pregnancy. The ha should be washed after applying the cream. Alternative: diclofenac gel (3 Solaraze®, use thinly twice-daily for ≤90d).

2 Bowen's disease Slow-growing red scaly plaque, eg on lower legs. ***Histolo*** Full-thickness dysplasia (carcinoma-*in-situ*). It infrequently progresses to squam cell cancer. Penile Bowen's disease is called Queyrat's erythroplasia. ***Treatme*** Cryotherapy, topical 5-flurouracil (as above) or photodynamic therapy.

Others

- **Secondary carcinoma** The most common metastases to skin are from brea kidney, and lung. The lesion is usually a firm nodule, most often on the scalp. S acanthosis nigricans (p546).
- **Mycosis fungoides** is a cutaneous T-cell lymphoma which is usually confined skin. It causes itchy, red plaques. (Sézary syndrome is a variant which is a associated with erythroderma).
- **Leukoplakia** This appears as white patches (which may fissure) on oral genital mucosa (where it may itch). Frank carcinomatous change may occur
- **Leprosy** Suspect in any anaesthetic hypopigmented lesion (p416).
- **Syphilis** Any genital ulcer is syphilis until proved otherwise. Secondary syphi papular rash—including, unusually, on the palms[1] (p419).
- **Also** Kaposi's sarcoma (p694); Paget's disease of the breast (p700).

1 *Other causes:* Stevens–Johnson syn.; hand, foot & mouth disease; palmar erythema in liver diseas

ABCDE criteria for diagnosis of melanoma
Asymmetry Border—irregular Colour—non-uniform Diameter >7mm Elevation

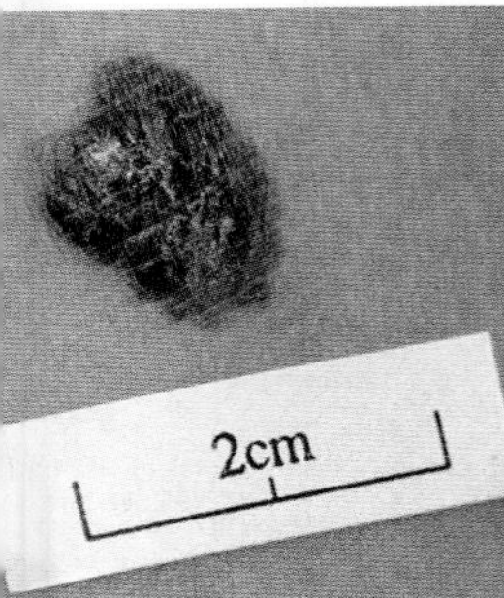

Fig 1. Melanoma

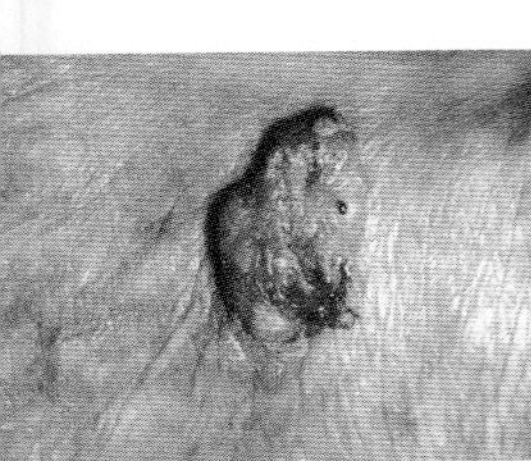

Fig 1. Squamous cell cancer

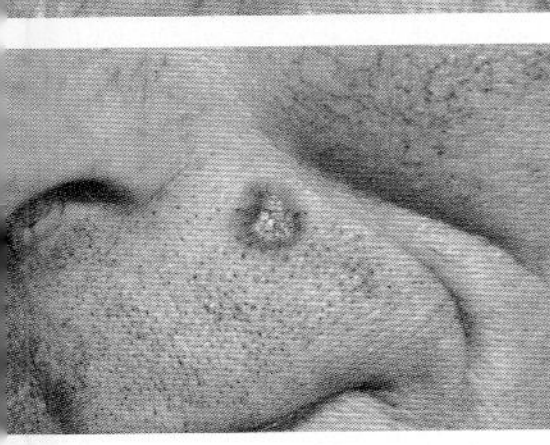

Fig 2. Basal cell carcinoma (BCC)

14 Surgery

Contents

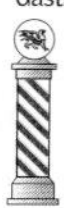

Relevant pages elsewhere: ►See **Gastroenterology** (p226) and **Dictionary of symptoms and signs** (p52).

Urology in other chapters: UTI/urine (p282); haematuria (p278); prostatism (p68); gynaecological urology (*OHCS* p306); stones (p284); GU obstruction (p286).

►►These are the three conditions where the promptest surgery is essential; ►notify the duty surgi registrar or consultant, and theatre, **at once** (urology, for torsion).

We thank Mr Ashok Handa who is our Specialist Reader for this chapter.

dominal areas:

1 Right upper quadrant (RUQ) or hypochondrium
2 Epigastrium
3 Left upper quadrant (LUQ) or hypochondrium
4 Right flank or loin
5 Peri-umbilical or central area
6 Left flank or loin
7 Right iliac fossa (RIF)
8 Suprapubic area
9 Left iliac fossa (LIF)

cisions:

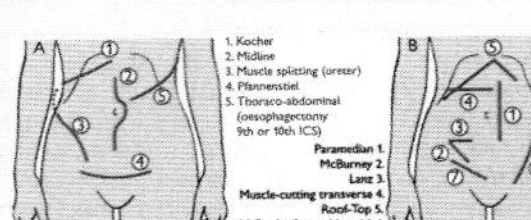

tomy	Cutting something out.
am	A radiological image.
exy	Anchoring of a structure to keep it in position.
asty	Surgical refashioning in order to regain good function.
copy	Procedure with instrumentation for looking into the body.
omy	An artifical union between a conduit and the outside world or another conduit (for **stoma care** see p568).
my	Cutting something open to the outside world.
ipsy	Fragementation of an object

gio-	Tube or vessel	**lith-**	Stone
pendic-	Appendix	**mast-**	Breast
ole-	Relating to gall/bile	**meso-**	Mesentery
lp-	Vagina	**nephr-**	Kidney
st-	Bladder/fluid-filled sac	**orchid-**	Testicle
och-	Ducts	**oophor-**	Ovary
ter-	Small bowel	**phren-**	Diaphragm
char-	Burn	**pyloromy-**	Pyloric sphincter
str-	Stomach	**pyel-**	Renal pelvis
pat-	Liver	**proct-**	Anal canal
ster-	Uterus	**salping-**	Fallopian tube
par-	Abdomen	**splen-**	Spleen

scess	A cavity containing pus. For different types consult the index. Remember the aphorism: *if there is pus about, let it out*.
stula	An abnormal connection between two epithelial surfaces. Fistulae often close spontaneously, but will not do so in the presence of malignant tissue, distal obstruction, foreign bodies, chronic inflammation, and the formation of a muco-cutaneous junction (eg stoma).
ernia	Any structure passing through another and so ending up in the wrong place.
eus	Used in this book as a term for adynamic bowel.
nus	A blind-ending tract, typically lined by epithelial or granulation tissue, which opens to an epithelial surface.
ent	An artificial tube placed in a biological tube to keep it open.
oma	(p568) An artificial union between conduits or a conduit and the outside.
cer	(p592) An abnormal break in an epithelial surface.
olvulus	(p595, p599) Twisting of a structure around itself. Common GI sites include the sigmoid colon and caecum, and more rarely the stomach.

pi-	Upon	**pan-**	Whole	**peri-**	Around
nd-	Inside	**para-**	Alongside	**sub-**	Beneath
ega-	Enlarged	**per-**	Going through	**trans-**	Across

Aims ►To ensure that, as far as possible, any fears are addressed and the pati understands the nature, aims, and expected outcome of surgery.
- Ensure that the right patient gets the right surgery. Have the symptoms a signs changed? If so, inform the surgeon.
- Get informed consent (p554).
- Assess/balance risks of anaesthesia, and maximize fitness. Is he a smok Optimizing oxygenation/perfusion **before** major surgery improves outcome.
- Check anaesthesia/analgesia type with anaesthetist. **Aim to allay anxiety & pa**

Pre-op checks Assess cardiorespiratory system, exercise tolerance, existi illnesses, drugs, and allergies. Is the neck unstable (eg arthritis complicati intubation)? Assess past history of: MI,[1] diabetes, asthma, hypertension, rheuma fever, epilepsy, jaundice. Assess any specific risks, eg is the patient pregnant? the neck/jaw immobile and teeth stable (intubation risk)? Has there been previ anaesthesia? Were there any complications (eg nausea, DVT)? ►Is DVT/PE propl laxis needed (p564)? ►If for 'unilateral' surgery, mark the correct arm/leg/kidn according to the recommendations of the UK National Patient Safety Agency.

Family history May be relevant eg in malignant hyperpyrexia (p558); dystrop myotonica (p502); porphyria; cholinesterase problems; sickle-cell disease.

Drugs Any drug/plaster/antiseptic allergies? ►Inform the anaesthetist about drugs even if 'over-the-counter'. For diabetes, see p576.
- ***Antibiotics: Tetracycline*** and ***neomycin*** may ↑neuromuscular blockade.
- ***Anticoagulants:*** ►**Tell the surgeon.** Avoid epidural, spinal, and regional bloc ***Aspirin*** should probably be continued unless there is a major risk of bleedi Discuss stopping ***clopidogrel*** therapy with the cardiologists/neurologists.
- ***Anticonvulsants:*** Give as usual pre-op. Post-op, give drugs IV (or by NGT) ur able to take orally. ***Valproate***: give usual dose IV. ***Phenytoin***: give IV slov (<50mg/min; monitor ECG). IM ***phenytoin*** absorption is unreliable.
- ***β-blockers:*** Continue up to and including the day of surgery as this preclude labile cardiovascular response.
- ***Contraceptive steroids:*** See *BNF*. Stop 4wks before major/leg surgery; ensu alternative contraception is used. Restart 2wks after surgery, provided mobi
- ***Digoxin:*** Continue up to and including morning of surgery. Check for toxic (ECG; plasma level); do plasma K^+ and Ca^{2+} (***suxamethonium*** can ↑K^+ and lead ventricular arrhythmias in the fully digitalized).
- ***Diuretics:*** Beware hypokalaemia, dehydration. Do U&E (and bicarbonate).
- ***Eye-drops:*** β-blockers get absorbed; anticholinesterases ↑[***suxamethonium***
- ***HRT:*** There may be an increased risk of DVT/PE. • ***Steroids:*** See p578.
- ***Levodopa:*** Possible arrhythmias when patient under GA.
- ***Lithium:*** Get expert help; it may potentiate neuromuscular blockade and cau arrhythmias. See *OHCS* p354.
- ***MAOIs:*** Get expert help as interactions may cause hypotensive/hypertensive cris
- ***Thyroid medication:*** see p579.
- ***Tricyclics:*** These enhance ***adrenaline*** (epinephrine) and arrhythmias.

Preparation ►Fast the patient; NBM for ≥2h pre-op (discuss with anaesthetist
- Is any bowel or skin preparation needed, or prophylactic antibiotics (p556)?
- Start DVT prophylaxis as indicated, eg graduated compression stockings (not there is peripheral arterial disease) + ***heparin*** 5000U SC 2h pre-op, then eve 8–12h SC for 7d or until ambulant. Low molecular weight heparin (LMWH, p17 eg ***enoxaparin*** 20mg/d SC, increased to 40mg/d in major-risk surgery.
- Write up the pre-meds (p558); book any pre-, intra-, or post-operati x-rays or frozen sections. Book post-operative physiotherapy.
- If needed, catheterize (p750) and insert a Ryle's tube (p747) before inductio These can reduce organ bulk, making it easier to operate in the abdomen.

1 If within the last 6 months, the peri-operative risk of reinfarction (up to 40%) makes m elective surgery too risky. ECHO & stress testing (+ exercise ECG or MUGA scan, p727) should be do

e-operative examination and tests—see NICE guidelines

Careful planning is the key to preventing perioperative death.[1] A good thought exercise is to imagine yourself at the next surgical *Mortality Meeting* and ask 'If I were looking back at the pre-op period, knowing that this patient had died, would I still consider that surgery was indicated?' The UK National Confidential Enquiry into Perioperative Deaths (NCEPOD) found that 'too many' operations are performed on moribund patients.
It is the anaesthetist's duty to assess suitability for anaesthesia. The ward doctor assists with a good history & examination, and can also reassure, inform, and get informed written consent (p558; ideally this should be from the surgeon herself).
Be alert to chronic lung disease, BP↑, arrhythmias, and murmurs (aortic stenosis; endocarditis prophylaxis needed?—see p136).

Pre-op checklist:
• Blood tests (inc. group & save or crossmatch)
• IV cannula
• ECG + CXR
• Drug chart
· Regular medications
· Analgesia + antiemetic
· Antibiotics
· LMWH/***heparin***
· Compression stockings
• Consent
• Marked site/side
• Anaesthetist informed
• Theatres informed
• Infection risk? (eg MRSA/
• HIV/HBV/HCV)
• NBM since when?
...not all will be required

Tests ►Be guided by the history and examination and local/NICE protocols.

U&E, FBC, and ward tests for blood glucose in most patients. If Hb <10g/dL tell anaesthetist. Investigate/treat as appropriate. U&E are particularly important if the patient is starved, diabetic, on diuretics, a burns patient, has hepatic or renal disease, has an ileus, or is parenterally fed.

Crossmatching: Examples: Group and save (G&S) for mastectomy or cholecystectomy. Crossmatch 2 units for Caesarean section; 4 units for a gastrectomy; 6 units for abdominal aortic aneurysm (AAA) surgery.

Specific blood tests: LFT in jaundice, malignancy, or alcohol abuse. Amylase in acute abdominal pain. Blood glucose if diabetic (p576). Drug levels as appropriate (eg ***digoxin, lithium***). Clotting studies in liver or renal disease, DIC (p336), massive blood loss, eg if on ***valproate***, ***warfarin***, or ***heparin***. HIV, HBsAg in high risk patients, after counselling. Sickle test in those from Africa, West Indies, or Mediterranean—and if origins are in malarial areas (including most of India). Thyroid function tests in those with thyroid disease.

CXR if known cardiorespiratory disease, pathology or symptoms, possible lung metastases, or >65yrs old. Remember to check the film prior to surgery.

ECG if >55yrs old or poor exercise tolerance, or history of myocardial ischaemia, hypertension, rheumatic fever, or other heart disease.

Echocardiogram may be performed if there is a suspicion of poor LV function.

Lateral cervical spine x-ray if history of rheumatoid arthritis, ankylosing spondylitis or Down's syndrome, to warn about difficult intubations.

MRSA screen: Rising above the frenzied media headlines, it is still important make every effort to reduce spread of MRSA. Colonisation is **not** a contra-indication to surgery, and if on balance surgery is appropriate, the case should be last on the list minimize transmission to others (with appropriate theatre protocol). Cover with appropriate antibiotic prophylaxis, eg ***vancomycin***.

American Society of Anesthesiologists (ASA) classification

Class I	Normally healthy.
Class II	Mild systemic disease.
Class III	Severe systemic disease that limits activity but is not incapacitating.
Class IV	Incapacitating systemic disease which poses a constant threat to life.
Class V	Moribund: not expected to survive 24h even with operation.

You will see a space for an ASA number on most anaesthetic charts. It is a health index **at the time of surgery**. The prefix **E** is used in emergencies.

Risk of mortality from elective surgery is currently about 1:100 000 to 1:150 000.

Surgery

Consent

In which of the following situations would you seek 'informed written consent' frc a patient? **1** Feeling for a pulse. **2** Taking some blood. **3** Inserting a central lir **4** Removing a section of small bowel during a laparotomy for division of adhesio **5** Orchidectomy after a failed operation for testicular torsion.

English law states that **any** intervention or treatment needs consent—ie all the above—yet, for different reasons, we know that, for some, informed forr consent is not regularly sought! In fact, **written** consent itself is not required law, but it does constitute 'good medical practice' in the best interests of t patient and practitioner. Sometimes actions and words can imply valid consent, by simply entering into conversation or holding out an arm. In these situations yo actions and their consequences are understood by the patient as a product of the knowledge, previous interactions with doctors and learning through experience However, if the consequences are not clear to the patient and they have t capacity to give consent (see below & BOX), you should seek informed writt consent, as this serves as a record of your conversation together.

For consent to be valid:

- It can be given any time before the intervention/treatment is initiated. Earlier better as this will give the patient time to think about the risks, benefits a alternatives—he may even bring forward questions on issues that you had n considered relevant. Think of consent as an ongoing process throughout t patient's time with you, not just the moment of signing the form.
- The proposed treatment or test must be clearly understood by the patier taking into account the benefits, risks (including complication rates if knowr additional procedures, alternative courses of action and their consequences.
- It must be given **voluntarily.** This can be difficult to evaluate—eg when li organ donation is being considered—see BOX for other difficult situations.
- The doctor who is providing treatment or undertaking the test needs to ensu that the patient has given valid consent. The act of seeking consent is ultimate the responsibility of the doctor looking after the patient, though the task may delegated to another health professional, as long as they are suitably trained ar qualified. Sometimes you may have be certified to get consent.
- The patient must have the **capacity** to give consent. UK law (case law rather th statute) implies that we are either fully competent or 'incompetent' but thin are not so clear-cut, so...

When taking consent:

- Think about whether you are the right person to be obtaining consent.
- Use words the patient understands and avoid jargon and abbreviations.
- Ensure that he believes your facts and can retain 'pros' and 'cons' long enough inform his decision. Fact sheets/diagrams for individual operations help.
- Make sure his choice is free from pressure from others, and explain that aft they have signed the form he is free to choose not to have the propose treatment (ie withdraw consent) at any time. Some patients may view th consent form as a contract from which they cannot *renege*.
- If the patient is illiterate, a witnessed mark does endorse valid consent. Similar if the patient is willing but physically unable to sign the consent form, then a entry into the medical notes stating so is valid.
- Remember to discuss further procedures that may become necessary during th proposed treatment. This avoids waking up to a nasty surprise (eg a missir testicle as in scenario **5** above).
- If you suspect the patient is not capable of giving consent then a form assessment needs to be documented in the medical notes.

Consent is complex, but remember that it exists for the benefit of the patient ar the doctor, giving you an opportunity to revisit expectations and involve th patient in his own care.

Special circumstances for consent...and who to ask

There are some areas of treatment or investigation for which it may be advisable to seek specialist advice if it is not part of your regular practice:

Who to ask if you are unsure?
Your team's senior/consultant
Your employing organisation
Legal defence organisation
National medical association
Local research ethics committee

- Photography of a patient.
- Innovative or novel treatment.
- Living organ donation.
- Storage, use or removal of human tissue (for any length of time), as regulated under the Human Tissue Act 2004.
- The storage, loss, or use of gametes, as regulated under the Human Fertilisation and Embryology Act 1990.
- The use of patient records or tissue in research or teaching.
- In the presence of an advanced directive or living will expressly refusing a particular treatment, investigation or action.
- Consent if <16yrs—consent form 3 in NHS. In the UK, those >16yrs can give valid consent. Those <16yrs can give consent for a medical decision provided they understand what it involves—the concept of *Gillick* competence. It is still good practice to involve the parents in the decision. If **<18yrs and refusing life-saving surgery**, talk to the parents and your senior; the law is unclear. You may need to contact the duty judge in the High Court.
- Consent in the incapacitated (NHS consent form 4). No one (parents, relatives, or even members of a healthcare team) is able to give consent on behalf of an adult in England, and the High Court may be required to give a ruling on the matters of lawfulness of a proposed procedure. Proceeding in a patient's best interest is decided by the clinician overseeing their care, although it is always good practice to involve family in the proposed course of treatment.

The right to refuse treatment

Their's not to make reply,
Their's not to reason why,
Their's but to do and die. **Alfred, Lord Tennyson from *The Charge of the Light Brigade*, 1854**

The rights of a patient are something of an antithesis to this military macabre of Tennyson, and it is our sacred responsibility to respect the legal and ethical rights of those we treat. We do this not only for the sake of the individual, but also for the sake of an enduring trust between the patient and doctor, remembering that is the patient's right to refuse treatment (if a fully competent adult) even when this may result in death of the patient, or even the death of an unborn child, whatever the stage of pregnancy. The only exception is in circumstances outlined by the Mental Health Act 1983.

Nil by mouth (NBM) before theatre

If in doubt about what is acceptable oral intake prior to induction for general anaesthesia (eg GI surgery), it is best to liaise with the anaesthetist concerned. However, guidelines have been published by the Royal College of Nursing to outline what is safe in the perioperative period. In **emergency surgery**, ≥6h NBM prior to theatre is best. For **adult elective surgery** in healthy patients without GI co-morbidity, water or clear fluids (eg black tea/coffee) are allowed up to 2h beforehand, with all other intake up to 6h beforehand.

In agreeing to a blood test, the patient understands that it may be an uncomfortable experience, perhaps with some bruising, but he also knows that the results of the test may help you in making a diagnosis and hopefully restore him to full health and vigour. But grey areas exist everywhere: when he extends his arm towards you, does he know that you could accidentally injure an artery or nerve, with all the complications that follow—does he need to know...?

Prophylactic antibiotics in surgery

Prophylactic antibiotics are given to counter the risk of wound infection (p5 which occurs in ~20% of elective GI surgery (up to 60% in emergency surge they are also given if infection elsewhere, although unlikely, would have sev consequences (eg when prostheses are involved). They are given 15–60min p to the procedure so that the skin concentration is maximised[10] and may be gi as a single dose, 3 doses, or more depending on local guidelines and contaminat at the site of surgery (see TABLE). A single dose given before surgery has b shown to be just as beneficial as more prolonged regimens in biliary surgery colorectal surgery.[11] [12] ►Wound infections are not necessarily trivial since se may lead to haemorrhage, wound dehiscence, and initiate a fatal chain of eve so take measures to minimise the risk of wound infection:

- Time administration correctly.
- Use antibiotics which will kill anaerobes and coliforms.
- Consider use of perioperative supplemental oxygen. This is a practical metho reducing the incidence of surgical-wound infections.[13]
- Practice strictly sterile surgical technique. (Ask for a hand with scrubbing u you are not sure—Sister will be more than pleased to help)!

Antibiotic regimens Check for local or personal preferences. Examples:

- ***Biliary surgery: Cefuroxime*** 1.5g, for 1 dose IV + metronidazole (below).
- ***Appendectomy:*** If uncomplicated, a single dose ***cefuroxime*** 1.5g IV is effective
- ***Colorectal surgery: Cefuroxime*** 1.5g/8h + ***metronidazole*** 500mg/8h, 1 doses IV. ***Tazocin***® 4.5g/8h, 1–3 doses IV can be used if there is heavy soilir
- ***Vascular surgery: Co-amoxiclav*** 1.2g IV on induction; if penicillin-aller ***cefuroxime*** 1.5g IV/IM + ***metronidazole*** 500mg IV. Anaerobic cover is not alw necessary. MRSA is an increasing concern, and so may warrant prophylaxis.

Bowel preparation in colorectal surgery

The place of bowel preparation in colorectal surgery has recently come under m scrutiny.[16] Whereas there are clear benefits when visualisation of the lumer required (eg colonoscopy), the intended benefit for elective open procedures minimizing post-operative infection may well be outweighed by the complications

- Liquifying bowel contents which are spilled during surgery
- Perforation
- Electrolyte loss leading to hyponatraemia and seizures[18]
- Dehydration
- A higher rate of post-operative anastomotic leakage[19]

Usually no laxatives are needed for right-sided operations (eg right he colectomy); the patient is just put on a 'low-residue' diet for a few days pre- then clear fluids the day before. For left-sided operations and rectal operations left hemicolectomy, anterior resection), laxatives and enemas may still be used. in doubt, check with the surgeon as to what preparation he prefers.

Example: 1 sachet of Picolax® (10mg ***sodium picosulfate*** + ***magnesium citra*** on the morning before surgery and 1 sachet during the afternoon before surge

Sutures

Sutures (stitches) are central to the art of surgery. The trainee may face seve long evenings practising knots over a pint of beer before they are allowed back tie at the table! In their broadest sense they are absorbable or non-absorbal synthetic or natural, and their structure may be divided into monofilame twisted, or braided. See TABLE opposite for some examples and their uses.

Monofilament sutures are quite slippery but minimize infection and produce l reaction (natural fibres of any type produce quite a vigorous reaction). Braid sutures have plaited strands and provide secure knots, but they may all infection to occur between their strands. Twisted sutures have 2 twisted strar and similar qualities to braided sutures. 3-0 or 4-0 (smaller) are the best sizes f skin closure.

assification of surgical procedures and wound infection risk

tegory	Description	Infection risk
ean	Incising uninfected skin without opening a viscus	<2%
ean-contaminated	Intraoperative breach of a viscus (but not colon)	8–10%
ntaminated	Breach of a viscus + spillage or opening of the colon	12–20%
ty	The site is already contaminated with pus or faeces, or from exogenous contagion eg trauma	25%

le after *MRCS Core Modules: Essential Revision Notes*, S. Andrews, Pastest, ISBN 1901198715

rgical drains in the post-operative period

e decision when to insert and remove drains may seem to be one of the great rgical enigmas—but there are basically 3 types to get a grip on.

Most are inserted to drain the area of surgery and are often put under suction or –ve pressure (Redivac® uses a 'high-vacuum'). These are removed when they stop draining. They protect against collection, haematoma and seroma formation (in breast surgery this can cause overlying skin necrosis).

The second type of drain is used to protect sites where leakage may occur in the post-operative period, such as bowel anastomoses. These form a tract and are removed after about 1 week.

The third type (eg Bellovac®) collects red blood cells from the site of the operation, which can then be autotransfused within 6h, protecting from the hazards of allotransfusion—it is used commonly in orthopaedics.

Shortening a drain' means withdrawing it (eg by 2cm/day). This allows the ct to seal up, bit by bit.

Evidence suggests that certain types of drain are not effective and may even d to more complications, such as when used to protect colorectal anastoses.[MET 20] ►Check the individual surgeon's preference before altering a drain.

me commonly encountered suture materials

e perfect suture material is monofilament, strong, easy to handle, holds knots ll, has predictable absorption and causes minimal tissue reaction. fortunately no single suture fits the bill for every occasion, and so suture ection (including size) depends on a the job in hand:

sorbable

ne	Material	Construction	Use
nocryl®	poliglecaprone	monofilament	subcuticular skin closure
S®	polydioxanone	monofilament	closing abdominal wall
ryl®	polyglactin	braided multifilament	tying pedicles; bowel anastomosis; subcutaneous closure
on®	polyglycolic acid	Braided multifilament	very similar to Vicryl®

-absorbable

ne	Material	Construction	Use
ilon®	polyamide	monofilament	closing skin wounds
lene®	polypropylene	monofilament	arterial anastomosis
silk®N	Silk	braided multifilament	securing drains
al	eg steel	clips or monofilament	skin wound/sternotomy closure

natural; other natural materials (eg cotton and catgut) are rarely used these days.

ing the removal of sutures

timing of suture removal depends on site and the general health of the ent. Face and neck sutures may be removed after 5d (earlier in children), p and back of neck after 5d, abdominal incisions and proximal limbs luding clips) after ~10d and those on the distal extremities after 14d. In ents with poor wound healing, eg on steroids, with malignancy, infection, nexia (p54), the elderly, or smokers, the sutures may need 14d or longer.

Before anaesthesia, explain to the patient what will happen and where he w wake up, otherwise the recovery room or ITU will be frightening. Explain that may feel ill on waking. The premedication aims to allay anxiety and to make t anaesthesia itself easier to conduct (see BOX). Typical regimens might include:

- ***Anxiolytics:*** Benzodiazepines eg ***temazepam*** 10–20mg PO. In childr ***midazolam*** 0.5mg/kg rectally 30min prior to procedure is effective.
- ***Analgesics:*** *See* p560. The patient should not be in pain prior to surge Opioids, local anaesthetic blocks, ***paracetamol*** and NSAIDs (beware bleeding ri are all used. In children or anxious adults, local anaesthetic cream (eg Eml Ametop®) may be used on a few sites for the anaesthetist's IVI (►they n prefer to site the cannula themselves!)
- ***Antiemetics:*** 5HT$_3$ antagonists (eg ***ondansetron*** 4mg IV/IM) are the most effect agents; others eg ***metoclopramide*** 10mg/8h IV/IM/PO are also used—see p233.
- ***Antacids: Ranitidine*** 50mg IV in patients at particular risk of aspiration.
- ***Antisialogues: Glycopyrronium*** (200–400μg in adults, 4–8μg/kg in childr given IV/IM 30–60min before induction) is sometimes used to decrea secretions that may cause respiratory obstruction in smaller airways.
- ***Antibiotics:*** *See* p556.

Give oral premedication 1–2h before surgery (1h if IM route used).

Side-effects of anaesthetic agents

- ***Hyoscine, atropine:*** Anticholinergic ∴ tachycardia, urinary retention, glauco sedation (especially in the elderly).
- ***Opioids:*** Respiratory depression, cough reflex↓, nausea & vomiting, constipat
- ***Thiopental:*** (For rapid induction of anaesthesia) laryngospasm.
- ***Propofol:*** Respiratory depression, cardiac depression, pain on injection.
- ***Volatile agents eg isoflurane:*** Nausea & vomiting, cardiac depress respiratory depression, vasodilation, hepatotoxicity (see *BNF*).

The complications of anaesthesia are due to loss of:

- ***Pain sensation:*** Urinary retention, diathermy burns, pressure necrosis, lc nerve injuries (eg radial nerve palsy from arm hanging over the table edge)
- ***Consciousness:*** Cannot communicate 'wrong leg/kidney'. **NB:** in some patie (eg 0.15%) ***retained*** consciousness is the problem. Awareness under GA sou like a contradiction of terms, but remember that anaesthesia is a process ra than an event. Such awareness can lead to ill-defined, delayed neuroses post-traumatic stress disorder (*OHCS* p347).
- ***Muscle power:*** Corneal abrasion (∴ tape the eyes closed), no respiration cough (leads to pneumonia and atelectasis—partial lung collapse caus shunting ± impaired gas exchange: it starts minutes after induction, and ma related to the use of 100% O_2, supine position, surgery and age as well as to of power). Cannot phonate (speak) and unable to impart vital information w paralysed—eg 'I am in pain ...'

Local/regional anaesthesia If unfit/unwilling to undergo general anaesthe local nerve blocks (eg brachial plexus) or spinal blocks (contraindica anticoagulation, local infection) using long-acting local anaesthetics such ***bupivacaine*** may be indicated. See TABLE for doses and toxicity effects.

Drugs complicating anaesthesia ►Inform anaesthetist. See p552 for list specific drugs, and actions to take.

Malignant hyperpyrexia This is a rare complication, precipitated by eg ***haloth*** or ***suxamethonium***, exhibiting autosomal dominant inheritance. There is a r rise in temperature (>1°C every 30min); masseter spasm may also be an e sign. Complications include hypoxaemia, hypercarbia, hyperkalaemia, metab acidosis, and arrhythmias. ►Get expert help immediately. Prompt treatment ***dantrolene***,[1] cooling and supportive care can reduce mortality significantly.

1 Give 1mg/kg every 5min IV—up to 10mg/kg in total (*OHCS* p628).

Surgery

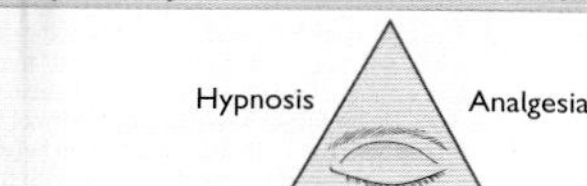

Muscle relaxation

The general principles of anaesthesia centre on the triad of hypnosis, ıalgesia, and muscle relaxation.

ıe conduct of anaesthesia typically involves:

Induction: Either intravenous (eg ***propofol*** 1.5–2.5mg/kg IV at a rate of 20–40mg every 10s; ***thiopental*** is an alternative) or, if airway obstruction or difficult IV access, gaseous (eg ***sevoflurane*** or ***nitrous oxide***, mixed in O_2).

Airway control: Either using a face mask, an oropharyngeal (Guedel) airway or by intubation. The latter usually requires muscle relaxation with a depolarizing/non-depolarizing neuromuscular blocker (*OHCS* p622).

Maintenance of anaesthesia: Either a volatile agent added to N_2O/O_2 mixture, or high-dose opiates with mechanical ventilation, or IV infusion anaesthesia (eg ***propofol*** 4–12mg/kg/h IVI).

End of anaesthesia: Change inspired gases to 100% oxygen only, then discontinue any anaesthetic infusions and reverse muscle paralysis. Once spontaneously breathing, place patient in recovery position and give oxygen by face mask.

r further details, see the chapter titled *Anaesthesia* in *OHCS* (p612)

cal anaesthetic toxicity and maximum doses

ter a few minutes conversation with an anaesthetist at work, it becomes parent that they are masters of the drug dose by weight! It is important to member the maximum doses for local anaesthetics, not least because we use em so frequently, but because the effects of overdose can be lethal.

Local anaesthetic toxicity starts with perioral tingling and paraesthesiae, ogressing to drowsiness, seizures, coma and cardiorespiratory arrest. If spected (the patient feels 'funny' and develops early signs) then stop ministration immediately and commence ABC resuscitation as required.

Handy to remember (though it can be worked out with a pen, paper and SI its) is that a 1% concentration is equivalent to 10mg/mL. Local anaesthetics e also basic, and so do not work well in acidic environments, eg abscesses.

gent	Total dose	Onset	Effective duration	Total dose with adrenaline*	Effective duration
idocaine	3mg/kg ≤200mg	Fast	½–2h	7mg/kg max 500mg	1–6h
evobupivacaine¶	2mg/kg	Medium	2–4h	not given	—
rilocaine#	6mg/kg	Fast	½–2h	6mg/kg max 400mg	1–6h

drenaline is effective at increasing the tissue $t_{½}$ of the anaesthetic and at reducing eeding at the site of administration—very useful eg when suturing the scalp.

Levobupivacaine (Chirocaine®) is replacing racemic ***bupivacaine*** in clinical practice cause it is less cardiotoxic.

Prilocaine can cause methaemoglobinaemia, especially in infants <6 months. This can be versed with IV ***methylene blue***.

Do not use ***adrenaline*** preparations in the fingers, toes, penis or nose because of the risk vasoconstriction of the end arteries and subsequent ischaemic necrosis.

ALWAYS CHECK THE VIAL. Adrenaline concentration should never be more than 1:80 000.

The control of pain

Humans are the most exquisite devices ever made for experiencing of pain: the ric our inner lives, the greater the varieties of pain there are for us to feel, and more resources we have for dealing with pain. If we can connect with patients ner lives we may make a real difference. **Never forget how painful pain is,** nor h fear magnifies pain. Try not to let these sensations, so often interposed betw your patient and his recovery, be invisible to you as he bravely puts up with th

Guidelines for success Review and chart each pain carefully and individuall

- Identify and treat the underlying pathology wherever possible.
- Give **regular** doses rather than on an as required basis.
- Choose the best route: PO, PR, IM, epidural, SC, inhalation, or IV.
- Explanation and reassurance contribute greatly to analgesia.
- Allow the patient to be in charge. This promotes well-being, and does not lea overuse. Patient-controlled continuous IV morphine delivery systems are use
- Liaise with the Acute Pain Service, if possible.

Non-narcotic (simple) analgesia ***Paracetamol*** 0.5–1.0g/4h PO (up to 4g da [15mg/kg/4h IV over ¼h in children >10kg; up to 60mg/kg/d]. Caution in impairment. NSAIDs, eg ***ibuprofen*** 400mg/8h PO [10mg/kg/8h in children >5kg ***diclofenac*** 50mg/8h PO, or 100mg PR/IM stat; these are good for musculoske pain and renal or biliary colic. CI: peptic ulcer, clotting disorders, anticoagula Cautions: asthma, renal or hepatic impairment, pregnancy, and the elderly. ***As*** is contraindicated in children due to the risk of Reye's syndrome (*OHCS* p652

Surgery

Opioid drugs for severe pain ***Morphine*** (eg 10–15mg/2–4h IV/IM) or ***diam phine*** (5–10mg/2–4h PO, SC, or slow IV, but you may need much more) are best These are 'controlled' drugs. For palliative care, see p520. ***Side-effects of opio*** These include nausea (so give with an antiemetic, eg ***prochlorperazine*** 12.5 stat IM), respiratory depression, constipation, cough suppression, urinary reten BP↓, and sedation (do not use in hepatic failure or head injury). Dependen rarely a problem. ***Naloxone*** (eg 100–200µg IV, followed by 100µg increments responsive) may be needed to reverse the effects of excess opioids (p826).

How effective are standard analgesics? Pain is subjective, but its measurer by patients is surprisingly consistent and reproducible. The table below g 'number needed to treat' (NNT, p650), ie the number of patients who nee receive the drug for one to achieve at least 50% pain relief over 4–6h (the ran 95% confidence intervals). For an index of analgesia meta-analyses see:

Codeine 60mg	11–48	Paracetamol 1000mg	3
Tramadol 50mg	6–13	Paracetamol 1000mg/codeine 60mg	2
Aspirin 650mg/codeine 60mg	4–7	Diclofenac 50mg or ibuprofen 400mg	2

Epidural analgesia Opioids and anaesthetics are given into the epidural spac infusion or as boluses. Ask the advice of the Pain Service. SE: thought to be le drug more localized: watch for respiratory depression; local anaesthetic-ind autonomic blockade (BP↓).

Adjuvant treatments Eg radiotherapy for bone cancer pain; anticonvuls antidepressants, ***gabapentin*** or steroids for neuropathic pain, antispasmodic ***hyoscine butylbromide***[1] (Buscopan® 10–20mg/8h PO/IM/IV) for intestinal, tract colic. If brief pain relief is needed (eg for changing dressings or explo wounds), try inhaled ***nitrous oxide*** (with 50% O_2—as Entonox®) with a demand' valve. Transcutaneous electrical nerve stimulation (TENS), local heat, or regional anaesthesia, and neurosurgical procedures (eg excision of neur may be tried but can prove disappointing. Treat conditions that exacerbate (eg constipation, depression, anxiety).

1 Not to be confused with ***hyoscine hydrobromide;*** used for drying secretions and in motion si

Why is controlling post-operative pain so important?

Psychological reasons: Pain control is a humanitarian undertaking.
Social reasons: Pain relief makes surgery less feared by society.
Biological reasons: There is evidence for the following sequence: pain → autonomic activation → increased adrenergic activity → arteriolar vasoconstriction → reduced wound perfusion → decreased tissue oxygenation → delayed wound healing → serious or mortal consequences.

Who is not suitable for day-case surgery?

Over the years peri-operative care has been devolved from the inpatient setting, with better results for the patient.[1] A number of operations are performed as day-cases, commonly including varicose vein surgery, cataracts and inguinal hernia repairs. Even traditionally more demanding surgery is now being performed as day-case (eg laparoscopic cholecystectomy) and theoretically any procedure is suitable, provided the time under general anaesthetic does not exceed ~1h. The use of regional anaesthesia also helps to avoid the SE of nausea and disorientation that may accompany a general anaesthetic, thus facilitating discharge. To avoid putting the patient at unnecessary risk, it is important to identify those who are **not** suitable for day case surgery.

This may include the following:

- Severe dementia.
- Severe learning difficulties.
- Living alone (and no helpers).
- Children if supervision difficult—changes in expectation, delays and pain relief can be problematic.
- BMI >32 (see p229).
- ASA category ≥III (see p553) and thus with potentially unstable co-morbidities—discuss with the anaesthetist as category III may be suitable with appropriate optimisation.
- Infection at the site of the operation.

Exclusions from local regional anaesthesia:

- Poor communication (eg deafness uncorrected by hearing aid) if co-operation is required during the anaesthetic procedure.
- Severe claustrophobia.

Discharging patients after day-case surgery

After day-case surgery, don't discharge until '**LEAP-FROG**' is established:

- Lucid, not vomiting, and cough reflex established.
- Easy breathing; easy urination.
- Ambulant without fainting.
- Pain relief + post-op drugs dispensed + given. Does he understand doses?
- Follow-up arranged.
- Rhythm, pulse & BP checked one last time. Is the trend satisfactory? Check no postural drop (collapsing at front doors tends to rip out your stitches).
- Operation site checked and explained to patient.
- GP letter sent with patient or carer; he/she *must* know what has happened.

1 Advantages: shorter waiting lists, fewer infections, fewer days off work, and ↑patient satisfaction.

General post-operative complications

Pyrexia Mild pyrexia in the first 48h is typically from atelectasis (needs prompt physio, not antibiotics), tissue damage/necrosis or even from blood transfusions, but you should still have a low threshold for infection screen. See MINIBOX for where to look for infection—also check the legs for DVT (causes ↑°C). Send blood for FBC, U&E, CRP, and cultures (±LFT). Dipstick the urine. Consider MSU, CXR, and abdominal ultrasound/CT depending on clinical findings.

Looking for infection

Check for signs of:
- Peritonism
- Chest infection
- UTI
- Wound infection
- Cannula site erythema
- Meningism
- Endocarditis

Confusion may manifest as agitation, disorientation, and attempts to leave hospital, especially at night. Gently reassure the patient in well-lit surroundings. See p476 for a full work-up. The common causes are:
- Hypoxia (pneumonia, atelectasis, LVF, PE)
- Drugs (opiates, sedatives, and many others)
- Urinary retention
- MI or stroke
- Infection (see above)
- Alcohol withdrawal (p274)
- Liver/renal failure

Occasionally, sedation is necessary to examine the patient; consider ***midazolam*** (see p761; antidote: ***flumazenil***) or ***haloperidol*** 0.5–2mg IM. Reassure relatives that post-op confusion is common (seen in up to 40%) and reversible.

Dyspnoea or hypoxia Any previous lung disease? Sit up and give O_2, monitor peripheral O_2 sats by pulse oximetry (p148). Examine for evidence of: • Pneumonia, pulmonary collapse or aspiration • LVF (MI; fluid overload) • Pulmonary embolism (p174); • Pneumothorax (p174; due to CVP line, intercostal block or mechanical ventilation). ***Tests*** FBC; ABG; CXR; ECG. Manage according to findings.

BP↓ If severe, tilt bed head down and give O_2. Check pulse & BP yourself; compare with pre-op values. Post-op ↓BP is often from hypovolaemia resulting from inadequate fluid input, so check fluid chart and replace losses. Monitor urine output (may need catheterization). A CVP line can help monitor fluid resuscitation (normal is 0–5cm H_2O relative to sternal angle). Hypovolaemia may also be caused by haemorrhage so review wounds and abdomen. If unstable, return to theatre for haemostasis. Beware cardiogenic and neurogenic causes and look for evidence of MI + PE. Consider sepsis and anaphylaxis. ***Management:*** p778.

BP↑ may be from pain, urinary retention, idiopathic hypertension (eg missed medication) or inotropic drugs. Oral cardiac medications (including antihypertensives) should be continued throughout the peri-operative period even if NBM. Treat the cause, consider increasing the regular medication, or if not absorbing orally try 50mg ***labetalol*** IV over 1 min (see p126).

Urine output↓ (oliguria) Aim for output of >30mL/h in adults (or >½mL/kg/h). **Anuria** means a blocked or malsited catheter (see p751) and never, we hope, an impending lawsuit from both ureters tied. Flush or replace catheter. **Oliguria** is usually due to too little replacement of lost fluid. Treat by increasing fluid input. ►Acute renal failure may follow shock, drugs, transfusion, pancreatitis or trauma.
- Review fluid chart and examine for signs of volume depletion.
- Urinary retention is also common, so examine for a palpable bladder.
- Establish normovolaemia (a CVP line may help here); you may need 1L/h IV for 2–3h. A 250–500mL bolus of colloid (eg Gelofusin®) over 30min may also help.
- Catheterize bladder (for accurate monitoring)—see p750; check U&E.
- If intrinsic renal failure is suspected, refer to a nephrologist early.

Nausea/vomiting Any mechanical obstruction, ileus, or emetic drugs (opiates, digoxin, anaesthetics)? Consider AXR, NGT, and an antiemetic (►**not *metoclopramide*** because of its prokinetic property). See p233 for choice of different anti-emetics.

↓Na^+ What was the pre-op level? SIADH (p666) can be precipitated by perioperative pain, nausea, and opioids as well as chest infection. Over-administration of IV fluids may exacerbate the situation. Correct slowly (p66…

›st-operative bleeding

Primary haemorrhage: Ie continuous bleeding, starting during surgery. Replace blood loss. If severe, return to theatre for adequate haemostasis. Treat shock vigorously (p778).

Reactive haemorrhage: Haemostasis appears secure until BP rises and oleeding starts. Replace blood and re-explore wound.

Secondary haemorrhage (caused by infection) occurs 1–2 weeks post-op.

lking about post-op complications...

ıen you are asked to give your thoughts on the complications of a particular eration—and this may be with an examiner or a patient—a good starting int is to divide them up accordingly:

From the anaesthetic: (see p558) eg respiratory depression secondary to nduction agents.

From surgery in general: (see opposite and BOX above) eg wound infection, ıaemorrhage, neurovascular damage, DVT/PE.

From the specific procedure: eg saphenous nerve damage in stripping of the ong saphenous vein.

lor the discussion towards the individual who, eg if an arteriopath, may have ignificant risk of cardiac ischaemia during hypotensive episodes whilst under anaesthetic. For some other post-op complications, see:

- Pain (p560)
- DVT (p564 & figs 1–4 below); pulmonary embolus (p174; massive, p802)
- Wound dehiscence (p566)
- Complications in post-gastric surgery (p636)
- Other complications of specific operations (p566).

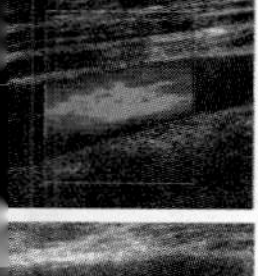

Fig 1. A normal duplex ultrasound of the superficial femoral vein (sagittal view). Compression ultrasound is the investigation of choice in suspected DVT: an acute thrombus within a vein will not show any intraluminal echo, and its presence is confirmed by lack of compression by the ultrasound probe (see fig 3 below).

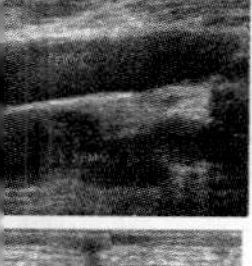

Fig 2. A sagittal view ultrasound of the femoral artery and vein. The vein (deep to the artery) has a ragged luminal edge with hyperechoic regions within the lumen. These are changes secondary to a propagating DVT.

ALL IMAGES COURTESY OF ADDENBROOKE'S HOSPITAL NHS TRUST

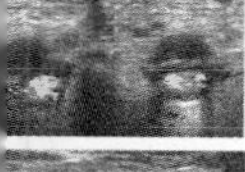

Fig 3. A duplex ultrasound showing a transverse view of the popliteal vein and artery, with (right) and without (left) compression. The vein (more superficial) is not collapsing under compression—a finding suggestive of DVT.

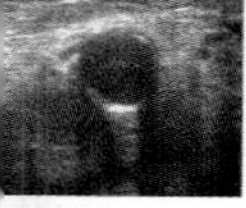

Fig 4. Ultrasound showing a transverse view of the femoral artery and vein. The lumen of the femoral vein (deep and medial to the artery) is occluded by thrombus, giving a hyperechoic signal compared to the arterial lumen.

Deep vein thrombosis (DVT)

See figs, p5

DVTs occur in 25–50% of surgical patients, and many non-surgical patients. 65% below-knee DVTs are asymptomatic; these rarely embolize to the lung.

Risk factors Age↑, pregnancy, synthetic oestrogen, surgery (especially pel orthopaedic), past DVT, malignancy, obesity, immobility, thrombophilia (p358

Signs • Calf warmth/tenderness/swelling/erythema • Mild fever • Pitting oede Homans' sign (↑resistance/pain on forced foot dorsiflexion) should not be tes for as it may dislodge thrombus.

ΔΔ: Cellulitis; ruptured Baker's cyst. Both may coexist with a DVT.

Tests ***D-dimer blood tests*** are sensitive but not specific for DVT (also ↑ in infect pregnancy, malignancy, and post-op). A –ve result, combined with a low pre clinical probability score (see BOX) is sufficient to exclude DVT. If D-dimer↑, or patient has a high/intermediate pretest clinical probability score, do ***compress US*** (fig 3, p563). If this is –ve, a repeat US may be performed at 1wk to ca early but propagating DVTs. ***Venography*** is rarely necessary. Do ***thrombophi tests*** (p358) before commencing anticoagulant therapy if there are predisposing factors, in recurrent DVT, or if there is a family history of DVT.

Prevention • Stop the Pill 4wks pre-op. • Mobilize early. • ***Heparin*** 5000U/12 until mobile; low molecular weight heparin (LMWH, eg ***enoxaparin*** 20mg/24h s to 40mg for high-risk patients, starting 2h pre-op, or ***dalteparin***) may be be (less bleeding, no monitoring needed). • Support hosiery (CI: ischaemia). • Ir mittent pneumatic pressure, until 16h post-op. • ***Fondaparinux*** (a factor inhibitor, approved in the EU) and ***ximelagatran*** may be better than LMWH

Treatment Meta-analyses have shown LMWH (eg ***enoxaparin*** 1.5mg/kg/24h s be superior to ***unfractionated heparin*** (dose guided by APTT, p334), but exter ileofemoral thrombi may still require unfractionated heparin as such patients v excluded from the trials. Start ***warfarin*** simultaneously with LMWH as prothrombotic for the first 48h, stopping heparin when INR is 2–3; treat f months if post-op (6 months if no cause is found; lifelong in recurrent DV thrombophilia). ***Inferior vena caval filters*** may be used in active bleedin when anticoagulants fails, to minimize risk of pulmonary embolus. ***Post-phle change*** can be seen in 10–30%. Prevention with thrombolytic therapy (to re damage to venous valves) and graduated compression stockings have both tried, but neither has been conclusively shown to be beneficial.

Swollen legs see also p66

Treatment—see

Bilateral oedema implies systemic disease with ↑venous pressure (eg right h failure) or ↓intravascular oncotic pressure (any cause of ↓albumin, so test the u for protein). It is **dependent** (distributed by gravity), which is why legs are affe early, but severe oedema extends above the legs. In the bed-bound, fluid mov the new dependent area, causing a sacral pad. The exception is the local increa venous pressure occurring in IVC obstruction: the swelling neither extends a the legs nor redistributes. ***Causes:*** • Right heart failure (p120); • Albumin↓ (p eg renal or liver failure); • Venous insufficiency: acute, eg prolonged sittin chronic, with haemosiderin-pigmented, itchy, eczematous skin ± ulcers; • V dilators, eg ***nifedipine;*** • Pelvic mass (p52); • Pregnancy—if BP↑ + protein diagnose pre-eclampsia (*OHCS* p48): find an obstetrician urgently. In all the ab both legs need not be affected to the same extent.

Unilateral oedema: Pain ± redness implies DVT or inflammation, eg celluli insect bites (any blisters?). Bone or muscle may be to blame, eg tum necrotizing fasciitis (p592); trauma (check for sensation, pulses and severe esp. on passive movement: ►a **compartment syndrome** with ischaemic nec needs prompt fasciotomy). Impaired mobility suggests trauma, arthritis, Baker's cyst (p686). **Non-pitting oedema** is oedema you cannot indent: see

retest clinical probability scoring for DVT: the Wells score

n patients with symptoms in both legs, the more symptomatic leg is used.

Clinical features	Score
Active cancer (treatment within last 6 months or palliative)	1 point
Paralysis, paresis, or recent plaster immobilization of leg	1 point
Major surgery or recently bedridden for >3d in last 4wks	1 point
Local tenderness along distribution of deep venous system	1 point
Entire leg swollen	1 point
Calf swelling >3cm compared to asymptomatic leg (measured 10cm below tibial tuberosity)	1 point
Pitting oedema (greater in the symptomatic leg)	1 point
Collateral superficial veins (non-varicose)	1 point
Alternative diagnosis as likely or more likely than that of DVT	−2 points

Vells score: ≥3 *points:* High pretest probability—treat as suspected DVT and erform compression US. ***1–2 points:*** Intermediate pretest probability—treat as uspected DVT and perform compression US. ***≤0 points:*** Low pretest probability f DVT—perform D-dimer test. If +ve then treat as suspected DVT and perform ompression US. If −ve, DVT reliably excluded.

ir travel and DVT

n 1954, Homans first reported an association between air travel and enous thromboembolism. Recently, the supposed risk of DVT and sub-sequent ulmonary emboli associated with air travel (the so-called 'economy-class yndrome') has been the subject of much public scrutiny. Factors such as ehydration, immobilization, decreased oxygen tension, and prolonged pressure n the popliteal veins resulting from long periods in confined aircraft seats have ll been suggested to be contributory factors. While the evidence linking air ravel to an increased risk of DVT is still largely circumstantial, the following acts may help answer questions from your patients, family, and friends:

- The risk of developing a DVT from a long distance flight has been estimated at 0.01–0.04% for the general population.
- The incidence of DVT in **high risk** groups has been shown to be 4–6% for flights >10h. Prophylaxis with one dose of LMWH **may** be justified.
- There is an increased risk of pulmonary embolus associated with long distance air travel.
- Compression stockings may decrease the risk of DVT, though they may also cause superficial thrombophlebitis.
- The role of prophylactic ***aspirin*** is still unclear and under investigation.
- Measures to minimize risk of DVT include leg exercises, increased water intake, and refraining from alcohol or caffeine during the flight.

questions to ask those with swollen legs

1 Is it **both** legs? 2 Is she pregnant? 3 Is she mobile?
4 Any trauma? 5 Any pitting? 6 Past diseases/on drugs?
7 Any pain? 8 Any skin changes? 9 Any oedema elsewhere?

reatment of leg oedema Treat the cause. Giving diuretics to everyone is not n answer. Ameliorate dependent oedema by elevating the legs (ankles higher han hips—do not just use foot stools); raise the foot of the bed. Graduated upport stockings may help (CI: ischaemia).

Specific post-operative complications

Laparotomy In the elderly, or the malnourished, the wound may break down fr a few days to a few weeks post-op, eg if infection or haematoma is present, or t is major surgery in a patient already compromised, eg by cancer, or this is a laparotomy. The warning sign of wound dehiscence (incidence ≈3.5%) is a p serous discharge. Always assume that the defect involves the whole of the wou Serious wound dehiscence may lead to a 'burst abdomen' with evisceration bowel (mortality 15–30%). If you are on the ward when this happens, put the g back into the abdomen, place a sterile dressing over the wound, give IV antibiot (eg **cefuroxime + metronidazole)** and call your senior. Allay anxiety, g parenteral pain control, set up an IVI, and return patient to theatre. ***Incisio hernia*** is a common problem (20%), repairable by mesh insertion.

Biliary surgery After exploration of the common bile duct (CBD), a T-tube is usu left in the bile duct draining freely to the exterior. A T-tube cholangiogram is d at 8–10d and if there are no retained stones, the tube may be pulled out.

Retained stones may be removed by ERCP (p728), further surgery, or instillat of stone-dissolving agents (via T-tube). If there is distal obstruction in the c fistula formation may occur with a chronic leakage of bile. Other complications biliary surgery are CBD stricture; cholangitis; bleeding into the biliary t (haemobilia) which may lead to biliary colic, jaundice, and haemateme pancreatitis; leak of bile causing biliary peritonitis. If jaundiced, it is importan maintain a good urine output as there is a danger of hepatorenal syndrome (p25 See TABLE for ***laparoscopic cholecystectomy***.

Thyroid surgery (also see p622) Recurrent (± superior) laryngeal nerve pa (→hoarseness) can occur permanently in 0.5% and transiently in 1.5%—warn patient that **their voice will be different** for a few days post-op because intubation and local oedema. **NB:** Pre-operative fibreoptic laryngoscopy should performed to exclude pre-existing vocal cord dysfunction); hypoparathyroid (p206), causing hypocalcaemia (p670) that is permanent in 2.5%; hypothyroid in the long term; thyroid storm (p816); tracheal obstruction due to haematom the wound may occur: ▸▸relieve by immediate removal of stitches or clips using cutter/remover that should remain at the beside; may require urgent surgery

Mastectomy Arm lymphoedema in up to 20% of those undergoing axillary n sampling or dissection—see BOX; skin necrosis.

Arterial surgery Bleeding; thrombosis; embolism; graft infection; MI; AV fist formation. ***Complications of aortic surgery:*** Gut ischaemia; renal fail respiratory distress; aorto-enteric fistula; trauma to ureters or anterior sp artery (leading to paraplegia); distal trash from dislodged thrombus.

Colonic surgery Sepsis; ileus; fistulae; anastomotic leak (10% for anterior rese ion); obstruction from adhesions (BOX); haemorrhage; trauma to ureters or sple

Small bowel surgery Short gut syndrome (best defined **functionally,** thou anatomically ≤250cm in the adult) may result from substantial resections of sr bowel. Diarrhoea and malabsorption (particularly of fats) lead to a numbe metabolic abnormalities including deficiency in vitamins A, D, E, K, & B_{12}, hyp oxaluria (causing renal stones), and bile salt depletion (causing gallstones).

Tracheostomy Stenosis; mediastinitis; surgical emphysema.

Splenectomy Acute gastric dilatation (a serious consequence of not using a NG to check that the one in place is working); thrombocytosis; sepsis. ▸Lifetime se risk is partly preventable with pre-op vaccines—ie *Haemophilus* type meningococcal, & pneumococcal (p381 & p152) and prophylactic penicillin (p3

Genitourinary surgery Septicaemia (from instrumentation in the presence infected urine)—consider a stat dose of ***gentamicin***; urinoma—rupture of a ure or renal pelvis leading to a mass of extravasated urine.

Gastrectomy See p636. **Prostatectomy** p603. **Haemorrhoidectomy** p626.

Adhesions—legacy of the laparotomy, bane of the surgeon

When re-operating on the abdomen, the struggle against adhesions tests the farthest and darkest boundaries of patience of the abdominal surgeon and the assistant. The skill and persistence required to gently and atraumatically tease apart these fibrous bands that restrict access and vision makes any progression, no matter how slight, cause for subdued celebration. Perseverance is the name of this game—also known as ***adhesiolysis***.

Any surgical procedure that breaches the abdominal or pelvic cavities can predispose to the formation of adhesions, which are found in up to 90% of those with previous abdominal surgery, hence why we do not rush to operate on small bowel obstruction: the operation predisposes to yet more adhesions. Handling of the serosal surface of the bowel causes inflammation, which over the period of weeks to years can lead to the formation of fibrous bands that tether the bowel to itself or adjacent structures—though adhesions can also form secondary to infection, radiation injury and inflammatory processes such as Crohn's disease. Their main sequelae are intestinal obstruction (the cause in ~60% of cases—see p598) and chronic abdominal or pelvic pain. Studies have shown that adhesiolysis may help relieve chronic pain, though for a small proportion of patients the pain never improves or even worsens after directed intervention.[41]

As far as prevention is concerned, the best approach is to avoid operating, though there is evidence to suggest that laparoscopy compared to laparotomy reduces the rate of local adhesions,[42] and that there may be a role for the insertion of synthetic films to prevent adhesions to the anterior abdominal wall.[43]

Lymphatic drainage of the breast

Risk of lymphoedema increases with the level of axillary dissection:

- **Level 1** dissection remains inferior to pectoralis minor
- **Level 2** goes behind pectoralis minor
- **Level 3** goes superior to pectoralis minor (rarely done).

The higher the dissection, the greater the risk of interference with lymphatic drainage of the arm and ∴ of lymphoedema.

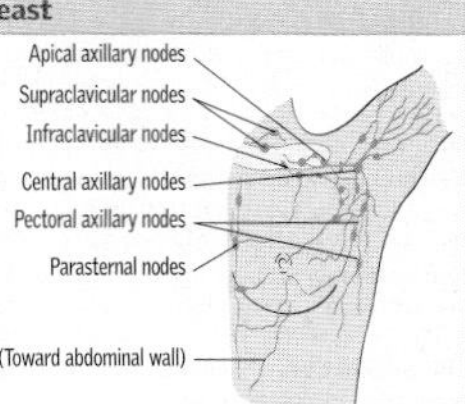

The complications of laparoscopic cholecystectomy

Complications that should be discussed include:	Risk
Conversion to open procedure	5%
CBD injury[1]	0.32%
Bile leak	0.2%
Post-operative haemorrhage	0.1%
Intra-abdominal abscess	0.07%
Mortality secondary to operative injury	0.04%

These complication rates are taken from one study that reviewed 39,238 cases.[44]
NB: Total operative mortality may be nearer 0.1%

1 The nasty long-term sequela of this is permanent CBD stricture and a life of misery along with it. CBD damage rate during laparoscopic surgery is twice that of open surgery.

Stoma care

A stoma (Greek στομα=mouth) is an artificial union made between 2 conduits (a choledochojejunostomy) or, more commonly, between a conduit and the outside eg a colostomy, in which faeces are made to pass through a hole in the abdomir wall into an adherent plastic bag, ideally as 1–2 formed motions/day.

The physical and psychological aspects of stoma care must not be undervalue Be alert to any vicious cycle in which a skin reaction leads to leakage→fear going out into the world→fear of eating→poor skin nutrition→further sl reactions→further leakage→more depression. These cycles can be circumvent by the ***stoma nurse***, who is **the** expert in fitting secure, odourless devices Ensure patients have her phone number for use before and after surgery. Her vis are more useful than any doctor's in explaining what is going to happen, what t stoma will be like, and in troubleshooting post-op problems. ►**Early direct se referral prevents problems.** Without her, a patient may reject his colostomy, nev attend to it, or even become suicidal.

Colostomies Pre-op, confirm that he is unsuited to one of the newer colostor avoiding operations (see below). Are they suitable for a laparoscopic operation?

- ***Loop colostomy:*** A loop of colon is exteriorized, opened, and sewn to the skin rod under the loop prevents retraction and may be removed after 7d. This can a defunctioning stoma (below), though faeces may pass beyond the loop. It often temporary, and more prone to complications than end colostomies.
- ***End colostomy:*** The bowel is divided; the proximal end brought out as a stoma; t distal end may be: 1 **resected**, eg abdominoperineal resection; 2 **closed** & left the abdomen (Hartman's procedure); 3 **exteriorized**, forming a 'mucous fistu
- ***Double-barrelled (Paul–Mikulicz) colostomy:*** The colon is brought out as double-barrel. It may be closed using an enterotome. See figs 1 & 3.

Incidence: 50,000 colostomies/yr[UK]. Most manage their colostomies well. The cc for appliances is ~£1300/yr (allowing for a bag-use rate of 1–3/d). If there is allergic-type reaction to the adhesive or other part of the device, a change device may be all that is needed. Contact the local specialist nurse. Avoid mc creams which can be troublesome if of an oily nature; Comfeel® is an exceptio

Ileostomies protrude from the skin and emit fluid motions which contain acti enzymes (so skin needs protecting). End ileostomy usually follows proctocolector typically for UC; loop ileostomies can also be formed. See fig 2.

Defunctioning stomas (eg loop colostomy/ileostomy) are used to relieve dis obstruction or to protect distal anastomoses. Although they do not reduce leaka rates, they probably minimise the severity of leakage when it does occur.

The alternatives to colostomy Total anorectal reconstruction uses grac muscle disconnected distally and wound around the anus and induced to contract b pulse generator implanted in the abdomen, with bowel action triggered by a har held radiofrequency controller. It is still rather experimental, but patients will a about it. Warn them that it is not without complications and that normal-qual continence will not be achieved because of lack of sensation of the arrival of stools **Posterior sagittal anorectoplasty (PSARP)** is also possible.

There is some evidence from non-randomized trials that sphincter-savi operations are not associated with poorer disease-free survival compared w abdominoperineal resection in those with rectal carcinoma near the anal verge

Urostomies are fashioned after total cystectomy, bringing urine from the urete to the abdominal wall via an **ileal conduit** that is usually incontinent. Formation a catherizable valvular mechanism may retain continence. Advances in urologic surgery have seen an increase in continence-saving procedures such as orthotoț neobladder reconstruction.

mplications of stomas

iaise with the stoma nurse, starting pre-operatively.

rly:

- Haemorrhage at stoma site
- Stoma ischaemia—colour progresses from dusky grey to black
- High output (can lead to $K^+\downarrow$)—consider ***loperamide*** ± ***codeine*** to thicken the output
- Obstruction secondary to adhesions (see p567)
- Stoma retraction.

layed:

- Obstruction (failure at operation to close lateral space around stoma)
- Dermatitis around stoma site (worse with ileostomy)
- Stoma prolapse
- Parastomal hernia (risk increases with time)
- Fistulae (p551)
- Psychological problems.

oosing a stoma site[1]

hen choosing the site for a stoma, avoid:

- Bony prominences (eg anterior superior iliac spine, costal margins)
- The umbilicus
- Old wounds/scars—there may be adhesions beneath
- Skin folds and creases
- The waistline.

e site should be assessed pre-operatively by the stoma nurse, with the patient th lying and standing.

When placing the first bag at the end of the operation, think about whether e patient will be sitting up or mobile (direct bag towards feet) or whether ey will be recumbent for a period (direct bag towards the flank). This will help e person looking after the bag in their task—which may not be the patient if ey are too unwell.

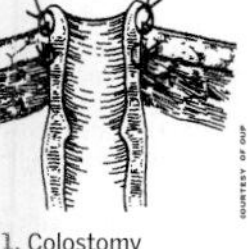

1. Colostomy

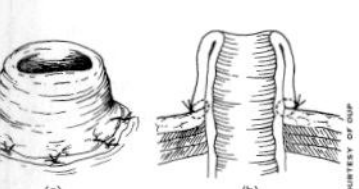

2. Ileostomy

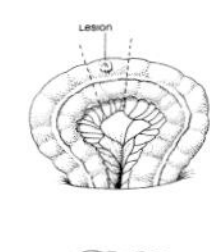

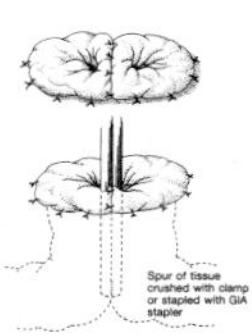

Fig 3. Paul–Mikulicz stoma

1 he same principles apply when choosing a drain site, though since they are usually only *in situ* for w days, pre-operative assessment is rarely required—see p557.

Blood transfusion and blood products

►Blood should only be given if strictly necessary.

- **Know and use** local procedures to ensure that the right blood gets to the r patient at the right time. See p553 for quantities to request.
- Take blood for crossmatching from only 1 patient at a time. Label immedia This minimizes risk of wrong labelling of samples.
- When giving blood, monitor TPR and BP every ½h.
- Do not use giving sets which have contained dextrose or Gelofusine®.

Group-and-save (G&S) requests Find out your local guidelines for elective surg Having crossmatched blood to hand may not be needed if a blood sample is alre in the lab, with group determined, with any atypical antibodies (ie G&S).

Products ***Whole blood:*** (rarely used) Indications: exchange transfusion; g exsanguination—use crossmatched blood if possible, but if not, use 'unive donor' group **O Rh−ve** blood, changing to crossmatched blood as soon as poss ►Blood >2d old has no effective platelets. ***Red cells:*** (packed to make haemato ~70%) Use to correct anaemia or blood loss. 1U ↑Hb by 1–1.5g/dL. In anae transfuse until Hb ~8g/dL. ***Platelets:*** (p348) Not usually needed if not bleedir count is $>20\times10^9$/L. 1U should ↑platelet count by $>20\times10^9$/L. Failure to d suggests refractoriness—discuss with haematologist. If surgery is planned, advice if $<100\times10^9$/L. ***Fresh frozen plasma (FFP):*** Use to correct clotting def eg DIC (p336); warfarin overdosage where **vitamin** K would be too slow; disease; thrombotic thrombocytopenic purpura (p300). It is expensive and ca all the risks of blood transfusion. Do not use as a simple volume expander. ***Hu albumin solution*** is produced as 4.5% or 20% protein solution and is for us protein replacement. 20% albumin can be used temporarily in the hypopro aemic patient (eg liver disease; nephrosis) who is fluid overloaded, without g an excessive salt load. Also used as replacement in abdominal paracentesis (p7 ***Others*** Cryoprecipitate (a source of fibrinogen); coagulation concentrates (injected in haemophilia); immunoglobulin (***anti-D***, *OHCS* p9).

Complications of transfusion ►**Management of acute reactions: see BO**

- ***Early (within 24h):*** Acute haemolytic reactions (eg ABO or Rhesus inc patibility); anaphylaxis; bacterial contamination; febrile reactions (eg from antibodies); allergic reactions (eg itch, urticaria, mild fever); fluid overl transfusion-related acute lung injury (TRALI)—basically ARDS due to a leucocyte antibodies in donor plasma.
- ***Delayed (after 24h):*** Infections (eg viruses: hepatitis B/C, HIV; bact protozoa; prions); iron overload (treatable with ***desferrioxamine***); graft-ver host disease; post-transfusion purpura—potentially lethal fall in platelet cour 7d post-transfusion requiring specialist treatment with IV immunoglobulin platelet transfusions.

Massive blood transfusion This is defined as replacement of an individual's er blood volume (>10U) within 24h. Complications: platelets↓; Ca^{2+}↓; clot factors↓; K^+↑; hypothermia.

Transfusing patients with heart failure If Hb ≤5g/dL with heart failure, tr fusion with packed red cells is vital to restore Hb to safe level, eg 6–8g/dL, must be done with great care. Give each unit over 4h with ***furosemide*** (eg 4 slow IV/PO; don't mix with blood) with alternate units. Check for ↑JVP and b lung crackles; consider CVP line. If CCF gets worse, and immediate transfusic vital, try a 2–3U exchange transfusion, removing blood at same rate as transfu

Autologous transfusion There is a role for patients having their own blood st pre-op for later use. ***Erythropoietin*** (***EPO***, p294) can increase the yield of autoloc blood in normal people. Intraoperative cell salvage with retransfusion is also b used more often, especially in cardiac, vascular and emergency surgery. C analysis shows that it may be worthwhile on an economic basis alone.

Surgery

[Tr]ansfusion reactions

[Al]l UK blood products are now leucocyte-depleted (white cells $<5\times10^6$/L) so as [to] reduce the incidence of complications such as alloimmunisation to HLA class I [an]tigens and febrile transfusion reactions.

[A]cute haemolytic reaction [(]eg ABO incompatibility) Agitat[i]on, T°↑ (rapid onset), ↓BP, flu[s]hing, abdominal/chest pain, [o]ozing venepuncture sites, DIC.	STOP transfusion. Check identity and name on unit; tell haematologist; send unit + FBC, U&E, clotting, cultures, & urine (haemoglobinuria) to lab. Keep IV line open with 0.9% saline. Treat DIC (p336).
[A]naphylaxis [B]ronchospasm, cyanosis, ↓BP, [s]oft tissue swelling.	SLOW or STOP the transfusion. Maintain airway and give oxygen. Contact anaesthetist. ➤➤See p780.
[B]acterial contamination [T]°↑ (rapid onset), ↓BP, and [r]igors.	STOP the transfusion. Check identity against name on unit; tell haematologist and send unit + FBC, U&E, clotting, cultures & urine to lab. Start broad-spectrum antibiotics.
[T]RALI (See OPPOSITE) [D]yspnoea, cough; CXR 'white out'	STOP the transfusion. Give 100% O_2. Treat as ARDS: ➤➤see p170. Donor should be removed from donor panel.
[N]on-haemolytic febrile trans[f]usion reaction Shivering and [f]ever usually ½–1h after [s]tarting transfusion.	SLOW or STOP the transfusion. Give an antipyretic, eg ***paracetamol*** 1g. Monitor closely. If recurrent, use leucocyte-depleted blood or WBC filter.
[A]llergic reactions [U]rticaria and itch.	SLOW or STOP the transfusion; ***chlorphenamine*** 10mg slow IV/IM. Monitor closely.
[F]luid overload [D]yspnoea, hypoxia, tachycardia, ↑JVP & basal crepitations.	SLOW or STOP the transfusion. Give oxygen and a diuretic, eg ***furosemide*** 40mg IV initially. Consider CVP line+exchange transfusion.

[B]lood transfusion and Jehovah's witnesses

[T]hese patients are likely to refuse even vital transfusions on religious grounds.[1] [T]hese views must be respected, but complex issues arise if the patient is a child, [or] (perhaps) an adult who lives a sheltered life, and may not be able to give, or [w]ithhold consent in an informed way—see p554. When in doubt, apply to the [c]ourt. Judges tend to take a narrow view on this, acting as if any immediate [b]enefit to life must trump putative benefits in any life hereafter.[2] How can [r]efusal be informed, it might be argued, if only the physical (and not the [m]etaphysical) consequences of transfusion can be foreseen?

Even if metaphysical considerations are put to one side, it is a question [w]hether giving a transfusion against consent could amount to a degrading act [or] torture, against which the European Convention on Human Rights gives [a]bsolute, inalienable protection. ►Some patients may not want to forsake their [p]rinciples but would not mind too much being told what to do, thereby not [b]eing the means of their child's destruction, while being true to their beliefs. It [is] possible to hold two incompatible beliefs at the same time.[1]

[1] Accepting transfusion implies **self-expulsion** from the church, but it is no longer a '**disfellowshipping [eve]nt**' with active expulsion. This tenet is based on (among others) the biblical verse "*no soul of you [sha]ll eat blood*" (Leviticus 17:12).
[2] V Wason 1998 Court Order (High Court Family Division) Re L (A Minor), June 1–10.

Nutritional support in hospital

►Over 25% of hospital inpatients may be malnourished. Hospitals can becom focused on curing disease that they ignore the foundations of good healt malnourished patients recover more slowly and experience more complicatio

Why are so many hospital patients malnourished?

1 Increased nutritional requirements (eg sepsis, burns, surgery).
2 Increased nutritional losses (eg malabsorption, output from stoma).
3 Decreased intake (eg dysphagia, sedation, coma).
4 Effect of treatment (eg nausea, diarrhoea).
5 Enforced starvation (eg prolonged periods nil by mouth).
6 Missing meals through being whisked off, eg for investigations.
7 Difficulty with feeding (eg lost dentures; no one available to give enough he
8 Unappetizing food: 'They feed me stuff I wouldn't give my cat'.

Identifying the malnourished patient

- ***History:*** Recent weight↓ (>20%, accounting for fluid balance); recent redu intake; diet change (eg recent change in consistency of food); nausea, vomit pain, diarrhoea which might have led to reduced intake.
- ***Examination:*** Examine for state of hydration (p664): dehydration can go ha in-hand with malnutrition, and overhydration can mask the appearance malnutrition. Evidence of malnutrition: skin hanging off muscles (eg over bice no fat between fold of skin; hair rough and wiry; pressure sores; sores at cor of mouth. Calculate the body mass index (p229); BMI <20kg/m² sugge malnourishment. Anthropomorphic indices, eg mid arm circumference, can a be used.
- ***Investigations:*** Generally unhelpful. Low albumin suggestive, but is affected many things other than nutrition. ↑Albumin can be helpful in monitoring recov

Surgery

Prevention of malnutrition Assess nutrition state and weight on admission, a eg weekly thereafter. Identify those at risk (see above). Ensure that meals uninterrupted, when possible. Provide appetizing food to the patient when wants to eat it. If patient requires nutritional support, seek help from dieticia

Calorie and nutritional requirements See TABLE.

Approximate energy contents See TABLE.

Enteral nutrition (ie nutrition given into gastrointestinal tract) If at all possi give nutrition by mouth. An all-fluid diet can meet requirements (but get advice fr dietician). If danger of choking or aspiration (eg after stroke), consider semi-s diet before abandoning food by mouth. Post-op enteral nutrition has been showr benefit patients (eg after surgery for gut perforation).[RCT 55]

Tube feeding: This is giving liquid nutrition *via* a tube, eg placed endoscopica radiologically, or surgically (directly into stomach, ie gastrostomy)—see BOX. nutritionally complete, commercially prepared feeds. Standard feeds (eg Nutri standard®, Osmolite®) normally contain ~1kCal/mL and 4–6g protein per 100r Most people's requirements are met with 2L/24h. Specialist advice from dieticia essential. Nausea and vomiting is less of a problem if feed given continuously w pump, but may have disadvantages compared with intermittent nutrition.

Guidelines for success

- Use fine-bore (9 Fr) nasogastric feeding tube when possible.
- Check position of nasogastric tube (pH testing, listening for *borborygmi*) nasoduodenal tube (x-ray) before starting feeding.
- Build up feeds gradually to avoid diarrhoea and distension.
- Weigh weekly, check blood glucose and plasma electrolytes (including phospha zinc, and magnesium, if previously malnourished).
- Treat underlying conditions vigorously—eg sepsis may impede +ve nitrogen balan
- ► Close liaison with a dietician is essential.

1 For an in depth guide to nutrition see *Manual of Dietetic Practice,3e*, Briony Thomas, Blackwell

teral tube feeding

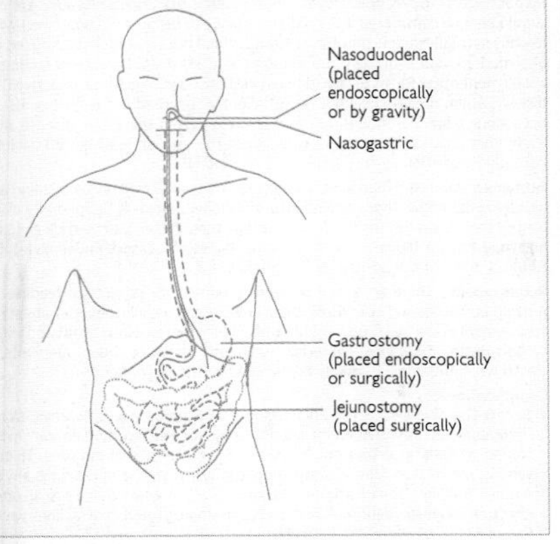

aily energy and nutritional requirements

ıbstance	Requirement (/kg/d)	Notes
ıergy	20–40kCal	Normal adult requirements will be 2000–2500kCal/d; even catabolic patients rarely require >2500kCal/d. Very high calorie diets (eg >4000kCal/d) can lead to a fatty liver.
	84–168kJ	Multiply kCal by a factor of 4.2.
trogen	0.2–0.4g	6.25g of enteral protein gives 1g of nitrogen. Considering nitrogen balance is important because although catabolism is inevitable, replenishment is vital.
rotein	0.5g	Contains 5kCal/g.
t	3g	Contains 10kCal/g.
ırbohydrate	2g	Contains 4kCal/g.
ater	30–35ml	+500ml/d for each °C of pyrexia.
a/K/Cl	1.0mmol each	Electrolytes need to be considered, even if not on IVI.

Parenteral (intravenous) nutrition

Do not undertake parenteral feeding lightly: it has risks. Specialist advice is vita should only be considered if the patient is likely to become malnourished with it—this normally means that the gastrointestinal tract is not functioning (eg bo obstruction), and is unlikely to function for at least 7d. Parenteral feeding supplement other forms of nutrition (eg in short bowel syndrome or active Cro disease, when nutrition cannot be sufficiently absorbed in the gut) or it car used alone (total parenteral nutrition—TPN). ►Even if there is GI disease, stu show that enteral nutrition is safer, cheaper, and at least as efficacious parenteral nutrition in the perioperative period.[1][56]

Administration Nutrition is normally given through a central venous line as usually lasts longer than if given into a peripheral vein. A peripherally inser central catheter (PICC line) is another option, though they can be trickier to ins and may have a higher rate of thrombophlebitis.[RCT 57] Insert under strict ste conditions and check position on x-ray—figs 1 & 2.

Requirements There are many different regimens for parenteral feeding. M provide 2000kCal and 10–14g nitrogen in 2–3L; this usually meets a patient's d requirements (see TABLE, p573). ~50% of calories are provided by fat and ~50% carbohydrate. Regimens comprise vitamins, minerals, trace elements, electrolytes; these will normally be included by the pharmacist.

Complications[2]

- ***Sepsis*** (Eg *Staphylococcus epidermidis* and *Staphylococcus aureus; Cand Pseudomonas;* infective endocarditis.) Look for spiking pyrexia and exam wound at tube insertion point. Take line **and** peripheral cultures. If cen venous line-related sepsis is suspected, the safest course of action is alway remove the line. Do not attempt to salvage a line when *S. aureus* or *Cand* infection has been identified. Antimicrobial-impregnated central lines decre the incidence of line-related infections.[58]
- ***Thrombosis*** Central vein thrombosis may occur, resulting in pulmonary emb or superior vena caval obstruction (p514). ***Heparin*** in the nutrient solution r be useful for prophylaxis in high-risk patients, though there is little clear- evidence in adult studies.
- ***Metabolic imbalance*** Electrolyte abnormalities—see BOX; deranged plas glucose; hyperlipidaemia; deficiency syndromes (TABLE, p273); acid-b disturbance (eg hypercapnia from excessive CO_2 production).
- ***Mechanical:*** Pneumothorax; embolism of IV line tip.

Guidelines for success

- ►Liaise closely with line insertion team, nutrition team and pharmacist.
- Meticulous sterility. Do not use central venous lines for uses other than nutrit Remove the line if you suspect infection. Culture its tip.
- Review fluid balance at least twice daily, and requirements for energy electrolytes daily.
- Check weight, fluid balance, and urine glucose daily throughout per of parenteral nutrition. Check plasma glucose, creatinine and electroly (including calcium and phosphate), and FBC daily until stable and then 3 time week. Check LFT and lipid clearance three times a week until stable and th weekly. Check zinc and magnesium weekly throughout.
- Do not rush. Achieve the maintenance regimen in small steps.
- Treat underlying conditions vigorously—eg sepsis may impede +ve nitrogen bala

1 Enteral feeding promotes integrity of the gut mucosal barrier, thus preventing bacterial and endot translocation across the gut wall, which can lead to multiple organ dysfunction syndrome (MODS) perpetuation of a systemic inflammatory response—even when the gut is not the primary source of pathol
2 For children, see Brit. Association for Parenteral and Enteral Nut. 2000 *Guidelines* ISBN 1899467

feeding syndrome

At risk with:
• Malignancy
• Anorexia nervosa
• Alcoholism
• GI surgery
• Starvation

s is a life-threatening metabolic complication of eeding *via* any route after a prolonged period of rvation. As the body turns to fat and protein tabolism in the starved state, there is a drop in the level circulating insulin (because of the paucity of dietary bohydrates). The catabolic state also depletes racellular stores of phosphate, although serum levels may nain normal (0.85–1.45mmol/L). When refeeding begins, level of insulin rises in ponse to the carbohydrate load, and one of the consequences is to increase lular uptake of phosphate.

A hypophosphataemic state (<0.50mmol/L) normally develops within 4d and nostly responsible for the features of '**refeeding syndrome**' which include: abdomyolysis; red and white cell dysfunction; respiratory insufficiency; hythmias; cardiogenic shock; seizures; sudden death.

Prevention requires at-risk patients to be identified, assessed and monitored sely during the period of refeeding (glucose, lipids, and electrolytes—sodium, tassium, phosphate, calcium, magnesium, and zinc). Close involvement of a tritionist is required.

Treatment is of the complicating features and includes parenteral phosphate ministration (eg 18mmol/d) in addition to oral supplementation.

e venous system at the thoracic outlet

nen trying to judge the position of a ntral venous line tip on CXR (see figs 1 2) it helps to know the anatomical ndmarks of the venous system. The bclavian veins join the internal jugular ins behind the sternoclavicular joints form the brachio-cephalic veins. ese come together behind the right sternocostal joint to form the perior vena cava (SVC), which runs om this point to the right 3rd ernocostal joint. The right atrium arts here.

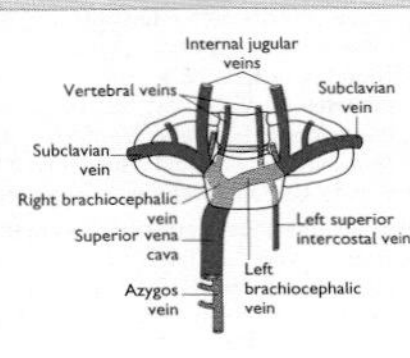

ter RCSI website

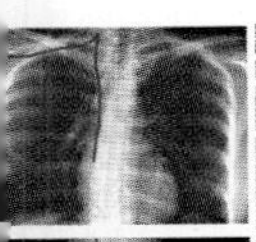

Fig 1. This is a CXR showing a correctly placed peripherally inserted central catheter (PICC) (red highlight). The catheter is placed under strict sterile conditions via the ante-cubital fossa, through the cephalic and subclavian veins, down into the SVC (compare with BOX above).

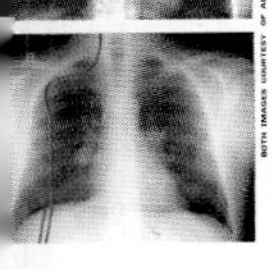

BOTH IMAGES COURTESY OF ADDENBROOKE'S HOSPITAL NHS TRUST

Fig 2. This is a CXR showing a malpositioned right subclavian central venous line (red highlight). Rather than passing inferiorly into the SVC and the right atrium, the catheter has passed up the right internal jugular vein towards the head (compare with BOX above). ►This line needs removal followed by re-insertion of a new line: see p762 for the technique.

Diabetic patients undergoing surgery

Insulin-dependent diabetes mellitus (eg Type 1 diabetes mellitus)

- Patients are often well informed about their diabetes; involve them fully v managing their diabetic care.
- Stress or intercurrent illness increases basal insulin needs (see p190).
- Always try to put the patient first on the list (surgery, endoscopy, bronchosc etc.). Inform the surgeon and anaesthetist early.
- Stop all long-acting insulin the night before. Get IV access before you nee urgently. If surgery is in the morning, stop all SC morning insulin. If surgery the afternoon, have the usual short-acting insulin in the morning at breakfast medium- or long-acting insulin. It may be feasible to continue ***glargine*** (p19 baseline therapy throughout the peri-operative period though there have bee large studies into this.
- Check blood glucose hourly. Aim for 7–11mmol/L during surgery.
- Check U&E pre-op. Start an IVI of 1L of 5% dextrose with 20mmol KCl, Dextrose saline can be given if Na^+ low, but do not give only saline; dextrose need constant infusion to maintain blood glucose.
- Start an infusion pump with 50U short-acting insulin (eg Actrapid®) in 50 0.9% saline. Give according to a sliding scale (see TABLE) adjusted in light of blood glucose.
- Post-op, continue IV insulin + dextrose until patient tolerating food. Ch fingerprick glucose every 2h. Switch to usual SC regimen around a meal.

Practical hints:

- Some centres prefer to control blood sugar with a glucose-potassium-ins (GKI) infusion—see BOX.
- If the patient is having minor surgery (ie will not be NBM for >6h) and definitely be able to eat post-op, IV insulin may not be necessary. Some advo giving the patient a small glucose drink early on the morning of surgery, delaying their morning insulin dose and breakfast until after the procedure.
- If in doubt, check with the anaesthetist and liaise with a diabetes specialist nur

Non-insulin-dependent diabetes mellitus (≈Type 2 diabetes)

- These patients are usually controlled on oral hypoglycaemics (p192). If diabe poorly controlled (eg fasting glucose >10mmol/L), treat as for type 1 diabe
- Do not give long-acting sulphonylureas (eg ***glibenclamide***) on the morning surgery, as they can cause prolonged hypoglycaemia on fasting.
- Beware lactic acidosis in patients on biguanides (eg ***metformin***), especiall using IV contrast agents and/or renal function poor (creatinine >150μmol/
- If the patient can eat post-operatively, simply omit tablets on the mornin surgery and give post-op with a meal.
- If the patient is having major surgery with restrictions to eating post-op, ch fasting glucose on the morning of surgery and start IV or SC insulin gi according to sliding scale. Post-op, consult the diabetic team as the patient r need a phase of insulin to supplement their oral hypoglycaemics.

Diet-controlled diabetes Usually no problem, though patient may briefly be ins dependent post-op. Monitor fingerprick glucose before meals and bedtime. Av giving 5% dextrose IVI as a fluid replacement as blood glucose will rise.

Peri-operative morbidity and mortality Diabetes mellitus is classed as intermediate risk factor for increased perioperative cardiovascular risk by American Heart Association, so screen for the presence of asymptomatic carc and renal disease (p553) and be aware of possible 'silent' myocardial ischaemia

One retrospective study on those undergoing major vascular surgery show that although long term survival was poorer for patients with diabe perioperative cardiovascular morbidity and mortality were only increased in presence of congestive heart failure and haemodialysis—ie **not** diabetes alon

An example of an IV sliding scale

Fingerprick glucose	IV soluble insulin[1]	Alternative SC insulin[2]
<2 ➡See p816	None–50% glucose IV + Hypostop® PO	
2–5	No insulin	No insulin
5–10	1u/h	2u/h (rough guide only)
10–15	2u/h	5u/h
15–20	3u/h	7u/h
>20	6u/h–get urgent diabetic review	

NB: this is a guide only: individual scales may vary between institutions

GKI infusions (glucose, K⁺ & insulin)

►A problem when giving IV insulin and IV dextrose simultaneously through separate intravenous lines is that if one cannula becomes blocked, the patient may become hypo- or hyperglycaemic. If the glucose and insulin are given through the same cannula, however, and the 3-way converter becomes blocked, the syringe driver may retrogradely fill the infusion set with insulin. When the cannula is subsequently resited and the infusion restarted, the patient will receive this large accumulated dose of insulin. This has caused lethal hypoglycaemia, so some centres now use GKI infusions instead of sliding scales.

- A 500mL bag of 5 or 10% dextrose ± KCl is given over 6h, with a short-acting insulin (eg Actrapid®) added according to blood glucose:[64]

Blood glucose (mmol/L)	Insulin dose (units/bag)	Serum K⁺ (mmol/L)	KCl to be added (mmol/bag)
<4	None	<3	20
4–6	5	3–5	10
6–10	10	>5	None
10–20	15		
>20	20		

- Check blood glucose every 3h. If levels too high or low, start a new 500mL bag of 5% dextrose with the correct insulin dose.
- Check U&E daily.

GKI infusions are useful when close monitoring of blood glucose is not possible, but are not be suitable in poorly controlled diabetes. If the patient is under a fluid restriction then it is possible to halve the bag volume and double the dextrose concentration (eg 250 mL of 10–20% dextrose), dosing the insulin per bag just as before. If the patient is ***hyponatraemic*** then a concomitant infusion of 0.9% saline should be considered.

NB: regimens vary and sometimes more insulin will be required; eg if shocked, severely ill, or if on steroids or sympathomimetics, 2–4 times as much insulin may be needed. See *BNF* section 6.1.

Surgery

1 Check glucose hourly and adjust insulin accordingly.
2 ►Only use SC route if IV route is problematic as it is associated with much variability; check finger prick glucose every 2–4h if NBM, or pre-meals if using SC insulin to supplement other hypoglycaemics.

Jaundiced patients undergoing surgery

Patients with obstructive jaundice are particularly prone to developing renal failu after surgery, perhaps from the toxic effect of bilirubin and any concomitant sep (see hepatorenal syndrome—p251). In practice this means that good urine outp must be maintained in such patients around the time of surgery.

Pre-operative preparation Avoid ***morphine*** in the premedication.

- Give antibiotic prophylaxis (p556) and treat sepsis to ↓ risk of endotoxaemia
- Insert IV line and give 1L of 0.9% saline over ½–1h following pre-med (unle the patient has heart failure), to produce a moderate diuresis peri-operatively loop diuretic (eg ***furosemide***) may be needed to ensure diuresis. Pre-op manni is no longer routine in jaundiced patients—it may even be deleterious.[RCT 66]
- Insert a urinary catheter.
- A 'renal' dose ***dopamine*** (2–5μg/kg/min) IVI **may** be indicated. See [RCT 67] but also
- Remember there may be side-effects from any central line used, and from the dru
  - Sepsis (immune dysfunction) · Arrhythmias · Gut + myocardial perfusion
  - Diuresis when hypovolaemic · Catabolism↑ · Gastric motility decreased
  - Pulmonary hypertension · Impaired hypoxic ventilatory responses[69]
- Check clotting and consider giving prophylactic ***vit K*** (p330), even if normal

During surgery

- Measure urine output hourly and give 0.9% saline IV to match the urine outp

For 48h after surgery

- Measure urine output every 2h; measure U&E daily.
- Give 0.9% saline at rate to match urine output and fluid lost eg through NGT; gi 2L of dextrose–saline every 24h.
- Consider ***furosemide*** if urine output is poor despite adequate hydration.
- Give 20mmol of K^+/L of fluid after 24h post-op if urine output good.

Surgery in those on steroids

Patients on steroid therapy need extra cover to cope with the stress of surgery their endogenous adrenal hormone levels will be suppressed, even for a peri after cessation of a course of treatment. The amount of extra cover need depends on the extent of the surgery and the pre-op dose of steroids. For routi surgery, aim to reduce the dose of steroid as much as possible. Consider stero cover for anyone who has had high-dose glucocorticoid therapy in the last yea ***Major surgery:*** Typically give ***hydrocortisone*** 50–100mg IV with the pre-med ar then every 6-8h IV/IM for 3d, then wean to previous medication. ***Minor surger*** Prepare as for major surgery except that ***hydrocortisone*** is given for 24h only.

The major risk with adrenal insufficiency is hypotension, so if this is encountere without an obvious cause, it may be worthwhile giving a STAT dose of 50m ***hydrocortisone*** IV. See BNF section 6.3 for steroid dose equivalences.

Surgery in those on anticoagulants

►Contact your lab, and inform the surgeon and anaesthetist. ***Very minor surge*** has been undertaken without stopping ***warfarin*** (do INR within 24h: it may be sa to proceed if <3.5). In ***major surgery***, drugs may be stopped for 2–5d pre-o Risks and benefits are individual to each patient, so exact rules are impossibl Discuss these issues when arranging consent. ***Vitamin K*** (eg 10mg IV) ± ***FFP*** may b needed in emergency surgery. ►**Monitor clotting meticulously.**

One elective option is conversion to ***heparin*** (stop 6h prior to surgery, ar monitor APTT perioperatively): unfractionated heparin's short $t_{½}$ allows swi reversal with ***protamine*** (p334). When rewarfarinizing, don't stop heparin cove until the INR is therapeutic, as warfarin is prothrombotic in the early stages.

The bleeding tendency effects of ***aspirin*** are reversed by 5d after stopping, b check with local policy to see if cessation is required.[RCT 72] The alteration of antiplatel agents (and NSAIDs) is a complex business and is best discussed with an expert.

Thyroid disease and surgery

Thyroid surgery for hyperthyroidism If severe, give ***carbimazole*** until euthyroid (p202). Arrange operation date and 10–14d before this, start aqueous iodine oral solution (Lugol's solution), 0.1–0.3mL/8h PO well diluted with milk or water. Continue until surgery.

Mild hyperthyroidism Start ***propranolol*** 80mg/8h PO and Lugol's solution as above at the 1st consultation. Stop Lugol's solution on the day of surgery but continue ***propranolol*** for 5d post-op.

▶**Thyrotoxic storm** A rare but potentially fatal consequence of thyroid surgery (mortality 50%). See p817.

Non-thyroid surgery ***Thyroxine*** has a long $t_{1/2}$ (~7d) so omitting a dose while nil by mouth will not have any major effects.

Surgery in the obese

It has long been believed that obesity increases the risk of post-operative complications.[1] Indeed, 50 years ago obesity was considered a contraindication to elective surgery.

One study has suggested, however, that obesity in itself may not be a risk factor for most complications. Overall incidence of complications after elective general surgery did not differ significantly between obese and non-obese patients, though only 1.7% of the 6336 patients in the trial had a BMI >40kg/m². The only post-operative complication found to have an increased incidence in the obese was wound infection after open surgery. Overall it would seem that the practice of forcing patients to lose weight prior to elective general surgery may be inappropriate.

Surgery for obesity Bariatric surgery has become very successful at weight reduction **and** symptom resolution (eg sleep apnoea), especially in the extremely obese. Common procedures include Roux-en-Y gastric bypass, stomach stapling, and laparoscopic banding. ***Complications:*** Dumping syndrome, wound infection, hernias, malabsorption, diarrhoea, and a mortality of ~0.5% (at experienced centres).

One prospective study on the effects of laparoscopic banding showed that at one year the mean **excess** weight loss was 45.7%, with improvement of quality of life. Whether or not the weight remains off in the long-term is yet to be firmly established.

Obesity has been shown to increase risks of cardiac and spinal surgery.

The acute abdomen

Someone who becomes acutely ill and in whom symptoms and signs are chie related to the abdomen has an acute abdomen. Prompt laparotomy is sometim essential: **repeated examination is the key to making the decision.**

Clinical syndromes that usually require laparotomy:

1 ***Rupture of an organ*** (Spleen, aorta, ectopic pregnancy) Shock is a leading sign see TABLE for assessment of blood loss. Abdominal swelling may be seen. Any histo of trauma: blunt trauma → spleen; penetrating trauma → liver. **Delayed** rupture the spleen may occur weeks after trauma. Peritonism may be mild.

2 ***Peritonitis*** (Perforation of peptic ulcer, diverticulum, appendix, bowel, or g bladder) Signs: prostration, shock, lying still, +ve cough test (p40), tenderne (± rebound/percussion pain, p70), board-like abdominal rigidity, guarding, a no bowel sounds. Erect CXR may show gas under the diaphragm (fig NB: Acute pancreatitis (p582) causes these signs, but does **not** require laparotomy so don't be caught out and ►ALWAYS CHECK SERUM AMYLASE.

Syndromes that may not require a laparotomy:

1 ***Local peritonitis:*** Eg diverticulitis, cholecystitis, salpingitis, and appendicitis (t latter **will** need surgery). If abscess formation is suspected (swelling, swingi fever, and WCC↑) do ultrasound or CT. Drainage can be percutaneous (ultrasou or CT-guided), or by laparotomy. Look for 'a sentinel loop' on plain AXR (p717

2 ***Colic*** is a regularly waxing and waning pain, caused by muscular spasm in hollow viscus, eg gut, ureter, salpinx, uterus bile duct, or gall bladder (in t latter pain is often dull and constant). Colic, unlike peritonitis, causes restlessne and the patient may well be pacing around when you go to see him!

Surgery

Obstruction of the bowel See p598.

Tests U&E; FBC; amylase; LFT; CRP; ABG (is there mesenteric ischaemia?); urinalysis. Laparoscopy may avert open surgery. CT can be helpful provided it is readily available and causes no delay; ultrasound is becoming more popular and may identify perforation or free fluid immediately, but appropriate performer training is important.

Pre-op care ►Don't rush to theatre. **Anaesthesia compounds shock**, so resuscitate properly first (p779) unless blood is being lost faster than it can be replaced, eg in ruptured ectopic pregnancy, (*OHCS* p262), leaking aneurysm (p586) or trauma.

Plan: Put to bed—then:
- Treat shock (p778)
- Crossmatch, eg 2U or jus group and save
- Blood culture; then...
- Antibiotics[1]
- Relieve pain (p560)
- IVI (0.9% saline)
- Plain abdominal film
- CXR if peritonitic or >50y
- ECG if >50yrs
- Consent
- NBM for 2h pre-op

The medical acute abdomen Irritable bowel syndrome (p268) is the chief caus so always ask about episodes of pain associated with loose stools, relieved b defecation, bloating, and urgency (but **not** blood—this may be UC). Other cause

►►Myocardial infarction	Pneumonia (p152)	Sickle-cell crisis (p326)
Gastroenteritis or UTI	Thyroid storm (p816)	Phaeochromocytoma (p818)
Diabetes mellitus (p190)	Zoster (p388)	Malaria (p382)
Bornholm disease (p55)	Tuberculosis (p386)	Typhoid fever (p414)
Pneumococcal peritonitis	Porphyria (p684)	Cholera (p414)
Henoch–Schönlein (p694)	Narcotic addiction	*Yersinia enterocolitica* (p41
Tabes dorsalis (p419)	PAN (p543)	Lead colic

Hidden diagnoses ►►Mesenteric ischaemia (p594), ►►acute pancreatitis (p584) ar ►►a leaking AAA (p586) are the *Unterseebooten* of the acute abdomen- unsuspected, undetectable unless carefully looked for, and underestimated deadly. They may have non-specific symptoms and signs that are surprisingly mil so always think of them when assessing the acute abdomen and hopefully you w 'spot' them! ►Finally: ALWAYS EXCLUDE PREGNANCY IN FEMALES.

1 Give antibiotics if peritonitic, eg *cefuroxime* 1.5g/8h IV + *metronidazole* 500mg/8h IV/PR.

auses of abdominal pain

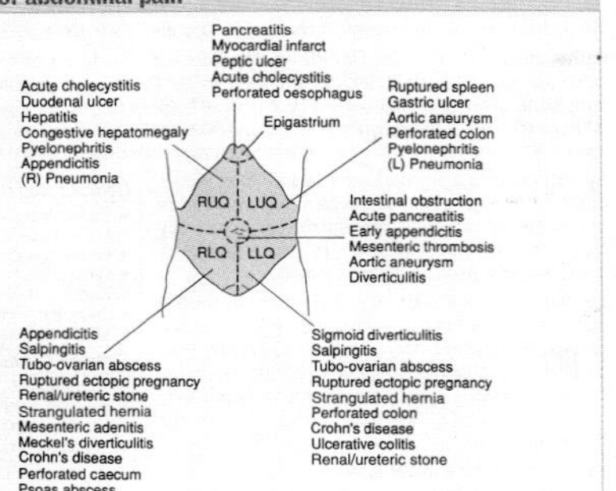

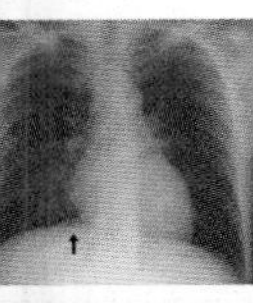

Fig 1. Erect CXR showing a sliver of air beneath the right hemidiaphragm (arrow), indicating presence of a pneumoperitoneum. ***Causes:***
- Perforation of the bowel (visible only in 75%)
- Gas-forming infection eg *Clostridium perfringens*
- Iatrogenic eg open or laparoscopic surgery[1]
- *Per vaginam* (water ski-ing; prolonged intercourse)
- Interposition of bowel between liver & diaphragm

ssessing hypovolaemia from blood loss

he most likely cause of shock in a surgical patient is hypovolaemia (but don't orget the other causes—p778). The most important physiological parameters or the assessment of shock assess target organ perfusion rather than the direct neasurement of BP and pulse, which may be 'normal' in one individual and yet otally abnormal for another. The most perfused organs in a normal state are the idney, brain, and skin, so check **urine output**, GCS and **capillary refill** (CR).

Of course, BP, pulse, and respirations are still **vital** signs, but the message here : ►treat suspected shock rather than wait for BP to fall. When there is any lood loss (eg a trauma situation), assess the status of the following:

arameter	Class I	Class II	Class III	Class IV
lood loss	>750mL >15%	750–1500mL 15–30%	1500–2000mL 30–40%	>2000mL >40%
ulse	<100bpm	>100bpm	>120bpm	>140bpm
P	↔	↔	↓	↓
ulse pressure	↔ or ↑	↓	↓	↓
espirations	14–20/min	20–30/min	30–40/min	>35/min
rine output	>30mL/h	20–30mL/h	5–15mL/h	Negligible
ental state	Slightly anxious	Mildly anxious	Confused →	Lethargic
luid to give	Crystalloid	Crystalloid	Crystalloid + blood	

ssumes a body mass of 70kg and a circulating blood volume of 5L.

American Col. of Surgeons' Committee on Trauma, Advanced Trauma Life Support® for Doctors (ATLS®) Student Manual 7e, Chicago: Am. Col. Surg, 2004.

Gas under the diaphragm can be still detected on CXR up to 10 days post-op.

Acute appendicitis

This is the most common surgical emergency (lifetime incidence = 6%).

Pathogenesis Gut organisms invade the appendix wall after lumen obstruction b lymphoid hyperplasia, faecolith, or filarial worms—or there may be impaired abili to prevent invasion, brought about by improved hygiene (so less exposure to g pathogens). This 'hygiene hypothesis' explains the rise in appendicitis rates in th early 1900s and its later decline (as pathogen exposure dwindles further).

Symptoms Classically periumbilical pain that moves to the RIF (see BOX). Anorexia is an important feature and vomiting is rarely prominent—pain normally precedes vomiting in the surgical abdomen. Constipation is usual. Diarrhoea may occur.

Special tests: Rovsing's sign (pain more in the RIF than the LIF when the LIF is pressed). In women, do a vaginal examination: does she have salpingitis (+ve cervical excitation, *OHCS* p286)? CT (if diagnosis unclear: reduces –ve appendicectomy rate, but may cause fatal delay). See BOX for evaluation of the ***Alvarado score***.

General signs
• Tachycardia
• Fever 37.5–38.5°C
• Furred tongue
• Lying still
• Foetor ± flushing
• Coughing hurts (p40)
• Shallow breaths
Signs in the RIF
• Guarding (p60)
• Rebound + percussion tenderness (p70)
• PR painful on right

Variations in the clinical picture

- The infant with watery diarrhoea and vomiting.
- The boy with vague abdominal pain who will not eat his favourite food.
- The shocked, confused octogenarian who is not in pain.

Surgery

Hints ►Don't rely on tests, eg WCC; CRP; urinoscopy; CT (may cause fatal delay).

- If the child is anxious, use his hand to press his belly—see also p601 for tips.
- Check for recent viral illnesses and lymphadenopathy—mesenteric adenitis?
- Don't **start** palpating in the RIF as this may make it difficult to illicit pain elsewher
- Do not ignore right-sided tenderness on rectal examination: it may be the only sig
- Expect your diagnosis to be wrong half the time. This means that those wh seem not to have appendicitis should be re-examined often.

Treatment Prompt ***appendicectomy***. Stump inversion at operation remains a topic of debate.[RCT 78] but also [RCT 79] ***Antibiotics: Metronidazole*** 500mg/8h + ***cefuroxime*** 1.5g/8h, 1 to 3 doses IV starting 1h pre-op, reduces wound infections. Give a longer course if perforated. ***Laparoscopy:*** Useful because of its diagnostic and therapeutic advantages (when performed by an experienced surgeon), especially in women and the obese. It is not recommended in cases suspected of gangrenous perforation because the rate of abscess formation may be higher.[MET 80]

ΔΔ
• Ectopic pregnancy
►►Do a pregnancy test!
• Mesenteric adenitis
• Cystitis
• Cholecystitis
• Diverticulitis
• Salpingitis/PID
• Dysmenorrhoea
• Crohn's disease
• Perforated ulcer
• Food poisoning
• Meckel's diverticulum

Complications

- ***Perforation*** (does not appear to cause later infertility in girls).[81] In childre perforation is commoner with decreasing age: this reflects diagnostic difficulty.
- ***Appendix mass*** May result when an inflamed appendix becomes covered wit omentum. US/CT may help with the diagnosis. Some advocate early surgery, bu initial management is usually conservative—NBM and antibiotics (eg ***cefuroxim*** 1.5g/8h IV and ***metronidazole*** 500mg/8h IV). Mark out the size of the mass an proceed to drainage if the mass develops into an abscess (see below). If the mas resolves, some perform an **interval** (ie delayed) **appendicectomy**. Exclude a coloni tumour (laparotomy or colonoscopy), which can present as early as the 4th decade
- ***Appendix abscess*** May result if an appendix mass fails to resolve. Signs includ enlargement of the mass or if the patient gets more toxic (pain↑; °C↑; pulse↑ WCC↑). ***Treatment*** usually involves drainage, either surgical or percutaneou (under US/CT-guidance). Antibiotics alone may bring resolution.

xplaining the pattern of abdominal pain in appendicitis

ne classic pattern in acute appendicitis is early periumbilical pain that then igrates to rest in the RIF. But why does this pattern occur?

The chief aspect to consider is the difference in innervation between the sceral and parietal peritoneal layers. A viscus and its visceral peritoneum have) somatic innervation, so the brain attributes the visceral (splanchnic) signals a physical location whose dermatome corresponds to the same entry level in ne spinal cord. Importantly, there is no laterality to the visceral unmyelinated -fibre pain signals, which enter the cord bilaterally and at multiple levels. ivision of the gut according to embryological origin is the important eterminant here:

ut	Division points	Somatic referral	Arterial supply
ore	Proximal to 2nd part of duodenum	Upper abdomen	Coeliac axis
Mid	Above to ⅔ along transverse colon	Middle abdomen	Superior mesenteric
lind	Distal to above	Lower abdomen	Inferior mesenteric

Early inflammation irritates the structure and walls of the appendix, so a olicky pain is referred to the mid-abdomen—classically periumbilical. As the flammation progresses and irritates the parietal peritoneum (especially on xamination!) the somatic, lateralized pain settles at McBurney's point, ⅔ of the ay along from the umbilicus to the right anterior superior iliac spine.

hese principles also help us understand patterns of ***referred pain***. In neumonia, the T9 dermatome is shared by the lung and the abdomen. Also, ritation of the underside of the diaphragm (sensory innervation is from above rough the phrenic nerve, C3–5) by an inflamed gallbladder or a subphrenic bscess refers pain to the right shoulder: dermatomes C3–5!

ppendicitis in pregnancy

ppendicitis occurs in ~1/1000 pregnancies. It is not commoner, but nortality is higher, especially from 20wks gestation. Perforation is commoner 15–20%), and increases fetal mortality from ~1.5% (for simple appendicitis) to 30%. As pregnancy progresses, the appendix migrates, so pain is often less vell localized, and signs of peritonism less obvious. ►Prompt assessment is vital; aparotomy should be performed by an experienced surgeon (*OHCS* p38).

he Alvarado score—what does it add up to?

he diagnosis of appendicitis has always been a clinical challenge. In 1986, Alvarado published a scoring system that was designed to identify those with uspected appendicitis who needed an operation.[83] The principle was to ninimise the number of –ve operations without missing messy perforated lisease, which holds a much worse prognosis. The scoring system was:

Feature	Score	Feature	Score
Migration of pain	1	Rebound pain	1
Nausea/vomiting	1	Temperature >37.3°C	1
Anorexia	1	WCC $>10\times10^9$/L	2
RIF tenderness	2	Neutrophil count ≥75%	1
Total score: if ≤4 = diagnosis unlikely; 5–6 = observe; ≥7 = operation required.			

However, the score alone has proven inadequate for diagnosis on account of poor sensitivity.[84] One study combined the scoring system with US imaging to see f this improved diagnostic yield, but the results showed that, apart from reduced time to operation, it was no better than independent clinical judgement.[RCT 85]

So where does that leave us? The scoring system clearly incorporates mportant features of appendicitis, but its application remains hindered by variable group demographics (eg it is more accurate in children and men) and the lack of an appropriate balance between specificity and sensitivity for a threshold score.[86] The ambiguity is in where to draw this line, but at least knowing the score may help—and forces us to get a full-data set of variables.

Acute pancreatitis

Causes 'GET SMASHE
Gallstones(38%)
Ethanol(35%)
Trauma(1.5%)
Steroids
Mumps
Autoimmune (PAN)
Scorpion venom
Hyperlipidaemia, hypothermia, ↑Ca^{2+}
ERCP(5%) and emboli
Drugs
also pregnancy or no cause found(10-

This unpredictable disease (mortality ~12%) is managed on the surgical wards, but because surgery is often not involved, it is easy to think that there is no acute problem: **there is**—due to self-perpetuating pancreatic inflammation (and of other retroperitoneal tissues). Litres of extracellular fluid are trapped in the gut, peritoneum, and retroperitoneum. There may be rapid progression from a phase of mild oedema to necrotizing pancreatitis. In fulminating cases, the pancreas is replaced by black fluid. Contributory factors to demise include protease-induced activation of complement, kinin, and the fibrinolytic and coagulation cascades. Evidence is accumulating that oxidant stress is important, and congenital abnormality (eg *pancreas divisum* an annular pancreas) is known to predispose to pancreatitis.

Symptoms Gradual or sudden severe **epigastric** or **central abdominal** p (radiating to the back); vomiting is prominent. Sitting forward may relieve pa

Signs may be mild in serious disease! Tachycardia, fever, jaundice, shock, ileus, r abdomen ± local/generalized tenderness and periumbilical discolouration (Cull sign) or in the flanks (Grey Turner's sign).

Tests Raised serum ***amylase*** (>1000U/mL); cholecystitis, mesenteric infarct and GI perforation can cause lesser rises (usually). It is excreted renally so re failure will ↑ levels. ►**Amylase may be normal even in severe pancreatitis** (le starts to fall within the 1st 24–48h). Serum ***lipase*** is more sensitive and specific pancreatitis, and may eventually replace amylase measurement. ***ABG*** to mon oxygenation and acid-base status. ***AXR:*** No psoas shadow (retroperitoneal fluid 'sentinel loop' of proximal jejunum (solitary air-filled dilatation). ***Erect CXR*** he exclude other causes (eg perforation). ***CT*** to assess severity—***MRI*** may be e better. ***US*** (if gallstones + AST↑). ***ERCP*** if LFT worsen (may mean duct obstructi

Management Get expert help. Nil by mouth and likely to need an NGT (p747).

1 Set up IVI and **give lots of 0.9% saline**, to counter third space sequestration, u vital signs are satisfactory and urine flows stays at >30mL/h. Insert a urin catheter and consider CVP monitoring. Think about nutrition early on (p572).
2 Analgesia: ***pethidine*** 75–100mg/4h IM, or ***morphine*** (may cause Oddi's sphinc to contract more, but it is a better analgesic and not contraindicated).
3 Hourly pulse, BP, and urine output; daily FBC, U&E, Ca^{2+}, glucose, amylase, AB
4 If worsening, take to ITU. O_2 if P_aO_2↓. In suspected abscess formation pancreatic necrosis (on contrast-enhanced CT), consider parenteral nutritio laparotomy & debridement. Antibiotics may help in specific severe disease.
5 ERCP + gallstone removal may be needed if there is progressive jaundice.
6 Repeat imaging (usually CT) is performed in order to monitor progress.

ΔΔ: Any acute abdomen (p580), myocardial infarct. **Prognosis** See BOX.

Early complications: Shock, ARDS (p170), renal failure (►**give lots of fluid!**), [sepsis, Ca^{2+}↓, (10mL of 10% ***calcium gluconate*** IV slowly is, rarely, need ***albumin*** replacement has also been tried), glucose↑ (transient; 5% need insul

Late complications (>1wk) ***Pancreatic necrosis*** & ***pseudocyst*** (fluid in lesser s fig 1), with T°↑, a mass ± persistent ↑amylase/LFT; it may resolve or need draina externally, or into stomach (eg laparoscopically). ***Abscesses*** need draining. ***Bleedi*** from elastase eroding a major vessel (eg splenic artery); embolization may be li saving. ***Thrombosis*** may occur in the splenic/gastroduodenal arteries, or in t colic branches of the superior mesenteric artery, causing bowel necrosis. ***Fistu*** normally close spontaneously. If purely pancreatic they do not irritate the sk Some patients suffer ***recurrent oedematous pancreatitis*** so often that near-to pancreatectomy is contemplated. ►It can all be a miserable course.

odified Glasgow criteria for predicting severity of pancreatitis

3 or more positive factors detected within 48h of onset suggest severe ncreatitis, and should prompt transfer to ITU/HDU. Mnemonic: **PANCREAS.** 95

P_aO_2	<8kPa
Age	>55yrs
Neutrophils:	WBC >15 x 10^9/L
Calcium	<2mmol/L
Renal function:	Urea >16mmol/L
Enzymes	LDH >600iu/L; AST >200iu/L
Albumin	<32g/L (serum)
Sugar	blood glucose >10mmol/L

ese criteria have been validated for pancreatitis caused by gallstones and cohol; Ranson's criteria are valid for alcohol-induced pancreatitis, and can only fully applied after 48h, which does have its disadvantages.

her methods of severity assessment: Severity can be assessed with the help CT.[1] CRP can also be a helpful marker. 96

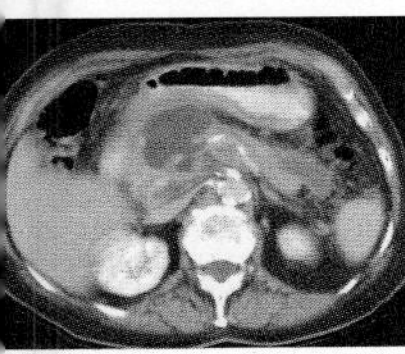

Fig 1. Axial CT of the abdomen (with IV and PO contrast media) showing a pancreatic pseudocyst occupying the lesser sac of the abdomen posterior the stomach. It is called a 'pseudocyst' because it is not a true cyst, rather a collection of fluid in the lesser sac. It develops at ≥6wks. The cyst fluid is of low attenuation compared to the stomach contents because it has not been enhanced by the contrast media.

[1] For a useful exposition on imaging in pancreatitis see www.emedicine.com/radio/topic521.htm

Aneurysms and dissections of arteries

The definition of an arterial aneurysm is dilatation to >150% of the ori diameter; remember that this is an ongoing process. ***True*** aneurysms are abno dilatations of arteries. ***False*** aneurysms (pseudoaneurysms) are collections of b around a vessel wall (eg after trauma) that communicate with the vessel lu Aneurysms may be fusiform or sac-like (eg circle of Willis Berry aneurysms; p fig 2) and on palpation (be gentle!) they are **expansile** (it expands and contr swellings that are pulsatile just transmit the pulse, eg nodes overlying arteri

Common sites Aorta, iliac, femoral & popliteal arteries. Pathophysiology: see

Complications Rupture; thrombosis; embolism; pressure on other structures

Ruptured abdominal aortic aneurysm (AAA) Death rates/year from rupt AAAs rise with age: 125/million in those aged 55–59; 2728/million if over 8

Symptoms & signs: Intermittent or continuous abdominal pain (radiates to b iliac fossae, or groins→don't dismiss this as renal colic), collapse, an **expa** abdominal mass, and shock. If in doubt, assume a ruptured aneurysm.

Management: ▸▸Summon a vascular surgeon and an experienced anaesthe Warn theatre. Put up 2 large IVIs. Treat shock with ORh−ve blood (if desper but keep systolic BP ≤100mmHg (but note: **raised** BP is common early on). D ECG, and take blood for amylase, Hb, crossmatch (10–40U may eventuall needed). Take the patient straight to theatre. Do not waste time doing x-rays: delay may result, though CT can be helpful in a stable patient with an uncer diagnosis. Catheterize the bladder. Give prophylactic antibiotics eg ***cefurox*** 1.5g + ***metronidazole*** 500mg IV. Surgery involves clamping the aorta above leak, and inserting a Dacron® graft (eg 'tube graft' or, if significant iliac aneur also, a 'trouser graft' with each 'leg' attached to an iliac artery). Mortali treated: 41% and improving; untreated: 100%.[MET 97]

Unruptured AAA Prevalence: 3% of those >50yrs. Often symptomless, they cause abdominal/back pain, and **may** be discovered incidentally on abdom examination (see BOX). The UK Small Aneurysm Trial suggested that aneury <5.5cm across might safely be monitored by regular examination ultrasound/CT,[RCT 98] though endovascular repair for these may be better surveillance.[99] Risk of rupture below this size is <1%/yr, compared with ~25% for aneurysms >6cm across. Aneurysms larger than this, rapidly expan (>1cm/yr) or symptomatic should be considered for elective surgery. It shoul noted that ~75% of aneurysms monitored in this way will eventually need re Elective operative mortality is ~5% and complications include spinal or mesen ischaemia and distal trash from dislodged thrombus debris.[100] Studies show age >80yrs is **not** a reason to decline surgery. ***Stenting*** Big operations sometimes be avoided by inserting an endovascular stent via the femoral ar When successfully positioned, such stents can lead to a shorter hospital stay fewer transfusions than with conventional surgery, but see fig 1 and its footr

Thoracic aortic dissection Blood splits the aortic media with sudden tea chest pain (± radiation to back). As the dissection unfolds, branches of the a occlude sequentially leading to hemiplegia (carotid artery), unequal arm pulses BP or acute limb ischaemia, paraplegia (anterior spinal artery), and anuria (r arteries). Aortic incompetence and inferior MI may develop if dissection mo proximally. ***Type A*** dissections involve the ascending aorta, irrespective of site of tear, whilst if the ascending aorta is not involved it is called ***type B***. ▸▸**All patie with type A thoracic dissection should be considered for surgery: get urg cardiothoracic advice.** ***Management:*** • Crossmatch 10U blood; ECG & CXR (expar mediastinum is rare). • CT/MRI or transoesophageal echocardiography (TOE).[101] to ITU; hypotensives: keep systolic at ~100–110mmHg: ***labetalol*** (p126) or ***esm*** (p112; $t_{½}$ is ultra-short) by IVI is helpful here. Acute operative mortality: <25

ː pathophysiology of aneurysmal disease

ᵢtheromatous degeneration is the main contrib-ʳ to the formation of true arterial aneurysms. er risk factors include connective tissue ɔrders (eg Marfan's, Ehlers–Danlos), and ːction (mycotic aneurysms, eg SBE/IE; tertiary hilis). For AAAs, degenerative processes leading ːystic medial necrosis include:

ımmune responses
iomechanical wall stress
hifts in the balance of remodelling causing proteo-ʏtic degradation of aortic wall connective tissue, g from ↑matrix metalloprotease activity
nflammation: increased lymphocyte and macro-hage infiltration
Molecular genetics: eg extracellular matrix rotein degradation.

Remember the cardio-vascular risk factors:

- Smoking
- Family history
- Diabetes mellitus
- Hypertension
- Hyperlipidaemia

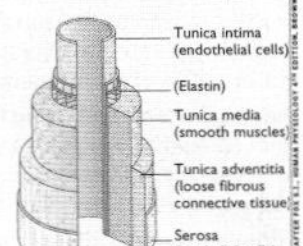

ɔulation screening for AAAs

umber of studies have looked at the screening of asymptomatic patients in risk' groups for AAAs. A multi-centre study showed that ultrasound screening 65–74yr old men decreases mortality related to AAAs. Cost per life-year ned was £28,400 after 4yrs, and is expected to drop to a quarter of this ıre after 10yrs. [102] A Danish study in 64–73yrs old men showed that the nber needed to screen with ultrasound to save one life was 352. [RCT 103]

Ɔne aspect of screening for AAA that is easily overlooked is the ~5% elective ːrative mortality. This makes informed consent (the Rees' rules, *OHCS* p486), a ᵛ issue in developing ultrasound-based screening of 'healthy' people.

Ɔther than screening, AAAs are picked up in a number of ways:

Symptomatic with abdominal pain
ncidentally on physical examination (though may miss ⅓ of AAAs)
ncidentally on radiological examination (especially ultrasound)
An abdominal mass noticed by the patient
Symptomatic distal shedding of mural thrombus
Rupture: see OPPOSITE.

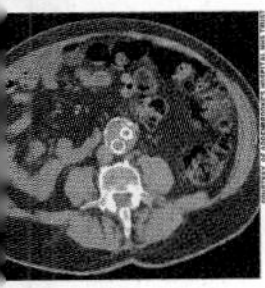

Fig 1. Axial CT of the abdomen showing position of an endovascular stent in the aorta, anterior to the vertebral column. The 'trousers' of the stent are seen within the calcified wall of the aorta. Although less invasive, many are unsuited to this method, owing to the anatomy of their aneurysms. Lifelong monitoring is needed: stents may leak and the aneurysm progress. [104] Safety and efficacy of endovascular stenting may not be better than open repair.[1]

ɑrly detection and surveillance of AAAs do not increase suitability for endovascular repair; this ːars to be determined early in an aneurysm's life (well below the 5.5cm diameter currently ɪpting referral from AAA surveillance programs). Hafez H 2006 *J Vasc Surg* 43 265.

Diverticular disease

A GI **diverticulum** is an outpouching of the gut wall. **Diverticulosis** means diverticula are present, and **diverticular disease** implies they are symptom **Diverticulitis** refers to inflammation of a diverticulum. Although diverticula ma congenital or acquired and can occur in any part of the gut, by far the r important type are acquired colonic diverticula, to which this page refers.

Pathology Most occur in the sigmoid colon with 95% of complications at this but right-sided and massive single diverticula can occur. Lack of dietary fib thought to lead to high intraluminal pressures which force the mucosa to herr through the muscle layers of the gut at weak points adjacent to penetra vessels. 30% of Westerners have diverticulosis by 60 years of age.

Diagnosis ***PR examination*** (may reveal a pelvic abscess, or colorectal cancer, chief competing diagnosis); ***sigmoidoscopy***; ***barium enema***; ***colonoscopy*** (fi p249); *CT* may be more useful than ***ultrasound***, and ***plain films*** may only be us in showing vesical fistulae (air in the bladder).

Complications of diverticulosis There may be altered bowel habit ± left-si colic relieved by defecation; nausea and flatulence. A high-fibre diet (wholen bread, fruit and vegetables) may be tried. Antispasmodics, eg ***mebeve*** 135mg/8h PO may help. Surgical resection is occasionally resorted to. Others

1 ***Diverticulitis***—with features above + pyrexia, WCC↑, CRP/ESR↑, a tender colo localized or generalized peritonism. Treatment: analgesia, NBM, IV fluids, antibiotics: see BOX. ►Beware diverticulitis in immunocompromised patients on steroids) who often have few symptoms, and may present late.
2 ►►***Perforation*** There is ileus, peritonitis ± shock. Mortality: 40%. Manage as an acute abdomen. At laparotomy a Hartman's procedure may be perforr (temporary colostomy + partial colectomy). It is possible to do colonic lavage the appendix stump, then immediate primary anastomosis (so avoiding rep surgery to close the colostomy). Neither is yet proven to be better.[105]
3 ***Haemorrhage*** is usually sudden and painless. It is a common cause of big re bleeds. ►See BOX. Bleeding usually stops with bed rest. Transfusion may needed. Embolization or colonic resection may be necessary after locat bleeding points by angiography or colonoscopy (here diathermy ± lc ***adrenaline*** injections may obviate the need for surgery).
4 ***Fistulae*** Enterocolic, colovaginal, or colovesical (pneumaturia ± intractible U Treatment is surgical, eg colonic resection.
5 ***Abscesses*** eg with swinging fever, leucocytosis, and localizing signs eg bo rectal mass (pelvic abscess—drain rectally). If no localizing signs, remember aphorism: *pus somewhere, pus nowhere = pus under the diaphragm.* subphrenic abscess is a horrible way to die, so do an urgent ultrasou Antibiotics ± ultrasound-guided drainage may be needed.
6 ***Post-infective strictures*** may form in the sigmoid colon.

Surgery

Angiodysplasia

Angiodysplasia refers to submucosal arteriovenous malformations that typic present as fresh PR bleeding in the elderly. The underlying cause is unknov ***Pathology:*** 70–90% of lesions occur in the right colon, though angiodysplasia affect anywhere in the GI tract. ***Diagnosis:*** PR examination, barium ener colonoscopy (fig 4, p248) may exclude competing diagnoses; ^{99m}Tc radionucl labelled red cell imaging (p725) is useful for identifying lesions during act bleeding (if >0.1mL/min). Mesenteric angiography is very helpful in diagnos angiodysplasia (shows early filling at the site of the lesion, then extravasation), a allows therapeutic embolization during active bleeding—it detects bleed >1mL/min. CT angiography offers a non-invasive alternative. ***Treatment optio*** Embolization, endoscopic laser electrocoagulation, resection.

anaging diverticulitis[106]

itial management

Mild attacks can be treated at home with bowel rest (fluids only) + *co-amoxiclav* (p368, or *metronidazole* 400mg/8h PO, or *ciprofloxacin*).

If oral fluids cannot be tolerated or pain cannot be controlled, admit to hospital for analgesia, NBM, IV fluids and antibiotics eg *cefuroxime* 1.5g/8h IV with *metronidazole* 500mg/8h IV/PR, until the results of cultures are available. Most settle on this regimen but there may be abscess formation (necessitating drainage) or perforation—see OPPOSITE for management.

naging: Ultrasound can detect perforation, free fluid, and collections, though with contrast is probably more accurate, especially in complicated disease. If contrast enema is performed, then water-soluble contrast should be used (see '34). ►In an acute attack colonoscopy should not be done.[107]

rgery: The need for surgery is reflected by the degree of infective complications:

tage 1	Small confined pericolonic abscesses	**Surgery rarely needed**
tage 2	Larger abscesses	**May resolve without surgery**
tage 3	Generalized suppurative peritonitis	**Surgery required**
tage 4	Faecal peritonitis	**Surgery required**

For severe or recurrent diverticulitis ~20% will require surgery.

Elective sigmoid resection after medical management as a 1-stage open procedure has been performed (also laparoscopically),[108] although interestingly no evidence currently exists to support elective surgery after ≥2 acute attacks of diverticulitis.[109]

For emergency colonic resection see OPPOSITE.

ctal bleeding—an acute management plan

e causes of rectal bleeding are covered elsewhere (MINIBOX). Here let's make an **acute management plan** for this common surgical event:

Typical causes

- Diverticulitis, p588
- Colorectal cancer, p612
- Haemorrhoids, p628
- Crohn's, UC, P264
- Perianal disease, p626
- Angiodysplasia, p588
- Rarities—trauma, also:
  - ischaemic colitis, p594
  - radiation proctitis
  - aorto-enteric fistula

ABC resuscitation, if necessary.

History and **examination**.

Blood tests: FBC, U&E, LFT, clotting, amylase (always thinking of pancreatitis), CRP, group & save serum—await Hb result before cross-matching unless unstable and bleeding.

Imaging May only need plain AXR, but if there are signs of perforation (eg sepsis, peritonism) or if there is cardiorespiratory co-morbidity, then request an erect CXR. See OPPOSITE for more imaging options (under **angiodysplasia**).

Fluid management Insert 2 cannulae (≥18G) into the ante-cubital fossae. Insert a urinary catheter if there is a suspicion of haemodynamic compromise—there is no absolute indication, but remember that you are weighing up the risks and benefits. Give crystalloid as replacement and maintenance IVI. Transfusion is rarely needed in the acute setting.

Antibiotics may occasionally be required if there is evidence of sepsis or perforation, eg *cefuroxime* 1.5g/8h IV + *metronidazole* 500mg/8h IV.

PPI Consider *omeprazole* 40mg/d IV—around 15% are UGI bleeds (p244).

Keep bed-bound The patient may feel the need to get out of bed to pass stool, but this could be another large bleed, resulting in collapse if they try to walk. ►Don't allow them to mobilise and inform the nursing staff of this.

Start a stool chart to monitor volume and frequency of motions. Send a sample for MC+S (3 if known to have compromising co-morbidity such as IBD).

Diet Keep on clear fluids so that they can have something, yet the colon will be clear for colonoscopy (which is of little value until bleeding has stopped).

Surgery The main indication for this is unremitting, massive bleeding.

Gallstones

Bile contains cholesterol, bile pigments (from broken down Hb), and phospho If the concentrations of these vary, different kinds of stones may be forr ***Pigment stones:*** Small, friable, and irregular. Causes: haemolysis. ***Choles stones:*** Large, often solitary. Causes: ♀, age, obesity. ***Mixed stones:*** Fa (calcium salts, pigment, and cholesterol). ***Gallstone prevalence:*** 8% of those 40yrs. 90% remain asymptomatic. Risk factors for stones becoming sympto smoking; parity. Stones may cause: acute or chronic cholecystitis, biliary pancreatitis (p584), or obstructive jaundice (p242).

Acute cholecystitis follows stone or sludge impaction in the neck of the bladder (GB), which may cause continuous epigastric or RUQ pain (referred t right shoulder—see p583), vomiting, fever, local peritonism, or a GB mass. The difference from biliary colic is the inflammatory component (local perito fever, WCC↑). If the stone moves to the common bile duct (CBD), obstru jaundice and cholangitis may occur—see BOX for complications. **Murphy's sign** 2 fingers over the RUQ. Ask the patient to breathe in. This causes pain and arre inspiration as an inflamed GB impinges on your fingers. It is only +ve if the test in the LUQ does not cause pain. ***Tests:*** WCC↑, ultrasound (a thick-w shrunken GB, pericholecystic fluid, stones, CBD—dilated if >6mm), HIDA choles igraphy (useful if diagnosis uncertain after US). Plain AXR only shows ~10 gallstones; it may identify a 'porcelain' GB. ***Treatment:*** NBM, pain relief, IVI antibiotics (eg ***cefuroxime*** 1.5g/8h IV). In suitable candidates, do cholecystec (laparoscopic if no question of GB perforation) within 72h; mortality: <1 delayed, relapse occurs in 18% and may be associated with more complicatio early surgery is generally recommended. Otherwise, operate after 6–12w elderly or high-risk/unsuitable for surgery, consider percutaneous cholecystost cholecystectomy can still be performed at a later date. Cholecystostomy is als preferred treatment for acalculous cholecystitis, though removal can be dor

Chronic cholecystitis Stones cause chronic inflammation ± colic. Vague abdo discomfort, distension, nausea, flatulence, and fat intolerance may also be ca by reflux, ulcers, irritable bowel syndrome, relapsing pancreatitis, or tur (stomach, pancreas, colon, GB). US is used to image stones and to assess diameter. MRCP (p729) is increasingly used to check for CBD stones. ℞: C cystectomy. If US shows a dilated CBD with stones, ERCP (p728) + sphinctero for stone removal, usually before surgery. No comparative trials favour lithotr

Biliary colic occurs when gallstones become symptomatic with cystic obstruction or by passing into the CBD—it is part of the spectrum of galls disease—giving RUQ pain (radiates → back) ± jaundice. ℞: Pain control: ***morp*** (see p584) ~5–10mg/4h IM + antiemetic. Elective cholecystectomy. **ΔΔ:** Ha the above may overlap. Urinalysis, CXR, and ECG help exclude other diseases.

Other presentations:

- ***Obstructive jaundice with CBD stones***—if LFT worsening, ERCP sphincterotomy ± biliary trawl, then cholecystectomy may be needed, or surgery with CBD exploration. If CBD stones are suspected pre-operatively, intraoperative fluoroscopic cholangiography can be done, though they can be successfully identified with pre-operative MRCP, p734.
- ***Cholangitis*** (bile duct infection) causing RUQ pain, jaundice, and rigors. T with eg ***cefuroxime*** 1.5g/8h IV and ***metronidazole*** 500mg/8h IV/PR.
- ***Gallstone ileus:*** A stone perforates the GB, entering the duodenum; it may obstruct the terminal ileum. X-ray: air in CBD (=pneumatobilia), small bowel levels, and a stone. Duodenal obstruction is rarer (Bouveret's syndrome).
- ***Pancreatitis*** (p584) • ***Empyema:*** The obstructed GB fills with pus.
- ***Silent stones:*** Some advise elective surgery. Dissolution of cholesterol stone oral ***ursodeoxycholic acid*** is expensive, and often causes diarrhoea.

nplications of gallstones

n the gall bladder:
- Biliary colic
- Acute and chronic cholecystitis
- Empyema
- Mucocoele
- Carcinoma

In the bile ducts:
- Obstructive jaundice
- Pancreatitis
- Cholangitis

In the gut:
- Gallstone ileus

eases having biliary complications

ıses of cholecystitis and biliary symptoms, other than gallstones, are rare, eg:
nfections:
- Typhoid
- Brucellosis
- Ascariasis
- Cryptosporidiosis, p380
- Opisthorchiasis

:omplications of parenteral nutrition
'olyarteritis nodosa (p543)
ormonal: release of cholecystokinin
tructural abnormality of the cystic duct
ligh pressure sphincter of Oddi.

e anatomy of the gallbladder and extrahepatic biliary tree

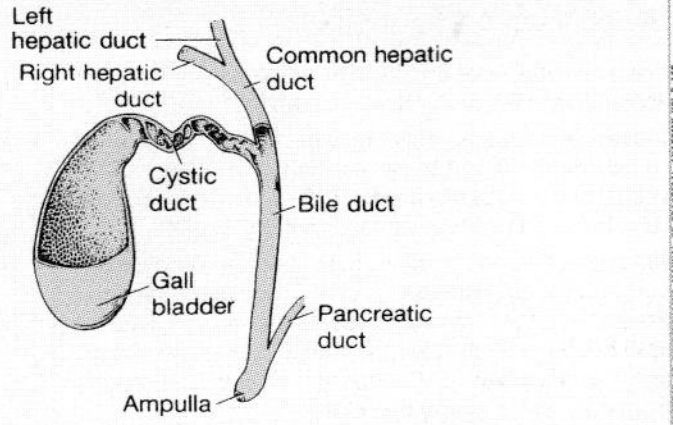

COURTESY OF CUNNINGHAM'S MANUAL OF PRACTICAL ANATOMY VOL 2 13E

it possible to perform double-blind RCTs in surgery?

2005 a double-blinded randomized controlled trial (RCT) looked at the ferences between open and laparoscopic cholecystectomy.[RCT 116] This raises ues on both the place and validity of double-blinded RCTs in surgery.

Overcoming established treatments always has difficulties, as when faced :h either surgery or a non-operative management, everyone's preference uld be to avoid surgery (with the complications of pain, scarring, etc.), becially if there is equipoise about which treatment is superior. Operations are o technically complex, and the skill required to perform them well has to be rned. The negative influence of the learning curve for a new treatment must considered and this may take time to overcome (p641). Furthermore, ntrolling the bias introduced by interperformer and patient variance is oossible (both in the trial and the 'real world'), not least because each patient different. There are also inherent difficulties in double-blinding surgical atment, though the imaginative extents to which researchers will go are nirable. 'Sham' surgery remains an contentious issue.[117]

Incidentally, the trial showed that laparoscopic patients were discharged oner, albeit on the same 2nd day of the stay, with no other major differences.

Gangrene and necrotizing fasciitis

Definitions Gangrene is death of tissue from poor vascular supply and is a sig critical ischaemia (see p596). Tissues are black and may slough. ***Wet gangre*** tissue death and infection occurring together (p707, fig 1). ***Dry gangrene*** m no infection. ***Pregangrene*** is a term used to describe tissue that is on the brir gangrene. Note a line of demarcation between living and dead tissue.[1]

Management Take cultures; look out for group A β-haemolytic streptococc cause of Fournier's (male genitalia) or Meleney's gangrene (post-opera ulceration), both a form of rapidly progressive necrotizing fasciitis or myos Other pathogens can be involved, eg *S. aureus*. **►In any atypical cellulitis, prompt surgical help.** Radical debridement (eg preserving a skin flap amputation is needed, always covered by antibiotics, including eg 5 day ***benzylpenicillin*** 600mg/6h IV starting 1h pre-op, to prevent gas gangren ***clindamycin*** 0.6–1.2g/6h IV/IM). Get the help of a plastic surgeon. Rememb consider mycobacteria in any necrotizing infection.[118]

Gas gangrene is a *Clostridium perfringens* myositis. Risk factors: diabetes; trau malignancy. Toxaemia, delirium, and haemolytic jaundice occur early. Ther oedema, crepitus from surgical emphysema and bubbly brown pus. Treatm Remove all dead tissue (eg amputation); ***benzylpenicillin***; ***hyperbaric*** ***clindamycin*** & ***metronidazole*** have a role.[119]

Surgery

Skin ulcers

see also OHCS, p

Causes
• Venous disease
• Arterial disease
· Large vessel
· Small vessel
• Neuropathy
• Diabetes
· Neuropathic, arterial or both
• Lymphoedema
• Vasculitis
• Malignancy (p54
• Infection
· TB, syphilis
• Trauma (pressure
• Pyoderma gangrenosum
• Drugs

Ulcers are abnormal breaks in an epithelial surface. Leg ulcers affect ~2% in developed countries.

Causes: see MINIBOX—there may be multiple causes. For leg ulcers, venous disease accounts for 70%, mixed arterial and venous disease for 15% and arterial disease alone for 2%. For pressure sores, see fig 1, p465.

History Ask about number, pain, trauma. Go over co-morbidities—eg varicose veins, peripheral arterial disease, diabetes, vasculitis etc. Is the history long or short? Is the patient taking steroids? Is the patient a bit odd? (remember self-induced ulcers: *dermatitis artefacta*). Has a biopsy been taken?

Examination Note features such as site, number, surface area, depth, edge, base, discharge, lymphadenopathy, sensation, and healing. See BOX. If in the legs, note features of venous insufficiency or arterial disease and if possible, apply a BP cuff to perform ankle—brachial pressure index (ABPI).

Tests Skin and ulcer biopsy may be necessary—eg to assess for vasculitis (need immunohistopathology) or malignant change in an established ul (Marjolin's ulcer). If ulceration is the first presentation of a suspected syste disorder then further screening tests will be required accordingly.

Management Managing ulcers is often difficult and expensive. Treat the caus and focus on prevention. Optimize nutrition. Are there adverse risk factors (d addiction, or risk factors for arteriopathy, eg smoking etc)? Get expert nurs care. Consider referral to community nurse, varicose leg ulcer clinic: 'Charing-cr 4-layer compression bandaging may help (only if arterial pulses OK: ABPI shoulc > 0.8) and is better than standard bandages. Treating ulcers with syste antibiotics rarely helps, though topical agents such as ***silver sulfadiazine*** ***gentamicin*** may be effective.[120]

1 'The first sign of his approaching end was when one of my old aunts, while undressing removed a toe with one of his old socks'. Graham Greene, *A Sort of Life*, 1971, Simon & Schus

atures of skin ulceration to note on examination

te Above the medial malleolus is the favourite place for ***gravitational ulcers*** nostly related to superficial venous disease, but may reflect venous pertension via damage to the valves of the deep venous system, eg 2° to DVT). enous hypertension leads to the development of superficial varicosities and in changes (***lipodermatosclerosis*** = induration, pigmentation, and flammation of the skin). Minimal trauma to the leg leads to ulceration which ten takes many months to heal. Ulcers on the sacrum or greater trochanter, or eel suggest ***pressure sores*** (*OHCS* p605), particularly if the patient is bed-bound ith suboptimal nutrition.

emperature The ulcer and surrounding tissues are cold in an ischaemic ulcer. If e skin is warm and well perfused then local factors are more likely.

urface area Draw a map of the area to quantify and time any healing (a ound >4weeks old is a chronic ulcer as distinguished from an acute wound).

hape Oval, circular (cigarette burns), serpiginous (*granuloma inguinale*, p404); nusual morphology can be secondary to myocbacterial infection, eg cutaneous berculosis or scrofuloderma (*tuberculosis colliquativa cutis*, where an infected mph node ulcerates through to the skin).

dge Eroded ≈ active and spreading; shelved/sloping ≈ healing; punched-ut ≈ syphilis or ischaemic; rolled/everted ≈ malignant; undermined ≈ TB.

ase Any muscle, bone, or tendon destruction (malignancy; pressure sores; chaemia)? There may be a grey-yellow slough, beneath which is a pale pink ase. **Slough** is a mixture of fibrin, cell breakdown products, serous exudate, ucocytes and bacteria—it need not imply infection, and can be part of the ormal wound healing process. **Granulation tissue** is a deep pink gel-like matrix ontained within a fibrous collagen network and is evidence of a healing wound.

epth If not uncomfortable for the patient (eg in neuropathic ulceration) a robe can be used gauge how deep the ulceration extends.

ischarge Culture before starting any antibiotics (which usually don't work). A atery discharge is said to favour TB; bleeding can ≈ malignancy.

ssociated lymphadenopathy suggests infection or malignancy.

ensation Decreased sensation around the ulcer implies neuropathy.

osition in phases of extension/healing Healing is heralded by granulation, car formation, and epithelialization. Inflamed margins ≈ extension.

Mesenteric ischaemia

►AF with abdominal pain should always prompt thoughts of mesenteric ischaem

Acute mesenteric ischaemia[122] almost always involves the small bowel and may follow superior mesenteric artery (SMA) thrombosis or embolism, mesenteric vein thrombosis, or non-occlusive disease (see MINIBOX). Arterial thrombosis is becoming the commonest cause of acute ischaemia as embolism becomes rarer. Venous thrombosis is more common in younger patients with hypercoagulable states and tends to affect smaller lengths of bowel. Non-occlusive ischaemia occurs in low flow states and usually reflects poor cardiac output, though there may be other factors such as recent cardiac surgery or renal failure.[123] Presentation is **a classical clinical triad:** ►Acute severe abdominal pain; no abdominal signs; rapid hypovolaemia → shock. Pain tends to be constant and central, or around the right iliac fossa. The degree of illness is often far out of proportion with clinical signs.

Acute ischaemia
- Arterial
  - Thrombotic (35%)
  - Embolic (35%)
- Non-occlusive (20%)
- Venous (5%)
- Other
  - Trauma
  - Vasculitis (p542)
  - Radiotherapy
  - Strangulation eg volvulus or hernia

Chronic ischaemia
- Usually a combination of a low flow state with atherosclerosis. Classified as either small or large bowel.

- ***Tests:*** There may be Hb↑ (due to plasma loss), WCC↑, modestly raised plasm amylase, and a persistent metabolic acidosis. Early on the abdominal x-ray shov a 'gasless' abdomen. Arteriography (fig 1) helps but many diagnoses are made laparotomy with the finding of nasty necrotic bowel on opening up. CT/M angiography may provide a non-invasive alternative to simple arteriography.
- ***Treatment:*** The main life-threatening complications secondary to acu mesenteric ischaemia are **1** septic peritonitis and **2** progression of a system inflammatory response syndrome (SIRS) into a multi-organ dysfunction syndron (MODS), that is mediated by bacterial translocation across the dying gut wa Resuscitation with fluid replacement, antibiotics (***gentamicin*** + ***metronidazo*** p371) and, usually, ***heparin*** are required. If arteriography is performe thrombolytics may be infused locally via the catheter. At surgery dead bowel mu be removed. Revascularization may be attempted on potentially viable bowel but is a difficult process and often needs a second laparotomy.
- ***Prognosis:*** Poor for arterial thrombosis and non-occlusive disease (<40 survive), though not so bad for venous and embolic ischaemia.[125]

Chronic small bowel ischaemia This presents quite a different picture to acu ischaemia, with severe, colicky post-prandial abdominal pain ('gut claudicatior with PR bleeding ± ↓weight (food hurts) and malabsorption. It is difficult diagnose but, following angiography, surgery may be helpful. Angioplasty is a appropriate treatment if the bowel is viable.

Chronic colonic ischaemia This usually follows low flow in the inferior mesenter artery (IMA) territory. ***Presentation:*** Lower left-sided abdominal pain and blooc diarrhoea. There may be pyrexia, tachycardia, PR bleeding, and a leucocytosi Usually this 'ischaemic colitis' resolves, but it may progress to gangrenou ischaemic colitis with the development of peritonitis and hypovolaemic shoc ***Tests:*** Barium enema may show 'thumb-printing' indentation of the barium due t submucosal swelling. MR angiography is being used increasingly.[126] ***Treatment:*** Th is usually conservative with fluid replacement and antibiotics. Most recover bu strictures are common. Percutaneous transluminal angioplasty and endovascul stent insertion are alternatives to revascularization surgery that show good resul with lower mortality.[127] Gangrenous ischaemic colitis requires prompt resuscitatic followed by resection of the affected bowel and stoma formation.

The arterial supply to the colon

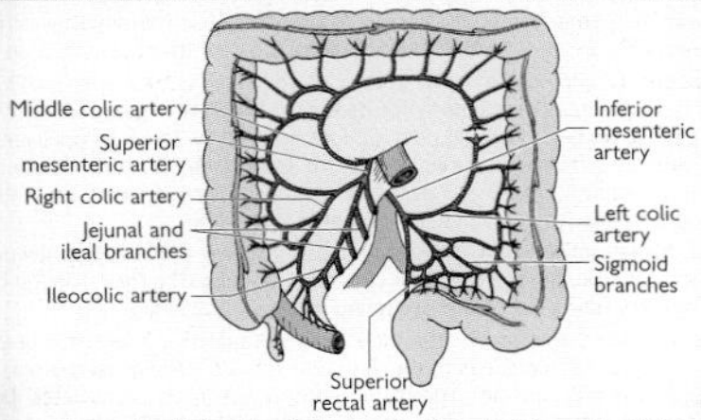

There are two **potential watershed areas** in the arterial supply of the colon. The first is at the splenic flexure where the SMA and the IMA circulations meet as the 'Marginal artery of Drummond'—it has also been called Griffith's point. The significance of good blood flow at this point to ensure adequate colonic supply after surgical ligation of the IMA has long been a point of debate. [128] The 2nd contentious watershed area is at the origin of the superior rectal artery—also known as Sudeck's point (fig 1). When ligated, flow to the rectum is maintained by the sigmoidal branches that arise from the left colic artery. [129] Remember that the arterial supply to the gut does have a large number of anatomical variations.

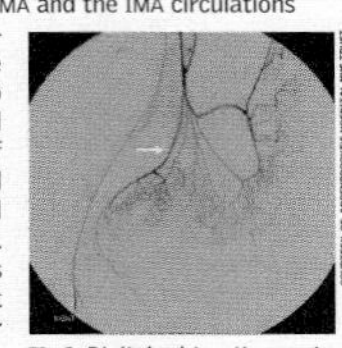

Fig 1. Digital subtraction angiogram (DSA) of the IMA and the superior rectal artery (arrow).

Volvulus of the stomach

If the stomach twists, the classical triad of gastro-oesophageal obstruction may occur: vomiting (then non-productive retching), pain, and failed attempts to pass an NG tube. Regurgitation of saliva also occurs. Dysphagia and noisy gastric peristalsis (relieved by lying down) may occur in chronic volvulus.

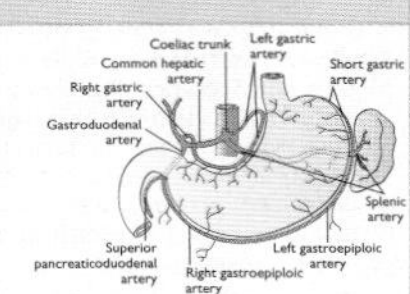

Risk factors ***Congenital:*** Paraoesophageal hernia; congenital bands; bowel malformations; pyloric stenosis. ***Acquired:*** Gastric/oesophageal surgery.

Tests Look for gastric dilatation and a double fluid level on erect films.

Treatment If acutely unwell (obstruction, peritonism, necrosis) arrange prompt resuscitation and laparotomy. In organoaxial volvulus, rotation is typically 180° left to right, about a line joining the relatively fixed pylorus and oesophagus. Mesenteroaxial rotation is at right angles to this line (and is from right to left). Laparoscopic management may be possible. [130]

Chronic ischaemia This is 'always' due to atherosclerosis (fibromuscular dyspla and vasculitis are very rare). Its chief feature is intermittent claudication.

Symptoms Cramping pain is felt in the calf, thigh, or buttock after walking fo fairly fixed distance (the **claudication distance**). **Ulceration**, **gangrene** (p592), a foot pain **at rest**—eg burning pain at night relieved by hanging legs over side bed—are the cardinal features of ***critical ischaemia***. Buttock claudication impotence imply Leriche's syndrome (p696). Young, heavy smokers are at risk fr Buerger's disease (thromboangiitis obliterans, p688).[131]

Signs: Absent pulses; cold, white leg(s); atrophic skin; punched out ulcers (of painful); postural/dependent colour change; a vascular (Buerger's) angle[1] of <2 and capillary **filling** time >15s are found in severe ischaemia.

Tests: Exclude DM, arteritis (ESR/CRP). Do FBC (anaemia, infection); U&E (re disease); lipids (dyslipidaemia); syphilis serology; ECG (cardiac ischaemia). Ch platelets, clotting and U&E (problems with IV contrast exacerbated by re disease) and do group & save if planning arteriography. ***Ankle–brachial press index (ABPI):*** Normal ≥ 1. Claudication ≈ 0.9–0.6. Rest pain ≈ 0.3–0.6. Impend gangrene ≤0.3 or ankle systolic pressure <50mmHg. Beware falsely h measurements from the incompressible vessels found in severe atherosclerosis, and chronic renal failure. Do ***contrast arteriography***, ***digital subtracti arteriography*** (**DSA**, fig 2**)** or ***colour duplex imaging*** to assess the extent a location of stenoses and the quality of distal vessels (*'run off'*). Remember to s ***metformin*** before angiography to avoid metabolic acidosis. ***MR angiography*** ha developing role (p721).[132] If only distal obliterative disease is seen, and lit proximal atheroma, suspect arteritis, previous embolus, or DM.

Management More conservative measures are undervalued—ie quit smoki ↓weight, exercise programmes.[RCT 133] ~ ⅓ of claudicants improve with exercise, remain the same, and ⅓ deteriorate. Results may be better with a supervis exercise programme.[RCT 134] The mainstay of treatment is energetic risk factor r uction: encourage cessation of smoking, and treat diabetes, hypertension (avoid blockers) and dyslipidaemia. Antiplatelet agents have a role (usually ***aspirin***).

Percutaneous transluminal angioplasty is good for short stenoses in big arter (a balloon is inflated in the narrowed segment). Stents maintain artery pater after angioplasty, and are beneficial for iliac artery disease.

Surgical reconstruction If atheromatous disease is extensive but distal run of good (ie distal arteries filled by collateral vessels), he may be a candidate arterial reconstruction by a bypass graft. Procedures include above knee femor popliteal bypass, femoral–femoral crossover and aorto–bifemoral bypass graf Vein grafts are often used but prosthetic grafts (eg polytetrafluoroethylene, PT are an option.[135] ***Aspirin*** helps prosthetic grafts to remain patent; ***warfarin*** may better after vein grafts and in high-risk patients.[RCT 136]

Sympathectomy (chemical or surgical) may help relieve rest pain if revascul ization is impossible. It may not be wise in diabetic patients with neuropathy.

Amputation may relieve intractable pain and death from sepsis and gangrene. T decision to amputate must be made by the patient, usually against a background failed alternative strategies. The level of amputation must be high enough ensure healing of the stump. Above knee amputation (AKA) tends to heal better, b has worse rehabilitation potential, whereas the reverse is true of below kn amputation (BKA). Having to perform the above knee procedure can also be herald of a much poorer overall prognosis—the 5 year survival for AKA in c retrospective study was 22.5% compared to 37.8% for BKA.[137] Rehabilitati should be started early with a view to limb fitting. ***Gabapentin*** (regimen on p49 can be used to treat the gruelling post-operative complication of phantom lir pain.[RCT 138] It may be more effective if started prior to surgery.

1 Leg goes pale when raised eg by 20° off the couch; compare sides

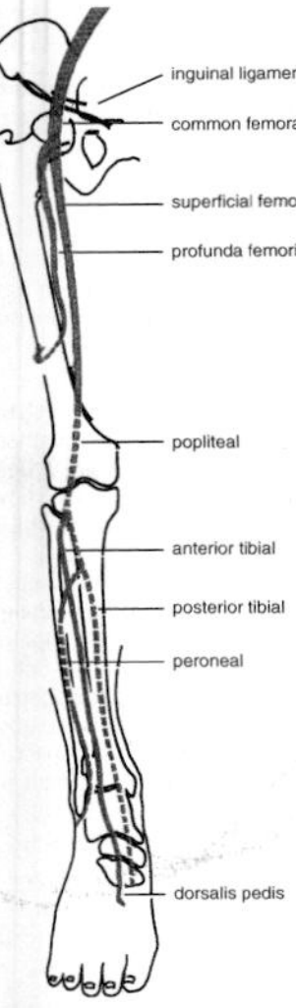

1. The arterial supply to the leg.

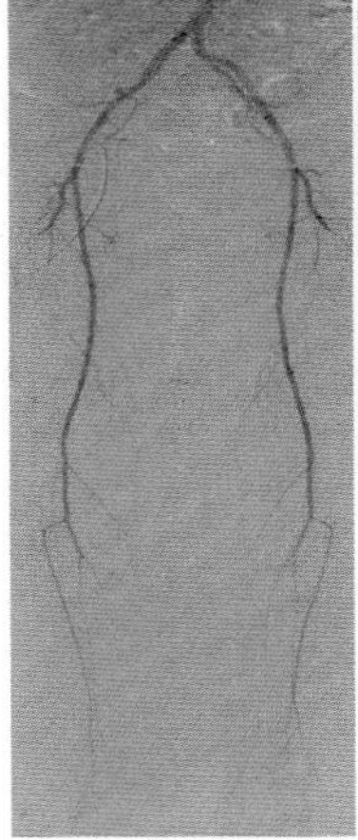

Fig 2. Digital subtraction angiogram (DSA) of the legs showing bilateral occlusive disease in the posterior tibial arteries. This patient had gangrene in his toes.

cute limb ischaemia

cute ischaemia This may be due to thrombosis *in situ* (~40%), emboli (38%), raft/angioplasty occlusion (15%), or trauma. There is little difference in resenting signs. Mortality: 22%. Amputation rate: 16%.

ymptoms & signs: 6 Ps—the part is pale, pulseless, painful, paralysed, araesthetic, and 'perishing with cold'. Onset of fixed mottling implies reversibility. Emboli commonly arise from the heart (infarcts, AF) or an neurysm (aorta, femoral, or popliteal). ►The limb may be red, but only when ependent, leading to disastrous misdiagnosis of gout or cellulitis.

lanagement: ►This is an emergency and may require urgent open surgery or ngioplasty. If diagnosis is in doubt, do urgent arteriography. If the occlusion is mbolic, the options are surgical embolectomy (Fogarty catheter) or local nrombolysis, eg ***tissue plasminogen activator*** (t-PA, p331), balancing the risks f surgery with the haemorrhagic complications of thrombolysis.[MET 139]

Anticoagulate with ***heparin*** after either procedure. Later, look for the emboli's ource: echocardiogram; ultrasound of aorta, popliteal and femoral arteries. schaemia following trauma and acute thrombosis may require urgent econstruction. ►Always be aware of the possibility of post-operative **eperfusion injury** and subsequent **compartment syndrome** (*OHCS*, p736).

Obstruction of the bowel

Cardinal features o intestinal obstructi
• Vomiting • Colic • Constipation • Distension

Features of obstruction Vomiting with relief, nausea and anorexia. Fermentation of the intestinal contents in established obstruction causes 'faeculent' vomiting ('faecal' vomiting is found when there is a colonic fistula with the proximal gut). **Colicky** abdominal pain is seen in early obstruction and may be absent in long-standing complete obstruction. **Constipation** need no absolute (ie no faeces or flatus passed) if obstruction is high, though in d obstruction nothing will be passed. Abdominal **distension** becomes more ma as the obstruction progresses. There are active, 'tinkling' bowel sounds.

The key decisions:

1 ***Is the obstruction of the small or large bowel?*** In small bowel obstruc vomiting occurs earlier, distension is less, and pain is higher in the abdomen. **AXR plays a key role in diagnosis**—see p716. In small bowel obstruction, shows central gas shadows and no gas in the large bowel. Small bow identified by *valvulae conniventes* that completely cross the lumen (large b haustral folds do **not** cross all the lumen's width).

In large bowel obstruction, pain is more constant; AXR shows gas proximal tc blockage (eg in caecum) but not in the rectum, unless you have done examination ►which is always essential! If the ileocaecal valve is competer doesn't allow reflux) pain may be felt over a distended caecum (see below

2 ***Is there an ileus or mechanical obstruction?*** In ileus (functional obstruc due to reduced bowel motility) there is no pain and bowel sounds are abse

3 ***Is the bowel strangulated?*** The patient is more ill than you would expect. T is a sharper and more constant pain than the central colicky pain of obstruction and it tends to be localized. Peritonism is the cardinal sign. T may be fever + WCC↑ along with other signs of mesenteric ischaemia (p59

Management

Typical causes
• Constipation (p240 • Hernias (p630) • Adhesions (p567) • Tumours (p612)
Rarer causes

• Crohn's disease
• Gallstone ileus (p59
• Intussusception (p6C
• Diverticular stricture
• TB (developing worl
• Volvulus
  · Gastric (p595)
  · Caecal
  · Sigmoid (see BOX)
• Foreign body

- ***General principles:*** The site, speed of onset, and completeness of obstruction determine definitive therapy: strangulation and large bowel obstruction require surgery soon, while ileus and incomplete small bowel obstruction can be managed conservatively, at least initially.
- ***Immediate action:*** ►'Drip and suck'—NGT and give IV fluids to rehydrate and correct electrolyte imbalance, see p656. Simply being nil by mouth does not give adequate rest for the bowel because the intestine can produce up to 9L of fluid/d.
- ***Further imaging:*** There is a case for investigating the cause by colonoscopy in some instances of suspected mechanical obstruction, though there is a danger of inducing perforation. A water-soluble contrast (eg Gastrografin®) follow-through study may be helpful in determi the level of obstruction—it also has some therapeutic action against mechanical obstruction. CT may show dilated, fluid-filled bowel and a transi zone at the site of obstruction (figs 1 & 2).
- ***Surgery:*** ►Strangulation requires emergency surgery, as does 'closed l obstruction'—large bowel obstruction with tenderness over a grossly dila caecum (>12cm requires urgent decompression), which occurs when ileocaecal valve remains competent despite bowel distension. For less urg large bowel obstruction, there is time for a water-soluble enema to try to c the obstruction and to correct fluid imbalance. Small bowel obstruc secondary to adhesions should rarely lead to surgery—see BOX, p567.

ıralytic ileus or pseudo-obstruction?

ıralytic ileus The cause of obstruction is known to be adynamic bowel due to ɐ absence of normal peristaltic contractions. Contributing factors include dominal surgery, pancreatitis (or any localized peritonitis), spinal injury, pokalaemia, hyponatraemia, uraemia, peritoneal sepsis and drugs (eg tricyclic tidepressants).

eudo-obstruction is like mechanical GI obstruction but with no cause for struction found. **Acute** colonic pseudo-obstruction is called Ogilvie's syndrome 700), and clinical features are similar to that of mechanical obstruction.[140] edisposing factors: puerperium; pelvic surgery; trauma; cardiorespiratory sorders. ***Treatment:*** Manage conservatively. ***Neostigmine*** or colonoscopic compression are sometimes useful. In **chronic** pseudo-obstruction weight loss om malabsorption is a problem.[141]

gmoid volvulus

gmoid volvulus occurs when the bowel twists on its mesentery, which can oduce severe, rapid, strangulated obstruction. There is a characteristic AXR th an 'inverted U' loop of bowel that looks a bit like a coffee bean. It tends to cur in the elderly, constipated and co-morbid patient, and is often managed by gmoidoscopy and insertion of a flatus tube. Sigmoid colectomy is sometimes quired. ►If not treated successfully, it can progress to perforation and fatal ritonitis. For ***gastric volvulus*** see p595.

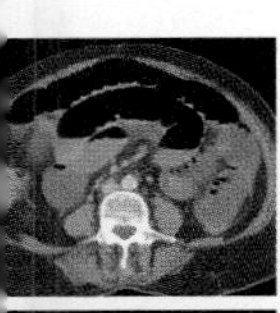

Fig 1. Axial CT of the abdomen post IV contrast medium. There are multiple loops of dilated and fluid filled small bowel in a patient with small bowel obstruction. There is no large bowel visible in this image because the patient has had a colectomy and formation of an ileoanal pouch (a prodecure done in ulcerative colitis).

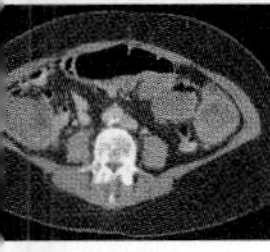

Fig 2. Axial CT of the abdomen post IV contrast medium showing dilated loops of fluid and air filled large bowel. The cause or level of obstruction is not discernable from this image. A 'transition zone' from dilated to non-dilated bowel may be present at the point of obstruction.

Some paediatric surgical emergencies

Congenital hypertrophic pyloric stenosis ►See *OHCS* p172. This usually prese not at birth but in the first 3–8wks as projectile vomiting (4 in1000 live birth ♂:♀≈4:1. The baby is malnourished and always hungry and the diagnosis is made palpating a pyloric mass in the RUQ during a feed. There may also be visible gast peristalsis passing from the LUQ. The baby can be severely alkalotic and depleted water and electrolytes because of the vomiting. This needs correcting **bef** surgery. Experienced operator US may be useful in assessment. Pass a NGT (p74 ***Treatment:*** Ramstedt's pyloromyotomy, which involves incision of the muscle do to the mucosa.

Intussusception The small bowel telescopes, as if it were swallowing itself invagination (see BOX). ***Presentation:*** Patients may be any age (usually 5– months) presenting with **episodic** intermittent inconsolable crying, with draw the legs up (colic) ± bilious vomiting. He may (but need not) pass blood PR (l redcurrant jam or cranberry sauce: 142 do a PR). A sausage-shaped abdominal m may be felt. He may become shocked and moribund. ***Tests/Management:*** The le invasive approach is US with reduction by air enema (preferred to bariu Pneumatic reduction, by passing a balloon catheter PR under radiographic cont is another option that is effective in up to 80%. If reduction by enema fa surgical reduction is needed. Prompt treatment is required to avoid the m complication of necrosis of the intussuscepting bowel, which if present, will need be excised at surgery. ***Pre-op care:*** ►►Resuscitate, crossmatch blood, pass NGT

NB: Children >4yrs present differently: rectal bleeding is less common, and th are more likely to have a long history (>3wks) and some sort of contribut pathology, eg Henoch–Schönlein purpura, cystic fibrosis, Peutz–Jeghers' syndro or tumours, eg lymphomas—in the latter, obstructive symptoms caused intussusception are the chief mode of presentation. Recurrence rate: ~5%.

Midgut malrotation During embryonic development, the mid-gut undergoes 27 of anticlockwise rotation. If this is faulty (malrotation) then the gut is prone undergo volvulus upon its abnormally-pedicled mesentery. This usually presents the neonatal period with dark green bilious vomiting, distension, and rec bleeding, though it can be asymptomatic for years before an acute presentati ***Treatment:*** ►►Resuscitation, then surgical correction of the malrotation involv broadening of the mesentery and replacing the bowel in a non-rotated positio

Torsion of the testis

The aim is to recognize this condition before the cardinal signs and symptoms a fully manifest, as prompt surgery saves testes. ►If in any doubt, surgery required. ***Symptoms:*** Sudden onset of pain in one testis, which makes walki uncomfortable. Pain in the abdomen, nausea, and vomiting are common. ***Sig*** Inflammation of one testis—it is tender, hot, and swollen. The testis may lie hi and transversely. Torsion may occur at any age but is most common at 11–30y ***Tests:*** Doppler USS (may demonstrate lack of blood flow to testis) and isoto scanning may be useful, but must not delay surgical exploration. ***Treatment:*** ►A consent for possible orchidectomy + **bilateral** fixation (orchidopexy)—see p5 At surgery expose and untwist the testis. If its colour looks good, return it to t scrotum and fix **both** testes to the scrotum ΔΔ: The main one is epididymo-orch (p618) but with this the patient tends to be older, there may be symptoms urinary infection, and more gradual onset of pain. Also consider tumour, traur and an acute hydrocele. NB: **Torsion of the hydatid of Morgagni**—a remnant of t Müllerian duct—occurs a little earlier, and causes less pain (fig 1). Its tiny bl nodule may be discernible under the scrotum. It is thought to be due to the sur in gonadotrophins which signal the onset of puberty. **Idiopathic scrotal oedema** a benign condition usually between ages 2–10yrs, and is differentiated fr torsion by the absence of pain and tenderness.

Tips on examining the abdomen in children

Examining the abdomen of a child or infant can prove extremely difficult and requires patience, practice and opportunism. So:

- An age-directed approach will help develop your relationship with the child.
- Remember that the parents will be closely involved in what you do.
- Play specialists may be able to provide distraction.
- Examining the abdomen may require an unorthodox approach, eg whilst sitting in mum's lap.
- There is no hope of eliciting any signs whilst the child is crying and tensing their tummy—everyone will be better off if you return when the child has settled down!
- Examining for rebound tenderness in young children is probably of little use for us and definitely uncomfortable for them.
- You should always examine the scrotum and inguinal regions in young boys to exclude the possibility of testicular torsion or a strangulated hernia.
- Performing a PR examination, if required, is best left to a specialist.
- Unless you have a magical way with children, don't be surprised to get the cold shoulder once in a while!

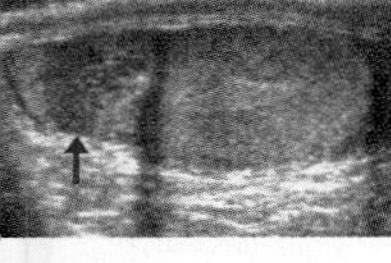

Fig 1. Ultrasound of the testis showing a torsion of a hydatid Morgagni (appendix of the testis). This is a hypoechoic area at the superior pole separate from the normal head of the epididymis (arrow).

Intussusception

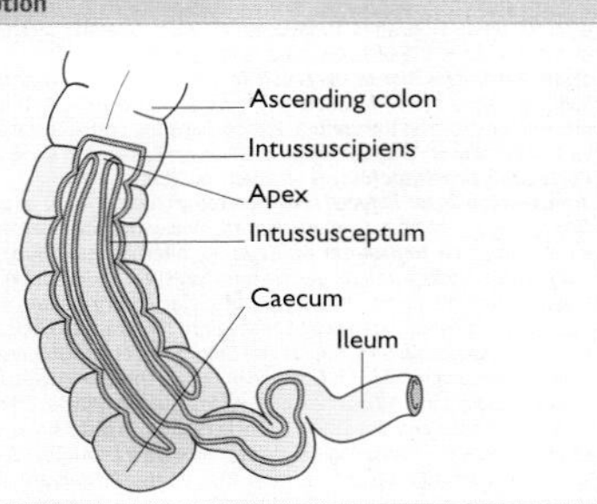

Urinary retention & benign prostatic hypertrophy

Retention means not emptying the bladder (∵ **obstruction** or ↓**detrusor power**

Acute retention The bladder is usually tender, containing ~600mL of urine. Th cause in men is usually prostatic obstruction, eg precipitated by anticholinergic 'holding on', constipation, pain, anaesthetics, alcohol, infection (p282). Questions t detect obstruction: see p40. ***Examine:*** Abdomen, PR, perineal sensation (cauda ec uina compression). ***Tests:*** MSU, U&E, FBC, and prostate-specific antigen (PSA, p681) Renal ultrasound if renal impairment. ***Tricks to aid voiding:*** Analgesia, privacy o hospital wards, ambulation, standing to void, voiding to the sound of runnin taps—or in a hot bath. ***If the tricks fail:*** Catheterize (p750) and try a prostat procedure (below). After eg 7 days, trial without catheter may work (esp. if <75yr old and <1L drained or retention was triggered by a passing event, eg genera anaesthesia), p751. ***Prevention: Finasteride*** reduces prostate size and retentio risk. ***Tamsulosin*** reduces risk of needing recatheterization after acute retention.

Chronic retention is more insidious. Bladder capacity may be >1.5L. Presentatio overflow incontinence, acute on chronic retention, a lower abdominal mass, UTI, o renal failure eg in the form of bilateral obstructive uropathy—see EMERGENCY BO Prostatic enlargement is the common cause. Others: pelvic malignancy; recta surgery; DM; CNS disease eg transverse myelitis/MS; zoster (S2–S4). ►Onl catheterize the patient if there is pain, urinary infection, or renal impairment (e urea >12mmol/L). Institute definitive treatment promptly. Intermittent sel catheterization is sometimes required (p751).

Catheters and catheterization See p750. **Prostate cancer** p606.

Benign prostatic hypertrophy (BPH) is common (24% if aged 40–64; if olde 40%). ↓Urine flow (eg <15mL/s) is associated with frequency, urgency (►p40) an voiding difficulty. ***Managing BPH:*** Assess severity of symptoms and impact on lif PR exam. Tests: MSU; U&E; ultrasound (residual volume↑, hydronephrosis—see fig 1 Rule out cancer: PSA,[1] transrectal ultrasound ± biopsy. Then consider:

1 ***Transurethral resection of the prostate*** (TURP, a common operation; ≤14% become impotent—see BOX). Crossmatch 2U. Consider perioperative antibiotic eg ***cefuroxime*** 1.5g/8h IV, three doses. Beware excessive bleeding post-op an clot retention. ~20% of TURPs need redoing within 10yrs.
2 ***Transurethral incision of the prostate*** (TUIP) involves less destruction than TUR and less risk to sexual function, but gives similar benefit. It achieves this b relieving pressure on the urethra. It is perhaps the best surgical option for thos with small glands <30g—ie ~50% of those operated on in some areas.
3 ***Retropubic prostatectomy*** is an open operation.
4 ***Transurethral laser-induced prostatectomy*** (TULIP) may be as good as TURP.
5 ***Drugs*** may be useful in mild disease, and while awaiting TURP, eg:
   - α-blockers: eg ***tamsulosin*** 400μg/d PO; alternatives: ***alfuzosin, doxazosi terazosin***. These ↓smooth muscle tone (prostate *and* bladder). SE: drowsines depression; dizziness; BP↓; dry mouth; ejaculatory failure; extra-pyramid signs; nasal congestion; weight↑. They are the drugs of choice.
   - 5α-reductase inhibitors: ***finasteride*** 5mg/d PO (↓testosterone's conversion t dihydrotestosterone).[2] It is excreted in semen, so warn to use condoms; female should avoid handling crushed pills. SE: impotence; ↓libido. Effects on prostat size are limited and slow, so, if α-blockers fail, many try surgery next.
6 ***Phytotherapy*** (pharmacological use of plants) **Saw palmetto** (*Sereona repens*) said to help symptoms of BPH (no more than drugs); trials are disappointing.
7 ***Wait and see*** is an option, but risks incontinence, retention, and renal failure

1 Do venepuncture for PSA **before** PR, as PR can ↑total PSA by ~1ng/mL (free PSA ↑by 10%). It is difficu to evaluate whether acute retention raises PSA, but we know that relieving obstruction causes it to drop!
2 ***Finasteride*** can prevent retention but has odd effects on risk of prostate cancer. The PCPT tri showed a ↓risk of indolent cancers, but ↑risk of Gleason >7 (p607).

Advice for patients concerning transurethral prostatectomy

Pre-op consent issues may centre on risks of the procedure, eg:

- Haematuria/haemorrhage
- Haematospermia
- Hypothermia
- Urethral trauma/stricture
- Post TURP syndrome (T° ↓; Na^+ ↓)
- Infection; prostatitis
- Impotence ~10%
- Incontinence ≤10%
- Clot retention near strictures
- Retrograde ejaculation (common)

Post-operative advice:

- Avoid driving for 2wks after the operation.
- Avoid sex for 2wks after surgery. Then get back to normal. The amount ejaculated may be reduced (as it flows backwards into the bladder—harmless, but may cloud the urine). It means you may be infertile. Impotence may be a problem after TURP, but do not expect this: in some men, erections improve. Rarely, orgasmic sensations are reduced.
- Expect to pass blood in the urine for the first 2 weeks. A small amount of blood colours the urine bright red. Do not be alarmed.
- At first you may need to urinate **more** frequently than before. Do not be despondent. In 6 weeks things should be much better—but the operation cannot be guaranteed to work (8% fail, and lasting incontinence is a problem in 6%; 12% may need repeat TURPs within 8yrs, compared with 1.8% of men undergoing open prostatectomy).
- If feverish, or if urination hurts, take a sample of urine to your doctor.

Obstructive uropathy

In someone with chronic urinary retention, an episode of **acute** retention may go unnoticed for several days and, because of their background symptoms, may only present when overflow incontinence becomes a nuisance—pain is not necessarily a feature.

After making the diagnosis of acute on chronic retention and inserting a catheter, the bladder residual can be as much as 1.5L of urine. Don't be surprised to be called by the biochemistry lab to be told that the serum creatinine is 1500 µmol/L! The good news here is that renal function usually returns to the baseline after a few days, (remembering that there may be some mild background impairment). Request an urgent US of the renal tract (fig 1) and consider the following in the acute setting to ensure a safe course:

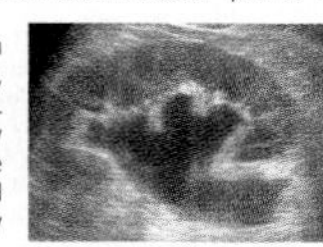

Fig 1. Ultrasound of an obstructed kidney showing hydronephrosis. The renal pelvis and ureter are dilated and the calyces are clubbed.

- **Hyperkalaemia:** Treat accordingly (p821).
- **Metabolic acidosis:** On ABG there is likely to be a respiratory compensated metabolic acidosis. Concerns should prompt discussion with a renal specialist (a good idea anyway), in case haemodialysis is required (p296).
- **Post-obstructive diuresis:** In the acute phase after relief of the obstruction, the kidneys produce a **lot** of urine—as much as a litre in the first hour. It is vital to provide resuscitation fluids and then match input with output. ►Fluid depletion rather than overload is the danger here.
- **Sodium and bicarbonate-losing nephropathy:** As the kidney undergoes diuresis, Na^+ and bicarbonate are lost in the urine in large quantities. Replace 'in for out' (as above) with isotonic 1.26% sodium bicarbonate solution—this should be available from ITU. Some advocate using 0.9% saline, though the chloride load may exacerbate acidosis. Withhold any nephrotoxic drugs.
- **Infection:** Treat infection, bearing in mind that the WCC↑ and CRP↑ may be part of the stress response. Send a sample of urine for MC+S.

Urinary incontinence

►Think twice before inserting a urinary catheter.
►Carry out rectal examination to exclude faecal impaction.
►Is the bladder palpable after voiding (retention with overflow)?
►Is there neurological co-morbidity: eg MS; Parkinson's disease; stroke; spinal traum

Anyone might 'wet themselves' on a long coach ride (we all would if the journ was long enough). Do not think of people as either dry or incontinent but incontinent in certain circumstances. Attending to these circumstances is important as focusing on the physiology.

Incontinence in men Enlargement of the prostate is the major cause incontinence: urge incontinence (see below) or dribbling may result from the part retention of urine. TURP & other pelvic surgery may weaken the bladder sphinc and cause incontinence. Troublesome incontinence needs specialist assessmen

Incontinence in women (See also **Voiding difficulty**, *OHCS* p307.)

1 ***Functional incontinence,*** ie when physiological factors are relative unimportant. The patient is 'caught short' and too slow in finding the toi because of immobility or unfamiliar surroundings, for example.

2 ***Stress incontinence:*** Leakage of urine due to incompetent sphincter, typica occuring when intra-abdominal pressure rises (eg coughing, laughing). There m be slippage of the proximal ⅓ of the urethra and the bladder neck out of t abdominal cavity. Increasing age and obesity are risk factors. The key diagnosis is the loss of small (but often frequent) amounts of urine wh coughing, etc. Examine for pelvic floor weakness/prolapse.[149] Look for cough le with the patient standing and with full bladder. Stress incontinence is commor pregnancy and following birth. It occurs to some degree in about 50% of pos menopausal women. In elderly women, pelvic floor weakness, eg with uteri prolapse or urethrocele (*OHCS* p290) is the commonest cause.

3 ***Urge incontinence*** (also known as 'overactive bladder syndrome') is the ch type seen in hospital practice. The urge to urinate is quickly followed by unco rollable and sometimes complete emptying of the bladder as detrusor contrac Large amounts of urine flow down the patient's legs. In the elderly it is usua related to **detrusor instability** (a urodynamic diagnosis—see BOX) or orga brain damage. Look for evidence of: stroke; Parkinson's; dementia. Other caus urinary infection; diabetes; diuretics; 'senile' vaginitis; urethritis.

In both sexes incontinence may result from diminished awareness due to confusi or sedation. Occasionally incontinence may be purposeful (eg preventing admissi to an old people's home) or due to anger.

Management ***Check for:*** UTI; DM; diuretic use; faecal impaction. Do U& ***Stress incontinence:*** Pelvic floor exercises may help. Intravaginal electri stimulation may also be effective, but is not acceptable to many women. A ri pessary may help uterine prolapse, eg while awaiting surgical repair. ***Duloxeti*** 40mg/12h PO is a new treatment; the main SE is nausea.[RCT 150] Surgical options inclu **Burch colposuspension** and **sling procedures**.[MET 151] A variety of minimal acce techniques (eg tension-free vaginal tape) are also available. ***Urge incontinen*** Examine for spinal cord and CNS signs (including cognitive test, p47); and f vaginitis—treat with ***estriol*** 0.1% cream (eg Ovestin®, one applicator dose twi weekly for a few months)—consider cyclical ***progesterone*** if for prolonged use a no hysterectomy, to avoid risk of uterine cancer. The patient (or carer) shou complete an 'incontinence' chart for 3 days to define the pattern of incontinen Maximize access to toilet; advise on toileting regimen (eg every 4h). The aim is keep bladder volume below that which triggers emptying. Drugs may help redu night-time incontinence (see BOX) but are generally disappointing. Consider ai (absorbent pad; Paul's tubing if ♂).

►Do urodynamic assessment (cystometry & urine flow rate measurement) bef any surgical intervention to exclude detrusor instability or sphincter dyssynergi

Managing detrusor instability

Agents for detrusor instability:	Symptoms that they may improve:
Tolterodine 1–2mg/12h PO; SE: dry mouth, eyes, and skin; drowsiness, abdominal pain, urinary retention.[RCT 152]	Frequency, urgency (alternative: ***oxybutynin***, but more SE).[MET 153] Avoid in myasthenia, and if glaucoma or UC are uncontrolled.
Solifenacin 5mg/24h (max 10mg)	Urinary frequency, urgency, and urge incontinence. SE: gastro-oesophageal reflux; altered taste; fatigue; oedema.
Imipramine 50mg PO at night	Nocturia, enuresis, coital incontinence
Oestrogens	Post-menopausal urgency, frequency + nocturia may be improved by raising the bladder's sensory threshold.
Surgery, eg clam ileocystoplasty	Usually reserved for troublesome or intractable symptoms. The bladder is bisected, opened like a clam, and 25cm of ileum is sewn in.
Neuromodulation via transcutaneous electrical stimulation[154]	(Stimulates afferent nerve fibres to modulate bladder reflexes, suppressing involuntary detrusor contractions.)
Hypnosis, psychotherapy, bladder training	(These all require good motivation.)

NB: ***desmopressin*** nasal spray 20µg as a night-time dose may have a role in ↓urine production, but not suitable in the elderly (SEs: fluid retention, heart failure, hyponatraemia).

A reminder about urinary symptoms

See also p40

Filling/storage symptoms
- Nocturia
- Urgency
- Urge incontinence
- Frequency

Voiding symptoms
- Poor stream
- Terminal dribbling
- Strangury
- Hesitancy
- *Pis en deux*=going twice.

Urinary tract malignancies

Renal cell carcinoma (hypernephroma, Grawitz tumour) arises from the proximal renal tubular epithelium. ***Epidemiology:*** 90% of renal cancers; mean age; 55yrs ♂:♀=2:1. 15% of those on haemodialysis develop renal cell carcinoma. ***Clinical features:*** 50% are incidental findings during abdominal imaging for other symptoms. Haematuria, loin pain, abdominal mass, anorexia, malaise, weight loss and PUO may all occur—often in isolation. Rarely, invasion of left renal vein compresses the left testicular vein causing a left varicocele. Spread may be direct (renal vein), via lymph nodes, or haematogenous (bone, liver, lung). ***Tests:*** **Blood** FBC (polycythaemia from erythropoietin secretion); ESR; U&E, alk phos (bony mets?) **Urine:** RBCs; cytology. **Imaging:** US (p730); CT/MRI (including 3D, fig 1); renal angiography (if partial nephrectomy or palliative embolization are being considered; angiography can also be done by CT/MR); IVU (filling defect in kidney ± calcification); CXR ('cannon ball' metastases). ***Treatment:*** Radical nephrectomy has been the gold-standard, though there may be a role for nephron-sparing surgery in small tumours (≤4cm). Metastatic disease is reason to consider immunotherapy with interferon-α and interleukin-2. ***Prognosis:*** 5yr survival: 45%

Transitional cell carcinoma (TCC) may arise in the bladder (50%), ureter, or renal pelvis. ***Epidemiology:*** Age >40yrs; ♂:♀ = 4:1. ***Risk factors:*** p608. ***Presentation*** Painless haematuria; frequency; urgency; dysuria; urinary tract obstruction. ***Diagnosis:*** Urine cytology; IVU; cystoscopy + biopsy; CT/MRI scan. ***Treatment:*** See **Bladder tumours**, p608. ***Prognosis:*** Varies with clinical stage/histological grade 10–80% 5yr survival.

Wilms' tumour (nephroblastoma, *OHCS* p133) is a childhood tumour of primitive renal tubules and mesenchymal cells. ***Prevalence:*** 1:100 000; the chief abdominal malignancy in children. It presents with an abdominal mass and haematuria. Check for associated syndromes (eg Beckwith–Wiedemann, *OHCS* p638). ***Tests:*** Urine cytology; US; IVU; renal angiography; CT/MRI scan. Avoid biopsy. ***Treatment*** Nephrectomy; radiotherapy; chemotherapy. ***Prognosis:*** 90% 5yr survival.

Prostate cancer is the 2nd commonest malignancy of men. ***Incidence:*** Rises with age: 80% in men >80yrs (in autopsy studies). ***Associations:*** ↑testosterone, +ve family history (p512). Most are adenocarcinomas arising in the peripheral prostate. Spread may be local (seminal vesicles, bladder, rectum) via nodes, or haematogenously (sclerotic bony lesions). ***Symptoms:*** May be asymptomatic or nocturia, hesitancy, poor stream, terminal dribbling, or urinary obstruction. Weight↓ ± bone pain suggests metastases. ***PR exam:*** May show a hard, irregular prostate. ***Diagnosis:*** ↑PSA (p681; normal in 30% of small cancers); transrectal ultrasound and biopsy; bone x-rays; bone scan; CT/MRI. ***Staging:*** MRI. If contrast-enhancing magnetic nanoparticles are used, sensitivity for detecting affected nodes rises from 35% to 90%. ***Treatment:*** **Local disease:** Which is better: radical prostatectomy (+ immediate ***goserelin*** if node +ve; a widely used regimen), radiotherapy or watchful waiting with serial PSA monitoring? The follow up to one trial found that at 10 years, radical prostatectomy significantly improved disease-specific mortality and local progression when compared with watchful waiting. (But radical surgery does double rates of erectile dysfunction and incontinence.) Radiotherapy combined with hormone therapy improves survival in advanced local disease. D transurethral resection for obstruction. Brachytherapy is being assessed for local disease. **Metastatic disease:** Hormonal drugs may give benefit for 1–2yrs Gonadotrophin-releasing analogues, eg 12-weekly ***goserelin*** (10.8mg SC as Zoladex LA®) first stimulate, and then inhibit pituitary gonadotrophin output. Alternatives: ***cyproterone acetate***; ***flutamide***; ***diethylstilboestrol***. ***Symptomatic treatment*** Analgesia; treat hypercalcaemia; radiotherapy for bone metastases or spinal cord compression. ***Prognosis:*** 10% die in 6 months, but 10% live >10yrs. ***Screening*** Rectal exam; PSA; transrectal ultrasound. There are problems with all (p681).

Advice to asymptomatic men asking for a PSA test

The prostate lies below the bladder, and surrounds the tube taking urine out. Prostate cancer is common in older men. Many men over 50 (to whom this advice applies) consider a PSA blood test to detect prostatic cancer. *Is this wise?*

- The test is not very accurate, and we cannot say that those having the test will live longer—even if they do turn out to have prostate cancer. This is because the cancer is often very lazy, so that, in most men with prostate cancer, death is from an unrelated cause.
- The test itself has no side-effects, provided you don't mind giving blood and time. But if the test is falsely positive, you may needlessly have more tests, such as sampling the prostate by the back passage (which may cause bleeding and infection in 1–5% of men).
- Only one in three of those with a high PSA level will have cancer.
- You may also be worried needlessly if later tests put you in the clear.
- Even if a cancer is found, there is no way to tell *for sure* if it will impinge on your health. Treatment may be recommended—and then you might end up having a bad effect from treatment which was not even needed.
- There is much uncertainty on treating those who **do** turn out to have prostate cancer: options are radical surgery to remove the prostate (this treatment may be fatal in 0.2–0.5% of patients), radiotherapy, or hormones.
- There is indirect evidence of benefit of screening from the USA where fewer radical prostatectomies reveal cancer-affected lymph nodes than those done before widespread PSA-based screening. Intensive screening and treatment for prostate cancer does not, however, appear to be associated with lower prostate-specific mortality in retrospective studies.[163]

► Ultimately, you must decide for yourself what you want.

Prognostic factors in prostate cancer

A number of prognostic factors help determine if 'watchful waiting' or aggressive therapy should be advised: • Age • Pre-treatment PSA level • Tumour stage (as measured by the TNM system),[164] and tumour grade—as measured by its Gleason score. Gleason grading is from 1 to 5, with 5 being the highest grade, and carrying the poorest prognosis. A pathologist determines Gleason grades by analysing histology from two separate areas of tumour specimen, and adding them to get the total Gleason score for the tumour, from 2 to 10. 8–10 suggest an aggressive tumour; 5–7 suggest intermediate grade; 2–4 is indolent. In one recent (provisional) study, 15yr prostate cancer mortality for conservative management of PSA-detected cancers was 0–2% for Gleason <7, 9–31% for Gleason score 7, and 28–72% for Gleason scores >7.[165]

Patients with high Gleason scores are more likely to be treated aggressively, (eg if younger and/or have higher stage disease). If 55–59yrs old at diagnosis, the predicted absolute 15yr survival benefit from radical (curative) treatment is about 0, 12, and 26% for Gleason scores <7, 7, and >7, respectively.[166]

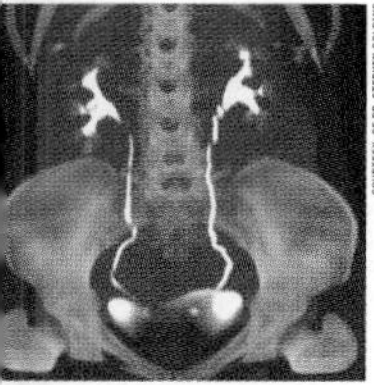

Fig 1. 3D CT urography of the urinary tract.

Bladder tumours

What appear as benign papillomata rarely behave in a purely benign way. They ꞔ almost certainly indolent transitional cell (urothelial) malignancies. Adenocarc omas and squamous cell carcinomas are rare in the West (the latter may foll schistosomiasis). UK incidence ≈ 1 : 5000/yr. ♂:♀ ≈ 4:1. Histology is important prognosis: **Grade 1**—differentiated; **Grade 2**—intermediate; **Grade 3**—poo differentiated. 80% are confined to bladder mucosa, and only ~20% penetra muscle (increasing mortality to 50% at 5yrs).

Presentation Painless haematuria; recurrent UTIs; voiding irritability.

Associations Smoking; aromatic amines (rubber industry); chronic cysti schistosomiasis (↑risk of squamous cell carcinoma); pelvic irradiation.

Tests
- Urine: microscopy/cytology (cancers may cause sterile pyuria).
- IVU may show filling defects ± ureteric involvement.
- Cystoscopy with biopsy is diagnostic.
- Bimanual EUA helps assess spread.
- CT/MRI or lymphangiography may show involved pelvic nodes.

Staging: See TABLE.

Treatment of transitional cell carcinoma (TCC) of the bladder
- ***Tis/Ta/T1:*** (80% of all patients.) Diathermy via transurethral cystosco Consider intravesical chemotherapeutic agents (eg ***mitomycin C***) for multi small tumours or high-grade tumours. Immunotherapy with intravesical *B* (which stimulates a non-specific immune response) is useful in high-gra tumours and carcinoma-*in-situ,* and may be better at preventing tumc progression than **mitomycin C** in superficial disease.[167] 5yr survival ≈ 95%.
- ***T2–3:*** Radical cystectomy is the 'gold standard'. Radiotherapy gives worse 5 survival rates than surgery, but preserves the bladder. 'Salvage' cystectomy c be performed if radiotherapy fails, but yields worse results than primary surge Post-op chemotherapy (eg M-VAC: ***methotrexate***, ***vinblastine***, ***adriamycin***, a ***cisplatin***) is toxic but effective, and there may also be a role for neoadjuva chemotherapy.[168] Methods to preserve the bladder with transurethral resectic partial cystectomy + systemic chemotherapy have been tried, but long-te results are disappointing. If the bladder neck is not involved, orthotopic recons uction rather than forming a urostoma is an option (both using ~40cm of t patient's ileum), but adequate tumour clearance must not be compromised. ►T patient should have all these options explained by a urologist and an oncologi
- ***T4:*** Usually palliative chemo/radiotherapy. Chronic catheterization and urina diversions may help to relieve pain.

Follow up History, examination, and regular cystoscopy: • ***High-risk tumou*** Every 3 months for 2yrs, then every 6 months; • ***Low-risk tumours:*** First follo up cystoscopy after 9 months, then yearly.

Tumour spread Local → to pelvic structures; lymphatic → to iliac and para-aor nodes; haematogenous → to liver and lungs.

Survival This depends on age at surgery. For example, the 3yr survival af cystectomy for T2 and T3 tumours is 60% if 65–75yrs old, falling to 40% if 7 82yrs old (in whom the operative mortality is 4%). With unilateral pelvic no involvement, only 6% of patients survive 5yrs. The 3yr survival with bilateral para-aortic node involvement is nil.

Complications: Cystectomy can result in sexual and urinary malfunction. Mass bladder haemorrhage may complicate treatment; consider ***alum*** solution bladc irrigation (safer than formalin): it is an in-patient procedure.[169]

NM staging of bladder cancer

is	Carcinoma-*in-situ*	Not felt at EUA
a	Tumour confined to epithelium	Not felt at EUA
1	Tumour in lamina propria	Not felt at EUA
2	Superficial muscle involved	Rubbery thickening at EUA
3	Deep muscle involved	EUA: mobile mass
4	Invasion beyond bladder	EUA: fixed mass

JA = examination under anaesthetic

s asymptomatic microscopic haematuria significant?

ipstick tests are often done routinely for new admissions. If microscopic aematuria is found, but the patient has no related symptoms, what does this iean? Before rushing into a barrage on investigations, consider:

ne study found incidence of urogenital disease (eg bladder cancer) was no igher in those with asymptomatic microhaematuria than those without.[170]

Asymptomatic microscopic haematuria is the sole presenting feature in only 4% of bladder cancers, and there is no evidence that these are less advanced than malignancies presenting with macroscopic haematuria.

When monitoring those with treated bladder cancer for recurrence, microscopic haematuria tests have a sensitivity of only 31% in those with superficial bladder malignancy, in whom detection would be most useful.

Although 80% of those with flank pain due to a renal stone have microscopic haematuria, so do 50% of those with flank pain but no stone.[171]

he conclusion is not that urine dipstick testing is useless, but that results should ot be interpreted in isolation. Take a holistic view. Smokers and those with +ve amily history for urothelial cancer may be investigated differently from those ith no risk factors (eg ultrasound, cystoscopy ± referral to a renal physician in ome patients), but in a young fit athlete, the diagnosis is more likely to be xercise-induced haematuria.[172] Wise doctors liaise with their patients. 'Shall we t sleeping dogs lie?' is a reasonable question for **some** patients. Give the facts nd let him decide, reserving to yourself the right to present the facts in certain ays, depending on your instincts, and those of a trusted colleague. Remember iat medicine is for gamblers (p646), and wise gamblers assess the odds against shifting set of circumstances.

Common lumps
• Fibroadenoma
• Cyst
• Cancer
• Fibroadenosis (foca diffuse nodularity)
Rare lumps
• Periductal mastitis
• Fat necrosis
• Galactocoele
• Abscess
• 'Non-breast' eg lipo or sebaceous cyst

►All solid lumps need histo-/cytological assessment.

History Previous lumps, family history, pain (rarely in cancer), nipple discharge or inversion, change in size related to menstrual cycle, number of pregnancies, first/last/latest period, drugs (eg HRT). Don't forget that 1% of all breast cancers are found in men.

Examination Inspect (arms up and down). Note position, size, consistency, mobility, fixity, and local lymphadenopathy. Any nipple discharge/inversion? Is the skin involved: dimpling; ulceration; *peau d'orange*?

Investigation All lumps should undergo ***'quadruple' assessment:*** Clinical examination (above) + histology/ cytology + mammography + ultrasound; see flow chart.

Breast cancer *Risk factors:* Risk is related to family history, age and unir rupted oestrogen exposure, hence: nulliparity; 1st pregnancy >30yrs old, e menarche; late menopause; HRT; obesity; BRCA genes (p512); not breast-feeding; Pill (possibly); past breast cancer (metachronous rate ≈2%, synchronous ≈1%). ***TNM staging:*** **T1** <2cm. **T2** 2–5cm. **T3** >5cm. **T4** Fixity to chest wall or *p d'orange*. **N1** Mobile ipsilateral nodes. **N2** Fixed nodes. **M1** Distant metastas

Treating early cancer • ***Surgery:*** Wide local excision (WLE) or mastecton breast reconstruction + axillary node sampling or surgical clearance. Local exci followed by radiotherapy gives equal survival, but higher local recurrence ra than mastectomy. • ***Radiotherapy:*** For tumours at high risk of local recurre post-mastectomy radiotherapy to the chest wall ↓local recurrence and ↑overall survival.[MET 173] Radiotherapy to the breast following WLE ↓local recurrenc Radiotherapy to the axilla is used if lymph node +ve on sampling and comp surgical clearance was not performed. SE: pneumonitis, pericarditis, rib fractu lymphoedema, brachial plexopathy. • ***Chemotherapy*** improves survival (es younger and node +ve), eg an anthracycline (***epirubicin*** is less cardiotoxic t ***doxorubicin***) + ***5FU*** + ***cyclophosphamide*** ± ***methotrexate***. ***Trastuzumab*** (Her tin®, below) also has a role. If these fail, ***vinorelbine*** or ***capecitabine*** + ***docet*** (a taxane) may be used. • ***Endocrine therapy*** aims to ↓oestrogen activity, ar used in all (o)estrogen receptor (ER) or progesterone receptor (PR) +ve disease. ER blocker ***tamoxifen*** is widely used, eg 20mg/d PO for 5yrs post-op (may ra cause uterine cancer so warn to report vaginal bleeding).[175] Aromatase inhibi (eg ***anastrozole***) targeting oestrogen synthesis can also be used, and may better tolerated than ***tamoxifen***. They are commonly used in post-menopa women. In pre-menopausal women with ER+ve tumours, ovarian ablation eithe surgery, radiotherapy, or GnRH analogues (p606, eg ***goserelin***) improves recurre and survival.[MET 176] • ***Support:*** Involve specialist breastcare nurses at from the sta they will have the closest contact with patients all the way through treatme

Treating distant disease Assess LFT, Ca^{2+}, CXR, skeletal survey, bone scan, live or CT. DXT (p518) to painful bony lesions. ***Tamoxifen*** is commonly used in ER+ve c ase; if relapse after initial success, consider chemotherapy. Tumours +ve for protein may respond to the monoclonal antibody ***trastuzumab*** (Herceptin®).

Preventing breast cancer deaths • Promote ***breast awareness*** • ***Mammogra*** every ~3yrs, eg if 50–70yrs old; screening ↓ breast cancer deaths by 25% in group. 2-view mammograms are used. Radiation risk is 'negligible'. Detection r are 6.4 cancers/1000 'healthy' women. Annual mammograms don't lower mort much further. NB: The fall in death rates from 51 to 35 per 100,000 during 19 2000 is largely attributed to wide use of ***tamoxifen***.[178] ***Raloxifene*** (used in p menopausal osteoporosis and similar to tamoxifen and has less risk of uterine cer & DVT) may have a role in preventing ER+ve cancers in women at ↑risk.[RCT 179 N=

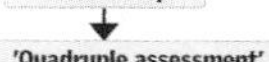

'Quadruple assessment'
linical examination
adiology: ultrasound for <35yrs old; mammography **and** ultrasound for >35yrs old[1]
istology/cytology (FNA or core biopsy: US-guided core biopsy is best for **new** lumps)

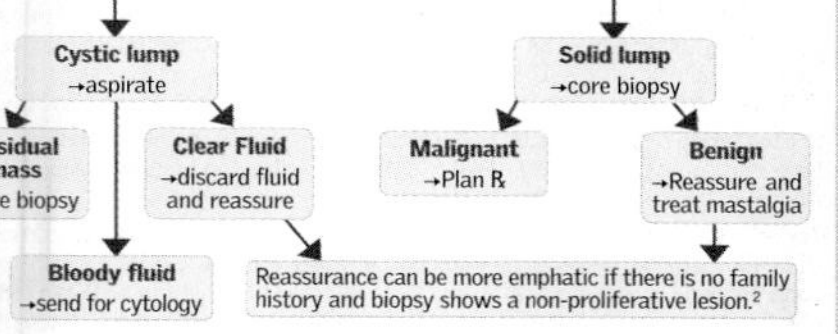

ple discharge

ses of discharge Duct ectasia (green/brown/red, often multiple ducts and teral), intraductal papilloma/adenoma/carcinoma (bloody discharge, often gle duct), lactation. ***Management:*** Diagnose the cause (mammogram, asound, ductogram); then treat appropriately. Cessation of smoking reduces charge from duct ectasia. Microdochectomy/total duct excision can be sidered if other measures fail, though may give no improvement in symptoms.

ntinel node biopsy

entinel node biopsy may reduce the number of needless axillary arances in lymph node –ve patients, thus decreasing post-op morbidity. RCT 180 In ping with the history of conservative breast surgery, it remains controversial. ypical procedure is as follows:
'atent blue dye (SE: anaphylaxis) and/or radiocolloid is injected perioperatively nto the periareolar area or the area of the primary tumour.
small incision is made in the axilla, and a gamma probe/visual inspection is sed to identify the sentinel node.
he sentinel node is biopsied and sent for histology ± immunohistochemistry.
lti-centre trials suggest that the sentinel node can be identified in 90% of ients. False negative rates of 9–14% are reported, though these drop to <5% surgeons become more experienced with the technique.

gnostic factors in breast cancer

ny factors help assess prognosis in breast cancer, including tumour size, grade, ph node status, ER/PR status, and presence of lympho-vascular invasion. The tingham Prognostic Index (NPI) is widely used to predict survival and risk of apse, and thus help select appropriate adjuvant systemic therapy:[3]

NPI = 0.2 × tumour size (cm) + histological grade + nodal status

reated with surgery alone, the 10yr survival rates are: NPI <2.4: 95%; 2.4–3.4: 85%; NPI 3.4–4.4: 70%; NPI 4.4–5.4: 50%; NPI >5.4: 20%.

has become more accurate at detecting invasive breast cancer, though mammography remains accurate at detecting ductal carcinoma-*in-situ* (DCIS). MRI is used in the assessment of ocal/bilateral disease and patients with cosmetic implants who are identified as high risk.
ere is a relatively ↑risk of malignancy if there is atypical hyperplasia or a proliferative lesion.
dal status is scored 1–3: **1** = node –ve; **2** = 1–3 nodes +ve; **3** = >3 nodes +ve for breast cancer.
ogical grade is also scored 1–3.

This is the 2nd most common cause of cancer deaths in the UK (19,000 deaths/ 56% of presentations are in those >70yrs old. Synchronous tumours are founc ~2.5% and metachronous tumours in ~1%. See BOX for tumour sites.

Predisposing factors Neoplastic polyps (see below), UC, Crohn's, fami adenomatous polyposis, HNPCC (p512), previous cancer, and low-fibre diet. NSAIDs and ***aspirin*** may be protective.[182] ***Genetics:*** No close relative affect colorectal cancer risk is 1:50. One 1st degree relative affected: risk=1:17; i affected, 1:10 (refer when 10yrs younger than the youngest affected relative

Presentation depends on site: ***Left-sided:*** Bleeding/mucus PR; altered bowel ha tenesmus; mass PR (60%). ***Right:*** Weight↓; Hb↓; abdominal pain. ***Eith*** Abdominal mass; obstruction; perforation; haemorrhage; fistula.

Tests FBC (microcytic anaemia); faecal occult blood (FOB); proctosco sigmoidoscopy, barium enema or colonoscopy (see figs 1 & 2, p248), which car done 'virtually' by CT—fig 6, p729); LFT, CT/MRI (fig 1); liver ultrasound. CEA (p6 may be used to monitor disease and effectiveness of treatment (p680). If polypo in family, refer for DNA testing once a patient is >15yrs old. Genetic testing m also help determine who will benefit from chemotherapy—see p512.

Staging: see TABLE.

Spread Local, lymphatic, by blood (liver, lung, bone) or transcoelomic.

Treatment[183] ***Surgery*** aims to cure. Exact technique may ↑survival times by up 50% (eg in TME[1]): so expert training is vital. • **Right hemicolectomy** is for cae ascending or proximal transverse colon tumours. • **Left hemicolectomy** is tumours in the distal transverse or descending colon. • **Sigmoid colectomy** is tumours of sigmoid colon. • **Anterior resection** is for low sigmoid or high rec tumours. Anastomosis is achieved at the first operation—stapling devices are s and effective.[184] • **Abdomino-perineal (A-P) resection** is for tumours low in rectum (≤8cm from anal canal): permanent colostomy and removal of rectum a anus (but see p568 for total anorectal reconstruction).

Radiotherapy may be used pre-op in rectal cancer to ↓local recurrence and ↑ survival.[185] It may be associated with a higher rate of post-operative complicat eg DVT, pathological fractures, fistulization.[186] Pre-op radiotherapy ± ***5-FU*** is a used to downstage initially unresectable rectal tumours. Post-op radiotherap only used in patients with rectal tumours at high risk of local recurrence.

Chemotherapy: There is good evidence that ***5-FU*** ± other agents (eg ***folinic a levamisole***) reduce Dukes' C mortality by ~25%.[187] The role of chemotherap Dukes' B tumours is under investigation. Chemotherapy is also used in palliatio metastatic disease; newer agents (eg ***irinotecan***, ***oxaliplatin***) may provide m options. Patients with single-lobe hepatic metastases and no extrahepatic spre may be suitable for curative surgery with liver resection.[188]

Prognosis 60% are amenable to radical surgery, and 75% of these will be aliv 7yrs (or will have died from other causes). Post-op anastomotic leakage has b shown to ↓survival rates in otherwise potentially curative operation Investigation for a suspected leak (↑T°, abdominal pain, peritonism) is with wa soluble contrast enema or CT with rectal contrast.

Polyps are lumps that appear above the mucosa. There are 3 types:

1 ***Inflammatory:*** Ulcerative colitis, Crohn's, lymphoid hyperplasia.
2 ***Hamartomatous:*** Juvenile polyps, Peutz–Jeghers' syndrome (p700).
3 ***Neoplastic:*** Tubular or villous adenomas: malignant potential, esp. if >2cm

Symptoms of polyps: Passage of blood/mucus PR. They should be biopsied a removed if they show malignant change. Most can be reached by the flex colonoscope and diathermy can avoid the morbidity of partial colectomy. Ch resection margins are clear of tumour.

1 TME = total mesorectal excision. It entails sharp dissection to yield an intact mesorectal envelo

cation of cancers of the large bowel

These are averages: black females tend to have re proximal neoplasms. White men tend to have re distal neoplasms.

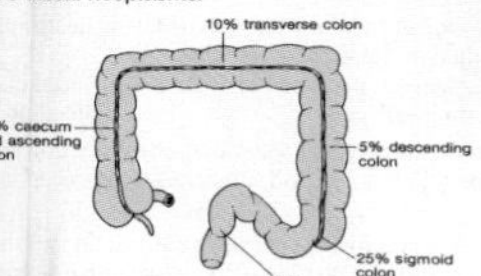

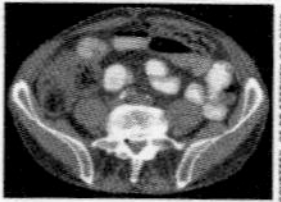

Fig 1. Axial CT of the abdomen with PO contrast medium showing thickening of the wall of the caecum (lying in the right iliac fossa) from adenocarcinoma.

kes' classification for the staging of colorectal cancer

ge	Description	Treated 5yr survival rate (%)
	Confined to beneath muscularis mucosae	~90
	Extension through muscularis mucosae	~65
	Involvement of regional lymph nodes	~30
	Distant metastases	<10

amples of scenarios prompting urgent referral for surgeon's sessment within 2 weeks

- ectal bleeding and a persistent change in bowel habit for >6wks.
- ersistent rectal bleeding without anal symptoms in those over 45yrs, with no bvious external evidence of benign anal disease.
- ron-deficiency anaemia without an obvious cause and Hb <10g/dL.
- palpable abdominal or rectal mass.
- ecent onset of looser stools and/or ↑frequency of defecation, persisting for 6wks. See p525 for review of the logic behind '2-week rules'.

iversal adult screening for colorectal cancer

number of screening methods have been proposed.

OB screening every 2yrs with home tests reduces mortality by 15–33%, but alse +ve rates are high (up to 10% of those screened) and there are problems vith acceptability. The patient has to be on a special diet while 2 out of 3 onsecutive stool samples are tested. Sample rehydration improves sensitivity ut increases false +ves.

igmoidoscopy can be used to screen for left-sided lesions with 90% ensitivity and 99% specificity within the region of the scope. One recent RCT eported good tolerability and a pick-up rate of any cancer or adenoma of up o 8% in women and up to 12% in men. RCT 191 Limitations include acceptability, ost, and not picking up right-sided lesions.

olonoscopy examines the **entire** colon and is the most accurate test. It is lready used in those at ↑risk of colorectal cancer due to personal or family istory, adenoma, or IBD. Perforation rate is higher than sigmoidoscopy (0.2% s 0.01%) and limitations include cost, need for sedation, acceptability to atients, and the availability of trained endoscopists.

Carcinoma of the stomach

Incidence of adenocarcinoma at the gastro-oesophageal junction is increasir
the West, though incidence of distal & body gastric carcinoma has fallen sharp
remains a tumour notable for its gloomy prognosis and non-specific presenta

Incidence 23/100,000/yr in the UK, but there are unexplained wide geograph
variations, being especially common in Japan. Associations:

- Blood group A
- *H. pylori* (p234)
- Atrophic gastritis; pernicious anaemia
- Adenomatous polyps
- Social cla
- Smoking

Pathology The adenocarcinoma may be polypoid, ulcerating, or leather bottle
(*linitis plastica*). Some are confined to mucosa and submucosa—so-called 'e
gastric carcinoma.

Presentation ***Symptoms:*** Often non-specific. Dyspepsia (p234) lasting >1 m
in patients aged ≥55yrs demands GI investigation. Others: weight ↓, vomi
dysphagia; anaemia. ***Signs*** suggesting incurable disease: epigastric m
hepatomegaly; jaundice, ascites (p624); large left supraclavicular (Virchow's) r
(=Troisier's sign); acanthosis nigricans (p546). ***Spread*** is local, lymphatic, bl
borne, and transcoelomic eg to ovaries (Krukenberg tumour).

Tests Gastroscopy + multiple ulcer edge biopsies. ►**Aim to biopsy all ga**
ulcers as even malignant ulcers may appear to heal on drug treatm
Endoscopic ultrasound (EUS) and CT/MRI are useful for staging. Staging laparos
is recommended for locally advanced tumours if metastases are not detecte
other investigations.[192]

Treatment See p636 for a description of surgical resections. For tumours ir
distal ⅔, a partial gastrectomy may suffice, but, if more proximal, total g
rectomy may be needed. Combination chemotherapy (eg ***epirubicin***, ***cisplatin***
5-fluorouracil) appears to increase survival in advanced disease.[193] Endosc
mucosal resection is used for early tumours confined to the mucosa.[194]

Palliation is often needed for obstruction, pain, or haemorrhage. In metast
disease, chemotherapy increases quality of life and survival. Judicious us
surgery and radiotherapy may also be useful.

5yr survival <10% overall, but nearly 20% for patients undergoing ra
surgery. The prognosis is much better for 'early' gastric carcinoma.

Carcinoma of the oesophagus

Incidence Australia <5/100,000/yr; UK <9; Brittany >50; Iran >100.
factors: Diet, alcohol excess, smoking, achalasia, Plummer–Vinson syndr
(p232), obesity, reflux oesophagitis ± Barrett's oesophagus (p686; there is a
fold ↑risk of adenocarcinoma if severe reflux for >10 years).

Site 20% occur in the upper part, 50% in the middle, and 30% in the lower
They may be squamous cell or adenocarcinomas (incidence rising).

The patient Dysphagia; weight ↓; retrosternal chest pain; lymphadenopathy (r
Signs from upper from the upper third of the oesophagus: Hoarseness; co
(may be paroxysmal if aspiration pneumonia). **ΔΔ:** See **Dysphagia**, p232.

Tests Barium swallow, CXR, oesophagoscopy with biopsy/brushings/EUS, CT,
Staging laparoscopy if significant infra-diaphragmatic component. ***Staging:*** T

Treatment Survival rates are poor with or without treatment. If localized T
disease, radical curative oesophagectomy may be tried. Transhiatal oesop
ectomy causes less morbidity than extended transthoracic resection, though
latter may be associated with ↑long-term survival. Pre-op chemotherapy (***cisp***
+ 5-FU) improves survival but causes some morbidity.[195] Surgery alone ma
preferable.[196] If surgery is **not** indicated, then chemo-radiotherapy may be b
than radiotherapy alone.[197] Palliation in advanced disease aims to res
swallowing with chemo/radiotherapy, stenting, and laser use.

e multi-disciplinary cancer meeting

er recent years there has been development of the multi-disciplinary meeting an essential part of the care for patients with cancer. They are a result of the orm of cancer services across the UK, which aimed to improve quality of life cancer sufferers by standardising and optimising screening, early detection d treatment of cancer. At any meeting you should be able to spot:

- Paired surgeons and physicians (eg upper GI surgeon and gastroenterologist).
- Radiologists
- Pathologists
- Oncologists
- Specialist care nurses
- Meeting administrators

s expert forum aims to provide the most up-to-date and relevant options for atment for each individual patient. However, despite everyone's best efforts, re can still remain an inherent uncertainty as to what is **exactly** the best atment for the patient—something which in the end may only be known to patient themselves when given the options.

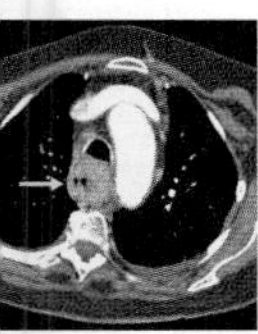

COURTESY OF DR. STEPHEN GOLDING

Fig 1. Axial CT of the chest after IV contrast medium showing concentric thickening of the oesophageus (arrow); the diagnosis here is oesophageal carcinoma. Loss of the fatty plane around the oesophagus suggests local invasion. Anterior to the oesophagus is the trachea and next to it is the arch of the aorta.

M staging in oesophageal cancer

read of oesophageal cancer is direct, by submucosal infiltration and local read—or to nodes, or, later, via the blood.

carcinoma-*in-situ*	**Nx**	nodes cannot be assessed
invading lamina propria/submucosa	**N0**	no node spread
invading muscularis propria	**N1**	regional node metastases
invading adventitia	**M0**	no distant spread
invasion of adjacent structures	**M1**	distant metastasis

►Examine the regional lymph nodes as well as the lump. If the lump is a r examine its area of drainage.

History How long has it been there? Does it hurt? Any other lumps? Is it ge bigger? Ever been abroad? Otherwise well?

Physical exam Remember the '6 S's: site, size, shape, smoothness, surface surroundings. ***Other questions:*** Does it transilluminate (see below)? Is it fix skin or underlying structures (see BOX)? Is it fluctuant? Lumps in certain site to mind particular pathologies (see lumps in groin and scrotum, p618). Remer to feel if a lump is pulsatile; this may seem to be a minor detail until faced w surprise on a minor operations list—assessment with US duplex may help.

Transilluminable lumps After eliminating as much external light as possible, a bright, thin 'pencil' torch on the lump, from behind, so the light is shining thr the lump towards your eye. If the lump glows red it is said to transillumina fluid-filled lump such as a hydrocele is a good example.

Lipomas These benign fatty lumps, occurring wherever fat can expand (ie scalp or palms), have smooth, imprecise margins, and a hint of fluctuance. only cause symptoms via pressure. Malignant change is very rare (suspect if growth, hardening, or vascularization). Multiple scattered lipomas, which m painful, occur in Dercum's disease, typically in postmenopausal women.

Surgery

Sebaceous cysts These are intradermal, so you cannot draw the skin over t Look for the characteristic punctum marking blocked sebaceous outflow. Infe is quite common, and foul pus exits through the punctum. ***Treatment:*** Sh them out whole can be tricky: learn from an expert.

Causes of lymph node enlargement ***Infection:*** Glandular fever; brucellosi HIV; toxoplasmosis; actinomycosis; syphilis. ***Infiltration:*** Malignancy (carcin lymphoma); sarcoidosis.

Cutaneous abscesses Staphylococci are the most common organisms. Haem *Streptococci* are only common in hand infections. *Proteus* is a common cau non-staphylococcal axillary abscesses. Below the waist faecal organisms common (aerobes and anaerobes). ***Treatment:*** Incision and drainage alone us cures. ***Boils (furuncles)*** are abscesses which involve a hair follicle an associated glands. ***A carbuncle*** is an area of subcutaneous necrosis w discharges itself on to the surface through multiple sinuses. Think of ***hidrade suppuritiva*** if there are recurrent inguinal or axillary abscesses.

Rheumatoid nodules are collagenous granulomas which appear in establi rheumatoid arthritis on the extensor aspects of joints—especially the elbow

Ganglia These are degenerative cysts from an adjacent joint or synovial sh commonly seen on the dorsum of the wrist or hand and dorsum of the foot. may transilluminate. 50% will disappear spontaneously. Aspiration ma effective, especially when combined with instillation of steroid hyaluronidase. For the rest, the treatment of choice is excision rather tha traditional blow from your bible (the *Oxford Textbook of Surgery!*).

Fibromas These may occur anywhere in the body, but most commonly unde skin. These whitish, benign tumours contain collagen, fibroblasts, and fibro

Dermoid cysts contain dermal structures; found at the junction of embr cutaneous boundaries eg in the midline or lateral to the eye.

Malignant tumours of connective tissue include the fibrosarcoma, liposar leiomyosarcoma (smooth muscle), and rhabdomyosarcoma (striated mu Sarcomas are staged using a modified TNM system which includes tumour g Needle-core (Trucut®) biopsies of large tumours precede excision. Any l suspected of being a sarcoma should not be simply enucleated in what r wrongly be considered a 'conservative' procedure. ►Refer to a specialist.

n or under the skin?

Intradermal	Subcutaneous
• Sebaceous cyst	• Lipoma
• Abscess	• Ganglion
• Dermoid cyst	• Neuroma
• Granuloma	• Lymph node

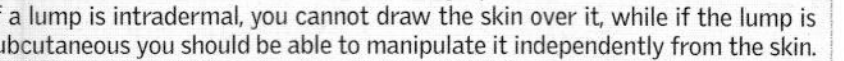

f a lump is intradermal, you cannot draw the skin over it, while if the lump is ubcutaneous you should be able to manipulate it independently from the skin.

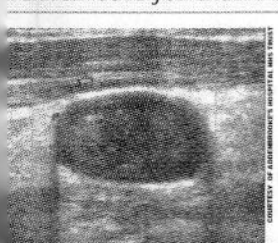

Fig 1. Ultrasound of a malignant lymph node. A sign of malignant infiltration is loss of the fatty hilum. Power Doppler (within the green box) shows loss of the normal hilar vascularity.

'alivary gland pathology

'here are 3 pairs of major salivary glands: parotid, submandibular, and ublingual (there are also numerous minor glands).

listory: Lumps; swelling related to food; pain; taste; dry eyes.

:xamination: Note external swelling; look for secretions; bimanual palpation for tones. Examine VIIth nerve and regional lymph nodes.

:ytology: This may be ascertained by FNA.

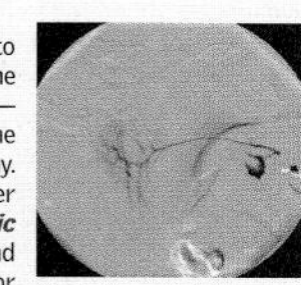

Fig 1. Normal sialogram of the parotid gland. The parotid duct (Stensen's duct) opens into the mouth opposite the 2nd upper molar.

'ecurrent unilateral pain and swelling is likely to e due to a stone. 80% are submandibular. The lassical story is of pain and swelling on eating—vith a red, tender, swollen, but uninfected gland. The tone may be seen on plain x-ray or by sialography. 'istal stones are removed via the mouth but deeper tones may require excision of the gland. ***Chronic ilateral symptoms*** may coexist with dry eyes and 1outh and autoimmune disease, eg Mikulicz's or jögren's syndrome (p698 & p702). ***Fixed swellings*** 1ay be from tumour, sarcoid, or are idiopathic.

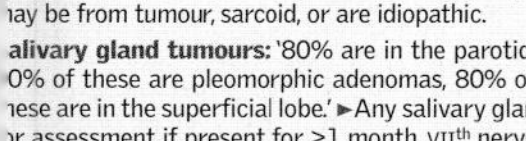

alivary gland tumours: '80% are in the parotid, 0% of these are pleomorphic adenomas, 80% of 1ese are in the superficial lobe.' ►Any salivary gland swelling must be removed)r assessment if present for >1 month. VIIth nerve palsy signifies malignancy.

Benign or malignant	Malignant	Malignant
Cystadenolymphoma	Mucoepidermoid	Squamous or adeno Ca
Pleomorphic adenoma	Acinic cell	Adenoid cystic Ca

leomorphic adenomas often present in middle age and grow slowly. emove by superficial parotidectomy. Adenolymphomas: usually older men; soft; 'eat by enucleation. Carcinomas: rapid growth; hard fixed mass; pain; facial alsy. Treatment: surgery + radiotherapy. Surgery complications:

1 Facial palsy. Have a facial nerve stimulator in theatre to aid identification.
2 Salivary fistula (often close spontaneously).
3 Frey's syndrome (gustatory sweating);[1] interposition of a soft-tissue flap at surgery may be preventative. 201 Tympanic neurectomy may also help.

On eating a lemon wedge, one cheek sweats and flushes (aberrant parasympathetic cholinergic ervation of cutaneous sympathetic receptors)

Lumps in the groin and scrotum

►Any lump within the tunica vaginalis is cancer until proved otherwise.
►Acute, tender enlargement of the testis is torsion (p600) until proved otherwis

Diagnosing groin lumps: See BOX.

Diagnosis of lumps in the scrotum:

1 ***Can you get above it?*** If not, it is an inguinoscrotal hernia (inguinal hernia ex ending into scrotum, p632), or a hydrocoele extending proximally (see belov
2 ***Is it separate from the testis?***
3 ***Is it cystic or solid?*** (Does it transilluminate? See p616.)
- Separate and cystic—epididymal cyst.
- Separate and solid—epididymitis (may also be orchitis).
- Testicular and cystic—hydrocele.
- ► Testicular and solid—**tumour**, orchitis, granuloma (p178), gumma (p41

Ultrasound may help in sorting out testis tumours from other lumps (**fig 1**). Do r assume that an injured testis was normal before the injury: this is not a rare mode tumour presentation; ultrasound may help here.

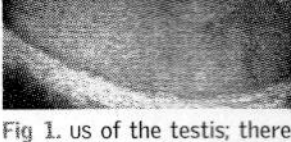
Fig 1. US of the testis; there heterogeneity (arrow) at t lower pole suggesting a tumo

Epididymal cysts usually develop in adulthood and contain clear or milky (spermatcele) fluid. They lie above and behind the testis. Remove if symptomatic.

Hydroceles (fluid within the tunica vaginalis) may be ***primary*** (associated with a patent processus vaginalis, which typically resolves during the 1st year of life) or ***secondary*** to testis tumour, trauma, or infection. Primary hydroceles are more common, larger, and usually develop in younger men. Treat by surgery or aspirati (may need repeating) ►Is the testis normal after aspiration? If *any* doubt, ultrasound.

Epididymo-orchitis Causes: *Chlamydia* (eg if >35yrs); *E. coli*; mumps; *N. gonorrho* TB. The area is usually tender. Take a urine sample; look for urethral discharge '1st catch' may be more helpful than an MSU. Consider a GUM screen. Warn abc possible infertility[202] and that symptoms worsen before they improve. ***R:*** <35yrs; ***doxycycline*** 100mg/12h PO for 10d (covers chlamydia; treat sexual pa ners).[203] If >35yrs old, associated UTI is common so try ***ofloxacin*** 300mg/12h for 10d.[204]

Testis tumours are the commonest malignancies in males aged 15–44. ***Varieti*** Seminoma (30–65yrs);[205] teratoma (20–30yrs); tumours of Sertoli or Leydig ce lymphoma. ~10% of malignancies occur in undescended testes, even af orchidopexy. A contralateral tumour is found in 5%. ***Typical presentation:*** Painl testicular lump, noticed after trauma or infection. ***Risk factors:*** Undescenc testis; infant hernia; infertility. ***Staging*** is essential: 1 No evidence of metastasis Infradiaphragmatic node involvement (spread is via the para-aortic nodes and r inguinal nodes). 3 Supradiaphragmatic node involvement. 4 Lung involveme (haematogenous). ***Tests:*** (To allow staging) CXR, CT, excision biopsy. α-fetoprot (eg >3iu/mL)[1] and β-human chorionic gonadotrophin (β-HCG) are useful tumc markers and help monitor treatment; check **before** and **during** treatme ***Treatment:*** Orchidectomy (inguinal incision; occlude the spermatic cord befc mobilization to ↓risk of intra-operative spread). Options are constantly upda (surgery, radiotherapy, chemotherapy). Seminomas are exquisitely radiosensiti Stage 1 seminomas: orchidectomy + radiotherapy gives a cure rate of ~95%. close follow-up to detect relapse. Cure of teratomas, even if metastases a present, is achieved by 3–4 cycles of ***bleomycin*** + ***etoposide*** + ***cispla*** Prevention of late presentation: self-examination. 5yr survival >90% in all grou

1 AFP is **not** ↑ in pure seminoma; may also be ↑ in: hepatitis, cirrhosis, liver cancer, open neural tube def

›iagnosing groins lumps: lateral to medial thinking

Psoas abscess—may present with back pain, limp and swinging pyrexia
Neuroma of the femoral nerve
Femoral artery aneurysm
Saphena varix—like a hernia, it has a cough impulse
Lymph node
Femoral hernia
Inguinal hernia
Hydrocele or varicocele[1]
›lso consider an undescended testis (cryptorchidism).

›he layers of fascia in the scrotum

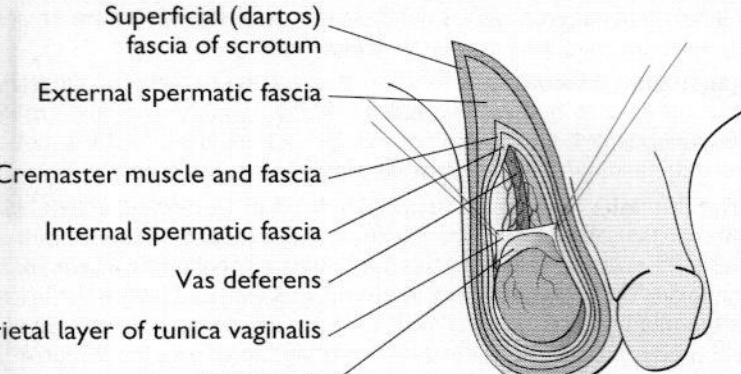

›iagnosis of scrotal masses[1]

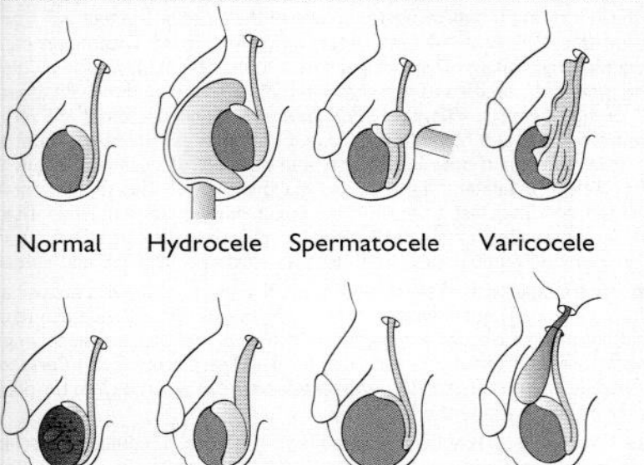

›A varicocele is formed by dilated veins in the pampiniform plexus of the spermatic cord, often visible ›istended scrotal blood vessels that feel like 'a bag of worms'. They are associated with subfertility, but ›ir (via surgery or embolization) seems to have little effect on subsequent pregnancy rates.

Lumps in the neck

►Don't biopsy lumps until tumours within the head and neck have been excluded an ENT surgeon. Culture all biopsied lymph nodes for TB.

Diagnosis First of all, ask how long the lump has been present. If <3wks, se limiting infection is the likely cause and extensive investigation is unwise. Next a yourself where the lump is. Is it intradermal—eg sebaceous cyst with a cent punctum (p616)? Is it a lipoma (p616)? If the lump is not intradermal, and is r of recent onset, you are about to start a diagnostic hunt over complicated terra

Midline lumps: • If patient is <20yrs old, the likely diagnosis is a ***dermoid cy*** (p616). • If it moves **up** on protruding the tongue and is below the hyoid, it is lik to be a ***thyroglossal cyst*** (fluctuant lump developing in cell rests in thyroi migration path; treatment: surgery; they are the commonest congenital cervi cystic lump). • In patients >20yrs old, it is probably a ***thyroid isthmus*** mass. • I is bony hard, the diagnosis may be a ***chondroma***.

Submandibular triangle: (Below jaw; above anterior belly of digastric.) • <20yrs, self-limiting lymphadenopathy is likely. If >20yrs, exclude ***malignc lymphadenopathy*** (eg firm, and non-tender). ►Is TB likely? • If it is not a no think of submandibular ***salivary stone***, ***sialadenitis***, or ***tumour***.

Anterior triangle: (Below digastric and in front of sternocleidomastoid.) Noc are common (see above): examine the areas which they serve (skin, mouth, thro thyroid; is the spleen enlarged?—this may indicate lymphoma). • ***Branchial cys*** emerge under the anterior border of sternocleidomastoid where the upper th meets the middle third (age <20yrs). They are due to non-disappearance of t cervical sinus (where the 2nd branchial arch grows down over the 3rd and 4th). Lir by squamous epithelium, their fluid contains cholesterol crystals. Treat by excisi There may be communication with the pharynx in the form of a fistula. • ***Cys hygromas*** arise from the jugular lymph sac and transilluminate brightly. Treat surgery or hypertonic saline sclerosant injection. Recurrence can be troublesor • If the lump is in the supero-posterior area of the anterior triangle, is it a ***paro tumour*** (more likely if >40yrs)? • ***Laryngoceles*** are an uncommon cause anterior triangle lumps. They are painless and may be made worse by blowi These cysts are classified as external, internal, or mixed, and may be associat with laryngeal cancer. • ***Carotid body tumours*** (chemodectoma) are very ra move from side to side but not up and down, and splay out the carotid bifurcati It is usually firm and occasionally soft and pulsatile. It does not usually cau bruits. It may be bilateral, familial, and malignant (5%). This tumour should suspected in masses just anterior to the upper third of sternomastoid. Diagno either by duplex ultrasonography (looking for splaying at the carotid bifurcation) digital computer angiography. Treatment is extirpation by a vascular surgeon

Posterior triangle: (Behind sternocleidomastoid, in front of trapezius, above clavic • If there are many small lumps, think of ***nodes***—TB, viruses such as HIV or E (infectious mononucleosis), any chronic infection or, if >20yrs, consider lympho or metastases eg from GI or bronchial or head and neck neoplasia.[1] • ***Cervical r*** may intrude into this area. • ***Pharyngeal pouches*** can protrude into the poster triangle on swallowing—see fig 1.

Tests Ultrasound shows lump consistency: cystic, solid, complex, vascular. defines masses in relation to their anatomical neighbours. Do virology and Manto test. CXR may show malignancy or reveal bilateral hilar lymphadenopathy; here y should consider sarcoid. Consider fine-needle aspiration (FNA)—►but remember opening caveat.

See BOX on p617 for ***Salivary gland pathology***.

1 In young Asian women **Kikuchi's disease** (necrotising lymphadenitis) is a rare and benign cause cervical lymphadenopathy. Diagnosis is made on excision biopsy.

he distribution of lymph nodes in the head and neck

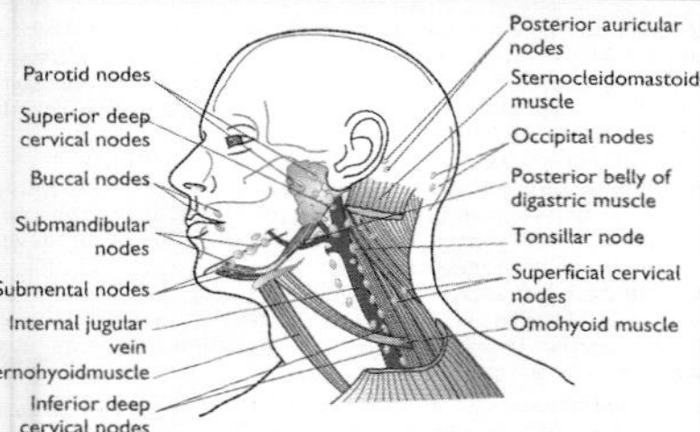

nportant relations to the carotid artery and internal gular vein in the neck

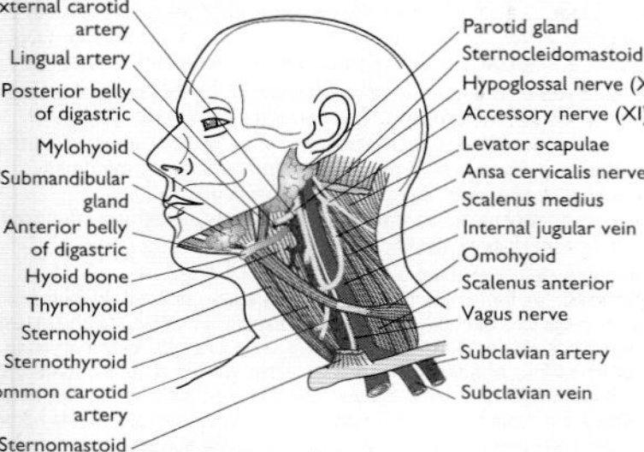

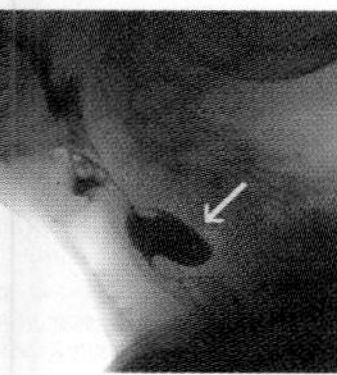

Fig 1. Contrast swallow study showing a pharyngeal pouch (arrow). It is a pulsion diverticulum that protrudes between the fibres of the inferior pharyngeal constrictor muscle. The patient may have a history of halitosis, sore throats and regurgitation of undigested food. As the pouch enlarges, there may be dysphagia as it presses against the oesophagus. These symptoms usually precede a palpable swelling in the neck which, if felt, would emanate from behind the trachea and sternocleidomastoid.

Lumps in the thyroid

Examination Watch the neck whilst the patient swallows water. Stand behind feel thyroid for size, shape (smooth?, one or many nodules?), tenderness, mobility. Ask the patient to swallow again. Percuss for retrosternal extension. lymph nodes or bruits? If the thyroid is enlarged (goitre), ask yourself 3 questic

1 Is the thyroid smooth or nodular?

2 Is the patient euthyroid, thyrotoxic (p202), or hypothyroid (p204)?
Smooth, non-toxic goitre: Endemic (iodine deficiency); congenital; goitrog thyroiditis; physiological; Hashimoto's thyroiditis (an autoimmune dise thought to be due to apoptosis induced by lymphocytes bearing Fas liga combining with thyrocytes bearing Fas).
Smooth, toxic goitre: Graves' disease—see fig 1.

3 Any nodules? Many or one? If >4cm across, malignancy is more likely. *Mu nodular goitre:* Usually euthyroid but hyperthyroidism may deve Hypothyroidism and malignancy are rare.

Single thyroid lump
• Cyst • Adenoma • Malignancy • Discrete nodule in multi-nodular goitre

Single thyroid lump is a common problem; ~10% will be malignant. First ask: Is he/she thyrotoxic? • Do T3 & T4. • Ultrasound (fig 2), to see if the lump is solid, cystic, complex or part of a group of lumps. • Radionuclide scans may show malignant lesions as hypofunctioning or 'cold', whereas a hyper-functioning 'hot' lesion suggests adenoma. • FNA (fine needle aspiration) and do cytology on fluid. ►No clinical/lab test is good enough to tell for sure if follicular neopla found on FNA are benign, so such patients are normally referred for surgery.

What should you do if high-resolution ultrasound shows impalpable nodul
Such thyroid nodules can usually just be observed provided they are:

- <1cm across (which is most; ultrasound can detect lumps <2mm; s 'incidentalomas' occur in 46% of routine autopsies) and asymptomatic.
- There is no past history of thyroid cancer or radiation.
- No family history of medullary cancer. (If any present, do ultrasound-guided excise if cytology is malignant.)

Thyroid neoplasia There are 5 types:

1 ***Papillary:*** 60%. Often in young. Spread: nodes & lung. ℞: total thyroidectom remove non-obvious tumour ± node excision ± radioiodine (^{131}I) to ablate resic cells may all be needed. Give T4 to suppress TSH. Prognosis: better if young &

2 ***Follicular:*** ≤25%. Middle-aged, spreads early via blood (bone, lungs). W differentiated. ℞: total thyroidectomy + T4 suppression + radioiodine ablat

3 ***Medullary:*** 5%. Sporadic (80%) or part of MEN syndrome (p207). May prod calcitonin. They do not concentrate iodine. ►Perform a phaeochromocyto screen pre-op. Do thyroidectomy + node clearance. External beam radiother should be considered to prevent regional recurrence.

4 ***Lymphoma:*** 5%. ♀:♂≈3:1. May present with stridor or dysphagia. Do staging pre-treatment (chemoradiotherapy). Assess histology for mucc associated lymphoid tissue (MALT) origin (associated with a good prognosis

5 ***Anaplastic:*** Rare. ♀:♂≈3:1. Elderly, poor response to any treatment. In absence of unresectable disease, excision + radiotherapy may be tried.

Thyroid surgery *Indications:* Pressure symptoms, hyperthyroidism, carcino cosmetic reasons. Render euthyroid pre-op with antithyroid drugs anc ***propranolol***. Check vocal cords by indirect laryngoscopy pre- and post-op.

Complications: Also see p566. ***Early:*** Recurrent laryngeal nerve pa haemorrhage (►►if compresses airway, instantly remove sutures for evacuatio clot); hypoparathyroidism (check plasma Ca^{2+} daily; there is commonly a trans drop in serum concentration); thyroid storm (symptoms of severe hy thyroidism—treat by ***propranolol*** PO or IV, antithyroid drugs, and iodine, p8 ***Late:*** Hypothyroidism; recurrent hyperthyroidism.

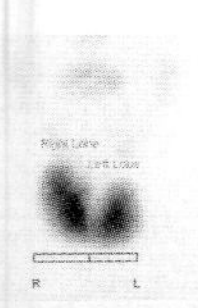

Fig 1. Radionuclide study of the thyroid showing changes consistent with Graves' disease (see also **Nuclear Medicine**, p724). There is increased uptake of the radionuclide trace throughout both lobes of the gland (right>left in this image).

BOTH IMAGES COURTESY OF ADDENBROOKE'S HOSPITAL NHS TRUST

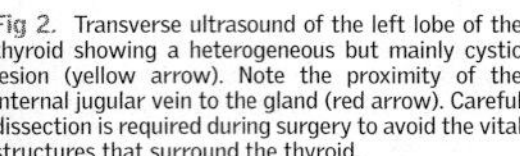

Fig 2. Transverse ultrasound of the left lobe of the thyroid showing a heterogeneous but mainly cystic lesion (yellow arrow). Note the proximity of the internal jugular vein to the gland (red arrow). Careful dissection is required during surgery to avoid the vital structures that surround the thyroid.

'he anatomy of the region of the thyroid gland

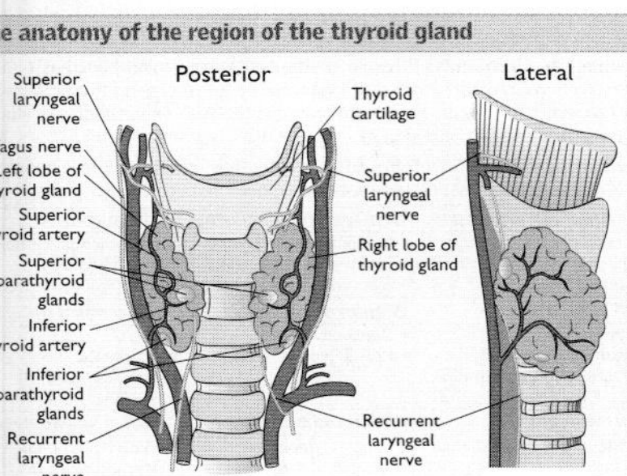

'he important structures that must be considered when operating on the hyroid gland include:

- Recurrent laryngeal nerve
- Superior laryngeal nerve
- Parathyroid glands
- Trachea
- Common carotid artery
- Internal jugular vein (not depicted–see fig 2).

Abdominal masses

As with any mass, determine size, site, shape, and surface. Find out if it is pulsat and if it is mobile. Examine supraclavicular and inguinal nodes. Is the lun ballottable (like bobbing an apple up and down in water)?

Right iliac fossa masses:		
• Appendix mass/abscess • Caecal carcinoma • Crohn's disease • Pelvic mass (see below)	• Intussusception • TB mass • Amoebic abscess • Actinomycosis (p409)	• Transplanted kidney (fig 1 • Kidney malformation • Tumour in an undescended testis

Abdominal distension Flatus, fat, fluid, faeces, or fetus (p52)? Fluid may outside the gut (ascites) or sequestered in bowel (obstruction; ileus). demonstrate ascites elicit signs of a fluid thrill and/or shifting dullness (p41).

Causes of ascites:		*Ascites with portal hypertensio*
• Malignancy★ • Infections★—esp TB • ↓Albumin (eg nephrosis)	• CCF; pericarditis • Pancreatitis★ • Myxoedema	• Cirrhosis • Portal nodes • Budd–Chiari syndrome★ (p688) • IVC or portal vein thrombosis

Tests: Aspirate ascitic fluid (paracentesis, p753) for cytology, culture, & prote level (≥30g/L in diseases marked★) with a 21G needle in RIF (p752); ultrasour Protein level rarely helps diagnostically; it tends to rise with diuretic therapy.

Left upper quadrant mass Is it spleen, stomach, kidney, colon, pancreas, or a ra cause (eg neurofibroma)? Pancreatic cysts may be true (congenital; cystadenom retention cysts of chronic pancreatitis; cystic fibrosis) or pseudocysts (fluid lesser sac from acute pancreatitis).

Splenomegaly Causes are often said to be **infective**, **haematological**, **neoplast** etc., but grouping by **associated feature** is more useful clinically:

Splenomegaly with fever	*With lymphadenopathy*	*With purpura*
• Infection[HS] (malaria, SBE/IE hepatitis,[HS] EBV,[HS] TB, CMV, HIV) • Sarcoid; malignancy[HS]	• Glandular fever[HS] • Leukaemias; lymphoma • Sjögren's syndrome	• Septicaemia; typhus • DIC; amyloid[HS] • Meningococcaemia
With arthritis	***With ascites***	***With a murmur***
• Sjögren's syndrome • Rheumatoid arthritis; SLE • Infection, eg Lyme (p418) • Vasculitis/Behçet's (p542)	• Carcinoma • Portal hypertension[HS]	• SBE/IE • Rheumatic fever • Hypereosinophilia • Amyloid[HS] (p354)
With anaemia	***With weight↓ + CNS signs***	***Massive splenomegal***
• Sickle-cell;[HS] thalassaemia[HS] • Leishmaniasis;[HS] leukaemia[HS] • Pernicious anaemia (p320) • POEM (p204)	• Cancer; lymphoma • TB; arsenic poisoning • Paraproteinaemia[HS]	• Malaria; leishmaniasis • Myelofibrosis; CML[HS] • Gaucher's syndrome[HS]

See webmentorlibrary.com for a full list of causes by any association; HS=causes of hepatosplenomega

Smooth hepatomegaly Hepatitis, CCF, sarcoid, early alcoholic cirrhosis (a sm liver is typical later); tricuspid incompetence (→ pulsatile liver).

Craggy hepatomegaly Secondaries or 1° hepatoma. (Nodular cirrhosis typically causes a small, shrunken liver, not an enlarged craggy one.)

Pelvic masses
• Fibroids • Fetus • Bladder • Ovarian cysts or malignancies

Pelvic masses *Is it truly pelvic?*—Yes, if by palpation you cannot get 'below it'.

Investigating lumps There is much to be said for performing an early ***CT*** to save time and money compared with leaving the test to the last in a long chain. If unavailable, ***ultrasound*** is the first test (transvagi approach may be useful—fig 2). ***Others:*** IVU; liver and spleen radioisotope sca Mantoux test (p386). Routine tests: FBC (with film); ESR; U&E; LFT; proteins; Ca^{2+}; C AXR; biopsy tests—a tissue diagnosis may be made using a fine needle guided ultrasound or CT control. MRI also has a role.

Surgery

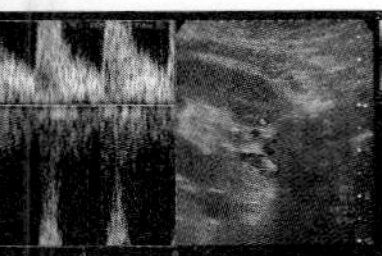

IMAGES COURTESY OF ADDENBROOKE'S HOSPITAL NHS TRUST

Fig 1. Ultrasound of a transplanted kidney with colour duplex imaging (on the right) and Doppler mode (on the left) showing flow in the graft vessels. Vascular thrombosis is a serious early post-operative complications in organ transplantation and ultrasound assessment is an invaluable investigative tool.

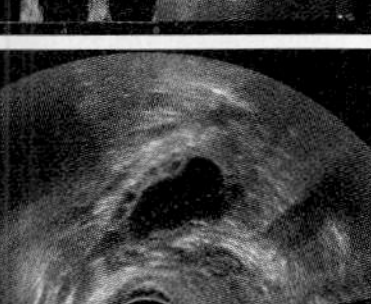

Fig 2. Transvaginal ultrasound showing a cystic lesion in the right ovary. Ovarian masses can grow to fill the abdomen and therefore may be seen in general surgical clinics. The fan shaped view of this ultrasound image is produced by the curved footplate of the probe.

In 1809 an American surgeon by the name of Ephraim McDowell performed an astonishing operation: the first successful elective laparotomy for an abdominal tumour. It was an ovariotomy for an ovarian mass in a 44-year ld who, prior to physical examination by McDowell, was believed to be gravid. ot only was this feat performed in the age before anaesthesia and antisepsis, ut it was also performed on a table in the front room of McDowell's Kentucky ome, at that time on the frontier of the West in the United States. His account the operation makes fascinating reading.[1] Whilst the strength of his agnostic convictions combined with his speed and skill at operating is to be dmired (the operation took 25 minutes), there is an even more laudable part ayed in this story. The patient, Mrs Jane Todd-Crawford, was fully willing to be volved with what can only be described as experimental surgery in the face of ncertainty. She defied pain simply by reciting psalms and hymns, and was back home within 4 weeks with no complications. We would be well served in membering commitment of Mrs Todd-Crawford as most exceptional. In the ush and hurry of our daily tasks perhaps it is all to easy to forget that the ndertaking of surgery today may be no less fear-provoking for patients than it as 200 years ago.

History of Surgery, H. Ellis, Greenwich Medical Media Limited, 2001, ISBN 1841100234

Around the anus

Pruritus ani Itch occurs if the anus is moist or soiled, eg fissures, incontine poor hygiene, tight pants, threadworm, fistula, dermatoses, lichen sclerosis, anx contact dermatitis (eg perfumed goods). ***Treatment:***

- Careful hygiene
- Moist wipe post-defecation
- Try anaesthetic cre
- No spicy food
- No steroid/antibiotic creams
- Capsaicin may help

Fissure-in-ano This is a midline longitudinal split in the squamous lining of lower anal canal—often, if chronic, with a sentinel mucosal tag at the exte aspect. 90% are posterior (anterior ones follow parturition). ♂:♀ is 1>1.

- Most are due to hard faeces, which makes defecation very painful—'like pas glass'. Spasm may constrict the inferior rectal artery, causing ischaemia, ma healing difficult and perpetuating the problem.[209]
- Rare causes (multiple ± lateral): Syphilis; herpes; trauma; Crohn's; anal Ca; psori
- Examine with a bright light. Do a PR ± sigmoidoscopy, if tolerated. Groin nc suggest a complicating factor (eg immunosuppression from HIV).
- Try 5% ***lidocaine*** ointment, extra dietary roughage and fluids + good anal tc ***Glyceryl trinitrate*** (GTN) ointment (0.2–0.3%) relieves pain and ischae caused by chronic fissures and spasm, and can prevent need for surgery, but cause headache. Trials suggest that ***botulinum toxin*** injection (eg 20U) is r effective than GTN.[210] If conservative measures fail, try day-case ***lateral par internal sphincterotomy***; ***manual anal dilatation*** (under GA) is also used, has fallen out of favour due to the greater risk of post-op anal incontinenc Pre-operative assessment with anorectal ultrasound and manometry recommended, especially for postpartum fissures.

Fistula-in-ano The fistula track communicates between the skin and the anal c or rectum. Blockage of deep intramuscular gland ducts is thought to predispos abscess formation, which then discharge to form the fistula. ***Goodsall's*** determines the path of the fistula track between openings: if anterior, the tra in a straight line; if posterior, the internal opening is **always** at the 6 'o' c position. ***Causes:*** Abscesses (see below); Crohn's disease, TB, diverticular dise ***Tests:*** MRI;[212] endoanal US scan.[213] ***Treatment:*** Fistulotomy + excision if ≤low tr sphincteric; tight or loose seton insertion. Staged sphincter repair may be requ

Anorectal abscesses are usually caused by gut organisms (rarely staphs or ♂:♀≈1.8. ***Location:*** Perianal (~45%), ischiorectal (≤30%), intersphincteric (>2 supralevator (~5%). Redness and swelling may spread well into the buttock. PR be too painful. Do incision & drainage, eg under GA (+ fistulotomy if, eg in Crc disease). ***Associations:*** DM, Crohn's, malignancy. Don't rely on antibiotics.

The perianal haematoma (also called a thrombosed external pile—see BOX, p6 Strictly, both names are wrong because it is actually a clotted venous saccul appears as a 2–4mm 'dark blue berry' under the skin. It may be evacuated v small incision under local anaesthesia or left alone if present for >1d.

Pilonidal sinus Obstruction of natal cleft hair follicles ~6cm above the anus, ingrowing of hair, excites a foreign body reaction, and may cause dev secondary tracks which open laterally ± abscesses, with foul-smelling disch (Barbers get these sinuses between their fingers.) ♂:♀≈10:1. ***Treatmen*** excision of the sinus tract ± primary closure, but is unsatisfactory in 10%. Cons pre-op ***cefuroxime*** 1.5g + ***metronidazole*** 500mg IV. Complex tracks can be open and packed individually, or skin flaps can be used to cover the defect.

Rectal prolapse The mucosa, or rectum in all its layers, may descend througl anus. This leads to incontinence in 75%. It is due to a lax sphincter and prolo straining. ***Treatment*** is by fixing the rectum to the sacrum (rectopexy) ± r insertion ± rectosigmoidectomy, or encircling the anus with a Thiersch wire.

Anal ulcers are rare. Consider Crohn's disease, anal cancer, TB, and syphilis.

Skin tags seldom cause trouble but are easily excised. **Piles** See p628.

[E]xamination of the rectum and anus

[I]t is necessary to have a chaperone present for the examination. Explain what [yo]u are about to do. Make sure curtains are pulled and doors are closed. The [pa]tient (and passers-by!) will appreciate it. Have the patient on his left side, his [kn]ees brought up towards the chest. Use gloves and lubricant. Part the buttocks [an]d inspect the anus. Press your index finger against the side of the anus. Ask [th]e patient to breathe deeply and insert your finger slowly; press with the pad [of] the finger first then twist and push in the tip. Feel for masses (haemorrhoids [ar]e not palpable) or impacted stool. Twist your arm so that the pad of your [fin]ger is feeling anteriorly. Feel for the cervix or prostate. Note consistency and [si]ze of prostate. Obliteration of its midline sulcus is a sign (unreliable) of [pr]ostate cancer. If there is a concern about the spinal cord, ask the patient to [sq]ueeze your finger and note the tone; also check perineal sensation. Note stool [or] blood on the glove and test for occult blood. Wipe the anus. Consider [pr]octoscopy (for the anus) or sigmoidoscopy (which mainly inspects the [re]ctum).

[A]natomy of the anal canal

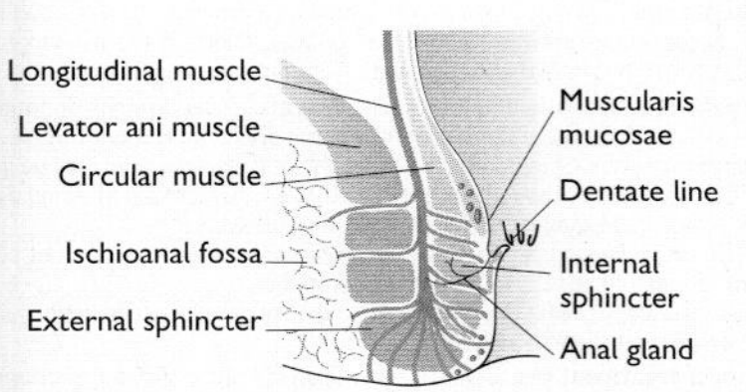

[A]nal cancer

[U]K *incidence:* 300/yr. ***Risk↑:*** Syphilis, anal warts (HPV 16, 6, 11, & 18 implicated), [an]oreceptive homosexuals (often young). ***Histology:*** Squamous cell (80%); [ra]rely basaloid, melanoma, or adenocarcinoma. ***The patient*** may present with [bl]eeding, pain, bowel habit change, pruritus ani, masses, stricture. ***ΔΔ:*** Condyl[om]a acuminata (warts[1]) or lata (syphilis, p419); leucoplakia; lichen sclerosis; [Bo]wen's disease; Crohn's disease. ***Treatment:*** Radiotherapy + ***5-fluorouracil*** + [m]***itomycin/cisplatin*** is usually preferred to anorectal excision & colostomy; 75% [re]tain normal anal function.[216]

[1 Pi]nk or grey soft, moist, cauliflower-like papules on moist surfaces with many discrete projections on a [broa]d base—or just simple small bumps. Confluent nodules (giant *condylomata acuminata* of Buschke & [Lo]wenstein) may evolve into verrucous cancers (a low grade non-metastasizing squamous type).

Haemorrhoids (piles)

The anus is lined mainly by discontinuous masses of spongy vascular tissue–anal cushions, which contribute to anal closure. Viewed from the lithot position, their positions are at 3, 7, & 11 o'clock. They are attached by smo muscle and elastic tissue, but are prone to displacement and disruption, ei singly or together. The effects of gravity (our erect posture), increased anal (?stress), and the effects of straining at stool may make them become both b and loose, and so to protrude to form piles (Latin *pila*, meaning a ball). They vulnerable to trauma and bleed readily from the capillaries of the underl lamina propria, hence their other name, haemorrhoids, (≈*running blood* in Gre Because loss is from capillaries, it is bright red. NB: Piles are **not** varicose vei

As there are no sensory fibres above the dentate line (squamomucosal junct piles are not painful unless they thrombose when they protrude and are grippe the anal sphincter, blocking venous return.

Differential diagnosis: Perianal haematoma; anal fissure; abscess; tum *proctalgia fugax* (idiopathic, intense, stabbing rectal pain). ►Never ascribe re bleeding to piles without adequate examination or investigation.

Causes Constipation with prolonged straining is a key factor. In many the bo habit may be normal. Congestion from a pelvic tumour, pregnancy, CCF, or po hypertension are important in only a minority of cases.

Pathogenesis There is a vicious circle: vascular cushions protrude through a t anus, become more congested, so hypertrophying to protrude again more rea These protrusions may then strangulate. See TABLE for classification.

The patient notices bright red rectal bleeding, often coating stools or dripping the pan after defecation. There may be mucous discharge and *pruritus ani*. Se anaemia may occur. Symptoms such as weight loss, tenesmus and change in bo habit should prompt thoughts of other pathology. In all rectal bleeding do:

- An abdominal examination to rule out other diseases.
- PR exam: prolapsing piles are obvious. Internal haemorrhoids are not palpa
- Proctoscopy to see the internal haemorrhoids.
- Sigmoidoscopy to identify rectal pathology higher up (you can get no highe than the rectosigmoid junction).

The best treatment Unknown, as meta-analyses differ. ***Infra-red coagula*** applied for 1.5–2s, 3–8 times to localized areas of piles works by coagula vessels, and tethering mucosa to subcutaneous tissue. Doing all the piles may a few sessions. ***Sclerosants:*** 2mL of 5% ***phenol*** in oil is injected into the pile ab the dentate line; SE: impotence; prostatitis). ***Rubber band ligation:*** SE: bleed infection. Do <3 band-treatments per session; a cheap treatment, but needs Banding produces an ulcer to anchor the mucosa (SE: bleeding, infection; pa infra-red coagulation is as successful and may be less painful).[RCT 217] ***Cryother*** (freezing) is also used but can produce a lot of watery discharge after procedure. A high-fibre diet may also help.

In all but 4th degree piles, these measures may obviate need for ***haem rhoidectomy*** (excision of piles ± ligation of vascular pedicles, as day-case surg needing ~2wks off work). SE: haemorrhage or stenosis. Stapled haemorrhoidect may result in less pain, a shorter hospital stay and quicker return to normal act than conventional surgery, provided the surgeon has the technical experience 1 week's ***lactulose*** + ***metronidazole*** (p371) starting pre-op reduces pain and off work.[RCT 219]

Complications: Constipation; infection; stricture; bleeding.

Prolapsed, thrombosed piles are treated with analgesia, ice packs and bed Pain usually resolves in 2–3 weeks and surgery is seldom necessary.

assification of haemorrhoids

st-degree	Remain in the rectum
nd-degree	Prolapse through the anus on defecation but spontaneously reduce
rd-degree	As for second-degree but require digital reduction
th-degree	Remain persistently prolapsed

ternal and external haemorrhoids

External haemorrhoid

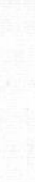

Origin below dentate line (external rectal plexus)

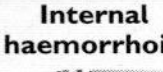

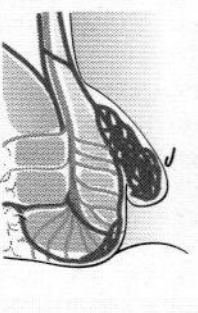

Origin above dentate line (internal rectal plexus)

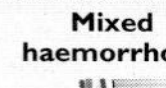

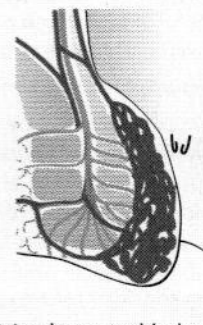

Origin above and below dentate line (internal and external rectal plexus)

AFTER CRAIG, J.A., NOVARTIS

hen 'thrombosed', an external pile is also sometimes (wrongly) called a rianal haematoma—see p626.

Definition Any structure passing through another so ending up in the wrong is a **hernia**. Hernias involving bowel are said to be **irreducible** if they cann pushed back into the right place. This does not mean that they are e necessarily obstructed or strangulated. **Incarceration** implies that the conter the hernial sac are stuck inside by adhesions. Gastrointestinal hernias **obstructed** if bowel contents cannot pass through them—the classical featu intestinal obstruction soon appear (p598). They are **strangulated** if ischa occurs—the patient becomes toxic and requires urgent surgery. Care mus taken when attempting reduction (see p632 for the technique) as it is possib perform **reduction *en masse***, pushing the strangulated bowel and hernial sac into the abdominal cavity, but giving the initial appearance of successful redu

Inguinal hernia The commonest kind, described on p632.

Femoral hernia Bowel enters the femoral canal, presenting as a mass in the u medial thigh or above the inguinal ligament where it points down the leg, unli inguinal hernia which points to the groin. They occur as often in women than (inguinal hernias are far more common in men) and are likely to be irreducible to strangulate. ***Anatomy:*** The neck of the hernia is felt inferior and lateral t pubic tubercle (inguinal hernias are superior and medial to this point). boundaries of the femoral canal are **anteriorly** and **medially** the inguinal ligar **laterally** the femoral vein and **posteriorly** the pectineal ligament and pecti The canal contains fat and Cloquet's node. ***Treatment:*** Repair is recommen

Surgery

Paraumbilical hernias These occur just above or below the umbilicus. Risk fa are obesity and ascites. Omentum or bowel herniates through the defect. Su involves repair of the rectus sheath. Also see BOX.

Epigastric hernias These pass through *linea alba* above the umbilicus.

Incisional hernias These follow breakdown of muscle closure after pre surgery (seen in 11–20%). If obese, repair is not easy. A randomized trial of re favoured mesh over suture techniques. RCT 220

Spigelian hernias These occur at the lateral edge of the rectus sheath, below lateral to the umbilicus.

Lumbar hernias These occur through 1 of the 2 lumbar triangles.

Richter's hernia This involves bowel wall only—not the whole lumen.

Maydl's hernia This involves a herniating 'double loop' of bowel. The strangu portion may reside as a single loop **inside** the abdominal cavity.

Littre's hernia This is a hernial sac containing a strangulated Meckel's divertic

Obturator hernias These occur through the obturator canal. Typically there is along the medial side of the thigh in a thin woman.

Other examples of hernias:

- Of the nucleus pulposus into the spinal canal (slipped disc).
- Of the uncus and hippocampal gyrus through the tentorium (tentorial hern space-occupying lesions.
- Of the brainstem and cerebellum through the foramen magnum (Arnold–C malformation, p686).
- Of the stomach through the diaphragm (hiatus hernia, p236).
- Of the terminal (intravesical) portion of the ureter into the bladder, with c ballooning between the mucosa and muscle layers. This is a ***ureterocele*** (*k* Greek for hernia), and results from stenosis of the ureteral meatus. Causes be congenital (eg persistence of Chawalla's membrane), or rarely schistoson or phaeochromocytoma. This intra-bladder hernia may cause obstruction ± or even herniate into the urethra and present as an interlabial mass. Mar ment may involve endoscopic meatotomy or ureterocelectomy ± reimplant

me examples of hernias

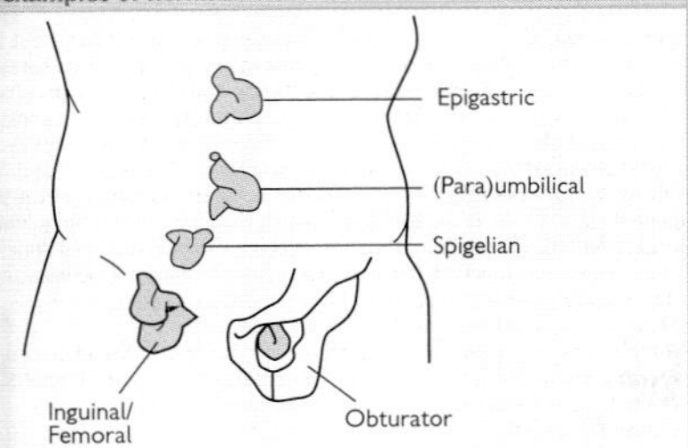

dominal wall defects in children (see OHCS, p130)

ring embryonic development, the testis is led down from its original position on ɜ posterior abdominal wall into the scrotum by the gubernaculum. If the nnection between the peritoneal cavity and the tunica vaginalis fails to close hind the testis, then there is a ***patent processus vaginalis***. It is through this at an indirect inguinal hernia occurs. About 4% of all male infants have an direct inguinal hernia (prematurity is a risk factor), whereas it is very common in female infants and, if found, should prompt thoughts of testicular ninisation. If the patent *processus vaginalis* contains peritoneal fluid only, then is a ***communicating hydrocele***. Repair is the same for both, involving high ation and division of the protruding peritoneal sac. Reinforcement of the sterior wall (eg with a mesh) is not required because the internal ring has not en chronically dilated.

True umbilical hernias (3% of live births) are a result of a persistent defect the transversalis fascia—the umbilical ring, through which the umbilical ssels passed to reach the foetus—whereas ***paraumbilical hernias*** are found in ults in a canal bordered by the umbilical fascia posteriorly, the linea alba teriorly and the rectus sheath laterally. True umbilical hernias can recur in ulthood eg in pregnancy (3rd trimester) or gross ascites (fig 2, p253). Surgical oair is rarely needed in children (3 in 1000) as most resolve by the age of 3.

Protrusion of the abdominal contents through a defect in the anterior dominal wall to the right of the umbilicus is seen in ***gastroschisis***, with the otruding bowel covered by a thin 'peel'. Prompt surgical repair is performed ter fluid resuscitation. Concomitant congenital abnormalities are rare.

Exomphalos (also called ***omphalocele***),[1] however, is associated with other ngenital abnormalities, such as anencephaly, cardiac defects, hydrocephalus d spina bifida. In this condition the abdominal contents are found outside the domen, covered in a three layer membrane consisting of peritoneum, harton's jelly and amnion. Surgical repair is less urgent than in gastroschisis cause the bowel is protected by these membranes. The challenge of surgery is fit the contents back into the relatively small abdominal cavity without mpromising venous return and lung ventilation. ***Meckel's diverticulum:*** p698.

1e *omphalos* is the centre-stone at the Temple of Apollo in Delphi, centre of the ancient world—hence mbilical association. Here Apollo persuaded Pan (the god of wild places, music, and syrinxes, p508) veal the art of prophesy, without which we would be without our most mysterious tool: *prognosis*.

Inguinal hernias

Indirect hernias pass through the internal inguinal ring and, if large, out thro the external ring—see BOX, p631 for the embryological story. Direct hernias p their way directly forward through the posterior wall of the inguinal canal, in defect in the abdominal wall. Predisposing conditions: chronic cough, constipat urinary obstruction, heavy lifting, ascites, previous abdominal surgery (eg dam to the iliohypogastric nerve during appendicectomy). There are 2 landmarks identify: ***The internal ring*** may be defined as being the **mid-point of the ingui ligament**, ~1½ cm above the femoral pulse (which crosses the **mid-inguinal poi** ***The external ring*** is a split in the external oblique aponeurosis just superior medial to the pubic tubercle (the bony prominence forming the medial attachm of the inguinal ligament). Relations of the inguinal canal are:

- ***Floor:*** Inguinal ligament and lacunar ligament medially.
- ***Roof:*** Fibres of transversalis, internal oblique and conjoint tendon medially.
- ***Front:*** External oblique aponeurosis + internal oblique for the lateral ⅓.
- ***Back:*** Laterally, transversalis fascia; medially, conjoint tendon.
- ***Contents:*** see BOX.

Examination Look for previous scars; feel the other side; examine the exte genitalia. Then ask: • Is the lump visible? If so, ask the patient to reduce it—i cannot, make sure that it is not a scrotal lump. Ask him to cough. Inguinal her appear inferomedial to the external ring. • If no lump is visible, feel for a co impulse. • Repeat the examination with the patient standing. ***Distinguishing dir from indirect hernias:*** This is loved by examiners but is of little clinical use— least because repair is the same for both (see below). The best way is to reduce hernia and occlude the internal ring with two fingers. Ask the patient to coug stand—if the hernia is restrained, it is indirect, if it pops out, it is direct.

Indirect hernias:	*Direct hernias:*	*Femoral hernias:*
• Common (80%)	• Less common (20%)	• More frequent in females
• Can strangulate	• Reduce easily	• Frequently irreducible
	• Rarely strangulate	• Frequently strangulate

Irreducible hernias You may be called because a long-standing hernia is n irreducible and painful. It is always worth trying to reduce these yourself- prevent strangulation and bowel necrosis (a grave event, demanding pror laparotomy). Learn how to do this from an expert—ie one of your patients who been reducing his hernia for years—then you will be well-equipped to act corre when the incipient emergency presents. Notice that such patients use the fla the hand, directing the hernia from below, up towards the contralateral shoul Sometimes, as the hernia obstructs, reduction requires perseverance, which ma rewarded by a gurgle from the retreating bowel and a kiss from the attend spouse who had thought that surgery was inevitable.

Repairs Advise to diet (if over-weight) and stop smoking pre-op. Mesh techniq (eg Lichtenstein repair) have replaced older methods such as the 'Shouldice' rep with its multilayered suture involving both anterior and posterior walls of inguinal canal. In mesh repairs, a polypropylene mesh reinforces the posterior w Recurrence rate is less than with other methods (eg <2% *vs* 10%). Lo anaesthetic techniques and day-case 'ambulatory' surgery may halve the price surgery. This is important because this is one of the most common operati (>100,000 per year in the UK). ***Laparoscopic repair*** is also possible, and gi similar recurrence rates, but is not currently recommended as standard practice Benefits include less post-operative pain, an earlier return to work indentification of undiagnosed contralateral hernias, though the set-up may c more than conventional surgery (p640).

Return to work: We used to advise 4wks' rest and convalescence over 10w but with new mesh (or laparoscopic) repairs, if comfortable, return to manual w (& driving) after ≤2wks is OK; explain this pre-operatively.

e anatomy of the inguinal canal

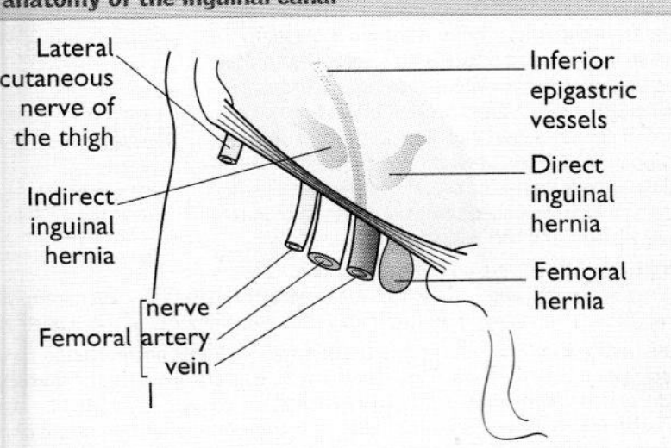

guinal hernia mesh repair

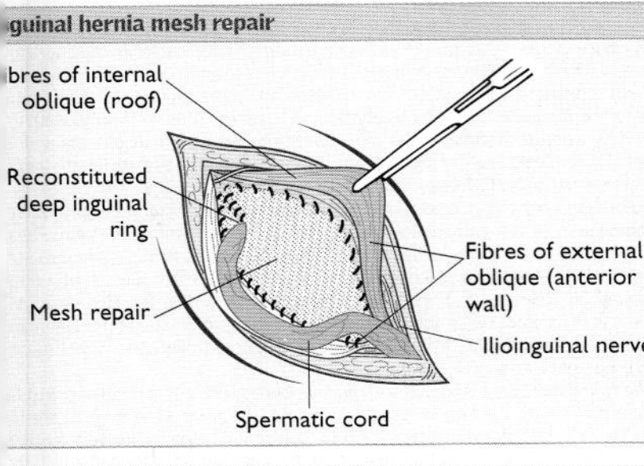

e contents of the inguinal canal in the male

The cremasteric fascia and internal spermatic fascia
The spermatic cord:
- Vas deferens, obliterated processus vaginalis, and lymphatics
- Arteries to the vas, cremaster, and the testis
- The pampiniform plexus and the venous equivalent of the above
- The genital branch of the genitofemoral nerve and sympathetic nerves

The ilioinguinal nerve, which enters the inguinal canal via the anterior wall and runs anteriorally to the cord.

B: In the female the round ligament of the uterus is in place of the male tructures. A hydrocele of the Canal of Nuck is the female equivalent of a ydrocele of the cord.

Varicose veins (VVS)

Primary causes (95%)
• Unknown
• Congenital valve absence (very rare)
Secondary causes (5
• Obstruction: DVT, fetus, ovarian tumour
• Valve destruction: DV
• Arteriovenous malformation (↑pressure

Blood from superficial veins of the leg passes into the deep veins by means of perforator veins (perforating deep fascia) and at the sapheno femoral and sapheno-popliteal junctions. Valves prevent blood from passing from deep to superficial veins. If they become incompetent there is venous hypertension and dilatation (**varicosities**) of the superficial veins occurs. Risk factors include prolonged standing, obesity, pregnancy, family history, and the 'pill'.[223]

Symptoms 'My legs are ugly'. Note that pain, cramps, tingling, heaviness, and restless legs are often attributed to VVS, but careful stud show these common symptoms are only slightly commoner in those with VVS.

Signs Oedema; eczema; ulcers; haemosiderin skin staining; haemorrhage; phlebi *atrophie blanche* (white scarring around a healing ulcer); lipodermatosclerosis (s hardness from subcutaneous fibrosis caused by chronic inflammation and necrosis). On their own VVS don't cause DVTs (***proximally spreading phlebitis*** the long saphenous vein in the thigh may be an exception).

Method of examination (Start with the patient standing.)

1 Note signs of poor skin nutrition: ulcers usually above the medial malleo (varicose ulcers, *OHCS* p604) with deposition of haemosiderin causing brov edges, eczema, and thin skin. Inspect the legs from anterior thigh to medial c (long saphenous vein) and the back of the calf (short saphenous vein). Palpa veins for tenderness (due to phlebitis) and hardness (due to thrombosis).

2 Feel for a ***cough impulse*** at the sapheno femoral junction (≈ incompetence). ***T percussion test:*** Tap the top of a vein and feel how far down its length you c feel repercussions (interrupted by competent valves).

3 ***Trendelenburg's test*** assesses if the saphenofemoral junction (SFJ) valve competent: lie the patient down and raise the leg to empty the vein. Place fingers on the SFJ (5cm below and medial to femoral pulse). Ask him to sta keeping the fingers in place. If the varicosities are controlled, they will r rapidly fill. Release the fingers to confirm that they then fill. This shows th there is SF incompetence and the operation of SF disconnection (Trendelenbur operation) should help. If the varicosities are not controlled, then there must incompetence at a lower level.

4 ***The tourniquet test*** is similar to Trendelenburg's test, but instead of controlli varicosities with the fingers, use a tourniquet tied around the thigh at the lev of the SFJ. If the varicosities are not controlled, repeat the test with t tourniquet just above and then just below the knee, until the level at which the is incompetence is identified.

5 ***Perthes' test*** determines if the deep femoral veins are competent. With t patient standing and veins filled, a tourniquet is placed around the mid-thigh a the patient walks for 5min. If the saphenous veins collapse below the tourniqu the deep veins are patent and the communicating veins are competent; unchanged, both saphenous and communicating veins are incompetent; if t veins increase in prominence and pain occurs, the deep veins are occluded.

6 ***Doppler ultrasound probes*** have overtaken the above tests. They listen for flo in incompetent valves, eg the SFJ, or the short saphenous vein behind the knee (t calf is squeezed: flow on release lasting over ½–1 second indicates significa reflux). If incompetence is not identified and treated, varicosities will return.

►Before surgery and after venous mapping, ensure that all varicosities are indelib marked **to either side** (to avoid tattooing if the incision is made through inked skin).

Saphena varix This is a dilatation (varicosity) in the saphenous vein at i confluence with the femoral vein (the SFJ). It is one of the many causes of a lump the groin (p619). Because it transmits a cough impulse, it may be mistaken for a inguinal or femoral hernia, but on closer inspection it may have a bluish tinge.

The superficial veins of the leg

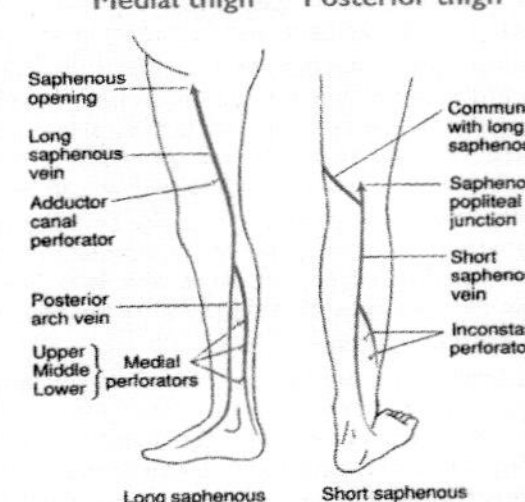

Treating varicose veins

►NICE guidelines suggest that the criteria for specialist referral of patients with VVs should be bleeding, pain, ulceration, superficial thrombophlebitis, or 'a severe impact on quality of life'.

- ***Education:*** Avoid prolonged standing; support stockings (compliance is a problem); lose weight; regular walks (calf muscle action aids venous return).
- ***Injection sclerotherapy:*** Especially for varicosities below the knee if there is no gross sapheno-femoral incompetence. Sclerosant (eg ***ethanolamine***) is injected at multiple sites and the vein compressed for a few weeks to avoid thrombosis (intravascular granulation tissue obliterates the lumen). It is unsuitable for perforation sites. A novel development of this technique involves mixing the sclerosant with air to form a foam that is injected at a single site, and spreads rapidly throughout the veins. Ultrasound monitoring prevents inadvertent spread of foam into the femoral vein.[224]
- ***Surgery:*** There are several choices, depending on vein anatomy and surgical preference, eg saphenofemoral ligation; multiple avulsions; stripping from groin to upper calf (stripping to the ankle is not needed, and may damage the saphenous nerve). ***Post-op:*** Bandage legs tightly, and elevate for 24h. Then encourage regular walking eg 3miles/d, taken as many short walks. Surgery is more effective than sclerotherapy in the long-term.[225]

When do varicose veins become an illness?

The obvious answer is that they do so when they hurt, but for some patients, this is too simple. Thanks to Albert Camus, we know that 'certain illnesses are desirable: they provide a compensation for a functional disorder which, in their absence, would express itself in a more serious disturbance'; this is common with VVs.[226] Perhaps many opt for surgery as a displacement activity to confronting deeper problems. ►We adopt the sickness role when we want sympathy. Somatization is hard to manage: here is one general approach to consider: Give time; don't dismiss these patients as 'just the "worried well"'.

- Explore the factors perpetuating illness behaviour (disordered physiology, misinformation, unhelpful 'coping' behaviour, social stressors).
- Agree a plan that makes sense to the patient's holistic view of himself.

Treat any underlying depression (drugs & cognitive therapy, OHCS p372).

Surgery

Gastric surgery and its aftermath

►Indications for gastric surgery include gastric cancer (p614) and peptic ul[c]er though medical therapy (p234) has made elective surgery for the latter rare.

Operations for benign gastric ulceration Those near the pylorus may [be] considered similarly to duodenal ulceration (p638). Away from the pylorus, elec[tive] operation is rarely needed as ulcers respond well to medical treatment, stop[ping] smoking, and avoidance of NSAIDs. In patients who are unable to tolerate med[ical] treatment, a laparoscopic highly selective vagotomy (HSV) can be done (p6[38]).

►►***Emergency surgery*** may be needed for haemorrhage or perforation. Haem[or]rhage is usually treated by underrunning the bleeding ulcer base or excision of [the] ulcer. If the former is done, then a biopsy should be taken to exclude maligna[ncy]. Perforation is usually managed by excision of the hole for histology, then clos[ure].

Operations for duodenal ulceration See p638.

Gastric carcinoma Localized disease may be treated by curative gastrecto[my]: either D_1 resection (excision of tumour and perigastric nodes) or D_2 resec[tion] (basically a D_1 resection extended to include nodes around the coeliac axis—BOX for the lymphatic drainage of the stomach). There is considerable controve[rsy] as to which should be performed, as some studies have shown worse morbidity [and] mortality for D_2 resections performed in Western countries. It is likely that [these] results reflect the lack of dedicated specialists such as those in Japan, wh[ere] gastric carcinoma is particularly common. D_2 resections should therefore only [be] performed in specialist centres. MET 227

Partial gastrectomy (the Billroth operations—see BOX)

- ***Billroth I:*** Partial gastrectomy with simple re-anastomosis (rejoining).
- ***Billroth II (Polya gastrectomy):*** Partial gastrectomy. The duodenal stum[p is] oversewn (leaving a blind loop), and anastomosis is achieved by a longitudi[nal] incision further down (into the proximal jejunum).

Physical complications of gastrectomy and peptic ulcer surgery

►As peptic ulcer surgery is largely obsolete, these complications are mainly [of] historical interest only.

- ***Recurrent ulceration:*** Symptoms are similar to those experienced p[re]operatively but complications are more common and response to medi[cal] treatment is poor. Further surgery is difficult.
- ***Abdominal fullness:*** Feeling of early satiety (± discomfort and distensio[n]) improving with time. Advise to take small, frequent meals.
- ***Bilious vomiting:*** This is difficult to treat—but often improves with time.
- ***Diarrhoea:*** May be disabling after vagotomy. ***Codeine phosphate*** may help.
- ***Gastric tumour:*** A rare complication of any surgery which ↓acid productio[n].
- ***Amylase↑:*** If with abdominal pain, this may indicate afferent loop obstructi[on] after Billroth II surgery and requires emergency surgery. 228

Metabolic complications

- ***Dumping syndrome:*** 229 Fainting and sweating after eating due to food of hi[gh] osmotic potential being dumped in the jejunum, causing oligaemia from rap[id] fluid shifts. 'Late dumping' is due to rebound hypoglycaemia and occurs 1–[3h] after meals. Both tend to improve with time but may be helped by eating le[ss] sugar, and more guar and pectin (slows glucose absorption). ***Acarbose*** may al[so] help to reduce the early hyperglycemic stimulus to insulin secretion. 230
- ***Weight loss:*** Often due to poor calorie intake.
- ***Bacterial overgrowth ± malabsorption*** (blind loop syndrome) may occur.
- ***Anaemia:*** Usually from lack of iron hypochlorhydria and stomach resection. B[12] levels are frequently low but megaloblastic anaemia is rare.
- ***Osteomalacia:*** There may be pseudofractures which look like metastases.

Surgery

›mplications of peptic ulcer surgery

	Partial gastrectomy	Vagotomy & pyloroplasty	Highly selective vagotomy
›currence	2%	7%	>7%
›mping	20%	14%	6%
›arrhoea	1%	4%	<1%
›etabolic	++++	++	0

›ese values are approximate and depend on the skill of the surgeon.)

›e Billroth operations

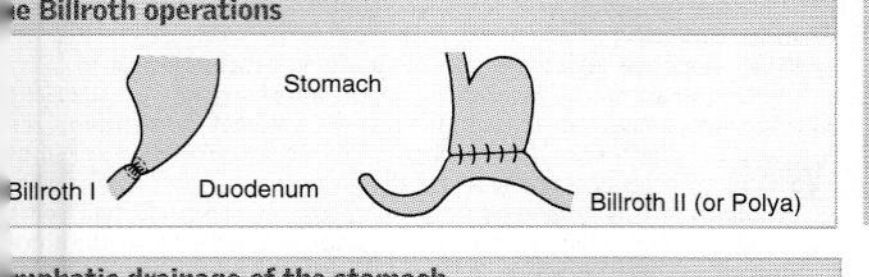

›mphatic drainage of the stomach

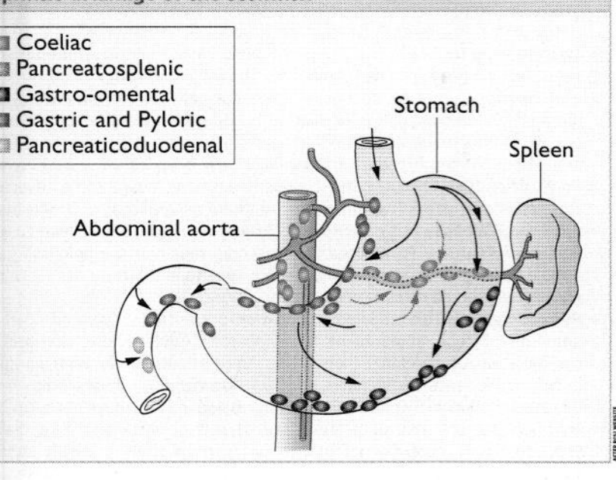

Theodor Billroth was a surgeon of German-Austrian origin, whose name lives on as a set of operations on the stomach (see BOX, The Billroth operations). He was a pioneer of abdominal surgery and the use of aseptic ›chniques, performing the first Billroth I procedure in 1881 for the resection ›f a pyloric gastric carcinoma. Among the many of his remarkable achievements included the first laryngectomy. He was also a talented musician (a close ›iend of Brahms) and a dedicated educator with something of a realist's view ›f the world:

›he pleasure of a physician is little, the gratitude of patients is rare, and even ›rer is material reward, but these things will never deter the student who feels ›e call within him. Theodor Billroth (1829–94) 231 232

Operations for peptic ulcers

Peptic ulcers usually present as epigastric pain and dyspepsia (p234). There is reliable method of distinguishing clinically between gastric and duodenal ulce Although management of both is usually medical in the 1st instance (eg with *pylori* eradication, p235), surgery still has a role.

Surgery is usually only required for complications such as ***haemorrhag perforation***, and ***pyloric stenosis***, though may be considered for the f patients who are not responsive to or tolerant of medical therapy.

Several types of operation have been tried but, as whenever considering operation, one must consider efficacy, side-effects, and mortality.

1 **Elective surgery:**
- ***Highly selective vagotomy:*** May be useful in patients unable to toler medical treatment. The vagus supply is denervated only where it supplies t lower oesophagus and stomach. The nerve of Latarget to the pylorus is l intact; thus, gastric emptying is unaffected (see BOX). The results of surg are greatly dependent on the skill of the surgeon.
- ***Vagotomy and pyloroplasty:*** A vagotomy reduces acid production from t stomach body and fundus, and reduces gastrin production from the antru However, it interferes with emptying of the pyloric sphincter and so a draina procedure (eg pyloroplasty) must be added. This operation is now alm obsolete, and is only performed in exceptional circumstances.
- ***Gastrectomy*** (p636) is rarely required (eg Zollinger–Ellison syndrome, p7C

2 **Emergency surgery** may be required for the following complications:
- ***Haemorrhage*** may be controlled endoscopically by ***adrenaline*** injecti diathermy, laser coagulation, or heat probe. Operation should be considered severe haemorrhage or rebleeding, especially in the elderly—see p246 indications. At surgery, the bleeding ulcer base is underrun or oversewn.
- ***Perforation*** (Fig 1) Most patients undergo surgery, though some advocate initial conservative approach in patients without generalized peritonitis (NBM, tube, IV antibiotics—this can prevent surgery in up to 50% of such cases) emergency surgery is required, laparoscopic repair of the hole will usua suffice (though has a worse recurrence rate than open repair). *H. pyl* eradication should be commenced post-op (p234).
- ***Pyloric stenosis*** This is a late complication, presenting with vomiting of la amounts of food some hours after meals. (Adult pyloric stenosis is complication of duodenal ulcers, and has nothing to do with congen hypertrophic pyloric stenosis, p600.) ***Treatment:*** Endoscopic ballc dilatation, followed by maximal acid suppression (p234), may be tried in the instance (**NB:** 5% risk of perforation). If this is unsuccessful, a drain procedure (eg gastro-enterostomy or pyloroplasty) ± highly select vagotomy may be performed, often laparoscopically. The operation should done on the next available list, after correction of the metabolic defect hypochloraemic, hypokalaemic metabolic alkalosis.

Fundoplication for gastro-oesophageal reflux

The goal This is to re-establish lower oesophageal sphincter tone.

The procedure Involves wrapping the gastric fundus around the lo oesophagus, closing the hiatus, and securing the wrap in the abdomen—see B There are various types of procedure eg Nissen (360° wrap), Toupet (27 posterior wrap), Watson (anterior hemifundoplication).

Access Usually laparoscopic, which in specialist centres is at least as effective controlling reflux as open surgery but with a lower mortality. Wound infecti and respiratory complications are also more common in open surgery, though incidence of dysphagia is similar for the two procedures—but see p640.

Surgery

ighly selective vagotomy

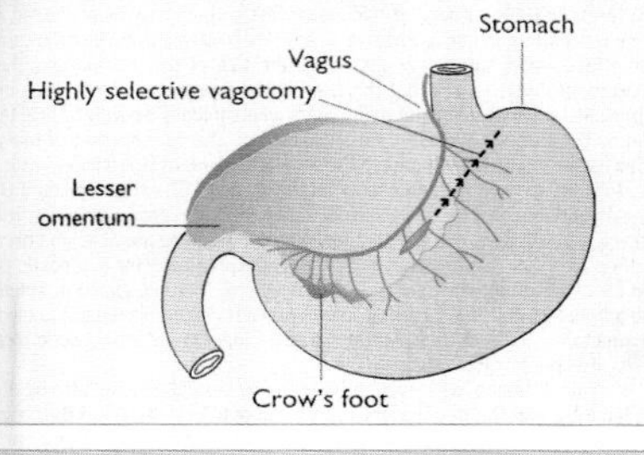

issen fundoplication

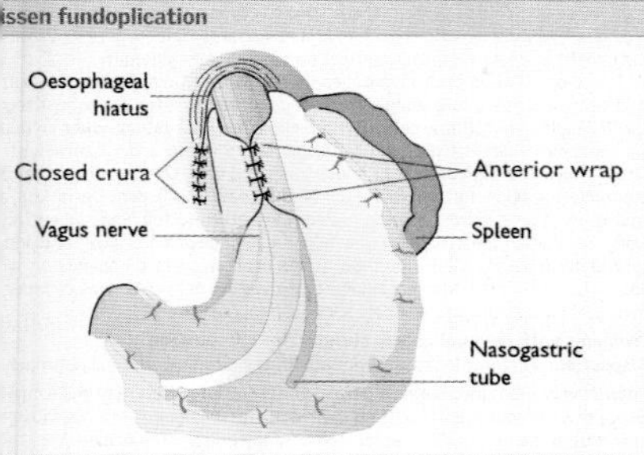

Minimally invasive surgery

The terms 'keyhole surgery' or minimal access surgery may be preferred, bec these procedures can be as invasive as any laparotomy, having just the same s side-effects—plus some new ones. It is the size of the incision and the us laparoscopes which marks out this branch of surgery. Laparoscopy has been established in gynaecology for many years where initially a purely optical telesc held by the surgeon, was used for visualization. The development of miniatu video cameras was the impetus to the widespread use of laparoscopy, as it allo an assistant to have the same view as the surgeon. The surgeon could there operate with both hands, while his assistant held the laparoscope and retracted viscera. Laparoscopic cholecystectomy was shown to be possible, and became method of choice. Laparoscopy is now in widespread use for diagnostic purp and for other conditions, such as appendicectomy,[MET 235] fundoplication, splenect and adrenalectomy. It is currently under evaluation for hernia repair,[MET 236] colecton nephrectomy (in renal transplants), parathyroidectomy, sentinel node biopsy, perforated peptic ulcer repair.[MET 238]

As a rule of thumb, whatever can be done by laparotomy can also be done the laparoscope. This does not mean that it **should** be done, but if the patient better sooner, has less post-operative pain, and can return to work earlier, have fewer complications, then these specific techniques will gain ascenden provided hospitals can afford the equipment. Laparoscopic surgery may also the benefit of a less suppressive effect on the immune system.[239]

It is worth noting that advantages do not include time. In upper GI surg laparoscopic surgery takes longer than open procedures. Also, the patient nee spend a night in hospital, usually. This has economic implications when compa laparoscopic inguinal hernia repair with open surgery done under local anaesth (after which the patient can go home the same day). On the other side of economic equation for hernia repair is that pain >24h post-op is less a laparoscopic procedures, and the patient can return to full employment aft week. In addition, laparoscopic repair allows detection of a previously undiagn contralateral hernia. Which method makes economic sense depends on wh doing the calculation; NICE concluded that open hernia repair was cheaper, their calculations did not include out of hospital costs.[240]

Surgery

Problems with minimal access surgery: for the surgeon

Inspection: Anatomy looks different due to the different surgical approach.

Palpation is impossible during laparoscopic procedures. This may make it har locate colon lesions prior to cutting them out. This means that pre-operative t may need to be more extensive (eg colonoscopy **and** barium enema).

Skill: Here the problem is not just that a new skill has to be learned and taught skills may become attenuated if operations are performed laparoscopically, and surgeons may not achieve quite the level of skill in either sphere if they try to do b

Problems for patients and GPs

Post-operative complications: What may be easily managed on a well surgical ward (eg haemorrhage) may be a challenge for a GP and terrify patient, who may be all alone after early discharge.

Loss of tell-tale scars: Afterwards there may only be a few abdominal wound future carers have to guess at what has been done. The answer here is to communi carefully with the patient, so that he knows what has been done—see BOX.

Problems for hospitals Just because minimal access surgery is often cost-effec it does not follow that hospitals can afford the procedures. Instruments continuously being refined, and quickly become obsolete—so that many are produced in disposable single-use form. Because of budgeting boundaries, hosp cannot use the cash saved, by early return to work or by freeing-up bed use, to for capital equipment and extra theatre time that may be required.

:posing patients to our learning curves. The jury is still out...

l surgeons, indeed all doctors, get better over time (for a while), as they rform new techniques with increasing ease and confidence. Mortality rates evitably vary. When Wertheim did his first radical hysterectomies, his first zen patients died—but then someone survived, and he assumed it was a good eration, and pressed ahead. He was a brave man, and thousands of women ve their lives to him. But if he had tried to do this today, he would have been opped. The UK's General Medical Council (GMC), and other august bodies nstantly tell us that we must protect the public by reporting doctors whose tients have low survival rates. The reason for this is partly ethical, and partly attempt to preserve self-regulation.

The defining feature of any profession lies, the GMC assumes, in self-gulation. To preserve this, we have the toughest professional codes of actice and disciplinary procedures of any group of workers. It is assumed at doctors are loyal to each other out of self-interest, and that this loyalty is d. This has never been tested formally, and is not evidence-based. We can agine two clinical worlds: one of constant 'reportings' and recriminatory dits, and another of trust and team-work. Both are imperfect, but we should t assume that the first world would be better for our patients.

It is easy to say that our patients demand honesty, and so long as we are ing our best, and referring where needed, all will be well. But honesty is aque at the bedside. We never know the **whole** truth about our past rformance. (All our patients with such-and-such a colostomy left hospital ive—but perhaps they all committed suicide later?) Should we tell our tient that this is the first time we have done this sort of operation supervised? When patients are sick with fear, they do not, perhaps, want to ow everything. We may tell to protect ourselves. We may **not** tell to protect rselves. Perhaps what we should do is, in the privacy of our own hearts, to peal to those 12 dead women-of-Wertheim—a jury as infallible as crificial—and try to hear their reply. And to those who complain that in ing so we are playing God, it is possible to reply with some humility that, hatever it is, it does not seem like play.

'It is amazing what little harm doctors do when one considers all the opportunities they have'—Mark Twain

15 Epidemiology

Contents

See also *QALY*

An example of epidemiology at work

Some decades ago, epidemiologists tested the hypothesis that smoking hypertension were associated with cardiovascular disease. Painstaking cc studies confirmed that these were indeed ***risk markers*** (a term that does imply causality). Over the years, as evidence accumulates, the term 'risk ma may give way to ***risk factor***, which implies causation, and the separate that risk-factor modification will cause a reduction in disease. Demonstrat dose–response relationship (with the correct time sequence) is good eviden a causal relationship—eg showing that the greater the number of cigar smoked, the greater the risk, or the higher the blood pressure, the greate cardiovascular mortality. It is still possible that BP is a risk marker of s other phenomenon, but this is less likely if the relationship between BP cardiovascular mortality is found to correlate *while keeping other known factors constant*. The work of the epidemiologist does not stop here. He o can use actuarial statistics to weigh the relative merits and interactions number of risk factors, to give an overall estimate of risk for an individual. then possible to say things like: 'If the 5-yr risk of a serious cardiac eve people with no overt cardiac disease is >15%, then drug treatmer hyperlipidaemia may begin to be cost-effective—and a 10% 5-yr risk may sufficient point to trigger antihypertensive treatment in someone with, say, of 150/90'. These figures are a guide only: only ~60% of those in the top of the risk distribution will have an adverse coronary event in the 5-yr pe Nevertheless, this is more accurate than taking into account risk fac singly—and so we are led to our first important conclusion: ***epidemic improves and informs our dialogue with our patients***. We can give pat good evidence on which to base their choices.

Risk equations (ideally as part of computerized medical records) ma given as follows (a, m, μ, and σ are variables relating risk factors):

If $a = 11.1122 - [0.9119 \times \ln(\text{BP})] - (0.2767 \times \text{SMO}) - [0.7181 \times \ln(\text{FAT})] - (0.5865 \times$

and for males $m = a - [1.4762 \times \ln(\text{AGE})] - 0.1759 \times \text{DIAB}$

and for females $m = a - 5.8549 + [1.8515 \times \ln(\text{AGE}/74)^2] - (0.3758 \times \text{DIAE}$

and $\mu = 4.4181 + m$

and $\sigma = e^{-(0.3155 - 0.278m)}$ and $v = [\ln(5) - \mu/\sigma]$

then **5-yr risk ≈ 1–(e–(ev))** if AGE is 30–74yrs, BP is the mean systolic, readings—and SMO, DIAB, and LVH are each 1 if a patient is a smoker, has diabetes (ventricular hypertrophy on ECG; if not present, each is 0. FAT is the ratio of total esterol to HDL. This is the EMIS formulation of the 'Dundee equations'; see J Rc 1997 *BMJ* ii 277 & corrected Sheffield tables for primary prevention of heart disease

►Note that results from these equations are approximations only: bew spurious accuracy. Also, populations differ: figures taken from Ame cohorts in the past underestimated risk by as much as 48% in UK ma workers and 31% for non-manual workers. Very many more underprivil people are eligible for preventive treatment if UK data are used.

essence of epidemiology

demiology is the study of the distribution of clinical phenomena in ulations. Its chief measures are prevalence and incidence.

initions The *period prevalence* is the number of cases, at any time during study period, divided by the population at risk. If the population at risk is lear, then the population must be specified—eg the prevalence of uterine cer varies widely, depending on whether you specify the general ulation (men, women, boys, and girls) or only women, or women who have already had a hysterectomy.

he *incidence* is the number of new cases within the study period which st be specified, eg annual incidence. *Point prevalence* is the prevalence a point in time. The *lifetime* prevalence of hiccups is ~100%; the (UK) dence is millions/year—but the point prevalence may be 0 at 3AM today if one is actually having hiccups.

ociation Epidemiological research is concerned with comparing rates disease in different populations, eg rates of lung cancer in a population of n who smoke, compared with men who do not. A difference in rates points an association (or dissociation) between the disease and factors which inguish the populations (in this case, smoking or not). If the rates are al, association is still possible, with a confounding variable (eg both ups share the same smoky environment).

ys of accounting for associations: *A* may cause *B*; *B* cause *A*; a 3rd nown agent, *P*, causes *A* and *B*; or it may be a chance finding.

here are 2 types of studies which explore causal connections:

se-control (retrospective) studies: The study group consists of those h the disease (eg lung cancer); the control group consists of those without disease. The previous occurrence of the putative cause (eg smoking) is npared between each group. Case–control studies are retrospective in t they start after the onset of the disease (although cases may be ected prospectively).

hort (prospective) studies: The study group consists of subjects osed to the putative causal factor (eg smoking); and the control group sists of subjects not exposed. The incidence of the disease is compared ween the groups over time. ►A cohort study generates incidence data, ereas a case–control study does not.

tching An association between *A* and *B* may be due to another factor To eliminate this possibility, matching for *P* is often used in case–control dies. One powerful, but unreliable (if numbers are small), way to do s in clinical trials is for the subjects to be allocated to groups randomly; eck important *P*s have been distributed evenly between groups.

ermatching If unemployment causes low income, and low income causes ression, then matching study and control groups for income would mask genuine causal link between unemployment and depression. ►Avoid tching factors which may intervene in the causal chain linking *A* and *B*.

nding If the subject does not know which of two trial treatments is having, the trial is single blind. To further reduce risk of bias, the erimenter should also not know (double blind).

n a good treatment trial, the blind lead the blind.

Epidemiology

er reading: D Sackett *Clinical Epidemiology*, Little, Brown, Boston; and D Sackett *Evidence-based ine: How to Practise and Teach EBM*, Churchill.

Evidence-based medicine (EBM)

This is the conscientious and judicious use of current best evidence from clir research in the management of individual patients.

The problem More than 2,000,000 papers are published each year. Pati benefit directly from a tiny fraction of these papers. How do we find them?

A partial solution 50 or so leading journals are scanned not by experts specialized field, but by searchers trained to identify papers which have a dir message for clinical practice, and meet predefined criteria of rigour (belc Summaries are then published, eg in *Evidence-based Medicine.*

Questions used to evaluate papers:

- Are the results valid? Randomized? Blinded? Were all patients accounted who entered the trial? Was follow-up complete? Were the groups similar at start? Was everyone treated equally, apart from the experimental interventi NB: randomized trials are now recognised as blunt instruments: adap (Bayesian) designs may sometimes be a more efficient way to get to the truth
- What are the results? How large (and precise) was the treatment effect?
- Will the results help my patients (cost/benefit sum).

Problems with the solution ►*The concept of scientific rigour is opaque.* W do we want? The science, the rigour, the truth, or what will be most usefu patients? These may overlap, but they are not the same.

- Will the best be the enemy of the good? Are useful papers rejected due some blemish? Answer: appraise *all* evidence (often impossible).
- By reformulating in terms of answerable questions, EBM risks missing patie reason for consulting. He may only want to express his fears, rather thar used as a substrate for an intellectual exercise.
- Is the standard the same for the evidence for *all* changes to our practice? might avoid prescribing drug X for constipation if there is any chance tha might cause colon cancer, as the choice of drugs is wise. More rob evidence is needed to persuade us to do something rather counterintuitive giving heparin in DIC (p336). There is no science to tell us how robust the d need to be: we decide off the top of our head (albeit a wise head, we hope)
- What about the correspondence columns of the journals from which winning papers are extracted? It takes years for unforeseen but fatal flaws surface, and be reported in correspondence columns.
- There is a danger that by always asking 'What is the evidence...' we divert resources from hard-to-prove areas (eg physiotherapy, which may very valuable) to easy-to-prove services. The unique personal attributes of therapist may be as important as the objective regimen.
- EBM is never 100% up-to-date, and reworking meta-analyses takes time a money, so specialists may ostensibly reject a new trial due to a tiny flaw, w the real reason is that they dread it might flip their once-perfect formulatic
- 'My increased knowledge gradually permeated or repressed the world intuitive premonitions...' (*Carl Jung*). These premonitions may be vital!
- If EBM is prescriptive, patient choice declines: not all patients are amenable rational dialogue. Does our zeal for EBM make us arrogant and inflexible?
- The patient before us may not quite fit the type of patient who provided research basis—and we may be tempted to ignore these small differen which may then have major unforeseen adverse effects.

Advantages of EBM This is mainly that patients get better faster—also:

- Our reading habits improve, and we can offer more rational choices to patier
- EBM leads us to ask questions, and then to be sceptical of the answers.
- As taxpayers, we should like it (wasteful practices can be abandoned).

EBM may not have as much impact as we hope, as gaining evidence is tir consuming and expensive, and sometimes impossible. Despite these caveats, is here to stay, so we may as well subscribe to its ideals—and to its journals.

Six to five against

Your surgical consultant asks whether Gobble's disease is more common in me or women. You have no idea, and make a guess. What is the chance of getting right? Common sense decrees that it is even chances; 'Sod's Law' predicts tha whatever you guess, your answer will always be wrong. A less pessimistic vie is that the balance is slightly tipped against you: according to Damon Runyo 'all life is six to five against'.

Do new symptoms suggest a new disease or are they from an existing disease The answer is often counter-intuitive. Suppose S is quite a rare symptom c Gobble's disease (seen in 5% of patients), but that it is a very commo symptom of disease A (seen in 90%). If we have a man whom we already kno has Gobble's disease and who goes on to develop symptom S, is not S mo likely to be due to disease A, rather than Gobble's disease? The answer usually no: *it is generally the case that* S *is due to a disease which is alrea known, and does not imply a new disease.*

The 'odds ratio' makes this clearer, ie the ratio of [the probability of th symptom, given the known disease] to [the probability of the symptom give the new disease × *the probability of developing the new disease*]. This ratio i usually, vastly in favour of the symptom being due to the old disease because c the prior odds of the two diseases.

Doctors as gamblers To the average mind it is distasteful to learn that docto gamble with patients' lives. One of us (JML) has just finished consulting with 2 patients. Not too many, perhaps: it might be argued that each of symptor especially if *serious*, should be investigated until the cause is found.

Let us look at this critically. What counts as a serious symptom? One tha might mean death, disfigurement, or disability. Some of these patients offered symptom groups before being dissuaded from going on. During elucidation c these symptoms others emerged, yielding a potentially endless cycle of investing ation. Certainly some of their symptoms might not seem serious ('this pain in m toe...'). But toe pain might be mortal if caused by emboli or osteomyeliti Fingernail problems with a slight rash might mean arsenic poisoning; letharg may mean cancer, and so on. So medicine is not for pessimists—almost anythin can be made to seem fatal, so that a pessimistic doctor would never get an sleep at night for worrying about the meanings of his patients' symptoms.

Medicine is not for blind optimists either, who too easily embrace a fool paradise of false reassurance. Rather, ***medicine is for gamblers***: Gamblers wh are happy to use subtle clues to change their outlook from pessimism t optimism and vice versa. Sometimes the gambling is scientific, rational, an methodical (odds-ratio analysis): sometimes it is not, as when the gambling based on prior knowledge (vital but ill-defined) of one's patient, or the fair apprehension of terror in this new patient's eyes which shows you that there something wrong, and that you don't yet know what it is.

Being lucky in both types of gambling is a requisite for being a successfu doctor: after all we would all rather have a lucky doctor than a wise one. In th game, especially when it gets deadly serious, the chips are not just financial (th most cost-effective next step). They betoken time (for you are spending yourse as surely as you are spending money, as you walk the wards), your reputatio and the health or otherwise of your patient. So do not worry about the fact c gambling: ***gambling is your job***. If you cannot gamble you cannot cure. But mak sure you assemble sufficient evidence to maximize your chances of being lucky.

An example of the odds ratio at work

A 50-yr-old man with known carcinoma of the lung has some transient neurological symptoms and a normal CT scan. Are these symptoms due to secondaries in the brain or to transient ischaemic attacks (TIAs)?

- The chance of secondaries in the brain which cause transient neurological symptoms is 0.045 given carcinoma of the lung.
- The chance of such secondaries not showing up on a CT scan is 0.1. Therefore the chance of this cluster of symptoms is 0.0045 (ie 0.045 × 0.1).
- The chance of a normal CT + transient CNS symptoms given a TIA is 0.9.
- The chance of a 50-yr-old man developing TIA is 0.0001. Therefore the odds ratio is 0.0045/(0.9 × 0.0001). This equals 50.

That is, the odds ratio is ~50 to 1 in favour of secondaries in the brain.

NB: It is only very rarely that the prior odds of a new disease are so high that the new disease is more likely, eg someone presenting with anaemia already known to have breast cancer, who lives in an African community where 50% of people have hookworm-induced anaemia, is likely to have anaemia due to hookworm *as well as* breast carcinoma.

Investigations change the odds

Only rarely does a single test provide a definitive diagnosis. More often te alter the odds of a diagnosis. When taking a history and examining patients, make various wagers with ourselves (often barely consciously) as to how lik various diagnoses are. Further test results simply affect these odds. A test worthwhile if it alters diagnostic odds in a clinically useful way.

The effect of an investigation on the diagnostic odds To work this out y need to know the *sensitivity* and *specificity* of the test. All tests have fa positive and false negative rates, as summarized below:

Test result	Patients with the condition	Patients without the condition
Subjects appear to have the condition	True +ve (*a*)	False +ve (*b*)
Subjects appear *not* to have condition	False −ve (*c*)	True −ve (*d*)

Specificity: How reliably is the test −ve in health? *d/d+b*. ***Sensitivity:*** Ho reliably is the test +ve in the disease? *a/a+c*. Screening tests need to have high sensitivity: we know that 3–6% of chest pain patients sent home fro casualty departments on the basis of a single ECG actually have myocard infarction (MI). A single ECG is specific (77–100%), but not very sensitive for (56%). Troponin tests (p104) are more sensitive. So a doctor might u sensitivity/specificity data to act as follows. If history and ECG suggest admit (thrombolysis, p782). If story and ECG are not typical of MI, do a tropo test 6h after onset of chest pain—only send home if 'normal'.[1] This strate reduces inappropriate discharge to ~1%.[2] Note that studies showing the effects are *very* dependent on the local prevalence of MI. A few more MIs in 'troponin normal' group would radically alter these results.

Suppose we have a test of sensitivity 0.8 and specificity 0.9. The *likeliho ratio* of the disease given a positive result (LR+) is the ratio of the chance having a positive test if the disease is present to the chance of having a posit test if the disease is absent [0.8/(1–0.9)]; ie 8:1 in the above example.

In general: LR+ = sensitivity/(1–specificity)

LR–(likelihood ratio of the disease given a negative result) (1–sensitivity)/specificity. (1–0.8/0.9, ie 2:9 in the above example.)

Is there any point to this test? Work out the 'posterior odds' assuming first a +ve and then a −ve test result—via the equation: *posterior odds* = (*pr odds*) × (*likelihood ratio*). If your clinical assessment of a man with exercis induced chest pain is that the odds of this being due to coronary artery disea (CAD) are 4 : 1 (80%), is it worth his doing an exercise tolerance test (sensitiv 0.72; specificity 0.8)? If the test were positive, the odds in favour of C would be 4 × (0.72)/(1–0.8) = 14:1 (93%). If negative, they would be 4 (1 – 0.72)/0.8 = 1.4 : 1 (58%), so the test has not in any way 'ruled out' CAD.

Experienced doctors are likely to have higher prior odds for the most like diagnosis. The above shows that with high prior odds, a test must have hi sensitivity and specificity for a negative result to bring the odds below 50%.

Another example is John, who is a 40-yr-old (not on NSAIDs, with no pr peptic ulcer) referred for '?endoscopy' because of dyspepsia. Before the result a bedside test for *Helicobacter pylori* is known, he has a 50% chance harbouring this organism, which, if present, is the probable cause of an ulcer The likelihood ratio for a −ve test result is 0.13 (sensitivity 0.88, specific 0.91). ***If the test is negative***, the chance of John having *H. pylori* is <11%—a it may be OK to send him home with symptomatic treatment (eg ranitidir without endoscopy—if there are no 'cancer (alarm) symptoms' (weight lo dysphagia, etc, p235). ***If the test is +ve***, the probability of *H. pylori* is >90 strongly suggesting the need for specific anti-ulcer (anti-helicobacter) thera p235 and endoscopy if this does not cure his symptoms.

1 Troponin T (TnT) ≤0.1μg/L (or troponin I ≤0.2μg/L; labs vary); what is normal is itself a statist issue, p652—as is what counts as an MI.

2 Sensitivity: 97%; specificity: 93%; –ve predictive value: 99.6%; +ve predictive value: 66%; LR+: 13.9; LR–: 0

Epidemiology

Number needed to treat (NNT)

If the risk of dying from an MI after 'standard treatment' is 10%, and a r treatment reduces this to 8%, then the **absolute risk reduction** is 2% (1 8%). The effect of the new drug is often made to look more impressive quoting the **relative risk reduction**, ie 20% [(10 – 8/10) × 100%]. Howeve 100 people with MI receive the drug, only ~2 would be expected to derive benefit. In terms of **numbers needed to treat**, we might say that 50 patie would need treating to save one additional life ([1/absolute risk reductior 100). NNTs provide a useful way of quantifying benefit, but do not take i account treatment costs or the degree of potential benefit. The converse of is number needed to harm. This is the number of people who must receiv treatment in order to produce one adverse event.

In some preventive studies of mild hypertension in the young, ~800 pe may need treating according to a certain regimen to prevent one stroke. W expressed like this, the treatment seems less wonderful.

One of the strengths of NNT is that it is context-dependent. If a r antihypertension regimen is being compared with an old regimen where the was 800 and the new regimen is only marginally better, the NNT to prevent death or stroke *by adopting the new regimen in place of the old* may run i many thousands, as will your drugs bill if the new drug is more expensive.

One problem with NNTs occurs if there is a large placebo effect, eg in p relief. Say the placebo response rate is 40% and that of a new analgesi 60%. NNT is 5. Perhaps it is better to say to patients starting the new drug t 60% respond. Also, one needs to be clear whether the mean or median is gi as the length of follow-up. For further examples, see www.nntonline.net.

Screening

Modified Wilson criteria for screening (1–10 spells ***iatrogenic***[1]—to rem us that in treating healthy populations we have an especial duty to do no har

1 The condition screened for should be an **i**mportant one.
2 There should be an **a**cceptable treatment for the disease.
3 Diagnostic and **t**reatment facilities should be available.
4 A **r**ecognizable latent or early symptomatic stage is required.
5 **O**pinions on who to treat as patients must be agreed.
6 The test must be of *high discriminatory power* (see below), *valid* (measuri what it purports to measure, not surrogate markers which might not correlate with reality), and be *reproducible*—with safety **g**uaranteed.
7 The **e**xamination must be acceptable to the patient.
8 The untreated **n**atural history of the disease must be known.
9 A simple **i**nexpensive test should be all that is required.
10 Screening must be **c**ontinuous (ie not a 'one-off' affair).

Summary: screening tests must be cost-effect

Problems *All screening programs do harm; some do good as well.* J Muir Gray *Brit J Gen Pr* 54

1 Those most at risk do not present for screening, thus increasing the gap between the healthy and the unhealthy—the *inverse care law* (p12).
2 The 'worried well' overload services by seeking repeat screening.
3 Services for investigating those testing positive are inadequate.
4 Those who are false positives suffer stress while awaiting investigation, a remain anxious about their health despite reassurance.

►Before screening, the chances of harming a patient (by anxiety or subseque invasive tests), as well as any benefits must be quantified: this is ***Rees' rule***

1 From Greek: iatros (physician) + genic, denoting illness caused by us doctors. You will find this w etched on all our soles producing a malign imprint however lightly we try to tread. ***Ways to red iatrogenic illness:*** • Use EBM if possible • Involve patients in all decisions • Check drug labels/dosa by reading them aloud • Be aware of drug interactions: look it up—don't assume you know • Exp to patients how to tell if things are going wrong, and what action to take ('if ... tell me ...').

[Ex]amples of NNTs

[St]udy	Outcome	NNT
[St]atins (p101) for primary prevention[1]	Death (MI)	931 (78) for 5yrs
[St]atins for secondary prevention (4S)	Death (MI)	30 (15) for 5.4yrs
[M]ild hypertension (MRC trial)	Stroke	850 for 1yr
[S]ystolic hypertension in elderly (SHEP)	Stroke	43 for 4.5yrs
[A]spirin in acute MI (ISIS-1)	Death	40
[S]treptokinase in acute MI (ISIS2)	Death	40
[A]CE-i for CCF (NYHA class IV (p121))	Death	6 for 1yr

[K]eep your eye on the question NNTs can vary markedly if the question is [sli]ghtly rephrased—eg from being about primary prevention to being about [se]condary prevention (as in the statin example above).[15]

[NN]T confidence intervals Get these by taking reciprocals of the values [de]fining the confidence interval for the absolute risk reduction (ARR). [If] ARR ≈ 10% with a 95% confidence interval of 5–15%, NNT ≈ 10 (ie [1]00/10) and the 95% NNT-confidence interval ≈ 6.7–20 (ie 100/15 to [1]00/5). Non-significant treatment effects are problematic as NNTs can only [b]e positive; here, give NNT *without* confidence intervals (Altman's rule).[16]

[Ex]amples of effective screening	*Unproven/ineffective screening*
[C]ervical smears for cancer	Mental test score (dementia)
[M]ammography for breast cancer	Urine tests (diabetes; kidney disease)
[F]inding smokers (+quitting advice)	Antenatal procedures (*OHCS* p8)
[L]ooking for malignant hypertension	PSA screening (prostate cancer, p607)

[N]B: Screening for cervical cancer (*OHCS* p272) and mammography (p610) are [fa]r from perfect: both are liable to false negatives, and a negative result is [in]terpreted as 'I'm fine' (and may be seen as a licence to take risks). So signs [o]f interval cancers (arising between screenings) may be wished away by [p]atients who assume they are in the clear.

1 [M]eta-analysis *Bandolier* 17(7), 41(3), 50(8)

16 Clinical chemistry

Contents

Relevant pages in other sections: Reference intervals (p736); acute renal failure (p292–3).

On being normal in the society of numbers

Laboratory medicine reduces our patients to a few easy-to-handle numbers: thi the discipline's great attraction—and its greatest danger. The normal rar (reference interval) is usually that which includes 95% of patients. If variatior randomly distributed, 2.5% of our results will be 'too high', and 2.5% 'too low' on average day, when dealing with apparently normal people. This statistical definit of normality is the simplest. Other definitions may be *normative*—ie stating w an upper or lower limit *should* be. Eg the upper end of the reference interval plasma cholesterol may be given as 6mmol/L because this is what biochemi state to be the *desired* maximum, while the risk of CHD increases above 5.2mmo 40% of people in some populations will have a plasma cholesterol greater th 6mmol/L and thus may be at increased risk. The WHO definition of anaemia pregnancy is an Hb of <11g/dL, which makes 20% of mothers anaemic. This 'I criterion has the presumed benefit of triggering actions which result in few deaths by haemorrhage. So do not just ask 'What is the normal range?'—a enquire about who set the range, for what population, and for what reason.

►Normal values can have hidden historical, social, and political desiderata—just l the normal values novelists ascribe to their characters: '...*Conventions a traditions, I suppose, work blindly but surely for the preservation of the norm type; for the extinction of proud, resolute and unusual individuals... Society must on, I suppose, and society can only exist if the normal, if the virtuous, and t slightly deceitful flourish, and if the passionate, the headstrong, and the too-truth are condemned to suicide and to madness. Yes, society must go on; it must bre like rabbits. That is what we are here for ... But, at any rate, there is always Leon to cheer you up; I don't want to sadden you. Her husband is quite an economic person of so normal a figure that he can get quite a large proportion of his clot ready-made. That is the great desideratum of life...*'

Ford Maddox Ford 1915 *The Good Soldier*, Penguin, p214 & p2

1 We thank Dr Paul Flynn who is our Specialist Reader for this chapter.

ıe essence of laboratory medicine

ıly do a test if the result will influence management. Make sure you look at the sult! Explain to the patient where this test fits in to his or her overall plan of anagement. ►Do not interpret laboratory results except in the light of clinical sessment (unless forced to by examiners).

:f there is disparity: trust clinical judgement and repeat the test. Reference :ervals (normal ranges) are usually defined as the interval, symmetrical about e mean, containing 95% of results on the population studied. The more tests u run, the greater the probability of an 'abnormal' result of no clinical ŋnificance: see p737.

rtefacts Delayed analysis for plasma potassium (p654).

ıion gap (AG) Reflects unmeasured anions (p658).

ochemistry results major disease patterns (↑ = raised, ↓ = lowered)

ehydration: Urea↑, albumin↑ (useful to plot change in a patient's condition). ıematocrit (PCV)↑, creatinine↑; also urine volume↓; skin turgor↓.

enal failure: Creatinine↑, urea↑, AG↑, K^+↑, PO_4^{3-}↑, HCO_3^-↓.

hiazide and loop diuretics: Sodium↓, potassium↓, HCO_3^-↑, urea↑.

:one disease	*Ca^{2+}*	*PO_4^{3-}*	*Alk phos*
›steoporosis	Normal	Normal	Normal
›steomalacia	↓	↓	↑
'aget's	Normal	Normal	↑↑
Ʌyeloma	↑	↑, normal	Normal
ɜone metastases	↑	↑, normal	↑
° Hyperparathyroidism	↑	↓, normal	Normal, ↑
ɦypoparathyroidism	↓	↑	Normal
?enal failure (low GFR)	↓	↑	Normal, ↑

epatocellular disease: Bilirubin↑, AST↑ (alk phos slightly↑, albumin↓). For ɜtails of the differences between AST and ALT, see p275.

holestasis: Bilirubin↑, γGT↑↑, alk phos↑↑, AST↑.

ɦyocardial infarction: troponin T/I ↑, CK↑, AST↑, LDH↑ (p105).

iabetes mellitus: Glucose↑, (HCO_3^-↓ if acidotic).

ddison's disease: Potassium↑, sodium↓.

ushing's syndrome: May show potassium↓, HCO_3^-↑, sodium↑.

onn's syndrome: May present with potassium↓, HCO_3^-↑ (and high blood 'essure). Sodium normal or ↑.

iabetes insipidus: Sodium↑, plasma osmolality↑, urine osmolality ↓ (both ʏpercalcaemia and hypokalaemia may cause nephrogenic diabetes insipidus).

ıappropriate ADH secretion: Na^+↓ with normal or low urea and creatinine, asma osmolality↓. Urine osmolality ↑ (and > than plasma osmolality), urine Na (>20mmol/L).

xcess alcohol intake: Evidence of hepatocellular disease. Early evidence γGT ↑, MCV↑, ethanol in blood before lunch.

ome immunodeficiency states: Normal serum albumin but *low* total protein ow as immunoglobulins are missing—also making cross-matching difficult ɛcause expected haemagglutinins are absent; *OHCS* p198).

ife-threatening biochemical derangements See p655.

►Laboratory staff like to have contact with you.

A laboratory decalogue

1 Interest someone from the laboratory in your patient's problem.
2 Fill in the request form fully.
3 Give clinical details, not your preferred diagnosis.
4 Ensure that the lab knows who to contact.
5 Label specimens as well as the request form.
6 Follow the hospital labelling routine for cross-matching.
7 Find out when analysers run, especially batched assays.
8 Talk with the lab before requesting an unusual test.
9 Be thoughtful: at 1630h the routine results are being sorted.
10 Plot results graphically: abnormalities show sooner.

Artefacts and pitfalls in laboratory tests

- Do not take blood sample from an arm which has IV fluid running into it.
- Repeat any unexpected result before acting on it.
- For clotting time do not sample from a heparinized IV catheter.
- Serum K^+ is overestimated if sample is old or haemolysed (this occurs if ve puncture is difficult).
- If using Vacutainers, fill *plain* tubes first—otherwise, anticoagulant cont ination from previous tubes can cause errors.
- Total calcium results are affected by albumin concentration (p670).
- INR may be overestimated if citrate bottles are under-filled.
- Drugs may cause *analytic* errors (eg prednisolone cross-reacts with cortisol suspicious if results are unexpected.
- Food may affect result, eg bananas raise urinary HIAA (p270).

Using dipsticks Store dipsticks in a closed container in a cool, dry place, refrigerated. If improperly stored, or past expiry date, do not use. For urine te dip the dipstick briefly in urine, run edge of strip along container and hold s horizontally. **Read at the specified time**—check instructions for the type of st For haematuria, proteinuria, etc., see p278.

Urine specific gravity (SG) can be measured by dipstick. It is not a good meas of osmolality. Causes of low SG (<1.003) are: diabetes insipidus, renal fail Causes of high SG (>1.025) are: diabetes mellitus, adrenal insufficiency, l disease, heart failure, acute water loss. Hydrometers underestimate SG by 0.0 per 3°C above 16°C.

Sources of error in interpreting dipstick results

Bilirubin: False +ve: phenothiazines. False –ve: urine not fresh, rifampicin.

Urobilinogen: False –ve: urine not fresh. Normally present in urine due metabolism of bilirubin in the gut by bacteria and subsequent absorption. Exc may give a false +ve test for prophobilinogen.

Ketones: L-dopa affects colour (can give false +ve). 3-hydroxybutyrate gi a false –ve.

Blood: False +ve: myoglobin, profuse bacterial growth. False –ve: ascorbic ac

Urine glucose: Depends on test. Pads with glucose oxidase are not affected other reducing sugars (unlike Clinitest®) but can give false +ve to perox chlorine; and false –ve with ascorbic acid, salicylate, L-dopa.

Protein: Highly alkaline urine can give false +ve.

Blood glucose: Sticks use enzymatic method and are glucose specific. A ma source of error is applying too little blood (a large drop to cover the pad necessary), and poor timing. Reflectance meters increase precision but introd new sources of error.

ıboratory results: when to take action NOW

On receiving a dangerous result, first check the name and date.
Go to the bedside. If the patient is conscious, turn off any IVI (until fluid is checked: a mistake may have been made) and ask the patient how he or she is. *Any fits, faints, collapses, or unexpected symptoms?*
Be sceptical of an unexpectedly wildly abnormal result with a well patient. Compare with previous values. Could the specimens have got muddled up? Is there an artefact? Was the sample taken from the 'drip' arm? Is a low calcium be due to a low albumin (p670)? Perhaps the lab is using a new analyser with a faulty wash cycle? ►*When in doubt, repeat the test.*

ıe values chosen below are somewhat arbitrary and must be taken as a guide ıly. Many results less extreme than those below will be just as dangerous if the ıtient is old, immunosuppressed, or has some other pathology such as ıeumonia.

asma biochemistry (beware electrocardiological ± CNS events, eg fits)
alcium (corrected for albumin) >3.5mmol/L. *If shortening* Q–T *interval on* ECG (p82), *then dangerous hypercalcaemia.* See p672.
alcium (corrected for albumin) <2.0mmol/L + symptoms such as tetany or long Q–T = *Dangerous hypocalcaemia.* See p670.
lucose <2mmol/L = *Hypoglycaemia. Glucose 50mL 50% IV if coma.*
lucose >20mmol/L = *Severe hyperglycaemia. Is parenteral insulin needed?* See p814.
otassium <2.5mmol/L = *Dangerous hypokalaemia, esp. if on digoxin.*
otassium >6.5mmol/L = *Dangerous hyperkalaemia.* See p668.
odium <120mmol/L = *Dangerous hyponatraemia.* See p666.
odium >155mmol/L = *Dangerous hypernatraemia.* See p666.
ood gases
O_2 <8.0kPa = *Severe hypoxia. Give O_2.* Go to p172.
H <7.1 = *Dangerous acidosis. Go to* p658 *to determine the cause.*
aematology results
b <7g/dL with low mean cell volume (<75fL) or history of bleeding.
This patient may need urgent transfusion (no spare capacity). See p570.
atelets <40×10^9/L *May need a platelet transfusion; call a haematologist.*
***asmodium falciparum* seen** *Start antimalarials now.* See p384.
SR >30mm/h + headache *Could there be giant cell arteritis?* See p542.
SF results
1 neutrophil/mm^3 *Is there meningitis: usually >1000 neutrophils?* See p806.
ram stain *Talk to a microbiologist; urgent blind therapy.* See p806.
onflicting, equivocal, or inexplicable results ►Get prompt help.

Intravenous fluid therapy

(See also p664 & p6

If fluids cannot be given orally, they are normally given intravenously. Alternat are via a central venous line or subcutaneously. However, remember that cannulae carry a risk of MRSA infection: femoral > jugular > subclavian > periph

Three principles of fluid therapy

1 **Maintain normal daily requirements** About 2500mL fluid containing roug 100mmol sodium and 70mmol potassium per 24h are requi A good regimen is 2L of 5% dextrose and 1L of 0.9% saline every 30h w 20–30mmol of potassium per litre of fluid. Post-operative patients may n more fluid and more saline depending on operative losses. If the se sodium is rising, then more dextrose and less saline is required.

2 **Replace additional losses** The amount and type of fluid lost is a guide (ch fluid charts, drainage bottles, etc.). Remember that febrile patients h increased insensible losses. In practice, the problem is usually whether to g saline or dextrose. Most body fluids (eg vomit) contain salt, but less t plasma, and thus replacement will require a mixture of saline and dextr Shocked patients require resuscitation with saline, or a colloidal plas expander, eg Dextran® or Haemaccel®, but not dextrose (caution in liver fail see below). Note that Dextran® interferes with platelet function and n prolong bleeding. Patients with acute blood loss require transfusion w packed cells or whole blood. As a holding measure, colloid or saline may be u while blood is being cross-matched. If more than 1L is required then gr O-negative or group-specific blood should be used (see p778).

3 **Special cases** Patients with ***heart failure*** and the ***elderly*** are at greater ris pulmonary oedema if given too much fluid. They also tolerate saline less w since Na^+ retention accompanies heart failure. If IV fluids must be given, with care. Patients with ***liver failure***, despite being oedematous and of hyponatraemic, have increased total body sodium, and saline should **not** used in resuscitation; salt-poor albumin solution or blood should be given. F maintenance for ***children*** is calculated as: 100mL/kg for the first 10 50mL/kg for the next 10kg; and 20mL/kg thereafter—all per 24hrs. Usu given as dextrose-saline (4% dextrose 0.18% saline).

Types of fluid ***0.9% saline ('normal saline')*** has about the same sodium cont as plasma (150mmol/L) and is isotonic with plasma. ***5% dextrose*** is isotonic, only contains 278mmol/L glucose, ie 50g/L (dextrose is glucose), and is a way giving water, since the liver rapidly metabolizes all the glucose leaving only wa It provides little energy. More concentrated glucose solutions exist, and may used in the treatment of hypoglycaemia. They are hypertonic and irritant to ve Therefore, care in their use is needed, and infusion sites should be inspec regularly, and flushed with saline after use. ***Dextrose-saline (one-fifth norm saline)*** is also isotonic, containing 0.18% saline (30mmol/L of sodium) and glucose (222mmol/L). It has roughly the concentration of saline required normal fluid maintenance, when given 10 hourly. Hypertonic and hypotonic sal solutions are available, but are for specialist use only. ***Hartmann's solut*** contains: Na^+ 131mmol/L, Cl^- 111mmol/L, lactate 29mmol/L, K^+ 5mmol/L, HC 29 mmol/L, and Ca^{2+} 2mmol/L. Some consider it more 'physiological'.

►The maximum concentration of K^+ that is safe to infuse via a peripheral lin 80mmol/L, at a maximum rate of 40mmol/h. Higher concentrates risk phlebi and faster rates dysrhythmias. Give more concentrated solutions via a central l

►Examine patients regularly to assess fluid balance: look for signs of heart fail (p120)—excess fluid given? Excess dextrose iv may lead to water overload (p66

►Daily weighing helps to monitor overall fluid balance, as will fluid balance cha

IV fluids on the surgical ward

Pre-op fluids Avoid rushing dehydrated patients to theatre before adequate resuscitation. Anaesthesia compounds shock by causing vasodilatation and depressing cardiac contractility. Exceptions are exsanguination from a ruptured ectopic pregnancy, major trauma, a ruptured aortic aneurysm, or severe upper GI haemorrhage, where blood is lost faster than it can be replaced.

Post-operative fluids A normal requirement is 2–3L/24h which allows for urinary, faecal, and insensible loss.

A standard regimen: (One of many) 2L 5% dextrose with 1L 0.9% saline/24h. Add K^+ post-op (20mmol/L). See p656 for other examples. More K^+ is needed if losses are from the gut (eg diarrhoea, vomiting, intestinal fistula, high output stoma). More saline is appropriate for those at risk of hyponatraemia: ►See BOX.

When to increase the above regimen:

- Dehydration: this may be ≥5L if severe. Replace this slowly.
- Shock (all causes, except for cardiogenic shock).
- Operative losses: check operation notes for extent of bleeding in theatre.
- Losses from gut: replace NGT aspirate volume with 0.9% saline.
- Transpiration losses: feverish patients and burns.
- Pancreatitis: large pools of sequestered fluid which must be considered.
- Losses from surgical drains: check fluid charts and replace significant losses.
- Low urine output (the night after surgery) is almost always due to inadequate infusion of fluid. Check JVP, and review for signs of cardiac failure. Treat by increasing IVI rate unless patient is in heart or renal failure, or profusely bleeding (when blood should be transfused). If in doubt, a fluid challenge may be indicated: 200mL of colloid (eg Gelofusine®) over 30–60 min, with monitoring of urine output. Then you may increase IVI rate to 1L/h of 0.9% saline for 2–3h. Only if output does not increase should a diuretic be considered; a CVP line may be needed if estimation of fluid balance is difficult. A normal value is 0–5cm of water relative to the sternal angle. Measuring urinary Na^+ may also help.

If not catheterized exclude retention, but otherwise do not catheterize until absolutely necessary.

When to decrease the above regimen: *Renal failure*—give 500mL plus the previous day's output (►with no K^+). *Heart failure*—halve the volume (1–1.5L/24h).

Guidelines for success (see also p664)

- Be simple. Chart losses and replace them. Know the urine output. Aim for 60mL/h; 30mL/h is the minimum in adults (½mL/kg/h).
- Measure plasma U&E if the patient is ill. Regular U&Es are not needed on young, fit people with good kidneys.
- Start oral fluids as soon as possible.

What fluids to use ►***Haemorrhagic/hypovolaemic shock*** (see p778): Insert 2 large IV cannulae, for fast fluid infusion. Start with crystalloid (eg 0.9% saline) or colloid (eg Gelofusine®) until blood is available. The advantage of crystalloids is that they are cheap—but they do not stay as long in the intravascular compartment as colloids, as they equilibrate with the total extracellular volume (dextrose is useless for resuscitation as it rapidly equilibrates with the enormous intracellular volume). In practice, the best results are achieved by combining crystalloids and colloids. Aim to keep the haematocrit at ~0.3, and urine flowing at >30mL/h. Monitor pulse and BP often.

Septicaemic shock: Use a plasma-like substance (eg Gelofusine®).

Heart or liver failure: Avoid sodium loads: use 5% dextrose.

Excessive vomiting: Use 0.9% saline: replace losses, including K^+.

Arterial blood pH is closely regulated in health to 7.40 ± 0.05 by vario mechanisms including bicarbonate, other plasma buffers, and the kidney. Acid–bas disorders needlessly confuse many people, but if a few simple rules are applie then interpretation and diagnosis are easy.

- pH <7.35 is an acidosis; pH >7.45 is an alkalosis.
- CO_2 is an acidic gas (normal concentration 4.7–6.0kPa).
- HCO_3^- alkaline (normal concentration 22–28mmol/L).
- 1° changes in HCO_3^- are termed ***metabolic,*** and of CO_2 ***respiratory.***
  1. Look at the pH: is there an acidosis or alkalosis?
  2. Is the CO_2 abnormal? If so, is the change in keeping with the pH (ie if the is an acidosis, is CO_2 raised)? If so it is a ***respiratory*** problem. If there is no change, or an OPPOSITE one, then the change is compensatory.
  3. Is the HCO_3^- abnormal, and if so, is the change in keeping with the pH? If so the problem is a ***metabolic*** one.

An example

pH 7.05, CO_2 2.0kPa, HCO_3^- 8.0mmol/L.
There is an *acidosis*, and the CO_2 is low, and so is a compensatory change. The HCC is low, and is thus the cause; ie a *metabolic acidosis*.

Metabolic acidosis pH↓, HCO_3^-↓

To help diagnosis, work out the anion gap (AG)—this estimates unmeasured anior (they are hard to measure directly). It is calculated as the difference betwe plasma cations (Na^+ & K^+) and anions (Cl^- & HCO_3^-). Normal range: 10–18mmol/L. is a measure of 'fixed' or organic acids—eg phosphate, ketones, and lactate.

Causes of metabolic acidosis and increased anion gap:
Due to increased production of fixed/organic acids. HCO_3^- falls and unmeasure anions associated with the acids accumulate.

- Lactic acid (shock, infection, hypoxia).
- Urate (renal failure).
- Ketones (diabetes mellitus, alcohol).
- Drugs/toxins (salicylates, biguanides, ethylene glycol, methanol).

Causes of metabolic acidosis and normal anion gap:
Due to loss of bicarbonate or ingestion of H^+ ions (Cl^- is retained).

- Renal tubular acidosis.
- Diarrhoea.
- Drugs (acetazolamide).
- Addison's disease.
- Pancreatic fistulae.
- Ammonium chloride ingestion.

Metabolic alkalosis *pH*↑, HCO_3^-↑

- Vomiting.
- K^+ depletion (diuretics).
- Burns.
- Ingestion of base.

Respiratory acidosis *pH*↓ *CO_2*↑

- Any lung, neuromuscular, or physical cause of respiratory failure (p172).

►Look at the P_aO_2. It will probably be low. Is oxygen therapy required?
►Use O_2 with care if chronic obstructive pulmonary disease (COPD) is th underlying cause, as too much oxygen may make matters worse (p168).

Respiratory alkalosis *pH*↑, *CO_2*↓

A result of hyperventilation.
CNS causes: Stroke; subarachnoid bleed; meningitis. ***Others:*** Anxiety; altitude T°↑; pregnancy; pulmonary emboli (reflex hyperventilation); drugs, eg salicylates

Terminology To aid understanding, we have used the terms acidosis and alkalosis where a purist would sometimes have used acid-, alkal-aemia.

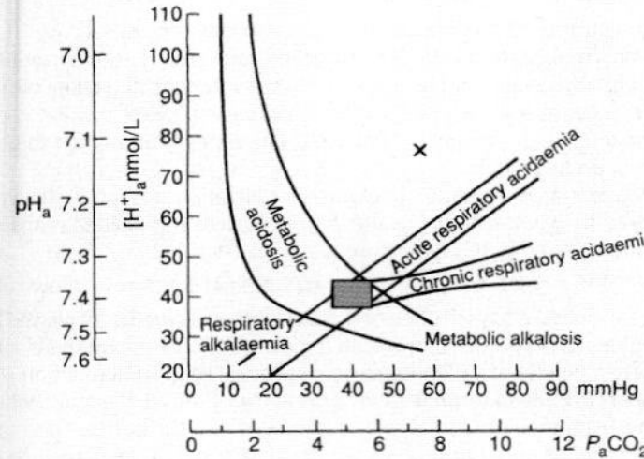

The shaded area represents normality. This method is very powerful. The result represented by point ×, eg indicates that the acidaemia is in part respiratory and in part metabolic. Seek a cause for each.

Kidney function

The kidney controls the elimination of many substances. It also mak erythropoietin, renin, and 1,25-dihydroxycholecalciferol. Filtered sodium exchanged with potassium and hydrogen ions by exchanges and channels in t distal tubule. Glucose spills over into urine when plasma concentration is abo renal threshold for reabsorption (≈10mmol/L, but varies from person to pers and is lower in pregnancy).

Creatinine clearance is a measure of glomerular filtration rate (GFR)—the volu of fluid filtered by glomeruli per minute. About 99% of this fluid is reabsorb Creatinine once filtered is only slightly reabsorbed. Thus:

$[\text{Creatinine}]^{\text{plasma}} \times \text{creatinine clearance} = [\text{creatinine}]^{\text{urine}} \times \text{urine flow rate}$

GFR can also be measured by injection of a radioisotope followed by repeated blo sampling (eg Cr^{51}EDTA) or an isotope scan (eg DTPA Tc^{99}). These methods allow more accurate estimate of GFR and may also provide split renal function.

To measure creatinine clearance Collect urine over 24h. At the start, void a discard urine; from then on, and at end of 24h, void into the bottle. Take samp for plasma creatinine once during 24h. Use formula above. Take care with uni Major sources of error are calculation (eg units) and failure to collect all uri Normal value is ≈125mL/min. The conversion factor from μmol/L to mg/dL f creatinine is 88.4; i.e. mg/dL = μmol ÷ 88.4.

Estimating kidney function 24hr urine collection is often unreliable, and a alternative approach is to estimate creatinine clearance or GFR using either t Cockcoft–Gault or MDRD equations (see BOX). The protein : creatinine ratio in a sp morning urine is an alternative way to monitor chronic renal decline: see p278.

Abnormal kidney function

There are three major biochemical pictures.

- **Low GFR** (classic acute renal failure)

  Plasma biochemistry: The following are raised: urea, creatinine, potassiu hydrogen ions, urate, phosphate, anion gap.

  The following are lowered: calcium, bicarbonate.

  Other findings: Oliguria.

  Diagnosis: Low GFR (creatinine clearance).

  Causes: Early acute oliguric renal failure (p292), long-standing chronic ren failure (p294).

- **Tubular dysfunction** (damage to tubules)

  Plasma biochemistry: The following are lowered: potassium, phosphate, urat bicarbonate. There is acidosis. Urea and creatinine are normal.

  ***Other findings** (highly variable):* Polyuria with glucose, amino acids, protei (lysozyme, β_2-microglobulin), and phosphate in urine.

  Diagnosis: Test renal concentrating ability (p224).

  Cause: Recovery from acute renal failure. Also: hypercalcaemia, hyperuri aemia, myeloma, pyelonephritis, hypokalaemia, Wilson's disease, galactosaemi heavy metal poisoning.

- **Chronic renal failure:** As GFR reduces, creatinine, urea, phosphate and urate a increase. Bicarbonate (and Hb) decrease(s). Eventually potassium increases an pH decreases. There may also be osteomalacia.

Assessment of renal failure may need to be combined with other investigations t reach diagnosis, eg urine microscopy (p278), radiology (p280), or renal biopsy (i glomerulonephritis), or ultrasound.

eatinine clearance: a worked example

ppose: urine creatinine concentration = **u** mmol/L;
plasma creatinine concentration = **p** μmol/L;
24h urine volume = **v** /mL.

ere are 1440min/24h (used below to convert urine flow rate from volume/24h
o volume per min). **p**/1000 is used to convert micromoles to millimoles.

eatinine clearance = **u** × **v**/1440 ÷ **p**/1000mL/min
u × **v**/**p** × 0.7.

us, if: **u**=5mmol/L; **p** =120μmol/L; **v** = 2500mL;

eatinine clearance = 5 × (2500/120) × 0.7
= 73mL/min.

timating GFR

lculating GFR is useful because it is easy to underestimate the degree of renal pairment if just serum creatinine is measured—especially in the elderly and men. Subjects with low muscle mass can have a 'normal' serum creatinine, spite a significant reduction in GFR eg 70mL/min. This can be particularly portant when potentially toxic drugs that are largely excreted by the kidney, renotoxic drugs are prescribed.

A number of formulae can be used. The **MDRD** (*Modification of Diet in Renal sease Study Group*) equation provides an estimate of GFR from 4 simple rameters: ***serum creatinine, age, gender and race (black/non-black)***, and is e of the best validated.[3] Many labs are now routinely reporting estimated GFR FR) on all U&E reports. However, the confidence intervals can be wide (90% of lues are within 30% of the true value, and 98% within 50%), and care should taken in unusual situations eg rapidly changing renal function, very low iscle mass. It is also better in subjects with a low GFR.

ckcroft-Gault equation provides an estimate of creatinine clearance:[4]

$$\text{reatinine clearance (mL/min)} = \frac{(140 - \text{age in years}) \times (\text{wt in kg})}{72 \times \text{serum creatinine in mg/dL}}$$

r women, multiply above by 0.85. Unreliable if: unstable renal function; very ese; oedematous. For an example adjusting for ideal body weight, see p434.

assifying renal impairment in chronic kidney disease (CKD)

ronic kidney disease can be classified based on the presence of kidney damage d the GFR, irrespective of the diagnosis.[1]

tage	GFR (mL/min)	Notes
1	>90	Normal or ↑GFR with other evidence of renal damage
2	60–89	Slight ↓GFR with other evidence of renal damage
3	30–59	Moderate ↓GFR with(out) evidence of renal damage
4	15–29	Severe ↓GFR with(out) evidence of renal damage
5	<15	Established renal failure

her evidence of renal damage = proteinuria, haematuria, or evidence of renal sease. One reason to classify renal impairment is to motivate secondary evention, eg to 'mandate' ACE-i or ARA if BP >140/85 especially if proteinuria is esent or stage ≥3. ***Problems using MDRD formula to grade renal disease:***

The MDRD formula was validated for patients with *established* renal failure: its use for screening *general* populations is questionable.

The formula is less accurate the milder the CKD. In one unpeer-reviewed study using ^{51}Cr-EDTA measured GFR (n=178), only 79% were correctly placed in stage 3, and 59% in stage 2.[5] ►Remember that the eGFR is only a screening test and, especially in mild renal impairment, may err on the side of pessimism.

ased on kidney disease outcomes quality initiative chronic kidney disease (K/DOQI CKD) USA classification

Urate and the kidney

Causes of hyperuricaemia High levels of urate in the blood (hyperuricaemia) result from increased turnover or reduced excretion of urate. Either may be c induced.

- ***Drugs:*** Cytotoxics; thiazides; pyrazinamide.
- ***Increased cell turnover:*** Lymphoma; leukaemia; psoriasis; haemolysis; mu death (rhabdomyolysis, p299 *Tumour lysis syndrome:* See p514.
- ***Reduced excretion:*** Primary gout (p534); chronic renal failure; nephropathy; hyperparathyroidism; pre-eclampsia (OHCS p48).
- ***In addition:*** Hyperuricaemia may be associated with hypertension hyperlipidaemia. Urate may be raised in disorders of purine synthesis such a Lesch–Nyhan syndrome (OHCS p648).

Hyperuricaemia and renal failure Severe renal failure from any cause ma associated with hyperuricaemia, and very rarely this may give rise to g Sometimes the relationship of cause and effect is reversed so that it is hyperuricaemia that causes the renal failure. This can occur following cytot treatment (***tumour lysis syndrome***), eg in leukaemia; and in muscle necrosi

How urate causes renal failure In some instances, ureteric obstruction urate crystals occurs. This responds to retrograde ureteric catheterization lavage. More commonly, urate precipitates in the renal tubules. This may occu plasma levels ≥1.19mmol/L.

Prevention of renal failure Before starting chemotherapy, ensure good hydra consider alkalinization of the urine; and initiate allopurinol (a xanthine oxi inhibitor), which prevents a sharp rise in urate following chemotherapy. F specific dosage regimen, see p514. There is a remote risk of inducing xant nephropathy.

Treatment of hyperuricaemic acute renal failure Prompt rehydration alkalinization of the urine after excluding bilateral ureteric obstruction. oliguria is established, haemodialysis is required and should be used in prefere to peritoneal dialysis.

Gout See p534.

Electrolyte physiology

Most sodium is extracellular and is pumped out of the cell by the sodium pum exchange for K^+ (ratio of 3:2) which requires energy from ATP.
Osmolarity is the number of osmoles per *litre* of solution.
Osmolality is the number of osmoles per kilogram of solvent (*normal:* 280–3
A mole is the molecular weight expressed in grams.

To estimate plasma osmolality: $2(Na^+ + K^+)$ + Urea + Glucose. If the measu osmolality is greater than this (ie an osmolar gap of >10mmol/L), consi diabetes mellitus, high blood ethanol, methanol, mannitol, or ethylene glycol.

Fluid compartments For 70kg man: *total fluid* = 42L (60% body weig *Intracellular fluid* = 28L (67% body fluid), *extracellular fluid* = 14L (33% b fluid). *Intravascular component* = 5L of blood (3L plasma).

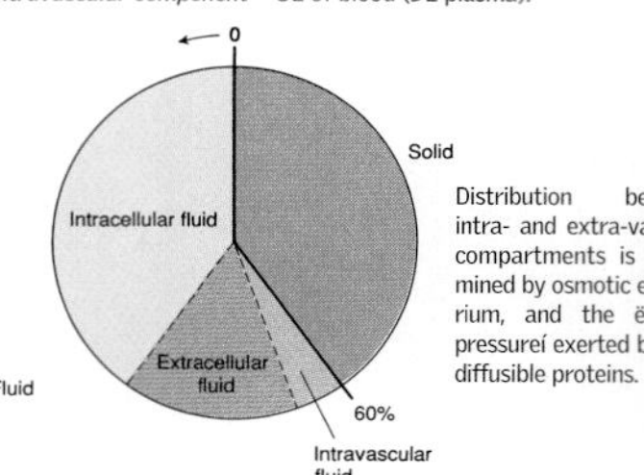

Distribution between intra- and extra-vascular compartments is determined by osmotic equilibrium, and the ëoncotic pressureí exerted by non-diffusible proteins.

Fluid balance over 24h is roughly:

Input (mL water)	*Output (mL water)*
Drink: 1500	Urine: 1500
In food: 800	Insensible loss: 800
Metabolism of food: 200	Stool: 200
Total: **2500**	Total: **2500**

Control of sodium *Renin* is produced by the juxtaglomerular apparatus in respo to decreased renal blood flow, and catalyses the conversion of *angiotensinoge* peptide made by the liver) to *angiotensin I*. This is then converted by angioten converting enzyme (ACE), which is located in the lung and blood vessels *angiotensin II*. The latter has several important actions including efferent re arteriolar constriction (so increasing perfusion pressure); peripheral va constriction; and stimulation of the adrenal cortex to produce *aldosterone*, wh activates the sodium pump in the distal renal tubule leading to reabsorptio sodium and water from the urine, in exchange for potassium and hydrogen io

High GFR *(p660) results in high sodium loss.*

High renal tubular blood flow and haemodilution decrease sodium reabsorptic the proximal tubule.

Control of water Controlled mainly by sodium concentration. ↑Plasma osmola causes thirst, and the release of antidiuretic hormone (ADH) from the poste pituitary which increases the passive water reabsorption from the renal collect duct, by opening water channels to allow water to flow from the hypotonic lum fluid into the hypertonic renal interstitium.

atriuretic peptides

ecretory granules have long been known to exist in the atria, and if omogenized atrial tissue is injected into rats, their urine volume (and Na^+ xcretion) rises. This is evidence of endocrine action via the effects of atrial atriuretic peptide (ANP). BNP is a similar hormone originally identified from pig rain (hence the B), but most BNP is secreted from ventricular myocardium. lasma BNP is closely related to left ventricular pressure.

In myocardial infarction and left ventricular dysfunction, these hormones can e released in large quantities. Secretion is also increased by tachycardia, lucocorticoids, and thyroid hormones. Vasoactive peptides (endothelin-1, ngiotensin II) also influence secretion. ANP and BNP both increase GFR and ecrease renal Na^+ resorption; they also decrease preload by relaxing smooth ıuscle. ANP partly blocks secretion of renin and aldosterone.

NP as a biomarker of heart failure[1] As plasma BNP reflects myocyte stretch, NP is used to diagnose heart failure. ↑BNP distinguishes heart failure from other auses of dyspnoea more accurately than left ventricular ejection fraction, ANP, nd N-terminal ANP (sensitivity: >90%; specificity: 80–90%). BNP is highest in ecompensated heart failure, intermediate in left ventricular dysfunction but no cute heart failure exacerbation, and lowest if no heart failure or LV dysfunction.

Vhat BNP threshold for diagnosing heart failure? If BNP >100ng/L, this liagnoses' heart failure better than other clinical variables or clinical judgement n on-call settings (history, examination, and CXR). BNP can be used to 'rule out' eart failure if <50ng/L—negative predictive value (PV) 96%, ie the chance of NP being <50ng/L given that heart failure is absent in 96%, see p646. In those vith heart failure, BNP is higher in systolic dysfunction than in isolated diastolic lysfunction (eg hypertrophic or dilated cardiomyopathy), and is highest in those vith systolic *and* diastolic dysfunction.

Threshold (ng/L)	Sensitivity (%)	Specificity (%)	Positive PV	Negative PV	Accuracy (%)
≥50	97	62	71	96	79
≥80	93	74	77	92	83
≥100	90	76	79	89	83
≥125	87	79	80	87	83
≥150	85	83	83	85	84[2]

NP increases in proportion to right ventricular dysfunction, eg in primary pulmonary hypertension, cor pulmonale, PE, and congenital heart disease, but ises are less than in left ventricular disorders.

Prognosis in heart failure: The higher the BNP, the higher the cardiovascular nd all-cause mortality (independent of age, NYHA class p121, previous MI and LV ejection fraction). ↑BNP in heart failure is also associated with sudden death. Serial testing may be important: persistently high BNP levels despite vigorous nti-failure treatment predict adverse outcomes. In one study, those with heart ailure randomized to get N-terminal BNP-guided (rather than symptom-guided) herapy had fewer adverse events.

Prognosis in angina and MI: BNP has some prognostic value here (adverse left ventricular remodelling;[3] LV dysfunction; death post-MI).

Prognosis in cor pulmonale/primary pulmonary hypertension: BNP is useful.

Cautions with BNP: A BNP >50ng/L does not exclude other co-existing diseases such as pneumonia. Also, assays vary, so liaise with your lab.

Clinical chemistry

Lemos J 2003 *Lancet* **362** 316 & Fuat A 2006 *BJGP* 56 3272 Maisel A *N Engl J Med* 2002 **347** 161

Abnormal remodelling (cell slippage producing a more spherical LV + systolic dysfunction) is seen on no or CT/MRI; it is measured as the *wall motion index* or the *left ventricular end-diastolic volume index* DVI, mL/m²). If EDVI is ≥5mL/m² ~6 months post-MI (compared with an initial post-MI value), remodel-g has occurred. *Sustained* ↑BNP reflects progressive ventricular remodelling long after acute MI. normal remodelling is preventable in CCF by ACE-i and exercise training.

Sodium: hyponatraemia

Signs & symptoms depend on severity and rate of change in serum sodium, a include: confusion, seizures, hypertension, cardiac failure, oedema, anorexia, naus muscle weakness.

Diagnosis See tree in diagram OPPOSITE. The key question is: Is the patie dehydrated? History and urine analysis are your guides.

Causes of hyponatraemia (For a full list, see the diagram OPPOSITE.)

- *Diuretics*, especially thiazides.
- *Water excess*, either orally, or as excess 5% dextrose IV.
- *Pseudohyponatraemia:* (1) If serum volume↑ from high lipids or protein, Na^+ fa but plasma osmolality is ↔. (2) If plasma glucose ≥20mmol/L, make correction.[1] (3) Na^+ will be ↓ if blood is from an arm with a dextrose IVI.

Management ►Don't base treatment on plasma Na^+ concentration alone. T presence of symptoms, duration, and state of hydration influence treatment. possible, correct the underlying cause. If chronic: fluid restriction, or cautio rehydration with saline if dehydrated, is often sufficient if asymptomatic, althou demeclocycline may be required. If symptomatic, saline may be given, but do n correct chronic changes rapidly (max 15mmol/d rise in serum sodium). Acu hyponatraemia may be treated with saline infusion and furosemide.

Hypervolaemic hyponatraemia (cirrhosis, CCF) treat the underlying disorder. ***emergency*** (seizures, coma), consider IVI of 0.9% saline or hypertonic saline (1.8% saline) at 70mmol Na^+/h. Aim for a gradual increase in plasma sodium ≈125mmol/L. Can combine with furosemide. Watch for heart failure, and cent pontine myelinolysis. ►Seek expert help.

Syndrome of inappropriate ADH secretion (SIADH) An important, but ove diagnosed, cause of hyponatraemia. The diagnosis requires concentrated uri (sodium >20mmol/L and osmolality >500mosmol/kg) in the presence of hyp natraemia (<125mmol/L) or low plasma osmolality (<260mosmol/kg), and t absence of hypovolaemia, oedema, or diuretics.

Causes: *Malignancy*, eg lung small-cell; pancreas; prostate; lymphoma.
CNS disorders: Meningoencephalitis; abscess; stroke; subarachnoid, subdu haemorrhage; head injury; Guillain–Barré; vasculitis, p542, eg SLE.
Chest disease: TB; pneumonia; abscess; aspergillosis.
Metabolic disease: Porphyria; trauma.
Drugs: Opiates; psychotropics; SSRIs; cytotoxics.
Treatment: Treat the cause, fluid restrict, occasionally demeclocycline.

Hypernatraemia

Signs & symptoms Look for thirst, confusion, coma, and fits—with signs dehydration: dry skin, ↓skin turgor, postural hypotension, and oliguria if wat deficient. Laboratory features: ↑PCV, ↑albumin, ↑urea.

Causes Usually due to water loss in excess of sodium loss:

- Fluid loss without water replacement (eg diarrhoea, vomit, burns).
- Incorrect IV fluid replacement (excessive saline).
- Diabetes insipidus (p224). Suspect if large urine volume. This may follow hea injury, or CNS surgery, especially pituitary.
- Osmotic diuresis (for diabetic coma, see p814).
- Primary aldosteronism: suspect if BP↑, K^+↓, alkalosis (HCO_3^-↑).

Management Give water orally if possible; if not, dextrose 5% IV slowly (~4L/24 guided by urine output and plasma Na^+. Some authorities recommend 0.9% sali (esp. if hypovolaemic) as this causes less marked fluid shifts and is hypotonic in hypernatraemic patient. Avoid hypotonic solutions.

1 Add ~4.3mmol/L to plasma Na^+ for every 10mmol/L rise in glucose above normal.

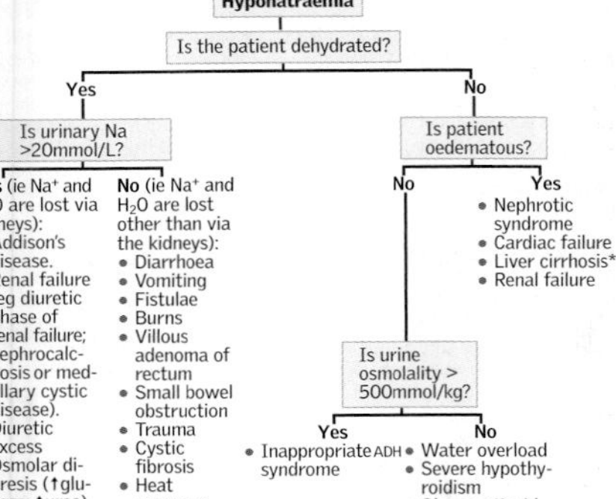

*: in cirrhosis, hyponatraemia may precede oedema

Hyponatraemia: it matters—and it is preventable

If 5% dextrose is infused post-operatively, the dextrose is quickly used, rendering the fluid hypotonic. This causes hyponatraemia (nausea, headaches, weakness, cognition↓, coma, death)—especially in those at risk: on excessive doses of thiazide diuretics, females (especially pre-menopausal) and those undergoing physiological stress, which causes inappropriate ADH secretion, hence the low Na^+. In some individuals, only marginally low plasma Na^+ levels cause serious effects (eg ~128mmol/L). Risk of harm is minimized by following these rules:

- Know the pre-op U&E.
- Don't infuse dextrose without saline.
- Do a post-op U&E. Look at the result (Obvious, and so forgettable).
- Don't attribute odd CNS signs to non-existent strokes/TIAs if Na^+↓.
- Don't ignore low sodiums. Get help if you don't know what to do.

Treatment: (►p666) 0.9% saline IVI; do U&E every 2h; aim to bring Na^+ up to 130mmol/L by 1–2mmol/L per hour. Diuretics eg furosemide may be useful in acute hyponatraemia, or if the patient is symptomatic. Hypertonic saline (eg 1.8% saline) should only be used in emergencies when the patient has profound neurological symptoms (seizures, coma).

Potassium

General points Most potassium is intracellular, and thus serum potassium lev are a poor reflection of total body potassium. The concentrations of K^+ and H^+ ic in extracellular fluid tend to vary together. This is because these ions compete w each other in the exchange with sodium which occurs across most cell membra (sodium is pumped out of the cell) and in the distal tubule of the kidney (sodium reabsorbed from the urine). Thus, if H^+ ion concentration is high, fewer K^+ ions w be excreted into the urine. Similarly K^+ will compete with H^+ for exchange acro cell membranes and extracellular K^+ will accumulate. Insulin and catecholamin both stimulate K^+ uptake into cells by stimulating the Na^+/K^+ pump.

Hyperkalaemia

►A plasma potassium >6.5mmol/L needs urgent treatment (p821) but first ensu that this is not an artefact (eg due to haemolysis inside the bottle).

Signs & symptoms Cardiac arrhythmias. Sudden death. ECG: Tall tented T wav small P wave; wide QRS complex becoming sinusoidal, VF. (see OPPOSITE)

Causes
- Oliguric renal failure
- K⁺-sparing diuretics
- Rhabdomyolysis (p299), burns
- Metabolic acidosis (DM)
- Excess K⁺ therapy
- Addison's disease (see p210)
- Massive blood transfusion
- Drugs, eg ACE-i, suxamethonium
- Artefact. Haemolysis of sample; delay in analysis—K⁺ leaks out of RB thrombocythaemia—platelets leak K⁺ as sample clots in tube.

Treatment Treat underlying cause. ►In emergency, see p821.

Hypokalaemia

If K^+ <2.5mmol/L, urgent treatment is required. Note that hypokalaem exacerbates digoxin toxicity.

Signs & symptoms Muscle weakness, hypotonia, cardiac arrhythmias, cramps, a tetany. *ECG:* Small or inverted T waves; prominent U wave (after T wave); prolong P–R interval; depressed ST segment.

Causes
- Diuretics
- Vomiting and diarrhoea
- Pyloric stenosis
- Villous adenoma rectum
- Intestinal fistulae
- Cushing's syndrome/steroids/ACTH
- Conn's syndrome
- Alkalosis
- Purgative and liquorice abuse
- Renal tubular failure (p660).

If on diuretics, then ↑bicarbonate is the best indication that hypokalaemia is like to have been long-standing. Magnesium may be low, and hypokalaemia is oft difficult to correct until magnesium levels are normalized. In hypokalaemic perioc paralysis, intermittent weakness lasting up to 72h appears to be caused by shifting from extra- to intracellular fluid. See *OHCS* p652. Suspect Conn's syndrom if hypertensive, hypokalaemic alkalosis in someone not taking diuretics (p212)

Treatment ***If mild:*** (>2.5mmol/L, no symptoms) give oral K^+ suppleme (≥80mmol/24h, eg Sando-K® 2 tabs/6–8h). If taking a thiazide diuret hypokalaemia >3.0mmol/L rarely needs treating. ***If severe:*** (<2.5mmol/L, and/ dangerous symptoms) give IV potassium cautiously, not more than 20mmol/h, a not more concentrated than 40mmol/L. Do not give potassium if oligur ►**Never** give potassium as a fast 'stat' bolus dose.

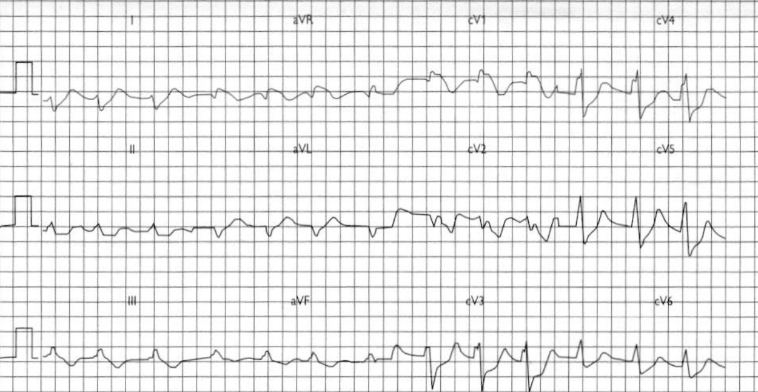

ECG 13—hyperkalaemia—note the flattening of the P-waves, prominent T-waves, and widening of the QRS complex.

Calcium: physiology

General points About 40% of plasma calcium is bound to albumin. Usually it total plasma calcium which is measured, although it is the unbound, ionized porti which is important. Therefore, *adjust total calcium level for albumin as follows:* A 0.1mmol/L to calcium concentration for every 4g/L that albumin is below 40g and a similar subtraction for raised albumin. However, many factors affect bindi (eg other proteins in myeloma, cirrhosis, individual variation) so be cautious in yc interpretation. If in doubt over a high calcium, take blood specimens uncuff (remove tourniquet after needle in vein, but before taking blood sample), and w the patient fasted.

The control of calcium metabolism

- ***Parathyroid hormone* (PTH):** A rise in PTH causes a rise in plasma Ca^{2+} anc decrease in plasma PO_4^{3-}. This is due to ↑Ca^{2+} and ↑ PO_4^{3-} reabsorption from bo and ↑Ca^{2+} but ↓ PO_4^{3-} reabsorption from the kidney. PTH secretion enhanc active vitamin D formation. PTH secretion is itself controlled by ionized plası calcium levels.
- ***Vitamin D:*** Calciferol (Vit D_3), and ergocalciferol (Vit D_2) are biologically identi in their actions. Serum Vit D is converted in the liver to 25-hydroxy Vit D (25(O Vit D). In the kidney, a second hydroxyl group is added to form the biologica active 1,25-dihydroxy Vit D (1,25$(OH)_2$ vit D), also called calcitriol, or the mu less active 24,25$(OH)_2$ Vit D. Calcitriol production is stimulated by ↓Ca^{2+}, ↓ PC and PTH. Its actions include ↑Ca^{2+} and ↑ PO_4^{3-} absorption from the gut; ↑Ca^{2+} a ↑ PO_4^{3-} reabsorption in the kidney; enhanced bone turnover; and inhibition of P release. Disordered regulation of 1,25$(OH)_2$ Vit D underlies familial normoca aemic hypercalciuria which is a major cause of calcium oxalate renal sto formation (p284).
- ***Calcitonin:*** Made in C-cells of the thyroid, this causes a decrease in plasr calcium and phosphate, but its physiological role is unclear. It is a marker detect recurrence or metastasis in medullary carcinoma of the thyroid.
- ***Thyroxine:*** May ↑plasma calcium although this is rare.
- ***Magnesium:*** ↓Mg^{2+} prevents PTH release, and may cause hypocalcaemia.

Hypocalcaemia

►Apparent hypocalcaemia may be an artefact of hypoalbuminaemia (above).

Signs & symptoms Tetany, depression, perioral paraesthesiae, carpo-pedal spa (wrist flexion and fingers drawn together) especially if brachial artery occlud with blood pressure cuff (*Trousseau's sign*), neuromuscular excitability, eg tappi over parotid (facial nerve) causes facial muscles to twitch (*Chvostek's sig* Cataract if chronic Ca^{2+}↓. **ECG**: Q–T interval↑.

Causes It may be a consequence of thyroid or parathyroid surgery. *If phospha raised,* then either chronic renal failure (p294), hypoparathyroidism, pseuc hypoparathyroidism (p206), or acute rhabdomyolysis. If phosphate ↔ or ↓ th either osteomalacia (high alkaline phosphatase), over-hydration or pancreatitis. respiratory alkalosis, the total Ca^{2+} may be normal, but ionized Ca^{2+}↓ and t patient may have symptoms because of this.

Treatment If *symptoms are mild,* give calcium 5mmol/6h PO. Do daily plasr calcium levels. ►For chronic renal failure, see p294. If necessary add alfacalcid start at 0.5–1µg/24h PO. If *symptoms are severe,* give 10mL of 10% calciu gluconate (2.25mmol) IVI over 30min (bolus injections are only needed very rare Repeat as necessary. If due to respiratory alkalosis, correct the alkalosis.

Hypercalcaemia

Signs & symptoms 'Bones, stones, groans, and psychic moans'. Abdominal pa vomiting; constipation; polyuria; polydipsia; depression; anorexia; weight lo tiredness; weakness; hypertension, confusion; pyrexia; renal stones; renal failu corneal calcification; cardiac arrest. ***ECG:*** Q–T interval↓.

Causes and diagnosis Most commonly malignancy (myeloma, bone metastas PTHrP↑, p353) and 1° hyperparathyroidism. Others include sarcoidosis, vit intoxication, and familial benign hypocalciuric hypercalcaemia (rare; defect calcium-sensing receptor). Pointers to malignancy are: ↓albumin, ↓Cl^-, ↓K^+, alk osis, ↓PO_4^{3-} ↑alk phos. Other investigations (eg isotope bone scan, CXR, FBC) may a be of diagnostic value.

Treat the underlying cause. If Ca^{2+} >3.5mmol/L, and severe abdominal pa vomiting, pyrexia, or confusion, aim to reduce calcium as follows:

- ***Blood tests:*** Measure U&E, Mg^{2+}, creatinine, Ca^{2+}, PO_4^{3-}, alk phos.
- ***Fluids:*** Rehydrate with IVI 0.9% saline, eg 4–6L in 24h as needed. Corre hypokalaemia/hypomagnesaemia (mild metabolic acidosis needs no treatmer This will reduce symptoms, and ↑renal Ca^{2+} loss. Monitor U&E.
- ***Diuretics:*** Furosemide 40mg/12h PO/IV, once rehydrated. Avoid thiazides.
- ***Bisphosphonates:*** A single dose of pamidronate (see table, p515) will low Ca^{2+} over 2–3d. Maximum effect is at 1wk. It inhibits osteoclast activity, and bone resorption.
- ***Steroids:*** Occasionally used, eg prednisolone 40–60mg/d for sarcoidosis.
- ***Salmon calcitonin:*** Now rarely used (8U/kg/8h IM). More side effects th bisphosphonates, but quicker onset. Again inhibits osteoclasts.
- ***Other:*** Chemotherapy may ↓Ca^{2+} in malignant disease, eg myeloma.

Magnesium

Magnesium is distributed 65% in bone and 35% in cells; plasma concentrati tends to follow that of Ca^{2+} and K^+. Magnesium excess is usually caused by re failure, but rarely requires treatment in its own right.

Magnesium deficiency causes paraesthesiae, fits, tetany, arrhythmias. Digita toxicity may be exacerbated. ***Causes:*** Severe diarrhoea; ketoacidosis; alcohol; to parenteral nutrition (monitor weekly); accompanying hypocalcaemia; accompar ing hypokalaemia (especially with diuretics) and hypophosphataemia. ***Treatme*** If needed, give magnesium salts, PO or IV (dose example: 8mmol $MgSO_4$ IVI ov 3min to 2h, depending on severity; monitor Mg^{2+} often).

Hypermagnesaemia is usually iatrogenic, or excessive antacids. ***Featur*** Neuromuscular depression, ↓BP, CNS depression, coma.

Zinc

Zinc deficiency This may occur in parenteral nutrition or, rarely, from a poor d (too few cereals and dairy products; anorexia nervosa; alcoholism). Rarely it is d to a genetic defect. ***Signs & symptoms:*** Look for red, crusted skin lesio especially around nostrils and corners of mouth. ***Diagnosis:*** Therapeutic trial zinc (plasma levels are unreliable as they may be low, eg in infection or traum without deficiency).

Selenium

An essential element present in cereals, nuts, and meat. Low soil levels in some pa of Europe and China cause deficiency states. Required for the antioxidant glutathic peroxidase, which ↓harmful free radicals. It is also antithrombogenic, and is requir for sperm motility proteins. Deficiency may increase the frequency of neoplasia a atheroma, and may lead to a cardiomyopathy or arthritis. Serum levels are a pc guide. Toxic symptoms may also be found with over-energetic replacement.

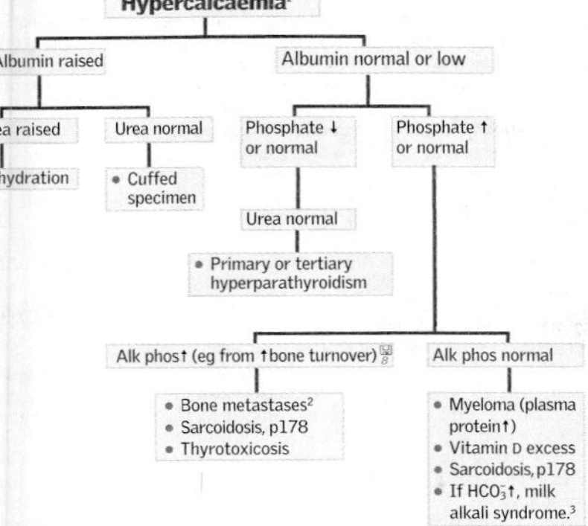

:: To distinguish bone metastases from hyperparathyroidism (the two main causes hypercalcaemia) look for a low albumin, low chloride, and an alkalosis: all suggest tastases. Raised plasma PTH indicates hyperparathyroidism.

his diagram is only a guide: take in conjunction with the clinical picture.
Most common primary: breast, kidney, lung, thyroid, prostate, ovary, colon.
ngesting too much calcium and alkali (eg in milk) can cause hypercalcaemia with metastatic ification and renal failure. Thyrotoxicosis causes alkalaemia because of hyperventilation.

Metabolic bone diseases 1. Osteoporosis

Osteoporosis implies reduced bone density. If trabecular bone is mostly affec crush fractures of vertebrae are common (accounting for the 'littleness' of littl ladies—and their dowager's hump); if cortical bone is mostly affected, fracture long bone is more likely, eg femoral neck: *the* big cause of death and orthopa expense, especially in older women. ***Prevalence:*** 35% of over 50s ♀:♂≈4:1.

Risk of future osteoporotic fracture is increased if:

• Slender or anorectic	• Early menopause	• Osteoporosis in family
• Smoker or alcoholic	• Cushing's syndrome	• Primary biliary cirrhosis
• Prolonged rest; old age	• Malabsorption	• Rheumatoid arthritis
• Hyperparathyroidism	• Thyrotoxicosis	• Hypogonadism
• >5mg/d prednisolone	• Myeloma	• Past low-trauma fractur
• Vertebral deformity	• Amenorrhoea	• Mastocytosis (*OHCS* p61(

Diagnosis: *X*-ray (easier with hindsight afforded by bone fracture), but sensitivity and specificity. Bone densitometry (OPPOSITE). Serum Ca^{2+}, PO_4^{3-}, anc phos normal. Biopsy specimens may be unrepresentative.

Prevention: Exercise; good, Ca^{2+}-rich diet; avoid smoking and excess alc For those at ↑risk, eg on corticosteroids (eg >7.5mg/d of prednisolc bisphosphonates ↓risk. **NB:** hormone replacement therapy (HRT) can prev osteoporosis, but the UK Committee on Safety of Medicines (CSM) says that ov to HRT's propensity to cause breast cancer (and other problems) it should no lor be a first-line option for preventing osteoporosis. ***Treatment:*** • Ca^{2+}-rich diet

- *Bisphosphonates* are used for the prevention and treatment of osteoporosis Alendronic acid 10mg/d (SE: abdo pain; nausea; photosensitivity, oesophag ulcers). ►Explain the need to swallow the pill while remaining upright >30min) with plenty of water 20min before breakfast (and any other dru stop if dysphagia or pain. A single weekly dose is available (70mg). Or didrc PMO® (14d of etidronate 400mg/d and 76d of calcium carbonate 1.25g in day cycles). It is important to maintain a good calcium and vit. D intake consider adding a daily supplement.
- *Others:* ***Vitamin D*** is effective (watch serum Ca^{2+}). ***Raloxifene*** (a selec oestrogen receptor modulator 'SERM') may also ↓ breast cancer risk. Its rol unclear. ***Calcitonin*** may be considered; reduces pain post vertebral fracture (r available intra-nasally). ***Recombinant PTH*** (teriparatide) stimulates new bone is effective in preventing fractures; NICE recommends it to prevent recurr fractures in those intolerant of bisphosphonates. ***Strontium ranelate*** conta 2 atoms of strontium (same periodic group as calcium) and seems to incre bone formation and reduce reabsorption. Effective in reducing fractures.

2. Paget's disease of bone

There is increased bone turnover associated with increased numbers of osteobla and osteoclasts with resultant remodelling, bone enlargement, deformity, a weakness. Rare in the under-40s. Incidence rises with age (3% over 55yrs c Commoner in temperate climes, and Anglo-Saxons. It may be asymptomatic or ca pain and enlargement of skull, femur, clavicle—and bowed (*sabre*) tibia—a pathological fractures, nerve deafness (bone overgrowth), and high-output CCF.

X-rays: Localized enlargement of bone. Patchy cortical thickening with sclerc osteolysis, and deformity (*osteoporosis circumscripta* of the skull). Affinity for a skeleton, long bones, and skull.

Blood biochemistry: Ca^{2+} and PO_4^{3-} normal; alk phos markedly raised.

Complications: Bone sarcoma (1% of those affected for >10yrs). Symptoms nerve compression, eg deafness. ***Treatment:*** If analgesia fails, alendronic acid (above) may be tried, to reduce pain and/or deformity. It is more effective th etidronate or calcitonin, and as effective as IV pamidronate. Follow expert adv

derstanding Dexa bone scan results: WHO osteoporosis criteria

ical sites examined are the lumbar spine (preferably 3 vertebrae) and hip. ne mineral density (BMD, in g/cm²) is compared with that of a young healthy ılt. The 'T-score' relates to the number of standard deviations the BMD is from average. If the T-score is:

>0	BMD is better than the reference.
) to −1	BMD is in the top 84%: no evidence of osteoporosis.
-1 to −2.5	Osteopenia, with risk of later osteoporotic complication, so consider preventive measures (see OPPOSITE).
-2.5 or worse	BMD is ≥2.5 standard deviations below the mean value for young adults: osteoporosis is present—severe if there is 1 or more fragility fracture.

example of a suitable indication for densitometry is before embarking on ednisolone treatment (>6 months, at >7.5mg/d; steroids contribute osteoporosis by promoting osteoclast bone resorption, and decreasing muscle ss and ↓GI calcium absorption).

Benefits of universal screening for osteoporosis are unproven.

3. Osteomalacia

In osteomalacia there is a normal amount of bone but its mineral content is (there is excess uncalcified osteoid and cartilage). Rickets is the result if process occurs during the period of bone growth; osteomalacia is the result occurs after fusion of the epiphyses.

Forms

- ***Vitamin D deficiency:*** Due to malabsorption (p272), poor diet, or lack of sunli
- ***Renal osteomalacia:*** Renal failure leads to 1,25-dihydroxycholecalcifer [1,25(OH)$_2$vitamin D] deficiency (p294).
- ***Drug-induced:*** Anticonvulsants may induce liver enzymes, leading to increased breakdown of 25-hydroxycholecalciferol.
- ***Vitamin D resistance:*** A number of mainly inherited conditions in which osteomalacia responds to high doses of vitamin D (see below).
- ***Liver disease:*** Reduced production of 25-hydroxy vitamin D (25(vitamin D), and malabsorption of vitamin D, eg cirrhosis (p252).

Investigations

Plasma: Mildly ↓Ca^{2+}; ↓ PO_4^{3-}; alk phos↑; PTH high; 25(OH)vitamin D↓, excep resistant cases; in renal failure 1,25(OH)$_2$vitamin D↓ (p294).

Biopsy: Shows incomplete mineralization.

X-ray: Cupped, ragged metaphyseal surfaces (in rickets). In osteomalacia there loss of cortical bone; also, apparent partial fractures without displacement ma seen especially on the lateral border of the scapula, inferior femoral neck medial femoral shaft (Looser's zones).

Signs & symptoms

Rickets: Knock-kneed; bow-legged. Features of hypocalcaemia—usually r (p694). Children with rickets are ill.

Osteomalacia: Bone pain; fractures (neck of femur); proximal myopathy (wadc gait), due to ↓ PO_4^{3-} and vitamin D deficiency *per se*.

Treatment Calcium-with-vitamin D (400U) tablets: 1–2 tablets/d.

- If due to malabsorption, give calciferol tablets, up to 1mg (=40,000U) dail parenteral calciferol, eg 7.5mg monthly.
- If vitamin-D-resistant, give calciferol 10,000 units/24h PO.
- If due to renal disease, give alfacalcidol (1α-hydroxy vitamin D) 1μg/24h PO adjust dose according to plasma calcium.
- Monitor plasma calcium, initially weekly, and if nausea/vomiting.

►Vitamin D therapy (esp. alfacalcidol) can cause dangerous hypercalcaemia.

Vitamin D-resistant rickets exists in 2 forms. Type I with low renal 1α-hydro lase activity, and type II with end organ resistance to 1,25(OH)2vitamin d, due point mutation in the receptor. Both are treated with large doses 1,25(OH)2vitamin d (calcitriol).

X-linked hypophosphataemic rickets Dominantly inherited—due to a defec renal phosphate handling (due to mutations in the PEX or PHEX genes which enc an endopeptidase). Rickets develops in early childhood and is associated with p growth. Plasma phosphate is low, alkaline phosphatase high, and there phosphaturia. Treatment is with high doses of oral phosphate, 1,25(OH)$_2$vitamin D. Hypophosphataemic osteomalacia may develop in patie consuming phosphate binders, eg aluminium hydroxide, or some rare tumour, ar accompanied by severe muscle weakness.

See also ***Renal bone disease***, p294.

Plasma proteins

Electrophoresis distinguishes a number of bands (see figure OPPOSITE).

Albumin is synthesized in the liver; $t_{½} \approx 20$d. It binds *bilirubin, free fatty acids,* Ca^{2+} and some *drugs*. ***Low albumin*** results in oedema. *Causes:* Liver disease, nephrotic syndrome, burns, protein-losing enteropathy, malabsorption, malnutrition, late pregnancy, artefact (eg from arm with IVI), posture (5g/L higher if upright), genetic variations, malignancy. ***High albumin—Causes:*** Dehydration; artefact (eg stasis).

α1 zone: α_1-antitrypsin, thyroxine-binding globulin, and high-density lipoprotein (HDL). α_1-antitrypsin deficiency (autosomal recessive) leads to cirrhosis and emphysema: unopposed phagocyte proteases. Accelerated age-related decline in FEV_1 from a normal of ~35mL/yr to 80mL/yr, exacerbated by smoking. Signs: dyspnoea, weight↓; cor pulmonale; PCV↑; LFT↑ (hepatocytes cannot secrete the protein).

α2 zone: α_2-macroglobulin, caeruloplasmin, very low density lipoprotein (VLDL, p682), and haptoglobin (p322).

β zone: Transferrin, low-density lipoprotein (LDL), fibrinogen, C3 and C4 complement. Reduced in active nephritis, glomerulonephritis, and SLE.

γ zone: Immunoglobulins, factor VIII, C-reactive protein (CRP), and α-fetoprotein. *Diffusely raised* in: chronic infections, liver cirrhosis, sarcoidosis, SLE, RA, Crohn's disease, TB, bronchiectasis, PBC, hepatitis, and parasitaemia. It is *low* in nephrotic syndrome, malabsorption, malnutrition, immune deficiency (severe illness, diabetes mellitus, renal failure, malignancy, or congenital).

Paraproteinaemia See p354.

Acute phase response The body responds to a variety of insults with, amongst other things, the synthesis, by the liver, of a number of proteins (normally present in serum in small quantities)—eg α_1-antitrypsin, fibrinogen, complement, haptoglobin and CRP. An increased density of the α_1- and α_2-fractions, often with a reduced albumin level, is characteristic of conditions such as infection, malignancy (especially α_2-fraction), trauma, surgery, and inflammatory disease.

CRP Levels help monitor inflammation/infection. Normal <8mg/L. Like the ESR, it is raised in many inflammatory conditions, but changes more rapidly; increases in hours and falling within 2–3d of recovery. Therefore, it can be used to follow the response to therapy (eg antibiotics) or disease activity (eg Crohn's disease). CRP values in mild inflammation 10–50mg/L; active bacterial infection 50–200mg/L; severe infection or trauma >200mg/L; see OPPOSITE. CRP levels also predict outcome in patients with cardiovascular disease if measured using a highly sensitive assay: Low risk <1mg/L; moderate risk 1–3; and high risk >3mg/L.

Urinary proteins

If urinary protein loss >0.15g/24h, then pathological. See p278.

Albuminuria Usually caused by renal disease. Microalbuminuria (protein excretion between 3 and 300mg/d may be seen with diabetes or hypertension).

Bence Jones protein consists of light chains excreted in excess by some patients with myeloma (p352). They are not detected by dipsticks and may occur with normal serum electrophoresis.

Haemoglobinuria p324. ***Myoglobinuria*** (rhabdomyolysis) p299. ***Microalbuminuria*** (seen in DM; ↑BP; SLE; glomerulonephritis)—see p301 for role in diabetes.

C-reactive protein (CRP)

Marked elevation	***Normal-to-slight elevation***
Bacterial infection	Viral infection
Abscess	Steroids/oestrogens
Crohn's disease	Ulcerative colitis
Connective tissue diseases (except SLE)	SLE
Neoplasia	Atherosclerosis
Trauma	
Necrosis (eg MI)	

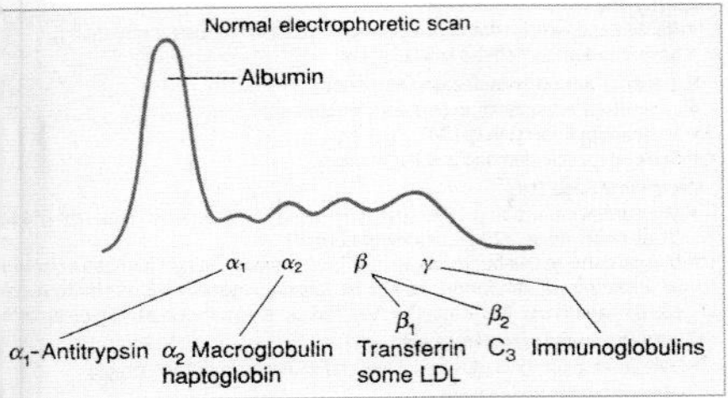

Normal electrophoretic scan

Albumin

α_1 α_2 β γ

β_1 β_2

α_1-Antitrypsin

α_2 Macroglobulin haptoglobin

Transferrin some LDL

C_3

Immunoglobulins

Plasma enzymes

►Reference intervals vary between laboratories.
Raised levels of specific enzymes can be a useful indicator of a disea However, remember that most can be raised for other reasons too. The ma causes of ***raised enzymes*** are given below. Normal values: see p742.

Alkaline phosphatase

- Liver disease (suggests cholestasis).
- Bone disease (isoenzyme distinguishable, reflects osteoblast activity) especi Paget's, growing children, healing fractures, osteomalacia, metasta hyperparathyroidism, and renal failure.
- Pregnancy (placenta makes its own isoenzyme).

Alanine-amino transferase (ALT; SGPT)

- Liver disease (suggests hepatocyte damage). Also raised in shock.

α-Amylase

- Acute pancreatitis (not chronic pancreatitis as little tissue remaining).
- Severe uraemia, diabetic ketoacidosis.

Aspartate-amino transferase (AST; SGOT)

- Liver disease (suggesting hepatocyte damage).
- Myocardial infarction (p104).
- Skeletal muscle damage and haemolysis.

Creatine kinase (CK)

- Myocardial infarction (p104; isoenzyme 'CK-MB'. MI diagnosed if CK-MB>6% to CK, or CK-MB mass >99 percentile of normal).
- Muscle damage (rhabdomyolysis, p299; prolonged running; haematoma; seizur IM injection; defibrillation; bowel ischaemia; myxoedema; dermatomyosi p538)—and *drugs* (eg statins). ►A raised CK does not necessarily mean an M

Gamma-glutamyl transferase (GGT, γGT)

- Liver disease (particularly alcohol-induced damage, cholestasis, drugs).

Lactate dehydrogenase (LDH)

- Myocardial infarction (p104).
- Liver disease (suggests hepatocyte damage).
- Haemolysis, pulmonary embolism, and tumour necrosis.

Troponin

- Myocardial infarction (p104).
- Pericarditis, myocarditis, PE, sepsis, renal failure (elevation less marked).

Clinical chemistry

Tumour markers

Tumour markers are rarely sufficiently specific to be of diagnostic value. Their m value is in monitoring the course of an illness and the effectiveness of treatme Reference ranges vary between laboratories.

Alpha-fetoprotein ↑In hepatocellular Ca (p262), germ cell tumours (not pu seminoma) hepatitis; cirrhosis; pregnancy; open neural tube defects.

CA 125 Raised in carcinoma of the ovary, uterus, breast, and hepatocellu carcinoma. Also raised in pregnancy, cirrhosis, and peritonitis.

CA 15-3 Raised in carcinoma of the breast and benign breast disease.

CA 19-9 Raised in colorectal and pancreatic carcinoma, and cholestasis.

Carcino-embryonic antigen (CEA) ↑In gastrointestinal neoplasms, especia colorectal CA. Also cirrhosis, pancreatitis, and smoking.

Human chorionic gonadotrophin Raised in pregnancy and germ cell tumours. F hydatidiform moles and choriocarcinoma, see *OHCS* p264.

Neurone specific enolase (NSE) ↑in small-cell lung cancer and neuroblastoma

Placental alkaline phosphatase (PLAP) ↑ in: pregnancy, ca, seminoma, smokin

Prostate specific antigen (PSA)

As well as being a marker of prostate cancer, PSA is (unfortunately) raised in benign prostatic hypertrophy. See prostate cancer (p606) and p607 for advising men who ask for a PSA test. 25% of large benign prostates give PSA up to 10 μg/L; levels may be higher if recent ejaculation; therefore, avoid ejaculation for 24h prior to measurement. Other factors causing raised PSA: recent rectal examination, prostatitis, and UTI (PSA levels may not return to base-line for some months after the latter).[1] Plasma reference interval is age specific, an example of the top end of the reference interval for total PSA is:

Healthy males of age (yrs)	*PSA μg/L*
40–50	2.5
50–59	3.5
60–69	5.0
70–79	6.5
80–89	7.5

The above is a rough guide only; different labs have different reference ranges, and populations vary. More specific assays, such as free PSA/total PSA index, and PSA density, are also becoming available, which may partly solve these problems. It is shown to illustrate the common problem of interpreting a PSA of ~8—and as a warning against casual requests for PSAs in the (vain) hope of simple answers. The following indicates the proportion of patients with a raised PSA and benign hypertrophy or carcinoma.

	PSA μg/L	
Benign prostatic hypertrophy	<4 in 91%	PSA will be ~50% lower after 6 months on 5α reductase inhibitors (to ↓prostate size, see p602)
	4–10 in 8%	
	>10 in 1%	
Prostate carcinoma	<4 in 15%	
	4–10 in 20%	
	>10 in 65%	

Enzyme Inducers and Inhibitors

Liver enzymes, including those involved in the metabolism of drugs (eg the cytochrome P450 enzyme family), may be either induced or inhibited by a range of commonly used drugs and food substances:

Enzyme inducers	**Enzyme Inhibitors**
Phenytoin	SSRIs
Rifampicin	Ciprofloxacin
Carbamazepine	Cimetidine
Omeprazole	Erythromycin
Alcohol	Ketoconazole
St John's wort	Grapefruit juice

This can lead to important interactions or side-effects. For example phenytoin reduces the effectiveness of the Pill due to more rapid oestrogen metabolism, and ciprofloxacin retards the metabolism of methylxanthines (aminophylline) which leads to higher plasma levels and potentially more side-effects. The *BNF* contains a list of the major interactions between drugs.

1. Up to six months in one study. G Aus 2003 *Urology* **62** 278

Hyperlipidaemia

Cholesterol is a major risk factor for coronary heart disease (CHD). Half the population have a serum cholesterol putting them at significant risk of CHD. Do treat in isolation, assess other risk factors: smoking, BP↑, DM, family history— ***risk equation***, p642. Benefits of treatment must be set against cost, a imposition of diets and tablet-taking (with expensive follow-up plans).

Trial evidence that treating hypercholesterolaemia is worthwhile

- *'4S' study.*[14] Secondary prevention trial (patients with ischaemic heart disea using simvastatin ≥20mg/d PO *nocte* in 4444 men aged 35–70 (cholesterol 5 8.0mmol/L). Number needed to treat (NNT, p650) to prevent 1 fatal MI was (over 6yrs), and 14 for non-fatal events.
- *WOSCOPS.*[15] Primary prevention trial in Scotland with over 6500 men (choleste >6.5mmol/L), pravastatin 40mg/24h PO *nocte*. NNT to prev 1 fatal MI was 142 (over 5yrs), and for all cardiac events was 55.
- *CARE study.*[16] Secondary prevention trial with 40mg of pravastatin/24h PC >4000 people, post-MI, with 'normal' cholesterol (<6.2mmol/L). NNT for fatalit was 91 (over 5yrs), and for non-fatal MI was 38.
- *HEART PROTECTION STUDY.*[17] Secondary prevention trial with 40mg simvastatir patients irrespective of cholesterol. NNT for death = 55. No evidence of 'thresh of cholesterol' for benefit.

Who to screen

- CHD or risk↑, eg DM, BP↑.
- Family history of hyperlipidaemia, or CHD before 65yrs old.
- Xanthomata or xanthelasmata.
- Corneal arcus before 50yrs old.

Management[18]

- Exclude familial or 2° hyperlipidaemias. Treat as appropriate.
- Lifestyle advice. Aim for BMI of 20–25. Diet with <10% of calories fr saturated fats; ↑fibre, fresh fruit & vegetables, omega-3 fatty acids . ↑Exerci
- Treat those with known CHD.
- If *no CHD*, risk tables (p642). ℞ when MI risk is >3%/yr, eg cholesterol >5.5 50-yr-old ♂ smoker with DM, LVH & BP↑, but cholesterol >6.9 if no LVH or DM.
- 'Statins' (p101) are first choice; they ↓cholesterol synthesis in the liv (eg ***simvastatin*** 40mg PO at night). CI: porphyria, LFT↑. SE: myositis (stop if CK↑ ≥10-fold. If any muscle aches, check CK; risk is 1/100,000 treatment yrs abdominal pain; LFT↑ (stop if AST ≥100U/L).
- 2nd-line therapy: fibrates, eg bezafibrate (useful in familial mix hyperlipidaemias); cholesterol absorption inhibitors eg ezetimibe (useful combination with a statin to enhance cholesterol reduction); anion exchar resins, eg cholestyramine; also consider nicotinic acid (HDL↑; LDL↓; SE: seve flushes—aspirin 300mg ½h pre-dose helps this).
- Hypertriglyceridaemia responds best to fibrates, nicotinic acid, or fish oil.

Familial or primary hyperlipidaemias *Risk of CHD*↑↑. Lipids travel in blo packaged with proteins as lipoproteins. There are four classes: chylomicro (mainly triglyceride); LDL (mainly cholesterol, the lipid correlating most stron with CHD); VLDL (mainly triglyceride); HDL (mainly phospholipid, correlating *invers* with CHD). See table OPPOSITE.

Secondary hyperlipidaemias A result of diabetes mellitus; alcohol abuse; T4 renal failure, nephrosis, and cholestasis.

Xanthomata These yellowish lipid deposits may be: eruptive (itchy nodules crops in hypertriglyceridaemia); tuberous (yellow plaques on elbows and knee planar—also called palmar (orange-coloured streaks in palmar creases), virtua diagnostic of remnant hyperlipidaemia; or deposits in tendons p76, eyeli (xanthelasmata p101), or cornea (arcus p76).

mary hyperlipidaemias

ɔl = plasma cholesterol mmol/L Trig = plasma triglyceride (mmol/L); **coloured** **merals** = WHO phenotype			
nilial ɔerchylomicronaemia ɔoprotein lipase ficiency or apoCII ficiency)[I]	Chol <6.5 Trig 10–30 Chylomicrons ↑		Eruptive xanthomata; lipaemia retinalis; hepatosplenomegaly (HSM)
nilial hyperchol-erolaemia[II] ɩL receptor defects)	Chol 7.5–16 Trig <2.3	LDL↑	Tendon xanthoma; corneal arcus; xanthelasma
nilial defective oprotein B-100[IIa]	Chol 7.5–16 Trig <2.3	LDL↑	Tendon xanthoma; arcus; xanthelasma
lygenic hyper-olesterolaemia[IIa]	Chol 6.5–9 Trig <2.3	LDL↑	*The commonest 1° lipidaemia* xanthelasma; corneal arcus
milial combined ıyperlipidaemia[IIb, IV or V]	Chol 6.5–10 Trig 2.3–12	LDL↑VLDL↑ HDL↓	*Next commonest 1° lipidaemia;* xanthelasma; arcus
sbetalipoproteinae-a (remnant particle sease)[III]	Chol 9–14 Trig 9–14	IDL↑ HDL↓ LDL↓	Palmar striae; tubero-eruptive xanthoma
milial hypertri-ɣceridaemia[IV]	Chol 6.5–12 Trig 3.0–6.0	VLDL↑	
pe V ʼperlipoproteinaemia	Trig 10–30; chylomicrons		Eruptive xanthoma; lipaemia retinalis; HSM

ımary HDL abnormalities

ɣperalphalipoproteinaemia ↑HDL chol >2

ɣpoalphalipoproteinaemia (Tangier disease) ↓HDL chol <0.92

ımary LDL abnormalities

ɔetalipoproteinaemia Trig<0.3, Chol<1.3, missing LDL, VLDL and chylomicrons, ıd fat malabsorption, retinopathy, and acanthocytosis

ɣpobetalipoproteinaemia chol<1.5 LDL↓, HDL ↓. Increased longevity

What are the priorities in treating diet-resistant hyperlipidaemia?

ɔp priority: *Treat those with known cardiovascular disease.*

ⁿᵈ priority: *Treat those with DM if risk of CV disease* >2% per year.

ʳᵈ priority: Those with a risk of CV disease >2% per year.

ɔreviations *IDL* = intermediate-density lipoprotein (*HDL* and *LDL* denote high and low density, ɔectively); chol = cholesterol; trig = triglyceride.

The porphyrias

The acute porphyrias are rare genetic diseases caused by errors in the pathway haem biosynthesis resulting in the toxic accumulation of porphobilinogen and aminolaevulinic acid (porphyrin precursors). Characterized by acute neurovisce crises, due to the increased production of porphyrin precursors, and th appearance in the urine. Some forms have cutaneous manifestations. Prevalen 1–2/100,000.

Acute intermittent porphyria A low-penetrant autosomal dominant conditi (porphobilinogen deaminase gene); 28% have no family history (*de nc mutations*). ~10% of those with the defective gene have neurovisceral symptor Attacks are intermittent, more common in women, and may be precipitated many drugs (see below). Urine porphobilinogens are raised during attacks a often (50%) between them (the urine may go deep red on standing). Fae porphyrin levels are normal. There are no skin manifestations.

Variegate porphyria and hereditary coproporphyria Autosomal domina characterized by photosensitive blistering skin lesions and/or acute attacks. T former is prevalent in Afrikaners in South Africa. Porphobilinogen high only in an attack, and other metabolites may be detected in faeces.

Features of an acute attack Colic ± vomiting ± fever ± WCC↑—so mimicking acute abdomen (anaesthesia can be disastrous here)—also:

- Hypertension
- Hyponatraemia
- Hypokalaemia
- Hypotonia
- Proteinuria
- Psychosis/odd behaviour[1]
- Peripheral neuritis
- Paralysis
- Seizures
- Sensory impairment
- Sight may be affected
- Shock (± collapse).

Drugs to avoid in acute intermittent porphyria are legion (they may precipita above symptoms ± quadriplegia, see *BNF/OTM*), they include: *alcohol*; *sever anaesthetic agents* (barbiturates, halothane); *antibiotics* (chloramphenic sulfonamides, tetracyclines); *painkillers* (pentazocine); *oral hypoglycaemic contraceptive pill*.

Treatment of an acute attack
- Remove precipitants, then:
- IV fluids to correct electrolyte imbalance.
- High carbohydrate intake (eg Hycal®) by NG tube if necessary.
- IV haematin is probably the treatment of choice in most centres now.
- Nausea controlled with prochlorperazine 12.5mg IM.
- Sedation if necessary with chlorpromazine 50–100mg PO/IM.
- Pain control with: aspirin, dihydrocodeine, or morphine.
- Seizures can be controlled with diazepam.
- Treat tachycardia and hypertension with propranolol.

Non-acute porphyrias

Porphyria cutanea tarda, erythropoietic protoporphyria, and ***congenit erythropoietic porphyria*** are characterized by cutaneous photosensitivity alor as there is no overproduction of porphyrin precursors, only porphyrins.

►Alcohol, lead, and iron deficiency cause abnormal porphyrin metabolism.

►Offer genetic counselling (*OHCS* p154) to all patients and their families.

1 Be sure I looked at her eyes
Happy and proud; at last I knew
Porphyria worshipped me; surprise
Made my heart swell, and still it grew
While I debated what to do.
That moment she was mine, mine, fair,
Perfectly pure and good: I found
A thing to do, and all her hair
In one long yellow string I wound
Three times her little throat around,
And strangled her ...
[From Porphyria's Lover, Robert Browning]

Clinical chemistry

17 Eponymous syndromes

See also *OHCS* p638

Alice in Wonderland syndrome (Todd's syndrome) Disturbance of one's vie oneself ± fast-forwarding of intrapsychic time. Can occur in epilepsy, migrair infectious mononucleosis.

Arnold–Chiari malformation The cerebellar tonsils and medulla are malfor congenitally and herniate through the foramen magnum. This may cause infa hydrocephalus with mental retardation, optic atrophy, ocular palsies and sp paresis of the limbs. Spina bifida, syringomyelia (p508), or focal cerebellar brainstem signs may occur eg ataxia, dysphagia, oscillopsia, nystagmus (p44). T may be bony abnormalities of the base of the skull (basilar impression). M better than CT in aiding diagnosis.

Baker's cyst This is when fluid from a knee effusion escapes to form a pop cyst, often swollen and painful. ***Differential:*** A ruptured Baker's cyst may mi DVT. Ultrasound can differentiate the two. ***Treatment:*** Aspiration is possible recurrence is common.

Barrett's oesophagus In chronic reflux oesophagitis (p236), columnar ga epithelium extends upwards replacing normal oesophageal squamous epith (the squamocolumnar junction migrates upwards). Intestinal metaplasia occ these cells. The length affected may be a few cm only or all the oesophagus can be continuous or patchy. The changes are visible on endoscopy. There is fold ↑risk of oesophageal adenocarcinoma. Once diagnosed, endoscopic survei programmes vary depending on age and general health; there is little evidence these programmes have reduced deaths from oesophageal cancer. ***Manage*** depends on what histology is found on biopsy. If pre-malignant changes (grade dysplasia) are found, oesophageal resection is generally advocated, espe in younger, fit patients; endoscopic mucosal ablation by epithelial lase photodynamic ablation is used in others. Photodynamic therapy (PDT) involves induced activation of an orally administered photosensitizer such a aminolaevulinic acid which causes the accumulation of protoporphyrin IX mucosal cells. Local laser light then causes necrosis, which is confirmed by fi squamous re-epithelialization. PDT remains experimental. If no pre-malig changes are found, regular endoscopy + biopsy, and intensive antireflux mea including long-term proton pump inhibitors are used. Exactly who to scree how often is not clear.

Bazin's disease Localized areas of fat necrosis with ulceration and an indu rash, characteristically on adolescent girls' calves. Originally thought to be a of skin TB, but cases unrelated to tuberculosis have been seen.

Behçet's disease A systemic vasculitis of unknown cause, associated with HL It is most commonly found in Turkey, the Mediterranean and Japan. ***Feat*** recurrent oral and genital ulceration, ocular inflammation (eg anterior or pos uveitis), skin lesions (eg erythema nodosum, papulopustular lesions), neurol (eg aseptic meningitis, encephalitis, CN palsies, confusion), vasculitis, joints erosive large joint oligoarthropathy), GI: diarrhoea, colitis. ***Diagnosis*** is n clinical. Pathergy test: needle prick leads to papule formation within 48 hou Steroids, ciclosporin, azathioprine or cyclophosphamide are used in severe d eg with ocular involvement. Colchicine may be effective in treating ulcera

Berger's disease (IgA nephropathy) p288. The commonest glomerulonep causing episodic haematuria, often coinciding with viral infections. Seco causes include alcoholic liver disease, ankylosing spondylitis, coeliac disease

Bickerstaff's brainstem encephalitis This disease is related to Miller– syndrome (p695): in addition to ophthalmoplegia, ataxia and areflexia, the extensor plantars and reduced consciousness—a reversible brain death pictu occur (no structural damage has been demonstrated). Plasmapheresis may

ɔnyms are so-called because they take their names from their chief tagonists (either doctors or patients). They are the sole route to medical fame: ıne was a drunkard and one's name was Johnny Walker one could form a society ed *Alcoholics Eponymous*'.

Alan Bennett

ısult the index for eponymous covered in other chapters.
biographical details, see www.whonamedit.com

:G of Brugada syndrome

ɔte right bundle branch block and the ıusual morphology of the raised ST gments in V1–3. This inherited ndition causing a faulty sodium annel predisposes to fatal rhythmias, eg ventricular fibrillation, pically in young males, which is eventable by using an implantable fibrillator. ►*Consider primary* ectrical cardiac disease in all those ith unexplained syncope. Relatives of ose with sudden unexplained death ay undergo unmasking of rhythmias by IV ajmaline tests—but me results are false +ve. Use dgment in subjecting those with ST normalities but no symptoms to ectrophysiological tests, right ntricular myocardial biopsy, and MRI. quencing SCN5A loci may identify the 67H missense mutation in affected milies.[1]

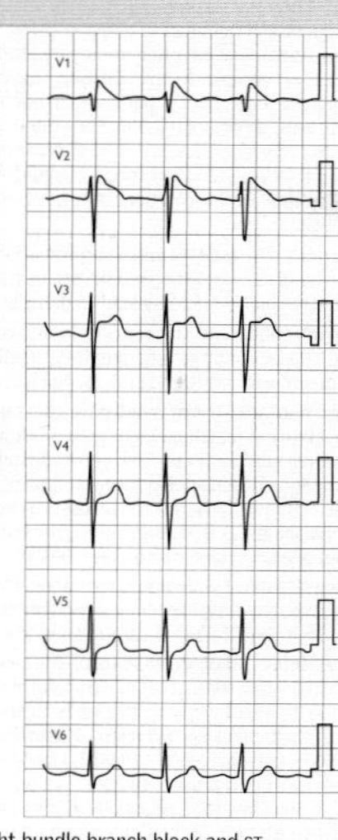

G 14—Brugada syndrome. Note right bundle branch block and ST ɔrphology in leads V1–3.

Ahn 2004 *Circulation* **109** 1463; ECG by kind permission of Dr Shayashi.

Brown-Séquard syndrome A lesion in one half of the cord (due to hemisection unilateral cord lesion) causes • Ipsilateral UMN weakness below the lesion (sever corticospinal tract, causing spastic paraparesis, brisk reflexes, extensor plant reflex) • Ipsilateral loss of proprioception and vibration (severed dorsal colum and • Contralateral loss of pain and temperature sensation (severed spinothalan tract which has crossed over; see fig 1, p508). ***Causes:*** Trauma, tumo degenerative disease (eg disk herniation, cervical spondylosis), MS.

Budd–Chiari syndrome Hepatic vein obstruction by thrombosis or tumour caus ischaemia and hepatocyte damage, presenting with liver failure, or insidious c rhosis. Abdominal pain, hepatomegaly, ascites and ↑ALT occur. Portal hypertensi occurs in chronic forms. ***Causes:*** include hypercoagulable states (the F pregnancy, malignancy, paroxysmal nocturnal haemoglobinuria, polycythaem rubra vera, thrombophilia) or liver, renal or adrenal tumour. ***Tests:*** Ultrasound hepatic vein Dopplers, CT or MRI. Angioplasty, transjugular intrahepatic port systemic shunt (TIPS) or a surgical shunt may be needed. Anticoagulate (lifelor unless there are varices. Consider liver transplant in fulminant hepatic necrosis cirrhosis.

Buerger's disease (thromboangiitis obliterans) This is inflammation of arteri veins, and nerves with thrombosis in the middle sized arteries, often in ma cigarette smokers. It may lead to gangrene. The underlying cause is unknown.

Caplan's syndrome This is multiple lung nodules in coal workers with rheumat arthritis, caused by an inflammatory reaction to the external allergen. CXR: bilate peripheral nodules (0.5–5cm). ***R̸:*** None are specific—treat symptoms (p184).

Charcot–Marie–Tooth syndrome (peroneal muscular atrophy) This inherit neuropathy starts in puberty with weak legs and foot drop, with variable loss sensation and reflexes. The peroneal muscles atrophy, leading to an invert champagne bottle appearance. Atrophy of hand and arm muscles also occurs. T most common form, CMT1A (caused by mutations in the PMP22 myelin gene chromosome 17), is inherited in an autosomal dominant manner. It is seldom *tot* incapacitating. Hand pain/paraesthesiae may respond to nerve release.

Churg–Strauss syndrome is a triad of asthma (often late-onset), eosinophilia a vasculitis, affecting the lungs, peripheral nerves and skin. Glomerulonephritis m occur, but renal failure is rare. ANCA is +ve. Most respond to steroids.

Creutzfeldt–Jakob disease (CJD) The cause is a prion (PrPSC): an altered form c normal protein (PrPC), that can transform other normal proteins into prion prote (hence its infectivity). ↑PrPSC leads to spongiform changes (tiny cavities) in t brain. Most cases are ***sporadic***. ***Variant CJD*** (vCJD; only 183 cases worldwide 2006) is transmitted via meat contaminated by CNS tissue affected by bov spongiform encephalopathy BSE; see BOX). In ***inherited*** forms (incidence: 1 10^6/yr, worldwide, eg as the Gerstmann–Sträussler syndrome), the 'norm protein is abnormally unstable and readily transforms to PrPSC. ***Iatrogenic*** cau may include: contaminated neurosurgical/dental instruments, corneal transpla hormones from human pituitaries (eg growth hormone) and ?blood products. Pr protein is resistant to sterilisation. ***Signs:*** Progressive dementia, focal CNS sig myoclonus, depression, eye signs (diplopia, supranuclear palsies, complex vis disturbances, homonymous field defects, hallucinations cortical blindness). ***Tes*** Tonsil/olfactory biopsy; CSF gel electrophoresis. ***Treatment***: None proven. De occurs within 6 months in sporadic and iatrogenic forms. ***Prevention:*** Regulati aimed at limiting the spread of BSE, the transmission of BSE prions to humans, a iatrogenic transmission, will hopefully limit the spread of this disease.

Crigler–Najjar syndrome An inherited cause of unconjugated hyperbilirubinae presenting in the first days of life with jaundice ± CNS signs. Cause: mutat leading to abolition of bilirubin UDP-glucuronosyltransferase (UGT) activity. ***R̸:*** Li transplant before irreversible kernicterus (*OHCS* p115) develops. Phototherapy keep bilirubin levels down while awaiting transplant.

he fine line between fame and infamy

fter his neurological experiments. Charles Brown-Séquard 1817–94 oclaimed that he had discovered the secret of perpetual youth after injecting mself with a concoction of testicular blood, seminal fluid, and testicular tracts from dogs and guinea pigs. In the 1880s over 12,000 doctors were ueuing up for his special extracts, which they used on their patients in various ays. He gave the extracts away free, provided that results of their use were ported back to him. 314 out of 405 cases of tabes were improved, and his own inary flow rate improved by 25%. Endocrinologists never forgave him for inging their science into disrepute—but, to this day, no one really knows hether he discovered anything of any practical use.[9]

gns which may distinguish variant CJD from sporadic CJD (sCJD)

- An earlier age at presentation (median 29yrs vs 60yrs in sporadic CJD).
- Longer survival (median 14 months vs 4 months in sporadic CJD).
- Psychiatric features are an early sign (anxiety, withdrawal, apathy, agitation, a permanent look of fear in the eyes, depression, personality change, lack of awareness of surroundings, insomnia). Hallucinations and delusions may occur—before akinetic mutism.
- Painful sensory symptoms are commoner (eg foot pain hyperaesthesia).
- Dementia is often delayed (occurs early in sporadic CJD).
- Normal EEG (sporadic CJD has a characteristic spike and wave pattern).
- MRI *may* show a characteristic signal in the posterior thalamic area. CT is normal in both forms of the illness, and CSF tests detecting 14-3-3 protein cannot be relied on (may be +ve in both variant and sporadic CJD).
- Mean CSF tau-pT181/tau protein ratio is 10-fold higher in vCJD than in sCJD.[10]
- Homozygosity for methionine at codon 129 of the PRP gene is typical.
- NB: as the incubation period may be up to several decades, predictions of incidence of vCJD may be underestimations.

Curtis-Fitz-Hugh syndrome is inflammation of the liver capsule (perihepatit due to chlamydial or gonococcal infection, often with pelvic inflammatory disea (in women). Right upper quadrant pain occurs.

Devic's syndrome (neuromyelitis optica) This is a variant of multiple scleros (with distinguishing features on MRI). There is demyelination of the optic nerv chiasm, and the cord. ***Treatment:*** Azathioprine is often used to suppress attacks, opposed to treatments such as β-interferon in MS. ***Prognosis*** is variable, a complete remission may occur.

Dressler's syndrome This develops 2–10wks after an MI or heart surge It is thought that myocardial necrosis stimulates the formation of autoantibodi against heart muscle. ***The Patient:*** He or she may suffer recurrent fever and ch pain ± pleural or pericardial rub (from serositis). Cardiac tamponade may occur, avoid anticoagulants. ***℞:*** Aspirin, NSAIDs or steroids.

Dubin–Johnson syndrome An autosomal recessive disorder, causing defecti hepatocyte excretion of conjugated bilirubin. It is caused by a point mutation ir gene coding for a canalicular transport protein. There is intermittent jaundice w pain in the right hypochondrium. There is no hepatomegaly. ***Tests:*** Alk phos bilirubinuria on dipstick. Liver biopsy: diagnostic pigment granules.[11]

Dupuytren's contracture Palmar fascia contracts so that the fingers (often finger) cannot extend. There is nodular thickening of the connective tissue over t 4th & 5th fingers. ***Prevalence:*** ~10% of ♂ >65yrs (↑ if +ve family histor ***Associations:*** Smoking, alcohol use, heavy manual labour, trauma, DM, phenytc HIV. Peyronie's may co-exist (p700). It is thought to be caused by local hypox ischaemia (the primary event) → increased xanthine oxidase activity → reduc oxygen → superoxide free radicals → fibroblast proliferation → Type III collager palmar fibrosis. Surgery may be needed.

Ekbom's syndrome (Restless legs) There is an irresistible desire to move the le when in bed, ± unpleasant leg sensations. The mechanism is unclear. It is usua idiopathic; secondary causes include iron deficiency, uraemia, pregnancy, polyneuropathy and rheumatoid arthritis. ***Treatment:*** Dopamine agonists a commonly used; benzodiazepines eg clonazepam (1–4mg PO nocte) may also he Ekbom also described delusional parasitosis: 'I am invaded by parasites'.[12]

Fabry's disease An X-linked recessive disorder of glycolipid metabolism, due ↓levels of lysosomal α-galactosidase A. There is accumulation of glycosphingolip in the skin (angiokeratoma corporis diffusum), eyes (lens opacities), heart (L conduction defects, infarction), kidneys (progressive renal failure), CNS (stroke) a peripheral nerves (neuropathy). Most die in the 5th decade due to renal failu stroke or MI. ***Treatment:*** Biweekly infusions of recombinant human α-galactosid A are safe: long term data are awaited.[13]

Fanconi anaemia is an autosomal recessive disorder with defective stem repair, leading to aplastic anaemia (with increased susceptibility to acute myel leukaemia), skin pigmentation, skeletal malformation (eg absent radii, short statu microcephaly, syndactyly), neurological deficits (congenital deafness, IQ↓), a cryptorchidism. Several genes have been implicated.[14]

Felty's syndrome Rheumatoid arthritis + splenomegaly + WCC↓. There hypersplenism (anaemia ± platelets↓), recurrent infections, also skin ulcers a lymphadenopathy. Rh factor: ↑↑. Splenectomy may improve neutropenia.

Foster Kennedy syndrome Optic atrophy of one eye with papilloedema of t other, due respectively to optic nerve compression and ↑ICP from a mass (meningioma, hydatid, plasmacytoma) on the side of the optic atrophy.

Friedreich's ataxia This is an autosomal recessive disorder, with expansions of trinucleotide repeat GAA in the X25 (frataxin) gene. There is degeneration of ma nerve tracts: spinocerebellar tracts degenerate causing cerebellar atax dysarthria, nystagmus, and dysdiadochokinesis. Loss of corticospinal tracts occ

Features distinguishing Devic's disease from multiple sclerosis

	Devic's disease	Multiple sclerosis
Course	May be monophasic or relapsing	Relapsing usually; see p488
Attack severity	Usually severe	Often mild
Respiratory failure	~30% of cases, due to cervical myelitis	Rare
MRI head	Usually normal	Many periventricular white-matter lesions
MRI cord	Multiple, small, peripheral lesions	Extensive central lesions
CSF oligoclonal bands	Absent	Present
Permanent disability	Usually attack-related	Usually in late progressive disease
Co-existent autoimmune disease	Present in up to 50%	Uncommon

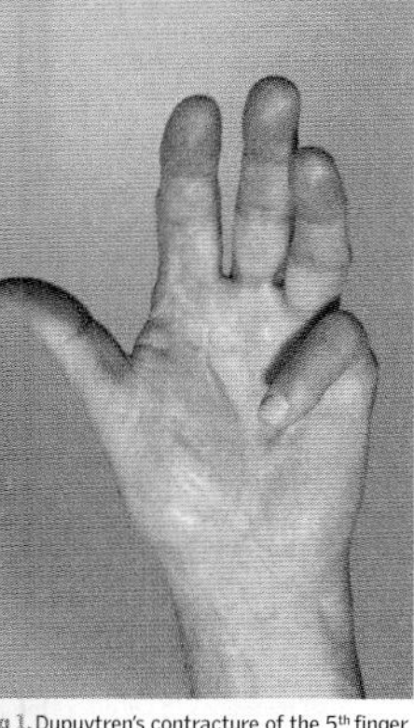

g 1. Dupuytren's contracture of the 5th finger

(weakness and plantars ↑↑) with peripheral nerve damage, so tendon reflexes paradoxically depressed (differential diagnosis p459). There is also dorsal colu degeneration, hence loss of positional and vibration sense. Pes cavus and scoli occur. Cardiomyopathy may cause CCF. Typical age at death: ~50yrs. **℞:** There is cure; surgery may provide symptomatic relief for musculoskeletal problems.

Froin's syndrome CSF protein↑ and xanthochromia with normal cell count, a sig blockage in CSF flow in the spine, eg from a spinal tumour. *[Georges Froin, 18*

Gardner's syndrome (Autosomal dominant) Variant of familial adenomat polyposis, caused by mutations in the APC gene (5q21). Features include hundr of malignant colon polyps (which 'inevitably', given time, become malignar typically before 40yrs old), benign bone osteomas, epidermal cysts, derm tumours, fibromas, and neurofibromas. ***Fundoscopy:*** Black spots (conger hypertrophy of retinal pigment epithelium); this helps detect carriers of the g before symptoms develop. ***Onset:*** 2–70yrs, eg mass effect (eg obstructed urete or bloody diarrhoea. Careful follow-up is needed. Subtotal colectomy + remova polyps may prevent malignancy. Endoscopic polypectomy with long-term sulin therapy has been tried to postpone prophylactic colectomy. *[EJ Gardner 19*

Gélineau's syndrome (narcolepsy) The patient, usually a young man, succumb irresistible attacks of inappropriate sleep ± vivid hallucinations, cataplexy (sud hypotonia), and sleep paralysis (paralysis of speech + willed movement on wak while fully alert, *OHCS* p393). ***Putative mechanism:*** Genetic mutations lead to of hypothalamic hypocretin-containing neurones, possibly via autoimmune c truction. 95% are +ve for HLA DR2. **℞:** Stimulants (eg methylphenidate, *c* p211, 10mg PO after breakfast and lunch) may cause dependence ± psycho Modafinil (~200mg PO as a single daily dose before noon) may be better. SE: anx aggression, dry mouth, euphoria, insomnia, BP↑, dyskinesia, alk phos↑.

Gerstmann's syndrome Finger agnosia (inability to identify fingers by nar left/right disorientation, agraphia (inability to write), acalculia (to calculate alexia (to read). These symptoms together suggest a dominant parietal lesior

Gilbert's syndrome This inherited metabolic disorder is a common cause *unconjugated* hyperbilirubinaemia, due to decreased bilirubin UDP-glucurono transferase activity. Prevalence is estimated at 1–2%. The onset is shortly a birth, but it may be unnoticed for many years. Jaundice occurs during intercur illness, and bilirubin rises on fasting. Liver biopsy is normal, but should rarely required clinically. It is a benign condition. *[Nicolas Gilbert, 1*

Gilles de la Tourette syndrome ***Presentation:*** (♂:♀≈4:1) Waxing and waning m and phonic tics (p460; mean age of onset: 6yrs), blinking, nodding, stuttering ± ir ressible, explosive, occasionally obscene verbal ejaculations ± anger control probl and attention-deficit disorder. There may be a witty, innovatory, phantasmag picture, 'with mimicry, antics, playfulness, extravagance, impudence, audacity, dr atizations, surreal associations, uninhibited affect, speed, 'go', vivid imagery memory, and hunger for stimuli'; also grunting, sniffing, throat-clearing, twir nipping people, obscene gestures (copropraxia), repeating self and others (pali echolalia), repeating others' movements (echopraxia). More prosaic forms commoner. ***Pathogenesis:*** Probably an inherited developmental disorder of b ganglia disinhibition. Group A β-haemolytic streps may trigger these symptom in Sydenham's chorea (p128; unproven, see BOX). ***MRI:*** Large left thalamu ***Associations:*** Obsessive–compulsive/attention-deficit disorder. **℞:** Haloper ~1.5mg/8h PO, pimozide, olanzapine, or risperidone—if the patient wants help

Goodpasture's syndrome Acute glomerulonephritis + lung symptoms (haem tysis/diffuse pulmonary haemorrhage) caused by antiglomerular basement m brane antibodies (binding kidney's basement membrane and alveolar membra ***Tests:*** CXR: infiltrates due to pulmonary haemorrhage, often in lower zones. Kic biopsy: crescentic glomerulonephritis. ***Treatment:*** ⏩Treat shock. Vigorous ir unosuppressive treatment and plasmapheresis; see p288. *[Ernest Goodpasture, 1*

ataplexy is highly specific for narcolepsy/Gélineau's syndrome

aytime sleepiness has many causes, but if it occurs with cataplexy the agnosis 'must' be narcolepsy. Cataplexy is bilateral loss of tone in antigravity uscles provoked by emotions such as laughter, startle, excitement, or anger. ssociated phenomena include: falls, mouth opening, dysarthria, mutism, and hasic muscle jerking around the mouth. Most attacks are brief, but injury can ccur (eg if several attacks per day). It is comparable to the atonia of rapid eye novement sleep *but without loss of awareness.* **ΔΔ:** Bradycardia, migraine, tonic/akinetic epilepsy,[20 21] delayed sleep phase syndrome, conversion disorder, alingering, and psychosis.[22]

Don't confuse capa***plex***y with cata***leps***y—a waxy flexibility where involuntary atue-like postures are effortless maintained (frozen) despite looking most ncomfortable (this motor-perceptual dissociative phenomenon may be induced y hypnosis, psychosis, antipsychotics, or a thalamic lesion).[23] Catalepsy is one of ne signs of ***catatonia***[24]—a neuropsychiatric syndrome of catalepsy, negativism, utism, muscular rigidity, mannerisms, autonomic instability, and fever.[25]

ost-streptococcal autoimmune CNS disorders (eg Tourettism)

roup A streptococci can (rarely) induce autoimmune diseases of the heart, ints, and brain, eg movement disorders (chorea, tics/Tourettism, dystonia, and arkinsonism), emotional disorders, and sleep disorders. MRI and pathological udies suggest that the most vulnerable CNS region is the basal ganglia. nmunopathogenesis is poorly understood: there is some support for utoantibody-mediated disease, but studies are conflicting.[26]

he lung and its various vasculitides (eg Goodpasture's)

ung vasculitis is most commonly seen with the primary idiopathic, small-vessel ANCA (p539) associated vasculitides (Wegener's granulomatosis, microscopic olyangiitis, and Churg–Strauss syndrome).[27] Medium-vessel vasculitis (classic olyarteritis nodosa), large-vessel vasculitis (Takayasu arteritis), primary nmune complex-mediated vasculitis (Goodpasture's syndrome), and secondary asculitis (SLE) can all affect the lung.

Guillain–Barré syndrome ***Incidence:*** 1–2/100,000/yr. ***Signs:*** A few weeks af 'flu vaccine, gastroenteritis or URTI, a symmetrical ascending muscle weakne occurs. Common triggers are *Campylobacter jejuni*, CMV, mycoplasma, zoster, H EBV. The pathogen causes antibody formation, which attack nerve cells. In 40%, cause is found. It may advance quickly, affecting all limbs at once, and can lead paralysis. There is a progressive phase of up to 4 weeks, followed by recove Unlike other neuropathies, *proximal* muscles are more affected, and tru respiratory, and cranial nerves (esp. VII) may be involved. Pain is common (eg ba limb) but sensory signs may be absent. Autonomic dysfunction may occur sweating, ↑HR, BP changes, dysrhythmias. Progressive respiratory involvement the chief danger. ***Tests:*** Nerve conduction studies: slowing of conduction. C protein↑ (often >5.5g/L), normal CSF white cell count. ***Treatment:*** *Respirato involvement requires transfer to* ITU. Check forced vital capacity (FVC) 4 hou ►*Ventilate sooner rather than later*, eg if FVC <1.5L, P_aO_2 <10kPa, P_aCO_2 >6k Specific treatment is with IV immunoglobulin 0.4g/kg/24h for 5d or plas exchange; they are equally effective. Corticosteroids have no role. ***Prognosis:*** Go ~85% make a complete or nearly complete recovery. 10% are unable to walk alo at 1yr. *Complete paralysis is compatible with complete recovery*. ***Mortality:*** 10

Henoch–Schönlein purpura (HSP) is a small vessel vasculitis, which presents w purpura (purple nodules which do not disappear on pressure—signifyi intradermal bleeding) often over buttocks and extensor surfaces, typically affecti young ♂. There may be glomerulonephritis (p288), joint involvement, abdomi pain (±intussusception), which may mimic an 'acute abdomen'.

Horner's syndrome Pupil constriction (*miosis*), sunken eye (*enophthalmos*), *pto.* and ipsilateral loss of sweating (*anhidrosis*) due to interruption of the fac sympathetic supply, eg at the brainstem (demyelination, vascular disease), co (syringomyelia), thoracic outlet (Pancoast's tumour, p700), or on the sympathe nerves' trip on the internal carotid artery into the skull (carotid aneurysm), a thence to the orbit. *[Johann Horner, 18*

Huntington's chorea is an autosomal dominant condition (gene on chromosome with full penetrance, due to expansions of a CAG trinucleotide repeat. Onset usually in middle age, so the child of an affected parent lives under a Damocl sword, having a 50% chance of becoming affected. Genetic tests are availab Signs are insidious, then progressive: chorea → irritability → dementia ± seizures death. ***Pathology:*** Cerebral atrophy with loss of corpus striatum GABA-nergic cholinergic neurones. ***Treatment:*** (p54) None prevents progression. Of counselling to patient and family. *[George Huntington, 18*

Jervell–Lange-Nielsen syndrome An autosomal recessive inherited disorder ventricular repolarization, causing a prolonged QTc interval (p82), associated w bilateral deafness. There is predisposition to syncope, seizures, Torsade de point sudden death. Mutations in a K^+ channel subunit may be responsible.

Kaposi's sarcoma (KS) This sarcoma is derived from capillary endothelial cells from fibrous tissue, and is associated with a serologically identifiable human herp virus (KSHV = HHV-8). It presents as purple papules or plaques on skin and muco (any organ). It metastasizes to lymph nodes. 3 types: **1** Classic, especially elde Mediterranean or Jewish males. **2** Endemic (Central Africa). In these two forr peripheral, slow-growing skin lesions are found, visceral involvement is rare, a lymph node involvement may lead to oedema. **3** KS in immunosuppression eg H organ transplant recipients. This can be aggressive, with multiple skin lesions a visceral involvement (eg lungs, bowel). In HIV, KS occurs particularly in homosex men, where it is diagnostic of AIDS (p396), and carries a poor prognosis. Pulmonary may present as breathlessness. Bowel KS may cause nausea, abdominal pa ***Diagnosis*** is by biopsy. ***R:*** Skin lesions are treated with radiotherapy or intralesio TNF-α. Chemotherapy is used for widespread disease. *[Moricz Kaposi, 18*

Diagnostic criteria in typical Guillain–Barré polyneuritis[1]

Features required for diagnosis:	**Features supporting diagnosis:**
Progressive weakness of all 4 limbs	Progression over days, up to 4wks
Areflexia	Near symmetry of symptoms
	Sensory symptoms/signs only mild
Features excluding diagnosis:	CN involvement (eg bilateral facial weakness)
Purely sensory symptoms	
Diagnosis of: • Myasthenia	Recovery starts ~2wks after the period of progression has finished
• Botulism	
• Poliomyelitis	Autonomic dysfunction
• Diphtheria	Absence of fever at onset
• Porphyria	CSF protein ↑ with CSF WCC <10×10⁶/L
• Toxic neuropathy	Typical electrophysiological tests

Variants of Guillain–Barré syndrome include:

- ***Chronic inflammatory demyelinating polyradiculopathy:*** (CIDP) characterized by a slower onset and recovery.
- ***Miller-Fisher syndrome*** which comprises of ophthalmoplegia, ataxia and areflexia. Associated with anti-GQ1b antibodies in the serum.

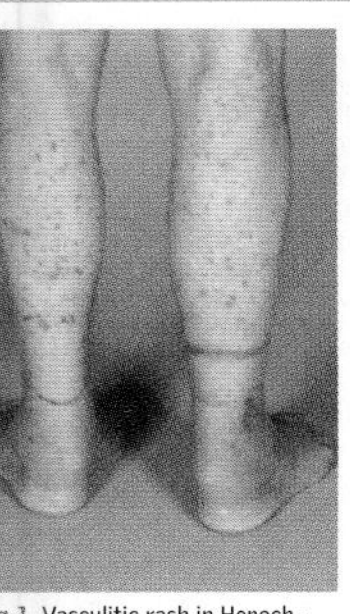

Fig 1. Vasculitic rash in Henoch–Schönlein purpura

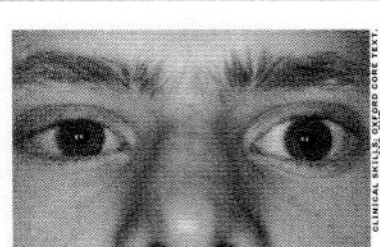

CLINICAL SKILLS, OXFORD CORE TEXT, 410, OUP.

Fig 2. Miosis in Horner's syndrome, affecting the patient's right eye.

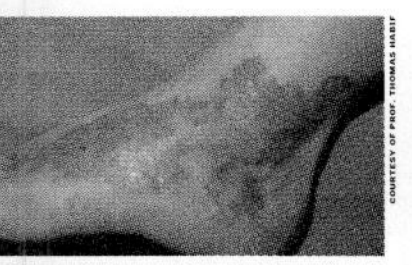

COURTESY OF PROF. THOMAS HABIF

Fig 3. Kaposi's sarcoma. [31]

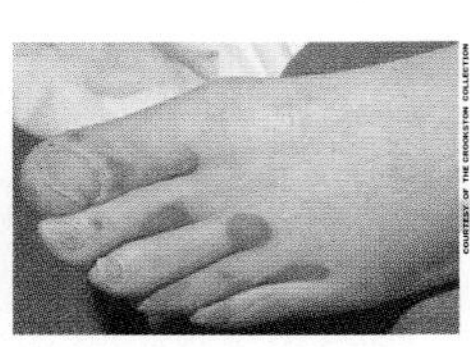

COURTESY OF THE CROOKSTON COLLECTION

Fig 4. Another patient with Kaposi's sarcoma. [30]

1 See M Bersudsky 2000 *Neuromuscul Disord* **10** 182 & A Hahn 1998 *Lancet* **352** 635

Klippel–Trénaunay syndrome A triad of port-wine stain, varicose veins, and li hypertrophy, due to vascular malformation. Usually sporadic, though a few famil exhibiting autosomal dominant inheritance have been reported.[32]

Korsakoff's syndrome ↓Ability to acquire new memories, eg after Wernicke's encep alopathy, due to thiamine deficiency (eg in alcoholics). The patient may have relive his grief each time he hears of the death of a friend. He confabulates to fil gaps in his memory owing to retrograde amnesia. **℞:** See *Wernicke's*, p706. Dc epezil may have a role.[33] *[Sergei Korsakoff (more accurately transliterated Korsakov), 18*

Langerhans'-cell histiocytosis (Histiocytosis X) A group of disorders involvi single- or multi-organ infiltration by granulomatous lesions containing dendri (Langerhans') cells. Lung and bone involvement is most common; skin, pituita thyroid, liver, spleen and lymph nodes may be affected. Lung disease is associat with smoking, and causes interstitial fibrosis. CXR shows nodular changes honeycomb pattern. ***Diagnosis:*** Biopsy (eg skin, lung) shows characteristic Birbe granules on electron microscopy. ***Treatment:*** This involves local excision steroids, vinblastine ± etoposide in severe disease. *OHCS* p644.[34]

Leriche's syndrome Absent femoral pulses, intermittent claudication of butto muscles, pale cold legs, and erectile dysfunction due to distal aortic occlusive d ease (eg a saddle embolus at its bifurcation); surgery may help.[35] *[René Leriche, 19*

Löffler's eosinophilic carditis Restrictive cardiomyopathy + eosinophilia (eg 1 × 10^9/L). It may be an early stage of tropical endomyocardial fibrosis and overla with idiopathic hypereosinophilic syndrome (HES), but is distinct from eosinophi leukaemia. ***Signs:*** increasing heart failure (75%) ± mitral regurgitation (49%) heart block. ***Treatment:*** Digoxin + diuretics often only help if the eosinophilia suppressed, eg by prednisolone or hydroxycarbamide (=hydroxyurea).[36]

Löffler's syndrome (pulmonary eosinophilia) An allergic infiltration of the lun by eosinophils. Allergens include: *Ascaris lumbricoides, Trichinella spiralis, Fascic hepatica, Strongyloides, Ankylostoma, Toxocara, Clonorchis sinensis,*[37] sulfonamid hydralazine, and nitrofurantoin. Often symptomless with incidental CXR (diffuse fa shaped shadows), or cough, T°↑, eosinophilia (in ~20%) & larval migrans (p430). Eradicate cause (eg p433). If idiopathic, steroids are effective. *[Wilhelm Löff 1887–1972]*

Lown–Ganong–Levine syndrome A pre-excitation syndrome, similar to Wol Parkinson–White (WPW, p112), characterized by a short P–R interval (<0.12 sec) normal QRS complex (as opposed to the δ-waves of WPW), and risk supraventricular tachycardia (but not AF/flutter). The cause is not complete understood, but may be due to paranodal fibres that bypass all or part of t atrioventricular node. The patient may complain of intermittent palpitations.[38]

McArdle's glycogen storage disease (Type V) Caused by the absence of glycolytic enzyme, muscle phosphorylase. Inheritance: autosomal recessive. Fatig and cramps follow exercise. Strenuous exercise may provoke rhabdomyolysis a myoglobinuria. Muscle biopsy is diagnostic, showing necrosis and atrophy. **℞:** Mo erate aerobic exercise is beneficial, but avoid heavy exertion. Creatini supplements and pre-exercise sucrose have been tried.[39]

Mallory–Weiss tear Vomiting *causes* haematemesis via an oesophageal tear.

Marchiafava–Bignami syndrome Alcohol-induced corpus callosum necro (±extrapontine myelinolysis) causing left-handed deficit of constructional abili agraphia, mutism, ataxia, poor bimanual co-ordination, gaze apraxia/pseud hallucinated look, dysarthria, epilepsy, paucity of vocal and facial expressi modulation,[40] ↓consciousness, coma. **Δ:** MRI.[41] **℞:** as *Wernicke's*, p706.

Marchiafava–Micheli syndrome (paroxysmal nocturnal haemoglobinuria, PN an acquired clonal expansion and of a multi-potent stem cell carrying a somat mutation in the X-linked PIG-A gene. Glycosylphosphatidylinositol (GPI)-anchor proteins are lacking on blood cells derived from these mutated stem cel predisposing to haemolysis, thrombosis, sepsis, and marrow failure.[42] See p32

Fatal effects of alcohol on the CNS
• Inhibitions↓ (unsafe sex↑ etc etc)
• Wernicke's encephalopathy
• Hepatic encephalopathy
• Cerebral atrophy (dementia)
• Central pontine myelinolysis
• Cerebellar atrophy (falls etc)
• Stroke (all varieties)
• Seizures
• Marchiafava–Bignami syndrome

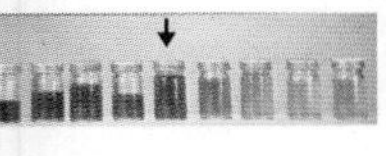

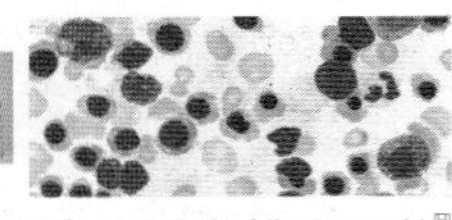

ig 1. **PNH.** As always, the darkest hour is before dawn (in this 24h urine sample).
3: this phenomenon is not all that reliable. A much better test even than a marrow opsy (Fig 1, right, showing a clone of PNH cells) is flow cytometric analysis of GPI-nchored proteins on peripheral blood cells. This can determine the size of the PNH one and type of GPI deficiency (complete or partial). **℞:** Most benefit from ipportive measures—but allogeneic stem cell transplantation is the only cure.

Marfan's syndrome is an autosomal dominant connective tissue disease. I caused by fibrillin-1 (15q21.1) gene mutations, which ↓extracellular microf formation, normally required to maintain elastic fibres. NB: ~25% of cases oc with no family history. ***Major criteria*** (diagnostic if >2): Lens dislocation (*ecto lentis*); aortic dissection or dilatation; dural ectasia; skeletal featu arachnodactyly (long spidery fingers), armspan > height, pectus deforr scoliosis, pes planus. ***Minor signs:*** Mitral valve prolapse, high-arched palate, j hypermobility. Diagnosis is clinical; MRI for dural ectasia (enlargement of the ne canal) may be helpful. ℞: The danger is aortic dissection: beta-blockers are use slow dilatation of the aortic root. Annual echocardiogram should be perforr with elective surgical repair when maximal aortic diameter is >5cm. In pregna the risk of dissection rises. Homocystinuria has similar skeletal deformities:

Marfan's autosomal dominant	*vs* ***Homocystinuria*** cystathione β-synthetase deficiency; a somal recessive with early vasculopatl
• Upwards lens dislocation	• Downwards lens dislocation
• Aortic valve incompetence	• Heart rarely affected
• *Normal* intelligence	• Mental retardation
• Scoliosis, flat feet, herniae	• Recurrent thromboses, osteoporosis
• Life expectancy is reduced from cardiovascular risks	• +ve urine cyanide-nitroprusside test
	• Response to pyridoxine

Meckel's diverticulum ***Prevalence:*** ≤2%. ≤2 inches long, and >2 feet from ileocaecal valve, it contains gastric and pancreatic tissue. There may be gastric a secretion, causing occult GI pain and bleeding. ***Diagnosis:*** Radionucleotide se laparotomy. Acute inflammation may present like appendicitis.

Meigs' syndrome The association of a pleural effusion (transudate, usually r sided) + benign ovarian fibroma (or thecoma) + ascites. *[Joseph Meigs, 1*

Ménétrier's disease consists of giant gastric mucosal folds up to 4cm high, ma involving the fundus, with atrophy of the glands and increased mucosal thickn The cause is unknown; CMV infection and *H. pylori* have been suggested. Ther excess mucous secretion, hyposecretion of gastric acid, and protein loss from stomach, causing peripheral oedema. There may be epigastric pain, vomiting, weight loss. It is a premalignant disease. ***Treatment:*** May respond to *H. py* eradication therapy. Some require surgery if intractable symptoms or concern c malignant change. *[Pierre Ménétrier, 18*

Meyer–Betz syndrome (Paroxysmal myoglobinuria) This idiopathic condi causes necrosis of exercising muscles. There is muscle pain, weakness, discoloured urine: pink→brown (as ↑myoglobin is excreted). Acute renal failure result from myoglobinuria (p299). DIC is associated. ***Tests:*** WCC↑, LFT↑, LDH↑, C urine myoglobin↑. ***Diagnosis:*** Muscle biopsy. Exertion should be avoided.

Mikulicz's syndrome A variant of Sjögren's syndrome, with symmetr enlargement of lacrimal and salivary glands, and blocking of ducts, with eyes/mouth. It may feature with TB, sarcoidosis or lymphoproliferative disease occur as a primary autoimmune disease. *[Johann von Mikulicz-Radecki, 18*

Milroy's syndrome (Lymphoedema praecox) An inherited malfunction of lymphatics causing asymmetric swelling of the legs (usually in young gi ***Management:*** • Reassure (it is benign; ≤10% progress to the other leg). • T any cellulitis actively. • Good foot hygiene. • If support stockings do not help, t Lymphapress® device for active compression at night. Surgery with skin graf very rarely needed for 'elephantiasis leg'.

Münchausen's syndrome The patient gains hospital admissions via decept feigning illness, hoping for a laparotomy (*laparotimophilia migrans*), or by bleec (*haemorrhagica histrionica*) or with curious fits (*neurologica diabolica*) or fa heart attacks (*cardiopathia fantastica*). Munchausen-by-proxy entails injury dependent person by his or her carer (eg mother) to gain medical attention. Co video surveillance is an ethically problematic tool which may be necessary diagnosis.

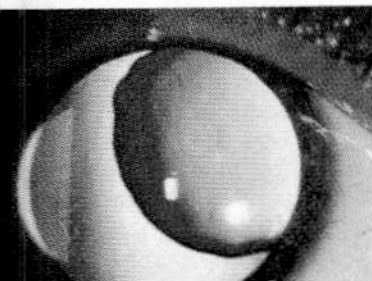

‹ 1. Lens dislocation in Marfan's
ndrome: here the lens is dislocated
periorly and medially.

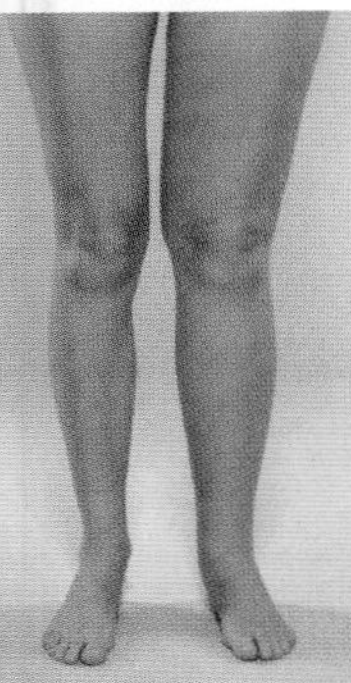

g 2. Milroy's syndrome.

Nelson's syndrome ↑skin pigmentation due to excess ACTH from an enlarg pituitary tumour, after bilateral adrenalectomy removes –ve feedback, p208.

Ogilvie's syndrome Acute functional ('pseudo') colonic obstruction caused malignant retroperitoneal infiltration, spine fracture, or electrolyte imbalance. Correct U&E, conservative measures. Contrast enema or colonoscopy allo decompression, and excludes mechanical causes. Neostigmine is also effecti suggesting parasympathetic suppression is to blame. Surgery is rarely neede

Ortner's cardiovocal syndrome Recurrent laryngeal nerve palsy from a large l atrium (eg from mitral stenosis) or aortic dissection.

Osler–Weber–Rendu syndrome (Hereditary haemorrhagic telangiectasi Telangiectasia on the skin and mucous membranes, which may cause epistaxis chronic GI bleeds, with iron deficiency anaemia. It is associated with pulmona hepatic and cerebral AVMs. Inheritance: autosomal dominant.

Paget's disease of breast is intra-epidermal spread of an intraductal cancer. A red, scaly lesion around the nipple should suggest Paget's disease: do a biop ►Never diagnose eczema of the nipple without a biopsy. ***Treatment:*** Mastectom lymph node clearance. *[Sir James Paget, 18*

Pancoast's syndrome Apical lung cancer + ipsilateral Horner's (p694), fr invasion of the cervical sympathetic plexus. Also shoulder/arm pain (brachial plex invasion C8–T2) ± hoarse voice/bovine cough (unilateral recurrent laryngeal ner palsy and vocal cord paralysis). *[Henry Pancoast, 19*

Parinaud's syndrome (Dorsal midbrain syndrome) Upward gaze palsy + pseu Argyll Robertson pupils (p70). Causes: hydrocephalus, pineal tumours, stroke.

Peutz–Jeghers' syndrome Germline mutations of gene LKB1 cause mucoc aneous dark freckles on lips, oral mucosa, palm and soles ± GI polyps (hamartoma causing obstruction or bleeds. ***Malignant change:*** ≤3%, typically duodenal poly ℞: Usually conservative or local excision. **NB:** hamartomas are excessive fo overgrowths of normal cells in an organ, composed of the same cell type.

Peyronie's disease Penile fibrosis leads to angulation, making coitus mo inconvenient. ***Associations:*** Dupuytren's (p690); atheroma. Erectile dysfuncti occurs in ~50%. ***Treatment:*** Surgery and prostheses aid penetration. Shock wa therapy, vitamin E, tamoxifen, colchicine, and intra-lesional verapamil or interfer α2α, have been used with variable success in early disease.

Pott's syndrome (spinal TB). Rare in the West, this is usually spread from an extr spinal source, most often the lungs. ***Features:*** Back pain, and stiffness of *all* ba movements. Fever, night sweats and weight loss may occur. Progressive bo destruction leads to vertebral collapse and gibbus (sharply angled curvature of t spine). Abscess formation may lead to cord compression, causing paraplegia, a bowel and bladder dysfunction (p458). ***X-rays:*** narrow disc spaces and vertebr osteoporosis early, leading to destruction with wedging of vertebrae. Lesions in t thoracic spine often lead to kyphosis. Abscess formation in the lumbar spine m track down to the psoas muscle, and erode through the skin. ℞: Anti-TB dru (p386). *[Sir Percival Pott, 177*

Prinzmetal (variant) angina Angina from coronary artery spasm: ECG: ST *elevati* ℞: Use Ca^{2+} channel-blockers (see angina p102) but not β-blockers. Associatio Circle of Willis occlusion from intimal thickening (moyamoya disease).

Raynaud's syndrome This is peripheral digital ischaemia due to vasospas precipitated by cold or emotion. Fingers or toes ache and change colour: pale → bl → red. It may be idiopathic (Raynaud's *disease*—prevalence: 3–20%; ♀:♂ >1:1), have an underlying cause (Raynaud's *phenomenon*). ***Tests:*** Exclude an underlyi cause (see BOX). ℞: Keep warm (eg electrically heated mittens); stop smokin Nifedipine 5–20mg/8h PO helps, as may losartan, prazosin, or fluoxetin Sympathectomy may help in those with severe disease. Iloprost, as a nebulize solution, may salvage digits with ulcers ± near-gangrene; effects last up to 16 wee Relapse is common.

'rinzmetal angina and vascular hyperreactivity

:oronary spasm plays an important role not only in Prinzmetal angina but also oronary heart disease in general, including acute coronary syndromes, specially in some populations (eg Japanese). Coronary spasm can be induced y a variety of stimuli with different mechanisms of action, including ergonovine, cetylcholine, and methacholine (the former is used diagnostically).[1] These ause vasodilatation by endothelium-derived relaxing factor when vascular ndothelium is functioning normally, whereas they cause vasoconstriction if the ndothelium is damaged. In the light of these facts, patients with coronary pasm are thought to have a disturbance in endothelial function as well as local yperreactivity of the coronary arteries.

If full anti-anginal therapy does not reduce symptoms, intracoronary radiation 20Gy brachytherapy) to vasospastic segments may be tried.

Prognosis is good (especially if non-smoker, no past MI, and no diabetes); there s some evidence that prognosis may be better with the new calcium channel lockers such as benidipine.

Prinzmetal angina is associated with vascular hyper-reactivity/vasospastic isorders such as Raynaud's phenomenon and migraine.

β-blockers and large doses of aspirin are contraindicated.

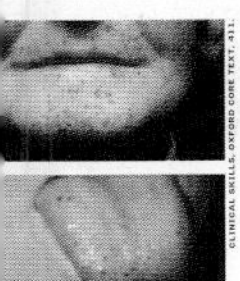

] 1. Telangiectasia in ler–Weber–Rendu ndrome.

Fig 2. Paget's disease of the breast.

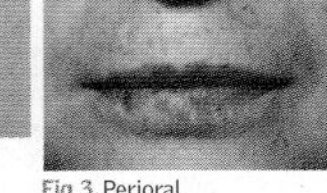

Fig 3. Perioral pigmentation, seen in Peutz–Jegher's syndrome.

:onditions in which Raynaud's phenomenon may be exhibited[2]

- ***Connective tissue disorders:*** Systemic sclerosis, SLE, rheumatoid arthritis, ermatomyositis/polymyositis.
- ***Occupational:*** Using vibrating tools.
- ***Obstructive:*** Thoracic outlet obstruction, Buerger's disease, atheroma.
- ***Haematological:*** Thrombocytosis, cold agglutinin disease, polycythaemia rubra vera (p350), monoclonal gammopathies.
- ***Drugs:*** β-blockers.
- ***Others:*** Hypothyroidism.

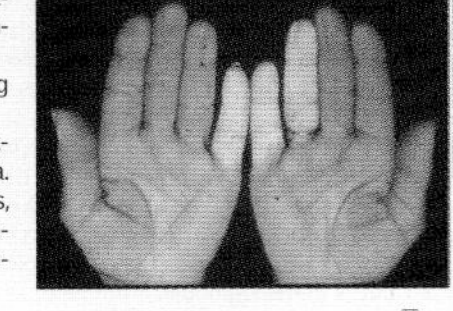

Fig 4. Raynaud's phenomenon in SLE.

Since Prinzmetal angina is not a 'demand-induced' symptom, but a supply (vasospastic) abnormality, ercise treadmill stress testing is of no diagnostic value. The most sensitive and specific test is IV gonovine. 50μg at 5min intervals is given in a specialist lab until a +ve result or 400μg is given. When sitive, the symptoms and ↑ST should be present. Nitroglycerin rapidly reverses the effects of gonovine if refractory spasm occurs.

Patient information on Raynaud's is available from www.raynauds.org.uk. For a review of Raynaud's enomenon, see FM Wigley 2002 *NEJM* **347** 100

Refsum's syndrome is an autosomal recessive disorder where there accumulation of phytanic acid in tissues, due to a mutation of the gene coding the peroxisomal enzyme phytanoyl-CoA hydroxylase. This leads to a sensorimo polyneuropathy, nerve deafness, night blindness (retinitis pigmentosa), cerebe ataxia, ichthyosis, anosmia, and can cause cardiomyopathy. ***Tests:*** Plasma phyta acid↑. ↑CSF protein with normal cell count. ***Treatment***: Restrict foods contain phytanic acid (animal fats, dairy products, green leafy vegetables); plasmaphere is used for severe or rapidly deteriorating clinical symptoms.

Romano–Ward syndrome (autosomal dominant) A mutation in a K^+ chan subunit causes congenital long QT syndrome, and a predisposition towa ventricular tachyarrythmias, torsades de pointes, syncope, and sudden death.

Rotor syndrome Defective excretion of conjugated bilirubin, producing cholest jaundice. Inheritance is probably autosomal recessive.

Sister Mary Joseph nodule An umbilical nodule, caused by a metastatic dep from an intra-abdominal malignancy.

Sjögren's syndrome is a chronic inflammatory autoimmune disorder. It may primary (♀:♂ 9:1, onset 4th–5th decade) or secondary, associated with connect tissue disease (eg RA, SLE, systemic sclerosis). There is lymphocytic infiltration a fibrosis of exocrine glands, especially lacrimal and salivary glands. ***Features:*** ↓t production (dry eyes, keratoconjunctivitis sicca), xerostomia (↓salivation— mouth, dental caries), parotid gland swelling. Other glands are affected caus vaginal dryness, dyspareunia, dry cough and dysphagia. Systemic features incl polyarthritis/arthralgia, Raynaud's, lymphadenopathy, vasculitis, lung, liver a kidney involvement, peripheral neuropathy, myositis and fatigue. It is associa with other autoimmune diseases (eg thyroid disease, autoimmune hepatitis, P and an ↑risk of non-Hodgkin's B-cell lymphoma. ***Tests:*** Measure conjuncti dryness using Schirmer's test: put a strip of filter paper under the lower lid a measure the distance along the paper that tears are absorbed; <5mm in 5mi +ve. Rose Bengal staining may show keratitis on slit-lamp examination. Anti (SSA) and anti-La (SSB) antibodies may be present. Rheumatoid factor is usu +ve; there may be +ve ANA and hypergammaglobulinaemia. Gland biopsy sho focal lymphocytic aggregation. ***℞:*** Treat sicca symptoms: eye drops eg hypror lose (artificial tears), gels, ointment, frequent drinks, sugar free pastilles/gum pilocarpine. NSAIDs and hydroxychloroquine are used for arthralgia, and immu suppressants may be indicated in severe systemic disease. *[Henrik Sjögren, 19*

Stevens–Johnson syndrome A severe form of erythema multiforme (p546), an variant of toxic epidermal necrolysis. It is caused by a hypersensitivity reacti usually to drugs (eg salicylates, sulfonamides, penicillin, barbitura carbamazepine, phenytoin), but is also seen with infections or cancer. There ulceration of the skin and mucosal surfaces (eg mouth, urethra, lungs, conjunctiv Typical target lesions develop, often on the palms or soles with blistering in centre. There may be a prodromal phase with fever, malaise, arthralgia, myalgi vomiting and diarrhoea. ***Treatment:*** The disease is usually self-limiting, so remov any precipitant and supportive care (eg calamine lotion for the skin) will usu suffice. Steroids (systemic and eye-drops) were used, but trials have been varia so ask a dermatologist and ophthalmologist. Ciclosporin and thalidomide have b used, but IV immunoglobulin is not helpful. ***Prognosis:*** Mortality ~5%. The illn may be severe for the first 10d before resolving over 30d. Damage to the eyes m persist and at worst, blindness may result.

Sturge–Weber syndrome (Encephalotrigeminal angiomatosis) The associat of a port wine stain on the face (often in trigeminal distribution) with contralat focal fits, due to a corresponding haemangioma in the brain. There may glaucoma, hemiplegia and learning impairment. ***Tests:*** Skull X-ray shows corti calcification, angiography is usually normal. MRI may show the angioma. ***℞:*** La therapy can remove facial port wine stains. Anticonvulsants are indicated seizures; hemispherectomy may be required if seizures are intractable.

uses of a long QT interval (eg Romano-Ward)

ıny conditions and drugs (check *BNF*) cause a long QT interval—and Brugada ıdrome, p687, is a similar syndrome predisposing to sudden cardiac death.

ngenital: Jervell-Lange-Nielsen syndrome: autosomal recessive with ;ociated deafness.[58] (Romano–Ward syndrome is autosomal dominant).

rdiac: Myocardial infarction or ischaemia; mitral valve prolapse.

/: May be a direct effect of the virus or from protease inhibitors.

etabolic: $K^+\downarrow$; $Mg^{2+}\downarrow$; $Ca^{2+}\downarrow$; starvation; hypothyroidism; hypothermia.

xic: Organophosphates.

ti-arrhythmic drugs: Quinidine; amiodarone; procainamide; sotalol.

tibiotics *et al*: Erythromycin; levofloxacin; pentamidine; halofantrine.

tihistamines: Terfenadine; astemizole.

otility drugs: Domperidone; droperidol in doses >1.25mg (also cisapride).

ychoactive drugs: Haloperidol; risperidone; tricyclics; SSRIs.

nnective tissue diseases: anti-Ro/SSA antibodies (p538).

rbalism: Ask about Chinese folk remedies (may contain unknown amounts arsenic).[59][60] Cocaine, quinine and artemisinins (and other antimalarials) are amples of herbalism-derived products which can prolong the QT interval.

HERBALISM IS NOT A BED OF ROSES

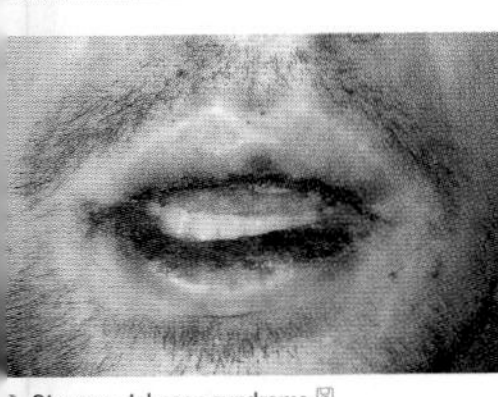

1. Stevens–Johnson syndrome.[61]

Takayasu's arteritis (Aortic arch syndrome, pulseless disease) Rare outside Japan, this systemic vasculitis affects the aorta and its major branches, causing stenosis and thrombosis. Acute inflammation causes dilatation and aneurysms; often affects ♀, 20–40yrs old. Symptoms depend on the arteries involved. The aortic arch is often affected, with cerebral, ophthalmological and upper limb symptoms eg dizziness, visual changes, weak arm pulses. Systemic features are common—eg fever, weight loss and malaise. ↑BP is often a feature, due to renovascular involvement. Complications include aortic valve regurgitation, aortic aneurysm and dissection; ischaemic stroke (↑BP and thrombus); and ischaemic heart disease. ***Diagnosis:*** ↑ESR & CRP; angiography of the aorta (invasive or CT/MR). ℞: Prednisolone (1mg/kg/day PO). Methotrexate or cyclophosphamide have been used in resistant cases. BP control is essential to ↓risk of stroke. Angioplasty, stenting, or bypass surgery are done for vascular complications. ***Prognosis:*** ~9 survival at 15 years. *[Mikito Takayasu, 19*

Tietze's syndrome (Idiopathic costochondritis) Localized pain/tenderness at the costosternal junction, enhanced by motion, coughing, or sneezing. The 2nd rib is most often affected. The diagnostic key is *localized* tenderness which is marked (flinches on prodding). ***Treatment:*** Simple analgesia, eg aspirin, NSAIDs. Its importance is that it is a benign cause of what at first seems to be alarming, cardiac pain. In lengthy illness, local steroid injections may be used.

Todd's palsy Limb weakness (eg hemiplegia) following a seizure. The patient seems to have had a stroke, but recovers in <24h. *[Robert Todd, 18*

Vincent's angina Mouth infection with ulcerative gingivitis from *Borrelia vincentii* (a spirochaete) + fusiform bacilli, often affecting young male smokers with poor oral hygiene. Try penicillin V 250mg/6h and metronidazole 400mg/8h PO, with chlorhexidine mouthwashes.

Von Hippel–Lindau syndrome is an autosomal dominant disorder, with germ-line mutation of a tumour suppressor gene on chromosome 3p (also implicated in sporadic renal cell carcinoma). It predisposes to bilateral renal cell carcinoma, retinal and cerebellar haemangioblastoma, and phaeochromocytoma. It may present with visual impairment or cerebellar signs (eg ataxia).

Von Willebrand's disease (VWD) Von Willebrand's factor (VWF) has 3 roles in clotting: to bring platelets into contact with exposed subendothelium, to make platelets bind to each other, and to bind to factor VIII protecting it from destruction in the circulation. There are >22 types of VWD, the commonest are:

- ***Type I:*** (commonest) Autosomal dominant deficiency (↓levels) of VWF.
- ***Type II:*** Abnormal VWF, with lack of high molecular weight multimers.
- ***Type III:*** Undetectable VWF levels (autosomal recessive with gene deletions).
- ***Type Normandy:*** Impaired VWF–factor VIII binding (mutations in VIII-binding domains of VWF; causes an *autosomal recessive* mimic of haemophilia A).

Signs are of a platelet type disorder (p330): bruising, epistaxis, menorrhagia, ↑bleeding post-tooth extraction. Symptoms are mild in Type I and II disease. ***Tests:*** APTT↑, bleeding time↑, Factor VIIIC↓ (clotting activity), VWF Ag↓; INR & platelets ↔. ℞: Get expert help. Vasopressin is used in mild bleeding, VWF rich Factor VIII concentrate for surgery or major bleed. Avoid NSAIDs.

Wallenberg's lateral medullary syndrome This relatively common syndrome comprises lesions to multiple CNS nuclei, caused by posterior inferior cerebellar artery occlusion leading to brainstem infarction. ***Features:*** • dysphagia, dysarthria (IX and X nuclei) • vertigo, nausea, vomiting, nystagmus (vestibular nuclei) • ipsilateral ataxia (inferior cerebellar peduncle) • ipsilateral Horner's syndrome (descending sympathetic fibres) • loss of pain and temperature sensation on the ipsilateral face (V nucleus) and contralateral limbs (spinothalamic tract). There is no limb weakness as the pyramidal tracts are unaffected.

In the rarer ***medial medullary syndrome***, vertebral or anterior spinal artery occlusion causes ipsilateral tongue paralysis (XII nucleus) with contralateral limb weakness (pyramidal tract, sparing the face) and loss of position sense.

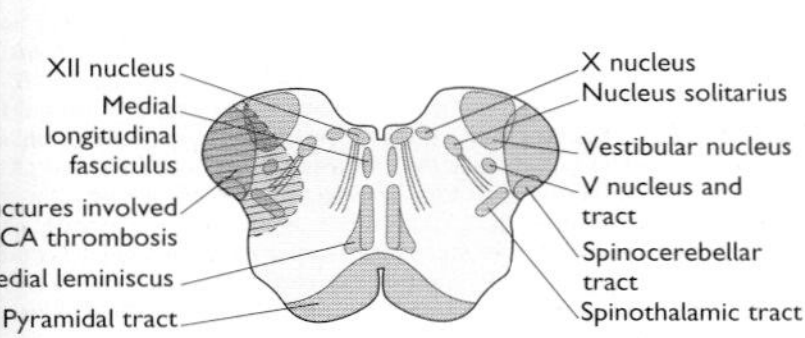

g 1. Cross section of the medulla showing structures involved in Wallenberg's teral medullary syndrome (posterior inferior cerebellar artery thrombosis).

Waterhouse–Friderichsen's (WhF) syndrome Bilateral adrenal cort haemorrhage, often occurring in rapidly deteriorating meningococcal seps alongside widespread purpura, meningitis, coma, and DIC. The meningococc endotoxin acts as a potent initiator of inflammatory and coagulation cascade Other causes include *H. influenzae*, pneumococcal, streptococcal, a staphylococcal sepsis. Adrenal failure causes shock, as normal vascular to requires cortisol to set activity of alpha and beta adrenergic receptors, a aldosterone is needed to maintain extracellular fluid volume. ***Treatmen*** ▸▸Antibiotics eg ceftriaxone 2g/12h IV (p806) and hydrocortisone 200mg/4h IV f adrenal support. ICU admission is usually indicated.

Weber's syndrome Ipsilateral 3rd-nerve palsy with contralateral hemiplegia, due infarction of one half of the midbrain, after occlusion of the paramedian branch of the basilar artery (which supply the cerebral peduncles).

Wegener's granulomatosis is a multisystem disorder of unknown cau characterised by necrotizing granulomatous inflammation and vasculitis of sm and medium vessels. It has a predilection for the upper respiratory tract, lungs a kidneys. ***Features:*** Upper airways disease is common, with nasal obstructic ulcers, epistaxis, or destruction of the nasal septum causing a characteris 'saddle-nose' deformity[1]. Sinusitis is often a feature. Renal disease causes rapic progressive glomerulonephritis with crescent formation, proteinuria or haematur Pulmonary involvement may cause cough, haemoptysis (severe if pulmona haemorrhage) or pleuritis. There may also be skin purpura or nodules, periphe neuropathy, mononeuritis multiplex, arthritis/arthralgia or ocular involvement keratitis, conjunctivitis, scleritis, episcleritis, uveitis, proptosis. ***Tests:*** cANC confirmed with a raised PR3 in the majority (p539). Urinalysis should be perform to look for proteinuria or haematuria. If these are present, consider a renal biop Do a CXR to look for evidence of pulmonary haemorrhage. Cytology fro sputum/BAL may show atypical cells that can be confused with bronch carcinoma. ***Treatment:*** Depends on the extent of disease. Severe disease (biopsy-proven renal disease) should be treated with corticosteroids a cyclophosphamide. Continuous oral cyclophosphamide may be more effective th pulsed IV regimens at inducing sustained remission, but may have more side effec Co-trimoxazole may be given as prophylaxis against *Pneumocystis carinii* a *Staphylococcal* colonisation. Patients with severe renal disease (eg creatinine 500µmol/L) may benefit from plasma exchange in addition. Azathioprine a methotrexate are used as maintenance therapies.

Wernicke's encephalopathy Thiamine (vitamin B_1) deficiency with a classical tri of ophthalmoplegia (nystagmus, lateral rectus or conjugate gaze palsies), atax (wide-based gait) and confusion. Always consider this diagnosis in alcoholics: it m also present with memory disturbance, hypotension, hypothermia, or reduc consciousness. Focal areas of brain damage occur, including periaqueduct punctate haemorrhages. ***Recognised causes:*** Alcoholism, eating disorde malnutrition, prolonged vomiting eg with chemotherapy, GI malignanc hyperemesis gravidarum. ***Tests:*** Red cell transketolase↓, (rarely done). ***Treatmen*** Urgent thiamine to prevent irreversible Korsakoff's syndrome (p696). Give thiamine (Pabrinex®) if there are any of the above features, 2–3 pairs of hig potency ampules/8h IV over 10min for up to 5d, then convert to oral thiamine. A IM (gluteal) preparation is available. Anaphylaxis may occur so have resuscitati facilities to hand. If there is co-existing hypoglycaemia (often the case in this gro of patients), make sure thiamine is given *before* glucose, as Wernicke's can precipitated by glucose administration to a thiamine-deficient patient. ***Prognosi*** Untreated, death occurs in 20%, and Korsakoff's psychosis occurs in 85%, quarter of whom will require long-term institutional care. *[Karl Wernicke, 187*

1 Common causes of a 'saddle-nose' deformity are trauma, and iatrogenic (eg post-rhinoplasty). Rar causes (popular with some finals examiners): Wegener's, relapsing polychondritis, syphilis, and lepros

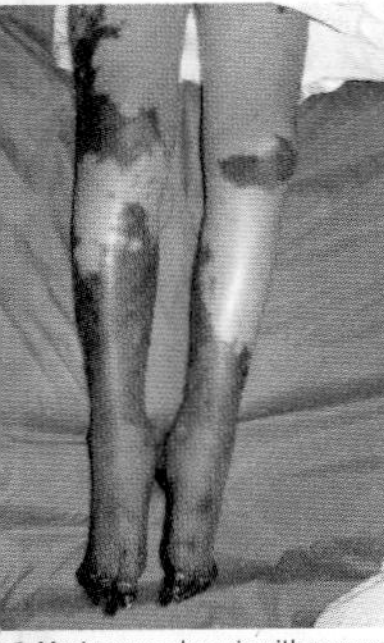

g 1. Meningococcal sepsis with purpura.

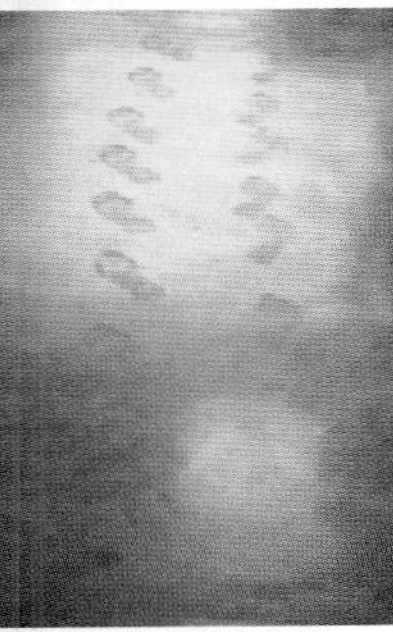

g 2. Wide based gait (footprints), seen in
Vernicke's encephalopathy.

Whipple's disease[1] A rare cause of GI malabsorption which usually occurs middle-aged white males, most commonly in Europe. It is caused by *Tropheryma whippelii*, which produces a systemic disease. ***Features:*** often starts insidiou with arthralgia (chronic, migratory, seronegative arthropathy affecting ma peripheral joints). GI symptoms commonly include weight loss, diarrhoea or colic abdominal pain, leading to malabsorption (p272). Systemic symptoms such fever, sweats, lymphadenopathy and skin hyperpigmentation also occur. Carc involvement may lead to endocarditis, which is typically blood culture negative. features include a reversible dementia, ophthalmoplegia, and facial myoclonus (if together, they are highly suggestive)—also hypothalamic syndrome (Hyperpha polydipsia, insomnia). NB: CNS involvement may occur without GI involvement. ***Tes*** Jejunal biopsy shows stunted villi. There is deposition of macrophages in the lam propria containing granules which stain positive for periodic acid-Schiff (PA Similar cells may be found in affected samples eg CSF, cardiac valve tissue, lym nodes, synovial fluid. The bacteria may be seen within macrophages on elect microscopy. MRI may demonstrate CNS involvement. ***R:*** should include antibiot which cross the blood-brain barrier. Current recommendations are IV ceftriaxo (or penicillin plus streptomycin) for 2wks then oral co-trimoxazole for 1yr. Shor courses risk relapse with CNS features. A rapid improvement in symptoms usua occurs. *[George Whipple, 19*

Zellweger syndrome (cerebrohepatorenal syndrome) A rare autosor recessive disorder characterized by absent peroxisomes. Peroxisomes a intracellular organelles, required for many cellular activities, including li metabolism. The syndrome is a severe form of infantile Refsum's syndrome, a exhibits similar biochemical abnormalities (p703). Clinical features inclu craniofacial abnormalities, severe hypotonia and mental retardation, glaucor cataracts, hepatomegaly and renal cysts. A number of causative genes (eg PE have been identified. Life expectancy is usually a few months only.

Zollinger–Ellison syndrome This is the association of peptic ulcers with a gastr secreting adenoma (gastrinoma). Gastrin excites excessive gastric acid producti which may produce multiple ulcers in the duodenum and stomach. The adenoma usually found in the pancreas, although it may arise in the stomach or duoden Most cases are sporadic; 20% are associated with Multiple Endocrine Neoplas type 1 (MEN1, p207). 60% are malignant, metastases are found in local lym nodes and the liver. ***Symptoms:*** Include abdominal pain and dyspepsia, from t ulcer(s), and chronic diarrhoea due to inactivation of pancreatic enzymes (a causes steatorrhoea) and damage to intestinal mucosa. ***Incidence:*** ~0.1% patients with peptic ulcer disease. Suspect in those with multiple peptic ulce ulcers distal to the duodenum, or a family history of peptic ulcers (or of islet c pituitary, or parathyroid adenomas). ***Tests:*** Raised fasting serum gastrin le (>1000pg/mL). Hypochlorhydria (reduced acid production eg in chronic atrop gastritis) should be excluded as this also causes a raised gastrin level: gastric should be <2. The secretin stimulation test is useful in suspected cases with o mildly raised gastrin levels (100-1000pg/mL). The adenoma is often small a difficult to image; a combination of somatostatin receptor scintigraphy, endosco ultrasound and CT is used to localise and stage the adenoma. ***R:*** High dose prot pump inhibitors (PPIs), eg omeprazole: start with 60mg/d and adjust according response. Measuring intragastric pH helps determine the best dose (aim to keep at 2–7). Surgical resection of the adenoma with lymph node clearance is genera recommended if >2cm in size, as this indicates malignant potential. Surgery usually avoided in MEN1, as adenomas are often multiple, and metastatic disease rare. Metastatic disease is treated with combination chemotherapy ± interferon Selective embolization may be undertaken for hepatic metastases. ***Prognosis:*** year survival: 80% if single resectable lesion, ~20% with hepatic metastases. patients should be screened for MEN1.

1 For a review of Whipple's disease, see T Marth 2003 *Lancet* **361** 239

18 Radiology

Contents

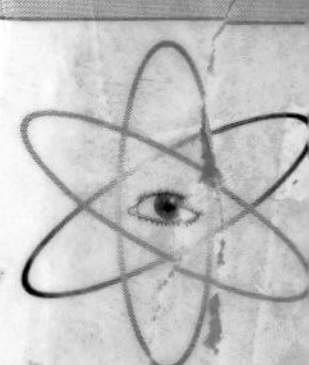

Fig 1. As in the natural world so it is in the physical: decay brings about new matter through a seemingly endless cycle. Yet the fragility of the human body reminds us that our own part in the cycle is fleeting. So how do we benefit? As humans, the answer may lie in the realm of the metaphysical rather than physical, but as doctors, at the nucleus of our work, we are given a vision not only into the inner workings of the body, but also into the colourful lives of those we treat.

Other relevant pages: Chest medicine (chapter 5); echocardiography (p98); further investigations in chest medicine (p150); x-ray findings in cestodes (p432) & trematodes (p433); cerebral artery territories (p440)

Images in other chapters: **CXR:** Cavitating Ca (p146); lung metastasis (p162); left lower lobe collapse (p163); sarcoidosis stages on CXR (p178); industrial dust diseases (p184); idiopathic pulmonary fibrosis (p183)

MRI: Pituitary adenoma (p219)

CT: Retroperitoneal fibrosis (p287); CVA (p441)

Enlarged images of chest and other x-rays are included before the index.

We thank Professor Peter Scally who is our Specialist Reader for this chapter.

Typical effective doses

The effective dose of an examination is calculated as the weighted sum of the doses to different body tissues. The weighting factor for each tissue depends on its sensitivity. The effective dose thus provides a single dose estimate related to the total radiation risk, no matter how the radiation dose is distributed around the body. This table is certainly not to be learnt; rather it serves as a reminder of the relative exposures to radiation that we prescribe in practice.

Procedure	Typical effective dose (mSv)	CXR equivalents	Approx. equivalent period of background radiation
X-ray examinations			
Limbs and joints	<0.01	<0.5	<1.5 days
Chest (PA)	0.02	1	3 days
Abdomen	1	50	6 months
Lumbar spine	1.3	65	7 months
CT head	2.3	115	1 year
IVU	2.5	125	14 months
Barium meal	3	150	16 months
Barium enema	7	350	3.2 years
CT chest	8	400	3.6 years
CT abdo/pelvis	10	500	4.5 years
Radionuclide studies			
Lung ventilation	0.3	15	7 weeks
Lung perfusion	1	50	6 months
Thyroid	1	50	6 months
Bone	4	200	1.8 years
PET head	5	250	2.3 years
Dynamic cardiac	6	300	2.7 years

Justifying exposure to ionising radiation

The very nature of ionising radiation that gives us vision into the human body also gives it lethal properties. The decision to expose patients to radiation must be made with the risks in mind, and even with strict guidelines we still have a tendency to over-exposure in medical practice. So when requesting an examination, the clinical benefits should far outweigh the risks of radiation sensitivity, cancer induction and genetic mutation.

The responsibility lies with us not to rely too heavily on radiological examinations and to restrain from the temptation of requesting examinations to comfort patients, or replace a lost film, or when the result will have no effect on management or clinical outcome. To give an idea of the relative doses involved, a CT examination of the abdomen and pelvis gives a typical effective dose of 500 times as much radiation as a CXR (see TABLE above). This important factor also tells us about the preference of ultrasound over CT when investigating abdominal and pelvic complaints such as acute appendicitis, especially given its youthful demographics.

►Unwitting exposure of the unborn fetus to radiation is inexcusable at any stage of gestation—unless the mother's life is in immediate danger—and it is the responsibility of the referring clinician to ensure that this is avoided. Discuss beforehand with the patient that you would like to do a pregnancy test, explaining why, being broad in your suppositions and tactful in your inquisitions.

The art of the request

One of the most nerve-wracking moments that you can encounter as a recent qualified doctor might be having to request a radiology investigation face-to-fa with a seasoned consultant radiologist. Imagine that you have been asked by yo team to request an ultrasound examination of the renal tract for one of yo patients who has a newly raised creatinine of 300 μmol/L. You explain that y aren't quite sure what to write on the request form, however they have alrea moved on to the next patient on the busy post-take ward round. What do yc write? How much do you write? Who do you ask? Below are some pointers th will aid you in making a successful request for a radiological investigation.

Before you start...

- Ensure that the investigation has not been done already or recently.
- *Is the patient fit to have the investigation?* An agitated or confused individual unlikely to stay still for a claustrophobic CT head examination!

The request form

- Include all relevant clinical information, blood tests and recent radiology findings on the request form. This is especially important given that there has been an increase in e-based request systems combined with a decrease in direct communication between the radiologist and the requesting clinician. Remember that the aim of radiology is to provide information in order to alter the management of the patient and the outcome of the disease. Think, therefore, what do I need to know?—see MINIBOX, Radiology can help.
- Include how the investigation will help resolve the clinical problem facing you.
- Include '± intervention' on the request form if you think it may take place (eg (abdomen ± drainage, for an abdominal collection).

Radiology can help:
• **Confirm** a suspecte diagnosis • **Exclude** somethin important • **Define** the extent of a disease • **Monitor** the progres of a disease

The verbal request

- Always **request** and never order an investigation.
- Know the case as fully as possible, but keeping your request brief and accurat
- Know what you need to confirm, exclude, monitor progress of or define.
- 'I was hoping to get your opinion about this interesting case...' is a potential successful opener to a request.
- Pre-empt by saying how the investigation will change your management (whi you will be invariably asked).
- Have any previous radiology of relevance with you when you make the reques eg a CXR if requesting a CT pulmonary angiogram (CTPA) or ventilation/perfusic ($\dot{V}/\dot{Q}$) scintigram.
- Inquire of the radiologist what he thinks is the correct investigation for the case.
- You may have an easier time requesting an investigation from a radiologist wl specialises in that particular technique (eg CT) or who is linked to your clinic team (eg he may lead your clinical x-ray meeting).

Stuck in the middle? You may find yourself a go-between, with your team on or side eagerly awaiting the investigation before the next move and the radiolog department on the other side trying to prioritise and fit the investigation into the already overscheduled timetable. It is in these situations it is important remember that the patient is also caught in the middle, completely unaware of tl goings-on around him. Take a few moments to lay out the progress plan and a expectations—it will make the experience of being swept away to the radiolog department without warning a far less scary experience!

Interpreting an image

It is not always possible to rely on a radiologist for the interpretation of an investigation, especially in an emergency or in the middle of the night. Remembering the following points may help hone your own interpreting skills:

- Take every passing opportunity to peruse examinations so that spotting both normal and abnormal variations comes more easily—the old idiom *practice makes perfect* is very apt here.
- Getting to grips with the science behind radiology makes interpretation easier and will explain the suitability of modalities to different clinical scenarios. Knowing how an investigation is done will also give practical clues to the result produced—eg a routine CXR is performed in the posteroanterior (PA) direction (the source posterior, the cassette anterior) so that the cardiac shadow is minimised.
- Use a systematic approach so that you don't pass anything unnoticed. Don't worry, though—some things can be notoriously difficult to spot.
- Virtually all investigations yield a 2D image from a 3D structure, though there have been recent developments in 3D imaging (fig 4, p719). A basic understanding of anatomical relationships of the area in question will help reconstruct the images in your mind into a clear representation of the reality before you.
- The standard orientation of all axial cross-sectional imaging is as if you are looking up at the supine patient from his feet. For images with non-conventional orientations (eg MRCP) look on the image for clue markings, or rely on your knowledge of anatomy—it can be tricky to visualise oblique sections!
- Don't rely solely on the investigation, but use it as part of the clinical work-up to help make an informed management decision.
- Go back to see the patient after looking at the investigation and reading the radiologist's report: you might picture them in a different light and notice something that you didn't before.

Presenting an image

Everyone has their own method for presenting, and the right way is **your own way**. As long as you cover everything systematically—because we all get 'hot-seat amnesia' at some point—the particulars will take care of themselves. Continue to polish your own method and remember a few extra tips for when an image is presented expectantly by your consultant/examiner and the floor is yours:

- A brief pensive silence with a thoughtful expression as you analyze the image is allowed—but not too long, otherwise it might look like you have been thrown!
- State the written details such as name, date of birth, where and how the imaging was taken. Look for clues: weighting of an MRI, a '**+ c**' indicating that contrast medium has been used, the phase of the investigation (arterial/venous/portal), or even the name of the organ printed on an ultrasound.
- State the type, mode and technical quality of investigation—not always easy!

Going through the above also gives you a bit of thinking time. Then:

- It is acceptable to start with any obvious abnormalities—they may be life-threatening—provided afterwards you move on systematically.
- Just like the bedside clues in a physical examination, there are clues in radiology examinations. Note oxygen masks, ECG leads, venous access, infusion apparatus, and invasive devices. Identifying what they are also helps you to look through what may otherwise appear to be a cluttered mess.
- Not everything on the image is inside the subject—some things may be on the surface/outside or not there at all, eg ring artefacts or 'stair-stepping' on CT.
- Stating a differential diagnosis is good practice, as not all findings are diagnostic.
- If there is additional clinical information that would help you to make a diagnosis, don't be afraid to ask. After all, we treat patients and not images!

Remember: X-ray=***radiodensity*** (lucency/opacity) CT=***attenuation***
US=***echogenicity/reflectivity*** MRI=***signal intensity***

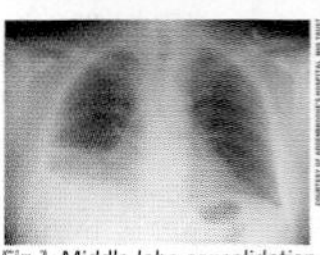
Fig 1. Middle lobe consolidation and a right pleural effusion.

Principles Images are usually taken on inspirat with the patient standing in front of the casse and the x-ray source behind (postero-anterio PA). Emergency images may be the other v (antero-posterior, AP), which magnifies heart s and supine, which alters the distribution of and fluid in the lungs and pleural cavities. Th are 4 radiographic densities: **air**, **fat**, **water/s tissue**, and **bone**. A border is only seen at interface of 2 densities, eg heart (soft tissue) lung (air); the 'silhouette' is lost if air in the lung is replaced by consolida (water). The silhouette sign localizes pathology (eg middle lobe pneumonia collapse causing loss of clarity of the right heart border, fig 1). When interpretin radiograph use a systematic approach that works for you—eg from outside inside, or inside-out—but start by assessing the technical qualities of the ima

- ***Rotation:*** The sternal ends of the clavicles should symmetrically overlie transverse processes of the 4th or 5th thoracic vertebrae.
- ***Inspiration:*** There should be 5 to 7 ribs visible anteriorly (or 10 posterio Hyperinflation can be abnormal, eg COPD.
- ***Exposure:*** An under-exposed image will be too white and an over-exposed im will be too black. Both cause a loss of definition and quality.
- ***Position:*** The entire lung margins must be visible, especially the costophrenic ang

Radiology

Trachea Should be central or just to the right. Deviated by collapse (towards side of the lesion), tension (away from the side of the lesion), or rotation of the f Also check heart position (below).

Mediastinum May be widened in many disorders: retrosternal thyroid; lymph node enlargement (sarcoidosis, lymphoma, metastases, TB); tumour (thymoma, teratoma, neurogenic tumours); aortic aneurysm; cysts (bronchogenic cyst, pericardial cyst); paravertebral mass (TB); oesophageal dilatation (achalasia, hiatus hernia). There are 4 'moguls' normally visible on the left border of the mediastinum that may help identify pathology if abnormal. From superior to inferior they are: 1 Aortic knuckle; 2 Pulmonary outflow tract; 3 Left auricle; 4 Left ventricle.

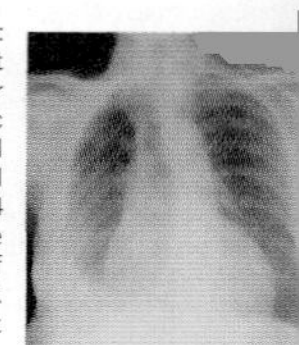
Fig 2. Cardiomegaly and los the right costophrenic a from a pleural effus consistent with heart failur

Hila The left hilum is higher than the right, but they should be the same size and density. May be pulled up or down by fibrosis or collapse. 1 ***Enlarged hila:*** Nodes; pulmonary arterial hypertension (± an enlarged second 'mogul'); bronchogenic carcinoma. 2 ***Calcification:*** Previous silicosis; histoplasmosis (p428). Sarcoidosis, TB and lymphoma can give bilate hilar + right paratracheal lymphadenopathy.

Heart Normally <15cm across—approximately 50% of the width of the thorax should lie to the right of the vertebral column, ⅔ to the left. It may app elongated if the chest is hyperinflated (COPD) or enlarged if the image is AP, ther failure (fig 2), or a pericardial effusion. Are there calcified valves?

The diaphragm The right side is usually slightly higher. ***Causes of a rais hemidiaphragm:*** Lung volume loss; stroke; phrenic nerve palsy (from: trauma; M p498; cancer); hepatomegaly; subphrenic abscess. Subpulmonic effusion a diaphragm rupture give apparent elevation. **NB:** Bilateral palsies (polio, muscu dystrophy) cause hypoxia.

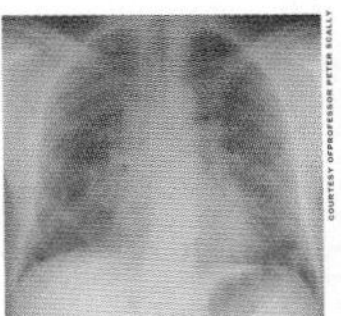

Fig 3. Diffuse reticular shadowing secondary to interstitial lung disease. The diagnosis was fibrosing alveolitis (UIP).

ıgs Shadowing is described as nodular, reticular twork of fine lines, interstitial), or alveolar ıffy). A single nodule can be described as an SOL.

dules:[1]

Neoplasia: lung carcinoma, adenoma, hamart-ɔma, metastases—often missed if small.

Infections (varicella pneumonia, hydatid, septic ɔmboli). An abscess can also appear as an SOL.

Granulomas (miliary TB, sarcoidosis, histo-ɔlasmosis, Wegener's granulomatosis, p706).

Pneumoconioses (except asbestosis), Caplan's syndrome (p688).

ticular shadows: (fig 3) Usually acute inter-ial changes (cardiac or noncardiac pulmonary erstitial oedema; atypical pneumonia, eg viral; or:

- Fibrosis; TB; histoplasmosis
- Sarcoidosis; silicosis; asbestosis
- Usual interstitial pneumonitis (UIP)
- Neoplasia (lymphangitis carcinomatosa)
- Fibrosing alveolitis; rheumatoid (p532)
- Wegener's (p706); SLE; PAN; CREST (p538)

veolar shadows: Usually pulmonary oedema from LVF (p786). Also:

- Pneumonia
- Haemorrhage
- Drugs (heroin, cytotoxics, p516)
- Smoke inhalation (p831)
- O_2 toxicity
- Fat emboli, ~7 days post-fracture
- Renal or liver failure (p294 & p250)
- ARDS (p170); DIC (p336)
- Head injury, or after neurosurgery
- Alveolar proteinosis
- Near-drowning (*OHCS* p724)
- Heat stroke (p778).

ʒ 4. Complete opacification the left hemithorax after eumonectomy; note the mediastinum is shifted to the left.

'Ring' shadows: Either airways seen end-on (air-bronchograms; bronchiectasis), or cavitating lesions, eg abscess (bacterial, fungal, amoebic), tumour, or pulmonary infarct (triangular with a pleural base).

Linear opacities: Septal lines (Kerley B lines, ie interlobular lymphatics seen with fluid, tumour, or dusts); atelectasis; pleural plaques (asbestosis). ***White-out*** of an entire hemithorax can occur in pneumonia, massive pleural effusion, ARDS, or after pneumonectomy (fig 4).

Air outside the lungs: Check for a pneumothorax ifficult to spot if apical or in a supine image), surgical emphysema (trauma, rogenic) and gas under the diaphragm (perforated viscus, trauma, surgery).

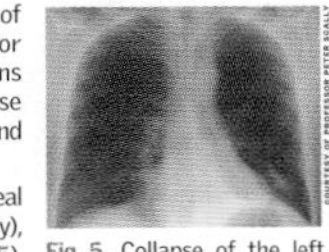

Fig 5. Collapse of the left lower lobe—the triangular opacity behind the heart. Also, the left main bronchus has been pulled down. ►Enlarged versions of these CXRs appear before the index.

ɔnes Check the ***clavicles*** for bone density (loss of ɪrtex in osteoporosis) or fracture, the ***ribs*** for actures, notching, absence (surgery) and lesions g metastases), the ***vertebral column*** for collapse destruction and the ***shoulders*** for fracture and thritis.

n apparently normal CXR? Check for tracheal mpression, absent breast shadow (mastectomy), uble left heart border (left lower lobe collapse, fig 5), id level behind the heart (hiatus hernia, achalasia), and ravertebral abscess (TB). ►Remember to check old nages for comparison: fig 3 could be acute terstitial oedema, but comparison with a previous nage showed that the changes were chronic.

1 Remember that the apex of the lower lobe rises up to the 4th rib posteriorly, so it is difficult to ascribe e true location of a lesion on a PA image without additional information from a lateral view. It may be tter to use the term 'zone' rather than lobe when localising a lesion.

Plain abdominal x-ray (AXR)

Enlarged images: p83

These are rarely diagnostic, and are non-contributory in most mild or moder instances of abdominal pain. Indications for AXR with acute abdominal symptoms a

- Acute abdominal pain warranting admission or surgery
- Suspicion of perforation or obstruction
- Acute exacerbation of inflammatory bowel disease
- Haematuria, renal failure, or renal colic
- Ingestion of a sharp or poisonous foreign body (eg lithium battery)
- Blunt or penetrating injury to the abdomen
- Intussusception in paediatrics.

Erect AXRs are rarely done, since bowel gas pattern is best seen on supine imag and free intraperitoneal gas (signifying perforation) is best seen on an erect c (fig 1, p581). The following routine covers most of the important aspects:

- **Gas patterns: Look for:** An abnormal quantity of gas in the stomach, sm intestine, or colon. Deciding whether you are looking at small or large bowel:

Small bowel:

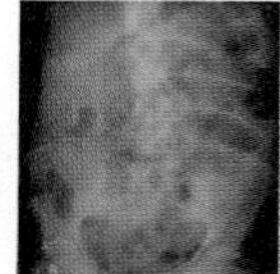

Fig 1. The pattern seen in small bowel obstruction.
- Smaller calibre
- Central; multiple loops
- *Valvuli conniventes:* folds that go from wall to wall, all the way across the lumen; more regular than *haustra*
- Grey (contains air & fluid)

Large bowel:

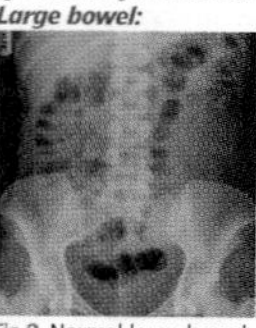

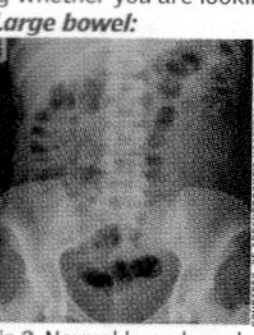

Fig 2. Normal large bowel gas pattern.
- Larger calibre
- Peripheral
- *Haustra:* do not go all the way across the lumen, but may appear to do so if viewed from an angle
- Blacker (contains gas)[1]

Ileus:

Fig 3. Multiple dilated a filled loops of large ar small bowel. This pattern seen in ileus.
- Both small and larg bowel visible
- There is no clear trans ition point that corres ponds to an obstructing lesion

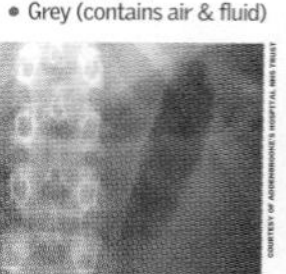

Fig 4. Part of the descending colon with mucosal thickening and loss of normal haustral pattern; seen in colitis

The small bowel's diameter is normally ~2.5cm, th colon ~5cm, and the caecum up to 10cm. Dilated sm bowel occurs in obstruction and paralytic ileu Dilated large bowel (≥6cm) occurs with both these, a also in toxic dilatation in someone who is really sick, ar in the elderly, benign hypotonicity. Grossly dilate segments of bowel occur in sigmoid and caec volvulus. Loss of normal mucosal folds, irregula mucosal islands, and bowel wall thickening can b seen in inflammatory colitis (eg IBD)—fig 4. 'Thum printing' is protrusion of rounded indentations thickened mural folds into the lumen and is seen large bowel ischaemia.

- **Gas outside the lumen:** You must explain any gas outside the lumen of th stomach, small intestine, and colon. It could be: 1 Pneumoperitoneum; sig visible on the supine AXR include: gas on both sides of the bowel wall (Rigler sign), a triangle of gas in the RUQ trapped beneath the falciform ligament, and football-shaped distribution of gas beneath the anterior abdominal wall. 2 Gas the urinary tract—eg in the bladder from a fistula. 3 Gas in biliary tre (pneumatobilia—see MINIBOX), or rarely 4 Intramural gas, found in bow

1 Also, the ascending colon contains liquid faeces, but the descending colon contains faecal pellets (*scybal*

►Enlarged versions of images appear before the index.

necrosis, clostridial infection, necrotizing enterocolitis (neonates) and pneumatosis cystoides intestinalis (a rare and benign condition).

Local peritoneal inflammation can cause localized ileus (a sentinel loop of intraluminal gas), giving a clue to the site of pathology. Roughly: *RUQ* ≈ cholecystitis, *LUQ* ≈ pancreatitis, *RLQ* ≈ appendicitis, *LLQ* ≈ diverticulitis.

Biliary tree Look for: Pneumatobilia (see MINIBOX) and calcification in the gall bladder (only ~10% of gallstones are visible on plain AXR). Calcification of the gallbladder wall (porcelain gallbladder) is a result of chronic inflammation secondary to gallstones or adenocarcinoma in 22% of cases.

Pneumatobilia:
• Post-ERCP • Post-surgery • Anaerobic cholangitis • Recent stone passage • Gallbladder–bowel fistula

The urinary tract The kidneys normally have an equivalent length of 2½–3½ vertebral bodies and slope inferolateraly, with the left sitting higher than the right. Their outlines can usually be discerned because they have a surrounding layer of perinephric fat—if this is or has been inflamed (eg perinephric abscess) then the outline is obliterated. The ureters pass near the tips of the lumbar transverse processes, cross the sacroiliac joints, down to the ischial spines, and turn medially to join the bladder. Check the kidneys and ureteric courses for calculi (visible in 90% of cases)—this requires practice! See p730 for intravenous urography (IVU).

Other soft tissues: Look for: Size/position of: liver, spleen and bladder. A grossly enlarged liver will push the bowel to the left side of the abdomen, spleen to the right, bladder superiorly. The liver and spleen should not extend below the level of the 12th rib on a correctly aligned image.

Other calcification: Calcification can be seen in the abdominal aorta, splenic artery, pancreas (chronic pancreatitis), mesenteric lymph nodes (fig 5), and granulomas in the liver and spleen. Phleboliths, recognised by their rounded shape and radiolucent centre, are harmless calcifications found in the perivesical veins.

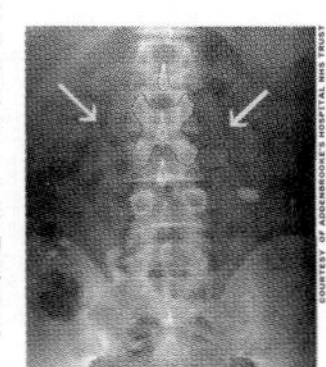

Fig 5. AXR showing calcified mesenteric lymph nodes. Also note; psoas lines (arrows); spinous process (green); transverse process (blue); pedicles (yellow): facet joint processes (outline in red); vertebral body (cyan).

Medical devices: Double-J and biliary stents, nephrostomy and gastrostomy tubes, intrauterine devices (eg coil), laparoscopic sterilisation clips, and chronic ambulatory peritoneal dialysis (CAPD) catheters (fig 6) can all be seen on AXR.

Bones and joints: In the lumbar spine, look for scoliosis and degenerative disease (osteophytes, joint space narrowing). Identify and compare the vertebral bodies, spinous processes (lack of arch closure in spina bifida), pedicles (can be destroyed in malignancy), facet joints, and transverse processes (fig 5). Be on the lookout for metastatic deposits (osteolytic or osteosclerotic) and Paget's disease (unusual patterns of bone expansion, sclerosis and/or lysis). Although not the preferred view, the sacroiliac joints can also be seen (sclerotic in early ankylosing spondylitis). In renal osteodystrophy (p294) there is a 'rugger jersey' spine of alternating bands of sclerosis (opacity) and osteopenia (lucency).

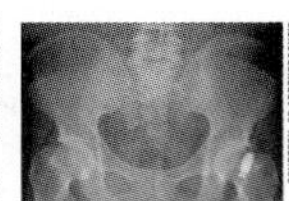

Fig 6. A CAPD catheter (for continuous ambulatory peritoneal dialysis). ►Enlarged images p839

Don't expect too many answers from plain abdominal images! Develop and rely on your clinical skills. At the end of the day the most common diagnosis for abdominal pain is abdominal pain of unknown origin: think of major pathologies.

Radiology

Computed tomography (CT)

Since its first use in Atkinson Morley Hospital in 1972, CT has become a speedy accurate aid to the clinician, with new systems producing whole body images in ur one breath (thanks to continuous, helical rather than sequential, axial data acquisit Within a single slice (eg 2–5mm thick) CT records the **attenuation**[1] of different tis to ionising radiation and calculates a mean value for a given volume of tissue, calle **voxel**, in a process called **volume averaging**. This value is represented in greys as a single point, called a **pixel**, in the final 2D image, usually 512 by 512 pixels. greyscale of the image is measured on the Hounsfield scale relative to attenuation of water, which has a value of 0 Hounsfield units (HU) and ranges f less than –1000 HU (low attenuation) to more than +1000 HU (high attenuati

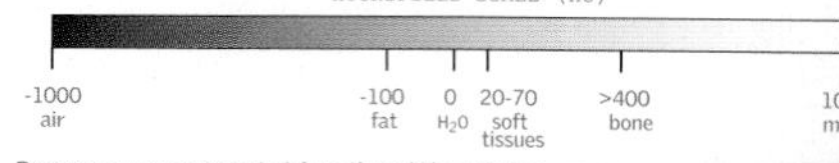

Because our eyes cannot pick up the subtle variation in attenuation of the tissues that CT can, there are different **windows** that can be used to look at tissues of different density, eg bone or lung (fig 1).

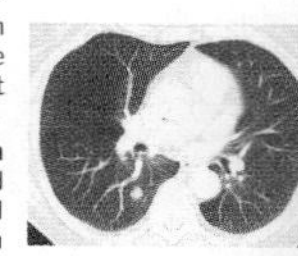

Fig 1. Axial CT chest on a lu window algorithm showing solitary pulmonary metastasi

CT with intravenous iodinated contrast medium gives the ability to image vascular anatomy and vascular structures in arterial, venous and delayed phases after the injection of contrast medium (fig 2). Contrast medium is usually given IV for examinations of the chest, abdomen and pelvis. CTs of the brain, spine, and musculoskeletal system are normally done without IV contrast. Enhancement of the colonic lumen can be achieved with oral contrast medium given 24h beforehand, or by rectal administration. Air is insufflated for CT colonography or 'virtual colonoscopy'—fig 6, p729). Oral contrast or water is administered 1h before an examination for definition of the stomach and small bowel. Also see **Contrast in imaging**, p734.

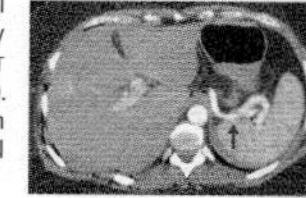

Fig 2. Axial CT of abdomen po IV contrast. The tortuous sple artery is well seen (arrow).

CT as the examination of choice: Staging and monitoring malignant disease; intracranial pathology, eg CVA, trauma, ↑ICP, and SOLs (especially when calcified, eg oligodendroglioma); trauma; pre-operative assessment of complex masses; obese patients (US in thinner individuals); most post-operative complications; visualisation of anatomy for drainage, biopsy and nerve blocks.

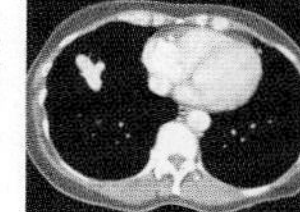

Fig 3. Axial CT of chest post contrast. The avidly enhancing middle lobe lesion was an arterio-venous malformation.[2]

1 Attenuation is the loss of energy of a wave due to absorption, refraction, reflection and divergence passes through a medium.
2 This emphasises the importance of building a 3D mental construct from the 2D axial slices.

efacts and interference **Remember that the CT** image is a matrix representation of the nuation produced by rotating the system around patient—this explains some of the artefacts that be produced. High attenuation items such as al fillings, clips and prostheses (and even bone) cause interference. This is one reason why the terior cranial fossa was not well imaged on CT—it etter now. 'Stair-stepping' and poorly defined es are caused by volume averaging (the partial me effect) and can be overcome by reducing the width for the desired sections.

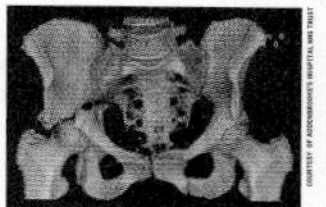

Fig 4. Surface rendered 3D CT reconstruction of the pelvis. There is a fracture through the superior acetabulum.

future of CT Multi-detector CT (MDCT) systems BOX $\dot{V}/\dot{Q}$ VS CTPA, p725) are an important ance. They image a volume of tissue, rather than vidual slices. Also by decreasing the thickness of ce, they increase volume averaging and thus ease resolution and reduce artefact. Multiplanar just axial) slices can be retrieved from one ep', giving thousands of images that are stored ally and reconstructed, eg into a 3D image (fig T angiography uses MDCT and digital modulation nology to enable 3D colour reconstructions. CT graphy is rapidly becoming the investigation of ce for the urinary tract. Perfusion CT scanning is veloping technique that maps cerebral blood by acquiring images over a period after a rapid IV bolus of contrast medium. ole is yet to be established in the investigation of acute stroke, though it does the advantages of being less invasive than angiography and more available MRI. CT combined with PET (see p730) has and increased sensitivity and ificity over each alone.

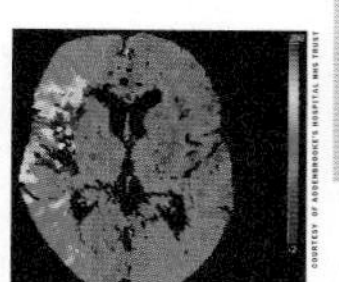

Fig 5. Head perfusion CT, with signs of ischaemia in the right middle cerebral artery territory.

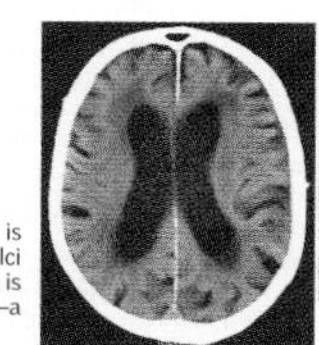

6. Axial non-enhanced CT of the brain. There is ricular dilatation with prominent cerebral sulci ating cerebral atrophy. But the degree of atrophy is not well-correlated with clinical symptoms—a nder that morphology does not reflect function.

o many CTs?

s tempting to think that we might be overusing such a valuable resource. en that CT examinations account for perhaps 40% of iatrogenic radiation osure it is sensible to consider if usage is appropriate. Yet in one review, the litors were unable to account for any substantial group of patients that were dergoing unnecessary CT examination.

When deciding to request a CT, it is still important to consider the need and benefit of CT over other imaging investigations. MRI is becoming more able as an alternative, especially in younger patients, and is even preferable circumstances where we regularly use CT because of its greater availability imaging the liver). Ultrasound may also be an accurate and appropriate rnative. To get the best result, discuss the options with a radiologist.

Magnetic resonance imaging (MRI)

1 A large proportion of the human body is fat or water (~80%).
2 Fat and water contain a large number of hydrogen nuclei (unpaired protons
3 The spin of a positively charged hydrogen nucleus gives it magnetic polarity

Thus...

- Placing the human body in a magnetic field (clinically from 0.2–3 Tesla) aligns hydrogen nuclei either with (parallel) or against (anti-parallel) the field.
- A radiofrequency (RF) pulse at the resonant frequency flips nuclei away from th original alignment by an angle depending on the amount of energy they abso
- When the RF pulse stops, the nuclei flip back (or **relax**) into their original alig ment, emitting the energy (called an **echo**) that was absorbed from the RF fie
- Measuring and plotting the energy of the returning signal according to locati (provided the nuclei haven't moved) gives a picture of fat, tissue, and water distributed throughout the body.
- The hydrogen nuclei in flowing blood move after receiving the RF pulses. The ec is not detected, and so the vessel lumen appears black.

Rather than radiodensity or attenuation, the correct descriptive terminology for greyscale seen in MRI is **signal intensity**: high signal appears white and low sig black (see below). **Weighting** is a quality of MRI that is dependent on the length of period between the RF pulses (**repetition time, TR**) and the time between an RF pu and the echo (**echo time, TE**). MR images are most commonly T1-weighted (good visualising anatomy) or T2-weighted (good for visualising disease) but can also b mixture of both, called **proton density** (PD) weighting. **FLAIR** sequences produ heavily T2-weighted images. A good way to determine the weighting of an MR image is look for water—eg in the aqueous humour of the eye, CSF, or synovial fluid (see TAB

Radiology

	T1-WEIGHTED	T2-WEIGHTED
TR TE	short (<1000ms) short (<30ms)	long (>2000ms) long (>80ms)
LOW SIGNAL ■	**water** flowing Hb fresh Hb haemosiderin	bone flowing Hb deoxyHb haemosiderin melanin
HIGH SIGNAL □	bone fat cholesterol gadolinium (p734) metHb	**water** cholesterol fresh Hb metHb

Advantages MRI's great bonus is that it does not involve ionising radiation. It h no known long term adverse effects, though power is limited by controls on ener deposition into tissue. It is excellent for imaging soft tissues (water- and hen proton-dense). It is preferred over CT for intracranial, head and neck, spinal, a musculoskeletal disorders. Multiplanar acquisition of images can provide multip views and 3D reconstruction from one examination.

Disadvantages include poor imaging of lung parenchyma and GI mucosa, bei more claustrophobic and noisy than CT, and current high cost combined with po availability.

Contraindications ***Absolute:*** • Cardiac pacemakers and other cardiac electric devices. • Intra-ocular metallic foreign bodies. (You may need to request an X-r of the orbits to exclude a foreign body) ***Relative:*** • Intracranial aneurysm cli • Certain types of artificial heart valves. • If unable to complete the pre-sc questionnaire. • 1st trimester of pregnancy (not currently approved.) • Cochle implants. NB: Orthopaedic prostheses and extracranial metallic clips are generally sa ►If uncertain, discuss with a radiologist.

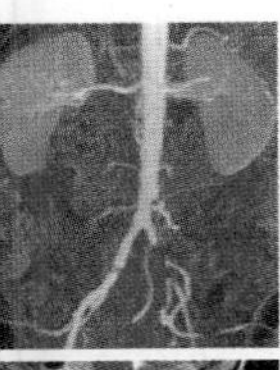

Fig 1. One of the many successful developments in MRI has been magnetic resonance angiography (MRA). It can accurately reconstruct vascular anatomy with or without IV gadolinium. This makes it a valuable in the assessment of vascular disease in patients with nephropathy. This also precludes the need for femoral puncture (the usual point of entry for conventional contrast angiography), which can have complications of haemorrhage, pseudoaneurysm formation and arterial thrombosis. This MRA shows complete occlusion of the left common iliac artery and focal stenosis of the right common iliac artery.

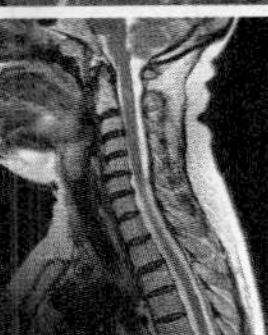

Fig 2. T2 weighted sagittal MRI of the cervical spine. There is impingement of the spinal cord at the C5/6 and C6/7 levels caused by degenerative disease. C2 (axis) is identifiable from the odontoid peg, that is embryologically derived from the body at C1 (atlas).

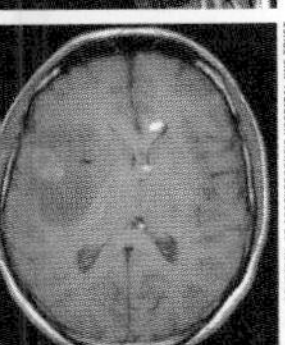

Fig 3. Axial T1 weighted MRI of the brain post IV gadolinium. In the right tempro-parietal region there is an area of low signal with a more central area of high signal. This is causing mass effect with effacement of the sulci and adjacent right frontal horn of the lateral ventricle. There is midline shift.

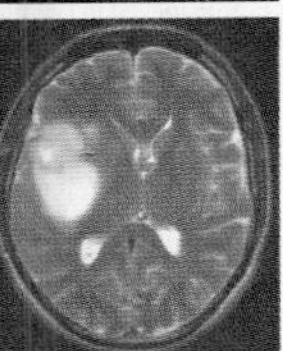

Fig 4. Axial T2 weighted MRI of the same patient at the same level. The high signal in the temporo-parietal region with more central focal high signal again shows mass effect. The diagnosis was of a cystic tumour. Note that on this T2 weighted image the cerebrospinal fluid within the ventricles and cortical sulci are of high signal due to their high water content.

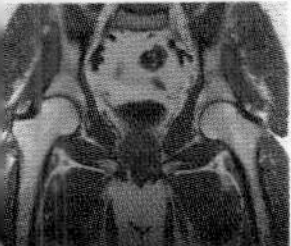

Fig 5. Coronal T1 weighted MRI of the hips. On T1 weighted imaging the normal adult bone marrow is high signal due to fatty yellow marrow, whilst red marrow gives a lower signal. MRI gives remarkable soft tissue contrast definition.

Ultrasound (US)

Unlike the other methods of imaging, ultrasound does not use electromagnetic radiation. Instead, it relies on the properties of longitudinal sound waves. This has made it a popular and safe form of diagnostic imaging. High frequency sound waves (3-15MHz) are produced from a piezo-electric quartz crystal, the size, shape and resonant frequency of which are important in determining tissue penetration and image quality. One of the interesting characteristics of ultrasound is that the transducer acts as both transmitter and receiver because of the piezo-electric properties of quartz crystal.[1]

The passage of sound waves through tissue is affected by **attenuation** and **reflection**. Attenuation disperses the waves out of the range of the receiver, whereas it is the waves reflected to the receiver that determine the image derived. The quality of this image is closely dependent on the difference in **acoustic impedance** between adjacent soft tissues.

With the help of software a real-time 2D image is produced. During processing an average attenuation value is assumed throughout the depth of the tissue examined. This means that if a higher-than-average attenuation structure is in the superficial tissues, then everything deep to it will be in a low intensity (black) **acoustic shadow**. If a lower-than-average attenuation object is in the superficial tissues then everything deep to it will be high intensity (white) or **enhanced**; see MINIBOX. If a tissue interface is strongly disparate, then all the waves are reflected back, making it impossible to image beyond it.

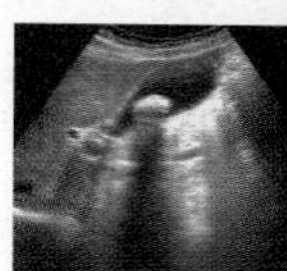

Fig 1. Abdominal US showing hyperechoic calcified gallstor causing a dense acoust shadow (black) posteriorl The hypoechoic gallbladde (bile) as a fluid structure ha echobright acoustic enhance ment (white). Different tissue have different acoustic impec ance values and therefor affect the velocity of th ultrasound wave as it trave through a tissue.

Acoustic shadow
• Fibrous tissue • Calcification • Gas
Acoustic enhancement
• Fluid-filled and cystic structures

Ultrasound techniques ***A-mode*** (standing for amplitude) gives a 1D trace tha depicts the depth of an interface and the strength of the reflected signal. ***B-mode*** (standing for brightness) is the most common technique, and gives 2D slices tha map the different magnitudes of echo in greyscale. ***M-mode*** (standing fo movement) displays a trace of the movement of structures within the line of th sound beam. It is used to effect in imaging eg heart valves (p98).

Duplex ultrasonography (flow and morphology) By combining the Doppler effec (the shift in wavelength caused by movement of a source or reflecting surface) wit B-mode ultrasound technology it is possible to determine flow characteristics of the circulation (fig 2). This is extremely useful ir arterial and venous studies, and echocardiography

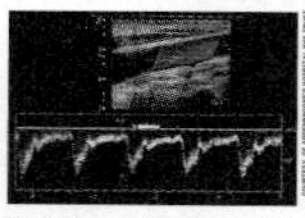

Fig 2. A normal Duplex US of the right common carotid artery. It can measure the flow rate in the artery (here 76cm/s). The Doppler trace (orange) is displayed below the main image.

Advantages of US Portable; quick; cheap; nonionising; real-time; can be used with intervention; car enter organs, eg anorectum, vagina, GI tract.

Disadvantages of US Inter-performer variance; poo quality in obese subjects; interference from bone bowel gas, calculi and other superimposed structures

Endoscopic US can be used to image structures from within the body. It is most commonly done as transoesophageal echocardiography (TOE, p98), but is also used to assess the depth of invasion of carcinomas eg pancreas, stomach.

1 When a voltage is applied to a piezo-electric crystal it changes shape, emitting a sound wave when it vibrates. In reverse, when a sound wave physically alters its shape an electrical current is induced.

Structures commonly imaged with ultrasound

The following structures should always be considered for imaging with ultrasound, given that it is non-invasive, non-ionising investigation:

Abdominal	Pelvic		Vascular	Other
Gall bladder	Uterus	Fetus	Carotid arteries[1]	Pleural effusion
Liver	Ovaries	Bladder	Abdominal aorta	Thyroid
Spleen	Salpinges		Portal system	Lumps & bumps
Appendix	Cervix		Peripheral arteries	Testes
Pancreas	Adnexae		Leg veins	Fistulae
Ascites	Appendix!			Musculoskeletal

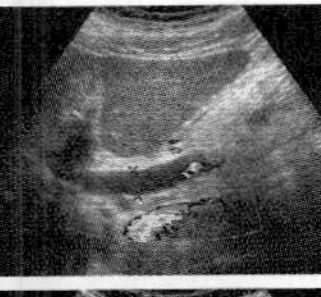

COURTESY OF ADDENBROOKE'S HOSPITAL NHS TRUST

Fig 3. Ultrasound of the liver showing the common bile duct to be dilated proximal to a presumed obstruction (a width >6mm if <60yrs old is abnormal). Duplex mode shows flow in the portal vein that lies (along with the hepatic artery) posterior to the duct in the lesser omentum's free edge. The next questions are 'what is causing the obstruction?' and 'where can I get that information?'.

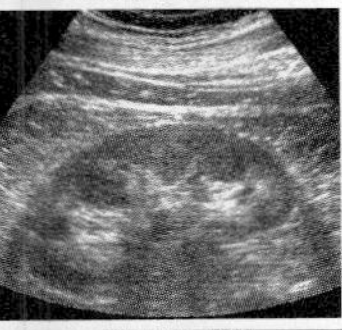

COURTESY OF ADDENBROOKE'S HOSPITAL NHS TRUST

Fig 4. Ultrasound of the kidney. On first inspection the image may appear normal but there is increased echogenicity predominantly within the medulla and some posterior acoustic shadowing associated with this. This is nephrocalcinosis of which there are many causes.

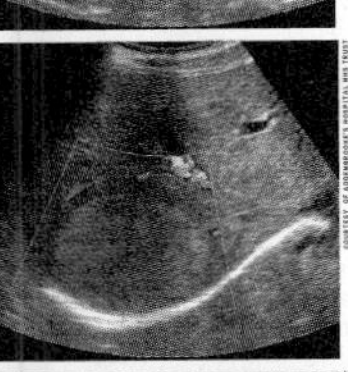

COURTESY OF ADDENBROOKE'S HOSPITAL NHS TRUST

Fig 5. Ultrasound of the liver showing a solitary round mass in the posterior aspect of the right lobe of the liver. This was a primary liver tumour. Duplex imaging shows a leash of vessels surrounding the lesion but not within it, suggesting it is not a highly vascular tumour.

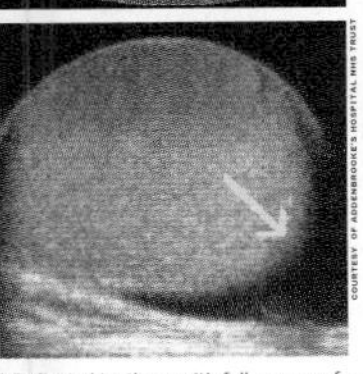

COURTESY OF ADDENBROOKE'S HOSPITAL NHS TRUST

Fig 6. Ultrasound of the testis showing a hydrocele (arrow). One of the great advantages of ultrasound that it does not use radiation, and so is ideal for imaging radiosensitive tissues such as the testis, thyroid, and fetus.

1 Indicated in: those with full recovery from stroke in whom endarterectomy is considered; suspected dissection; young patients with ischaemic stroke, and all patients with TIA.

Nuclear medicine

Nuclear medicine is a growing field with both diagnostic and therapeut applications. The latter is developing rapidly, but here we are mostly concerne with its diagnostic capabilities. The use of molecules labelled with a radioisoto means that there is exposure to ionising radiation, though doses are usually le than those from a CT abdomen (see TABLE, p711).

Positron emission tomography (PET) maps glucose metabolism in the body. F-1 fluorodeoxyglucose (FDG), a short half-life glucose analogue (λ=110min), is take up by metabolically active tissues. It decays rapidly to produce a positron tha after travelling a few mm through tissue, annihilates with an electron to produce pair of high energy photons (γ rays), which are subsequently detected. Neoplasm have a high uptake of FDG, but so do benign inflammatory and granulomatous le ions—if one is considering false +ves, consider sarcoidosis and TB. Non-pathologic high uptake of FDG in brain, liver, kidney, bladder, larynx and lymphoid tissue pharynx can interfere with interpretation leading to falsely –ve scans. Resolution lesions can be down to 4mm. 3D analysis greatly increases sensitivity compared 2D. ***Cancer:*** PET has a role when combined with MRI and CT. It is used in a colorect cancer for evaluation of local recurrence, treatment of liver metastases and in looking for extrahepatic metastases when considering hepatic resection. Also indicated for staging of: non-small cell lung cancer; lymphoma; melanoma; oesophageal cancer. ***Dementia:*** PET of no proven value, but is used in research. ***Radionuclide imaging in cardiology:*** p726.

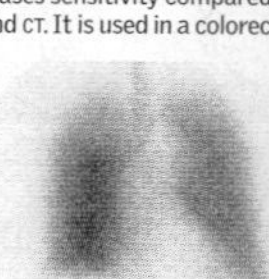

Fig 1. Ventilation scintigram.

Ventilation ($\dot{V}$) scintigraphy (fig 1) uses technetium (Tc) or xenon-133 (^{133}Xe). Requires a CXR within last 24h for comparison. You can sometimes discern it from a perfusion image by the presence of radioisotope in the upper airway.

Perfusion ($\dot{Q}$) scintigraphy (fig 2) uses 99m-technetium-labelled (^{99m}Tc) macroaggregates that block a small proportions of lung capillaries and thus lodge in the pulmonary circulation. Reported as high, intermediate, low probability, or normal according to findings. A normal perfusion scintigram excludes PE, hence its high sensitivity.

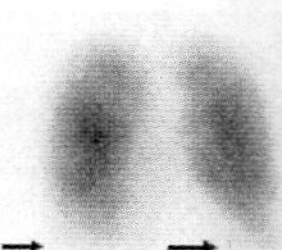

Fig 2. Perfusion scintigra showing mismatches with fig

Bone scintigraphy Important for primary and secondary bone tumours (often –ve in myeloma) and bone disorders such as osteomalacia, stress fractures, avascular necrosis, and the arthropathies. Uses bisphosphonates labelled with ^{99m}Tc. More sensitive than X-ray for finding metastases because some lesions may not appear on X-ray if less than 50% of the bone matrix has been destroyed.

Thyroid disease TcO_4 is commonly used. Studies can differentiate between Graves' disease, toxic multinodular goitre, and subacute thyroiditis (fig 3 and also fig 1, p623). Excellent for identifying ectopic tissue and functioning nodules, and also indicated for detecting residual or recurrent thyroid tissue after surgery. 10% of cold (non-functioning) nodules are malignant, whereas hot nodules are normally toxic adenomas. Iodine-131 (^{131}I) is used for therapeutic intervention in thyrotoxicosis.

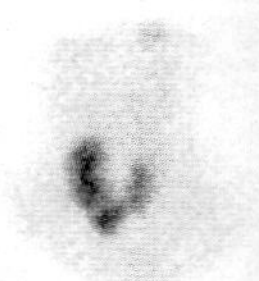

Fig 3. ^{131}I scintigram showing multinodular goitre.

Radiology

eochromocytoma Iodine-123 (^{123}I) metaiodo-ɛylguanide (MIBG) is taken-up by sympathetic ɪes, and indicates functioning, ectopic, and astatic adrenal medullary (and other neural crest) ours. ^{123}I-MIBG is also used for treatment.

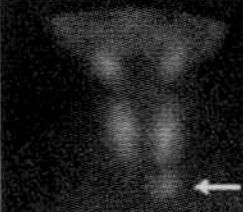

Fig 4. MIBI study showing a parathyroid adenoma.

erparathyroidism ^{99m}Tc-methoxyisobutyl isonitrile I) scans can detect parathyroid adenomas (fig 4).

enal cortical disease Radionuclide imaging is l to differentiate adenoma from diffuse hyperplasia.

aemorrhage Scans performed after endoscopy CT for ***acute bleeding***. Uses a red cell-labelled technique. More sensitive than ography and useful in cases of intermittent GI bleeding. In ***chronic bleeding***, e when all other investigations are negative, using red cell (^{99m}Tc-pertechnet- techniques if ectopic gastric mucosa or a Meckel's diverticulum is suspected.

hn's disease White cell-labelled technique (indium-111) can pinpoint areas of ll bowel activity and extent of disease in conjunction with barium studies. Also cated to assess acute flare-up of colonic disease for Crohn's and UC.

Radiology

al studies Chromium-51 (^{51}Cr) EDTA or DTPA Tc, p182) is used to assess GFR. ^{99m}Tc-mercapto-ɛyltriglycine (MAG3) technique assesses relative l function and renal transit time (eg in tructive nephropathy or renovascular disease). amic renal mapping gives quantifiable rmation about renal function and the degree of truction which is not available from other lalities. ^{99m}Tc-dimercaptosuccinic acid (DMSA) nning (fig 5) is the gold standard for evaluation of l scarring that occurs eg in reflux nephropathy.

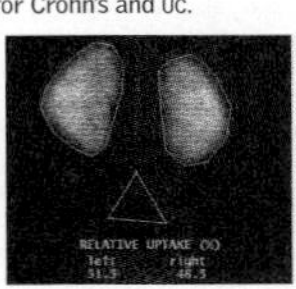

Fig 5. DMSA showing relative renal function of each kidney.

Q̇ scintigram or CTPA?[1]

is question continues to leave us without a finite answer. Standard investigation has been R then V̇/Q̇ scintigraphy: PPV of 96% if high obability, and reliable to exclude PE if 'normal'. PA (fig 6) is sensitive and specific (reported 0%) if the embolus lies in the pulmonary teries, but its bane has been the subsegmental (making CTPA only 60% sensitive and 70% ecific if included in total lung analysis). New ıltidetector CT (MDCT) systems have up to 64 tectors, giving thinner slices (0.6–1.25mm) d a faster scanning time that reduces spiratory motion artefacts and gives better bsegmental imaging. Faster data acquisition also requires less IV contrast edium, beneficial for patients with renal and cardiac impairment. Preliminary sults from the PIOPED II trial (an ongoing multicentre prospective study) gave PA alone a sensitivity and specificity of 83% and 96% respectively. The mpletion of the trial is awaited, but first-line investigation may be commended as CTPA and venous phase CT of the leg veins and pelvis. CTPA's vantages are that it is more readily available and that it can demonstrate her lesions.

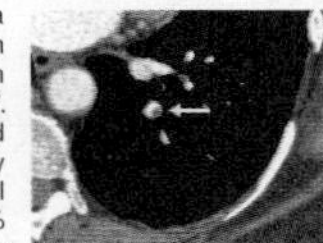

Fig 6. CT pulmonary angiogram (CTPA) showing a filling defect consistent with an embolus within a branch of a left pulmonary artery.

[1] Q̇=ventilation/perfusion; CTPA=CT pulmonary angiography.

Radionuclide imaging in cardiology

Myocardial perfusion imaging A non-invasive method of assessing reg myocardial blood flow and the cellular integrity of myocytes. The technique radionuclide tracers which cross the myocyte membrane and are tra intracellularly. Thallium-201 (^{201}Th), a K^+ analogue, is distributed via reg myocardial blood flow and requires cellular integrity for uptake. N technetium-99 (^{99}Tc) based agents are similar to ^{201}Th but have improved im characteristics, and can be used to assess myocardial perfusion an performance in the same study. Myocardial territories supplied by unobstru coronary vessels have normal perfusion whereas regions supplied by ster coronary vessels have poorer relative perfusion, a difference that is accentuat exercise. For this reason, exercise tests are used in conjunction with radionu imaging to identify areas at risk of ischaemia/infarction. Exercise scans compared with resting views: ***reperfusion*** (ischaemia, see BOX, 'Cardiac perf scintigraphy') or ***fixed defects*** (infarct) can be seen and the coronary a involved reliably predicted. Drugs (eg ***adenosine***, ***dobutamine*** and ***dipyridar*** can also be used to induce perfusion differences between normal underperfused tissues.

Myocardial perfusion imaging adds information in patients presenting acute MI (to determine the amount of myocardium salvaged by thrombolysis in diagnosing acute chest pain in those without classical ECG changes (to defin presence of significant perfusion defects).

Positron emission tomography (PET) Severely underperfused tissues, suc those supplied by a critically stenotic coronary artery, switch from fatty metabolism to glycolytic metabolism. Such altered cellular biochemistry ma imaged by PET using 18F-labelled fluorodeoxyglucose (FDG), which identifies glycolytically active tissue that is viable. This phenomenon, severe re ischaemia, occurs in up to 40% of fixed defects seen on ^{201}Th scans.

Cardiac CT and MRI

CT Recent improvements in CT technology have made routine cardiac ima possible. 16 or 64 slice CT, because of its speed and resolution, can image coro arteries and exclude significant disease with a NPV of 97–99%. It can also visu CABG patency, provide coronary artery Ca^{2+} scoring (a risk factor for coro artery disease), demonstrate cardiac anatomy including congenital anomalies estimate ventricular function. With undiagnosed significant chest pain, CT increasingly be used for the 'triple rule out', an enhanced study of the ches simultaneously exclude coronary artery occlusion, pulmonary emboli, and a dissection. This comes at the cost of radiation exposure.

MRI has less resolution than CT but its lack of ionising radiation make it a choice for congenital heart disease in children and adults. MRI is superior to C functional assessment although resolution limits its imaging of coronary ar disease. Flow velocities can be measured and because the flow is proportion the pressure differences, degrees of stenosis and regurgitation across heart va can be calculated. Myocardial infarction, perfusion and viability can also be im with the use of IV gadolinium contrast medium. Both CT and MR use ECG-gatir acquire the imaging data and relate it to the position in the cardiac cycle, minimising the movement artefact. This only works when the patient is in s rhythm.

·rdiac ^{99m}technetium MUGA scintigram

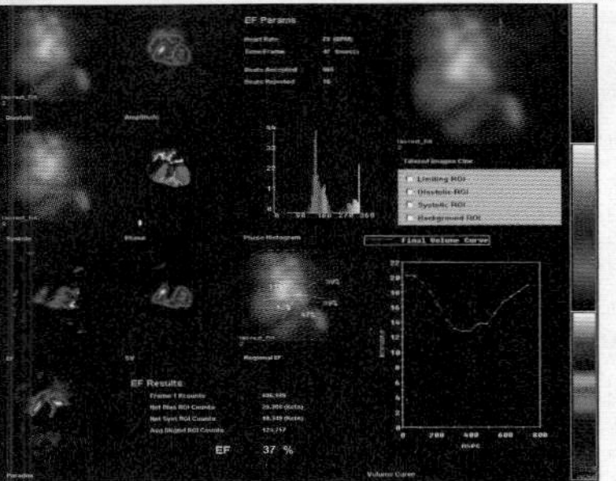

ltiple gated acquisition (MUGA) scanning is a non-invasive method of asuring left ventricle ejection fraction (EF, 37% in the study shown above). er injection of ^{99}Tc, a dynamic image of the left ventricle is obtained over eral hundred heartbeats by gamma camera. A widespread use for MUGA nning has been in the pre-operative assessment of patients for vascular gery. However one review suggested it was an accurate predictor of long-n prognosis but not of operative risk. Stress echocardiography and fusion scintigraphy may have more clinical relevance in this role.

·rdiac perfusion scintigraphy

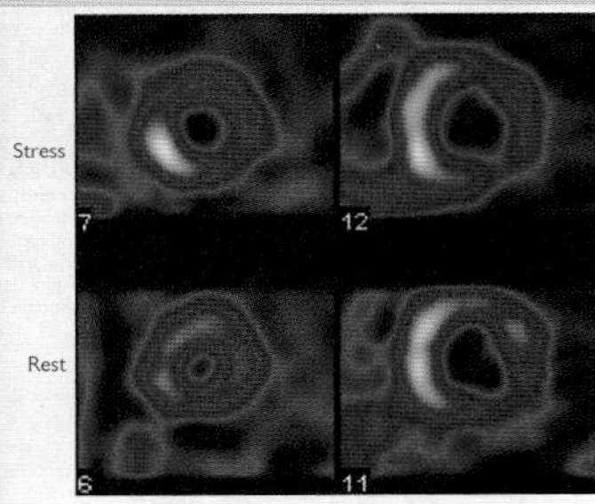

: perfusion study showing perfusion defect in the left ventricle anterior & lateral lls at stress which is reversible (difference between stress and rest images).

Abdominal ultrasound (US) (fig 1) is used for the investigation of abdominal pain, abnormal LFT, jaundice, hepatomegaly and abdominal masses. Patients should be nil by mouth for 4h before the scan in order to allow visualization of the gall bladder (fig 1, p722). Pelvic ultrasound requires the bladder to be full. Ultrasound may also be used to guide diagnostic biopsy or therapeutic aspiration.

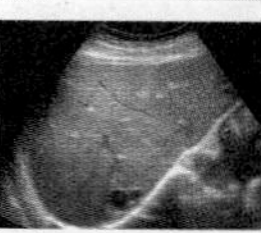

Fig 1. Liver US scan: a cy lesion is seen in the right lo

Endoscopic retrograde cholangiopancreatography (ERCP, fig 2) ***Diagnostic indications:*** Cholangitis; jaundice with dilated intrahepatic ducts; jaundice with normal calibre ducts and a non-diagnostic liver biopsy; recurrent pancreatitis; post-cholecystectomy pain. Also useful when MRCP (below) is unavailable. ***Therapeutic indications:*** Sphincterotomy for common bile duct stones; stenting of malignant strictures. ***Pre-procedure:*** Check LFT, clotting and platelet count. Prescribe antibiotic prophylaxis (eg ***ciprofloxacin*** 750mg PO 2h before), analgesia (eg ***morphine*** 5mg and ***metoclopramide*** 10mg IV 1h before) and sedation (eg ***midazolam*** 2.5–10mg IV). ***Procedure:*** A catheter is advanced from a side-viewing duodenoscope via the ampulla into the common bile duct. Contrast medium is injected and x-rays taken to show lesions in the biliary tree and pancreatic ducts. ***Complications:*** Pancreatitis; bleeding; cholangitis; perforation. Mortality <0.2% overall; 0.4% if performing stone removal.

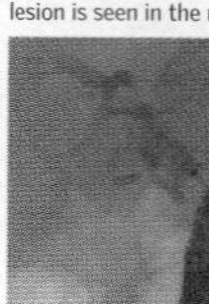

Fig 2. The ERCP shows dil intra- and extrahepatic du The multiple filling def relate to calculi within obstructing the ducts. Note cholecystectomy clips.

Contrast swallows (fig 3) can help in dysphagia (p232). Real-time fluoroscopic imaging studies are used to assess swallowing function.

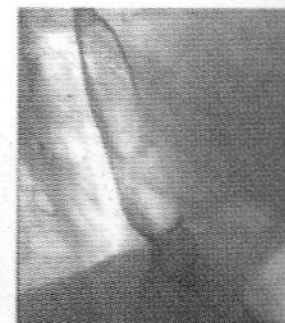

Fig 3. Double contrast sw showing a Schatski or B ring a benign circumferential str pathognomonic of a hiatus h as it marks the junction bet squamous & columnar epith

Small bowel follow through (fig 4) After bowel prep, barium is ingested and images taken every ~½h until barium reaches the caecum. Spot images are taken of areas of interest, eg the terminal ileum.

Small bowel enema After bowel prep, the duodenum is intubated and barium is introduced. Although technically more demanding than barium follow-through, it gives better mucosal definition.

Barium enema Always do a PR first ± rigid sigmoidoscopy and biopsy. Preparation is as in colonoscopy (p248). For a double contrast barium enema (fig 5), barium and air or CO_2 are introduced per rectum. Iodinated contrast medium may be used instead of barium in suspected colonic obstruction. The enema may show diverticular disease or cancers (eg an irregular 'apple-core' narrowing of the lumen). In Crohn's disease, look for 'cobblestoning', 'rose thorn' ulcers, and colonic strictures with rectal sparing. ***Disadvantages:*** Significant radiation dose; no biopsy possible.

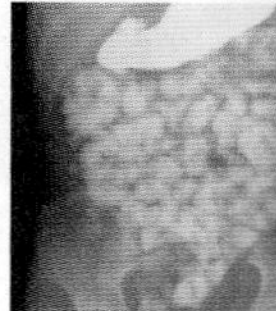

Fig 4. A normal small b follow through, at 45 mins.

mputed tomography (CT) (figs 6 & 7) is licated if ultrasound is difficult or nondiagnostic. allows better visualization of the GI tract roperitoneal structures. Oral or IV contrast dium enhances definition (p734). The big disad-ntage is the high radiation dose. CT colonography irtual colonoscopy') is being used increasingly: it es excellent mucosal definition but interpretat-takes time and has inter-observer variability.[10] polyps >9mm specificity is 97% but sensitivity 35% and drops to 48% if <6mm.[MET 11]

agnetic resonance imaging (MRI) gives superior t tissue imaging and enables the distinction of any benign and malignant lesions. It has become reasingly popular for imaging of the liver.

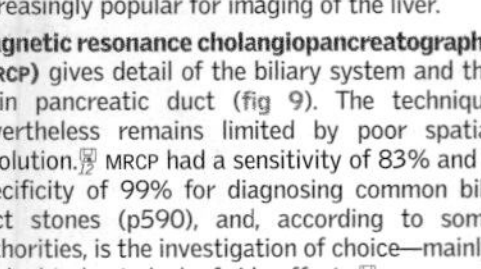

agnetic resonance cholangiopancreatography RCP) gives detail of the biliary system and the ain pancreatic duct (fig 9). The technique vertheless remains limited by poor spatial solution.[12] MRCP had a sensitivity of 83% and a ecificity of 99% for diagnosing common bile ct stones (p590), and, according to some thorities, is the investigation of choice—mainly, doubt, due to lack of side-effects.[13]

ireless capsule endoscopy (See p248).

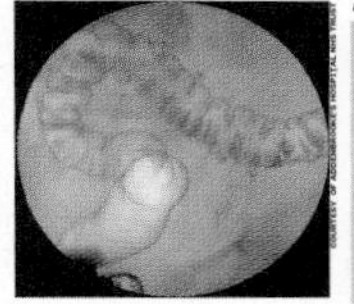

Fig 5. Double contrast enema showing diverticulosis of the sigmoid colon. This method improves mucosal definition.

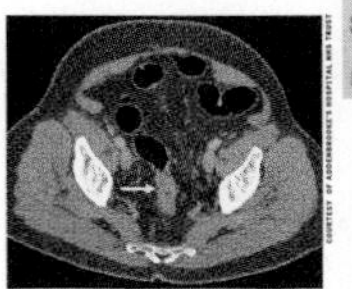

Fig 6. Axial CT colonogram: rectal thickening & stenosis (arrow) consistent with a rectal tumour.

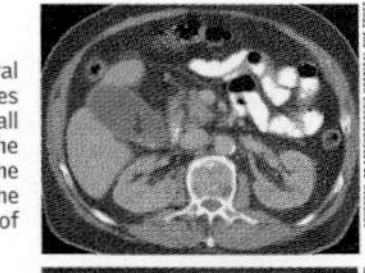

7. Axial CT of the abdomen post IV and oral ntrast medium. The gallbladder contains gallstones row). Oral contrast medium is seen within the small wel but not the large bowel. Lateral to the rtebral column are the psoas muscles and the dneys. Anterior to the vertebrae are the IVC and the rta. Anterior to the IVC is the uncinate process of e pancreas.

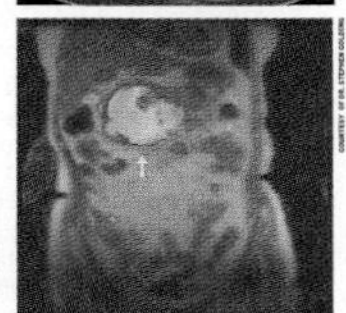

8. Coronal T2-weighted abdominal MRI showing a ncreatic pseudocyst. Note how the **high signal** cyst cupies the lesser sac (arrow), abutting the eromedial edge of the liver.

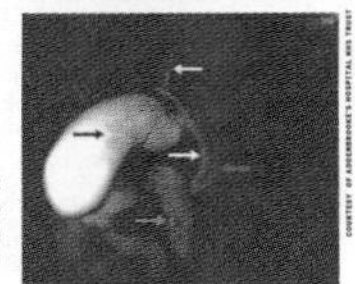

9. MRCP of the biliary system showing: left hepatic ct (yellow arrow); multiple gallstones in the llbladder (black arrow); common bile duct (white row); pancreatic duct (red arrow); duodenum (green row).

AXR Look at kidneys, paths of the ureters, and bladder. Note any abnormal calcification—related to which of these 3 processes?

1 Calculi; only 90% are seen on plain films.
2 Dystrophic calcification, eg in carcinomas or TB.
3 Nephrocalcinosis (parenchymal, rare, fig 4, p723).

Ultrasound is best initial image, showing:

- Renal size—**small** in chronic renal failure, **large** in renal masses, benign cysts,[1] hypertrophy if other kidney missing, polycystic kidney disease (fig 1), and rarities such as amyloidosis (p354).
- Hydronephrosis, which may indicate ureteric obstruction or reflux (fig 1, p683).
- Perinephric collections (trauma, post-renal biopsy).
- Transplanted kidneys (collections, obstruction, perfusion—fig 1, p625).
- Bladder residual volume: useful in assessment of the need to catheterise.
- Prostate: transrectal ultrasound enables US-guided biopsy of focal lesions. NB: Prostate size does not correlate with symptoms.

Advantages: Fast; cheap; independent of renal function; no IV contrast medium or radiation risk. ***Disadvantages:*** Intraluminal masses (eg transitional cell carcinomas) in the upper tracts may not be seen; not a functional study; only suggests obstruction if there is dilatation of the collecting system (~5% of obstructed kidneys have non-dilated systems).

Computed tomography (CT) has revolutionized renal colic imaging. Unenhanced images are 97% sensitive for calculi, and show many other pathologies (fig 2). CT has a similar radiation dose to IVU. CT allows detailed delineation of: masses (solid or cystic, contrast enhancement, calcification, local/distant extension, renal vein involvement); renal trauma (2 kidneys, haemorrhage, devascularization, laceration, urine leak); retroperitoneal lesions.

Intravenous urogram/pyelogram (IVU = IVP) is a study for defining anatomy (esp. pelvicalyceal), and for finding pathology distorting the collecting system.[2] It yields some functional information. Abdominal images are taken before and after IV contrast, which is filtered by the kidney, reaching the renal tubules at ~1min (***nephrogram phase***). At this stage look for indentations (scarring) and protrusions (cysts, tumour). Try to decide which kidney is normal if there is a difference in size or a delay in the nephrogram. The smaller kidney may be normal (other side enlarged) or abnormal (chronic disease). The larger kidney may be normal (compensatory) or abnormal (eg tumour, cysts, obstruction). Later

1 Cysts may be inherited, developmental, or acquired—eg polycystic kidney disease, medullary sponge kidney, multicystic dysplastic kidney, medullary cystic disease, tuberous sclerosis, renal sinus cysts, von Hippel-Lindau's disease.

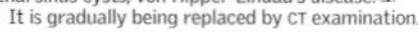

2 It is gradually being replaced by CT examination.

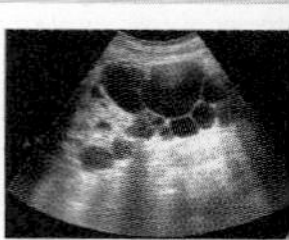

Fig 1. Renal US showing m iple simple cysts with poste acoustic enhancement.

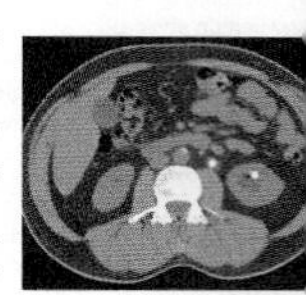

Fig 2. Axial unenhanced CT the abdomen. There is a l proximal ureteric calcu (anterior to the left psoas) a a left calyceal calculus. The l ureteric calculus is causing m obstruction of the left kidney bone window algorithm m help highlight calcium der objects within the abdomen. <7mm diameter, a calculus likely to pass spontaneously.

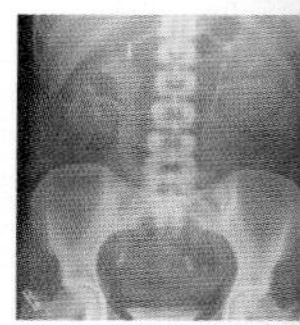

Fig 3. IVU: bilateral dup ureters. The superior ure moiety (arrowed) is ectopic a enters the bladder, urethra vagina more inferiorly than normally placed inferior ure moiety. The superior ureter m be associated with a ureteroc and is more likely to obstru The inferior ureter may associated with reflux neph pathy & scarring.

ages show contrast medium in the pelvis (pyelogram), ureters, and bladder. Look r filling defects (fig 7) and evidence of obstruction (fig 8).

trograde pyelography is good at showing pelvilyceal and ureteric anatomy, and at detecting thology such as transitional cell carcinoma (TCC). ntrast is injected via a ureteric catheter.

rcutaneous nephrostomy The renal pelvis is nctured with imaging guidance. Diagnostic ages are obtained following contrast injection ntegrade pyelogram, fig 4). A nephrostomy tube ay then be placed to allow drainage.

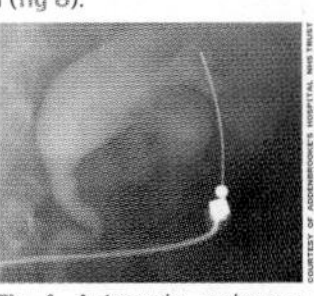

Fig 4. Antegrade pyelogram showing percutaneous puncture of a dilated renal pelvis by a fine co-axial needle. Contrast is injected to outline the calices.

nal arteriography (fig 5) Still the final arbiter of nal artery stenosis. Therapeutic indications: gioplasty; stenting and selective embolization eeding tumour, trauma, or AV malformation).

agnetic resonance imaging (MRI), with its good soft tissue resolution, may be ed to clarify equivocal CT findings. Magnetic resonance angiography (MRA) is eful in imaging renal artery anatomy and identifying stenosis (fig 6).

adionuclide imaging See p730.

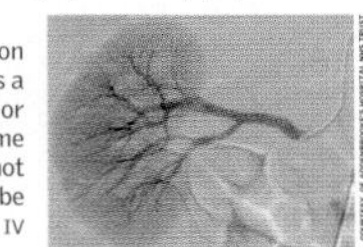

g 5. Normal renal artery digital subtraction giogram (DSA). It is possible to tell that this is a A as no other structure has any definition or ntrast in the image. There is, however, some terference from overlying bowel gas, which is not uncommon problem. GI tract peristalsis can be minished during the examination by using IV *yscopan* or *glucagon*.

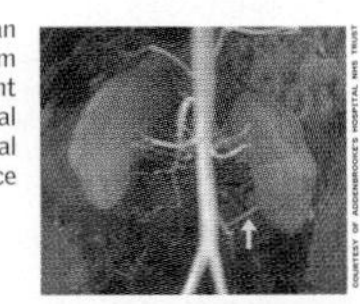

g 6. Coronal 3D MRA of the kidneys showing an omalous left renal artery (arrow) arising from e same level as the IMA. This is important formation pre-transplant. Anomalous renal teries are common and, like the normal renal teries, are end arteries, hence the consequence infarction if tied at surgery.

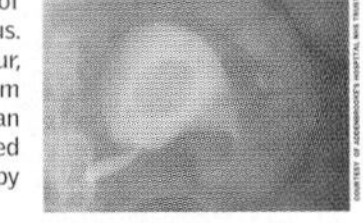

g 7. IVU showing a filling defect in the centre of e renal pelvis corresponding to a renal calculus. lling defects can also be caused by tumour, ematoma, fungal balls or sloughed papillae from nal papillary necrosis. The filling defect can metimes have the impressive multi-faceted pearance of a staghorn calculus that can occupy e entire pelvicalyceal system.

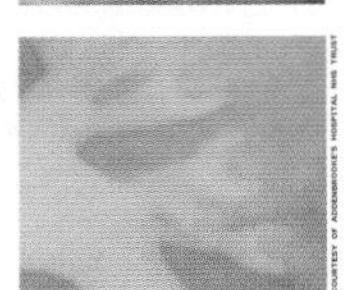

g 8. Magnified IVU showing blunting of the lyces, an early sign of urinary tract obstruction. equentially in obstruction there is calyceal unting → clubbing → ballooning, as hydronephsis develops.

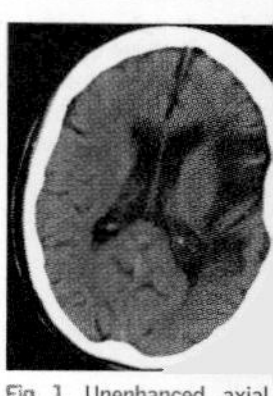

Fig 1. Unenhanced axial head: note the old stroke in left middle cerebral art territory.

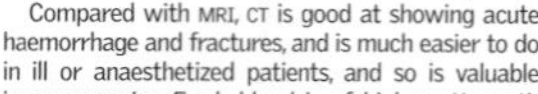

Computed tomography (CT) The attenuation of biological soft tissues is in a narrow range from about +80 for blood and muscle, to 0 for CSF, and down to −100 for fat (see p718 for the Hounsfield scale). IV contrast medium may be given, initially demonstrating an angiographic effect as the high attenuation contrast in the vessels makes them appear white. Later, if there is a defect in the blood–brain barrier, as with neoplasms or infection, contrast medium will opacify the margins of a lesion, giving an enhancing, white area in the cerebrum or cerebellum. Some intracranial components do not have a blood–brain barrier and enhance normally: eg pituitary gland and choroid plexus.

Compared with MRI, CT is good at showing acute haemorrhage and fractures, and is much easier to do in ill or anaesthetized patients, and so is valuable in emergencies. Fresh blood is of higher attenuation (∴ whiter) than brain tis Attenuation of haematomas declines as Hb breaks down so that a subacute subd haematoma at 2wks may have an attenuation the same as adjacent brain, makin difficult to detect. A chronic subdural haematoma will be of relatively low attenuat

CT is commonly performed in acute stroke to exclude haemorrhage (eg p anticoagulation). The actual area of infarction/ischaemia will not show up for a day so, and will be low-attenuation **cytotoxic oedema** (intracellular oedema including b white and grey matter—look for loss of grey matter definition).

Tumours and abscesses can have common features, eg a ring enhancing m surrounding vasogenic oedema, and mass effect. **Vasogenic oedema** extracellular and spreads through the white matter. Mass effect causes compressio the sulci and ipsilateral ventricle, and may also cause herniation, (subfalc transtentorial, or tonsillar). ►On p475 there are images of this.

One indication for CT is acute, severe headache. If there is concern ab subarachnoid haemorrhage, a non-contrast CT may show acute blood. Even if it does it will show if the basal cisterns are normal and therefore lumbar puncture is proba safe.

Cranial CT perfusion is a developing technique that assesses cerebral blood f without the need for invasive angiographic techniques (fig 5, p719). ***3D CT angiogra*** gives excellent mapping of the cerebral circulation (fig 4).

Magnetic resonance imaging (MRI) See p720. Example of stroke on MRI: p4 The chief image sequences are:

- ***T1-weighted images:*** Give good anatomical detail to which the T2 image can compared. Fat is brightest (signal intensity↑); other tissues are darker to vary degrees. Flowing blood is low signal. Gadolinium-DTPA contrast medium (p7 usually results in an increase in signal intensity.
- ***T2-weighted images:*** These provide the best detection of most lesions as th usually contain some oedema fluid and therefore appear white (eg fig 4, p72 Fat and fluid appear brightest. Flowing blood is again low signal.

Magnetic resonance angiography (MRA) can map the carotid, vertebrobasilar a cerebral arterial circulations. ***Functional MRI*** can image regional blood flow.

Contrast angiography (fig 4) is less common as a diagnostic tool since the adve of MRA and CT angiography and perfusion techniques, though it has the advanta of being therapeutic—eg coil embolization of saccular aneurysms.

Radionuclide imaging See p724. PET is mostly used as a research tool in demen but perfusion scintigraphy can be used in the assessment of Alzheimer's disea other dementias (fig 5), and localising epileptogenic foci. Dopamine scintigrap can be used to assess local cerebral uptake in Parkinson's disease.

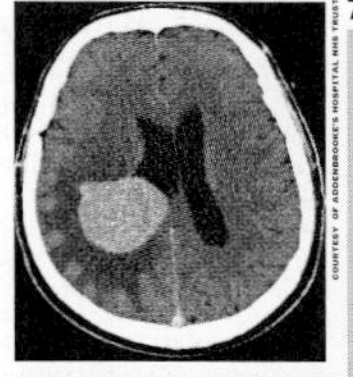

2. Axial contrast enhanced CT of the brain. There homogenously enhancing well defined mass in the t cerebral hemisphere that is protruding into the y of the right lateral ventricle. There is mild mass ct (the corpus callosum is displaced to the left), low attenuation vasogenic oedema surrounds the s.

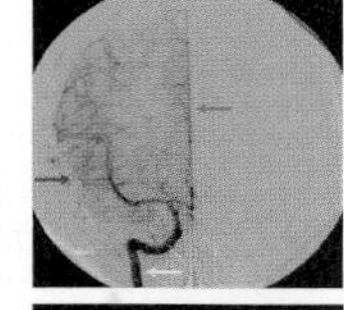

3. Digital subtraction angiogram (DSA). The right rnal carotid artery (yellow arrow), anterior ebral artery (green arrow) and middle cerebral ery (red arrow) are shown.

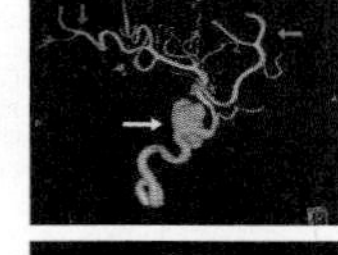

4. 3D DSA showing an internal carotid artery urysm (yellow arrow) viewed from the right. The erior cerebral artery circulation is marked by the en arrow and the middle cerebral artery ulation by the red arrow.

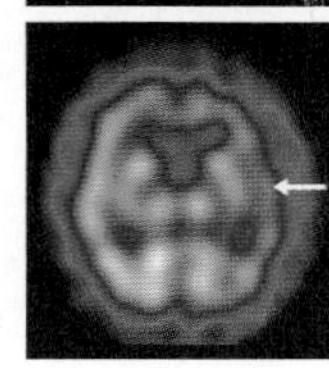

5. Selected axial image from a cerebral perfusion CT' study showing hypoperfusion in the left ietal frontal lobes.

Contrast in imaging

The use of x-irradiation in imaging relies on the principle that tissues of differ electron densities produce different degrees of attenuation. Two adjacent tissues a similar electron density are indistinguishable on plain x-ray. Increasing elect density increases attenuation and makes tissues appear more radio-opaq Although this can occur pathophysiologically (eg calcification in chro pancreatitis or malignancy) it can be induced artificially by the use of a contr medium and thus create a visible interface. Most of the body consists of hydrog (1 electron), oxygen (8), and carbon (6) atoms. Conventional contrast age contain iodine (53 electrons) or barium (56). Contrast medium is usu administered by the following routes:

- PO: barium or iodine based agents for swallow, meal, or follow through.
- PR: eg barium or iodine based agent enema.
- Inhaled: technetium or xenon used in ventilation scintigraphy.
- IV: iodine or gadolinium based contrast agents.

IV contrast medium has the most widespread clinical application. The id intravenous contrast medium should be non-ionic, hydrophilic, iso-osmolar and n chemotoxic and should have no adverse reactions.

Iodine based contrast agents Iodine is used because of its relatively high elect density and good physiological tolerance. When used with CT, the examinatior said to be **contrast enhanced**—look for '+ **c**' amongst the scan details. Caut should be taken in patients with the following because of the increased risk adverse reactions (have latest renal function to hand): renal or cardiac impairme atopy; myeloma; diabetes; sickle cell disease; the elderly and infants; a history allergy. Minor reactions include nausea, vomiting and a sensation of warm Moderate reactions include urticaria, bronchospasm, angioedema and ↓BP (1:25 theoretical risk of death for 1:150 000 ►***Metformin*** must be withheld before a for 48hrs after IV contrast administration because of risk of lactic acidosis. ►Av iodine-based agents in patients with active hyperthyroidism.

Barium sulphate is the most common contrast medium used in examination of GI tract. Water-insoluble particles of 0.6–1.4μm diameter are mixed with la organic molecules such as pectin and gum to promote good flow, mucosal adherer and high density in thin layers. Risks: chemical pneumonitis or peritonitis.

Water-soluble **iodine based** contrast agents (eg Gastrografin®) are used instead barium where there is a risk of peritoneal contamination (eg fistula, megacol ulceration, diverticulitis, bowel anastomosis, acute intestinal haemorrhage). It high osmolarity. ►Contains iodine so establish allergy history and thyroid stat

Air In a double contrast enema, air (or CO_2) is insufflated as a **negative contr medium** after barium administration to enhance mucosal definition (fig 5, p72

Gadolinium is a lanthanide series element with paramagnetic qualities that administered intravenously (as gadolinium-DTPA) to enhance the contrast of cert structures in MRI. It works by reducing the time to relaxation (TR) of hydrog nuclei in its proximity and appears as high signal on T1 weighted scans. It does r cross the blood-brain barrier and is therefore useful in enhancing isointense ext axial tumours such as meningiomas. It can also highlight areas where the blo brain barrier has broken down secondary to inflammatory or neoplastic process It is renally excreted and well tolerated, because only small doses are used. Adve reactions do include headache, nausea and local irritation at the site of injecti with idiosyncratic reaction reported in less than 1%.

maging the acutely unwell patient

sking yourself '*Does this investigation need to be done right now?*' will often 'eld the answer '*no!*', yet there are a few occasions when early imaging can rovide vital diagnostic information and influence the prognosis for a patient:

- Acute cauda equina syndrome (p458): ▸▸MRI lumbar spine.
- Suspected thoracic aorta dissection (p586): ▸▸CT thorax + IV contrast medium, MRI or TOE. The mediastinum is rarely widened on CXR.
- Acute renal failure (p292 & p820): ▸▸US of renal tract should be performed to exclude an obstructive (∴ easily treatable) cause.
- Acute pulmonary oedema: ▸▸A portable CXR will help the clinical picture but should not delay definitive treatment (p786).
- Acute abdomen with signs of peritonism: ▸▸Erect CXR should be performed looking for intraperitoneal free gas (fig 1, p581), a sign of intestinal perforation. Remember that a patient who has had surgery will have gas (air/CO_2) in the abdominal cavity, detectable on plain radiography as late as day 10 post-op.[15] Early CT (<6h after onset of symptoms) in addition to plain radiography appears not to provide additional diagnostic information in gastroduodenal perforation.[16] In one study performing an US technique (the **scissors** manoeuvre) to look for sub-diaphragmatic free air had 94% sensitivity and 100% specificity.[17]
- Any patient with post-traumatic midline cervical spine tenderness—not just for the emergency department! ▸▸Hard collar and backboard immobilisation followed by a lateral C-spine x-ray, then full C-spine series. All the vertebrae down to the top of T1 must be visualised and cleared before it is safe to take the collar off. CT may be required if the plain radiographs are inadequate or inconclusive.
- Sudden onset focal neurology, **worst ever** headache, deteriorating GCS: ▸▸CT head, then LP if no evidence of ↑ICP. Once an examination has been reported as normal, the nursing team can take a rest from work-intensive 'neuro' observations.

emember that imaging—or re-imaging for a poor quality film—should never elay the definitive treatment of an emergency condition, eg:

- Tension pneumothorax (p798 and fig 1): ▸▸decompression **not** CXR.
- Intra-abdominal haemorrhage or viscus rupture (p580): ▸▸laparotomy.
- High clinical suspicion of torsion of testis (p600): ▸▸surgery **not** Doppler US.
- Collapse, acute abdomen, shock, moribund: ▸▸laparotomy. A ruptured aneurysm has an extremely poor prognosis that tails off by the minute (p586).

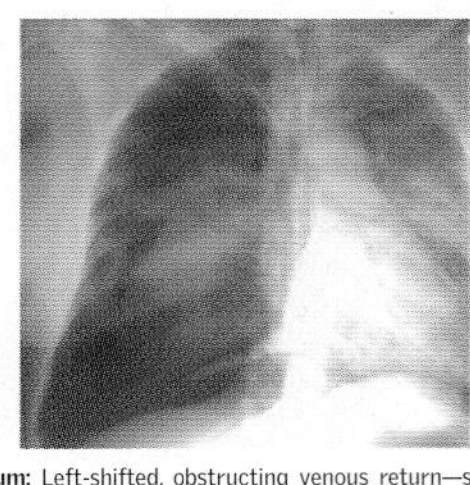

ig 1. This is a great educational ilm from the intensive care unit. The inexperienced doctor could be listracted by the poor quality, badly centred film: the technicians do the best they can under difficult conditions. To ask for a new film here would be a mistake. There is adequate information to make a ife-saving decision. After checking the name of the patient, see that the tubes and lines are well positioned—the endotracheal (ET) and NG tubes and the right subclavian venous line. **Lungs:** The left lung shows consolidation. The right is too black and the right hemidiaphragm is depressed. **Pleura:** The pleural recess is seen at the right base. **Mediastinum:** Left-shifted, obstructing venous return—so cardiac output↓, and a threat to life. Is it being pushed or pulled? Check **hila**, **bones** and **soft tissues**. Is the ET tube down the right main bronchus, inflating the right lung and collapsing the left? No. Is the right lung collapsed? Yes. ▸▸Right tension pneumothorax. Needle thoracocentesis decompression and a chest tube are needed now. The left lung consolidation could be a result of any of the causes of ARDS (p170). If intubated, consolidation/collapse often occurs at the left base: suction catheters pass down the ET tube and preferentially into the right main bronchus.

19 Reference intervals, etc.

Contents

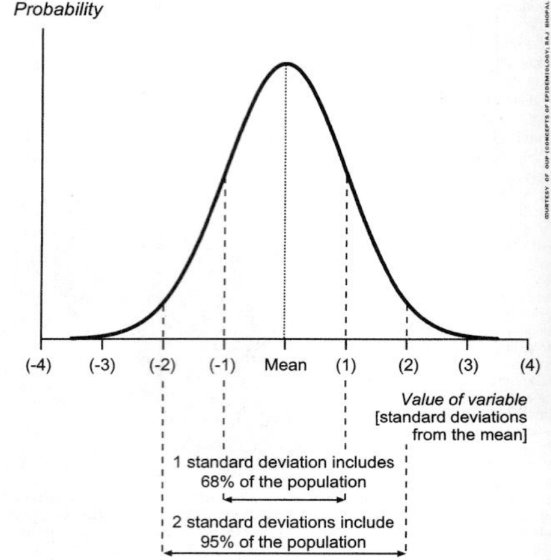

ne Gaussian ('Normal') distribution

:e upon a time, in a famous hospital named R— in the middle of England, ·e lived a crusty old surgeon and a brilliant young house officer. The surgeon ed infallible and peremptory edicts such as 'all my patients with a moglobin less than 10 must be transfused'. Everyone did as the surgeon said s was a long time ago) except for the wily house officer who understood :istics, sampling error, and the play of chance. One day she was rung up by haematologist who asked her "Why have you requested 3 blood counts on ; Wells today? One is enough. You are wasting our resources!" "Not so," said house officer. "The first Hb was 9.8; the second was 9.7 and the third was 1g/dL. I knew if I was persistent, I stood a good chance of preventing an ecessary transfusion. She is a patient of Mr X." The two conspirators smiled each other down the telephone, and no more was said. Of course the right / of dealing with this problem is through clinical governance, and dialogue 1 the surgeon. But the point remains: numbers are elastic, despite, on asion, being given to 3 decimal places. Don't believe in them as absolute ties, and don't believe that the normal range is anything other than itrary; think before you act: think statistically. *Think like Gauss.*

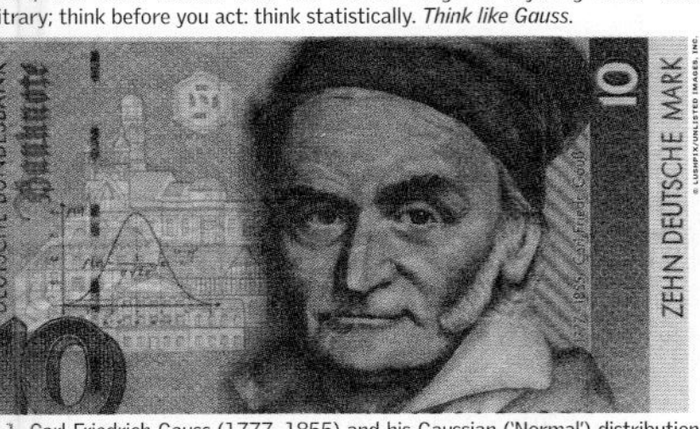

1. Carl Friedrich Gauss (1777–1855) and his Gaussian ('Normal') distribution. ; bell-shaped graph is the theoretical basis of reference intervals (normal ıes—see below). In some ways Gauss would have made an ideal handbook hor: he left behind him a tiny notebook of just 19 pages which solved 146 blems in mathematics including non-euclidean geometry—his motto being *ca sed matura* (few but ripe). His messages were brief and perhaps *too* much to point (not surprisingly, since he invented the first telegraph in 1833)—on being :urbed during deep thought to be told that his wife was dying it is reported that ·eplied "Tell her to wait a moment until I'm through..."[1]

ne definitions

ange: The lowest and highest value of all observations in the set being studied.

rithmetic mean: The sum of all observations ÷ by the number of observations.

1edian: The median is the middle value (eg 9 data points are higher and 9 are ›wer). If their distribution is Normal, then the median co-insides with the mean.

tandard deviation (SD): The square root of the variance (the average of the quare of the distance of each data point from the mean). When the istribution of the observations is Normal, 95% of observations are located in ne interval 'mean ± 1.96SD'. This is the basis of the reference interval.[2]

tandard error of the mean: This is the SD divided by the square root of the umber of observations. Suppose a population mean of serum urate is 5.4mg per 00mL and the standard deviation is 1. If you drew 100 samples of 25 people in ach sample and calculated 100 sample means, how many of those means would ou expect to fall within the range 5.4–1.96×1 to 5.4+1.96×1? Answer: 95.[3]

Gentamicin

The potential for oto- and nephro-toxicity is great if gentamicin is inappropriately, so use local expert advice/guidelines Although historically twice or 3-times daily, many now favour **once daily dosing**—fewer SEs, ± b bactericidal activity. Meta-analyses back this, provided there is no increa cardiac output (eg anaemia; Paget's disease), and the context is not ascites, b children, or pregnancy. The big problem is lack of information on calculating monitoring once-a-day regimens. The *Cooke & Grace* regimen provisio recommends, for feverish neutropenic adults with serum creatinine <300μmol starting dose of gentamicin 5mg/kg IVI over 30min. Measure serum trough later. If <1mg/L, then do twice weekly monitoring. If trough is 1–2mg/L, dose, and check trough after 24h. If trough >2mg/L, stop and switch drug. regimens also exist (D Nicolau 1995 *Antimicrob Agents Chemoth* **39** 650).

Nomogram for repeated dosing of gentamicin

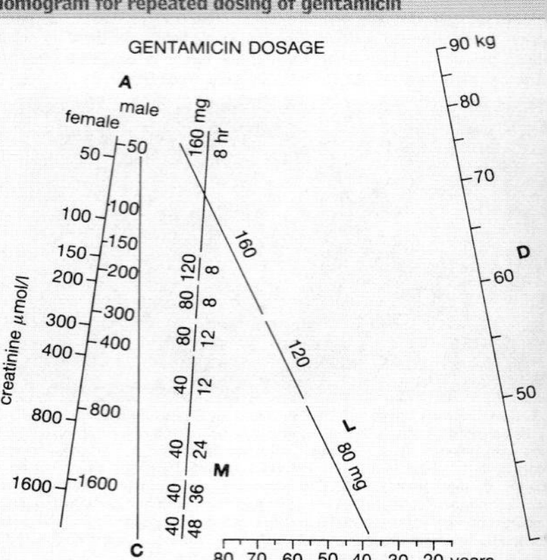

The above allows for thrice daily doses.

1 Join with a straight line the serum creatinine concentration appropriate to the se scale A and the age on scale **B**. Mark the point at which this line cuts line **C**.
2 Join with a line the mark on line **C** and the body weight on line **D**. Mark the point which this line cuts lines **L** and **M**, to get the loading and maintenance doses, respecti
3 Confirm the appropriateness of this regimen at an early stage by measuring serum le especially in severe illness and renal impairment.
4 Adjust **dose** if peak concentration (1h after IM dose; ½ after IV dose) outside the r 5–10mg/L. A trough concentration (just before dose) above 2mg/L indicates the need a longer **dosage interval**.

ıg therapeutic ranges in plasma

anges should only be used as a guide to treatment.

drug in an apparently too low concentration may still be clinically ful. Some patients require (and tolerate) levels in the 'toxic' range.

mikacin peak (1h post IV dose): 20–30mg/L. Trough: <10mg/L.

arbamazepine Optimal concentration: 20–50μmol/L [4–12mg/L].

lonazepam trough: 0.08–0.24μmol/L [0.025–0.075mg/L].

igoxin[1] (6–12h post dose) 1–2.6nmol/L [0.8–2μg/L]. <1.3nmol/L may be toxic if there is hypokalaemia. Signs of CVS toxicity: arrhythmias, heart block. CNS: confusion, insomnia, agitation, seeing too much yellow (xanthopsia), delirium. GI: nausea.

thosuximide trough: 300–700μmol/L [40–100mg/L].

entamicin[1] For single-dose regimen, see opposite. Peak—1h post IV dose:)–18μmol/L [5–10mg/L; 3–5mg/L in IE]. Trough (just before dose): <4.2μmol/L (<2mg/L; <1mg/L in IE). Toxic signs: tinnitus, deafness, nystagmus, vertigo, renal failure. See OPPOSITE.

hium[1] (12h post dose). Guidelines vary: 0.4–0.8mmol/L is reasonable. ***Early*** signs of toxicity (Li^+ ≤1.5mmol/L): tremor, agitation, twitching. ***Intermediate:*** lethargy. ***Late:*** (Li^+ >2mmol/L) spasms, coma, fits, arrhythmias, renal failure (haemodialysis may be needed). See *OHCS* p354.

ilmicin peak—1h post IV dose: 7–12mg/L. Trough <2mg/L.

henobarbital Trough: 60–180μmol/L [15–40mg/L].

henytoin[1] trough: 40–80μmol/L [10–20mg/L]. Signs of toxicity: ataxia, nystagmus, sedation, dysarthria, diplopia.

eophylline 10–20mg/mL (55–110μmol/L). (► see p795) Take sample 4–6h after starting an infusion (which should be stopped for ~15min just before the specimen is taken). Signs of toxicity: arrhythmias, anxiety, tremor, convulsions.

ramycin peak (1h post IV dose): 11–21μmol/L [5–10mg/L]. Trough: ≤4.3μmol/L [<2mg/L].

ncomycin trough: 5–10 mg/L (initiate monitoring 48 hr after first dose). In SBE/IE, the trough level is 10–15mg/L. Peak levels are now rarely checked.

ı time since the last dose should be specified on the form.

ıugh levels should be taken just before the next dose.

ıgs for which *routine* monitoring is indicated.

Some important drug interactions

▸see BNF www.bnf.

Note: '↑' means the effect of the drug in italics is increased (eg thro inhibition of metabolism or renal clearance). '↓' means that its effec decreased (eg through enzyme induction).

Adenosine ↓ by: aminophylline. ↑ by dipyridamole.

Aminoglycosides ↑ by: loop diuretics.

Anti-diabetic drugs (any) ↑ by: alcohol, β-blockers, monoamine oxidase in tors, bezafibrate. ↓ by: corticosteroids, diazoxide, diuretics, contracep steroids, (possibly also lithium).

Sulfonylureas ↑ by: azapropazone, chloramphenicol, bezafibrate, trimoxazole, miconazole, sulfinpyrazone.

Sulfonylureas ↓ by: rifampicin (nifedipine occasionally).

Metformin ↑ by: cimetidine. With alcohol: lactic acidosis risk.

Antiretroviral agents (HIV): See p402.

Angiotensin-converting enzyme (ACE) inhibitors ↓ effect by: oestrogens NSA

Antihistamines Avoid anything which ↑concentrations and risk of arrhythm eg erythromycin, other macrolides (eg azithromycin), antifungals, halofant tricyclics, antipsychotics, SSRIs (p442), protease inhibitors (p402), diuretic blockers, antiarrhythmics.

Azathioprine ↑ by: allopurinol.

β-blockers Avoid verapamil; ↓: NSAIDs. Lipophilic β-blockers (eg propranolol) metabolized by the liver, and concentrations are ↑ by cimetidine. This does happen with hydrophilic β-blockers (eg atenolol).

Carbamazepine ↑ by: erythromycin, isoniazid, verapamil.

Cimetidine: theophylline↑, warfarin↑, lidocaine↑, amitriptyline↑, proprano pethidine↑, phenytoin↑, metronidazole↑, quinine↑.

Contraceptive steroids ↓ by: antibiotics, barbiturates, carbamazep phenytoin, rifampicin.

Ciclosporin ↑ by: erythromycin, nifedipine, grapefruit juice. ↓ by: phenytoin.

Digoxin ↑ by: amiodarone, carbenoxolone and diuretics (as K^+ levels lower quinine, verapamil.

Diuretics ↓ by: NSAIDs—particularly indometacin.

Ergotamine ↑ by: erythromycin (ergotism may occur).

Fluconazole: Avoid concurrent astemizole .

Lithium ↑ by: thiazide diuretics.

Methotrexate ↑ by: aspirin, NSAIDs. Many antibiotics (check *BNF*).

Phenytoin ↑ by: chloramphenicol, cimetidine, disulfiram, isoniazid, sulfonami ↓ by: carbamazepine.

Potassium-sparing diuretics with ACE-inhibitors: Hyperkalaemia.

Theophyllines ↑ by: cimetidine, ciprofloxacin, erythromycin, contracep steroids, propranolol. ↓ by: barbiturates, carbamazepine, phenytoin, rifamp See p795.

Valproate ↓by: carbamazepine, phenobarbital, phenytoin.

Warfarin and ***nicoumalone*** (=acenocoumarol) ↑ by: alcohol, allopur amiodarone, aspirin, chloramphenicol, cimetidine, ciprofloxacin, co-trimoxaz danazol, dipyridamole, disulfiram, erythromycin (and broad-spect antibiotics), gemfibrozil, glucagon, ketoconazole, metronidazole, micona nalidixic acid, neomycin, NSAIDs, phenytoin, quinidine, simvastatin (but pravastatin), sulfinpyrazone, sulfonamides, tetracyclines, thyroxine.

Warfarin and ***nicoumalone*** ↓ by: aminoglutethimide, barbiturates, carban epine, contraceptive steroids, dichloralphenazone, griseofulvin, rifamp phenytoin, vitamin K.

Zidovudine (AZT) ↑ by: paracetamol (increased marrow toxicity).

IVI solutions to avoid *Dextrose:* Avoid furosemide, ampicillin, hydralaz insulin, melphalan, phenytoin, and quinine.

0.9% saline IVI: Avoid amphotericin, lignocaine, nitroprusside.

aematology—reference intervals

(For B_{12}, folate, Fe, and TIBC, see p742-3)

easurement	Reference interval	Your hospital
'hite cell count (WCC)	4.0–11.0 × 10^9/L	
ed cell count	♂ 4.5–6.5 × 10^{12}/L	
	♀ 3.9–5.6 × 10^{12}/L	
aemoglobin	♂ 13.5–18.0g/dL	
	♀ 11.5–16.0g/dL	
cked red cell volume (PCV)	♂ 0.4–0.54L/L	
or haematocrit	♀ 0.37–0.47L/L	
ean cell volume (MCV)	76–96fL	
ean cell haemoglobin (MCH)	27–32pg	
ean cell haemoglobin concentration (MCHC)	30–36g/dL	
eutrophils	2.0–7.5 × 10^9/L;	
	40–75% WCC	
'mphocytes	1.3–3.5 × 10^9/L;	
	20–45% WCC	
osinophils	0.04–0.44 × 10^9/L;	
	1–6% WCC	
asophils	0.0–0.10 × 10^9/L;	
	0–1% WCC	
onocytes	0.2–0.8 × 10^9/L;	
	2–10% WCC	
atelet count	150–400 × 10^9/L	
eticulocyte count	0.8–2.0%[1] 25–100×10^9/L	
'ythrocyte sedimentation rate	Depends on age (p356)	
'othrombin time (factors I, II, VII, X)	10–14s	
ctivated partial thrombo-plastin time (VIII, IX, XI, XII)	35–45s	
dimers[2]	<0.5mg/L	

'oposed therapeutic ranges for prothrombin time: See p335

nly use percentages as reference interval if red cell count is normal; otherwise, use the absolute e. Express as a ratio *vs* control.

·dimer assay may be useful as a screening test for thromboembolic disease see *Lancet* 1999 **353** . However, the reference range depends on the assay—**check** with your haematology lab.

Reference intervals (RI)—*biochemistry*

See p652 for the *philosophy of the normal range*; see *OHCS* p222 *for children* Drugs (and other substances) may interfere with any chemical method; as th effects may be method dependent, it is difficult for the clinician to be awar all the possibilities. If in doubt, discuss with the lab.

Substance	Specimen	Reference interval (labs vary, so a guide only)	Your hosp
Adrenocorticotrophic hormone	P	<80ng/L	
Alanine aminotransferase (ALT)	P	5–35iu/L	
Albumin	P[1]	35–50g/L	
Aldosterone	P[2]	100–500pmol/L	
Alkaline phosphatase	P	30–150u/L (adults)	
α-amylase	P	0–180 Somogyi u/dL	
α-fetoprotein	S	<10ku/L	
Angiotensin II	P[2]	5–35pmol/L	
Antidiuretic hormone (ADH)	P	0.9–4.6pmol/L	
Aspartate transaminase	P	5–35iu/L	
Bicarbonate	P[1]	24–30mmol/L	
Bilirubin	P	3–17μmol/L	
BNP (see p665)	P	<50ng/L	
Calcitonin	P	<0.1μg/L	
Calcium (ionized)	P	1.0–1.25mmol/L	
Calcium (total)	P[1]	2.12–2.65mmol/L	
Chloride	P	95–105mmol/L	
[3]Cholesterol (see p682)	P	<5.0mmol/L	
VLDL (see p682)	P	0.128–0.645mmol/L	
LDL	P	<2.0mmol/L	
HDL	P	0.9–1.93mmol/L	
Cortisol	P	A.M. 450–700nmol/L midnight 80–280nmol/L	
Creatine kinase (CK)	P	♂ 25–195iu/L ♀ 25–170iu/L	
Creatinine (∝ to lean body mass)	P[1]	70–≤150μmol/L	
Ferritin	P	12–200μg/L	
Folate	S	2.1μg/L	
Follicle-stimulating hormone (FSH)	P/S	2–8u/L in ♀ (luteal); >25u/L in menopause	
Gamma-glutamyl transpeptidase	P	♂ 11–51iu/L ♀ 7–33iu/L	
Glucose (fasting)	P	3.5–5.5mmol/L	
Growth hormone	P	<20mu/L	
HbA_{1c} (= glycosylated Hb)	B	<5.5%; <6.5≈good control in DM	
Iron	S	♂ 14–31μmol/L ♀ 11–30μmol/L	
Lactate dehydrogenase (LDH)	P	70–250iu/L	
Lead	B	<1.8mmol/L	
Luteinizing hormone (LH) (premenopausal)	P	3–16u/L (luteal)	
Magnesium	P	0.75–1.05mmol/L	

1 See *OHCS* p15 for reference intervals in pregnancy.
2 The sample requires special handling: contact the laboratory.
3 Desired upper limit of cholesterol would be <6mmol/L. In some populations, 7.8mmol/L i top end of the distribution.
P=plasma (eg heparin bottle); **S**=serum (clotted; no anticoagulant); **B**=whole blood (edetic acid EDTA bo

nolality	P	278–305mosmol/kg
athyroid hormone (PTH)	P	<0.8–8.5pmol/L
lactin	P	♂ <450u/L; ♀<600u/L
state specific antigen (PSA)	P	0–4µg/ml, age specific, see p681
tein (total)	P	60–80g/L
l cell folate	B	0.36–1.44µmol/L (160–640µg/L)
nin (erect/recumbent)	P[2]	2.8–4.5/ 1.1–2.7pmol/mL/h
lium	P[1]	135–145mmol/L
roid-binding globulin (TBG)	P	7–17mg/L
roid-stimulating hormone (TSH) widens with age, p200	P	0.5–5.7mu/L
roxine (T4)	P	70–140nmol/L
roxine (free)	P	9–22pmol/L
al iron-binding capacity	S	54–75µmol/L
glyceride	P	0.55–1.90mmol/L
iodothyroinine (T_3)	P	1.2–3.0nmol/L
ponin T (see p104)	P	<0.1µg/L
te	P[1]	♂ 210–480µmol/L ♀ 150–390µmol/L
a	P[1]	2.5–6.7mmol/L
amin B_{12}	S	0.13–0.68nmol/L (>150ng/L)

rial blood gases—reference intervals

.35–7.45 — P_aCO_2: 4.7–6.0kPa

>10.6kPa — Base excess: ±2mmol/L

: 7.6mmHg = 1kPa (atmospheric pressure ≈ 100kPa)

ne reference intervals	Reference interval	Your hospital
tisol (free)	<280nmol/24h	
droxyindole acetic acid	16–73µmol/24h	
droxymethylmandelic acid HMMA, VMA)	16–48µmol/24h	
tanephrines	0.03–0.69µmol/mmol creatinine (or <5.5µmol/day)	
nolality	350–1000mosmol/kg	
oxogenic steroids	♂ 28–30µmol/24h ♀ 21–66µmol/24h	
oxosteroids (neutral)	♂ 17–76µmol/24h ♀ 14–59µmol/24h	
osphate (inorganic)	15–50mmol/24h	
assium	14–120mmol/24h	
tein	<150mg/24h	
dium	100–250mmol/24h	

Useful addresses (for those in the UK)

For *addresses of disease-specific organizations,* see the Health Informa Line (below, or www.patient.org.uk/); for *poisons information services* see p8

Diabetes UK 10 Queen Ann St, London W1M 0BD (020 7323 1531)

British Medical Association (BMA) BMA House, Tavistock Square, Lor WC1H 9JP (020 7387 4499)

Bureau of Hygiene and Tropical Medicine Keppel St, London WC1E (020 7636 8636)

Central Public Health Lab 61 Colindale Av, London NW9 5HT (020 8200 44(

Committee on Safety of Medicines (part of the MHRA) freepost, London SW8

Communicable Disease Surveillance Centre (for up-to-date advice on tr health needs) 61 Colindale Avenue, London NW9 5HT (020 8200 6868)

Disabled Living Foundation (Advice on aids and equipment to help disabled) 380–384 Harrow Rd, London W9 2HU (020 7289 6111)

Evidence-based medicine Cochrane Centre (01865 516300)
NHS Centre for Reviews and Dissemination (01904 433707)
Central Health Outcomes Unit DOH (020 7972 2000)
Centre for Health Economics (01904 433645)
Centre for Evidence-based Medicine (01865 221321)
Bandolier (01865 226863); INTERNET: www.jr2.ox.ac.uk/Bandolier
UK clearing house—Health Outcomes (0113 233 3940)

General Medical Council 178 Great Portland St, London W1W (020 7580 76

Health Information Line (for a wide range of information for doctors patients, and addresses of disease-specific organizations) 0800 665544

Liverpool School of Tropical Medicine Pembroke Place, Liverpool L3 (0151 708 9393)

Malaria Reference Laboratory (for advice on malaria prophylaxis) 020 7636 8636 (for advice on treatment ring 020 7387 4411)

Medic-Alert Foundation 12 Bridge Wharf, 156 Caledonian Rd, London N1 (020 7833 3034)

Medical Defence Union (UK) 3 Devonshire Place, London W1N 2EA (020 7 6181 and 0800 716376, fax 0161 491 1420)

Medical & Dental Defence Union 144 West George St, Glasgow (0141 332 664

Medical Foundation for the Care of Victims of Torture 96–98 Grafton Kentish Town, London NW5 3EJ (020 7813 7777) www.torturecare.org.uk

Medical Protection Society 50 Hallam St, London W1N 6DE (020 7637 054

Multiple Sclerosis Society 25 Effie Road, London SW6 1EE (020 7736 6267

National Counselling Service for Sick Doctors (0870 241 0535)

NHS direct 0845 46 47

The Patients' Association (an advice service for patients) PO Box 9 Harrow (0845 608 4455)

Transplant service (UK) (Can these organs be used?) 0117 9507 777. To m your own organs available, add your name online at uktransplant.org.uk

ıternet addresses, and becoming a Knowledge Information fficer

ıe internet is older than most doctors, being of the same vintage as, say, enicillin—is used more often than penicillin, and is having just as profound fects on medicine. During the time it takes you to read this page, your better-onnected patients may have checked out your latest prescription and be ondering why it does not tally with the recommendations of Guatemalan uidelines on Gynaecomastia, or the National Institute for Health and Clinical xcellence's Treatise on Toxoplasmosis. Our patients have time and motivation, hereas we have little time and our motivation may be flickering. This can em threatening to the doctor who sees himself/herself as a dispenser of isdom and precious remedies. It is less threatening if we consider ourselves be in partnership with our patients. The evidence is that those who use the ternet to question their therapy receive a better service.

If all this makes you depressed don't give up. The chances are that someone your team is more familiar with the technology than you. Ask her if she will your Knowledge Information Officer for a while. The answer will probably 'Yes'. If everyone says 'No', then you are probably ahead of your team. So go your local librarian, and ask his advice, get some training, and then offer urself as your team's Knowledge Information Officer. If no one asks you y questions, your team is either sleeping or dead (all organisms and ganizations have information needs)—or you are not available at the right ne: get yourself an e-mail address and teach the team to send you messages.

ow to use a Knowledge Information Officer Their role is to answer your nical questions. Can tetanus toxoid cause purpura? Is there a connection etween knee pain and constipation? Frame your questions as simply as ossible. You are not asking him whether it is likely that this patient's purpura due to last week's tetanus vaccine, just if it is a reported happening. You aintain clinical responsibility and use the knowledge you are given to frame ppropriate management.

seful sources for Knowledge Information Officers *A basic starter kit:*

Drugs: eMIMS (more up to date than eBNF, but see the *What's new* section at www.bnf.org); *eMIMS* contains many Data-sheets; free and updated monthly.

Differential diagnoses (eg what causes chest pain, knee pain, and urea↑?) and *rare diseases*—try Mentor (www.webmentorlibrary.com)

Research: Medline is free at www.ncbi.nlm.nih.gov/entrez/query.fcgi?db=PubMed. Searches can be limited with nested commands: eg angina [therapy] **AND** (2005 [PDAT] **OR** 2004 [PDAT]) **AND** (new eng j med [JOURNAL] or lancet [JOURNAL]) **AND** human **AND** hasabstract **AND** randomized controlled trial [PTYP] Note use of upper case AND/OR, and no space in the phrase 'hasabstract'. This search yields 6 results, for example. Adding '**AND** buck g [AUTHOR]' narrows it down to one. For advanced advice on using Medline, see *OHCS* p504. Be careful. Missing out a close-bracket ')' before 'and human' gives 2220 results. Also, check your spelling carefully.

Meta-analyses: www.update-software.com (eg Cochrane library).

you *are* your team's Knowledge Information Officer, decide how to categor-e, store, and retrieve knowledge you import and export. Time-management urus tell us that the main time-waster is, for most organizations, chasing ems known to exist but currently lost. Manual systems and bursting filing abinets are not the answer: linked hard disks and searchable databases are.

20 Practical procedures

Contents

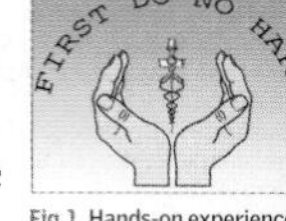

Fig 1. Hands-on experienc a vital part of the learni process in medicine—withc it we could never hope improve our skills, and tł would gently drift away fr us on a current of inadequa But a golden rule remember is: ►*first do harm.* We must know wh we are out of our depth call for senior help may one of the most importa that you ever make.

►Always keep your skills in emergency procedures well-honed by going on cours etc. It is often wiser to wait for someone else to come and carry out an urge procedure than to try for the first time by oneself (fig 1)—but some procedu must occasionally be performed at once—see EMERGENCY BOX, p749.

Relevant pages in other chapters: Arrhythmias (p110); bone marrow biop (p348); cardiogenic shock (p788); consent, (p554); enteral tube feeding (B p753); intravenous fluid therapy (p656); liver failure (p250); local anaesthet (TABLE, p559); meningitis (p806); pleural effusion (p176); pneumothorax (p17 p798); renal biopsy (p280); subarachnoid haemorrhage (p470); tensi pneumothorax (p798); the venous system of the thoracic inlet (BOX, p575).

We thank Dr Iain Wilson who is our Specialist Reader for this chapter.

asogastric (Ryle's) tubes

ıese tubes are passed into the stomach *via* the nose—orogastric if *via* the outh—and drain externally. Sizes: 16 = large, 12 = medium, 10 = small.

ses:

To empty the stomach: eg pre-op, acute pancreatitis, intestinal obstruction, paralytic ileus, gastric outflow obstruction, risk of aspiration.

Intra-operatively: eg to inflate/deflate the stomach to give easier access to the upper abdomen, to decompress the bowel or to test an anastomosis.

For irreversible dysphagia: eg motor neurone disease.

For feeding ill patients: use a special fine-bore tube.

assing the tube Nurses are experts and will ask you (who may never have assed one) to do so only when they fail—so the first question to ask is: 'Have ou asked the charge-nurse from the ward next door?'

Wear non-sterile gloves and an apron to protect from those 'rich encrustations' so often found on our clothes after a few days on the wards.

Explain the procedure. Take a new, cool (hence less flexible) tube. Have a cup of water to hand. Lubricate well with aqueous gel.

Use the tube, by holding it against the patient's head, to estimate the length required to get from the nostril to the back of the throat.

Place lubricated tube in nostril with its natural curve promoting passage down, rather than up. The right nostril is often easier than the left. Advance directly backwards (not upwards).

When the tip is estimated to be entering the throat, rotate the tube by ~180° to discourage passage into the mouth.

Advance the tube into the oesophagus during a swallow and thence into the stomach. It may be easier to swallow with a sip of water and easier to advance if rotating rather than pushing. **If this fails:** Try the other nostril, then oral insertion.

The tube should have distance markings along it: the stomach is at ~35–40cm in an adult, so advance to at least this distance, preferably 10–20cm beyond.

Secure with tape to the nose. Use pH paper to test that you are in the stomach—the gastric contents will be acidic. Using a CXR to check positioning is generally now regarded as an unnecessary exposure to radiation, though some may require it (eg fine bore tubes).

Either spigot the tube, or allow to drain into a dependent catheter bag secured to the patient's clothing (zinc oxide tape around tube to form a flap, safety pin through flap).

·Do not pass a tube nasally if there is any suspicion of a facial fracture.

·Get senior help if the patient has recently had upper GI surgery—it is not ood news to have pushed the tube through a fresh anastomosis!

omplications: • Pain, or, rarely: • Loss of electrolytes • Oesophagitis • Tracheal r duodenal intubation • Necrosis: retro- or nasopharyngeal • Perforation of the tomach.

Veaning When thinking about removing a nasogastric tube that is *in situ* for ecompression or relief of obstruction, it is a good idea to wean it so that the atient manages well without it:

First it should be on free drainage with eg 4hrly aspirations;

Then spigot with 4hrly aspirations;

Then spigot only. If this is tolerated along with oral intake then it is probably safe to remove the tube;

If progression is not tolerated then take a step backwards.

Placing IV cannulae (drips)

►Although siting a cannula has almost become *de rigueur* for hospital admiss try to avoid IVIs, as infections/MRSA at the IVI site can cause real proble especially in the elderly. Insertion skill is best shown at the bedside by an exp

1 **Set up a tray** Swab to clean skin; cannula(e); syringe + 1mL 1% *lidoca* cotton-wool/gauze swab to stop bleeding from unsuccessful attempts; ta Tegaderm® to fix cannula; elastoplast; saline flush; portable sharps bin: ►**ne lestick injuries do happen**. Take multiple items for brave but failed atten
2 **Set up a drip-stand** with first bag of fluid (carefully checked with a nurse); through' a giving-set (a nurse will show you how).
3 **Ask a nurse to help** until you are experienced. Nurses prefer helping ra than changing the bed clothes because of spilt blood.
4 **Explain** the procedure to the patient, including that only the tube and **not** needle remains in the arm. Place the tourniquet around the arm.
5 **Have the patient lying down** This prevents most faints and further probl when they do occur.
6 **Search hard for the best vein** (palpable, not merely visible). Don't be too ha Rest the arm below the level of the heart to aid filling. Ask them to clench unclench their fist. Feel with your most sensitive finger—a golden touch come with practice.
7 ►**Stay away from** arms with AV dialysis fistulae and the ipsilateral side axillary surgery. Also avoid sites crossing a joint, if possible.
8 **Get comfortable** It makes all the difference when learning.
9 **Place a paper towel** under arm to soak up any blood.
10 **Tap the vein** to make it prominent.
11 **Clean the skin** Use local anaesthetic (or *Emla*® cream or **tetrcaine** 4% gel it is kinder, it **does** work, but takes ~¾h to work. Consider using a fine needl raise a bleb of *lidocaine*, like a nettle sting, just to the vein's side. Wait 15

After it is in: 1 Take blood with a syringe or adapter, if you are going to. 2 Rem the tourniquet. 3 Flush the cannula. 4 Fix cannula firmly with tape; check f 5 Connect fluid tube. 6 Bandage a loop of the tube to the arm. If the drip is ac a joint, use a splint. 7 Check the flow speed. Write a fluid chart (p656). 8 W the drip comes down, remove the cannula. (A patient once asked at follow-up i still needed 'this green plastic thing in my hand'.) NB: Adding heparin to the IVI not been shown to maintain patency (unlike arterial lines).[MET 3]

If you fail after 3 attempts ►Shocked patients need fluid quickly: if you having trouble putting in a drip, call your senior. The advice below assumes that drip is not immediately life-saving. ►►If it is, see EMERGENCY BOX.

Experienced doctors can forget they had to learn. Ask to be taught and for when you need it. Is this the right needle for the right job? What is the drip for? If patient may need blood quickly, use a large size (eg grey; green is suitable for s IVIs—or even pink if the veins are fragile, see TABLE). Other measures:

- Explain to the patient that veins can be difficult. Take a break...
- Try submerging the arm in a bowl of warm water for 2min.
- Use a blood pressure cuff at 80mmHg as a tourniquet.
- Try putting a small amount of GTN paste over the vein.

If you still cannot get the drip in You are now downcast, so call your senic it may hurt your pride but perhaps this was not your time. Calling him could m him, you and your patient happy and not many things do that! If you are afrai ask your senior, ask another house officer—they are much more likely to succ than you at this juncture. If you cannot find anyone to help, have a coffee and ret an hour later. Veins are capricious: they come and go.

Resiting Inflamed drip sites need prompt resiting of the drip. If site is heal gently infuse a 5mL syringe of 0.9% saline through the cannula. If resista and/or pain prevents this, the drip needs resiting. If the drip has 'tissu (subcutaneous leakage), resiting is also required (see BOX).

ıe drip has tissued'

ʃou are called about the above, ask yourself: • Is there fluid in bag and giving-:? • Inspect the cannula: take bandage off. • Is the drip still needed? • Are the ıtrol taps open? • Are there kinks in the tube? • Is a venous valve blocking the ınula end?

travenous cannulae sizes and UK colour conventions

ıuge	Colour	Diameter (mm)	Length (mm)	Flow rate (mL/min[v])
.4G		2	45	250
.6G		1.7	42	170
.8G		1.2	40	90
20G		1	32	55
22G		0.28	25	25
24G		0.7	19	24

Maximum flow rate under gravity.

According to **Poiseuille's law**[1] the flow rate (Q) of a fluid through a tubular structure is inversely proportional to viscosity (η) and length (l) and proportional to the pressure difference across it (Pi – Po) and the radius to the **power of 4**. Hence: $Q \propto \frac{(Pi - Po)\,r^4}{\eta\, l}$

ast throw of the dice

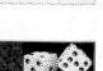

ıt once it may come down to you. For some, this is one of the challenges and ills in medicine. There may be no one else available to help when there is an olute and urgent indication for IV drugs/fluids/blood—and all of the above asures have been tried, and have failed. Think of lonesome night shifts, overrun ergency departments, a disaster scene, war, or medicine in the field. The owing measures are not recommended for non-life threatening scenarios.

on't worry. Have a good look again. Feet? Inside of the forearm? Upper arm? lave you really exhausted all of your options for help from a colleague? Maybe ne ITU registrar is approachable—they do have remarkable skills.

s the patient familiar with his/her own veins (eg previous IV drug abuser)?

there is only a small amount IV medication required and a small, short vein, ou may be able to gain access with a carefully placed butterfly needle that is aped down. Some drugs cannot be passed this way (eg amiodarone, K^+).

he external jugular vein may become prominent when the patient is head own (Trendelenberg) by 5–10° (►not in situations of fluid overload, LVF, ↑ICP) nly attempt cannulation of this vein if you are not going to jeopardise future entral line insertion, and if you can clearly determine the surrounding anatomy.

y do the following if you have had the appropriate training/experience:

ptions in children: **1** Inserting an intraosseous needle 2–3cm inferior and just ıedial to the tibial tuberosity (indicated after 2 failed peripheral cannulations an emergency). This is not generally done in adults (off the battle-field)[4] as ıe bone is far less forgiving and far more painful. **2** Cannulating a scalp vein.

entral venous catheterisation (p762). This may be just as hard in a rofoundly hypovolaemic arrest patient, and a good knowledge of local natomy and of the procedure (± ultrasound guidance) will be invaluable.

A cut down to the long saphenous vein may (must!) be attempted, in emis,[5] *even if you have no prior experience* (at this site you won't kill by ıg ham-fisted). ▸▸Make a transverse incision 1–2cm anterior and superior to the lial malleolus ▸▸Free the vein with forceps ▸▸Cannulate it under direct vision. ere, **'first do no harm'** is trumped by **'nothing ventured, nothing gained'**.

efully, it shouldn't ever have to come to these measures, but one day...

ɜeuille's law is a neat piece of physiology and worth remembering—it is applicable in form to almost every system in the body.

Catheterizing bladders

Catheters ***Size:*** (in French gauge): 12=small; 16=large; 20=very large (eg 3-w Use the smallest you can. Latex is soft (►ask about allergy); simplastic firme silastic (silicone) catheter may be used long term, but costs more. ***Shape:*** **Fole** typical (fig 1); ***coudé*** **(elbow)** catheters have an angled tip to ease aro prostates but are more risky; **Teeman** catheters have tapered ends for a sim reason; **3-way** catheters are used in clot or debris retention and have an ex separate lumen for irrigation fluid that is attached to the irrigation set via an e port on the distal end (fig 2)—call the urology ward for advice on how to set this **Condom** (Conveen®) catheters♂ (Paul's tubing) have no indwelling parts, and preferred by nurses and patients (less pain) even though they may leak and fall o

Catheter problems: • ***Infection*** (don't use antibiotics unless systemic unwell—discuss treatment with a microbiologist). Consider bladder irrigation 0.9% saline or chlorhexidine 0.02% (may irritate). • ***Bladder spasm*** may be pai —try reducing the water in the balloon or an anticholinergic drug eg ***oxybut***

Methods of catheterizing bladders

Checklist:
• Gloves
• Catheter
• ***Lidocaine*** jelly
• 10mL 0.9% salin
• Prep, eg Savlon®
• Drape
• Kidney dish
• Gauze swabs
• Forceps
• Drainage bag
• Specimen contai

1 ***Per urethram:*** This route is used to relieve urinary retention, to monitor urine output in critically ill patients, or to collect urine for diagnosis uncontaminated by urethral flora. ►It is contraindicated in urethral injury (eg pelvic fracture) and acute prostatitis. Catheterization introduces bacteria into the bladder, so **aseptic technique is vital.**[1] Women and men are often catheterized by nurses; you too should be able to catheterize both.

- Explain the procedure, and consider analgesia. If you don't have a catheterisation pack, make up your own (see BOX).
- Lie the patient supine in a well-lit area: women with knees flexed and abducted with heels together. Use a gloved hand to prep urethral meatus pubis-to-anus direction, holding the labia apart with the other hand. \ uncircumcised men (ask the patient beforehand if they have been circumcise make sure), retract the foreskin to 'prep' the glans; use a gloved hand to holc penis still and off the scrotum. The hand used to hold the penis or labia sh not touch the catheter (use forceps if needed). A sterile drape with a hole ir middle may help asepsis. **Remember:** left hand dirty, right hand sterile.
- Put sterile ***lidocaine*** 1–2% gel on the catheter tip and ≤10mL into the ure (≤5mL if ♀). In men, stretch the penis perpendicular to the body to eliminate urethral folds that may lead to false passage.
- Use steady **gentle** pressure to advance the catheter. ►**Never force the cath** In men, mild resistance in the first ~10cm may be from a urethral stricture previous catheterisation. Insert to the hilt; wait until urine emerges be inflating the balloon. Remember to check the balloon's capacity before infla (written on the outer end). Collect a sterile specimen and attach a drainage Pull the catheter back so that the balloon comes to rest at the bladder ne
- If you are having trouble getting past the prostate try: more lubrication; a la catheter; a *coudé* catheter—or call the urologists, who may use a guide-w

► Remember to reposition the foreskin in uncircumcised men after the cathet inserted to prevent massive oedema of the glans and paraphimos (see p6

2 ***Suprapubic catheterization*** Ensure the bladder is distended so that there risk of peritoneal penetration; you may have to wait for it to fill up. Clean the infiltrate with local anaesthetic down to the bladder, nick the skin, and then in trocar down vertically above the symphysis pubis. When urine is draining, adv the catheter over the trocar and tape it down securely.

►Have all the kit ready beforehand and a helping hand as it can get messy!

1 Routine antibiotic prophylaxis can be used at the time of insertion/removal of a urinary cathe prevent transient bacteraemia—eg ***gentamicin*** 2.5mg/kg IV stat. Evidence is scarce, so check local

;elf-catheterisation

This is a good, safe way of managing chronic retention from a neuropathic)ladder (eg in multiple sclerosis, diabetic neuropathy, spinal tumour or trauma). Never consider a patient in difficulties from a big residual volume to be too old, /oung, or disabled to learn. 5-yr-old children can learn the technique, and can 1ave their lives transformed—so motivation may be excellent. There may be 'ewer UTIs as there is no residual urine—and less reflux obstructive uropathy. Assessing suitability entails testing sacral dermatomes: a 'numb bum' implies ↓ ;ensation of a full bladder; higher sensory loss may mean catheterization will be)ainless. Get help from your continence adviser who will be in a position to 'each the patient or carer that catheterizations must be gentle (the catheter is of a much smaller calibre), particularly if sensation is lacking, and must number >4/d ('always keep your catheter with you; don't wait for an urge before :atheterizing'). See fig 3.

] 1. A size 14F latex ley catheter with the lloon inflated *via* the omost port of the outer d (green).[1] NB: These ages are not to scale.

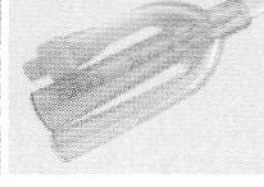

Fig 2. The external end of a size 20F 3-way catheter. The lowest port is for the bladder irrigation fluid and the uppermost port (yellow) is for balloon inflation.

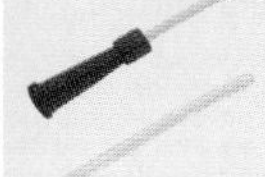

Fig 3. A size 10F catheter for self-catheterisation. They are usually much smaller than indwelling catheters eg 10F compared to 14F. Note that this catheter also has no balloon.

The catheter is not draining..."

'ou will be asked to check catheters that are not draining. Possibilities are:

- The catheter is bypassing: a condom catheter may be more appropriate.
- The catheter is blocked: with aseptic technique flush and withdraw 20mL of sterile 0.9% saline with a bladder syringe. This may get the flow going again. A 3-way catheter may be needed if there is clot or debris retention.
- The catheter has slipped into the proximal (prostatic♂) urethra, possible even if the balloon is fully inflated. This is may be the case if a flush enters but cannot be withdrawn: with aseptic technique deflate the balloon, advance and reinflate, then flush and withdraw again.
- Renal hypoperfusion: in a dehydrated/post-op patient a fluid challenge of 250mL Gelofusine® STAT (or slower if renal/cardiac co-morbidity) may help. Check all other parameters (eg pulse, BP, CVP) and increase rate of IV fluids if appropriate.
- Acute renal failure (p820): this is unlikely, though most probably from renal hypoperfusion (ie pre-renal failure), but there may be other factors involved causing acute tubular necrosis, eg nephrotoxic drugs.
- The catheter has perforated the lower urinary tract on insertion and is not lying in the bladder or urethra. If suspected, call the urologists immediately.

Remember: urine output should be >400mL in 24h or >0.5mL/kg/h (see p562).

'rial without catheter (TWOC)

When it is time to remove a catheter, the possibility of urinary retention must be :onsidered. If very likely, arrange for a urology outpatient TWOC in 2 weeks; otherwise remove the catheter first thing one morning. If retention does occur, nsert a long-term catheter (eg silicone) and arrange urology clinic follow-up.

We would like to thank Addenbrooke's Hospital Urology Department for supplying the catheters.

Tapping ascites

Ascites may be sampled to provide a cytological or bacterial diagnosis, eg exclude spontaneous bacterial peritonitis (SBP, see p252). Before starting ens that you know the patient's platelets + clotting times. If they are abnormal, s help before proceeding.

- Place the patient flat and tap out the ascites, marking a point where fluid been identified, avoiding vessels, stomas and scars (adhesions to the ante abdominal wall). The left side may be safer (less chance of nicking liver/sple
- Clean the skin. Infiltrate some local anaesthetic, eg 1% ***lidocaine*** (see p55
- Insert a 21G needle on a 20mL syringe into the skin and advance while aspirat until fluid is withdrawn.
- Remove the needle and apply a sterile dressing.
- Send fluid for ***microscopy***, ***culture***, ***chemistry*** (protein, see p176), and ***cytolo*** Call microbiology to forewarn them if urgent analysis of the specimen is requi

Diagnostic aspiration of a pleural effusion

- If not yet done, a CXR may help evaluate the side and size of the effusion.
- Percuss the upper border of the pleural effusion and choose a site 1 o intercostal spaces below it (usually posteriorly or laterally).
- Mark the spot and then clean the area with an antiseptic solution.
- Infiltrate down to the pleura with 5–10mL of 1% ***lidocaine*** (see p559).
- Attach a 21G needle to a syringe and insert it just above the upper border of rib below the mark to avoid the neurovascular bundle (see BOX). Aspirate wh advancing the needle. Draw off 10–30mL of pleural fluid.

Send fluid to the lab for ***chemistry*** (protein, glucose, pH, LDH, amyla ***bacteriology*** (microscopy and culture, auramine stain, TB culture); ***cytology*** an indicated, ***immunology*** (rheumatoid factor, ANA, complement).

Pleural biopsy

This is usually performed in patients with a pleural effusion when analysis pleural fluid has not provided an underlying diagnosis. It should not performed on the ward in patients without an effusion as this require different approach. This procedure requires some practice, so if you inexperienced, ask a senior doctor to assist you.

- Place the patient in an upright position on the edge of the bed, arms resting c pillow on a bed-table to provide support.
- Identify the upper border of the pleural effusion posteriorly or laterally and m an intercostal space 1–2 ribs below this.
- Clean the skin with an antiseptic solution and apply sterile drapes.
- Infiltrate down to the pleura with 5–10mL of 1% ***lidocaine*** (see p559).
- Check that you are in the correct space by aspirating pleural fluid.
- Make a deep skin incision 0.5cm wide immediately above the upper border of rib below the chosen intercostal space (avoids neurovascular bundle).
- Carefully advance the Abrams' needle through the incision until a 'give' is felt you enter the pleural space.
- Open the needle by twisting the trocar. Check that fluid can be aspirated.
- Manoeuvre the open needle so that the cutting notch is pointing inferiorly avoid the neurovascular bundle) and caught on the pleura—pull the needle b slightly at an angle to the chest wall—then close the needle and withdraw slight tug may be required at this stage.
- Withdraw the needle in expiration and repeat.
- Place the tissue samples in the appropriate media for histological and mi biological examination. Send to the lab for ***microscopy***, ***culture***, and ***histolog***
- Withdraw the needle, and apply a sterile dressing, occasionally a single sut may be required. Perform a post-procedure CXR.

›dominal paracentesis

r patients with tense, refractory or recurrent ascites that is symptomatic, it is ssible to drain the ascites using a Bonnano® catheter (initially designed for ›rapubic catheterisation). Paracentesis in such patients even in the presence ›ntaneous bacterial peritonitis may be safe. The procedure is best done ›ervised before attempting it alone. ***Contraindications:*** End-stage cirrhosis; agulopathy; hyponatraemia (≤126mmol/L); sepsis. The main complication of › procedure is severe hypovolaemia secondary to reaccumulation of the :ites, so intravascular replenishment with a plasma expander is required—eg 0mL 20% ***human albumin*** IV for each litre of ascites drained. You may need call the haematology lab to request this in advance.

Ensure you have good IV access—eg 18G cannula in the antecubital fossa.
Examine the abdomen carefully, evaluating the ascites and checking for ›rganomegaly. Mark where you are going to enter. Approach from the left side unless previous local surgery/stoma prevents this—call a senior for support and advice if this is the case.
Prepare the patient as if for an ascitic tap (see OPPOSITE), taking extra care to keep the procedure aseptic (use a sterile drape). Infiltrate the local anaesthetic.
Perform an ascitic tap first so that you know you are in the correct place.
Carefully thread the catheter over the (large and long) needle using the guide so that the pig-tail has been straightened out. Remove the guide.
With the left hand hold the needle ~1 inch from the tip—this will stop it from advancing too far (and from performing an aortic biopsy!). With the right hand, hold the other end.
Gently insert the needle perpendicular the skin at the site of the ascitic tap up to your hold with your left hand—ascites should now drain easily. If necessary advance the needle and catheter a short distance until good flow is achieved.
Advance the catheter over the needle with your left hand, keeping the needle in exactly the same place with your right hand. ►Do not re-advance the needle because it will go through the curled pig-tail and do not withdraw it because you won't be able to thread in the catheter.
When fully inserted, connect the catheter to a drainage bag (keep it below the level of the abdomen) and tape it down securely to the skin.
The patient should stay in bed as the ascites drains.
Replenish intravascular volume with human albumin (see above).
Ask the nursing staff to remove the catheter after 6h or after a pre-determined volume has been drained. (Up to 20L can come off in 6 hours!)
Send a sample of ascitic fluid to the lab for MC+S.
Check U&E after the procedure and re-examine the patient.

fe approach to entering the pleura by the intercostal route

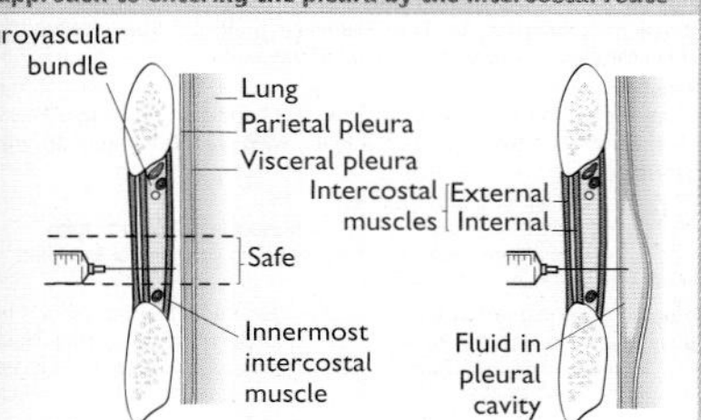

Inserting a chest drain

Indications:
- Pneumothorax: ventilated; tension; persistent/recurrent (eg <24h afte aspiration); large 2nd spontaneous pneumothorax if >50yrs old)
- Malignant pleural effusion
- Empyema or complicated parapneumonic effusion
- Traumatic haemopneumothorax; • Air transfer
- Post-operatively: eg thoracotomy; oesophagectomy; cardiothoracic surgery.

Sterile procedure:[9]
- Have the x-rays or CT scans available to confirm location for chest drain inser
- Preparation: Trolley with dressing pack; iodine; needles; 10mL syringe; 20mL ***lidocaine***; scalpel (№15); suture; chest drain (eg 10–14F, if traum haemothorax larger gauge eg 28–30F); underwater drainage bottle; conne tubes; sterile H_2O; tape. Incontinence pad under patient. Swab extensively
- Choose insertion site:[10] 4th–6th intercostal space, anterior- to mid-axillary li the 'safe triangle' (see BOX). A more posterior approach eg the 7th s posteriorly may be required to drain a loculated effusion, and occasionally th intercostal space in the mid-clavicular line may be used for a pneumothoraces—however, both approaches tend to be less comfortable.
- Infiltrate down to pleura with 10–20mL of 1% ***lidocaine***. Check that either air or can be aspirated from the proposed insertion site—if not **do not** proceed. Wait
- Make a 2cm incision above 6th rib, to avoid neurovascular bundle under **Bluntly** dissect down to the pleura. Puncture pleura with scissors or force large bore tube (>24F), then sweep a finger inside chest to clear adherent and exclude (eg in blunt abdominal trauma) stomach in the chest! **NB:** Some kits use a Seldinger technique for insertion.
- ► Before inserting the drain, remove the metal trochar completely; introdu the drain **atraumatically** using forceps to advance it.
- Advance the tip upwards to the apex (or base if draining an effusion). Sto meeting resistance. Then attach the drain via the tubing to the underwater Ensure that the longer tube within the bottle is underwater and bubbling respiration. If the patient is to be moved to another hospital, substitute Heir flutter valve or drainage bag with flap valve for underwater drain.
- ► You should never clamp chest drains inserted for pneumothoraces. Clamp is occasionally used when pleural effusions are being drained to control th rate of drainage and prevent expansion pulmonary oedema.[11]
- With large/medium bore tubes, the incision should be closed with a mat suture or suture across the incision. Purse string sutures are no-lo recommended as they may lead to increased scarring and wound pain.
- Fix the drain with a second suture tied around the tube like a 'Roman ga Secure the drain with tape (eg 'Sleek®') to prevent it from slipping.
- Request a CXR to check the position of the drain.

Complications:
- Thoracic or abdominal organ injury • Lymphatic damage ∴ chylothorax
- Damage to long thoracic nerve of Bell ∴ wing scapula • Rarely, arrhythmi

Watch out for:
- Retrograde flow back into the chest
- Persistent bubbling—there may be a continual leak from the lung
- Blockage of the tube from clots or kinking—no swinging or bubbling
- Malposition—check position with CXR.

Removal (in pneumothorax) should be considered when the drain is no-lo bubbling and the CXR shows reinflation. Smartly withdraw during expiratio Valsalva manoeuvre and close the hole immediately with the pre-placed su There is no need to clamp the drain beforehand as the for need reinserti unlikely.[RCT 13] Give analgesia beforehand, eg ***morphine*** or a strong NSAID.[14]

e 'safe triangle' for insertion of a chest drain

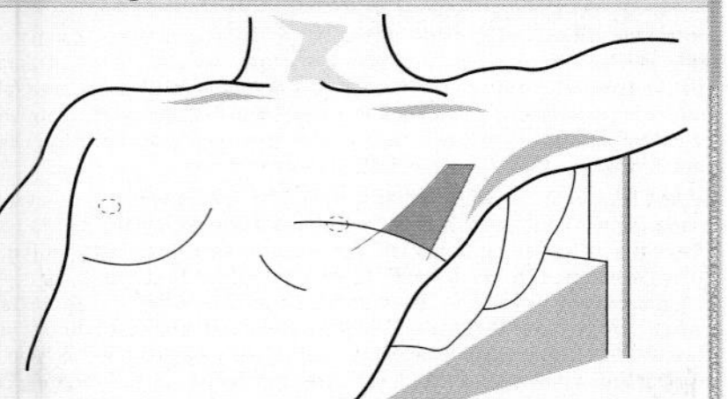

lieving a tension pneumothorax

mptoms: Acute respiratory distress, chest pain, ►►respiratory arrest.
ns: Hypotension; distended neck veins; asymmetrical lung expansion; chea and apex deviated away from side of reduced air entry and perresonance to percussion. ►►There is no time for a CXR (but see fig 1, p735).
n: To release air from the pleural space. In a tension pneumothorax air is wn into the intra-pleural space with each breath, but cannot escape due to alve-like effect of the tiny flap in the parietal pleura. The increasing ssure progressively embarrasses the heart and the other lung.
00% oxygen.
nsert a large bore IV cannula (eg Venflon®) usually through the 2nd ntercostal space in the mid-clavicular line or the 'safe triangle' for chest rain insertion (see BOX). Remove the stylet, which will allow the trapped ir to escape, usually with an audible hiss. The tension pneumothorax has ow been converted to an open pneumothorax. Tape securely. ►Don't re-over the cannula as tensioning will recur.
'roceed to formal chest drain insertion (see OPPOSITE).

piration of a pneumothorax

Identify the 2nd intercostal space in the midclavicular line (or 4–6th intercostal space in the midaxillary line) and infiltrate with 1% ***lidocaine*** down to the pleura overlying the pneumothorax.
Insert a 16G cannula into the pleural space. Remove the needle and connect the cannula to a 3-way tap and a 50mL syringe. Aspirate up to 2.5L of air (50mL×50). Stop if resistance is felt, or if the patient coughs excessively.
Request a CXR to confirm resolution of the pneumothorax. If successful, consider discharging the patient and repeating the CXR after 24h to exclude recurrence, and again after 7–10d. Advise to avoid air travel for 6 weeks after a normal CXR. Diving should be permanently avoided.
If aspiration is unsuccessful (in a significant, symptomatic pneumothorax), insert an intercostal drain (see OPPOSITE).

Lumbar puncture (LP)

Contraindications • Bleeding diathesis; • Cardiorespiratory comprom • Infection at site of needle insertion, and most importantly: • ↑Intracra pressure (suspect if very severe headache, ↓level of consciousness with fal pulse, rising BP, vomiting, focal signs, or papilloedema). Give urgent treatmen needed and discuss urgently with a relevant clinician with a view to CT scanning is not infallible, so be sure your indication for LP is strong.

Method Explain to the patient **what** sampling CSF entails, **why** it is needed, **co-operation** is vital, and that they can **communicate with you** at all stages
- Place the patient on his or her left side, with the back on the edge of the fully flexed (knees to chin). Avoid allowing the patient to slump.
- Landmarks: plane of iliac crests through the level of L3/4 (see BOX). In adults, spinal cord ends at the L1/2 disc. Mark L3/4 intervertebral space (or one sp below, L4/5), eg by a gentle indentation of a thumb-nail on the overlying s (better than a ballpoint pen mark, which might be erased by the sterilizing flu
- Wash hands. Don a mask and sterile gloves.
- Sterilize the back with tincture of iodine (unless allergic).
- Open the spinal pack. Check manometer fittings. Have 3 plain sterile tubes ar fluoride tube (for glucose) ready.
- Inject 0.25–0.5mL 1% ***lidocaine*** (p559) under skin at marked site.
- Wait 1min, then insert spinal needle (22G, stilette in place) through the m aiming towards umbilicus. Feel resistance of spinal ligaments, and then the d then a 'give' as the needle enters the subarachnoid space. **NB:** Keep the neec bevel facing **up**, parallel with dural fibres.
- Withdraw stilette. Wait for CSF.
- Measure CSF 'opening' pressure with a manometer.
- Catch fluid in three sequentially numbered bottles (<5–10mL total). Cons taking and privately reserving a labelled sample in case of an accident!
- Remove needle and apply dressing. Send CSF promptly for ***microscopy***, ***cult*** ***protein***, and ***glucose*** (do plasma glucose too)—call the lab to let them know applicable, also send for: cytology, fungal studies, TB culture, virology (incluc Herpes PCR), syphilis serology, oligoclonal bands (with serum sample comparison) if multiple sclerosis suspected. Is there xanthochromia (p692)?
- Lying flat for >1h is traditionally advised (probably unnecessary), checking observations and BP regularly. Post-LP headache is partly preventable reducing CSF leakage by using finer needles shaped to part the dura rather t cut it: see BOX.

CSF composition ***Normal values:*** Lymphocytes <5/mm^3; no polymorphs; pro <0.4g/L; glucose >2.2mmol/L (or ≥50% plasma level); pressure <200mmCSF ***meningitis:*** See p806. ***In multiple sclerosis:*** See p488.

Bloody tap: This is an artefact due to piercing a blood vessel, which is indica (unreliably) by fewer red cells in successive bottles, and no yellowing of (xanthochromia). To estimate how many white cells (*W*) were in the CSF before blood was added, use the following:

$$W = \text{CSF WCC} - [(\text{blood WCC} \times \text{CSF RBC}) \div \text{blood RBC}]$$

If the blood count is normal, the rule of thumb is to subtract from the total CSF (per μL) one white cell for every 1000 RBCs. To estimate the true protein le subtract 10mg/L for every 1000 RBCs/mm^3 (be sure to do the count and pro estimation on the same bottle). **NB:** High protein levels in CSF make it appear yell

Subarachnoid haemorrhage: Xanthochromia (yellow supernatant on spun C Red cells in equal numbers in all bottles (unreliable). RBCs will excite inflammatory response (eg CSF WCC raised), most marked after 48h.

Raised protein: Meningitis; MS; Guillain–Barré syndrome. ***Very raised CSF prot*** Spinal block; TB; or severe bacterial meningitis.

ost-LP headache

sk: ~30%, typically occurring within 24h of LP, with resolution over hours to wks (mean: 3–4d). Patients describe a constant, dull, ache bilaterally which is ore frontal than occipital. The most characteristic symptom is of **positional rthostatic) exacerbation**—worse when upright and usually pain-free when cumbent. There may be mild meningism or nausea. The pathology is thought to continued leakage of CSF from the puncture site and intracranial **hypo**tension, ough there may be other mechanisms involved.[15]

evention: Use the smallest spinal needle that is practical (22G) and keep the vel aligned as described OPPOSITE. **Blunt** needles (more expensive!) can reduce k, perhaps from 30% to 5%—and are recommended (ask an anaesthetist out supply).[16] Collection of CSF takes too long (>6min) if needles smaller than G are used.[17]

eatment: Despite years of anecdotal advice to the contrary, none of the llowing have ever been shown to be a risk factor: position during or after the ocedure; hydration status before, during, or after; amount of CSF removed; mediate activity or rest post-LP.[MET 18] Time is a consistent healer. For severe or olonged headaches, ask an anaesthetist about a **blood patch**.[RCT 19] This is a reful injection of 20mL of autologous venous blood into the adjacent epidural ace (said to 'clog-up the hole'). Immediate relief occurs in 95%.

: Post-LP brain MRI scans often show diffuse meningeal enhancement with dolinium. This is thought to be a reflection of increased blood flow secondary intracranial hypotension. Interpret these scans with caution and in the ntext of the patient's clinical situation.

efining the 3rd – 4th lumbar vertebral interspace

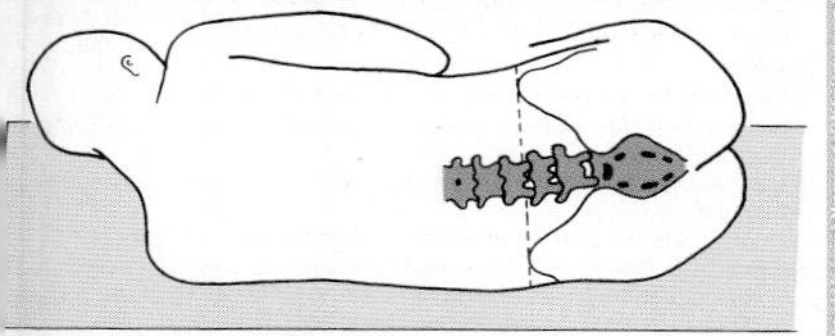

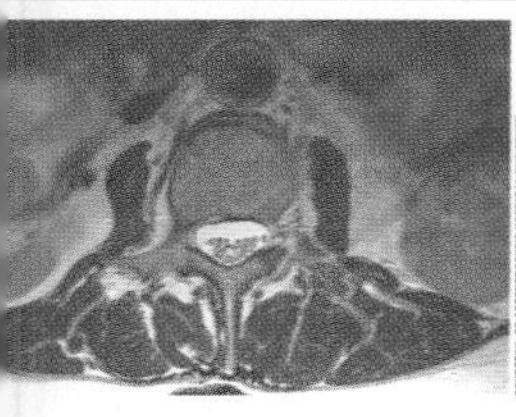

Fig 1. Axial T2 weighted MRI of the lumbar spine. The conus ends at the L1/L2 level with continuation of the cauda equina. Lumbar puncture below the L2 level will not damage the cauda equina as the nerve roots will part around an LP needle.

Cardioversion/defibrillation

►Do not wait for a crisis before familiarizing yourself with the defibrillator, as t several types. Day 1 on a new ward should include a visit to the 'defib trolley'.

Indications: VF/VT, fast AF (p116), supraventricular tachycardias if c treatments (p112) have failed or there is haemodynamic compromise.

Aim: To completely depolarize the heart using a direct current.

Procedure:

- Unless critically unwell, conscious patients require a general anaesthetic.
- Almost all defibrillators are now paddle-free and use 'hands free' pads instead (less chance of skin arc than jelly). Place the pads (eg Littmann™ Defib Pads) on chest, 1 over apex (p29) and 1 below right clavicle. The positions are often given by a diagram on the reverse of the pad.
- ***Monophasic defibrillators*** (fig 1)*:* Set the energy level at 360J for VF/VT; 100J for AF; 50J for atrial flutter.
- ***Biphasic defibrillators*** (fig 2)*:* Impedence is less with a biphasic shock and 150J is used for shocks for VF/VT. They use less energy and are just as effective as monophasic defibrillators in cardioversion of AF, if not better.[RCT 20] [RCT 21] One large retrospective study showed that biphasic cardioversion of atrial flutter was not as successful.[22]
- ***Automatic external defibrillators (AED):*** Can be used by anyone who can turn them on and apply the pads. Follow the instructions given by the AED.

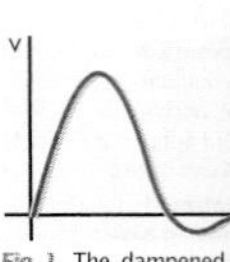

Fig 1. The dampened monophasic waveform.

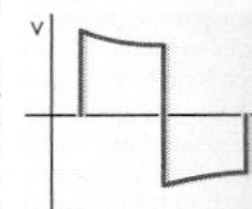

Fig 2. Rectilinear biph waveform with trunca exponential decay. M new external defibrilla use this waveform.

Shocking:

1. Clearly state that you are charging the defibrillator.
2. Make sure no one else is touching the patient, the bed, or anything in touching these.
3. Remove oxygen from the patient as it is flammable and could be ignited flash arc.
4. Clearly state that you are about to shock the patient.
5. Press the button(s) on the electrode(s) to give the shock. If there is a ch in rhythm before you shock and the shock is no longer required, turn the to 'discharge'. Do not allow anyone to approach until the reading has dro to 0J.
6. After a shock: watch ECG; repeat the shock (at 200J once again, then 3 subsequently if monophasic).
7. Consider anticoagulation, as the risk of emboli is increased.
8. Get an up-to-date 12-lead ECG.

NB: For AF and SVT, it is necessary to synchronize the shock on the R-wave o ECG (by pressing the 'SYNC' button on the machine). This ensures that the s does not initiate a ventricular arrhythmia. **If the sync mode is engaged in VF defibrillator will not discharge!**

►In children, use 2J/kg, then 4J/kg in VF/VT; if monophasic, and if >10kg, use a paddles; *OHCS* p239.

Practical procedures

ɪking arterial blood gas (ABG) samples[1]

ɪe reaction of a patient to ABG ɪmpling is often very different to ʻhen they are subjected to ɛnepuncture, so try to explain ɪat the blood sample you are ɔout to take is going to feel fferent and is for a different ɹrpose (p148 for indications & ɪalysis). The usual site is the ɪdial artery at the wrist. ►Don't ɜe this site if there is an ʻteriovenous fistula for ɪemodialysis.

ɪocedure:

- Get kit ready; include: portable sharps bin; pre-heparinized syringe; needle—blue size (23G) is good; gloves; alcohol swab; gauze swab; tape.
- Feel thoroughly for the best site. Look at both sides.

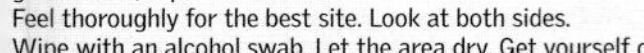

- Wipe with an alcohol swab. Let the area dry. Get yourself comfortable.
- Ask an assistant to hold the hand and arm with the wrist slightly extended.
- Before sampling, expel any excess heparin in the syringe. Infiltration over the artery with a small amount of 1% ***lidocaine*** (p559) through a 25G (orange) needle makes the procedure painless.
- Hold the syringe like a pen, with the needle bevel up. Let the patient know you are about to take the sample. Feel for the pulse with your other hand and enter at 45°, aiming **beneath** the finger you are feeling with.
- The syringe will fill up on its own in a pulsatile manner if you are in the artery. Rarely, entry into a vein next to the artery will give a similar result. Colour of the blood is no guide to its source!
- Remove the needle when enough blood has been taken (1–2mL to allow for spillage or a dud reading from the machine) and apply firm pressure until any leakage is stemmed to avoid a large lump followed by a massive bruise!
- Expel any air from the syringe as this will alter the oxygenation of the blood.
- Cap and label the sample, noting if the patient was on supplementary oxygen.
- Take the sample to the nearest analysis machine or send it by express delivery to the lab (which may be by your own feet). If it is going to stand for any foreseeable length of time then put the sample in a bag of ice.
- Syringes and analysis machines differ, so get familiar with the local nuances.

ʰe other site that is amenable to ɜG sampling is the femoral ʻtery. Surprisingly this may be ss uncomfortable as it is a ɪlatively less sensitive area and ɛcause when supine, the patient ɪnnot see the needle and thus ɪay feel less apprehensive. The ʻachial artery can also be used, ɪt be aware that median nerve ts closely on its medial side.

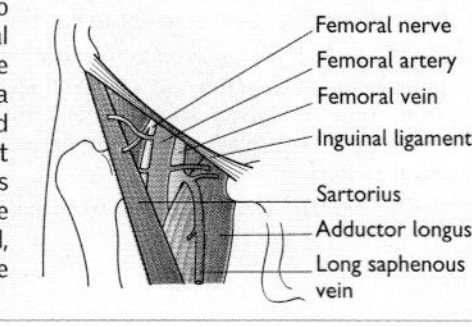

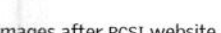
ɪmages after RCSI website

Cricothyroidotomy

Essence An emergency procedure to overcome airway obstruction above the le of the larynx.

Indications Upper airway obstruction when endotracheal intubation not possib eg irretrievable foreign body; facial oedema (burns, angio-oedema); maxillofa trauma; infection (epiglottitis).

Procedure Lie the patient supine with neck extended (eg pillow under shoulde unless there is suspected cervical-spine instability. Run your index finger down neck anteriorly in the midline to find the notch in the upper border of the thyr cartilage: just below this, between the thyroid and cricoid cartilages, is depression—the cricothyroid membrane.

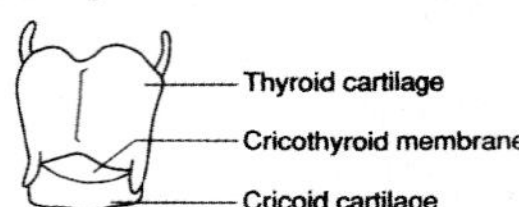

1 ***Needle cricothyroidotomy:*** Pierce the membrane with large-bore cannula (14 attached to syringe: withdrawal of air confirms position; ***lidocaine*** may or may be required). Slide cannula over needle at 45° to the skin superiorly in the sagit plane. Use a Y-connector or improvise connection to O_2 supply at 15L/min: u thumb on Y-connector to allow O_2 in over 1s and CO_2 out over 4s ('transtrach jet insufflation'). This is the preferred method in children <12yrs. This will o sustain life for 30–45min before CO_2 builds up.

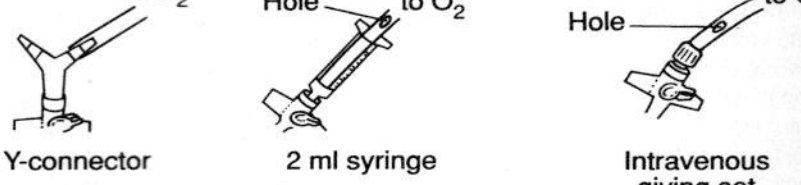

2 ***Mini-Trach II®:*** This contains a guarded blade, introducer, 4mm uncuffed tu (slide over introducer) with ISO connection and binding tape. The patient will ha to be ventilated via a bag, as the resistance is too high to breathe spontaneous This will sustain for 30–45min.

3 ***Surgical cricothyroidotomy:*** Smallest tube for prolonged ventilation is 6m Introduce high-volume low-pressure cuff tracheostomy tube through a horizor incision in membrane. Take care not to cut the thyroid or cricoid cartilages.

Complications Local haemorrhage ± aspiration; posterior perforation of trache oesophagus; subglottic stenosis; laryngeal stenosis if membrane over-incised childhood; tube blockage; subcutaneous tunnelling; vocal cord paralysis hoarseness (the recurrent laryngeal nerve runs superiorly in the trach oesophageal groove).

►NB: Needle and Mini-Trach® are temporary measures pending formal tracheosto

Emergency needle pericardiocentesis[1]

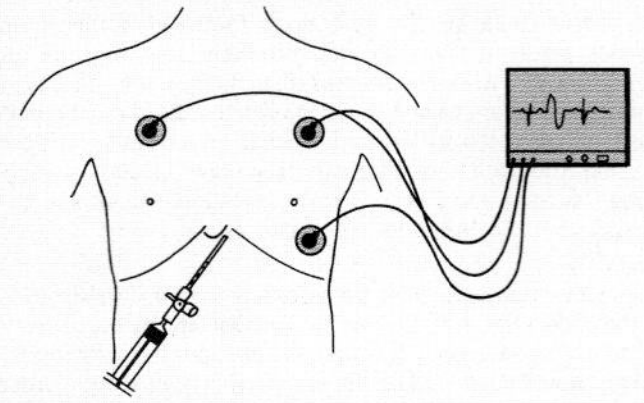

- Get your senior's help (for whom this may serve as an *aide-mémoire*).
- Equipment: 20mL syringe, long 18G cannula, 3-way tap, ECG monitor, skin cleanser.
- If time allows, use aseptic technique, and, if conscious, local anaesthesia and sedation, eg with ***midazolam***: titrate up to 0.1mg/kg IV—start with 2mg over 1min, 1mg in elderly—antidote: ***flumazenil*** 0.2mg IV over 15s, then 0.1mg every 60s, up to 1mg in total.
- Ensure you have IV access and full resuscitation equipment to hand.
- Introduce needle at 45° to skin just below and to left of xiphisternum, aiming for tip of left scapula. Aspirate continuously and watch ECG. Frequent ventricular ectopics or an injury pattern (ST segment↓) on ECG imply that the myocardium has been breached—withdraw slightly. As soon as blood is obtained through the needle, slide the cannula into place.
- Evacuate pericardial contents through the syringe and 3-way tap. Removal of only a small amount of fluid (eg 20mL) can produce marked clinical improvement. If you are not sure whether the fluid you are aspirating is pure blood (eg on entering a ventricle), see if it clots (heavily bloodstained pericardial fluid does not clot), or measure its PCV (though this may be difficult in the acute setting).
- You can leave the cannula *in situ* temporarily, for repeated aspiration. If there is reaccumulation, pericardiectomy may be needed.
- Send fluid for microscopy and culture, as needed, including tests for TB.

Complications: Laceration of ventricle or coronary artery (± subsequent haemopericardium); aspiration of ventricular blood; arrhythmias (ventricular fibrillation); pneumothorax; puncture of aorta, oesophagus (± mediastinitis), or peritoneum (± peritonitis).

Practical procedures

1 Procedures used by cardiologists for elective pericardiocentesis may differ, involving the use of guide-wires, screening, and catheters.

Subclavian venous cannulation

Subclavian venous cannulae may be inserted to provide a measurement of central venous pressure (CVP), to administer certain drugs (eg *amiodaro* chemotherapy), or for intravenous access (fluid therapy, TPN). They are not with hazards (see complications below), so decide whether the patient requires one fi and then ask for help if you are inexperienced. In an emergency the procedure be done using the landmark method (described below), though NICE n recommends that all central venous catheterisation should now be perforn using US guidance.[1] See TABLE for contraindications.

Procedure:

- If possible, get written consent for the procedure (p554). Check clotting + platel
- Position the patient flat, with 1 pillow. Head-down tilt may help if volume deplet
- ► This can compromise cardiac function and precipitate catastrophic acute LV
- Wash hands, don a gown and sterile gloves. This is an aseptic procedure.
- Clean the area with chlorhexidine or iodine solution (unless allergic to these), a apply sterile drapes.
- Assemble the catheter, and flush all the lumina with saline.
- Identify the insertion point: 1cm below the junction of the medial third a lateral ⅔ of the clavicle. Nick the skin with a scalpel.
- Using a green needle inject 5–10mL of 1–2% ***lidocaine*** (p559) under the s and into the subcutaneous tissues, down to the clavicle.
- Using the introducer needle, and an appropriate syringe partly filled with sal puncture the skin and advance the needle to the clavicle. Once you hit clavicle, move the needle under the clavicle and aim for the oppos sternoclavicular joint. This methods reduces the risk of puncturing the pleu Aspirate as you advance the needle and you should be able to cannulate subclavian vein. When in the vein you should be able to easily aspirate blood
- Remove the syringe, keeping the needle still and insert the guide-wire. Remove needle over the wire but **never** let go of the wire or it may all enter the vein, mak removal very difficult. The wire should advance with ease, if it does not, you will h to restart the procedure as you should not remove the wire through the nee
- Next, feed the dilator over the wire. Often twisting it slightly will facilitate insertion. **NB:** Always have one hand on the wire.
- Remove the dilator and feed the catheter over the wire, remembering to ha the end of the wire in your hand before the tip of the catheter enters the sl
- Feed the catheter into the vein, remove the wire, and check that blood can aspirated through each lumen.
- Flush each lumen, and then stitch the catheter in place.
- Order a CXR to check the position of the catheter and exclude a pneumothora
- If a cannula is found to be located in the internal jugular vein (fig 2, p574) must be withdrawn and another reinserted.

Complications (~20% in total):

- Haemorrhage; arterial puncture or cannulation; AV fistula formation.
- Internal jugular cannulation; air embolism.
- Pneumothorax; haemothorax; chylothorax (lymph).
- Phlebitis; thrombus formation on tip or in vein. In patients with a high risk of (eg malignancy), a continuous infusion of unfractionated ***heparin*** may reduce risk of thrombosis.[24]
- Bacterial colonisation; cellulitis; sepsis. ►If taking blood cultures in a febr patient with a central venous line, remember to take samples from the cent line and from a new peripheral site (ie not a pre-existing cannula).

Other sites of insertion include the femoral vein (see BOX, p759) and the inter jugular vein (see BOX, p31). There is evidence to suggest that the femoral approa is associated with a higher rate of line infection and thrombosis.[RCT 25]

1 This is more appropriate for the internal jugular route as the clavicle casts a shadow over the subclavian v

ight subclavian vein puncture—infraclavicular approach

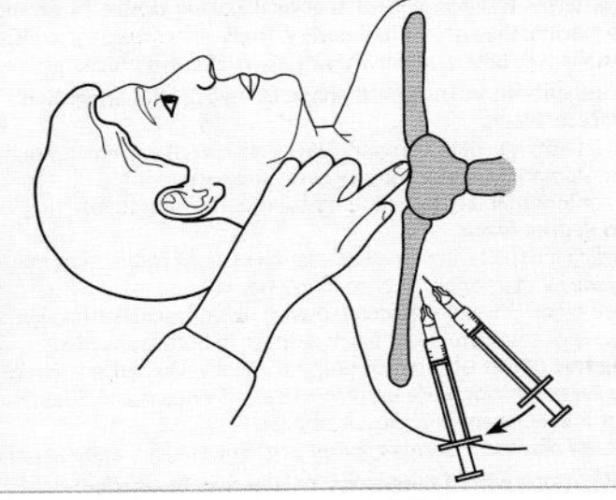

ontraindications to central venous cannulation

Absolute	Relative
nfection at insertion site	Coagulopathy
Significant tricuspid regurgitation	Ipsilateral carotid endarterectomy
Renal cell cancer involving the right atrium	Newly inserted cardiac pacemaker leads

Inserting a temporary cardiac pacemaker

Often it is wiser to liaise with a specialist pacing centre to arrange prom definitive pacing than to try temporary transvenous pacing, which often l complications (see below) which may delay a definitive procedure.

Possible indications in the acute phase of myocardial infarction:

- ***Complete AV block:***
  - With inferior MI (right coronary artery occlusion) pacing may only be need if symptomatic; spontaneous recovery may occur.
  - With anterior MI (representing massive septal infarction).
- ***Second degree block:***
  - Wenckebach (p111 implies decremental AV node conduction; may respond ***atropine*** in an inferior MI; pace if anterior MI.
  - Type 2 block is usually associated with distal fascicular disease and carr high risk of complete heart block, so pace in both types of MI.
- ***First degree block:*** Observe carefully: 40% develop higher degrees of block
- ***Bundle branch block:*** Pace prophylactically if evidence of trifascicular disea (p86) or non-adjacent bifascicular disease.
- ***Sino-atrial disease + serious symptoms:*** Pace unless responds to ***atropin***

Other indications where temporary pacing may be needed:

- Pre-op: if surgery is required in patients with type 2 or complete heart blc (whether or not MI has occurred); do 24h ECG; liaise with the anaesthetist.
- Drug poisoning, eg with β-blockers, digoxin, or verapamil.
- Symptomatic bradycardia, uncontrolled by ***atropine*** or ***isoprenaline***.
- Suppression of drug-resistant VT and SVT (overdrive pacing; do on ITU).
- Asystolic cardiac arrest with P-wave activity (ventricular standstill).
- During or after cardiac surgery—eg around the AV node or bundle of His.

Technique for temporary transvenous pacing Learn from an expert.

- ***Preparation:*** Monitor ECG; have a defibrillator to hand; check that radiographer with screening equipment is present.[1] Create a sterile field a ensure the pacing wire fits down the cannula easily. Insert a peripheral cannu
- ***Insertion:*** Place the cannula into the subclavian or internal jugular vein (p76 If this is difficult, access to the right atrium can be achieved *via* the femoral ve Pass the pacing wire through the cannula into the right atrium. It will either pa easily through the tricuspid valve or loop within the atrium. If the latter occu it is usually possible to flip the wire across the valve with a combined twisti and withdrawing movement. Advance the wire slightly. At this stage the wi may try to exit the ventricle through the pulmonary outflow tract. A furth withdrawing and rotation of the wire will aim the tip at the apex of the rig ventricle. Advance slightly again to place the wire in contact with t endocardium. Remove any slack to ↓risk of subsequent displacement.
- ***Checking the threshold:*** Connect the wire to the pacing box and set t 'demand' rate slightly higher than the patient's own heart rate and the output 3V. A paced rhythm should be seen. Find the pacing threshold by slowly reduci the voltage until the pacemaker fails to stimulate the tissue (pacing spikes are longer followed by paced beats). The threshold should be less than 1V, but slightly higher value may be acceptable if it is stable—eg after a large infarctic
- ***Setting the pacemaker:*** Set the output to 3V or over 3 times the thresho value (whichever is higher) in 'demand' mode. Set the rate as required. Suture t wire to the skin, and fix with a sterile dressing.
- Check the position of the wire (and exclude pneumothorax) with a CXR.
- Recurrent checks of the pacing threshold are required over the next few day The formation of endocardial oedema can raise the threshold by a factor of 2–

Complications Pneumothorax; sepsis; cardiac perforation; pacing failure: from lo of capture, loss of electrical continuity in pacing circuit, or electrode displacemer

1 Balloon-flotation techniques do not need radiographic guidance, have been shown to be quicker a easier to insert, with fewer complications compared to placement of semi-rigid electrode wires. RCT

Siting a temporary cardiac pacemaker

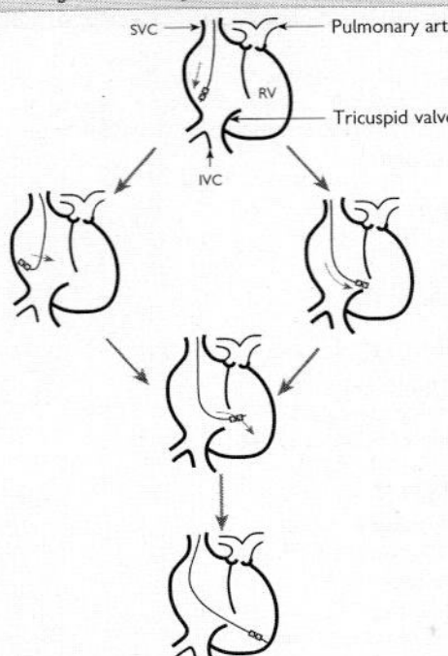

Non-invasive transcutaneous cardiac pacing

This method (performed through a defibrillator with external pacing facility) has the advantages of being quicker, less risky than the transvenous route, and easier to perform. Its main disadvantage is the pain caused by skeletal muscle contraction in the non-sedated patient. Indications for pacing via the transcutaneous route are as OPPOSITE, **plus** if transvenous pacing (or someone able to perform it) is unavailable or non-imminent in an emergency situation.

- ▸▸Give sedation and analgesia, eg ***midazolam*** + ***morphine*** IV titrated to effect.
- ▸▸Clipping chest hair may help improve electrical contact; ►don't shave the skin, as nicks can predispose to electrical burns. Ensure the skin is dry.
- ▸▸Almost all modern transcutaneous devices can function through defibrillation 'hands free' pads, and so these can be applied as for defibrillation (see p758). If necessary, the pads can be placed in an AP position: anteriorly over the V_2–V_3 electrode position and posteriorly at the same level, just below the scapula.
- ▸▸Select 'demand' mode, (which synchronises the stimulus with the R wave, so avoiding pacing on the T wave—which can provoke VF or VT) and adjust the ECG gain so that QRS complexes can be seen.
- ▸▸Select an appropriate pacing rate: eg 60–90bpm in an adult.
- ▸▸Set the pacing current at the lowest setting and turn on the pacemaker.
- ▸▸Increase the pacing current until electrical capture occurs (normally from 50–100mA), which can be confirmed by seeing a wide QRS complex **and** a T wave on the trace (ventricular electrical capture). This does not necessarily mean that there has been mechanical capture—one clinical trial has described using emergency cardiac ultrasound to assess for this.[26]
- ▸▸There will be some interference from skeletal muscle contraction on the ECG trace, as well as possible artefact, which could be mistaken for a QRS complex. The absence of a T wave is an important discriminator between the two.
- ▸▸CPR can continue with the pads in place, though only when the pacing unit is **off**.
- ▸▸Once adequate cardiac output has been maintained, seek expert help and arrange transvenous pacing.

21 Emergencies

Don't go so fast: we're in a hurry! Talleyrand to his coachm[illegible]

Many diseases may present as emergencies, but if you know about the followir[illegible] you will be very unlucky to lose a patient from a disease not listed here, on[illegible] general medical take, provided you remember to ask for help.

Emergencies covered in other chapters See inside front cover.

In OHCS—Paediatrics: Life support and cardiac arrest (OHCS p238–p239); is he[illegible] seriously ill? (*OHCS* p103); epiglottitis (*OHCS* p158). ***Adults:*** The major disaster (*OHC*[illegible] p806) Trauma (*OHCS* p718–p789); drowning (*OHCS* p724); ectopic pregnancy (*OHC*[illegible] p262); eclampsia (*OHCS* p48); amniotic fluid embolus (*OHCS* p89); obstetric shoc[illegible] (*OHCS* p55); glaucoma (*OHCS* p430); pre-hospital care/first aid (*OHCS* p790–p814)

Sources include: *BMJ*; *NEJM*; Oxford Handbook of Acute Medicine, OUP.

1 *We thank Dr S Haydock (Specialist Reader) & Specialist Readers from other chapters.*

Introduction to emergencies

There is nothing more intoxicating than spending a day saving lives, but as night creeps on, and you start losing more patients than you should, despair can hit with the force of ice. It is no comfort to know that you are now wiser and older (by 100yrs). So when you find yourself washing your hands between one death and the next, for one second be honest with yourself, and write of your errors and sorrows on the surface of the water—a few temporary ambiguous squiggles framing your thoughts and the life that is lost. This is not about audit and accountability (this comes later: now you need to fortify yourself to survive this onslaught)—so, in case a manager is looking over your shoulder, pull the plug, and as the water flows away, know that it mingles with the rising tide of our own failings at the bedside, through which we have surfaced—no doubt a little faster than we should. At your next bedside you may do better if you can buy time: time to take a history, time to think, and time to ask. To buy this precious time, support vital functions, as follows.

Preliminary assessment (primary survey)

Airway Protect cervical spine, if injury possible.
Assessment: any signs of obstruction? Ascertain patency
Management: establish a patent airway.

Breathing Assessment: determine respiratory rate, check bilateral chest movement, percuss and auscultate.
Management: if no respiratory effort, treat as arrest (see inside back cover), intubate and ventilate. If breathing compromised, give high concentration O_2, manage according to findings, eg relieve tension pneumothorax.

Circulation Assessment: check pulse and BP; is he peripherally shut-down?; check capillary refill; look for evidence of haemorrhage.
Management:
- if no cardiac output, treat as arrest (inside back cover)
- if shocked, treat as on p778.

Disability Assess 'level of consciousness' with AVPU score (alert? responds to voice? to pain? unresponsive?); check pupils: size, equality, reactions. *Glasgow Coma scale*, if time allows.

Exposure Undress patient, but cover to avoid hypothermia.

Quick history from relatives may assist with diagnosis: ***Events*** surrounding onset of illness, evidence of overdose/suicide attempt, any suggestion of trauma? ***Past medical history:*** Especially diabetes, asthma, COPD, alcohol, opiate or street drug abuse, epilepsy or recent head injury; recent travel. ***Medication:*** Current drugs. ***Allergies***.

Once ventilation and circulation are adequate, you may have bought enough time to carry out history, examination, investigations, and appropriate management in the usual way.

Headache: differential diagnosis

No signs on examination
- Tension headache
- Migraine
- Cluster headache
- Post-traumatic
- Drugs (nitrates, calcium channel antagonists)
- Carbon monoxide poisoning or anoxia

Signs of meningism?
- Meningitis (may not have fever or rash)
- Subarachnoid haemorrhage (examination may be normal)

Decreased conscious level or localizing signs?
- Encephalitis/meningitis
- Stroke
- Cerebral abscess
- Subarachnoid haemorrhage
- Tumour
- Subdural haematoma
- TB meningitis

Papilloedema?
- Tumour
- Malignant hypertension
- Benign intracranial hypertension
- Any CNS infection, if prolonged (eg >2wks)—eg TB meningitis

Others
- Temporal arteritis (ESR↑)
- Glaucoma
- Paget's disease (Alk Phos ↑↑)
- Sinusitis
- Altitude sickness
- Cervical spondylosis
- Venous sinus occlusion (focal neurological deficits)
- Vertebral artery dissection (neck pain and cerebellar/medullary signs)

Worrying features or 'red flags'[1]
- First and worst headache—*subarachnoid haemorrhage*
- Thunderclap headache—*subarachnoid haemorrhage;* (p470 for other causes
- Unilateral headache and eye pain—*cluster headache, acute glaucoma*
- Unilateral headache and ipsilateral symptoms—*migraine, tumour, vascular*
- Cough-initiated headache—*raised ICP/venous thrombosis*
- Persisting headache ± scalp tenderness in over 50s—*temporal arteritis*
- Headache with fever or neck stiffness—*meningitis*
- Change in the pattern of 'usual headaches'
- Decreased level of consciousness

Two other vital questions:
- Where have you been? (malaria)
- Might you be pregnant? (pre-eclampsia; especially if proteinuria and BP↑)

1 Adapted from C Hawkes 2002 *Hosp Med* **63** 732–42.

Breathlessness: emergency presentations

Wheezing?
- Asthma
- COPD
- Heart failure
- Anaphylaxis

Stridor? (Upper airway obstruction)
- Foreign body or tumour
- Acute epiglottitis
- Anaphylaxis
- Trauma, eg laryngeal fracture

Crepitations?
- Heart failure
- Pneumonia
- Bronchiectasis
- Fibrosis

Chest clear?
- Pulmonary embolism
- Hyperventilation
- Metabolic acidosis, eg diabetic ketoacidosis (DKA)
- Anaemia
- Drugs, eg salicylates
- Shock (may cause air hunger, p778)
- Pneumocystis pneumonia
- Central causes

Others
- Pneumothorax—pain, increased resonance
- Pleural effusion—'stony dullness'

Chest pain: differential diagnosis

First exclude any potentially life-threatening causes, by virtue of history, bri examination, and limited investigations. Then consider other potential causes. F the full assessment of cardiac pain, see p80 & p104.

Life-threatening

- Acute myocardial infarction
- Angina/acute coronary syndrome
- Aortic dissection
- Tension pneumothorax
- Pulmonary embolism
- Oesophageal rupture

Others

- Pneumonia
- Chest wall pain
  - Muscular
  - Rib fractures
  - Bony metastases
  - Costochondritis
- Gastro-oesophageal reflux
- Pleurisy
- Empyema
- Pericarditis
- Oesophageal spasm
- Herpes zoster
- Cervical spondylosis
- Intra-abdominal
  - Cholecystitis
  - Peptic ulceration
  - Pancreatitis
- Sickle-cell crisis

Before discharging patients with undiagnosed chest pain, be sure in your own mi that the pain is not cardiac (this pain is usually dull, may radiate to jaw, arm, epigastrium, and is usually associated with exertion). Do CXR, ECG, FBC, U&E, a 'cardiac' enzymes, including troponin T p104). Discuss options with a colleagu and the patient. Don't simply turn people out on to the street.

►Just because the patient's chest wall is tender to palpation, this doesn't mean t cause of the chest pain is musculoskeletal. Even if palpation reproduces the sar type of pain, ensure that you exclude all potential life-threatening causes. Althou chest wall tenderness has discriminatory value against cardiac pain, it may be feature of a pulmonary embolism.

Coma

Definition *Unrousable unresponsiveness.*

Causes of coma

Metabolic: Drugs, poisoning, eg carbon monoxide, alcohol, tricyclics
Hypoglycaemia, hyperglycaemia (ketoacidotic, or HONK, p816)
Hypoxia, CO_2 narcosis (COPD)
Septicaemia
Hypothermia
Myxoedema, Addisonian crisis
Hepatic/uraemic encephalopathy

Neurological: Trauma
Infection meningitis (p806); encephalitis, eg Herpes simplex give IV aciclovir if the slightest suspicion (p388), *tropical:* malaria (➡p385; do thick films), typhoid, rabies, trypanosomiasis
Tumour: cerebral/meningeal tumour
Vascular, subdural/subarachnoid haemorrhage, stroke, hypertensive encephalopathy
Epilepsy: non-convulsive status (p477) or post-ictal state

Immediate management see OPPOSITE (and coma CNS exam, p776)

- Assess airway, breathing, and circulation. Consider intubation if GCS <8. Support the circulation if required (ie IV fluids). Give O_2 and treat any seizures. Protect the cervical spine.
- Check blood glucose in all patients. Give 50mL 50% dextrose IV immediately if presumed hypoglycaemia.
- IV thiamine if any suggestion of Wernicke's encephalopathy.
- IV naloxone for opiate intoxication (may also be given IM or via ET tube); flumazenil for benzodiazepine intoxication if airway compromised (may precipitate seizures especially if tricyclic intoxication)

Examination

- Vital signs are vital—obtain full set, including temperature.
- Signs of trauma—haematoma, laceration, bruising, CSF/blood in nose or ears, fracture 'step' deformity of skull, subcutaneous emphysema, 'panda eyes'.
- Stigmata of other illnesses: liver disease, alcoholism, diabetes, myxoedema.
- Skin for needle marks, cyanosis, pallor, rashes, poor turgor.
- Smell the breath (alcohol, hepatic fetor, ketosis, uraemia).
- Meningism (p806) ►but do *not* move neck unless cervical spine is cleared.
- Pupils (p777) size, reactivity, gaze.
- Heart/lung exam for murmurs, rubs, wheeze, consolidation, collapse.
- Abdomen/rectal for organomegaly, ascites, bruising, peritonism, melaena.
- Are there any foci of infection (abscesses, bites, middle ear infection?)
- Any features of meningitis: neck stiffness, rash, focal neurology?
- Note the *absence* of signs, eg *no* pin-point pupils in a known heroin addict.

Quick history from family, ambulance staff, bystanders: Abrupt or gradual onset? How found—suicide note, seizure? If injured, suspect cervical spinal injury and do not move spine (*OHCS* p768). Recent complaints—headache, fever, vertigo, depression? Recent medical history—sinusitis, otitis, neurosurgery, ENT procedures? Past medical history—diabetes, asthma, ↑BP, cancer, epilepsy, psychiatric illness? Drug or toxin exposure (especially alcohol or other recreational drugs)? Any travel?

Taking stock The diagnosis may be clear, eg hyperglycaemia, alcohol excess, drug poisoning, uraemia, pneumonia, hypertensive, or hepatic encephalopathy (p251). If there are localizing CNS signs and no history of trauma, and there is no fever, the diagnosis is only probably stroke. In all undiagnosed coma patients or in those with focal neurological signs, a CT scan is very helpful. A lumbar puncture may be needed for meningitis (p806) or subarachnoid haemorrhage (p470).

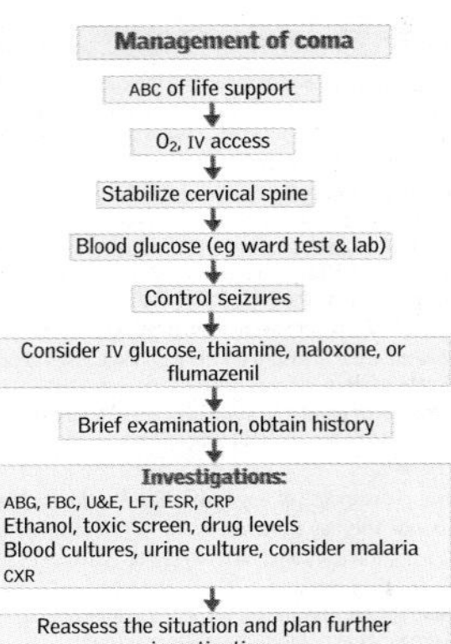

NB: check pupils every few minutes during the early stages, particularly if trauma is the likely cause. Doing so is the quickest way to find a localizing sign (so helpful in diagnosis, but remember that false localizing signs do occur)—and observing changes in pupil behaviour (eg becoming fixed and dilated) is the quickest way of finding out just how bad things are.

The Glasgow coma scale (GCS)

This gives a reliable, objective way of recording the conscious state of a person. can be used by medical and nursing staff for initial and continuing assessment. has value in predicting ultimate outcome. 3 types of response are assessed:

Best motor response This has 6 grades:

6 ***Carrying out request ('obeying command'):*** The patient does simple thin[g] you ask (beware of accepting a grasp reflex in this category).

5 ***Localizing response to pain:*** Put pressure on the patient's fingernail bed with pencil then try supraorbital and sternal pressure: purposeful movemen[t] towards changing painful stimuli is a 'localizing' response.

4 ***Withdraws to pain:*** Pulls limb away from painful stimulus.

3 ***Flexor response to pain:*** Pressure on the nail bed causes abnormal flexion limbs—decorticate posture.

2 ***Extensor posturing to pain:*** The stimulus causes limb extension (adductio internal rotation of shoulder, pronation of forearm)—decerebrate posture.

1 ***No response to pain.***

Note that it is the best response of any limb which should be recorded.

Best verbal response This has 5 grades:

5 ***Oriented:*** The patient knows who he is, where he is and why, the year, seaso and month.

4 ***Confused conversation:*** The patient responds to questions in a conversation manner but there is some disorientation and confusion.

3 ***Inappropriate speech:*** Random or exclamatory articulated speech, but r conversational exchange.

2 ***Incomprehensible speech:*** Moaning but no words.

1 ***None.***

Record level of best speech.

Eye opening This has 4 grades:

4 ***Spontaneous eye opening.***

3 ***Eye opening in response to speech:*** Any speech, or shout, not necessari request to open eyes.

2 ***Eye opening in response to pain:*** Pain to limbs as above.

1 ***No eye opening.***

An overall score is made by summing the score in the 3 areas assesse Eg: no response to pain + no verbalization + no eye opening = 3. Severe injury, GC ≤8; moderate injury, GCS 9–12; minor injury, GCS 13–15.

NB: An abbreviated coma scale, AVPU, is sometimes used in the initi assessment ('primary survey') of the critically ill:

- **A** = alert
- **V** = responds to **v**ocal stimuli
- **P** = responds to **p**ain
- **U** = **u**nresponsive

Some centres score GCS out of 14, not 15, omitting 'withdrawal to pai NB: The GCS scoring is different in young children; see *OHCS* p201.

Emergencies

The neurological examination in coma

This is aimed at locating the pathology in 1 of 2 places. Altered level of consciousness implies either **(1)** a diffuse, bilateral, cortical dysfunction (usually producing loss of awareness with normal arousal) or **(2)** damage to the ascending reticular activating system (ARAS) located throughout the brainstem from the medulla to the thalami (usually producing loss of arousal with unassessable awareness). The brainstem can be affected directly (eg pontine haemorrhage) or indirectly (eg compression from trans-tentorial or cerebellar herniation secondary to a mass or oedema).

- Level of consciousness; describe using *objective* words.
- Respiratory pattern—Cheyne–Stokes (p54), hyperventilation (acidosis, hypoxia, or rarely, neurogenic), ataxic or apneustic (breath-holding) breathing (brainstem damage with grave prognosis).
- Eyes—almost all patients with ARAS pathology will have eye findings.

Visual fields In light coma, test fields with visual threat. No blink in 1 field suggests hemianopsia and contralateral hemisphere lesion.

Pupils *Normal direct & consensual* = intact midbrain. *Midposition (3–5mm) non-reactive ± irregular* = midbrain lesion. *Unilateral dilated & unreactive* ('fixed') = 3rd nerve compression. *Small, reactive* = pontine lesion ('pinpoint pontine pupils') or drugs. *Horner's syndrome* (p694) = ipsilateral lateral medulla or hypothalamus lesion, may precede uncal herniation. Beware patients with false eyes or who use eye drops for glaucoma.

Extraocular movements (EOMs)—observe resting position and spontaneous movement; then test the vestibulo-ocular reflex (VOR) with either the *Doll's-head manoeuvre* (normal if the eyes keep looking at the same point in space when the head is quickly moved laterally or vertically) or *ice water calorics* (normal if eyes deviate towards the cold ear with nystagmus to the other side). If present, the VOR exonerates *most* of the brainstem from the VII nerve nucleus (medulla) to the III (midbrain). *Don't move the head unless the cervical spine is cleared.*

Fundi—papilloedema, subhyaloid haemorrhage, hypertensive retinopathy, signs of other disease (eg diabetic retinopathy).

- Examine for CNS asymmetry (tone, spontaneous movements, reflexes).

►►Shock

Essence Circulatory failure resulting in inadequate organ perfusion. *Generall* systolic BP is <90mmHg. Signs: pallor, pulse↑, capillary return↓ (press a nailbed air hunger, oliguria. Causes are either *pump failure* or *peripheral circulation failur*

Pump failure

- ***Cardiogenic shock***
- ***Secondary:*** *pulmonary embolism, tension pneumothorax, cardiac tamponade*

Peripheral circulation failure

- ***Hypovolaemia***
  Bleeding: trauma, ruptured aortic aneurysm, ruptured ectopic pregnancy. *Flui loss:* Vomiting (eg GI obstruction), diarrhoea (eg cholera), burns, pools (sequestered (unavailable) fluids ('third spacing', eg in pancreatitis). *Hea exhaustion* may cause hypovolaemic shock (also hyperpyrexia, oliguria, rhabdo myolysis, consciousness↓, hyperventilation, hallucination, incontinence, collaps coma, pin-point pupils, LFT↑, and DIC, p336).
- ***Anaphylaxis***
- ***Sepsis:*** Gram –ve (or +ve) septicaemic shock from endotoxin-induce vasodilatation may be sudden and severe, with shock and coma but no signs (infection (fever, WCC↑).
- ***Neurogenic:*** eg post-spinal surgery.
- ***Endocrine failure:*** Addison's disease or hypothyroidism; see p818.
- ***Iatrogenic:*** Drugs, eg anaesthetics, antihypertensives.

Assessment ►ABC.

- *ECG:* rate, rhythm, ischaemia?
- *General:* cold and clammy—cardiogenic shock or fluid loss. Look for signs (anaemia or dehydration—skin turgor, postural hypotension? Warm and we perfused, with bounding pulse—septic shock. Any features suggestive (anaphylaxis—history, urticaria, angio-oedema, wheeze?
- *CVS:* usually tachycardic (unless on β-blocker, or in spinal shock—*OHCS* p772) an hypotension. But in the young and fit, or pregnant women, the systolic BP ma remain normal, although the *pulse pressure* will narrow, with up to 30% bloo volume depletion. Difference between arms—aortic dissection?
- *JVP or central venous pressure:* If raised, cardiogenic shock likely.
- *Check abdomen:* any signs of trauma, or aneurysm? Any evidence of GI bleed?– check for melaena.

Management ►If BP unrecordable, call the cardiac arrest team.
See opposite for general management. Specific measures:

- ***Anaphylaxis:*** p780.
- ***Cardiogenic shock:*** p788.
- ***Septic shock:*** (if no clue to source, p372): IV cefuroxime 1.5g/6–8h (after bloo culture) or gentamicin (p738; do levels; reduce in renal failure) + antipseudo monal penicillin, eg ticarcillin (as Timentin®, p368, max dose 3.2g/4h IVI). Giv colloid, or crystalloid, by IVI. Refer to ITU if possible for monitoring ± inotropes aim for CVP 8–12mmHg, MAP >65mmHg. Urine >35ml/h. Low dose steroids ma help as may recombinant human activated Protein C.
- ***Hypovolaemic shock:*** Fluid replacement: saline or colloid initially; if bleeding us blood; risks and benefits: see p570. Titrate against BP, CVP, urine output. Trea the underlying cause. If severe haemorrhage, exsanguinating, or more than 1L o fluid required to maintain BP, consider using group-specific blood, or O Rh–v blood (p570). Correct electrolyte abnormalities. Acidosis often responds to flui replacement.
- ***Heat exposure (heat exhaustion):*** tepid sponging + fanning; avoid ice an immersion. Resuscitate with high-sodium IVI, such as 0.9% saline ± hydrocortisone 100mg IV. Dantrolene seems ineffective. Chlorpromazine 25mg IM may be used to stop shivering. Stop cooling when core temperature <39°C

Management of shock

If BP unrecordable, call the cardiac arrest team

↓

ABC (including high-flow O_2)

↓

Raise foot of the bed

↓

IV access × 2 (wide bore; get help if this takes >2min)

↓

Identify and treat underlying cause

↓

Infuse crystalloid *fast* to raise BP (unless cardiogenic shock)

↓

Seek expert help early

↓

Investigations
- FBC, U&E, ABG, glucose, CRP
- Cross-match and check clotting
- Blood cultures, urine culture, ECG, CXR
- *Others:* lactate, echo, abdominal CT, USS

↓

Consider arterial line, central venous line, and bladder catheter (aim for a urine flow >30mL/h)

↓

Further management
- Treat underlying cause if possible
- Fluid replacement as dictated by BP, CVP, urine output
- Don't overload with fluids if cardiogenic shock (exclude PE & RV infarct 1st)
- If persistently hypotensive, consider inotropes

NB: Remember that higher flow rates can be achieved through peripheral lines than through 'standard' gauge central lines.
If cause unclear: ℞ as hypovolaemia—most common cause, and reversible.
Ruptured abdominal aortic aneurysm: aim for a systolic BP of ~90mmHg.

SIRS, sepsis, and related symptoms

The pathogenesis of sepsis and septic shock is becoming increasingly understood. The 'systemic inflammatory response syndrome' (SIRS) is thought to be a central component, involving cytokine cascades, free radical production, and the release of vasoactive mediators. SIRS is defined as the presence of 2 or more of the following features:[4]
- Temperature >38°C or <36°C
- Tachycardia >90 bpm
- Respiratory rate >20 breaths/min or P_aCO_2 <4.3 kPa
- WBC >12×10⁹/L or <4×10⁹/L, or >10% immature (band) forms

Related syndromes include:

Sepsis: SIRS occurring in the presence of infection.

Severe sepsis: Sepsis with evidence of organ hypoperfusion eg hypoxaemia, oliguria, lactic acidosis, or altered cerebral function.

Septic shock: Severe sepsis with hypotension (systolic BP <90mmHg) despite adequate fluid resuscitation, or the requirement for vasopressors/inotropes to maintain blood pressure.

Septicaemia was used to denote the presence of multiplying bacteria in the circulation, but has been replaced with the definitions above.[5]

▸▸Anaphylactic shock

Type I IgE-mediated hypersensitivity reaction. Release of histamine and othe agents causes: capillary leak; wheeze; cyanosis; oedema (larynx, lids, tongue, lips urticaria. More common in atopic individuals. An *anaphylactoid reaction* result from direct release of mediators from inflammatory cells, without involvir antibodies, usually in response to a drug, eg acetylcysteine.

Common precipitants

- Drugs, eg penicillin, and contrast media in radiology
- Latex
- Stings, eggs, fish, peanuts, strawberries, semen

Signs and symptoms

- Itching, erythema, urticaria, oedema
- Wheeze, laryngeal obstruction, cyanosis
- Tachycardia, hypotension

Management of anaphylaxis

Secure the airway—give 100% O_2
Intubate if respiratory obstruction imminent

↓

Remove the cause; raising the feet may help restore the circulation

↓

Give adrenaline IM ***0.5mg (ie 0.5mL of 1 : 1000)***
Repeat every 5min, if needed as guided by BP, pulse, and respiratory function, until better

↓

Secure IV access

↓

Chlorphenamine 10mg IV and hydrocortisone 200mg IV

↓

IVI (0.9% saline, eg 500mL over ¼h; up to 2L may be needed)
Titrate against blood pressure

↓

If wheeze, treat for asthma (p794)
May require ventilatory support

↓

If still hypotensive, admission to ITU and an IVI of adrenaline may be needed ± aminophylline (p795) and nebulized salbutamol (p795): get expert help.

↓

Further management:

- Admit to ward. Monitor ECG.
- Continue chlorphenamine 4mg/6h PO if itching.
- Suggest a 'Medic-alert' bracelet naming the culprit allergen (p744).
- Teach about self-injected adrenaline (eg 0.3mg, Epipen®) to prevent a fatal attack.
- Skin-prick tests showing specific IgE help identify allergens to avoid.

NB: *⇥adrenaline (=epinephrine) is given IM and NOT IV unless the patient is severely ill, or has no pulse. The IV dose is **different:** 100µg per min—titrating with the response. This is 1mL of **1 : 10,000 solution** per minute. Stop as soon as a response has been obtained.*

If on a β-blocker, consider salbutamol IV in place of adrenaline.

Acute myocardial infarction*

A common medical emergency, and prompt appropriate treatment saves lives a myocardium. If in doubt, seek immediate help. Diagnosis: p104.

Pre-hospital management

Arrange an emergency ambulance. Aspirin 300mg PO (unless cle contraindication). Analgesia, eg morphine 5–10mg IV + metoclopramide 10mg (avoid IM injections, as risk of bleeding with thrombolysis). Sublingual GTN unle hypotensive.

Management See OPPOSITE for acute measures.

Thrombolysis effective in reducing mortality if given early. Greatest benefit is se if given <12h of the onset of chest pain, but some benefit up to 24h. The Briti Heart Foundation advises that the time from onset of pain to thrombolysis shou be <90min (<60min if possible).

Indications for thrombolysis: Presentation within *12h* of chest pain with:

- ST elevation >2mm in 2 or more chest leads or
- ST elevation >1mm in 2 or more limb leads or
- Posterior infarction (dominant R waves and ST depression in V_1–V_3)
- New onset left bundle branch block.

Presentation within *12–24h* if continuing chest pain and/or ST elevation.

Thrombolysis contraindications: (consider urgent angioplasty instead)

- Internal bleeding
- Prolonged or traumatic CPR
- Heavy vaginal bleeding
- Acute pancreatitis
- Active lung disease with cavitation
- Recent trauma or surgery (<2wks)
- Cerebral neoplasm
- Severe hypertension (>200/120mmHg)
- Suspected aortic dissection
- Previous allergic reaction
- Pregnancy or <18wks postnatal
- Severe liver disease
- Oesophageal varices
- Recent head trauma
- Recent haemorrhagic stroke

Relative CI: History of severe hypertension; peptic ulcer; history of CVA; bleedir diathesis; pregnancy; ≤18 weeks post-partum; anticoagulants.

Streptokinase (SK) is the usual thrombolytic agent. Dose: 1.5 million units 100mL 0.9% saline IVI over 1h. SE: nausea; vomiting; haemorrhage; stroke (1% dysrhythmias. Any hypotension usually responds to slowing down or stopping tl infusion. Also watch for allergic reactions and anaphylaxis (rare). Do not repea unless it is within 4d of the first administration.

Alteplase (rt-PA), followed by heparin, may be indicated if the patient ha previously received SK (>4d ago) or reacted to SK. Accelerated rt-PA has benefit given within 6h, especially in younger patients with anterior MI. ***Reteplase*** is give as 2 IV boluses 2h apart, and ***tenecteplase*** is given by bolus injection (over 10sec which in some cases may be an advantage.

Complications

- Recurrent ischaemia or failure to reperfuse (usually detected as persisting pai and ST-segment elevation in the immediate aftermath of thrombolysis analgesia, GTN, β-blocker, consider re-thrombolysis or angioplasty.
- Stroke.
- Pericarditis: analgesics, try to avoid NSAIDs.
- Cardiogenic shock: see p788 and heart failure: see p786.

Right ventricular infarction

- Confirm by demonstrating ST elevation in RV3/4, and/or echo. NB: RV4 means tha V_4 is placed in the right 5th intercostal space in the midclavicular line.
- Treat hypotension and oliguria with fluids.
- Avoid nitrates and diuretics.
- Intensive monitoring and inotropes may be useful in some patients.

*Refers to acute coronary syndrome with ST-segment elevation, new LBBB, or true posterior MI.

Management of an acute MI

Attach ECG monitor and record a 12-lead ECG

↓

High-flow O_2 by face mask (caution, if COPD)

↓

IV access
Bloods for FBC, U&E, glucose, lipids, cardiac enzymes (p105)

↓

Brief assessment
- History of cardiovascular disease; risk factors for IHD
- Contraindications to thrombolysis?
- Examination: pulse, BP, JVP, cardiac murmurs, signs of heart failure, peripheral pulses, scars from previous cardiac surgery

↓

Aspirin 300mg (unless already given by GP/paramedics)

↓

Morphine 5–10mg IV + antiemetic, eg metoclopramide 10mg IV

↓

GTN sublingually 2 puffs or 1 tablet as required

↓

Thrombolysis see OPPOSITE

↓

β-blocker, eg atenolol 5mg IV (unless asthma or left ventricular failure)

↓

CXR
Do not delay thrombolysis while waiting unless suspected aneurysm

↓

Consider glucose, insulin, and potassium infusion for patients with diabetes mellitus (DIGAMI **regimen**[1])

↓

Consider DVT prophylaxis

↓

Continue medication except calcium channel antagonists (unless specific indication)

↓

For further management: see p108

NB: ►*If pain is uncontrolled, especially if continuing ST elevation, consider re-thrombolysis with rt-PA (no bolus), tenecteplase, or rescue angioplasty.*

ote on the role of glucose, potassium, and insulin infusion (GKI) in acute MI. *GKI* in acute MI gone in and out of vogue. Evidence for insulin infusion in whatever form in diabetic patients is e clear, and this should probably be part of our 'best care' management. More recently, interest focused on the role of such infusions in non-diabetic patients. Some, but not all, studies/meta-yses suggest benefit: R Diaz 1998 *Circulation* **98** 2227 G Krljanac Am J Cardiol 2005 **96** 053

Acute coronary syndrome—without ST-elevation

Acute coronary syndrome (ACS) includes ***unstable angina***, evolving ***myocardi[al] infarction*** (MI), and non-Q wave or subendocardial MI. Although the underlyi[ng] pathology is similar, management differs and, therefore, ACS is usually divided in[to] 2 classes:

- ***ACS with ST segment elevation*** or new LBBB (acute MI see p782).
- ***ACS without ST segment elevation*** (unstable angina or non-Q wave MI).

ACS is associated with a greatly increased risk of MI (up to 30% in the 1st mont[h]). Patients should be managed medically until symptoms settle. They are th[en] investigated by angiography with a view to possible angioplasty or surgery (CAB[G]).

Assessment

Brief history: previous angina, relief with rest/nitrates, history of cardiovascu[lar] disease, risk factors for IHD.

Examination: pulse, BP, JVP, cardiac murmurs, signs of heart failure, periphe[ral] pulses, scars from previous cardiac surgery.

Investigations ECG: ST depression; flat or inverted T waves; or normal. FBC, U&[E], glucose, lipids, cardiac enzymes. CXR.

Measurement of cardiac troponins helps to predict which patients are at risk o[f] cardiac event, and who can be safely discharged early. Note that 2 differe[nt] forms of troponin are measured: troponin T and troponin I: they have differe[nt] reference intervals (consult your lab).

Emergencies

Management

►See OPPOSITE for acute management

►For management of ACS with ST-elevation, see p782.

The aim of drug therapy is twofold:

1. Anti-ischaemic, eg β-blocker, nitrate, calcium channel antagonist.
2. Antithrombotic, eg aspirin, low molecular weight heparin, abciximab, wh[ich] interfere with platelet activation, and so reduce thrombus formation.

Further measures:

- Wean off *glyceryl trinitrate* (GTN) infusion when stabilized on oral drugs.
- Stop heparin when pain-free for 24h, but give at least 3–5 days of therapy.
- Check serial ECGs and cardiac enzymes for 2–3d.
- Address modifiable risk factors: smoking, hypertension, hyperlipidaem[ia], diabetes.
- Gentle mobilization.

►*If symptoms recur, refer to a cardiologist for urgent angiography and angiopla[sty] or CABG.*

Prognosis Overall risk of death ~1–2%, but ~15% for refractory angina desp[ite] medical therapy. Risk stratification can help predict those most at risk and all[ow] intervention to be targeted at those individuals. The following are associated w[ith] an increased risk:

- Haemodynamic instability: hypotension, pulmonary oedema.
- T-wave inversion or ST segment depression on resting ECG.
- Previous MI.
- Prolonged rest pain.
- Older age.
- Diabetes mellitus.

Indications for consideration of invasive intervention:

- Poor prognosis, eg pulmonary oedema.
- Refractory symptoms.
- Positive exercise tolerance tests (ETT) at low workload.
- Non-Q wave MI.

Acute management of ACS without ST-segment elevation

Admit to CCU and monitor closely

↓

High-flow O_2 by face mask

↓

Analgesia: eg morphine 5–10mg IV + metoclopramide 10mg IV

↓

Nitrates: GTN spray or sublingual tablets as required

↓

Aspirin: 300mg PO (unless contraindicated) *reduces risk of MI and death*

↓

Oral β-blocker: eg metoprolol 50–100mg/8h or atenolol 50–100mg/24h
If β-blocker contraindicated (asthma, COPD, LVF, bradycardia, coronary artery spasm), give rate-limiting calcium antagonist (eg verapamil[1] *80–120mg/8h PO, or diltiazem 60–120mg/8h PO)*

↓

Low molecular weight heparin: (eg enoxaparin 1mg/kg/12h or dalteparin 120U/kg/12h SC)
Alternatively: unfractionated heparin 5000U IV bolus then IVI
Check APTT 6-hourly. Alter IVI rate to maintain APTT at 1.5–2.5 times control

↓

IV nitrate if pain continues
(eg GTN 50mg in 50mL 0.9% saline at 2–10mL/h)
titrate to pain, and maintain systolic BP >100mmHg

↓

Record ECG while in pain

High-risk patients
(persistent or recurrent ischaemia, ST-depression, diabetes, ↑troponin)
- Infusion of a GPIIb/IIIa antagonist (eg tirofiban)[9] and, ideally, urgent angiography.
- Addition of clopidogrel may also be useful

↓

Optimize drugs:
- β-blocker; Ca^{2+} channel antagonist; ACE-i; nitrate.
- Intensive statin regimens, *starting at top dosages*, may decrease long- *and* short-term mortality/adverse events, eg by stabilizing plaques.[2,3]

↓

►*If symptoms fail to improve, refer to a cardiologist for urgent angiography ± angioplasty or CABG*

Low-risk patients
(no further pain, flat or inverted T-waves, or normal ECG, ***and*** *negative troponin)*
- May be discharged if a repeat troponin (>12h) is negative.
- Treat medically and arrange further investigation eg stress test, angiogram.

1 Do not use verapamil and a β-blocker together (can cause asystole).
2 Comparing intensive & moderate lipid lowering with statins after ACS. N=4162. Cannon C *NEJM* 2004
3 Intensive statin therapy—a sea change in cardiovascular prevention. Topol E *NEJM* 2004.

➤Severe pulmonary oedema

Causes

- Cardiovascular—usually left ventricular failure—post-MI, or ischaemic hea disease. Also mitral stenosis, arrhythmias, and malignant hypertension.
- ARDS (p170, any cause, eg trauma, malaria, drugs), look for predisposing facto eg trauma, post-op, sepsis. *Is aspirin overdose or glue-sniffing/drug abuse likel* Ask friends/relatives.
- Fluid overload.
- Neurogenic, eg head injury.

Differential diagnosis Asthma/COPD, pneumonia, and pulmonary oedema are oft hard to distinguish, especially in the elderly, where that may co-exist. Do n hesitate to treat all 3 simultaneously (eg with salbutamol nebulizer, furosemide diamorphine, amoxicillin—p368).

Symptoms Dyspnoea, orthopnoea (eg paroxysmal), pink frothy sputum. NB: druç other illnesses (recent MI/COPD or pneumonia).

Signs Distressed, pale, sweaty, pulse↑, tachypnoea, pink frothy sputum, puls alternans, JVP↑, fine lung crackles, triple/gallop rhythm (p32), wheeze (cardi asthma). Usually sitting up and leaning forward. Quickly examine for possib causes.

Emergencies

Investigations

- CXR (p121)—cardiomegaly, signs of pulmonary oedema: look for shadowi (usually bilateral), small effusions at costophrenic angles, fluid in the lu fissures, and Kerley B lines (linear opacities).
- ECG—signs of MI.
- U&E; 'cardiac' enzymes, ABG.
- Consider echo.
- Plasma BNP may be helpful if diagnosis in question.

Management

Begin treatment before investigations. See OPPOSITE.

Monitoring progress: BP; heart rate; cyanosis; respiratory rate; JVP; urine outp ABG.

Once stable and improving:

- Daily weights; BP and pulse/6h. Repeat CXR.
- Change to oral furosemide or bumetanide.
- If on large doses of loop diuretic, consider the addition of a thiazide (bendroflumethiazide or metolazone 2.5–5mg daily PO).
- ACE-i if left ventricular failure. If ACE-i contraindicated, consider hydralazine a nitrate (may also be more effective in (Afrocaribbeans).
- Also consider β-blocker and spironolactone.
- Is the patient suitable for cardiac transplantation?
- Consider digoxin ± warfarin, especially if AF.

Nesiritide, recombinant human brain natriuretic peptide, may have a role in the short-term managem of decompensate cardiac failure as it improves haemodymanics in such patients. However, expensive and further data on safety and outcome are required before it is more widely adopted.

Management of heart failure

Sit the patient upright

↓

Oxygen
100% if no pre-existing lung disease

↓

IV access and monitor ECG
Treat any arrhythmias, eg AF (p110–p116)

↓

Investigations whilst continuing treatment
see OPPOSITE

↓

Diamorphine 2.5–5mg IV slowly
Caution in liver failure and *COPD*

↓

Furosemide 40–80mg IV slowly
Larger doses required in renal failure

↓

GTN spray 2 puffs SL or 2 × 0.3mg tablets SL
Don't give if systolic BP <90mmHg

↓

Necessary investigations, examination, and history

↓

If systolic BP ≥100mmHg, start a nitrate infusion
eg isosorbide dinitrate 2–10mg/h IVI; keep systolic BP ≥90mmHg

↓

If the patient is worsening: further dose of furosemide 40–80mg
Consider ventilation (invasive or non-invasive eg CPAP; get help) or increasing nitrate infusion
Alternatively venesect 500mL blood (rarely done)

↓

If systolic BP <100mmHg, treat as cardiogenic shock (p788),
ie consider a Swan-Ganz catheter and inotropic support

Notes

- If failure to improve, reassess and consider alternative diagnoses, eg hypertensive heart failure, aortic dissection, pulmonary embolism, pneumonia.
- There are logical reasons for considering using nitrates first-line rather than loop diuretics: nitrates reduce pre- and after-load and are coronary vasodilators. In contrast most of the acute beneficial effects of loop diuretics stem from venodilatation rather than diuresis. Only small randomized trials have compared the two therapies but nitrates seem as, if not more effective that loop diuretics.

⏩Cardiogenic shock

This has a high mortality. ►Ask a senior physician's help both in formulating exact diagnosis and in guiding treatment.

Cardiogenic shock is shock caused primarily by the failure of the heart to maint the circulation. It may occur suddenly, or after progressively worsening he failure.

Causes

- Myocardial infarction
- Arrhythmias
- Pulmonary embolus
- Tension pneumothorax
- Cardiac tamponade
- Myocarditis; myocardial depression (drugs, hypoxia, acidosis, sepsis)
- Valve destruction (endocarditis)
- Aortic dissection

Management

If the cause is myocardial infarction prompt revascularization (thrombolysis acute angioplasty) is vital; ⏩see p782[1] for indications and contraindications.

- Manage in Coronary Care Unit, if possible.
- Investigation and treatment may need to be done concurrently.
- See OPPOSITE for details of management.
- ***Investigations*** ECG, U&E, CK, ABG, CXR, echo. If indicated, CT thorax (ao dissection/PE) or V̇/Q̇ scan.
- ***Monitor*** CVP, BP, ABG, ECG; urine output. Do a 12-lead ECG every hour until diagnosis is made. Consider a Swan–Ganz catheter to assess pulmonary wec pressure and cardiac output, and an arterial line to monitor pressure. Catheter for accurate urine output.

Cardiac tamponade

Essence: Pericardial fluid collects → intra-pericardial pressure rises → heart can fill → pumping stops.

Causes: Trauma, lung/breast cancer, pericarditis, myocardial infarct, bacteria, TB. *Rarely:* Urea↑, radiation, myxoedema, dissecting aorta, SLE.

Signs: Falling BP, a rising JVP, and muffled heart sounds (Beck's triad); JVP↑ inspiration (Kussmaul's sign); pulsus paradoxus (pulse fades on inspiratio Echocardiography may be diagnostic. CXR: globular heart; left heart border conv or straight; right cardiophrenic angle <90°. ECG: electrical alternans (p140).

Management: This can be very difficult. Everything is against you: tir physiology, and your own confidence, as the patient may be too ill to give a histo and signs may be equivocal—but bitter experience has taught us not to equivoc for long.

⏩Request the presence of your senior at the bedside (do not make do w telephone advice). With luck, prompt pericardiocentesis (p761) brings swift rel While awaiting this, give O_2, monitor ECG, and set up IVI. Take blood for group a save.

1 SHOCK trial 2003 V Menon *Congest Heart Fail* 9 35. NNT for acute angioplasty = 5.

Management of cardiogenic shock

Oxygen
Titrate to maintain adequate arterial saturations

↓

Diamorphine 2.5–5mg IV for pain and anxiety

↓

Investigations and **close monitoring**
(see OPPOSITE)

↓

Correct arrhythmias (p110–p114), U&E abnormalities or acid–base disturbance

↓

Optimize filling pressure
if available measure pulmonary capillary wedge pressure (PCWP)

If PCWP <15mmHg fluid load
↓
Give a plasma expander 100mL every 15min IV Aim for PCWP of 15–20mmHg

If PCWP >15mmHg
↓
Inotropic support eg dobutamine 2.5–10μg/kg/min IVI. Aim for a systolic BP >80mmHg

↓

Consider 'renal dose' dopamine
2–5μg/kg/min IV (via central line only)

↓

Consider intra-aortic balloon pump if you expect the underlying condition to improve, or you need time awaiting surgery

↓

Look for and treat any reversible cause
MI or PE—consider thrombolysis;
surgery for: acute VSD, mitral, or aortic incompetence

▸▸Broad complex tachycardia

ECG shows rate of >100bpm and QRS complexes >120ms (>3 small squares on EC done at the standard UK rate of 25mm/s).

Principles of management

If in doubt, treat as ventricular tachycardia (the commonest cause).
Identify the underlying rhythm and treat accordingly.

Differential

- Ventricular tachycardia (VT) including torsade de pointes
- SVT with aberrant conduction, eg AF, atrial flutter
- Pre-excited tachycardias, eg AF, atrial flutter, or AV re-entry tachycardia wi underlying WPW (p112).

(NB: Ventricular ectopics should not cause confusion when occurring singly; but >3 together at a rate of >120, this constitutes VT.)

Identification of the underlying rhythm may be difficult, seek expert hel Diagnosis is based on the history: if IHD/MI the likelihood of a ventricular arrhyt mia is >95%, a 12-lead ECG, and the lack of response to IV adenosine (p112).

ECG findings in favour of VT:

- Fusion beats or capture beats (ECG p115).
- Positive QRS concordance in chest leads.
- Marked left axis deviation or rightwards axis.
- AV dissociation (occurs in 25%) or 2 : 1 or 3 : 1 AV block.
- QRS complex >160ms.
- Any atypical bundle-branch-block pattern.

Management Give high-flow O_2 by mask and monitor O_2 saturations.

- Connect patient to a cardiac monitor and have a defibrillator to hand.
- Correct electrolyte abnormalities.
- Check for adverse signs. Low cardiac output (clammy, consciousness↓, BP <9(oliguria; angina; pulmonary oedema.
- Obtain 12-lead ECG (request CXR) and obtain IV access.

If haemodynamically unstable

- Synchronized DC shock (see Resuscitation Guidelines inside back cover).
- Correct any hypokalaemia and hypomagnesaemia: 60mmol KCl at 30mmol/ and 5mL 50% magnesium sulphate over 30min).
- Follow with amiodarone 300mg IV over 20-60min.
- For refractory cases procainamide or sotalol may be considered.

If haemodynamically stable

- Correct hypokalaemia and hypomagnesaemia: as above.
- Amiodarone 300mg IV over 20–60 min. Alternatively lidocaine 50mg (2.5mL 2% solution) IV over 2min, repeated every 5min up to 200mg.
- If this fails, use synchronized DC shock.

After correction of VT

- Establish the cause (via the history and tests above)
- Maintenance anti-arrhythmic therapy may be required. If VT occurs after MI, gi IV amiodarone or lidocaine infusion for 12–24h; if 24h after MI, also start oı anti-arrhythmic: sotalol (if good LV function) or amiodarone (if poor LV functio
- Prevention of recurrent VT: surgical isolation of the arrhythmogenic area implantation of tiny automatic defibrillators may help.

Ventricular fibrillation (ECG p115 Use non-synchronized DC shock (there is no wave to trigger defibrillation, p758): see inside back cover.

Ventricular extrasystoles (ectopics) are the commonest post-MI arrhythmia b they are also seen in healthy people (often >10/h). Patients with frequent ectopi post-MI have a worse prognosis, but there is no evidence that antidysrhythr drugs improve outcome, indeed they may increase mortality.

orsade de pointes: A form of VT, with a constantly varying axis, often in the ›tting of long-QT syndromes (ECG p115); causes, p702. This can be congenital or cquired, eg from drugs (eg some anti-dysrhythmics, tricyclics, antimalarials, and ewer antipsychotics). Torsade in the setting of congenital long-QT syndromes can e treated with high doses of β-blockers.

In acquired long-QT syndromes, stop all predisposing drugs, correct ypokalaemia, and give $MgSO_4^{2+}$ (2g IV over 10 min). Alternatives include: overdrive acing or isoprenaline IVI to increase heart rate.

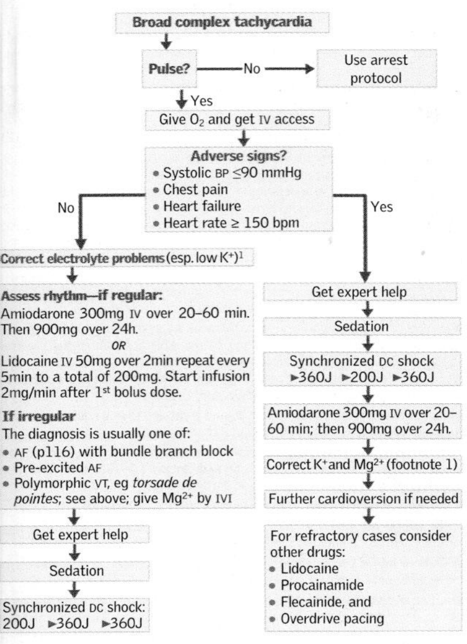

If potassium low: give **potassium chloride** by IVI, up to 60mmol, max. rate 30mmol/h. ›ive **magnesium sulfate** IVI 5mL 50% in 30min.

►►Narrow complex tachycardia

ECG shows rate of >100bpm and QRS complex duration of <120ms (<3 sm squares on ECGs done at the standard UK rate of 25mm/s).

Differential diagnosis

- ***Sinus tachycardia:*** normal P-wave followed by normal QRS.
- ***Atrial tachyarrhythmias:*** Rhythm arises in atria, AV node is a bystander.
  - Atrial fibrillation (AF): absent P-wave, irregular QRS complexes.
  - Atrial flutter: atrial rate ~260–340bpm. Saw-tooth baseline, due to continuo atrial electrical activity. Ventricular rate often 150bpm (2 : 1 block).
  - Atrial tachycardia: abnormally shaped P-waves, may outnumber QRS.
  - Multifocal atrial tachycardia: 3 or more P-wave morphologies, irregular Q complexes.
- ***Junctional tachycardia:*** AV-node is part of the pathway. P-wave either buried QRS complex or occurring after QRS complex.
  - AV nodal re-entry tachycardia.
  - AV re-entry tachycardia, includes an accessory pathway, eg WPW (p112).

Principles of management See algorithm OPPOSITE.

- If the patient is compromized, use DC cardioversion.
- Otherwise, identify the underlying rhythm and treat accordingly. The chief thi is to decide whether the rhythm is regular or not (likely AF).
- Vagal manoeuvres (carotid sinus massage, Valsalva manoeuvre) transient increase AV block, and may unmask an underlying atrial rhythm.
- If unsuccessful, give adenosine which causes transient AV block. It has a sho half-life (10–15s) and works in 2 ways:
  - by transiently slowing ventricles to show the underlying atrial rhythm,
  - by cardioverting a junctional tachycardia to sinus rhythm.

Give 6mg IV bolus into a large vein, followed by saline flush, while recording rhythm strip. If unsuccessful, give 12mg, then one further 12mg bolus. Warn abo SE: transient chest tightness, dyspnoea, headache, flushing. ***Relative CI:*** asthm 2nd/3rd-degree AV block or sinoatrial disease (unless pacemaker). ***Interaction*** potentiated by dipyridamole, antagonized by theophylline.

Specifics ***Sinus tachycardia:*** Identify and treat underlying cause.

Supraventricular tachycardia: If adenosine fails, use verapamil 2.5–5mg IV ov 2–3min. **NB:** NOT if on a β-blocker. If no response, a further 5mg IV over 3min age <60yrs). Alternatives: atenolol 5mg IV or sotalol 20–120mg IV (over 10mi or amiodarone. If unsuccessful, use DC cardioversion.

Atrial fibrillation/flutter: Manage along standard lines (p116).

Atrial tachycardia: Rare; may be due to digoxin toxicity: withdraw digox consider digoxin-specific antibody fragments. Maintain K^+ at 4–5mmol/L.

Multifocal atrial tachycardia: Most commonly occurs in COPD. Correct hypox and hypercapnia. Consider verapamil if rate remains >110bpm.

Junctional tachycardia: Where anterograde conduction through the AV no occurs, vagal manoeuvres are worth trying. Adenosine will usually cardiovert junctional rhythm to sinus rhythm. If it fails or recurs, β-blockers (or verapamil ***not*** with β-blockers, digoxin, or class I agents such as quinidine). If this does n control symptoms, consider radiofrequency ablation.

Wolff–Parkinson–White (WPW) syndrome (*ECG* p117) Caused by congeni accessory conduction pathway between atria and ventricles. Resting ECG show short P–R interval and widened QRS complex due to slurred upstroke or 'delta wav 2 types: WPW type A (+ve δ wave in V_1), WPW type B (–ve δ wave in V_1). Patier present with SVT which may be due to an AVRT, (p112) pre-excited AF, or pr excited atrial flutter. Risk of degeneration to VF and sudden death. ℞ flecainic propafenone, sotalol, or amiodarone. Refer to cardiologist for electrophysiology a ablation of the accessory pathway.

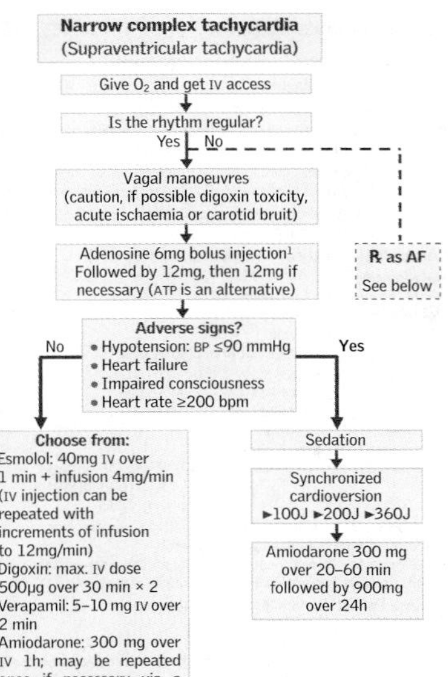

regular narrow complex tachycardia

Treat as AF—by far the most likely diagnosis.
Control rate with either β blocker or digoxin.
If onset <48h consider cardioversion with either amiodarone, 300mg in over 20–60 min, then 900mg over 24h; or DC shock, see p758.
Consider anticoagulation with heparin and/or warfarin to reduce the risk of stroke.

onsult *BNF* if on dipyridamole or has had a heart transplant
Resuscitation Council (UK) guidance for more details (www.resus.org.uk)

➡Acute severe asthma

►The severity of an attack is easily underestimated.

►An atmosphere of calm helps.

Presentation Acute breathlessness and wheeze.

History Ask about usual and recent treatment; previous acute episodes and t severity and best peak expiratory flow rate (PEF). Have they been admitted to

Differential diagnosis Acute infective exacerbation of COPD, pulmonary oede upper respiratory tract obstruction, pulmonary embolus, anaphylaxis.

Investigations PEF—but may be too ill; arterial blood gases; CXR (to excl pneumothorax, infection); FBC; U&E.

Assessing the severity of an acute asthmatic attack

Severe attack:

- Unable to complete sentences
- Respiratory rate >25/min
- Pulse rate >110 beats/min
- Peak expiratory flow <50% of predicted or best

Life-threatening attack:

- Peak expiratory flow <33% of predicted or best
- Silent chest, cyanosis, feeble respiratory effort
- Bradycardia or hypotension
- Exhaustion, confusion, or coma
- Arterial blood gases: normal/high P_aCO_2 >5kPa (36mmHg)
  P_aO_2 <8kPa (60mmHg)
  low pH, eg <7.35

Treatment ►Life-threatening or severe asthma, see OPPOSITE.

- Salbutamol 5mg **nebulized with oxygen**.
- If PEF remains <75%, repeat salbutamol and give prednisolone 30mg PO.
- Monitor oxygen saturation, heart rate, and respiratory rate.

Discharge Patients, before discharge, must have:

- Been on discharge medication for 24h.
- Had inhaler technique checked.
- Peak flow rate >75% predicted or best with diurnal variability <25%.
- Steroid and bronchodilator therapy.
- Own a PEF meter and have management plan.
- GP appointment within 1wk.
- Respiratory clinic appointment within 4wks.

Drugs used in acute asthma

Salbutamol (β_2-agonist) *SE:* Tachycardia, arrhythmias, tremor, K^+↓.

Hydrocortisone (steroid)

Aminophylline (Inhibits phosphodiesterase; ↑[cAMP]). *SE:* pulse↑; arrhythmia nausea, seizures. The amount of IVI aminophylline may need altering accordir to the individual patient: always check the *BNF*. Monitor ECG.

- ***Factors which may necessitate reduction of dose:*** Cardiac or liver fail drugs which increase the half-life of aminophylline, eg cimetidine, ciproflox erythromycin, contraceptive steroids.
- ***Factors which may require*** ↑*dose:* Smoking, drugs which shorten the half- eg phenytoin, carbamazepine, barbiturates, rifampicin.
- ►Aim for plasma concentration of 10–20μg/mL (55–110μmol/L). Serious t icity (BP↓, arrhythmias, cardiac arrest) can occur at concentrations ≥25μg/ Measure plasma K^+: theophyllines may cause K^+↓. Don't load patients already oral preparations. Stick with one brand (bioavailability varies).

Emergencies

[I]mmediate management of acute severe asthma[RCT 14]

[A]ssess severity of attack (see above). Warn ITU if attack severe.

[S]tart treatment immediately (prior to investigations).

- Sit patient up and give high-dose O_2 in: 100% via non-rebreathing bag.
- Salbutamol 5mg (or terbutaline 10mg) plus ipratropium bromide 0.5mg **nebulized with O_2.**
- Hydrocortisone 100mg IV or prednisolone 40-50mg PO or both if very ill.
- CXR to exclude pneumothorax.

[I]f life-threatening features (above) present:

- Inform ITU, and seniors.
- Add magnesium sulphate ($MgSO_4$) 1.2–2g IV over 20min.
- Give salbutamol nebulizers every 15min, or 10mg continuously per hour.

[F]urther management

[I]f improving
- 40–60% O_2.
- Prednisolone 40–50mg/24h PO.
- Nebulized salbutamol every 4h.
- Monitor peak flow and oxygen saturations.

If patient not improving after 15–30min
- Continue 100% O_2 and steroids.
- Hydrocortisone 100mg IV or prednisolone 30mg PO if not already given.
- Give salbutamol nebulizers every 15min, or 10mg continuously per hour.
- Continue ipratropium 0.5mg every 4–6h.

If patient still not improving
- Discuss with seniors and ITU.
- Repeat salbutamol nebulizer every 15min.
- $MgSO_4$ 1.2–2g IV over 20min, unless already given.
- Consider aminophylline; if not already on a theophylline, load with eg 5mg/kg IVI over 20min,[1] then 500µg/kg/h where kg is ideal body weight, p434—eg in a small adult: 750mg/24h; large adult 1200mg/24h. Adjust dose according to plasma theophylline, if available. Do levels if infusion lasts >24h. Alternatively, give salbutamol IVI, eg 3–20µg/min. IPPV may be required.

If no improvement, or life-threatening features are present, consider transfer to ITU, accompanied by a doctor prepared to intubate.

[M]onitoring the effects of treatment

- Repeat PEF 15–30min after initiating treatment.
- Pulse oximeter monitoring: maintain S_aO_2 >92%.
- Check blood gases within 2h if: initial P_aCO_2 was normal/raised or initial P_aO_2 <8kPa (60mmHg) or patient deteriorating.
- Record PEF pre- and post-β-agonist in hospital at least 4 times.

[O]nce patient is improving

- Wean down and stop aminophylline over 12–24h.
- Reduce nebulized salbutamol and switch to inhaled β-agonist.
- Initiate inhaled steroids and stop oral steroids if possible.
- Continue to monitor PEF. Look for deterioration on reduced treatment and beware early morning dips in PEF.
- Look for the cause of the acute exacerbation and admission.

1 [B]ritish Thoracic Society advice 2003 *Thorax* 58 sup 1 page 1.

Acute exacerbations of COPD

Common medical emergency especially in winter. May be triggered by vira bacterial infections.

Presentation Increasing cough, breathlessness, or wheeze. Decreased exer capacity.

History Ask about usual/recent treatments (especially home oxygen), smo status, and exercise capacity (may influence a decision to ventilate the patie

Differential diagnosis Asthma, pulmonary oedema, upper respiratory t obstruction, pulmonary embolus, anaphylaxis.

Investigations
- Peak expiratory flow (PEF)—but may be too ill.
- Arterial blood gases.
- CXR to exclude pneumothorax and infection.
- FBC; U&E; CRP.
- ECG.
- Blood cultures (if pyrexial).
- Send sputum for culture.

Management
- Look for a cause, eg infection, pneumothorax.
- See OPPOSITE for acute management.
- Prior to discharge, liaise with GP regarding steroid reduction, domiciliary oxy (p168), smoking, pneumococcal & 'flu vaccinations (p152).

Treatment of stable COPD: See p168 for further information.

Non-pharmacological:	Stop smoking, encourage exercise, treat poor nutrition or obesity, influenza, vaccination.
Pharmacological:	
• Mild	Short-acting β_2-agonist or ipratropium PRN.
• Moderate	Regular short-acting β_2-agonist and/or ipratropium. Consider corticosteroid trial.
• Severe	Combination therapy with regular short-acting β_2-agonist and ipratropium. Consider corticosteroid trial (p169). Assess for home nebulizers.

More advanced disease:
- Consider pulmonary rehabilitation in moderate/severe disease.
- Consider long-term oxygen therapy if P_aO_2 <7.3kPa (p168).
- Indications for surgery: recurrent pneumothoraces; isolated bullous disease; l volume reduction surgery (selected patients).
- Assess social circumstances and support required. Identify and t depression.
- Air travel may be hazardous if P_aO_2 <6.7kPa; check availability of O_2.

Management of acute COPD

Controlled oxygen therapy
Start at 24–28%; vary according to ABG.
Aim for a P_aO_2 >8.0kPa with a rise in P_aCO_2 <1.5kPa

↓

Nebulized bronchodilators
Salbutamol 5mg/4h and ipratropium 500µg/6h

↓

Steroids
IV hydrocortisone 200mg and oral prednisolone 30–40mg

↓

Antibiotics
Use if evidence of infection, eg amoxicillin 500mg/8h PO, p153

↓

Physiotherapy to aid sputum expectoration

↓

If no response
Repeat nebulizers and consider IV aminophylline[1]

↓

If no response
1. Consider nasal intermittent positive pressure ventilation (*NIPPV*) *if respiratory rate >30 or pH <7.35.*
It is delivered by nasal mask and a flow generator

↓

2. Consider intubation[2] & ventilation if pH <7.26 and P_aCO_2 is rising

↓

3. Consider a respiratory stimulant drug, eg doxapram 1.5–4mg/min IV *SE: agitation, confusion, tachycardia, nausea*
Only for patients who are not suitable for mechanical ventilation
A short-term measure only, and rarely used now NIPPV available

Oxygen therapy

- The greatest danger is hypoxia, which probably accounts for more deaths than hypercapnia. *Don't leave patients severely hypoxic.*
- However, in some patients, who rely on their hypoxic drive to breathe, too much oxygen may lead to a reduced respiratory rate, and hypercapnia, with a consequent fall in conscious level.
- Therefore, care is required with O_2, especially if there is evidence of CO_2 retention. Start with 24–28% O_2 in such patients. Reassess after 30min.
- Monitor the patient carefully. Aim to raise the P_aO_2 above 8.0kPa with a rise in P_aCO_2 <1.5kPa.
- In patients without evidence of retention at baseline use 28–40% O_2, but still monitor and repeat ABG.

1 Aminophylline: Do not give a loading dose to patients on maintenance methylxanthines (theophyllines/aminophylline). Load with 250mg over 20min, then infuse at a rate of ~500µg/kg/h. Check plasma levels if given for >24h. ECG monitoring is required.
2 A decision to ventilate will depend on the patient's premorbid state—exercise capacity, home oxygen, and comorbidity. Ask about this information before you need to make this decision.

▸▸Pneumothorax (see image p735)

▸▸**Tension pneumothorax** requires immediate relief (see below). Do not dela management by obtaining a CXR.

Causes Often spontaneous (especially in young thin men) due to rupture of subpleural bulla. Other causes: asthma; COPD; TB; pneumonia; lung absces carcinoma; cystic fibrosis; lung fibrosis; sarcoidosis; connective tissue disorder (Marfan's syndrome, Ehlers–Danlos syndrome); trauma; iatrogenic (subclavian CV line insertion, pleural aspiration or biopsy, percutaneous liver biopsy, positiv pressure ventilation).

Clinical features ***Symptoms:*** There may be no symptoms (especially in fit youn people with small pneumothoraces) or there may be sudden onset of dyspnoe and/or pleuritic chest pain. Patients with asthma or COPD may present with sudden deterioration. Mechanically ventilated patients may present with hypoxi or an increase in ventilation pressures. ***Signs:*** reduced expansion, hyper-resonanc to percussion and diminished breath sounds on the affected side. *With a tensio pneumothorax, the trachea will be deviated away from the affected side and th patient will be very unwell.*

Investigations ►*A* **CXR** *should not be performed if a tension pneumothorax i suspected, as it will delay immediate necessary treatment.* Otherwise, request a expiratory film, and look for an area devoid of lung markings, peripheral to th edge of the collapsed lung (see p735). *Ensure the suspected pneumothorax is not large emphysematous bulla.* Check **ABG** in dyspnoeic patients and those wit chronic lung disease.

Management Depends on whether it is a primary or secondary (underlying lun disease) pneumothorax, size and symptoms—see OPPOSITE.

- Pneumothorax due to trauma or mechanical ventilation requires a chest drair
- Aspiration of a pneumothorax, see p755
- Insertion and management of a chest drain, see p754.

Surgical advice: Arrange if: bilateral pneumothoraces; lung fails to expand afte intercostal drain insertion; 2 or more previous pneumothoraces on the same side or history of pneumothorax on the opposite side.

▸▸Tension pneumothorax (see p735)

This is a medical emergency.

Essence: Air drawn into the pleural space with each inspiration has no route o escape during expiration. The mediastinum is pushed over into the contralatera hemithorax, kinking and compressing the great veins. Unless the air is rapidl removed, cardiorespiratory arrest will occur.

Signs: Respiratory distress, tachycardia, hypotension, distended neck veins, trache deviated away from side of pneumothorax. Increased percussion note, reduced ai entry/breath sounds on the affected side.

Treatment:

To remove the air, insert a large-bore (14–16G) needle with a syringe, partiall filled with 0.9% saline, into the 2nd intercostal interspace in the midclavicular lin on the side of the suspected pneumothorax. Remove plunger to allow the trappe air to bubble through the syringe (with saline as a water seal) until a chest tub can be placed. Alternatively, insert a large-bore Venflon in the same location.
Do this *before* requesting a CXR.
Then insert a chest drain. See p754.

Acute management of pneumothorax

1° pneumothorax

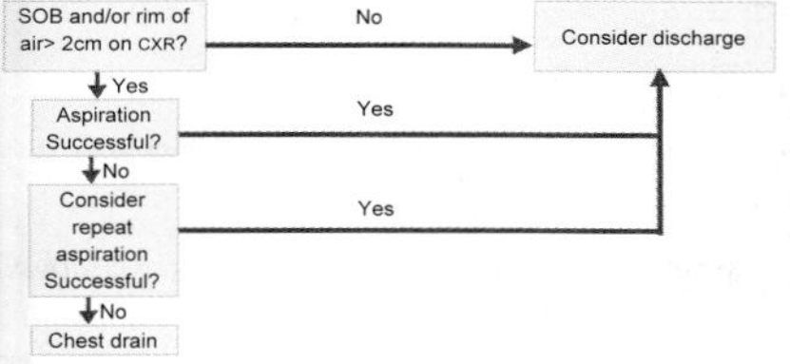

2° pneumothorax

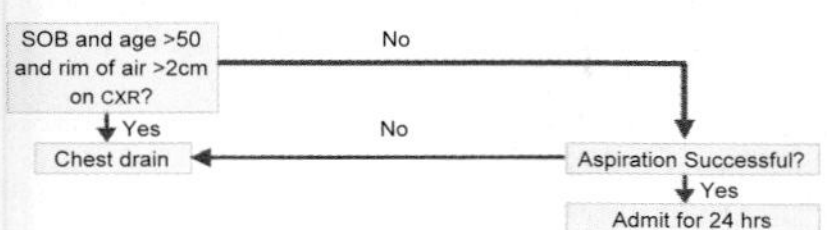

Aspiration of a pneumothorax: »see p755.

Intercostal tube drainage: For insertion, see p754.

- Use a small tube (10–14F) unless blood/pus is also present.
- Never clamp a bubbling tube.
- Tubes may be removed 24h after the lung has re-expanded and air leak has stopped (ie the tube stops bubbling). This is done during expiration or a Valsalva manoeuvre.
- If the lung fails to re-expand within 48h, or if there is a persistent air leak, specialist advice should be obtained, as suction or surgical intervention may be required.
- If suction is required, high volume, low pressure (–10 to –20cm H_2O) systems are required.

Pneumonia

An infection of the lung parenchyma. Incidence of community-acquired pneumoni is 12 per 1000 adults. Of these, 1 will require hospitalization, and mortality i these patients is still 10%.

Common organisms

- *Streptococcus pneumoniae* is the commonest cause (60–75%).
- *Mycoplasma pneumoniae* (5–18%).
- *Staphylococcus aureus.*
- *Haemophilus influenzae.*
- *Legionella* species and *Chlamydia psittaci.*
- Gram-negative bacilli, often hospital-acquired or immunocompromisec eg *Pseudomonas* especially in those with COPD.
- Viruses including influenza account for up to 15%.

Symptoms

- Fever, rigors, malaise, anorexia, dyspnoea, cough, purulent sputum (classicall 'rusty' with pneumococcus), haemoptysis, and pleuritic chest pain.

Signs

- Fever, cyanosis, herpes labialis (pneumococcus), confusion, tachypnoea, tachy cardia, hypotension, signs of consolidation (diminished expansion, dull percussio note, increased tactile vocal fremitus/vocal resonance, bronchial breathing), an a pleural rub.

Investigations

- CXR (X-ray images, fig 1 on p714).
- Oxygen saturation arterial blood gases if S_aO_2 <92% or severe pneumonia.
- FBC, U&E, LFT, CRP, atypical serology.
- Blood and sputum cultures.
- Pleural fluid may be aspirated for culture.
- Bronchoscopy and bronchoalveolar lavage if the patient is immunocompromise or on ITU.

Severity

Calculate the core adverse features 'CURB-65' score:

- **C**onfusion (abbreviated mental test ≤8);
- **U**rea >7mmol/L;
- **R**espiratory rate ≥30/min;
- **B**P <90/60mmHg).
- Age≥65

Score: 0–1 home treatment possible; 2 hospital therapy; ≥3 indicates sever pneumonia. Other features increasing the risk of death are: co-existing diseas bilateral/ multilobar involvement; P_aO_2 <8kPa/S_aO_2 <92%.

Management See OPPOSITE.

Complications

Pleural effusion, empyema, lung abscess, respiratory failure, septicaemi pericarditis, myocarditis, cholestatic jaundice, renal failure.

Management of pneumonia

Oxygen to maintain P_aO_2 >8kPa
caution if history of COPD

↓

Treat hypotension and shock: *see* p778

↓

Investigations
see OPPOSITE

↓

Antibiotics
see BELOW

↓

Intravenous fluids may be required
(anorexia, dehydration, shock)

↓

Analgesia for pleuritic chest pain, eg paracetamol 1g/6h or *NSAID*

↓

Some patients may need intubation
and a period of ventilatory support

Antibiotic treatment of pneumonia

Clinical setting	Organisms	Antibiotic (further dosage details: p368 & p369)
Community acquired		
Mild, no previous ℞	*Streptococcus pneumoniae* *Haemophilus influenzae*	Amoxicillin 500mg–1.0g/8h or erythromycin[1] 500mg/6h PO
Mild	*Streptococcus pneumoniae* *Haemophilus influenzae* *Mycoplasma pneumoniae*	Amoxicillin 500mg–1.0g/8h PO + erythromycin[1] 500mg/6h PO or fluoroquinolone if IV required: ampicillin 500mg/6h + erythromycin[1] 500mg/6h IVI
Severe	As above	Co-amoxiclav IV or cephalosporin IV (eg Cefuroxime 1.5g/8h IV) AND erythromycin[1] 1g/6h IVI
Atypical	*Legionella pneumophilia*	Clarithromycin 500mg/12h PO/IVI ± rifampicin
	Chlamydia species	Tetracycline
	Pneumocystis jiroveci	High-dose co-trimoxazole (see p398, p399)
Hospital acquired		
	Gram negative bacilli Pseudomonas Anaerobes	Aminoglycoside IV + antipseudomonal penicillin IV eg ticarcillin, p368 or 3rd gen. cephalosporin IV (p369)
Aspiration		
	Streptococcus pneumoniae Anaerobes	Cefuroxime 1.5g/8h IV + metronidazole 500mg/8h IV
Neutropenic patients		
	Gram positive cocci Gram negative bacilli	Aminoglycoside IV + antipseudomonal penicillin IV or 3rd gen. cephalosporin IV
	Fungi (p160)	Consider antifungals after 48h

3rd gen=3rd generation, eg cefotaxime, p369; gentamicin is an example of an aminoglycoside (p371).

1 Clarithromycin 500mg/12h PO/IVI may be used in place of erythromycin throughout the above.

▸▸Massive pulmonary embolism (PE)

▸Always suspect pulmonary embolism (PE) in sudden collapse 1–2wks after surgery. Death rate in England and Wales: 30,000–40,000/yr.

Mechanism Venous thrombi, usually from DVT, pass into the pulmonary circulation and block blood flow to lungs. The source is often occult.

Risk factors
- Malignancy.
- Surgery—especially pelvic.
- Immobility.
- The Pill (there is also a slight risk attached to HRT).
- Previous thromboembolism and inherited thrombophilia, see p358.

Prevention Early post-op mobilization is the simplest method; consider:
- Antithromboembolic (TED) stockings.
- Low molecular weight heparin prophylaxis SC.
- Avoid contraceptive pill if at risk, eg major or orthopaedic surgery.
- Recurrent PEs may be prevented by anticoagulation, vena caval filters are of limited use, and should be combined with anticoagulation.

Signs and symptoms
- Acute dyspnoea, pleuritic chest pain, haemoptysis, and syncope.
- Hypotension, tachycardia, gallop rhythm, JVP↑, loud P_2, right ventricular heave, pleural rub, tachypnoea, and cyanosis, AF.

Classically, PE presents 10d post-op, with collapse and sudden breathlessness while straining at stool—but PE may occur after any period of immobility, or with no predisposing factors. Breathlessness may be the only sign. Multiple small emboli may present less dramatically with pleuritic pain, haemoptysis, and gradually increasing breathlessness.

▸Look for a source of emboli—especially DVT (is a leg swollen?).

Investigations
- *U&E*, *FBC*, baseline clotting.
- *ECG* (commonly normal or sinus tachycardia); right ventricular strain pattern V1–3 (p84), right axis deviation, RBBB, AF, may be deep S-waves in I, Q-waves in III, inverted T-waves in III ('$S_I\ Q_{III}\ T_{III}$').
- *CXR*—often normal; decreased vascular markings, small pleural effusion. Wedge-shaped area of infarction. Atelectasis.
- *ABG:* hyperventilation + gas exchange↓: P_aO_2↓, P_aCO_2↓, pH often↑, p148.
- CT pulmonary angiography is sensitive and specific in determining if emboli are in pulmonary arteries. If helical CT is unavailable, a *ventilation-perfusion ($\dot{V}/\dot{Q}$) scan* can aid diagnosis. If $\dot{V}/\dot{Q}$ scan is equivocal, pulmonary angiography or bilateral venograms may help (MRI venography or plethysmography are alternatives).
- D-dimer blood test, ↑ if thrombosis present. May help in excluding a PE.

Management See OPPOSITE for immediate management.
- Try to prevent further thrombosis with compression stockings.
- Heparin concurrently with warfarin for ≥5d, and until INR >2. Then stop.
- If obvious remedial cause, 6wks' treatment with warfarin may be sufficient. Otherwise, continue for at least 3–6 months (long-term if recurrent emboli, or underlying malignancy).
- Is there an underlying cause, eg thrombophilic tendency (p358), malignancy (especially prostate, breast, or pelvic cancer), SLE, or polycythaemia?

▸If good story and signs, make the diagnosis. Start treatment (OPPOSITE) before definitive investigations: most PE deaths occur within 1h.

Management of massive pulmonary embolism

Oxygen, 100%

↓

Morphine 10mg IV with antiemetic if the patient is in pain or very distressed

↓

►If critically ill, consider immediate surgery

↓

IV access and start heparin
either unfractionated heparin ~10,000U IV bolus then ~18U/kg/h IVI as guided by APTT (p334)
or low molecular weight heparin, eg tinzaparin 175U/kg/24h SC

↓

What is the systolic BP?

<90 mmHg
Start rapid colloid infusion[1]

↓

If BP still↓ after 500mL colloid, dobutamine 2.5–10μg/kg/min IV; aim for systolic BP >90mmHg

↓

If BP still low, consider noradrenaline

↓

If the systolic BP <90mmHg after 30–60min of standard treatment, clinically definite PE and no CI (p782), consider thrombolysis.[2]

>90 mmHg
Start warfarin 10mg/24h PO (p334)

↓

Confirm diagnosis

1 Controversial, but some authorities say it is best to infuse plasma-expanding fluids even if CVP↑, to maintain BP & organ perfusion, see *Concise OTM* (*OUP*, 2000) page 151—but see Task Force on PE, European Society Cardiology *Eur Heart J* 2000 **21** 1301.
2 A standard regimen is: ***Loading dose:*** streptokinase 250,000U IVI over 30min.
Maintenance dose: streptokinase 100,000U/h IVI for 12–72h, according to response. **Or** rt-PA (alteplase) 10mg IV over 1–2min followed by 90mg IV over 2h; max 1.5mg/kg if patient <65kg.

▸▸Acute upper gastrointestinal bleeding

Causes

- Peptic ulcer ~40%.
- Mallory Weiss tear 15%.
- Gastroduodenal erosions ~10%.
- Oesophagitis ~10%.
- Varices ~7%.
- Other: malignancy, vascular malformations, haemoptysis (swallowed blood).

Signs & symptoms Haematemesis, or melaena, dizziness (especially postural) fainting, abdominal pain, dysphagia? Postural hypotension, hypotension, tachycardia (not if on β-blocker), ↓JVP, ↓urine output, cool and clammy, signs of chronic liver disease (p252); telangiectasia or purpura; jaundice (biliary colic + jaundice + melaena suggests haemobilia). NB: ask about previous GI problems, drug use, and alcohol intake.

Management:

Is the patient shocked?

- Cool & clammy to touch (especially nose, toes, fingers) ↓capillary refill.
- Pulse >100bpm.
- JVP <1cm H_2O.
- Systolic BP <100mmHg.
- Postural drop (>20mmHg on standing).
- Urine output <30mL/h.

If not shocked: Insert 2 big cannulae; start slow saline IVI to keep lines patent; check bloods and monitor vital signs + urine output. Aim to keep Hb >8g/dL. **NB:** Hb may not fall until circulating volume is restored.

If shocked: See OPPOSITE for management

CVP line: Consider for high risk patients eg ↑age, CV disease, on β-blockers.
Acute drug therapy: Following successful endoscopic therapy in patients with **major** ulcer bleeding, IV omeprazole (80mg stat followed by 8mg/h for 72h) is recommended. There is no firm evidence to support the use of somatostatin or antifibrinolytic therapy in the majority of patients.

Variceal bleeding: Resuscitate then proceed to urgent endoscopy for banding or sclerotherapy. Give octreotide 50μg/h IVI for 2–5d. Terlipressin may also be used. If massive bleed or bleeding continues, pass a Sengstaken–Blakemore tube p231. A bleed is the equivalent of a large protein meal so start treatment to avoid hepatic encephalopathy (p250). Esomeprazole 40mg PO may also be helpful in preventing stress ulceration.

Endoscopy: Within 4h if you suspect variceal bleeding; within 12–24h if shocked on admission or significant comorbidity. Endoscopy can identify the site of bleeding, estimate the risk of rebleeding (see opposite) and can be used to administer treatment. ***No site of bleeding identified:*** Bleeding site missed on endoscopy; bleeding site has healed (Mallory–Weiss tear or Dieulafoy's lesion); nose bleed (swallowed blood); site distal to 3rd part of the duodenum (Meckel's diverticulum, colonic site).

Rebleeds Serious event: 40% of patients who rebleed will die. If 'at risk' maintain a high index of suspicion. If a rebleed occurs, check vital signs every 15min and call senior cover. To prevent rebleeding in endoscopically-proven high risk cases, IVI omeprazole has been tried, eg 80mg followed by an infusion of 8mg/h for 72h, then 20mg/24h PO for 8wks.

Signs of a rebleed:

- Rising pulse rate.
- Falling JVP ± decreasing hourly urine output.
- Haematemesis or melaena.
- Fall in BP (a late and sinister finding) and decreased conscious level.

Emergencies

Immediate management if shocked

Protect airway and keep NBM
Insert two large-bore cannulae *14–16G*

↓

Draw bloods
FBC, U&E, LFT, glucose, clotting screen
Cross-match 6 units

↓

Give high-flow O_2

↓

Rapid IV colloid infusion
Up to 1L

↓

If remains shocked, give blood
Group specific or O Rh–ve until cross-match done

↓

Otherwise slow saline infusion[1]
To keep lines open

↓

Transfuse as dictated by haemodynamics

↓

Correct clotting abnormalities
Vitamin K, FFP, platelet concentrate

↓

Set up CVP line to guide fluid replacement
Aim for >5cm H_2O CVP may mislead if there is ascites or CCF
A Swan–Ganz catheter may help

↓

Catheterize and monitor urine output
Aim for >30mL/h

↓

Monitor vital signs every 15min until stable, then hourly

↓

Notify surgeons of all severe bleeds

↓

Urgent endoscopy for diagnosis ± control of bleeding

ockall scoring system for prognosis in acute GI bleeding

	Score			
ariable	0	1	2	3
ge	<60	60-80	>80	
hocked?	No	SBP >100 pulse >100	SBP <100, pulse >100	
o-morbidity?	None		Any major	Renal/liver failure, or malignancy
iagnosis	Mallory–Weiss or normal	All other diagnoses	Malignancy	
leeding isible?	None/spot		Visible blood/clot spurting vessel	

Score <3 means an excellent prognosis; >8 means a high risk of death

void saline in patients with decompensated liver disease (ascites, peripheral oedema) as it sens ascites, and despite a low serum sodium, patients have a high body sodium. Use whole od, or salt-poor albumin for resuscitation, and 5% dextrose for maintenance.

▸▸Meningitis[ND]

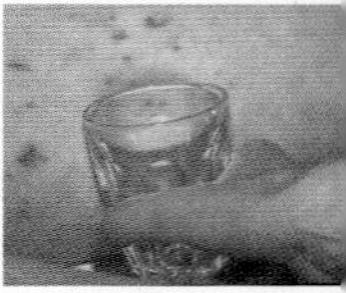

▸***Do not*** delay treatment, it may save a life.

▸Make sure the referring GP gives a dose of antibiotic (benzylpenicillin, eg 1.2g IM/IV) before sending the patient to you if possible.

Early features Headache, leg pains, cold hands and feet, abnormal skin colour.

Later signs
- Meningism: neck stiffness, photophobia, Kernig's sign (pain + resistance on passive knee extension with hip fully flexed).
- Conscious level ↓, coma.
- Seizures (~20%) ± focal CNS signs (~20%).
- Petechial rash (non-blanching—see fig 1; may only be 1 or 2 spots, or none
- Signs of galloping sepsis: slow capillary refill; DIC; BP↓. T° and pulse: ↑ or nor

Fig 1. Glass test for purpura

Common organisms
- Meningococcus
- Pneumococcus
- *Haemophilus influenzae*
- *Listeria monocytogenes*

Differential Malaria, encephalitis, septicaemia, subarachnoid bleed, dengue, teta

Management
- Careful examination: pay attention to neurology; look for rashes; assess GC
- If shocked, resuscitate with fluids and oxygen.
- If ICP raised, summon help immediately and inform neurosurgeons.
- Start antibiotics (below) immediately.

Investigations
- U&E, FBC, LFT, glucose, coagulation screen.
- Blood culture, throat swabs (1 for bacteria, 1 for virology), stool sample for vir
- Lumbar puncture (p756) if safe.[1] Don't forget to measure the opening press (7–18cm CSF is normal; in meningitis it may be >40; typically 14– **Contraindications** are: suspected intracranial mass lesion, focal signs, papill ema, trauma, middle ear pathology or major coagulopathy. Send samples MC&S, gram stain, protein estimation, glucose, and to virology.

CSF in meningitis	*Pyogenic*	*Tuberculous* (p387)	*Viral ('aseptic')*
Appearance	Often turbid	Often fibrin web	Usually clear
Predominant cell[1]	Polymorphs	Mononuclear	Mononuclear
Cell count/mm³	Eg 90–1000+	10–1000	50–1000
Glucose[†]	<½ plasma	<½ plasma	>½ plasma
Protein (g/L)	>1.5	1–5	<1
Bacteria	In smear & culture	Often none in smear	None seen or cultu

- CT head before LP if mass lesion or raised ICP suspected (eg conscious ↓).
- CXR.

Antibiotics Local policies vary. If in doubt ask. The following are suggestions where the organism is unknown:
- <55yrs: cefotaxime 2mg/6h slow IV.
- >55yrs: cefotaxime as above + ampicillin 2g IV/4h (for *Listeria*).
- Aciclovir if viral encephalitis suspected.
- Once organism isolated, seek urgent microbiological advice.

1 LP is generally safe without a prior CT if there are no clinical contra-indications such as CNS signs or papilloedema. If there are contra-indications, then do a CT scan first; but don't wa the scan before giving empirical antibiotic therapy. NB: ≤5 lymphocytes/mm³ may be norm long as there are no neutrophils. Normal protein: 0.15–0.45g/L. Normal CSF glucose: 4.2mmol/L: *Causes of* hypoglycorrhacia (↓CSF glucose): sepsis; parasitic meningitis eg from e snails (do CSF eosinophil count); also herpes encephalitis, hypoglycaemia, sarcoid, CNS vasculiti Predominant cell type may be lymphocytes in TB, listerial, and cryptococcal meningitis.

Meningitis ℞: If outside hospital, let *nothing* delay IV/IM benzylpenicillin 1.2g ıile awaiting transport. In hospital: ABCs; high-flow O_2. IVI + fluid resus. Ask a ırse to draw up cefotaxime 2g. **Do septicaemic or meningitic features predominate?**

See British Infection Society guideline 2005

ɪpticaemic signs to fore: eg ↓capillary refill time; ɪd hands + feet (occurs before BP falls); rash. 2006 data

→ Do not attempt LP
Cefotaxime 2g IV
Get help from critical care team
Signs of shock?

- ɪs → **ɪke to ITU for:** Fluid resuscitation; Pre-emptive intubation; Inotropes/vasopressors; Activated protein C[2]; Aim for systolic BP of >80mmHg and urine flow >30mL/h
- No → Careful monitoring → Repeat review

Meningitic signs predominate, ie neck stiffness; photophobia

→ **Dexamethasone** 4–10mg/6h IV[1]

→ If no shock, or ICP↑ signs, **Do** LP. If not sure, get senior help

→ 2g **cefotaxime** IV post-LP at once (pre-LP, if to be delayed by >½h)

→ If signs of ↑ICP, take to ITU; and do **not** do LP

→ Nurse at 30°; have low threshold for intubation. NB: don't rely on CT to rule out ↑ICP. Also, papilloedema is a late sign. → Repeat review

ɪmmunocompromized, get help; add **ampicillin** 2g/6h IV for *Listeria*, also if >55yrs old

ɪbsequent therapy: **Cefotaxime** 2–4g/8h IVI (eg for 10d); ↓dose in renal failure; see ɪ69 and *datasheet* (SPC). **Maintenance fluids:** avoid overhydration and underhydration espite ICP↑). **Isolate** for 1st 24h. If response to the above is poor consider preɪptive **intubation & ventilation** ± **inotropic/vasopressor** support (p778).

ffer prophylaxis to: • Household contacts (in droplet range). • Those who have kissed e patient's mouth. • Yourself (rarely needed). Give **rifampicin** (600mg/12h PO for 2 ɪys; children >1yr 10mg/kg/12h; <1yr 5mg/kg/12h) or **ciprofloxacin** (500mg PO, 1 ɪse child 5–12yrs: 250mg stat). Neither is guaranteed in pregnancy, but are commended (harm is unlikely).

mergency management of encephalitis[ND]

spect encephalitis whenever odd behaviour, ↓consciousness, cranial nerve lesıs, or paralysis is preceded by a prodrome (T°↑, rash, lymphadenopathy, cold ɪres, conjunctivitis, meningeal signs, seizures). It is often necessary to treat before e exact cause is known—often viral with no *specific* treatment (arboviruses; CMV, V; p389; measles; Japanese B or West Nile encephalitis) but as specific treatment available for herpes simplex encephalitis, aim to start **aciclovir** within 30min of e patient arriving (⏩10mg/kg/8h IVI over 1h) for 14–21 days. Specific therapies ɪo exist for CMV & toxoplasmosis (p392). ***Tests:*** Blood & viral culture (throat; CSF; ɪU)/PCR; enhanced CT (MRI if contrast-allergic) pre-LP; toxoplasma tests (p392). **Δ:** Malaria, rabies, TB, SLE, hypoglycaemia, beri-beri (give vit B1 if in doubt, p707). ***ɪpportive therapy:*** See ICP↑, p812; **dexamethasone** 10mg/6h IV has a role.

1 Dexamethasone 0.15mg/kg/6h IV eg from just *before* 1st antibiotic dose; evidence is now good-ish, ɪ. for pneumococcal meningitis and in children. Avoid dexamethasone in septic shock, known ɪningococcal disease, immunocompromized states, and in post-op meningitis. 2 *Drotrecogin alfa (activated)* is approved by NICE.

▸▸Status epilepticus

This means seizures lasting for >30min, or repeated seizures without interveni consciousness. Mortality and the risk of permanent brain damage increase with t length of attack. Aim to terminate seizures lasting more than a few minutes soon as possible (<20min).

Status usually occurs in known epileptics. If it is the 1st presentation epilepsy, the chance of a structural brain lesion is high (>50%). Diagnosis of ton clonic status is usually clear. Non-convulsive status (eg absence status continuous partial seizures with preservation of consciousness) may be mc difficult: look for subtle eye or lid movement. For other signs, see p477. An EEG c be very helpful. ►*Could the patient be pregnant* (any pelvic mass)? If so, eclamp (*OHCS* p48) is the likely diagnosis, check the urine and BP: call a sen obstetrician—immediate delivery may be needed.

Investigations

- Bedside glucose, the following tests can be done once ℞ has started: Gluco blood gases, U&E, Ca^{2+}, FBC, ECG.
- Consider anticonvulsant levels, toxicology screen, LP, culture blood and urine, E CT, carbon monoxide level.
- Pulse oximetry, cardiac monitor.

Treatment See OPPOSITE. Basic life support—and these agents:

1 ***Lorazepam*** ~4mg as a slow bolus (≤2min) into a large vein. Beware respiratc arrest during the last part of the injection. Have full resuscitation facilities hand for all IV benzodiazepine use. (Alternative: ***diazepam*** as ***Diazemuls***® but is less long-lasting—give 10mg IV over 2min; if needed, repeat at 5mg/min, ur seizures stop or 20mg given—or significant respiratory depression occurs.) T rectal route is an alternative for diazepam if IV access is difficult.[1] ***Buc midazolam*** (Epistatus®) is an easier to use oral alternative; dose for thc 10yrs old and older: 10mg (1mL); if 1–4yrs old, 0.5mL; if 6–12 months o 0.25mL; squirt half the volume between the lower gum and the cheek on ea side. While waiting for this to work, prepare other drugs. If fits continue ...

2 **Phenytoin infusion:** 15mg/kg IVI, at a rate of ≤50mg/min. (Don't p diazepam in same line: they don't mix.) Beware BP↓ and do not use bradycardic or heart block. Requires BP and ECG monitoring. 100mg/6–8h is maintenance dose (check levels). If fits continue ...

3 **Diazepam infusion:** 100mg in 500mL of 5% dextrose; infuse at about 40mL (3mg/kg/24h). Close monitoring, especially respiratory function, is vital. It most unusual for seizures to remain unresponsive following this. If they c allow the idea to pass through your mind that they could be pseudoseizur (p698), particularly if there are odd features (pelvic thrusts; resisting attemp to open lids and your attempts to do passive movements; arms and legs flailir around).

4 **Dexamethasone** 10mg IV if vasculitis/cerebral oedema (tumour) possible.

5 **General anaesthesia** This requires expert guidance on ITU.

As soon as seizures are controlled, start oral drugs (p484). Ask what the cau was, eg hypoglycaemia, pregnancy, alcohol, drugs, CNS lesion or infectio hypertensive encephalopathy, inadequate anticonvulsant dose (p482).

1 Diazepam Rectubes®: give 0.5mg/kg stat dose—eg ~3 10mg tubes PR (respiratory problems at th dose are *very* rare: all survived). If your back is still against the wall with no response after 10min, try last 10mg tube. Halve dose if elderly. *For children's Stesolid® regimen* (it is different), see *OHCS* p266

Management of status epilepticus

Open and maintain the airway, lay in recovery position
Remove false teeth if poorly fitting, insert oral/nasal airway, intubate if necessary

↓

Oxygen, 100% + suction (as required)

↓

IV access and take blood:
- U&E, LFT, FBC, glucose (eg BM test®), calcium
- Toxicology screen if indicated, anticonvulsant levels

↓

Thiamine 250mg IV over 10min if alcoholism or malnourishment suspected.
Unless glucose known to be normal, IV glucose 50mL 50%

↓

Correct hypotension with fluids

↓

Slow IV bolus phase—to stop seizures: eg lorazepam 4mg

↓

IV infusion phase: If seizures continue, start phenytoin, 15mg/kg IVI, at a rate of ≤50mg/min. Monitor ECG and BP. 100mg/6–8h is a maintenance dose (check levels).
Alternative: diazepam infusion:100mg in 500mL of 5% dextrose; infuse at ~40mL/h as opposite

↓

General anaesthesia phase: Continuing seizures require expert help with paralysis and ventilation with continuous EEG monitoring in ITU

B: ►**Never** spend longer than 20min on someone with status epilepticus ithout having help at the bedside from an anaesthetist.

erebral abscess

spect this in any patient with ICP↑, especially if there is fever or ↑WCC. It may llow ear, sinus, dental, or periodontal infection; skull fracture; congenital heart sease; endocarditis; bronchiectasis. It may also occur in the absence of systemic gns of inflammation.

gns: Seizures, fever, localizing signs, or signs of ↑ICP. Coma. Signs of sepsis sewhere (eg teeth, ears, lungs, endocarditis).

vestigations: CT/MRI (eg 'ring-enhancing' lesion); ↑WBC, ↑ESR; biopsy.

eatment: Urgent neurosurgical referral; treat ↑ICP (p812). If frontal sinuses or eth are the source, the likely organism will be *Strep. milleri* (microaerophilic), or opharyngeal anaerobes. In ear abscesses, *B. fragilis* or other anaerobes are most mmon. Bacterial abscesses are often peripheral; toxoplasma lesions (p392) are eeper (eg basal ganglia). NB: ask yourself: is there underlying immunosuppression?

▸▸Head injury

▸If the pupils are unequal, diagnose rising intracranial pressure (ICP), eg fr extradural haemorrhage, and summon urgent neurosurgical help (p474). Ret vein pulsation at fundoscopy helps exclude ICP↑.

Initial management (See OPPOSITE) Write full notes. Record times.

- Involve neurosurgeons at an early stage, especially with comatosed patients if raised ICP suspected.
- Examine the CNS. Chart pulse, BP, T°, respirations + pupils every 15min.
- Assess anterograde amnesia (loss from the time of injury, ie post-traumatic) retrograde amnesia—its extent correlates with the severity of the injury, an never occurs without anterograde amnesia.
- Nurse semi-prone if no spinal injury; meticulous care to bladder & airway.

Who needs a CT head?

- If any of the following are present, a CT is required immediately:
- GCS <13 at any time, or GCS 13 or 14 at 2h following injury
- Focal neurological deficit
- Suspected open or depressed skull fracture, or signs of basal skull fracture
- Post-traumatic seizure
- Vomiting >once
- Loss of consciousness AND any of the following
  - Age ≥65
  - Coagulopathy
  - 'Dangerous mechanism of injury' eg RTA, fall from great height
  - Antegrade amnesia of >30min.

When to ventilate immediately:

- Coma ≤8 on Glasgow coma scale (GCS; p776)
- P_aO_2 <9kPa in air (<13kPa in O_2) or P_aCO_2 >6kPa
- Spontaneous hyperventilation (P_aCO_2 <3.5kPa)
- Respiratory irregularity.

Ventilate before neurosurgical transfer if:

- Deteriorating level of consciousness
- Bilateral fractured mandible
- Bleeding into mouth, eg skull base fracture
- Seizures.

Risk of intracranial haematoma in adults

Fully conscious, no skull fracture = <1:1000
Confused, no skull fracture = 1:100
Fully conscious, skull fracture = 1:30
Confused, skull fracture = 1:4

Criteria for admission

- Difficult to assess (child; post-ictal; alcohol intoxication).
- CNS signs; severe headache or vomiting; fracture.
- Loss of consciousness does **not** require admission if well, and a responsible ad is in attendance.

Drowsy trauma patients (GCS <15 to >8) smelling of alcohol: Alcohol is unlikely cause of coma if plasma alcohol <44mmol/L. If unavailable, estimate blo alcohol level from the osmolar gap, p664. If blood alcohol ≈ 40mmol/L, osmol gap ≈ 40mmol/L. Never assume signs are just alcohol.

Complications ***Early:*** Extradural/subdural haemorrhage, seizures. ***Late:*** Subdu p474; seizures; diabetes insipidus; parkinsonism; dementia.

Indicators of a bad prognosis Old age, decerebrate rigidity, extensor spasm prolonged coma, ↑BP, P_aO_2↓ (on blood gases), T° >39°C. 60% of those with loss consciousness of >1 month will survive 3–25yrs, but may need daily nursing ca

For *Spinal cord injury & Persistent vegetative states*, see OHCS (p768–p776 & p77

Immediate management plan

ABC

↓

Oxygen, 100%
Intubate and hyperventilate if necessary
NB: beware of a cervical spine injury

↓

Stop blood loss and support circulation
Treat for shock if required (p778)

↓

Treat seizures with diazepam

↓

Assess level of consciousness (GCS)
Antegrade and retrograde amnesia

↓

Rapid examination survey

↓

Investigations:
U&Es, glucose, FBC, blood alcohol, toxicology screen, ABG & clotting

↓

Neurological examination

↓

Brief history
When? Where? How? Had a fit? Lucid interval? Alcohol?

↓

Evaluate lacerations of face or scalp
Palpate deep wounds with sterile glove to check for step deformity. Note obvious skull/facial fractures[1]

↓

Check for CSF leak, from nose (rhinorrhoea) or ear
Any blood behind the ear drum?
If either is present, suspect basilar skull fracture: do CT
Give tetanus toxoid, and refer at once to neurosurgeons

↓

Palpate the neck posteriorly for tenderness and deformity
If detected, or if the patient has obvious head injury, or injury above the clavicle with loss of consciousness, immobilize the neck and get cervical spine radiographs

↓

Radiology
As indicated: cervical spine, chest X-rays; CT of head

[1] Periorbital (raccoon sign), or postauricular (Battle sign) ecchymoses.

▸▸Raised intracranial pressure (ICP↑)

There are 3 types of cerebral oedema:

- Vasogenic: ↑ capillary permeability—tumour, trauma, ischaemia, infection.
- Cytotoxic: cell death, eg from hypoxia.
- Interstitial: eg obstructive hydrocephalus.

Because the cranium defines a fixed volume, brain swelling quickly results in ↑ which may produce a sudden clinical deterioration. Normal ICP is 0–10mmHg. T oedema from severe brain injury is probably both cytotoxic and vasogenic.

Causes

- Primary or metastatic tumours.
- Head injury.
- Haemorrhage (subdural, extradural, subarachnoid; intracerebral, intraventricular).
- Meningoencephalitis; brain abscess.
- Hydrocephalus; cerebral oedema; status epilepticus.

Signs & symptoms

- Headache; drowsiness; vomiting; seizures. History of trauma.
- Listlessness; irritability; drowsiness; falling pulse and rising BP (Cushir response); coma; Cheyne–Stokes respiration; pupil changes (constriction at fi later dilatation—do not mask these signs by using agents, such as tropicami to dilate the pupil to aid fundoscopy).
- Papilloedema is an unreliable sign, but venous pulsation at the disc may absent (absent in ~50% of normal people, but *loss* of it is a useful sign).

Investigations

- U&E, FBC, LFT, glucose, serum osmolality, clotting, blood culture, CXR.
- CT head.
- Then consider lumbar puncture if safe. Measure the opening pressure!

Treatment

The goal is to ↓ICP and avert secondary injury. Urgent neurosurgery is required the definitive treatment of ↑ICP from focal causes (eg haematomas). This achieved via a craniotomy or burr hole. Also, an ICP monitor (or bolt) may be plac to monitor pressure. Surgery is generally *not* helpful following ischaemic or ano injury.

Holding measures are listed OPPOSITE.

Herniation syndromes ***Uncal herniation*** is caused by a lateral supratento mass which pushes the ipsilateral inferomedial temporal lobe (uncus) through t temporal incisura and against the midbrain. The 3rd nerve, travelling in this spa gets compressed causing a dilated ipsilateral pupil, then ophthalmoplegia (a fix pupil localizes a lesion poorly but is 'ipsi-lateralizing'). This may be follow (quickly) by contralateral hemiparesis (pressure on the cerebral peduncle) a coma from pressure on the ascending reticular activating system (ARAS) in t midbrain.

Cerebellar tonsil herniation is caused by ↑pressure in the posterior fossa forci the cerebellar tonsils through the foramen magnum. Ataxia, VI nerve palsies, a +ve Babinskis (upgoing plantars) occur first, then loss of consciousness, irregu breathing, and apnoea. This syndrome may proceed very rapidly given the sm size of, and poor compliance in, the posterior fossa.

Subfalcian (cingulate) herniation is caused by a frontal mass. The cingula gyrus (medial frontal lobe) is forced under the rigid falx cerebri. It may be sil unless the anterior cerebral artery is compressed and causes a stroke— contralateral leg weakness ± abulia (lack of decision-making).

Immediate management plan

↓

Correct hypotension and treat seizures

↓

Brief examination; history if available
Any clues, eg meningococcal rash, previous carcinoma

↓

Elevate the head of the bed to 30°–40°

↓

If intubated, hyperventilate to ↓P_aCO_2 (eg to 3.5kPa)
This causes cerebral vasoconstriction and reduces ICP almost immediately

↓

Osmotic agents (eg mannitol) can be useful *pro tem* but may lead to rebound ↑ICP after prolonged use (~12–24h)
Give 20% solution 1–2g/kg iv over 10–20min (eg 5mL/kg). Clinical effect is seen after ~20min and lasts for 2–6h. Follow serum osmolality—aim for about 300mosmol/kg but don't exceed 310

↓

Corticosteroids are *not* effective in reducing ICP except for oedema surrounding tumours
eg dexamethasone 10mg IV and follow with 4mg/6h IV/PO

↓

Fluid restrict to <1.5L /d

↓

Monitor the patient closely, consider monitoring ICP

↓

Aim to make a diagnosis

↓

Treat cause or exacerbating factors
eg hyperglycaemia, hyponatraemia

↓

Definitive treatment if possible

▸▸Diabetic ketoacidosis (DKA)

Hyperglycaemic ketoacidotic coma only occurs in type I diabetes: it may be th mode of presentation, eg a 1–3-day history of gradual decline into dehydratio acidosis, and coma. Precipitants include: infection, surgery, MI, non-compliance, o wrong insulin dose. The diagnosis requires ketosis and acidosis (pH <7.3).

Signs & symptoms

- Polyuria, polydipsia, lethargy, anorexia, hyperventilation, ketotic breat dehydration, vomiting, abdominal pain, coma.

Investigations

- Lab glucose, U&E, HCO_3^-, amylase, osmolality, ABG, FBC, blood cultures.
- Urine tests: ketones, MSU; CXR.
- To estimate plasma osmolarity: 2[Na^+] + [urea] + [glucose] mmol/L.

Pitfalls in diabetic ketoacidosis

- ***Plasma glucose*** is usually high, but not always, especially if insulin continued
- ***High WCC*** may be seen in the absence of infection.
- ***Infection:*** often there is no fever. Do MSU, blood cultures, and CXR. Start broac spectrum antibiotics early if infection is suspected.
- ***Creatinine:*** some assays for creatinine cross-react with ketone bodies, so plasm creatinine may not reflect true renal function.
- ***Hyponatraemia*** is common, due to osmolar compensation for the hype glycaemia. ↑ or ↔ [Na^+] indicates severe water loss. As treatment commence Na^+ rises as water enters cells. Na^+ is also low due to an artefact; correcte plasma [Na^+] = Na^+ + 2.4[(glucose –5.5)/5.5].
- ***Ketonuria*** does not equate with ketoacidosis. Normal individuals may have up t ++ketonuria after an overnight fast. Not all ketones are due to diabetes– consider alcohol if glucose normal. Test plasma with Ketostix® or Acetest® t demonstrate ketonaemia.
- ***Recurrent ketoacidosis:*** blood glucose may return to normal long before ketone are removed from the blood, and a rapid reduction in the amount of insuli administered may lead to lack of clearance and return to DKA. This may be avoide by maintaining a constant rate of insulin, eg 4–5U/h IVI, and co-infusing dextros 10–20% to keep plasma glucose at 6–10mmol/L—the extended insulin regime
- ***Acidosis*** but without gross elevation of glucose may occur, but conside overdose (eg aspirin) and lactic acidosis (in elderly diabetics).
- ***Serum amylase*** is often raised (up to ×10) and non-specific abdominal pain i common, even in the absence of pancreatitis.

Management See OPPOSITE. Dehydration is more life-threatening than hype glycaemia—so its correction takes precedence.

- Monitor potassium, glucose, creatinine, HCO_3^-, hourly initially. Aim for a fall i glucose of 5mmol/h, and correction of the acidosis. The use of venous HCO_3^- as guide to progress, may prevent the need for repeated arterial blood ga sampling.
- Flow chart of vital signs, conscious level, urine output, and ketones; inse catheter if no urine passed for >4h. Monitoring CVP may sometimes be helpful i guiding fluid replacement.
- Find and treat infection (lung, skin, perineum, urine after cultures).
- Give heparin 5000U/8h (or low molecular weight version) SC until mobile.
- Change to SC insulin when ketones are ≤1+ and eating (p193).

NB: if acidosis is severe (pH <7), some give IV bicarbonate (eg 1mL/kg of 8.4% ove 1h, and recheck arterial pH); others never give it because of effects on the Hb dissociation curve and cerebral circulation—discuss with senior.

Complications Cerebral oedema, aspiration pneumonia, hypokalaemia, hypo magnesaemia, hypophosphataemia, thromboembolism.

►Talk with the patient: ensure there are no further preventable episodes.

Other emergencies: Hyperosmolar non-ketotic coma & hypoglycaemia: p816.

Management plan

IV access and start fluid (0.9% saline IVI) replacement immediately

↓

Check plasma glucose: usually >20mmol/L
if so give 4–8U soluble insulin IV

↓

Investigations

- Lab glucose, U&E, HCO_3^-, osmolality, blood gases, FBC, blood culture
- Urine tests: ketones, MSU; CXR

↓

NG tube only if nauseated/vomiting/unconscious

↓

Insulin sliding scale (below)

↓

Continue fluid replacement, K^+ replacement

↓

Check glucose and U&E, HCO_3^- regularly (hourly initially)

↓

What precipitated the coma?

Fluid replacement

- Give 1 litre (L) of 0.9% saline stat. Then, typically, 1L over the next hour, 1L over 2h, 1L over 4h, then 1L over 6h
- Use dextrose saline or 5% dextrose when blood glucose is <15mmol/L
- Those >65yrs or with CCF need less saline more cautiously

Potassium replacement

- Total body potassium is invariably low, and plasma K^+ falls as K^+ enters cells with treatment
- Don't add K^+ to the first bag, less will be required in renal failure or oliguria. Check U&E hourly initially, and replace as required:

Serum K^+ (mmol/L)	Amount of KCl to add per litre of IV fluid:
<3.0	40mmol
3–4	30mmol
4–5	20mmol

Sliding scale of insulin via IVI pump in diabetic ketoacidosis

Add 50U soluble insulin (Actrapid/Humulin-S) to 50mL saline in a syringe (1U/mL)

Hourly glucose result (mmol/L)	Soluble insulin	If infection or insulin resistance (p191)
0–3.9	0.5U/h	1U/h
4–7.9	1	2
8–11.9	2	4
12–16.0	3	6
>16	4	8

If no pump, load with 10U IM, then give 4–6U/h IM while glucose is >14mmol/L.

▸▸Other diabetic emergencies

Hypoglycaemic coma Usually *rapid* onset; may be preceded by odd behaviour (e aggression), sweating, pulse↑, seizures.

Management: Give 20–30g dextrose IV eg 200–300ml of 10% dextrose. This i preferable to 50–100mL 50% dextrose which harms veins. Expect promp recovery. Glucagon 1mg IV/IM is nearly as rapid as dextrose but will not work i drunk patients. Dextrose IVI may be needed for severe prolonged hypoglycaemia Once conscious, give sugary drinks and a meal.

Hyperglycaemic hyperosmolar non-ketotic (HONK) coma Only those with type-2 diabetes are at risk of this. The history is longer (eg 1wk), with marked dehydratio and glucose >35mmol/L. Acidosis is absent as there has been no switch to keton metabolism—the patient is often old, and presenting for the first time. Th osmolality is >340mosmol/kg. Focal CNS signs may occur. The risk of DVT is high, s give *full* heparin anticoagulation (p334).

Rehydrate over 48h with 0.9% saline IVI, eg at ½ the rate used in ketoacidosis Wait an hour before giving any insulin (it may not be needed, and you want t avoid rapid changes). If it is needed, 1u/h might be a typical initial dose. Look fo the cause, eg MI, or bowel infarct.

Hyperlactaemia is a rare but serious complication of DM (eg after septicaemia o biguanide use). Blood lactate: >5mmol/L. Seek expert help. Give O_2. Treat an sepsis vigorously.

Emergencies

▸▸Thyroid emergencies

Myxoedema coma ***Signs & symptoms:*** Looks hypothyroid (p204); >65yrs hypothermia; hyporeflexia; glucose↓; bradycardia; coma; seizures.

History: Prior surgery or radioiodine for hyperthyroidism.

Precipitants: Infection; myocardial infarction; stroke; trauma.

Examination: Goitre; cyanosis; heart failure; precipitants.

Treatment: Preferably in intensive care.

- Take venous blood for: T3, T4, TSH, FBC, U&E, cultures, cortisol.
- Take arterial blood for P_aO_2.
- Give high-flow O_2 if cyanosed. Correct any hypoglycaemia.
- Give T3 (triiodothyronine) 5–20µg IV slowly. Be cautious: this may precipitat manifestations of undiagnosed ischaemic heart disease.
- Give hydrocortisone 100mg/8h IV—vital if pituitary hypothyroidism is suspecte (ie no goitre, no previous radioiodine, no thyroid surgery).
- IVI 0.9% saline. Be sure to avoid precipitating LVF.
- If infection suspected, give antibiotic, eg cefuroxime 1.5g/8h IVI.
- Treat *heart failure* as appropriate (p122).
- Treat *hypothermia* with warm blankets in warm room. Beware complication (hypoglycaemia, pancreatitis, arrhythmias). See p832.

Further therapy: T3 5–20µg/4–12h IV until sustained improvement (eg ~2–3d then thyroxine (T4=levothyroxine) 50µg/24h PO. Continue hydrocortisone. Give I fluids as appropriate (hyponatraemia is dilutional).

Hyperthyroid crisis (thyrotoxic storm) ***Sign & symptoms:*** Severe hyper thyroidism: fever, agitation, confusion, coma, tachycardia, AF, D&V, goitre, thyroi bruit, 'acute abdomen' picture.

Precipitants: Recent thyroid surgery or radioiodine; infection; MI; trauma.

Diagnosis: Confirm with technetium uptake if possible, but do not wait for this i urgent treatment is needed.

Treatment: Enlist expert help from an endocrinologist. See OPPOSITE.

Management plan for thyrotoxic storm

IVI 0.9% saline, 500mL/4h. NG tube if vomiting.

↓

Take blood for: T3, T4, cultures (if infection suspected).

↓

Sedate if necessary (eg chlorpromazine 50mg PO/IM).

↓

If no contraindication, give propranolol 40mg/8h PO (maximum IV dose: 1mg over 1min, repeated up to 9 times at ≥2min intervals).

↓

High-dose digoxin may be needed to slow the heart, eg 1mg over 2h IVI.

↓

Antithyroid drugs: carbimazole 15–25mg/6h PO (or via NGT, if needed). After 4h give Lugol's solution 0.3mL/8h PO for 1wk to block thyroid.

↓

Hydrocortisone 100mg/6h IV or dexamethasone 4mg/6h PO.

↓

Treat suspected infection with eg cefuroxime 1.5g/8h IVI.

↓

Adjust IV fluids as necessary; cool with tepid sponging ± paracetamol.

↓

Continuing treatment: After 5d reduce carbimazole to 15mg/8h PO. After 10d stop propranolol and iodine. Adjust carbimazole (p202).

▸▸Addisonian crisis

Signs & symptoms: Patients may present in shock (tachycardia; peripher vasoconstriction; postural hypotension; oliguria; weak; confused; comatose)- typically (but not always!) in a patient with known Addison's disease, or someo on long-term steroids who has forgotten to take tablets. An alternati presentation is with hypoglycaemia.

Precipitating factors: Infection, trauma, surgery.

Management: If suspected, treat before biochemical results.

- Take blood for cortisol (10mL heparin or clotted) and ACTH if possible (10n heparin, to go straight to laboratory).
- Hydrocortisone sodium succinate 100mg IV stat.
- IVI: use a plasma expander first, for resuscitation, then 0.9% saline.
- Monitor blood glucose: the danger is hypoglycaemia.
- Blood, urine, sputum for culture.
- Give antibiotics (eg cefuroxime 1.5g/8h IVI).

Continuing treatment

- Glucose IV may be needed if hypoglycaemic.
- Continue IV fluids, more slowly. Be guided by clinical state.
- Continue hydrocortisone sodium succinate 100mg IV/IM every 6h.
- Change to oral steroids after 72h if patient's condition good. The tetracosact (=tetracosactide) test is impossible while on hydrocortisone.
- Fludrocortisone is needed only if hydrocortisone dose <50mg/d and t condition is due to adrenal disease.
- Search for the cause, once the crisis is over.

▸▸Hypopituitary coma

Usually develops gradually in a person with known hypopituitarism. Rarely, t onset is rapid due to infarction of a pituitary tumour (pituitary apoplexy)— symptoms include headache and meningism, subarachnoid haemorrhage is oft misdiagnosed.

Presentation: Headache; ophthalmoplegia; consciousness↓; hypotension; hyp thermia; hypoglycaemia; signs of hypopituitarism (p216).

Tests: T4; cortisol; TSH; ACTH; glucose. Pituitary fossa CT/MRI.

Treatment:

- Hydrocortisone sodium succinate 100mg IV/6h.
- Only after hydrocortisone begun: T3 10μg/12h PO.
- Prompt surgery is needed if the cause is pituitary apoplexy.

▸▸Phaeochromocytoma emergencies

Stress, abdominal palpation, parturition, general anaesthetic, or contrast me used in radiography may produce dangerous *hypertensive crises* (pallor, pulsati headache, hypertension, feels 'about to die').

Treatment ▸Get help.

- Phentolamine 2–5mg IV. Repeat to maintain safe BP.
- Labetalol is an alternative agent.
- When BP controlled, give phenoxybenzamine 10mg/24h PO (increase by 10mg as needed, up to 0.5–1mg/kg/12h PO); SE: postural hypotension; dizzine tachycardia; nasal congestion; miosis; idiosyncratic marked BP drop soon af exposure. The idea is to increase the dose until the blood pressure is control and there is no significant postural hypotension. A β_1-blocker may also be giv at this stage, usually to control any tachycardia (p100).

Surgery is usually done electively after a period of 4–6wks to allow full alp blockade and volume expansion. When admitted for surgery phenoxybenzamine dose is increased until significant postural hypotension.

Acute renal failure (ARF)—management

►Seek expert help promptly: BP, urinary sediment, serum K⁺, creatinine, ar ultrasound ***must*** be rapidly known. Have them to hand. See p292.

Definition Acute (over hours or days) deterioration in renal function, characterize by a rise in serum creatinine and urea, often with oliguric or anuria.

Causes

- Hypovolaemia.
- Low cardiac output.
- Sepsis.
- Drugs.
- Obstruction (p286).
- Other eg hepatorenal syndrome (p231), vasculitis (p542).

Investigations

- U&E, Ca^{2+}, PO_4^{3-}, FBC, ESR, CRP, INR, LFT, CK, LDH, protein electrophoresis, hepati serology, auto-antibodies (p539), blood cultures.
- Urgent urine microscopy and cultures. White cell casts suggest infection, but a seen in interstitial nephritis, and red cell casts an inflammatory glomerul condition (p288).
- USS of the renal tract.
- ECG, CXR.

Management See OPPOSITE for acute measures. Underlying principles are:

1. **Treat precipitating cause** Treat acute blood loss with blood transfusion, ar sepsis with antibiotics (p372). ARF is often associated with other diseases th need more urgent treatment. For example, someone in respiratory failure *a* renal failure may need to be managed on ITU, not a renal unit, to ensure optim management of the respiratory failure.
2. **Treat life-threatening hyperkalaemia** See OPPOSITE.
3. **Treat pulmonary oedema, pericarditis, and tamponade** (p788) Urge dialysis may be needed. If in pulmonary oedema, and no diuresis, consid removing a unit of blood, before dialysis commences.
4. **Treat volume depletion** if necessary. Resuscitate quickly; then match input output. Use a large-bore line in a large vein (central vein access can be risky obvious volume depletion).
5. **Treat sepsis.**
6. **Further care.**
   - Has obstruction been excluded? ►Examine for masses PR and *per vagina* arrange urgent ultrasound; is the bladder palpable? Bilateral nephrostomi relieve obstruction, provide urine for culture, and allow anterogra pyelography to determine the site of obstruction.
   - If worsening renal function but dialysis independent, consider renal biops
   - Diet: high in calories (2000–4000kcal/d) with adequate high-quality prote Consider nasogastric feeding or parenteral route if too ill.

Prognosis Depends on cause (ATN mortality: surgery or trauma—60%, medi illness—30%, pregnancy—10%). Oliguric ARF is worse than non-oliguric—more bleeds, sepsis, acidosis, and higher mortality.

Urgent dialysis if:

- K⁺ persistently high (>6.0mmol/L).
- Acidosis (pH <7.2).
- Pulmonary oedema and no substantial diuresis.
- Pericarditis. (In tamponade (p788), only dialyse *after* pressure on the heart relieved.)
- High catabolic state with rapidly progressive renal failure.

Management

Catheterize to assess hourly urine output, and establish fluid charts

↓

Assess intravascular volume BP, JVP, skin turgor, fluid balance sheet, weight, CVP, attach to cardiac monitor **consider inserting a central venous cannula**

↓

Investigations *(see OPPOSITE)*

↓

Identify and treat hyperkalaemia—see below
Use a cardiac monitor

↓

If dehydrated
Fluid challenge: 250–500mL of colloid or saline over 30min

↓

Reassess
Repeat challenge if still dehydrated. Aim for a CVP of 5–10cm

↓

Once fluid replete, continue fluids at 20mL + previous hour's urine output per hour

↓

If volume overloaded, consider urgent dialysis
A nitrate infusion, furosemide or 'renal dose' dopamine may help in the short term, especially to make space for blood transfusion etc. but does not alter outcome

↓

Correct acidosis with sodium bicarbonate, eg 50mL of 8.4% IV

↓

If clinical suspicion of sepsis, take cultures, then treat vigorously
Do not leave possible sources of sepsis (eg IV lines) in situ if not needed

↓

Avoid nephrotoxic drugs, eg NSAIDs, care with gentamicin. Check Data Sheet for all drugs given.

yperkalaemia

he danger is ventricular fibrillation. A K^+ >6.5mmol/L will usually require rgent treatment, as will those with ECG changes:

- Tall 'tented' T-waves ± flat P-waves ± increased P–R interval (see p669).
- Widening of the QRS complex—leading eventually, and dangerously, to a sinusoidal pattern and VF/VT.

reatment:

- 10mL calcium gluconate (10%) IV over 2min, repeated as necessary if severe ECG changes (may cause skin necrosis if extravasation: avoid injecting into small peripheral cannulae). This provides cardio-protection; it does not change serum potassium levels.
- Insulin + glucose, eg 20U soluble insulin + 50mL of glucose 50% IV. Insulin moves K^+ into cells.
- Nebulized salbutamol (2.5mg) also makes K^+ enter cells.
- Polystyrene sulfonate resin (eg Calcium Resonium®, 15g/8h in water) orally or, if vomiting makes the PO route problematic, as a 30g enema (followed by colonic irrigation, after 9h, to remove K^+ from the colon).
- Dialysis.

Acute poisoning—general measures

Diagnosis mainly from history. The patient may not tell the truth about what h been taken. Use *MIMS Colour Index*, *eMIMS* images, *BNF* descriptions, or t computerized system 'TICTAC' (ask pharmacy) to identify tablets and plan speci treatment. Clues may become apparent:

- ***Fast or irregular pulse:*** Salbutamol, antimuscarinics, tricyclics, quinine, phenothiazine poisoning.
- ***Respiratory depression:*** Opiate or benzodiazepine toxicity.
- ***Hypothermia:*** Phenothiazines, barbiturates.
- ***Hyperthermia:*** Amphetamines, MAOIs, cocaine, or ecstasy (p827).
- ***Coma:*** Benzodiazepines, alcohol, opiates, tricyclics, or barbiturates.
- ***Seizures:*** Recreational drugs, hypoglycaemic agents, tricyclics, phenothiazin or theophyllines.
- ***Constricted pupils:*** Opiates or insecticides (organophosphates, p827).
- ***Dilated pupils:*** Amphetamines, cocaine, quinine, or tricyclics.
- ***Hyperglycaemia:*** Organophosphates, theophyllines, or MAOIs.
- ***Hypoglycaemia:*** Insulin, oral hypoglycaemics, alcohol, or salicylates.
- ***Renal failure:*** Salicylate, paracetamol, or ethylene glycol.
- ***Metabolic acidosis:*** Alcohol, ethylene glycol, methanol, paracetamol, or carb monoxide poisoning—p826.
- ***↑Osmolality:*** Alcohols (ethyl or methyl); ethylene glycol. See p658.

Management See OPPOSITE for a general guide to management.

- ***Take blood*** as appropriate (p824). Always check paracetamol and salicyla levels.
- ***Empty stomach*** if appropriate (p824).
- ***Consider specific antidote*** (p826) or oral activated charcoal (p824).
- ***If you are not familiar with the poison*** get more information. The *Data She Compendium* SPC is useful. If in doubt how to act, phone the Poisons Informati Service: in the UK phone 0870 600 6266.

Continuing care Measure temperature, pulse, BP, and blood glucose regularly. U a continuous ECG monitor. If unconscious, nurse semi-prone, turn regularly, ke eyelids closed. A urinary catheter will be needed if the bladder is distended, renal failure is suspected, or forced diuresis undertaken. Take to ITU, eg respiration↓.

Psychiatric assessment Be sympathetic despite the hour! Interview relatives a friends if possible. Aim to establish:

- ***Intentions at time:*** Was the act planned? What precautions against bei found? Did the patient seek help afterwards? Does the patient think the meth was dangerous? Was there a final act (eg suicide note)?
- ***Present intentions.***
- ***What problems*** led to the act: do they still exist?
- ***Was the act*** aimed at someone?
- Is there a ***psychiatric disorder*** (depression, alcoholism, personality disord schizophrenia, dementia)?
- What are his ***resources*** (friends, family, work, personality)?

The assessment of suicide risk: The following increase the chance of futu suicide: original intention was to die; present intention is to die; presence psychiatric disorder; poor resources; previous suicide attempts; socially isolat unemployed; male; >50yrs old. See *OHCS* p338. There is an increased risk of dea in the first year following initial presentation.

Referral to psychiatrist: This depends partly on local resources. Ask advice presence of psychiatric disorder or high suicide risk.

Common law or the Mental Health Act: (in England and Wales) may provide the detention of the patient against his or her will: see *OHCS* p400.

Emergency care

ABC, clear airway

↓

Consider ventilation (if the respiratory rate is <8/min, or P_aO_2 <8kPa, when breathing 60% O_2, or the airway is at risk, eg GCS < 8)

↓

Treat shock (p778)

↓

If unconscious, nurse semi-prone

Further management

↓

Assess the patient

↓

History from patient, friends, or family is vital

↓

Features from the examination may help (see OPPOSITE)

↓

Investigations

- Glucose, U&E, FBC, LFT, INR, ABG, ECG, paracetamol, and salicylate levels
- Urine/serum toxicology, specific assays as appropriate

↓

Monitor

- T°, pulse & respiratory rate, BP, O_2 saturations, urine output ± ECG

↓

Treatment

- Supportive measures: may need catheterization
- ↓Absorption: consider gastric lavage ± activated charcoal, see p824

↓

Specific measures, see p824; for **antidotes**, see p826
Consider naloxone if ↓conscious level and pin-point pupils

Acute poisoning—specific points

Plasma toxicology For all unconscious patients, paracetamol and aspirin levels ar blood glucose are required. The necessity of other assays depends on the dru taken and the index of suspicion. Be guided by the poisons information servic More common assays include: digoxin; methanol; lithium; iron; theophyllin Toxicological screening of urine, especially for recreational drugs, may be of use some cases.

Gastric lavage Rarely used. Lavage after 30–60 min may make matters wors ►*Do not empty stomach* if petroleum products or corrosives such as acids, alkal bleach, descalers have been ingested (*exception:* paraquat), or if the patient unconscious or unable to protect their airway (unless intubated). ►Never indu vomiting.

Gastric emptying and lavage If comatosed, or no gag reflex, ask for a anaesthetist to protect airway with cuffed endotracheal tube. If conscious, g verbal consent.

- Monitor O_2 by pulse oximetry. See p148.
- Have suction apparatus to hand and working.
- Position the patient in left lateral position.
- Raise the foot of the bed by 20cm.
- Pass a lubricated tube (14mm external diameter) via the mouth, asking th patient to swallow.
- Confirm position in stomach—blow air down, and auscultate over the stomac
- Siphon the gastric contents. Check pH with litmus paper.
- Perform gastric lavage using 300–600mL tepid water at a time. Massage th left hypochondrium.
- Repeat until no tablets in siphoned fluid.
- Leave activated charcoal (50g in 200mL water) in the stomach unless alcoh iron, Li^+, or ethylene glycol ingested.
- When pulling out tube, occlude its end (prevents aspiration of fluid remaining the tube).

Activated charcoal reduces the absorption of many drugs from the gut whe given as a single dose of 50g with water, eg salicylates, paracetamol. It is given repeated doses (50g/4h) to increase elimination of some drugs from the blood, e carbamazepine, dapsone, theophyllines, quinine, digoxin, phenytoin, phenobarbita and paraquat. Lower doses are used in children.

Help on the web: UK GPs and other NHS workers and departments may register with ***toxbase*** www.spib.axl.co.uk for free up-to-date toxicological advice.

Some specific poisons and their antidotes

Benzodiazepines Flumazenil (for respiratory arrest) 200µg over 15s; then 100 at 60s intervals if needed. Usual dose range: 300–600µg IV over 3–6min (up 1mg; 2mg if on ITU). May provoke fits.

β-blockers Severe bradycardia or hypotension. Try atropine up to 3mg IV. Gi glucagon 2–10mg IV bolus + 5% dextrose if atropine fails (± an atropine infusi of 50µg/kg/h). If unresponsive, consider pacing or an aortic balloon pump.

Cyanide This fast-killing poison has affinity for Fe^{3+}, and inhibits the cytochro system, ↓aerobic respiration. ***3 phases:*** • Anxiety ± confusion • Pulse↑ or ↓ • Fits shock ± coma. ***Treatment:*** ➡100% O_2, GI decontamination; if consciousness either sodium nitrite + sodium thiosulfate, or dicobalt edetate 300mg IV over 5min, then 50mL 50% dextrose IV. (repeat up to twice); or hydroxocobalamin over 30 min (70mg/kg), repeated once is required. *Get expert help.* See p831.

Carbon monoxide Despite hypoxaemia skin is pink (or pale), not blue carboxyhaemoglobin (COHb) displaces O_2 from Hb binding sites. ***Symptom*** Headache, vomiting, pulse↑, tachypnoea, and, if COHb >50%, fits, coma, & cardi arrest. ➡Remove the source. Give 100% O_2. Metabolic acidosis usually responds correction of hypoxia. If severe, anticipate cerebral oedema. Give mannitol I (p813). Confirm diagnosis with a heparinized blood sample (COHb >10%) quick as levels may soon return to normal. Monitor ECG. *Hyperbaric O_2 may help: discu with the poisons service if is or has been unconscious, pregnant, COHb >20%, failing to respond.*

Digoxin *Symptoms:* Cognition↓, yellow-green visual halos, arrhythmias, nausea, anorexia. If serious arrhythmias are present, correct hypokalaemia, and inactiva with digoxin-specific antibody fragments (Digibind®). If load or level is unknow give 20 vials (800mg)—adult or child >20kg. Consult Data Sheet/SPC. Dilute water for injections (4mL/38mg vial) and 0.9% saline (to make a convenie volume); give IVI over ½h, via a 0.22µm-pore filter. If the amount of digox ingested is known, the data-sheet/SPC will tell you how many vials of Digibind® give, eg if 25 tabs of 0.25mg ingested, give 10 vials; if 50 tabs, give 20 vials; if 1C tabs, give 40 vials.

Heavy metals Enlist expert help.

Iron Deferoxamine 15mg/kg/h IVI; max 80mg/kg/d. **NB:** gastric lavage if ir ingestion in last hour; consider whole bowel irrigation.

Oral anticoagulants If major bleed, treat with vitamin K, 5mg slow IV; gi prothrombin complex concentrate 50U/kg IV (or if unavailable, fresh frozen plas 15mL/kg IVI). For abnormal INR with no (or minimal) bleeding, see BNF. If it is vit that anticoagulation continues, enlist expert help. Warfarin can normally restarted within 2–3d.

NB: coagulation defects may be delayed for 2–3d following ingestion.

Opiates (Many analgesics contain opiates.) Give naloxone eg 0.4–2mg IV; repe every 2min until breathing adequate (it has a short $t_{½}$, so it may need to be giv often or IM; max. 10mg). Naloxone may precipitate features of opiate withdrawal diarrhoea and cramps which will normally respond to diphenoxylate and atropi (Lomotil®—eg 2 tablets/6h PO). Sedate as needed (see p13). High-dose opia misusers may need methadone (eg 10–30mg/12h PO) to combat withdraw Register opiate addiction (*OHCS* p362), and refer for help.

Emergencies

ıenothiazine poisoning (eg chlorpromazine) No specific antidote. *Dystonia ɔrticollis, retrocollis, glossopharyngeal dystonia, opisthotonus):* try benzatropine -2mg IV/IM. Treat *shock* by raising the legs (± plasma expander IVI, or dopamine if desperate). Restore body temperature. *Monitor ECG.* Avoid lidocaine in rsrhythmias. Use diazepam IV for prolonged fits in the usual way (p808). *euroleptic malignant syndrome* consists of: hyperthermia, rigidity, extrapyramidal gns, autonomic dysfunction (labile BP, pulse↑, sweating, urinary incontinence), utism, confusion, coma, WCC↑, CPK↑; it may be treated with cooling. Dantrolene is been tried (p558).

ırbon tetrachloride poisoning this solvent, used in many industrial processes, uses vomiting, abdominal pain, diarrhoea, seizures, coma, renal failure, and nder hepatomegaly with jaundice and liver failure. IV acetylcysteine may improve ognosis. Seek expert help.

ʼganophosphate insecticides inactivate cholinesterase—the resulting increase in etylcholine causes the **SLUD** response: **s**alivation, **l**acrimation, **u**rination, and arrhoea. Also look for sweating, small pupils, muscle fasciculation, coma, spiratory distress, and bradycardia. ***Treatment:*** Wear gloves; remove soiled othes. Wash skin. Take blood (FBC & serum cholinesterase activity). Give atropine 2mg every 10min till full atropinization (skin dry, pulse >70, pupils dilated). Up 3 days' treatment may be needed. Also give pralidoxime 30mg/kg slowly IV (in e UK, the poisons information service will tell you how to get it; it is diluted with 10mL water for Injections). Repeat as needed every 30min; max 12g in 24h. ven if fits are not occurring, diazepam 5–10mg IV seems to help.

ıraquat poisoning (Found in weed-killers.) This causes D&V, painful oral ulcers, veolitis, and renal failure. Diagnose by urine test. Give activated charcoal *at once* 00g followed by a laxative, then 50g/3–4h, ± antiemetic). ►*Get expert help.* void O_2 early on (promotes lung damage).

:stasy poisoning Ecstasy is a semi-synthetic, hallucinogenic substance (MDMA, 4-methylenedioxymethamphetamine). Its effects range from nausea, muscle pain, urred vision, amnesia, fever, confusion, and ataxia to tachyarrhythmias, hyper-ermia, hyper/hypotension, water intoxication, DIC, K^+↑, acute renal failure, patocellular and muscle necrosis, cardiovascular collapse, and ARDS. There is no tidote and treatment is supportive. Management depends on clinical and lab ıdings, but may include:

Administration of activated charcoal and monitoring of BP, ECG, and temperature for at least 12h (rapid cooling may be needed).

Monitor urine output and U&E (renal failure p293), LFT, CK, FBC, and coagulation (DIC p336). Metabolic acidosis may benefit from treatment with bicarbonate.

Anxiety: diazepam 0.1–0.3mg/kg PO. Max IV does over 2min.

Narrow complex tachycardias in adults: consider metoprolol 5–10mg IV.

Hypertension can be treated with nifedipine 5–10mg PO or phentolamine 2–5mg IV. Treat hypotension conventionally (p778).

Hyperthermia: attempt to cool, if rectal T° > 39°C. Consider dantrolene 1mg/kg IV (may need repeating: discuss with your senior and a poisons unit, p822). Hyperthermia with ecstasy is akin to serotonin syndrome, and propranolol, muscle relaxation and ventilation may be needed.

ıakes (adders) ***Anaphylaxis*** p780. ***Signs of envenoming:*** BP↓ (vasodilatation, per cardiotoxicity) D&V; swelling spreading proximally within 4h of bite; bleeding ıms or venepuncture sites; anaphylaxis; ptosis; trismus; rhabdomyolysis; ılmonary oedema. ***Tests:*** WCC↑; clotting↓; platelets↓; U&E; urine RBC↑; CK↑; P_aO_2↓, :G. ***Management:*** Avoid active movement of affected limb (so use splints/slings). *void incisions and tourniquets.* ►Get help. Is antivenom indicated (IgG from ɜnom-immunized sheep)?—eg 10mL IV over 15min (adults ***and*** children) of *uropean Viper Antiserum* (from Farillon) for adder bites; have adrenaline to ınd—p780. Monitor ECG. For foreign snakes, see *BNF*.

Salicylate poisoning

Children: *OHCS* p1

Aspirin is a weak acid with poor water solubility. It is present in many over-th counter preparations. Anaerobic metabolism and the production of lactate a heat are stimulated by the uncoupling of oxidative phosphorylation. Effects a dose-related, and potentially fatal: • 150mg/kg: mild toxicity • 250mg/ moderate • >500mg/kg: severe toxicity.

Signs & symptoms Unlike paracetamol, many early features. Vomitir dehydration, hyperventilation, tinnitus, vertigo, sweating. Rarely; lethargy or con seizures, vomiting, ↓BP and heart block, pulmonary oedema, hyperthermia. Patier present initially with respiratory alkalosis due to a direct stimulation of the cent respiratory centres and then develop a metabolic acidosis. Hyper-hypoglycaemia may occur.

Management *General:* p822. Correct dehydration. Gastric lavage if within 1 activated charcoal (may be repeated, but is of unproven value).

- Paracetamol and salicylate level, glucose, U&E, LFT, INR, ABG, HCO_3^-, FBC. Salicyla level may need to be repeated after 2h, due to continuing absorption if potentially toxic dose has been taken.
- Levels over 700mg/L are potentially fatal.
- Monitor urine output, and blood glucose. If severe poisoning: salicylate leve blood pH, and U&E. Consider urinary catheter and monitoring urine pH. Bewa hypoglycaemia.
- Correct any metabolic acidosis with 1.26% HCO_3^- (sodium bicarbonate).
- If plasma level >500mg/L (3.6mmol/L), consider alkalinization of the urine, 1.5L 1.26% HCO_3^- with 40mmol KCl IV over 3h. Aim to make the **urine** pH 7.5 8.5. **NB:** monitor serum K^+ as hypokalaemia may occur.
- Consider dialysis if plasma level >700mg/L, and if renal or heart failure, seizur severe acidosis, or persistently ↑plasma salicylate. ECG monitor.
- Discuss any serious cases with the local toxicological service or national poiso information service.

Paracetamol poisoning

150mg/kg, or 12g in adults may be fatal. However, prompt treatment can preve liver failure and death. ►1 tablet of paracetamol = 500mg.

Signs & symptoms None initially, or vomiting ± RUQ pain. Later: jaundice a encephalopathy from liver damage (the main danger) ± renal failure.

Management *General measures* p822, lavage if >12g (or >150mg/kg) tak within 1h. Give activated charcoal if <8h since ingestion. Specific measures:

- Glucose, U&E, LFT, INR, ABG, FBC, HCO_3^-; blood paracetamol level at 4h post-ingestic
- If <8h since overdose and plasma paracetamol is above the line on the gra OPPOSITE, start acetylcysteine.
- If >8h and suspicion of large overdose (>7.5g) err on the side of caution a start acetylcysteine, stopping it if level below treatment line and INR/ALT norm
- Acetylcysteine is given by IVI: 150mg/kg in 200mL of 5% dextrose over 15m Then 50mg/kg in 500mL of 5% dextrose over 4h. Then 100mg per kg/16h in 1 of 5% dextrose. Rash is a common SE: treat with chlorphenamine, and obser do not stop unless anaphylatoid reaction with shock, vomiting, and whee (≤10%). An alternative is methionine 2.5g/4h PO for 16h (total: 10g), b absorption is unreliable if vomiting. Benefit is lessened by concurrent charco
- If ingestion time is unknown, or it is staggered, or presentation is >15h fro ingestion, treatment *may* help. ►Get advice.
- The graph may mislead if HIV+ve (hepatic glutathione↓), or if long-acti paracetamol has been taken, or if pre-existing liver disease or induction of liv enzymes has occurred. ►Beware glucose↓; ward-test hourly; INR/12h.
- Next day do INR, U&E, LFT. If INR rising, continue acetylcysteine until <1.4.
- If continued deterioration, discuss with the liver team. Don't hesitate to get he

riteria for transfer to a specialist unit:

Encephalopathy or *ICP*↑. Signs of CNS oedema: BP >160/90 (sustained) or brief rises (systolic >200mmHg), bradycardia, decerebrate posture, extensor spasms, poor pupil responses. ICP monitoring can help, p812.

INR >2.0 at <48h—or >3.5 at <72h (so measure INR every 12h). Peak elevation: 72–96h. LFTs are *not* good markers of hepatocyte death. If INR is *normal* at 48h, the patient may go home.

Renal impairment (creatinine >200μmol/L). Monitor urine flow. Daily U&E and serum creatinine (use haemodialysis if >400μmol/L).

Blood pH <7.3 (lactic acidosis → tissue hypoxia). • *Systolic BP* <80mmHg.

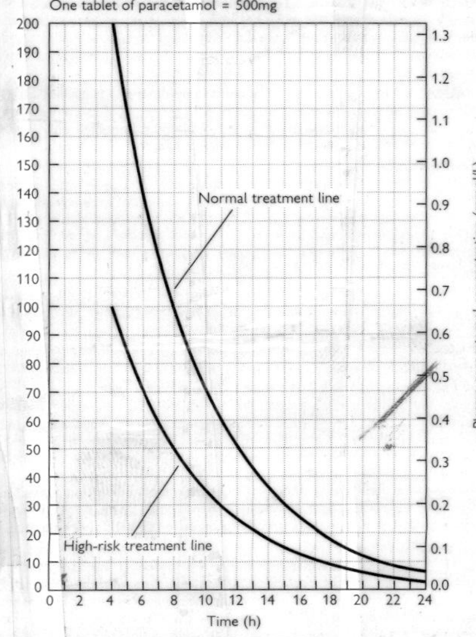

tients whose plasma-paracetamol concentrations are above the **normal eatment line** should be treated with acetylcysteine by intravenous infusion r, provided the overdose has been taken **within 10-12h**, with methionine mouth). Patients on enyzme-including drugs (eg carbamazepine, enobarbital, phenytoin, rifampicin, and alcohol) or who are malnourished g in anorexia, in alcoholism, or those who are HIV-positive) should be eated if their plasma-paracetamol concentrations are above the **high-risk eatment line**. (We thank Dr Alun Hutchings for permission to reproduce is graph.)

▸▸Burns

Resuscitate and arrange transfer for all major burns. (>25% partial thickness adult and >20% in children). Assess site, size, and depth of the burn. Referral is st warranted in cases of full thickness burns >5%, partial thickness burns >10% adults or >5% in children or the elderly, burns of special sites, chemical ar electrical burns and burns with inhalational injury.

Assessment *Burn size* is important to assess (see BOX) as it influences the size the inflammatory response (vasodilatation, increased vascular permeability) ar thus fluid shift from the intravascular volume. The size must be estimated calculate fluid requirements. Ignore erythema. *Burn depth* determines healir time/scarring; assessing this may be hard, even when experienced. The b distinction is whether the burn is partial thickness (painful, red, and blistered) c full thickness (insensate/painless; grey-white). **NB:** burns can evolve, particular over the 1st 48h.

Resuscitation *Airway:* Beware of upper airway obstruction developing if h gases inhaled. Suspect if history of fire in enclosed space, soot in oral/nasal cavi singed nasal hairs of hoarse voice. A flexible laryngo/bronchoscopy is usef Involve anaesthetists early and consider early intubation.

Breathing: Exclude life-threatening chest injuries (eg tension pneumothorax) ar constricting burns. Give 100% O_2 if carbon monoxide poisoning is suspecte (mostly from history, may have cherry-red skin, measure carboxyhaemoglob (COHb) and compare to nomograms). With 100% O_2 $t_{½}$ of COHb falls from 250m to 40min (consider hyperbaric O_2 if: pregnant; CNS signs; >20% COHb). SpO_2 (oxir etry) is unreliable. Decompress if chest burns impair thorax excursion (*OHCS* p73

Circulation: Partial thickness burns >10% in a child and >15% in adults requi IV fluid resuscitation. Put up 2 large-bore (14G or 16G) IV lines. Do not worry if yc have to put these through burned skin, intraosseous access is valuable in infan (see *OHCS*). Secure them well: they are literally lifelines.

Use a ***burns calculator*** flow chart or a formula, eg: ***Parkland formula*** (popula 4 × weight (kg) × % burn=mL Hartmann's solution in 24h, half given in 1st 8h.

Muir and Barclay formula: [weight (kg) × %burn]/2=mL colloid (eg Haemaccel per unit time. Time periods are 4h, 4h, 4h, 6h, 6h, and 12h. Either formula acceptable but must use appropriate fluid ie crystalloid for Parkland not colloi **NB:** A meta-analysis (somewhat flawed) suggests the use of colloid (albumin) c cause ↑ mortality (slightly); it is also expensive. Replace fluid from the time of bu not from the time first seen in hospital.

Formulae are only guides: adjust IVI according to clinical response and uri output; aim for >0.5mL/kg/h (>1mL/kg/h in children), ~50% more in electri burns and inhalation injury. Monitor T° (core & surface); catheterize the bladd

Treatment Do *not* apply cold water to extensive burns for long periods: this n intensify shock. Take care with circumferential full thickness burns of the limbs compartment syndrome may develop rapidly particularly after fluid resuscitatic Decompress the limbs (escharotomy and fasciotomy) as necessary. If transferrir to a burns unit, do not burst blisters or apply any special creams as this can hind assessment. Simple saline gauze or Vaseline® gauze is suitable; cling film is usef as a temporary measure and relieves pain. Use morphine in IV aliquots and titra for good analgesia. Ensure tetanus immunity. Antibiotic prophylaxis is not routir

Definitive dressings There are many dressings for partial thickness burns, eg bi logical (pigskin, cadaveric skin), synthetic (Mepitel®, Duoderm®) and silver sulfa azine cream alone (Flamazine®) or with cerium nitrate as Flammacerium® (on named-patient basis[UK]); it forms a leathery eschar which resists infection. Maj full thickness burns benefit from early tangential excision and split-skin grafts the burn is a major source of inflammatory cytokines causing SIRS (systen inflammatory response syndrome) and forms a rich medium for bacterial grow

Smoke inhalation

Initially there is laryngospasm that leads to hypoxia and straining (leading to petechiae), then hypoxic cord relaxation leads to true inhalation injury. Free radicals, cyanide compounds, and carbon monoxide accompany thermal injury. Cyanide compounds (generated eg from burning plastics) bind reversibly with ferric ions in enzymes, so stopping oxidative phosphorylation, causing dizziness, headaches, and seizures. Tachycardia and dyspnoea soon give way to bradycardia and apnoea. Carbon monoxide is generated later in the fire as oxygen is depleted. NB: COHb levels do not correlate well with the severity of poisoning and partly reflect smoking status and urban living conditions.

100% O_2 is given to elute both cyanide and CO.

Involve ICU/anaesthetists early: early ventilation may be useful, consider repeated bronchoscopic lavage.

Enlist expert help in cyanide poisoning: there is no one regimen suitable for all situations. Clinically mild poisoning may be treated by rest, O_2, and amyl nitrite 0.2–0.4mL via an Ambu® bag. IV antidotes may be used for moderate poisoning: sodium thiosulfate is a common first choice. More severe poisoning may require eg hydroxocobalamin, sodium nitrite, and dimethylaminophenol.

Lund & Browder charts[1]

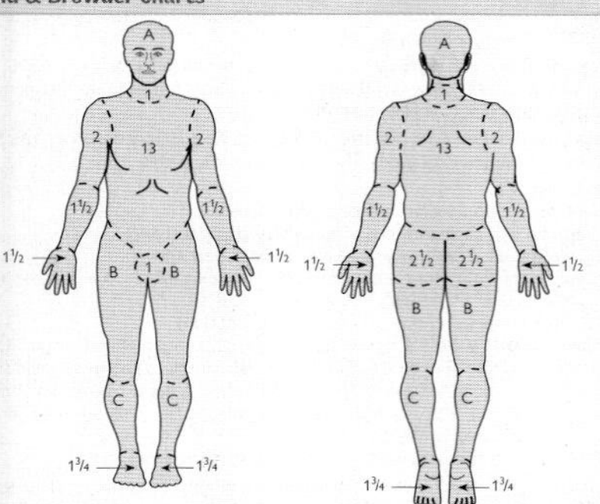

Relative percentage of body surface area affected by growth

Area	Age 0	1	5	10	15	Adult
A: half of head	9½	8½	6½	5½	4½	3½
B: half of thigh	2¾	3¼	4	4¼	4½	4¾
C: half of leg	2½	2½	2¾	3	3¼	3½

Accurate but time-consuming compared with the '**Rule of nines**': arm: 9%; front of trunk 18%; ead & neck 9%; leg 18%; back of trunk 18%; perineum 1%. The rule of nines generally verestimates burn area (better than underestimating). **A modified rule of nines for children:** om birth up to 1yr, surface area of head and neck is 18% and each leg is 14%. For each year ter, the head loses 1% and each leg gains 0.5%—so adult proportions are reached by age 10yrs. *'e thank Professor Tor Chiu for help in preparing this topic.*

Hypothermia

►*Have a high index of suspicion and a low-reading thermometer.* Most patients a elderly and do not complain, or feel, cold—so they have not tried to war themselves up. In the young, hypothermia is usually either from cold exposure (e near-drowning), or it is secondary to impaired level of consciousness (eg followir excess alcohol or drug overdose).

Definition Hypothermia implies a core (rectal) temperature <35°C.

Causes In the elderly hypothermia is often caused by a combination of:

- Impaired homeostatic mechanisms: usually age-related.
- Low room temperature: poverty, poor housing.
- Disease: Impaired thermoregulation (pneumonia, MI, heart failure).
- Reduced metabolism (immobility, hypothyroidism, diabetes mellitus).
- Autonomic neuropathy (p494, eg diabetes mellitus, Parkinson's).
- Excess heat loss (psoriasis). Cold awareness ↓ (dementia, confusion).
- Increased exposure to cold (falls, especially at night when cold).
- Drugs (major tranquillizers, antidepressants, diuretics). Alcohol.

The patient *How frozen I then became: I did not die, yet nothing of li remained.*[1] So don't assume that if vital signs seem to be absent, the patient mu be dead: rewarm (see below) and re-examine. If T° <32°C, this sequence may occu ↓BP → coma → bradycardia → AF → VT → VF. The abdomen can feel 'colder than cla If >32°C, there may simply be pallor ± apathy.

Diagnosis Check oral or axillary T°. If ordinary thermometer shows <36.5°C, use low-reading one PR. Is the rectal temperature <35°C? Infra-red ear thermomete can accurately reflect core temperature.

Tests Urgent U&E, plasma glucose, and amylase. Thyroid function tests; FBC; bloc cultures. Consider blood gases. The ECG may show J-waves.

Treatment

- Ventilate if comatose or respiratory insufficiency.
- Warm IVI (for access or to correct electrolyte disturbance).
- Cardiac monitor (both VF and AF can occur during warming).
- Consider antibiotics for the prevention of pneumonia (p153). Give these routine in patients over 65yrs with a temperature <32°C.
- Consider urinary catheter (to assess renal function).
- ***Slowly rewarm.*** Do not reheat too quickly, causing peripheral vasodilatatio shock, and death. Aim for a rise of ½°C/h. Old, conscious patients should sit in warm room taking hot drinks. Thermal blankets may cause too rapid warming old patients. The first sign of too rapid warming is falling BP. Treat by allowir patient to cool down slightly.
- Rectal temperature, BP, pulse, and respiratory rate every ½ hour.

NB: Advice is different for victims of sudden hypothermia from immersion. Here, e if there has been a cardiac arrest, and T° <30°C, mediastinal warm lavag peritoneal or haemodialysis, and cardiopulmonary bypass (no heparin if traum may be needed (*OHCS* p724).

Complications Arrhythmias (if there is a cardiac arrest continue resuscitating un T° >33°C, as cold brains are less damaged by hypoxia); pneumonia; pancreatit acute renal failure; intravascular coagulation.

Prognosis Depends on age and degree of hypothermia. If age >70yrs ar T° <32°C then mortality >50%.

Before hospital discharge Anticipate problems. Will it happen again? What is h network of support? Review medication (could you stop tranquillizers)? How progress to be monitored? Liaise with GP/social worker.

1 In the last round of the 9th circle of *Hell*, Dante tells how those betraying their benefactors a encased in ice (*canto XXXIV*) 'Com'io divenni allor gelato e fioco...Io non mori e non rimasi vivo

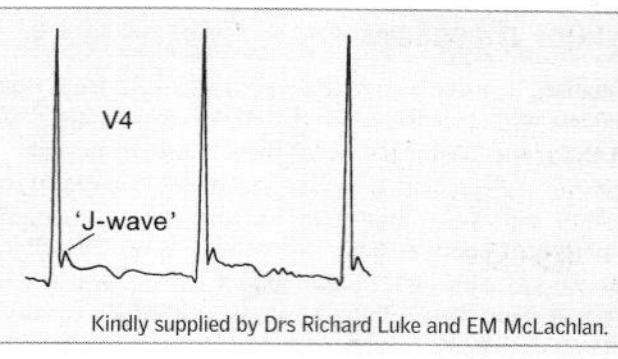

Kindly supplied by Drs Richard Luke and EM McLachlan.

Major disasters

Planning All hospitals have a detailed *Major Accident Plan*, but additionally the tasks of key personnel can be distributed on individual *Action Cards*.

At the scene Call the police; tell them to take command.

Safety: Is paramount—your own and others. Be visible (luminous monogrammed jacket) and wear protective clothing where appropriate (safety helmet; waterproofs; boots; respirator in chemical environment).

Triage: See OHCS p797. Label RED if will die in a few mins if no treatment. YELLOW = will die in ~2h if no treatment; GREEN = can wait. (BLUE = dead).

Communications: Are essential. Each emergency service will dispatch a control vehicle and will have a designated incident officer for liaison. Support medical staff from hospital report to the medical incident officer—he is usually the first doctor on the scene: his job is to assess then communicate to the receiving hospital the number and severity of casualties, to organize resupply of equipment and to replace fatigued staff. He must resist temptation to treat casualties as this compromises his role.

Equipment: Must be portable and include: intubation and cricothyrotomy set; intravenous fluids (colloid); bandages and dressings; chest drain (+flutter valve); amputation kit (when used, ideally 2 doctors should concur); drugs—*analgesic*: morphine; *anaesthetic*: ketamine 2mg/kg IV over >60s (0.5mg/kg is a powerful analgesic without respiratory depression); limb splints (may be inflatable); defibrillator/monitor; ± pulse oximeter.

Evacuation: Remember: with immediate treatment on scene, the priority for evacuation may be reduced (eg a tension pneumothorax—RED—relieved can wait for evacuation—becomes YELLOW), but those who may suffer by delay at the scene must go first. Send any severed limbs to the same hospital as the patient ideally chilled—but not frozen.

At the hospital a 'major incident' is declared. The *first receiving* hospital will take most of the casualties; the *support* hospital(s) will cope with overflow and may provide mobile teams so that staff are not depleted from the first hospital. A control room is established and the medical coordinator ensures staff have been summoned, nominates a triage officer, and supervises the best use of inpatient beds and ITU/theatre resources.

Blast injury may be caused by domestic (eg gas explosion) or industrial (eg mining) accidents or by terrorist bombs. Death may occur without any obvious external injury (air emboli). Injury occurs in 6 ways:

1. **Blast wave** A transient (milliseconds) wave of overpressure expands rapidly producing cellular disruption, shearing forces along tissue planes (submucosal/subserosal haemorrhage) and re-expansion of compressed trapped gas—bowel perforation, fatal air embolism.
2. **Blast wind** This can totally disrupt a body or cause avulsive amputations. Bodies can be thrown and sustain injuries on landing.
3. **Missiles** Penetration or laceration from missiles are by far the commonest injuries. Missiles arise from the bomb or are secondary, eg glass.
4. **Flash burns** These are usually superficial and occur on exposed skin.
5. **Crush** Injuries: beware sudden death or renal failure after release.
6. **Psychological injury** Eg post-traumatic stress disorder (OHCS p347).

Treatment Approach the same as any major trauma OHCS p726. Rest and observe any suspected of exposure to significant blast but without other injury. Gun-shot injury: see OHCS p720.

Source: I Greaves 1999 *Pre-hospital Medicine*, Arnold; S Mellor *Recent Advances in Surgery* 14, Churchill Livingstone, London 1991 p53–p68

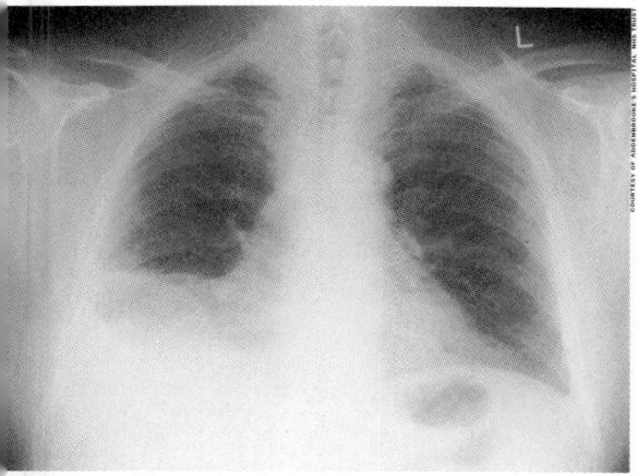

COURTESY OF ADDENBROOKE'S HOSPITAL NHS TRUST

Middle lobe consolidation and a right pleural effusion.

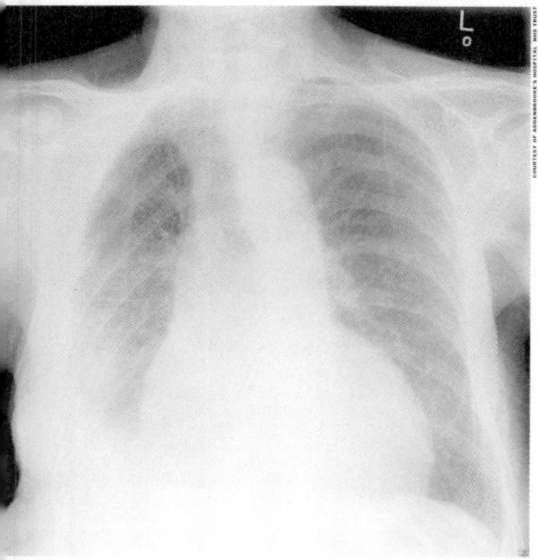

COURTESY OF ADDENBROOKE'S HOSPITAL NHS TRUST

There is cardiomegaly and loss of the right costophrenic angle from a pleural effusion: consistent with heart failure.

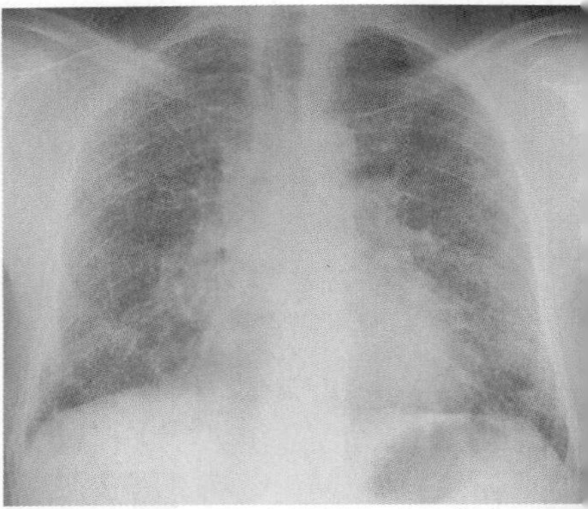

Diffuse reticular shadowing secondary to interstitial lung disease. The diagnosis was fibrosing alveolitis (UIP).

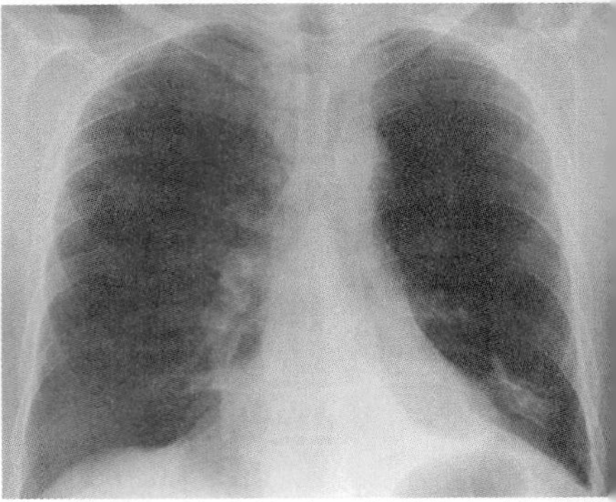

Collapse of the left lower lobe—the triangular opacity behind the heart. Also, the left main bronchus has been pulled down.

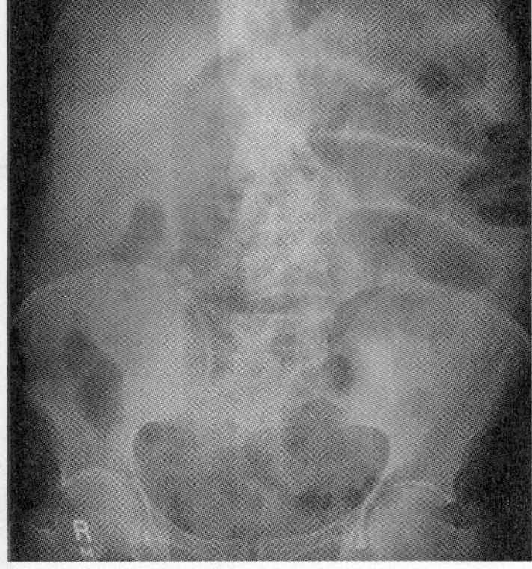

The gas pattern seen in small bowel obstruction.

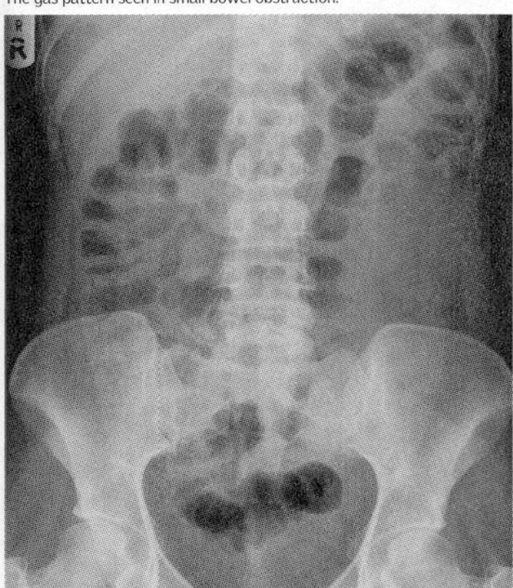

Normal large bowel gas pattern.

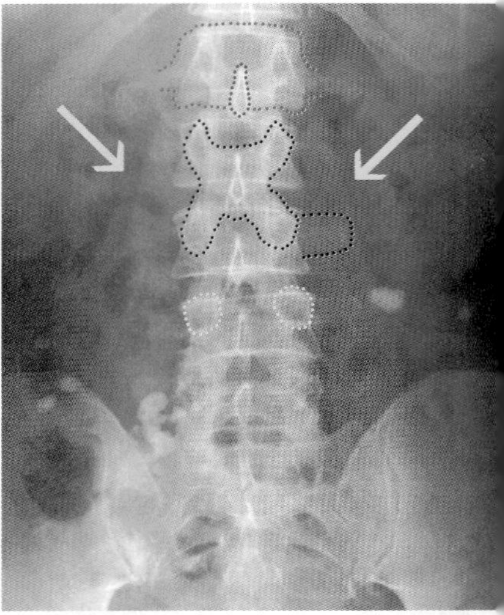

AXR showing calcified mesenteric lymph nodes. Also note; psoas lines (arrows); spinou process (green); transverse process (blue); pedicles (yellow): facet joint processe (outline in red); vertebral body (cyan).

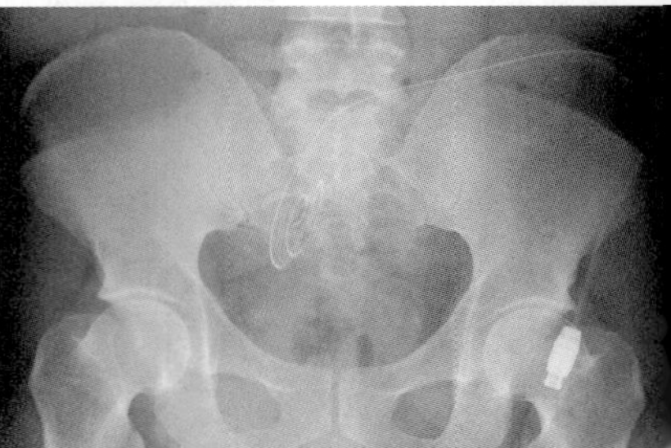

A CAPD catheter (for continuous ambulatory peritoneal dialysis).

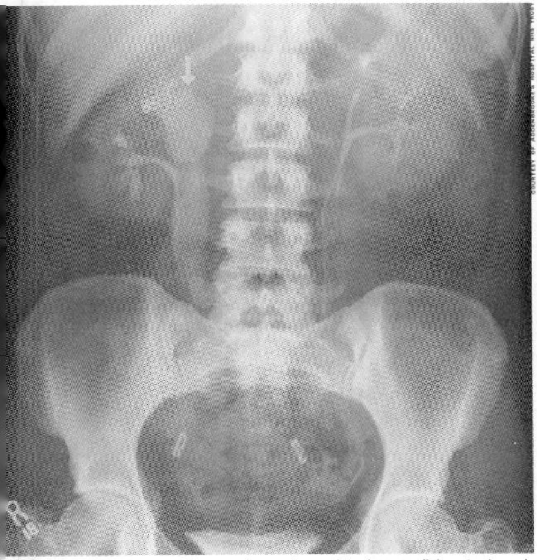

U: bilateral duplex ureters. The superior ureter moiety (arrowed) is ectopic and ters the bladder, urethra or vagina more inferiorly than the normally placed inferior eter moiety. The superior ureter may be associated with a ureterocele and is more ely to obstruct. The inferior ureter may be associated with reflux nephropathy and arring.

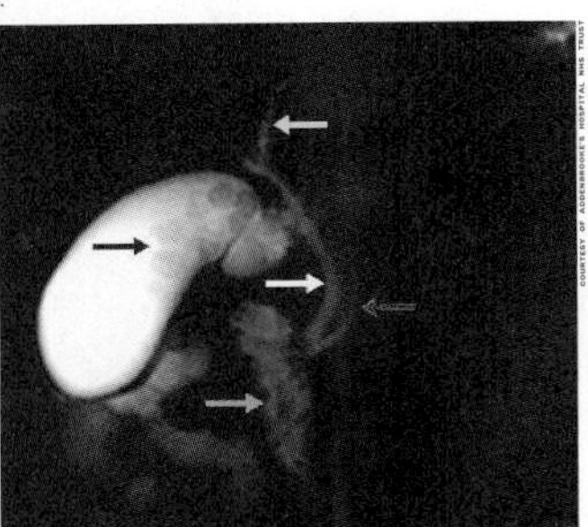

MRCP of the biliary system showing: left hepatic duct (yellow arrow); multiple gallstones in the gallbladder (black arrow); common bile duct (white arrow); pancreatic duct (red arrow); duodenum (green arrow).

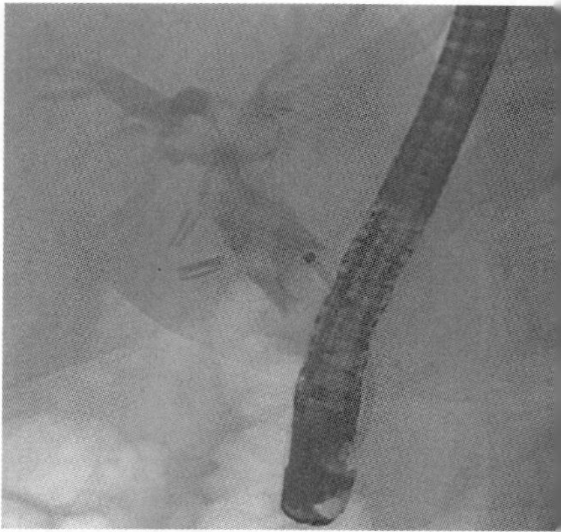

The ERCP shows dilated intra- and extrahepatic ducts. The multiple fill-ing defects relate t calculi within and obstructing the ducts. Note cholecystectomy clips.

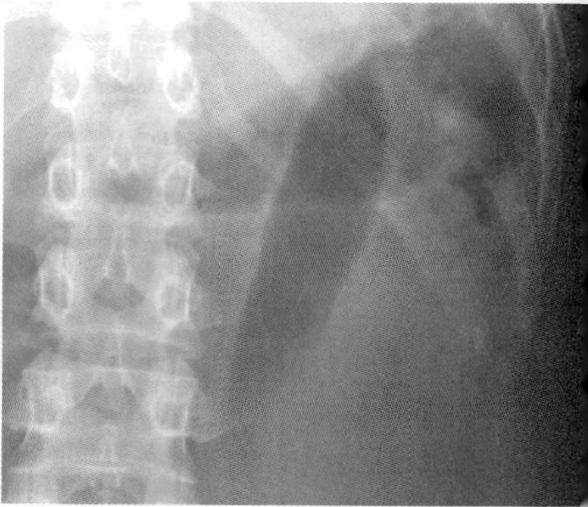

Part of the descending colon with mucosal thickening and loss of normal haustral pattern; seen in colitis.

breviations: F after a page number refers to a figure or image; syn=syndrome.

All indexes can be improved; tell us how at ohcm.index@oup.com

All indexes can be improved; tell us how by e-mailing ohcm.index@oup.com

All indexes can be improved; tell us how by e-mailing ohcm.index@oup.com

G

H

All indexes can be improved; tell us how by e-mailing ohcm.index@oup.com

J

K

L

All indexes can be improved; tell us how by e-mailing ohcm.index@oup.com

S

All indexes can be improved; tell us how by e-mailing ohcm.index@oup.com

T

U

V

Acknowledgments

Akira Fujii Image, **Courtesy of David Malin**; Author's stethoscope superimposed, Figure 1, p2; After
Clinical Examination; N Talley, **Blackwell**, Auscultating the heart, p29; Typical waveforms of common heart
murmurs, p35; After Clinical Examination, Macleod, **Churchill**, the jugular venous pressure wave, p31;
After Clinical Anatomy Principles, **L.H. Mathers** ISBN 0815189265, the jugular venous systems, p31;
After AIDS to undergraduate medicine, J Burton, **Churchill**, Arterial pulse waveforms, p31; After
P **Paoliel**, the cardiac cycle, p33; After **RCSI** www.rcsi.ie, Surface plural, lung and fissure markings, p37;
Courtesy of Addenbrooke's Hospital NHS Trust, Figure 1, p47; Figure 1, 2 p219; Figure 1, p529; Figure
1, 2, 3, 4 p563; Figure 1, 2, p575; Figure 1, p587, p595, p601, p617, p618, p621; Figure 2, p597; Figure 1,
2, p599; Figure 1, p603; Figure 1 (in 'Salivary gland pathology' colour box), p617; Figure 1, 2 p623; Figure
1, 2, p625; Figure 1, 2, p714; Figure 4, p715; Figure 1, 2, 3, 4, p716; Figure 5, 6, p717; Figure 1, 2, 3, p718;
Figure 1, 2, 3, p719; Figure 1, 2, 3, 4, 5, p721; Figure 1, 2, p722; Figure 3, 4, 5, 6, p723; Figure 1, 2, 3, p724;
Figure 4, 5, 6, p725; Cardiac MUGA scintigram, p727; Figure 1, 2, 3, 4, p728; Figure 5, 6, 7, 9, p729; Figure
1, 2, 3, p730; Figure 4, 5, 6, 7, 8, p731; Figure 1, p732; Figure 2, 3, 4, 5 p733; Figure 1, p757; Enlarged
Radiology Image: Middle lobe consolidation and a right pleural infusion, p836; Enlarged Radiology Image:
There is cardiomegaly and loss of right costophrenic angle, p836; Enlarged Radiology Image: The gas
pattern seen in small bowel obstruction, p838; Enlarged Radiology Image: Normal large bowel gas
pattern, p838; Enlarged Radiology Image: AXR showing calcified mesenteric lymph nodes, p839; Enlarged
Radiology Image: A CAPD catheter, p839; Enlarged Radiology Image: IVU: bilateral duplex ureters, p840;
Enlarged Radiology Image: Normal MRCP of the biliary system, p840; Enlarged Radiology Image: ERCP
showing dilated intra-and extrahepatic ducts, p841; Enlarged Radiology Image: Part of the descending
colon with mucosal thickening and loss of normal hautral pattern, p841; Image after **RCSI website**, the
contents of the cavernous sinus and the cranial nerve names, p49; Figure 2, p259; Figure 1, p263;
Courtesy of Professor Eric W. Fonkalsrud., Figure 1, p55; After KUMAR & CLARK, Internucleur
ophthalmoplegia (INO) and its causes, p65; Ted Hughes, Birthday Letters. **Faber & Faber**, by kind
permission., Palpitations, Russian roulette and hypochondrias, p67; Understanding Angina ©American
Heart Association; by kind permission, Coronary artery anatomy, p97; After R Hall **Med International** 17
'74., Echocardiography, p99; After PJ Kumar and ML Clark Clinical Medicine, Fungi and the lung, p161;
Courtesy of Yale University School of Medicine, Figure 1, p162; **Courtesy of Prof P Scally**, Figure 1,
p163; Figure 1, p183, After B Harrison Thoracic Medicine, ed P Emerson, **Butterworth**, London, Examples
of serial peak flow charts, p165; Figure 1, p463, p500; Figure 1, p735; ©Lushpix/Unlisted Images, Inc.,
Figure 1, p737; Figure 1, p581; American Col. of Surgeons' Committee on Trauma, Advanced Trauma Life
Support® for Doctors (ATLS®) Student Maunal 7e, Chicago: Am. Col. Surg, 2004., Figure Table: Assessing
hypovolaemia from blood loss, p581; Figure 3, 5, p715; Figure Enlarged Radiology Image: Diffuse reticular
shadowing secondary to interstitial lung disease, p837; Figure Enlarged Radiology Image: Collapse of the
left lower lobe, p837 **Courtesy of Professor Jonathan D. Trobe**, Figure 1,3, 4 p195; Oxford Textbook of
Medicine, **OUP.**, Figure 2, p195; Figure 1, 2, 3 p544; Differential diagnosis of 'red-eye', p545; Figure 1,
p699; Figure 1, p376; Figure 2, 3, 4 p393; Figure 2, p441; After http://www.patient.co.uk/
showdoc/pilsinl/043.gif, Figure 1, p506; **Courtesy of Dr. Stephen Golding**, Figure 1, p233; Figure 3, p237;
After **www.tiscali.co.uk**, Hiatus hernia- sliding and rolling, p237; Figure 1, p585; Image After Fox S.I.,
Human Physiology 4th edition, **Brown**, The pathophysiology of aneurysmal disease, p587; Figure 1, p607,
p613, p615; After **RCSI website**, The layers of fascia in the scrotum, p619; After RD Judge, GD Zuidema,
FT Fitzgerald Clinical Diagnosis 5th edn, **Little, Brown**, Boston, Diagnosis of scrotal masses, p619; After
RCSI website, The distribution of lymph nodes in the head and neck, p621; The anatomy of the region of
the thyroid gland, p623; After **RCSI website**, Figure Diagram: Anatomy of the anal canal, p627; After
Craig, J.A., **Novartis**, Internal and external haemorrhoids, p629; Reproduced with permission from
Surgery at a glance; P Grace; **Blackwell**, Figure Diiagram: Some examples of hernias, p631; After **RCSI
website**, Inguinal hernia mesh repair, p633; After **RCSI website**, Lymphatic drainage of the stomach,
p637; Highly selective vagotomy, p639; After **Sandone, C.**, Nissen fundoplication, p639; J Ahn 2004
Circulation 109 1463; ECG by kind permission of **Dr Shayashi.**, ECG 14, p687; Clinical Skills, Oxford Core
Text, 410, **OUP**, Figure 2, p695; 411., Figure 1, 3 p701; Figure 8, p729; Image and Commentary; **Courtesy
of Dr. Anthony Mee**, Figure 1, 2 p237; **Courtesy of Ian Herriott**, Figure 1, p243; After **www.rcsi.ie**, the
pathway of bilirubin metabolism, p243; Figure 1, 3 p249; Figure 1, p259; Figure 2, p267; **Courtesy of Dr.
Jon Simmons**, Figure 1, 2 p245; Figure 2, 4, 5 p249; **Courtesy of ST. Mark**; S Hospital Endoscopy Unit,
Figure 1, p248; **Courtesy of Dr. Roger Wagner**, Figure 1, p276; 'SILENCE'—**Courtesy of Tiago-Phelipe**,
Silence, p277; Principal source: Atlas of Bedside Microscopy ©JM Longmore; **RCGP**, Urine microscopy,
p279; **Courtesy of Dr. Ian Roberts**, Figure 1, 2, 4, 5 p280; **Courtesy of Dr. Tom Turmezei**, Figure 3, p280;
Oxford Textbook of Nephrology, 2465, Figure 1, p287; Figure 1, 2, 3, p751; After Clinically Oriented
Anatomy, K. Moore, Safe Approach to entering the pleura by the intercostal route, p753; Redrawn from
Thorax 2003 58 suppl II; ii55, with permission., The 'safe triangle' for insertion of a chest drain, p755;
Defining the 3rd-4th lumbar vertebral interspace, p757; after **www.ebme.co.uk**, Figure 1, 2, p758;
Images after **RCSI website**, Taking arterial blood gas (ABG) samples, p759; **Courtesy of The PKD
Foundation**, Figure 1, p305; **Courtesy of Prof. Krzysztof Lewandowski**, Figure 1, p309; Figure 3, p313;
Figure 4, p315; Figure 1, 2, 3, 4, 5 p317; **Courtesy of Professor Thomas Habif**, Figure 2, p313; Figure 2, 5,
p547; **RCSI website**, Lymphatic drainage of the breast, p567; the venous system at the thoracic outlet,
p575; Figure 3, p695; Figure 1, p703; **Courtesy of Dr. Nivaldo Medeiros**, Figure 1, 6 p315; Figure 7, p315;
Figure 2, p351; **Courtesy of Prof. Christine Lawrence & Crookston Col.**, Figure 5, p315; Figure 1, p301,
p303; Figure 4, 5 p313; Figure 3, p315; Figure 1, 2 p327; Figure 1, 2, 3, 4 p339; Figure 1,2, 3, 4 p341;
Figure 2, 4 p343; Figure 1, p345; Figure 3, p347, p351; Figure 1, p351, p353, p355; Figure 2, 3 p353;
Courtesy of Professor Barbara Bain ©2005 Massachusetts Medical Society, Figure 8, p315; Figure 1,
p319; Figure 2, 3, 4, 5, 6, 7 p325; Figure 2, p347; Figure 2, p315; **Courtesy of The Crookston Collection**,
Figure 9, p315; Figure 2, p329, p331, p337, p339, p345; Figure 4, p695, p701; Figure 1, p697; Figure 1 (in
Revised Criteria' colour box), p541; **Courtesy of Dr Erwin van Den Enden**, Figure 1, p329; **Courtesy of
Dr Tom D Thacher**, Figure 1, p347; **Courtesy of OTM**, Figure 2, p355; After Izabela Kurkiewicz, Figure 1,
p364; **Courtesy of Vincent A. Fischetti Ph.D.**, Figure 1, p365; ©**David Belnap**; University of Utah & James

Hogle; Harvard Med. School), Figure 2, p366; **Courtesy of Prof Donald Duszynski**, University of New Mexico, Figure 2, p379; **Courtesy of Prof Upton**; Kansas Univ, Figure 1, p380; After Paintings by Gertrude Nicholson, in Oatney Gr. The Primate Malarias; **U.S. Dept. of Health, Education and Welfare**, Figure 1 p383; Figure 5, p383; Figure 1, p404; Figure 1, p406; Author's Collection (JML); Stained at the Bedside Figure 2, p406; Figure 1, p410; Figure 1, 2 p424; Figure 1, p418; Figure 3, p423; Figure 1, 3 p425 **Nasjonalgalleriet** (National Gallery), OSLO, Figure 2, p425; After Expert Reviews in Molecular Medicine **CUP**, 1999, Figure 4, p425; Figure 1, 2, p426, p427, p428; Figure 2, p428; Figure 1, 2, 3 p430; Figure 1 p431, p432, p433; **Courtesy of Dr. Chi Wai L Eung**, FRCP, Figure 1, p388; **Courtesy of JML & Axel Schneider**, Figure 1, p389; After Murphy & Webster (in Fields Virology, **Lippincott**)., Figure 1, p391 **Courtesy of Prof Klaus Radsak**; Marburg, Figure 1, p392; after fernando monroy, Figure 1, p393 **Courtesy of Subhash K. Mohan**, Figure 1, p399; **Courtesy M. McGinnis**, Figure 20, p399; **Courtesy of Prof Arthur Huntley**, Figure 1, p408; Figure 5, 8, p429; **Courtesy of Centers for Disease Control & Prevention**, Figure 1, p413; **Courtesy of Prof. Jayakar Thomas**, Figure 1, p417; **Courtesy of Pro Spilatro**, Figure 1, p419; **Courtesy of Dbelnap (Utah) & J Hogle (Harvard)**, Figure 1, p421; **Courtesy of Pierre-Yves Guillaume**, Figure 3, 4, 6, 7 p429; **Courtesy of Danil Hamoundi**, MD, Figure 1, p440; Figure 1 p470; Figure 1, p457; **Courtesy of M Bhargava & J Hunter**, Figure 1, p526; Oxford Textbook of Rheumatology, **OUP**, Figure 1, 2 p531; **Courtesy of David F. Fiorentino**, MD, PHD. with kind permission from **Skin & Aging**., Figure 1, p541; **Courtesy of Amy McMichael**, MD. with kind permission from **Skin & Aging**., Figure 2, p541; **Courtesy of Dr. William Herring**., Figure 1, p543; Both Images **Courtesy of Cunningham's Manual of Practical Anatomy** vol 2 138, The anatomy of the gallbladder and extrahepatic biliary tree, p591; Image reproduced with kind permission from Clinical Anatomy, H. Ellis, **Blackwell**, The arterial supply to the colon, p595; Image after **RCSI website**., Volvulus of the stomach, p595; After McKee, C., **www.yoursurgery.com**, Intussusception, p601; **Courtesy Meningitis Research Foundation** Figure 1, p806.